D1423454

WITHDRAWN
FROM LIBRARY

WITHDRAWN
FROM LIBRARY

BRITISH MEDICAL ASSOCIATION

1000954

Audiology
Diagnosis

Second Edition

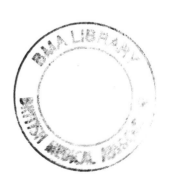

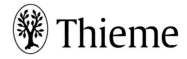

Audiology
Diagnosis

Second Edition

Ross J. Roeser, Ph.D.
Lois & Howard Wolf Professor in Pediatric Hearing
Executive Director Emeritus
School of Behavioral and Brain Sciences
University of Texas at Dallas/Callier Center for Communication Disorders
Dallas, Texas

Michael Valente, Ph.D.
Professor of Clinical Otolaryngology
Director of Adult Audiology
Division of Audiology
Department of Otolaryngology—Head and Neck Surgery
Washington University School of Medicine
St. Louis, Missouri

Holly Hosford-Dunn, Ph.D.
Managing Member
Arizona Audiology Network, LLC
President
TAI, Inc.
Tucson, Arizona

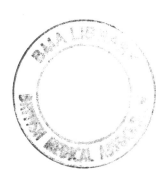

Thieme
New York · Stuttgart

Thieme Medical Publishers, Inc.
333 Seventh Ave.
New York, NY 10001

Medical Editor: Birgitta Brandenburg
Vice President, Production and Electronic Publishing: Anne T. Vinnicombe
Production Editor: Molly Connors, Dovetail Content Solutions
Associate Marketing Manager: Verena Diem
Sales Director: Ross Lumpkin
Chief Financial Officer: Peter van Woerden
President: Brian D. Scanlan
Compositor: Thomson Digital Services
Printer: CPI books, Birkach

Library of Congress Cataloging-in-Publication Data

Audiology. Diagnosis / edited by Ross J. Roeser, Michael Valente, Holly Hosford-Dunn. — 2nd ed.
    p. ; cm.
Companion v. to: Audiology : treatment, and Audiology : practice management.
Includes bibliographical references and index.
ISBN-13: 978-1-58890-542-0 (alk. paper)
ISBN-13: 978-3-13-116432-2 (alk. paper)
    1. Hearing disorders—Diagnosis. 2. Audiometry. I. Roeser, Ross J. II. Valente, Michael. III. Hosford-Dunn, Holly.
[DNLM: 1. Hearing Disorders—diagnosis. WV 270 A904 2007]
RF294.A824 2007
617.8'075—dc22

                                                 2007001684

Copyright © 2007 by Thieme Medical Publishers, Inc. This book, including all parts thereof, is legally protected by copyright. Any use, exploitation, or commercialization outside the narrow limits set by copyright legislation without the publisher's consent is illegal and liable to prosecution. This applies in particular to photostat reproduction, copying, mimeographing or duplication of any kind, translating, preparation of microfilms, and electronic data processing and storage.

Important note: Medical knowledge is ever-changing. As new research and clinical experience broaden our knowledge, changes in treatment and drug therapy may be required. The authors and editors of the material herein have consulted sources believed to be reliable in their efforts to provide information that is complete and in accord with the standards accepted at the time of publication. However, in view of the possibility of human error by the authors, editors, or publisher of the work herein or changes in medical knowledge, neither the authors, editors, nor publisher, nor any other party who has been involved in the preparation of this work, warrants that the information contained herein is in every respect accurate or complete, and they are not responsible for any errors or omissions or for the results obtained from use of such information. Readers are encouraged to confirm the information contained herein with other sources. For example, readers are advised to check the product information sheet included in the package of each drug they plan to administer to be certain that the information contained in this publication is accurate and that changes have not been made in the recommended dose or in the contraindications for administration. This recommendation is of particular importance in connection with new or infrequently used drugs.

Some of the product names, patents, and registered designs referred to in this book are in fact registered trademarks or proprietary names even though specific reference to this fact is not always made in the text. Therefore, the appearance of a name without designation as proprietary is not to be construed as a representation by the publisher that it is in the public domain.

Printed in Germany

5 4 3 2

US ISBN: 978-1-58890-542-0
GTV ISBN: 978-3-13-116432-2

Contents

Preface to the Second Edition

Harry Truman was a great leader and, some would say, an effective president. However, as is clearly evident in the second edition of our three volumes—*Audiology: Diagnosis, Audiology: Treatment,* and *Audiology: Practice Management*—he was off target when he said, "The only thing new in the world is the history you don't know." Since the publication of the first edition of our series just 7 years ago, there has been not only new information but also new technology, treatments, and trends in practice that have affected audiology in a way that has resulted in all areas of our profession growing exponentially. We now have better diagnostic procedures, more advanced technology and treatment programs, and additional practice strategies that allow audiologists to be more effective in diagnosing and treating their patients.

What's more exciting about the growth in the field of audiology that has occurred in the past few years is that we now have an expanding and maturing educational system for graduate students who choose to spend their lives in the profession. During the preparation of the first edition of our series, the doctor of audiology degree (Au.D.) was new. Yes, in 2000 there were programs in existence, and most universities at the time were in the planning stages of upgrading their programs to the doctoral level. However, at that time it was unclear how this shift in the educational model would impact the profession. Today, according to the Audiology Foundation of America, there are 70 university programs offering the Au.D. degree, 1500 residential students currently enrolled in Au.D. programs, and more than 3725 practicing doctors of audiology. So, we have an expanded body of knowledge that is being consumed by a growing and more sophisticated constituent body of professionals who have dedicated themselves to providing the best diagnosis and treatments to those with hearing disorders using more sophisticated practice procedures. All of these trends point to growth.

A novel thought is to consider the information in these three volumes as a mathematical equation:

$$X = D + T + P$$

where D is diagnosis, T is treatment, P is practice management, and X is the sum of all of the current knowledge in the three represented areas provided by the most knowledgeable experts in their respective fields. That is what we wanted these books to be.

People don't just decide one day that because there is more information and more individuals to consume it, they will devote a couple years of their lives to putting it together in a bundle of books. The three of us jointly arrived at the decision to publish a second edition of the "trilogy," as it has become known colloquially, because we felt a need to pay back to our profession a modicum of what it has given to us. We each have been very fortunate to be exposed to some of the best mentors, have been provided with tremendous support both psychologically and financially, and have been rewarded greatly in many other ways by being audiologists. We feel that we have been fortunate to practice audiology during the period of growth that the profession has experienced. We want to share those positive experiences with our readers.

We owe a special debt of gratitude to the authors of the chapters in these three volumes, who were willing to contribute their knowledge and experience as well as their valuable time in preparing the material. We thank them not only for all of their hard work and diligence in meeting a demanding publication schedule, but also for their tolerance in putting up with what we considered "constructive editorial comments." We realize that criticism is easy, but it is the science and art that are difficult. They were quite tolerant and gracious.

Finally, Thieme Medical Publishers provided us with the support of Ivy Ip. Ivy was our front-line representative with our authors once they agreed to be part of our team. We thank her for all of her efforts in making the second edition of our books a reality.

Ross J. Roeser—roeser@utdallas.edu
Michael Valente—valentem@ent.wustl.edu
Holly Hosford-Dunn—tucsonaud@aol.com

Preface to the First Edition

This book is on the topic of diagnostic audiology, and is one in a series of three texts prepared to represent the breadth of knowledge covering the multi-faceted profession of audiology in a manner that has not been attempted before. The companion books to this volume are *Treatment* and *Practice Management*. In total, the three books provide a total of 73 chapters covering material on the range of subjects and current knowledge audiologists must have to practice effectively. Because many of the chapters in the three books relate to each other, our readers are encouraged to have all three of them in their libraries, so that the broad scope of the profession of audiology is made available to them.

A unique feature of all three books is the insertion of highlighted boxes (pearls, pitfalls, special considerations, and controversial points) in strategic locations. These boxes emphasize key points authors are making and expand important concepts that are presented.

The 26 chapters in this book cover all aspects of diagnostic audiology. In the first chapter, we review diagnostic procedures as they relate to the profession of audiology. Included in Chapter 1 is a review of the scope of practice in audiology, specifically as it relates to diagnostic procedures; a review of the classical diagnostic audiological tests; and a presentation on the effectiveness of classical diagnostic audiological tests. Two additional topics in Chapter 1 are whether audiologists have the prerogative to diagnose hearing loss and the issue of how we refer to those we serve, whether it be "patients" or "clients."

Chapters 2 through 10 present basic and advanced information on fundamental principles in diagnostic audiology including: anatomy and physiology of the auditory and vestibular systems, disorders of the auditory system, radiology and functional brain imaging, pharmacology, acoustics and psychoacoustics, and instrumentation and calibration. An example of the expanding scope of practice for the profession of audiology is that the topics of radiology, brain imaging, and pharmacology have never been included in an audiology textbook.

Diagnostic audiological procedures are reviewed in Chapters 11 through 24. The diverse topics covered in these chapters include: pure tone tests, clinical masking, speech audiometry, central auditory tests in children and adults,

middle ear measures, clinical electrophysiology, otoacoustic emissions, neonatal hearing screening, intraoperative monitoring, and assessment of vestibular function.

In Chapter 25 a new dimension in diagnostic audiology, genetics, is reviewed. Finally, in Chapter 26 insights into the future of diagnostic audiological procedures are provided by several leading audiologists.

This book could not have been completed without the tireless efforts of Ms. Debbie Moncrieff and Dr. Jackie Clark. Ms. Moncrieff, a doctoral candidate at UTDallas/Callier Center, assisted as an editorial consultant in reading and editing chapters. Her suggestions added immensely to the quality of the material in the chapters. Dr. Clark co-authored a chapter and added many substantive comments to several chapters; her input was invaluable.

The three of us were brought together by Ms. Andrea Seils, Senior Medical Editor at Thieme Medical Publishers, Inc. During the birthing stage of the project Andrea encouraged us to think progressively—out of the box. She reminded us repeatedly to shed our traditional thinking and concentrate on the new developments that have taken place in audiology in recent years and that will occur in the next 5 to 10 years. With Andrea's encouragement and guidance, each of us set out what some would have considered to be the impossible—to develop a series of three cutting edge books that would cover the entire profession of audiology *in a period of less than 2 years*. Not only did we accomplish our goal, but as evidenced by the comprehensive nature of the material covered in the three books, we exceeded our expectations! We thank Andrea for her support throughout this 2-year project.

The authors who were willing to contribute to this book series have provided outstanding material that will assist audiologists in-training and practicing audiologists in their quest for the most up-to-date information on the areas that are covered. We thank them for their diligence in following our guidelines for preparing their manuscripts and their promptness in following our demanding schedule.

The consideration of our families for their endurance and patience with us throughout the duration of the project must be recognized. Our spouses and children understood our mission when we were away at editorial meetings; they were patient when we stayed up late at night and awoke in the wee hours of the morning to eke out a few more paragraphs; they tolerated the countless hours we were away from them. Without their support and encouragement we would never have finished our books in the timeframe we did.

Finally, each of us thanks our readers for their support of this book series. We would welcome comments and suggestions on this book, as well as the other two books in the series. Our email addresses are below.

Ross J. Roeser—roeser@utdallas.edu
Michael Valente—valentem@ent.wustl.edu
Holly Hosford-Dunn—tucsonaud@aol.com

Contributors

Prudence Allen, Ph.D.
School of Communication Sciences
and Disorders
National Centre for Audiology
University of Western Ontario
London, Ontario, Canada

Lynn S. Alvord, Ph.D.
Division of Audiology
Department of Otolaryngology
Henry Ford Hospital
Detroit, Michigan

Sally A. Arnold, Ph.D.
Associate Professor
Department of Speech-Language
Pathology
Buffalo, New York

Bopanna B. Ballachanda, Ph.D.
Director of Audiology
Premier Hearing Centers
Sante Fe, New Mexico

Robert B. Burr, Ph.D.
Adjunct Professor
Department of Neurosurgery
University of Utah
Spokane, Washington

Kathleen C.M. Campbell, Ph.D.
Professor and Director of Audiology
Research
Department of Surgery
Southern Illinois University
School of Medicine
Springfield, Illinois

Michael P. Castillo, M.D.
Resident
Department of Otolaryngology
UT Southwestern Medical Center
Dallas, Texas

Jackie L. Clark, Ph.D.
University of Texas at Dallas/Callier
Center for Communication
Disorders
Dallas, Texas
Research Associate
University of Witwatersrand
Johannesburg, South Africa

John A. Ferraro, Ph.D.
Professor and Chairman
Department of Hearing and Speech
University of Kansas Medical Center
Kansas City, Kansas

Tom Frank, Ph.D.
Professor
Department of Communication
Sciences and Disorders
Pennsylvania State University
University Park, Pennsylvania

Richard E. Gans, Ph.D.
Director
American Institute of Balance
Seminole, Florida

Theodore J. Glattke, Ph.D.
Professor
Department of Speech & Hearing
Sciences
University of Arizona
Tucson, Arizona

Linda Gray, M.D.
Associate Professor
Department of Radiology
Duke University Medical Center
Durham, North Carolina

Holly Hosford-Dunn, Ph.D.
Managing Member
Arizona Audiology Network, LLC
President
TAI, Inc.
Tucson, Arizona

Wafaa Kaf, M.D., Ph.D.
Assistant Professor
Department of Communications
Sciences and Disorders
Missouri State University
Springfield, Missouri

Robert W. Keith, Ph.D.
Professor of Audiology
Department of Otolaryngology—Head
and Neck Surgery
University of Cincinnati College
of Medicine
Cincinnati, Ohio

James N. Lee, Ph.D.
Department of Radiology
Center for Advanced Medical
Technologies
University of Utah
Salt Lake City, Utah

Edward Lobarinas, Ph.D.
Research Assistant Professor
Department of Communicative
Disorders and Sciences
State University of New York
at Buffalo
Buffalo, New York

Richard K. McHugh, Ph.D.
Research Scholar
Department of Cell and Molecular
Biology
House Ear Institute
Los Angeles, California

David L. McPherson, Ph.D.
Professor
Department of Communication
Disorders
Brigham Young University
Provo, Utah

Marissa Mendrygal, B.S.
Au.D. Student
School of Behavioral and Brian Sciences
University of Texas at Dallas/Callier
Center for Communication Disorders
Dallas, Texas

Aage R. Møller, Ph.D. (D.Med.Sci)
Professor of Neuroscience
School of Behavioral and Brain Sciences
University of Texas at Dallas
Richardson, Texas

Frank E. Musiek, Ph.D.
Director of Auditory Research
Department of Communication
    Disorders
University of Connecticut
Storrs, Connecticut

Victoria B. Oxholm, M.A.
Clinical Audiologist
Veterans Administration Hospital
White River Junction, Vermont

Cynthia McCormick Richburg, Ph.D.
Assistant Professor of Audiology
Department of Communication
    Sciences and Disorders
Missouri State University
Springfield, Missouri

Martin S. Robinette, Ph.D.
Professor
Department of Audiology
Mayo Clinic College of Medicine
Glendale, Arizona

Ross J. Roeser, Ph.D.
Lois & Howard Wolf Professor
    in Pediatric Hearing
Executive Director Emeritus
School of Behavioral and Brain Sciences
University of Texas at Dallas/Callier
    Center for Communication Disorders
Dallas, Texas

Peter S. Roland, M.D.
Professor and Chairman
Department of Otolaryngology—Head
    and Neck Surgery
UT Southwestern Medical Center
Dallas, Texas

Allyson D. Rosen, B.S.
Schreyer Honors College Scholar
Department of Communication
    Sciences and Disorders
Pennsylvania State University
University Park, Pennsylvania

Richard J. Salvi, Ph.D.
Professor
Department of Communicative
    Disorders and Sciences
State University of New York
    at Buffalo
Buffalo, New York

Nathan D. Schwade, M.D.
Associate Professor
UT Southwestern Medical Center
Los Alamos, New Mexico

Sonal S. Sheth, Ph.D.
Advanced Research Associate
Department of Cell and Molecular
    Biology
House Ear Institute
Los Angeles, California

Angela G. Shoup, Ph.D.
Assistant Professor
Director of Division of Communication
    and Vestibular Disorders
Department of Otolaryngology—Head
    and Neck Surgery
UT Southwestern Medical Center
Dallas, Texas

Lynn G. Spivak, Ph.D.
Director
Hearing and Speech Center
Long Island Jewish Medical Center
Assistant Professor
Department of Otolaryngology and
    Communicative Disorders
Albert Einstein College of Medicine
New Hyde Park, New York

Brad A. Stach, Ph.D.
Director
Division of Audiology
Henry Ford Medical Group
Detroit, Michigan

Wei Sun, Ph.D.
Assistant Professor
Department of Communicative
    Disorders and Sciences
State University of New York
    at Buffalo
Buffalo, New York

Linda M. Thibodeau, Ph.D.
Professor of Audiology
Department of Behavioral and Brain
    Science
University of Texas at Dallas
Dallas, Texas

Debara L. Tucci, M.D.
Associate Professor
Department of Surgery/Otolaryngology
Duke University Medical Center
Durham, North Carolina

Michael Valente, Ph.D.
Professor of Clinical Otolaryngology
Director of Adult Audiology
Division of Audiology
Department of Otolaryngology—Head
    and Neck Surgery
Washington University School
    of Medicine
St. Louis, Missouri

Julie Martinez Verhoff, Au.D.
Research Audiologist
Department of Hearing, Speech, and
    Language Sciences
Gallaudet University
Washington, District of Columbia

Jeffrey A. Weihing, M.A.
Ph.D. Student
Department of Communication
    Disorders
University of Connecticut
Storrs, Connecticut

Charles G. Wright, Ph.D.
Associate Professor
Department of Otolaryngology—Head
    and Neck Surgery
UT Southwestern Medical Center
Dallas, Texas

M. Wende Yellin, Ph.D.
Department of Speech Pathology and
    Audiology
Northern Arizona University
Flagstaff, Arizona

Acknowledgments

For the Book Series

The three editors of this book series came together in late 1990. Prior to the first meeting we had all known of each other, but only casually. However, during the first meeting there was an immediate recognition among us that, although we had very different backgrounds and professional orientations, a professional magnetism drew us together. Long hours together flew by during the many sessions where we discussed contents, possible contributors, and logistics. When asked to produce a second edition, each of us was very reluctant, but agreed because we knew that this would provide us with an opportunity to work together once again. So, strange as it may seem, each of us would like to thank our two other editorial colleagues for making the second edition a reality. We each said that the main reason for taking on this gargantuan task was that we had the support of the two other editors.

Each of us would like to thank the authors for the considerable time and effort they took from their private and professional lives to produce chapters reflecting the highest scholarship.

The staff of Thieme Medical Publishers, Brian Scanlan, President, Birgitta Brandenburg, Editor, and Ivy Ip, Assistant Editor, who worked so many hours during the entire production process deserve special recognition. These key individuals keep the machines running at the Thieme headquarters in the background so that authors and editors can carry out their writing, recruiting, and editorial tasks.

Ross J. Roeser—roeser@utdallas.edu
Michael Valente—valentem@ent.wustl.edu
Holly Hosford-Dunn—tucsonaud@aol.com

For this Book

As primary editor for *Audiology: Diagnosis*, I want to thank Dr. Jackie Clark, UTD/Callier fellow faculty member, and Marissa Mendrygal, a UTD/Callier Center Au.D. student, for their editorial suggestions and support. Not only did they coauthor several chapters, but they provided invaluable editorial suggestions and advice on many issues in this book. I also want to thank my long-time secretary Linda Sensibaugh, who was always there when I need her to help in the production process.

The book would not have been completed without the continuing support of my wife, Sharon, who for 44 years has always said, "That's O.K., I know you have important work to do." Whereupon I would reply, "Thank you sweetie—this is my last book project. NO MORE BOOKS." Now that the three books have been finished, it seems like there's just one more that I might think about, but, ". . . this will be the LAST one, sweetie, I promise."

Ross J. Roeser—roeser@utdallas.edu

Chapter 1

Diagnostic Procedures in Audiology

Ross J. Roeser, Michael Valente, and Holly Hosford-Dunn

Audiology is the science of hearing. Over the years, audiology has evolved into an autonomous profession, and today audiologists are the primary health care professionals involved in the identification or diagnosis, prevention, and evaluation of hearing, balance, and related disorders. In addition, audiologists are the most important resource for nonmedical habilitation/rehabilitation services for individuals with hearing disorders through the application of hearing aids, associated rehabilitation devices (assistive listening devices and implantable devices), and (re)habilitation programs for children and adults. Audiologists are also involved in related research pertinent to the prevention, identification, and management of hearing loss and related disorders.

for issues on service delivery, third-party reimbursement, legislation, consumer education, regulatory action, state and professional licensure, legal intervention, and interprofessional relations. In the 50 to 60 years that the profession of audiology has been in existence, the scope of practice has changed drastically. This metamorphosis has occurred gradually as a result of emerging clinical, technological, and scientific developments, which are now commonplace in our modern world. Whereas only 30 years ago audiologists were primarily performing behavioral tests of auditory function, today audiologists have a wide range of electrophysiological assessment tools to select from, and audiology is the primary discipline involved in hearing rehabilitation with hearing aids, implantable hearing instruments, assistive listening devices, and aural rehabilitative programs.

♦ Scope of Practice in Audiology

The scope of practice for a profession is defined by professional organizations, government agencies, and licensing laws. Scope of practice information is used as a reference

Pearl

- Audiology is defined as the science of hearing, the art of hearing assessment, and the (re)habilitation of individuals with hearing impairment.

Two professional organizations have developed scope of practice statements for audiology: the American Speech-Language-Hearing Association (ASHA) and the American Academy of Audiology (AAA). Copies of these documents can be found on respective Web sites. The activities listed range from the application of procedures for assessment, diagnosis, management, and interpretation of test results related to disorders of hearing, balance, and other neural systems to participation in the development of professional and technical standards. The ASHA Scope of Practice statement makes it clear that the list of activities is not intended to be exhaustive but reflects the current practice of the profession of audiology.

Scope of practice statements relate to what a profession does; they are also based on what a profession is. Audiology as a profession has been associated with hearing and disorders of hearing. Based on this, some have argued that audiologists should not be involved with procedures outside of assessment or rehabilitation of the auditory system. Their rationale is that to continue to be within the mainstream of the profession, audiology practice should focus exclusively on hearing and hearing disorders. However, it is clear that today audiologists are practicing in related areas, such as intraoperative monitoring and balance assessment. Chapters 23 and 24 of this text cover these topics.

The process for changing the scope of professional practice for any profession is either to change professional codes or state licensing laws that govern the profession or to extend the practice until it is challenged legally, then have the courts adjudicate the issue. Modifying the scope of practice by changing professional codes and state licensing laws is a time-consuming and expensive process. For example, before the mid-1970s, the ASHA Code of Ethics prohibited audiologists from dispensing hearing aids. It took years to make the necessary amendments to allow audiologists to engage in this critical practice. In addition, definitions contained in codes and licensure must be broad, so it is not appropriate to specify all functions or procedures. Professional preparation and clinical experience are the important criteria that define the limits within which a profession can operate.

It is not uncommon for a profession to extend its practice until legally challenged. The courts are constantly challenging professional boundaries. For example, after extended litigation, optometrists are now able to prescribe antibiotics for conjunctivitis. When challenged, audiologists must be prepared to defend their practices with evidence of their qualifications and competencies through documentation of adequate academic preparation and experience. Because the scope of practice in audiology is expanding, the necessary academic preparation is undergoing critical review, and the professional doctorate (AuD) has been accepted by ASHA and AAA as the minimum entry level for the profession.

The broad range of activities and services within the scope of practice for audiologists, as defined by the ASHA Task Force on Clinical Standards, is listed in **Table 1–1**. Most of the 23 procedures are broadly defined, requiring complex knowledge and years of experience for clinical

Table 1–1   Activities within the Scope of Practice for Audiologists*

Hearing screening
Speech screening
Language screening
Follow-up procedures
Consultation
Prevention
Counseling
Aural rehabilitation
Aural rehabilitation assessment
Product dispensing
Product repair/modification
Basic audiological assessment[†]
Pediatric audiological assessment
Comprehensive audiological assessment[†]
Electrodiagnostic test procedures[†]
Auditory evoked potential assessment[†]
Neurophysiological intraoperative monitoring[†]
Balance system assessment[†]
Hearing aid assessment
Assistive listening system/device selection
Sensory aids assessment[†]
Hearing aid fitting/orientation
Occupational hearing conservation

*Preferred practice patterns are available from the American Speech-Language-Hearing Association for each of these procedures.
[†]Diagnostic procedures.

competency. An important point made in this table, one that relates directly to this textbook, is that many of the activities include diagnostic procedures. Moreover, preferred practice patterns have been written for these and other diagnostic audiological procedures performed by audiologists and are available from ASHA (American Speech-Language-Hearing Association, 1995).

In the remaining portion of this chapter, traditional and current diagnostic tests are reviewed, the effectiveness and use of diagnostic audiological tests are discussed, and the role of audiologists in diagnostic testing is described.

◆ Diagnostic Audiological Tests

Table 1–2 lists traditional and current diagnostic audiological tests that have been developed through the years. In reading the chapters in this book, it is clear that major advances have been made in diagnostic audiology. Today, audiologists are performing diagnostic procedures that employ not only behavioral psychoacoustic tests with pure tones and speech but also radiology, brain imaging, middle ear measures, auditory electrophysiology, ear canal emissions, and sophisticated tests of vestibular function. More and more, tests are being developed to assess central auditory function in children and adults. Even genetics is becoming an important factor in diagnostic testing. These topics are covered in detail by the most prominent audiologists and audiology researchers in the country within the chapters of this text.

Table 1–2 Summary of Diagnostic Audiological Tests

Tuning fork tests
   Weber
   Schwabach*
   Bing
   Air conduction and bone conduction comparison
Loudness balancing
Békésy (self-recording) audiometry*
   Classical diagnostic Békésy audiometry
   Reverse sweep Békésy*
   Békésy comfort loudness*
Short increment sensitivity index*
Threshold tone decay tests
   Classical (Carhart) threshold tone decay test
   Owens threshold tone decay test
Suprathreshold adaptation test*
Speech audiometry
Middle ear/immittance measures (tympanometry)
   Tympanogram
   Ipsilateral/contralateral comparison
   Acoustic reflex decay
Auditory evoked potentials
Otoacoustic emissions
Tests for pseudohypoacusis
Tests for auditory processing disorders

Note: Tests marked with an asterisk are presented for historical purposes only.

In the remaining portion of this chapter, the traditional diagnostic audiological tests are reviewed, and their effectiveness is discussed. Some of these tests are still in use today, but many are not; they are presented primarily for historical purposes.

Pearl

- The term *retrocochlear* refers to areas in the auditory system beyond the cochlea, including the brainstem and higher levels. The word *central* refers to areas in the auditory system beyond the brainstem.

Tuning Fork Tests

The use of tuning forks provided the first assessment procedures for diagnosing the magnitude and type (conductive, sensorineural, or mixed) of hearing loss. With current sophisticated diagnostic equipment and procedures, tuning fork tests have limited application. However, because tuning forks are readily available and because it is possible to use a standard bone conduction vibrator to perform audiometric tuning fork tests, physicians and audiologists will find some of the procedures useful for patients in some situations. The most useful tuning fork test is the Weber, which is applied when patients present with unilateral hearing loss. Chapter 11 reviews tuning fork test procedures.

Air Conduction and Bone Conduction Comparison

Pure-tone threshold audiometry is the gold standard for diagnostic audiological testing. From pure-tone air conduction (A/C) and bone conduction (B/C) thresholds, the degree or magnitude (mild, moderate, severe, or profound), configuration (e.g., sloping, rising, flat), and type (conductive, mixed, or sensorineural) of hearing loss are determined. Results from pure-tone threshold testing are also used to determine parameters and help in interpreting results from additional diagnostic tests. As examples, the presentation levels for some behavioral diagnostic tests are set based on pure-tone thresholds, and the classification of speech recognition scores into "cochlear" or "retrocochlear" for a given patient is based on the pure-tone threshold sensitivity. Chapter 11 provides a comprehensive review of pure-tone A/C and B/C procedures.

The configuration of the audiogram is an important factor when interpreting diagnostic tests. It is not always possible to determine the cause of a hearing loss by reviewing the type and configuration of the hearing loss, but many conditions have stereotypical findings. A few classical examples are as follows:

- Meniere's syndrome (endolymphatic hydrops) is a condition in which there is increased pressure in the endolymph in the inner ear, which first presents with fluctuating, low-frequency, rising sensorineural hearing loss. As the disease process continues, the loss changes to a flat and then sloping configuration in the latter stages. Accompanying the hearing loss are the symptoms of low-frequency (roaring) tinnitus, vertigo, and nausea.

- Noise-induced hearing loss occurs gradually when ears are exposed to high-intensity sounds. The stereotypical finding for hearing loss caused by noise exposure is a reduction of hearing in the 4000 to 6000 Hz region, with improvement of hearing at 8000 Hz. Over time, if the ear continues to be exposed to high-intensity sounds, the hearing loss in the 4000 to 6000 Hz region increases and gradually spreads to lower frequencies.

- Presbycusis (or presbyacusia) is hearing loss caused by advancing age, beginning in the fourth or fifth decades of life. The loss is sensorineural and initially affects high frequencies only. As the loss progresses, it gradually invades the lower frequencies but continues to influence high frequencies the most.

- Otosclerosis is a condition in which a spongy material develops in the bony capsule of the inner ear and on the footplate of the stapes, which results first in a conductive hearing loss. As the condition progresses, the loss becomes mixed and sloping, with the classical "Carhart's notch"—an increased depression in B/C thresholds of 5 dB at 500 and 4000 Hz, 10 dB at 1000 Hz, and 15 dB at 2000 Hz. Bone conduction thresholds will improve by the amount of the Carhart's notch with successful surgery.

Loudness Balancing

Loudness balancing procedures were among the first diagnostic audiological tests to be developed. During loudness balancing tests, the loudness of stimuli presented to a patient's normal-hearing ear are compared with the loudness in the ear with hearing loss. Implicit in loudness balancing is the requirement that one ear have normal threshold sensitivity, at least at some frequencies.

Loudness balancing procedures are performed to determine whether "recruitment" is present or absent in an ear with hearing loss. Originally, the alternate binaural loudness balancing (ABLB) and the monaural loudness balancing (MLB) tests were developed. However, patient requirements used for the MLB were so difficult that the MLB procedure was not used clinically. The ABLB is performed by alternating a pure tone between the two ears, keeping the intensity in one ear (usually the ear with normal hearing) fixed and varying the intensity in the other ear until the two tones are judged equally loud by the patient. The test begins at 20 dB SL (sensation level) in the fixed (normal) ear. After equal loudness is judged, the intensity is increased in 20 dB increments until either the patient's tolerance level or the maximum limit of the audiometer is reached.

Pearl

- Recruitment is the rapid growth of loudness in an ear with sensorineural hearing loss. The presence of recruitment in an ear with sensorineural hearing loss suggests cochlear site of lesion. The absence of recruitment suggests a noncochlear (or retrocochlear) site of lesion.

Findings from the ABLB are plotted graphically with laddergrams, which are shown in **Fig. 1–1**. No recruitment is indicated if the decibel difference between the two ears remains constant (**Fig. 1–1A**). However, if the loudness difference between the two ears decreases, with less intensity increase in the abnormal ear required for equal loudness in the normal ear, then either partial or complete recruitment

is indicated. Partial recruitment is present when a decrease exists in the difference between the two ears, but equal intensities are not established (**Fig. 1–1B**). Complete recruitment is present if equal loudness occurs at equal intensities (**Fig. 1–1C**). In derecruitment an increase occurs in the intensity difference between the two ears to achieve equal loudness (**Fig. 1–1D**).

Recruitment was originally thought to be an abnormal finding, in that the loudness growth in the impaired ear appeared to be abnormally fast (**Fig. 1–1C**). That is, in ears showing recruitment, even though a loss of threshold hearing sensitivity exists, at high intensities no difference in loudness is found when compared with the normal loudness function. On the basis of this, recruitment was first defined as an abnormal growth of loudness in an ear with sensorineural hearing loss. However, several clinical research studies have changed this original concept, and it is now recognized that recruitment is not an abnormal or pathological finding, but rather represents the impaired ear's ability to respond normally to loudness at high intensities (Sanders, 1979).

The abnormal finding from tests of recruitment, such as the ABLB, is the absence of recruitment, or derecruitment, which is an unusually slow growth of loudness in an ear with sensorineural hearing loss. The presence of recruitment has been and continues to be associated with cochlear site of lesion. In an ear with sensorineural hearing loss, the absence of recruitment does not rule out a pathological cochlear condition but is considered a possible retrocochlear sign. The most abnormal finding on loudness balancing tests is derecruitment, which is a highly positive sign for retrocochlear involvement.

Békésy (Self-Recording) Audiometry

Békésy (1947) described what was then a revolutionary audiometer that allowed patients to track their own thresholds—a self-recording audiometer. Threshold testing is performed with the self-recording (Békésy) audiometer by instructing the patient to activate a handheld switch

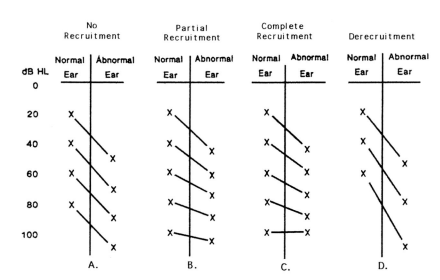

Figure 1–1 Laddergrams from the alternate binaural loudness balancing (ABLB) test. For each example, the normal ear has a 0 dB HL (hearing level) threshold and the abnormal ear a 30 dB HL threshold.

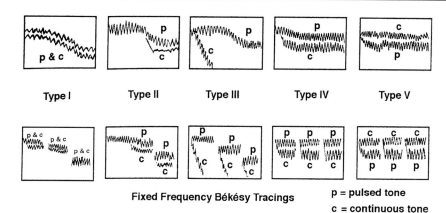

Type I   Type II   Type III   Type IV   Type V

Fixed Frequency Békésy Tracings

p = pulsed tone
c = continuous tone

Figure 1–2 Classical Békésy diagnostic patterns showing thresholds for pulsed (p) tones and continuous (c) tones. The top tracings are for sweep frequencies (100 to 10,000 Hz) and the bottom for the fixed frequencies of 250, 1000, and 4000 Hz.

when the test signals are just heard and release the switch immediately when the test signals become inaudible. As the patient is responding, the self-recording audiometer marks the responses on an audiogram form, and thresholds are calculated from the tracings. With this procedure, thresholds can be obtained for a variety of stimuli using sweep frequency (e.g., 100–10,000 Hz) or fixed frequency recordings and continuous or pulsed tones. The application of Békésy's technology allows for the classification of diagnostic results into several categories, as described here.

J. Jerger (1960) was among the first to research the use of the Békésy audiometer for diagnostic purposes. In the classical Békésy procedure, thresholds for a pulsed (p) pure tone are compared with those using a continuous (c) pure tone. The pulsed tone has a duration of 200 msec, a rise–fall time of 50 msec, and a 50% duty cycle. Originally, four patterns were described (types I–IV), but later Jerger and Herer (1961) added one more, type V. The five classical Békésy patterns are shown in **Fig. 1–2**. Results were consistent with the following:

- Type I—Normal hearing, conductive hearing loss, and sensorineural hearing loss of unknown origin

- Type II—Sensorineural hearing loss caused by a cochlear site of lesion

- Type III—Retrocochlear site of lesion oftentimes caused by an acoustic neuroma or cerebellopontine angle tumor

- Type IV—Cochlear or retrocochlear site of lesion

- Type V—Pseudohypoacusis

On the basis of results from numerous clinical studies using the classical Békésy procedure, several modifications to that procedure were developed; the most notable were reverse-sweep Békésy and Békésy comfort level.

Short Increment Sensitivity Index

The short increment sensitivity index (SISI) test (Jerger et al, 1959) is based on the differential intensity function of the ear (see Chapter 9). That is, the test determines the ability of the patient to detect a 1 dB change of intensity in a pure-tone stimulus when superimposed on a continuous tone presented at 20 dB SL. The classical SISI procedure is graphically illustrated in **Fig. 1–3**. During the test, a pure tone is presented continuously at 20 dB SL (a 20 dB pedestal), and 25 to 28 presentations of 1 to 5 dB are superimposed on it. The increases in intensity are 300 msec in duration, with a 50 msec rise–fall time and a 200 msec "on" time. One increment is presented every 5 seconds, and the patient is instructed to respond when the increments

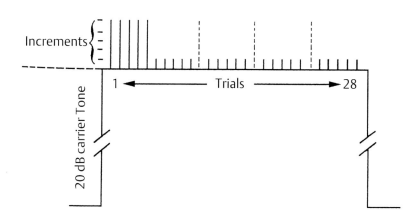

Increments

20 dB carrier Tone

1 ⟵ Trials ⟶ 28

Figure 1–3 Diagram of the procedure used in the short increment sensitivity index (SISI) test.

are detected. During the test, only the 1 dB increments are used to calculate the SISI score. The first five 5 dB increments are used for practice to see whether the patient can perform the task. During the 11th, 17th, and 23rd trials, the stimuli are changed. If the patient is not responding, 5 dB increments are presented to ensure that the patient is attending to the task. However, if a high rate of responding occurs for the 1 dB increments, the increments are removed during these trials to prevent rhythmic responding. The SISI score is calculated by multiplying the number of the 1 dB increments that are correctly detected by 5, giving a percentage of correct responses. Scores between 0 and 70% are negative for cochlear pathological conditions; scores of 75% and above are positive for cochlear pathological conditions. Modifications to the classical procedure included reducing the initial five 5 dB practice increments in 1 dB steps (i.e., 4, 3, and 2 dB) to eliminate the sudden reduction of the signal to 1 dB and reducing the number of 1 dB increments by half, from 20 to 10.

Through the years the classical SISI test was shown to be an accurate predictor of a cochlear pathological condition. A tendency exists for the test to be more predictive of cochlear hearing loss at higher frequencies (2000–4000 Hz) than at low frequencies (250–500 Hz).

A high-intensity modification of the classical procedure was introduced to detect retrocochlear pathological conditions. When the 20 dB SL pedestal is raised to 75 dB HL (hearing level), patients with normal hearing and cochlear hearing loss are able to detect the 1 dB increments, but patients with retrocochlear pathological conditions are not. As a result, patients with normal hearing and sensorineural hearing loss of cochlear origin will have high SISI scores, but those with a retrocochlear pathological condition will have low scores.

Threshold Tone Decay Tests

Threshold tone decay (TTD) tests quantify the amount of auditory fatigue present when stimuli are given at or near threshold sensitivity for each patient. The general procedure is to measure the ability of a patient to perceive and maintain a pure tone presented continuously. In the classical procedure, the patient is instructed to respond when the tone is perceived by raising a finger and continue to respond as long as the tone is heard (Carhart, 1957). The tone is initially presented below threshold and increased slowly in 5 dB steps until the patient first responds. As soon as the patient responds, timing begins, and if the tone is heard for a full minute, the test is terminated. If, however, the signal fades into inaudibility and the patient stops responding before the 1 minute period is over, the intensity is increased by 5 dB without interruption, and timing begins again. This procedure continues until the patient is able to sustain the tone for 1 full minute or until the signal reaches 30 dB SL.

The classical procedure can be time-consuming, possibly requiring as much as 4 to 5 minutes for each frequency tested. To shorten the test, Olsen and Noffsinger (1974) suggested that the initial stimulus be presented at 20 dB SL. Not only is this a time-saving procedure that maintains the

test's sensitivity, but it also makes the test easier for patients because stimuli are easier to perceive at the initial suprathreshold level.

The extent of the decay, both in the number of frequencies at which decay occurs and the intensity and rapidity of the decay, provides differential diagnostic information in the following areas: (1) slow tone decay is associated with cochlear pathological conditions, whereas marked or rapid decay is associated with retrocochlear pathological conditions; (2) tone decay in excess of 30 dB (SL) is very likely associated with retrocochlear pathological conditions, regardless of its rapidity; and (3) the greater the number of frequencies involved, the greater the likelihood of retrocochlear involvement.

Several modifications to the Carhart procedure were suggested. For example, to shorten the test, Rosenberg (1958) suggested that decay be measured only for a total of 60 seconds. Owens (1964) described a modification of the classical tone decay test that incorporates a 20 second rest period between each stimulus presentation. In the Owens procedure, each tone presentation begins at 5 dB SL; if the patient does not perceive the tone for 60 seconds, the stimulus is discontinued for 20 seconds before reintroduction at successive 5 dB increments. This procedure continues until the stimulus is perceived for 60 seconds or a level of 20 dB SL is reached. It is possible to differentiate between decay occurring with cochlear versus retrocochlear site of lesion with the Owens procedure. Patients with retrocochlear lesions characteristically show decay at all frequencies, and the rapidity of the decay does not change as the intensity is increased. Patients with cochlear pathological conditions, in contrast, show decay at one or two frequencies, and the decay is slower as the intensity of the test signal is increased.

TTD testing should continue to be considered as a viable screening diagnostic tool because of its high sensitivity and specificity. The procedure requires no special equipment and can be performed in a short time period.

Speech Audiometry

Pure tones are used in diagnostic audiology primarily because they are simple to generate and are capable of differentially assessing the specific effects of auditory system pathological conditions. However, pure-tone measurements provide only limited information concerning the communication difficulty a patient may experience and/or the diagnostic site of lesion. Speech audiometry assesses the patient's ability to respond to standardized material for threshold assessment (speech recognition threshold, SRT) and speech perception ability with words (word recognition scores) and/or sentences (speech recognition scores). The topic of speech audiometry is covered in detail in Chapter 14.

Speech audiometry provides data to assess the validity of pure-tone thresholds and obtain diagnostic information regarding site of lesion. Validation of pure-tone data is accomplished by comparing thresholds for speech materials, the SRT, to thresholds for pure tones in the 500 to 2000 Hz range (pure-tone average, PTA). Such comparison should reveal close agreement (within 6–8 dB). Whenever a difference exists between the SRT and the PTA, the validity of the

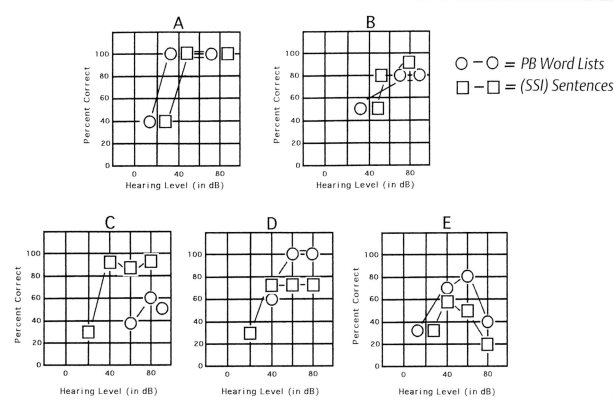

$\bigcirc - \bigcirc = PB$ Word Lists

$\square - \square = (SSI)$ Sentences

Figure 1–4 Examples of performance intensity (PI)/phonetically balanced (PB) functions for words (PI-PB) and sentences (Synthetic Sentence Identification, SSI; PI-SSI) for **(A)** normal-hearing, **(B–D)** cochlear hearing loss with different configurations, and **(E)** eighth nerve site. Patients with central site and presbycusis have configurations similar to example **(D)**.

results are in question, and the equipment, the procedures used to obtain the data, and patient cooperation must be checked (see Chapters 11 and 14).

Diagnostic information from speech audiometry can be obtained by comparing word and speech intelligibility scores at different intensities. The shape of the performance intensity (PI) function and the difference in the functions for words and sentences provide diagnostic information. **Figure 1–4** gives the classical results showing PI functions using words and sentences for different sites of lesions. The findings for this procedure were obtained with standard phonetically balanced (PB) word lists and sentences from the synthetic sentence identification (SSI) test (Jerger and Hayes, 1977).

Pearl

• A PI function compares percent of correct responses for speech materials with words (word intelligibility scores) or sentences (speech intelligibility scores) at various levels of presentation.

---

1. Normal findings: Patients have high speech recognition scores (between 90 and 100%) for both types of stimuli at low and high intensities (**Fig. 1–4A**).

2. Cochlear site: Patients with a cochlear site of lesion have PI functions that are predictable in the following ways:

   a. With flat audiometric configurations, identical or similar PI functions are obtained for words (PI-PB) and sentences (PI-SSI; **Fig. 1–4B**).

   b. With sloping high-frequency losses, the PI function for words (PI-PB) is reduced compared with the PI function for sentences (PI-SSI; **Fig. 1–4C**).

   c. With rising audiometric configurations, the PI function for words (PI-PB) is elevated compared with the PI function for sentences (PI-SSI; **Fig. 1–4D**).

3. Eighth nerve site: The direction and magnitude of the PI function is not predictable, but significant PI rollover occurs. Rollover is defined as a significant reduction in PI scores that occurs at high intensities. That is, scores reach a maximum in the midrange intensities; when the intensity is increased, a sharp decrease in performance occurs (**Fig. 1–4E**).

4. Central site: The PI function for words (PI-PB) is typically elevated compared with the PI function for sentences (PI-SSI), similar to cochlear losses with rising configurations (**Fig. 1–4D**).

5. Presbycusis: The PI functions for words (PI-PB) and sentences (PI-SSI) are below normal. Typically, the PI

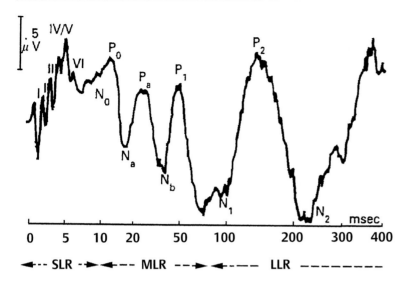

Figure 1–5 Example of the composite human auditory evoked response, including the short latency (electrocochleography) response (SLR), auditory brainstem response, middle latency response (MLR), and long latency response (LLR).

function for words is elevated compared with the PI function for sentences (**Fig. 1–4D**).

Pearl

- Rollover is observed on the PI function obtained during word/speech recognition testing when a significant reduction in scores occurs as the presentation level's intensity of the stimuli increases. Rollover is associated with retrocochlear involvement.

Middle Ear Measures

Middle ear measurement is performed with immittance instruments. Immittance instruments do not assess hearing—they provide objective information on the mechanical transfer function of sound in the outer and middle ear and, depending on the status of the outer and middle ear and cochlear function, provide data on the integrity of auditory nerve function at the level of the brainstem. With the immittance test battery, it is possible to obtain diagnostic information on the status of the outer and middle ear, cochlear function, and the integrity of the eighth nerve and brainstem by obtaining a tympanogram, as well as static measures of middle ear function and acoustic reflexes to ipsilateral and contralateral stimulation. Technological advances have automated the middle ear assessment technique to the point that microprocessor immittance equipment can now complete a middle ear assessment test battery for both ears in a matter of minutes. Chapter 18 is a comprehensive review of basic and advanced middle ear measurement procedures.

Auditory Evoked Potentials

Auditory stimuli are capable of evoking responses in the electrical activity of the central nervous system and, with

the use of computer technology, can be recorded from electrodes placed on the head. **Figure 1–5** provides an example of the composite auditory evoked response, including the short latency (electrocochleographic) response (SLR), auditory brainstem response (ABR), middle latency response (MLR), and long latency (LLR) response. Auditory evoked responses have been used in diagnostic audiology for more than 5 decades, and as more knowledge is being made available in this area, it is clear that auditory electrophysiological measures will become even more prominent diagnostic tools in audiology in the future. Topics related to auditory evoked potentials in diagnostic audiology are covered in Chapters 19 through 21.

Otoacoustic Emissions

Otoacoustic emissions (OAE) are recorded by introducing a brief acoustic signal into the ear canal and measuring the acoustic energy that is emitted. OAE were discovered only within the past 2 decades, but their use in studying auditory physiology and diagnostic audiology has already made a significant difference in everyday clinical practice. Chapter 22 presents an excellent review of OAE, and Chapter 23 discusses, among other issues, the application of OAE in neonatal hearing screening.

Tests for Pseudohypoacusis

Pseudohypoacusis literally means "falsely (*pseudo-*) reduced hearing (*hypoacusis*)" and is applied to cases where patients have exaggerated hearing loss. Some patients demonstrating pseudohypoacusis have no hearing loss. Generally, though, some hearing loss is present for most patients, although the degree of impairment is exaggerated. Through the years, other terms, including *nonorganic hearing loss, functional hearing loss, psychogenic hearing loss, hysterical deafness,* and *malingering,* have been used to describe patients whose hearing loss is questionable. Each of these terms has specific connotations, and for this reason they must be used with caution when describing these patients. The topic of pseudohypoacusis is covered in detail in Chapter 15.

Tests for Auditory Processing Disorders

What was once referred to as *central auditory processing* is now labeled *auditory processing* or *auditory processing disorders* (Jerger and Musiek, 2000). There is no question that diagnosing auditory processing disorders is a growing area of importance in diagnostic audiology and will provide audiologists with significant advances in the future. Although many of the current procedures involve behavioral tests, auditory electrophysiology and brain imaging are also proving to be of significant value in the clinical setting. Chapters 16 and 17 cover diagnosing auditory processing disorders in children and adults, respectively.

◆ The Effectiveness of Diagnostic Audiological Tests

All diagnostic procedures, whether for the auditory system or any other system, are designed to identify the presence of a disorder as early as possible. When indicated, diagnostic procedures can also help to identify the cause or nature of the disorder. The value of a diagnostic test depends on the ability to perform as intended. That is, the procedure must accurately identify those patients with the disorder while clearing those patients without the disorder. In diagnostic audiology, two processes have been used to assess the effectiveness of diagnostic procedures: clinical decision analysis (CDA)/information theory analysis and evidence-based practices (EBP).

Clinical Decision Analysis/Information Theory Analysis

Before any assessment of a diagnostic test's effectiveness can be made, the first step is to test the reliability. Reliability deals with consistency; if the test is administered and then repeated (test–retest) at a different time by the same (intraexaminer) or a different (interexaminer) individual, to what extent will the test results be the same? Without a high degree of reliability, the test is not effective because the results of the test will vary either from session to session or from tester to tester, or possibly both. Test reliability can be controlled and maintained at a high level by standardizing test administration, ensuring proper equipment calibration, and controlling patient variables. Careful attention to these matters will help ensure a high level of reliability, but it does not guarantee it.

Pearl

- Reliability measures the intraexaminer and interexaminer consistency of a test. Validity is a measure of the ability of a test to detect the disorder for which it was designed.

It is easy to see how poor reliability has serious consequences for diagnostic procedures; the reliability of a test must be high for it to be effective. However, just because a test is reliable, it still may not be effective if it fails to identify the problem for which it is being conducted. The validity of a test assesses its effectiveness in identifying the disorder for which it was designed.

CDA and information theory analysis are procedures that measure test validity based on mathematical models (S. Jerger, 1983; Turner and Nielsen, 1984). CDA allows for decisions to be made about tests when uncertainty exists: uncertainty is always present with diagnostic procedures because they are not perfect. That is, certain predictable errors always exist.

In applying CDA to audiological tests, assumptions must be made. Traditionally, one basic assumption has been made on the basis of whether tests are positive for retrocochlear disorder (a positive result) or negative for retrocochlear disorder (a negative result), with negative results for retrocochlear disorders being positive for cochlear disorder. By considering diagnostic procedures in this way, it is possible to model the outcomes in a matrix relating to the actual presence or absence of retrocochlear disorder.

Figure 1–6 provides a model for analyzing diagnostic test data. As shown, the diagnostic test results can be grouped by the number of test outcomes suggesting positive (fail) and negative findings (pass) and by the number of patients with retrocochlear (condition present) or cochlear (condition absent) site of lesion. With these parameters, classification of the data into four cells is possible: correct identification of the abnormal condition (cell A—sensitivity), correct identification of the normal condition (cell D—specificity), incorrect identification of the normal condition, or false-positive (cell B), and incorrect identification of the abnormal condition, or false-negative (cell C).

These four possible outcomes allow one to evaluate the effectiveness of a diagnostic test by calculating its sensitivity, specificity, predictive values (PV) of positive (PV1) and negative (PV2) results, and efficiency, as described in the following.

1. **Sensitivity**   The sensitivity of a test is its accuracy in correctly identifying disordered subjects; in the case of site of lesion tests, sensitivity is the ability to identify a retrocochlear disorder. Sensitivity is calculated by dividing the true-positive results by the total number of patients with retrocochlear disorder.

2. **Specificity**   The specificity of a test is its accuracy in correctly rejecting patients without retrocochlear disorder. That is, these patients would be classified as having cochlear site of lesion. Specificity is calculated by dividing true-negative results by the total number of patients with cochlear disorder. Sensitivity and specificity are generally related inversely; as one increases, the other decreases.

3. **Predictive value**   The PV of a test is related to the number of false-negative results in patients with retrocochlear disorders and the number of false-positive results in patients with cochlear disorders. PV is

	Condition Present	Condition Absent
Positive (Fail)	A Correct identification of abnormal condition (sensitivity) 21	B False-positive 6
Negative (Pass)	C False-negative 3	D Correct identification of normal condition (specificity) 586

A + B = 27

C + D = 589

(A + C = 24)   (B + D = 592)   616

Sensitivity = $\dfrac{A}{A+C} \times 100$ $\dfrac{21}{24} = 88\%$

False-negative = $\dfrac{C}{A+C} \times 100$ $\dfrac{3}{24} = 13\%$

Specificity = $\dfrac{D}{B+D} \times 100$ $\dfrac{586}{592} = 99\%$

False-positive = $\dfrac{B}{B+D} \times 100$ $\dfrac{6}{592} = 1\%$

Predictive value (positive results) = $\dfrac{A}{A+B} \times 100$ $\dfrac{21}{27} = 78\%$

Predictive value (negative results) = $\dfrac{D}{C+D} \times 100$ $\dfrac{586}{589} = 99\%$

Efficiency = $\dfrac{A+D}{A+B+C+D} \times 100$ $\dfrac{607}{616} = 99\%$

Figure 1–6 Hypothetical data analyzing the effectiveness of a diagnostic audiological test.

influenced by the prevalence of the disorder. However, the prevalence of retrocochlear disorders in patients with sensorineural hearing loss is unknown. Therefore, to calculate the PV of audiological tests, an estimate must be made regarding prevalence. Using the estimate makes it possible to calculate the PV of the PV1 and the PV of the PV2. The PV1 is calculated by dividing the true-positive findings by the total number of positive tests; the PV2 is calculated by dividing the true-negative findings by the total number of negative tests.

4. **Efficiency**   Efficiency specifies a test's overall accuracy. When applied to site of lesion procedures, it is the ability to accurately identify both cochlear and retrocochlear disorders. Efficiency is calculated by dividing the true-positive plus the true-negative findings by the total number of patients. In each case, the results of all the above measures are multiplied by 100 to derive a percentage.

In addition to these four measures, the false-negative rate (those with the disorder who are missed by the diagnostic test) and false-positive rate (those without the disorder but who are identified as having the disorder) can be calculated.

The ideal diagnostic audiological test is one that has high true-positive (sensitivity) and true-negative (specificity) rates and low false-positive and false-negative rates. The hypothetical data given in **Fig. 1–6** show sensitivity and specificity rates of 88 and 99% and false-negative and false-positive rates of 13 and 1%, respectively. In addition, the PV1 and PV2 are 78 and 99%, respectively, and the efficiency is 99%.

Whether the results from the test being evaluated in **Fig. 1–6** support routine clinical use depends on a variety factors, such as the possible use of other diagnostic tests, the consequences of incorrectly identifying or failing to identify the condition, and costs. Costs include not only the funding required to perform the tests but also other factors, such as time, inconvenience, and consequences if the test results are not accurate.

The preceding principles have been applied to diagnostic audiological test procedures by several investigators (S. Jerger, 1983; Turner and Nielsen, 1984). For example, Jerger and Jerger (1983) reported on the sensitivity, specificity, PV1 and PV2, and efficiency of six diagnostic audiological tests from data reported by Jerger and Jerger (1983) and Musiek et al (1983). Results have shown that the sensitivity of the six diagnostic tests (ABR, acoustic reflex, Békésy comfort loudness [BCL], Békésy, PI-PB, and the suprathreshold adaptation test [STAT]) ranges from 45 to 97%, with ABR audiometry being the most sensitive (97%) and Békésy and STAT being the least sensitive (50 and 45%, respectively). Specificity ranged from 70 to 100%, with Békésy and STAT having high specificity (90–100%) and acoustic reflexes and BCL the lowest specificity (70%). Although some variability exists, these results agree with reports of other investigators. The general inverse relationship between the sensitivity of a test and its specificity is demonstrated by Békésy audiometry. This procedure had next to the lowest sensitivity but the highest specificity. An exception to this trade-off is ABR, which has unusually high sensitivity and specificity.

The derived PVs were based on a prevalence rate of 50%. The PV for positive results ranged from 74 to 100%, whereas negative results ranged from 62 to 96%. As with sensitivity and specificity, generally a trade-off was present between the PV1s and PV2s. For example, Békésy audiometry had the highest PV1 (100%), indicating that no false-positive findings for any patient with cochlear disorder were present, but a low PV2 (67%) was present. Overall, PV1s were high for ABR, PI-PB, Békésy, and STAT. PV2s were high for ABR, acoustic reflex, and BCL. Of the six procedures evaluated, efficiency ranged from 68 to 91%. ABR had the highest efficiency at 91% and STAT the lowest at 68%. The remaining four procedures varied only slightly from 75 to 78%.

These types of data help to quantify the overall usefulness of diagnostic audiological tests performed in isolation. However, when a test battery approach is used, additional factors must be considered, such as the complex interactions between the various test procedures and the interpretation when discrepancies exist between test outcomes.

Two factors that have had an impact on diagnostic audiological tests and the diagnostic audiological test battery, especially with respect to identifying retrocochlear disorders, are the advancement of radiographic techniques, specifically magnetic resonance imaging (MRI), and an increased sensitivity to financial costs and reimbursement through managed care. Studies have reported the sensitivity of enhanced MRI in detecting acoustic neuromas, even those considered small, to be near 100% (Wilson et al, 1997). Coupled with data that show the cost of diagnostic audiological testing can exceed an MRI screening procedure, it is easy to see why MRI has become the gold standard for detecting acoustic neuromas (Hirsch et al, 1996). These are the types

of advances that have had a major impact on current diagnostic audiolological practice.

Evidence-Based Practice

Third-party payers and the increased sophistication of patients due to the instant and comprehensive availability of health-related information on the Internet has forced all health care providers to apply EBP to diagnostic and assessment procedures. One might assume that EBP refers only to the use of scientific methods to gather data on clinical practice. However, this notion is misleading in that the most widely accepted definition of EBP is the integration of the best research evidence with clinical expertise and patient values. Thus EBP involves a process by which the effectiveness of clinical practice is validated through thorough study and analysis. The general procedures followed in establishing EBP include framing the clinical question, finding the evidence, assessing the evidence, and making the decision.

Considerable attention has been given to EBP in recent years, and there is a growing literature on the processes used for EBP. Findings from studies on EBP are also being published regularly in a variety of areas. Up-to-date information on this expanding topic is available on the following Web sites, and it is certain that this area will grow considerably in the future:

- Academy of Neurologic Communication Disorders and Sciences
  http://www.ancds.org/practice.html
- American Academy of Pediatrics
  http://www.aap.org/policy/paramtoc.html
- American Speech-Language-Hearing Association (ASHA)
  http://www.asha.org
- National Electronic Library for Health (National Health Service of the UK)
  http://libraries.nelh.nhs.uk/guidelinesFinder
- Royal College of Speech-Language Therapists (UK)
  http://www.rcslt.org
- Scottish Intercollegiate Guidelines Network
  http://www.sign.ac.uk/guidelines/index/html
- The National Guideline Clearinghouse
  http://www.guideline.gov
- Veterans Administration
  http://www.oqp.med.va.gov/cpg.cpg.htm

◆ What Are Audiologists Doing?

In selecting a test battery, because of time and reimbursement constraints, that which is ideal may not be that which is real. The question arises as to which tests are preferred in clinical practice, and the answer has to do with efficiency. Two types of efficiency are in play when audiologists

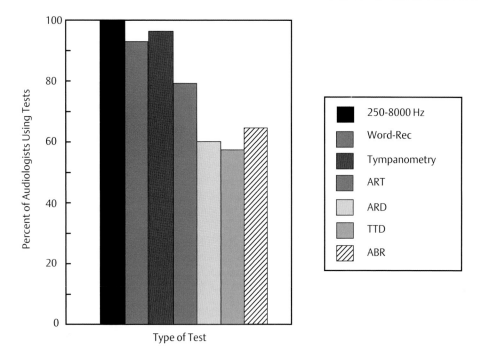

Figure 1–7 De facto audiometric test battery based on combined results from surveys of members of the American Academy of Audiology conducted by Chermak et al (1998) and Martin et al (1998). 250–8000 Hz, pure-tone audiometric testing; Word-Rec, word recognition testing; ART, acoustic reflex test; ARD, acoustic reflex decay; TTD, threshold tone decay; ABR, auditory brainstem response.

construct a test battery for clinical use. Besides its definition as a measure of validity, as discussed above, efficiency can also refer to functionality and serviceability. In practical application, some tests are easier for patients to manage and faster for audiologists to perform. Some tests lend themselves to quick interpretation and to modifications that reduce test time. Such tests have practical efficiency.

In the absence of widely accepted published practice guidelines for audiology, two trends are at work to establish standard diagnostic audiological test batteries. First, audiologists in busy practice settings tend to gravitate toward test protocols that allow rapid testing, especially if clinic scheduling allows only 30 minutes for a "comprehensive" audiometric evaluation. Second, managed care organizations and other third-party payers allow reimbursement for only certain procedural codes, which effectively eliminates noncovered tests from the audiological batteries applied to patients under those plans.

As to which tests are "popular," two surveys of AAA members reported on current audiological practices in the United States. Martin et al (1998) surveyed 218 audiologists on specific procedures they used most often. Chermak et al (1998) surveyed 185 audiologists, asking them to identify and rank the "central auditory tests" they used. **Figures 1–7** to **1–9** combine and summarize portions of findings from these two surveys, yielding de facto test batteries that reflect the present standard of care for audiology in the United States.

Figure 1–7 shows that most practicing audiologists (80%) currently apply a combination of pure-tone audiometry, speech audiometry, acoustic immittance, and the acoustic reflex test (ART) in their daily routine. Acoustic reflex decay (ARD), TTD,

and ABR also are used but by fewer audiologists (~60% of respondents). This does not mean that every patient receives the de facto battery suggested by **Fig. 1–7** but that those tests are available in many practices and are used to evaluate patients. A few audiologists (10%) eschew tympanometry and seem to get by with only pure-tone and speech audiometry. Of the available site-of-lesion tests, only ABR and TTD appear to be used by more than 60% of audiologists **(Fig. 1–7)**.

According to Martin et al (1998), it is not only the test protocols that are pared down in actual practice, but also the test procedures. The following shortcuts and percentage of respondents surveyed were reported:

♦ Bone conduction testing performed only if acoustic immittance results are abnormal (6% of respondents)

♦ Use of monitored live-voice presentation in SRT and word/speech recognition tests (94 and 91%, respectively)

♦ Elimination of familiarization component in SRT and word recognition tests (42 and 82%, respectively)

♦ Use of 5 dB step sizes for SRT determination (90%)

♦ SRT criterion based on "two out of three correct" SRT criterion (60%)

♦ Use of half lists for word-recognition testing (56%)

♦ Masking levels set for speech, independent of speech presentation level

Not all trends suggested compromise. Martin et al (1998) also found that more audiologists are testing 3000 and 6000 Hz

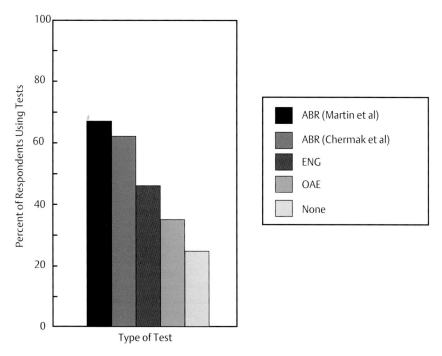

Figure 1–8 Popularity of electrophysiological and electroacoustic tests, based on percent of respondents to surveys by Chermak et al (1998) and Martin et al (1998). ABR, auditory brainstem response; ENG, electronystagmography; OAE; otoacoustic emissions.

thresholds than in the past. Also, 24% of the respondents reported the use of insert earphones in clinical evaluations.

Figure 1–8 details data for (electro)physiological tests, including ABR, electronystagmography (ENG), and OAE. Between 50 and 70% of the audiologists surveyed reported using ABR, ENG, or both; 30 to 35% reported using OAE;

and 25 to 30% reported no use of the procedures. This situation is likely to change as ABR equipment ages, OAE equipment becomes more accessible, and the OAE procedures are recognized for reimbursement.

Figure 1–9 compares the percent of audiologists using site of lesion tests over time, from 1972 to 1997. As shown, a

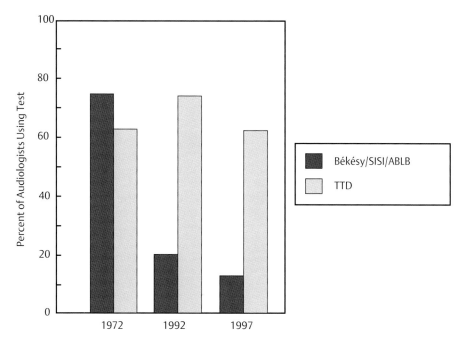

Figure 1–9 Comparison of use of behavioral site of lesion tests by audiologists in a 25-year period. Békésy/SISI/ABLB percentages are averages of percent use reported for respondents for each of the three tests (Data from Martin FN, Champlin CA, Chambers JA. Seventh Survey of Audiometric Practices in the United States. Journal of the American Academy of Audiology 1998; 9(2),95–104).

significant decline occurred in the general use of site of lesion testing. Compared with 75 to 80% of audiologists using Békésy, SISI, and ABLB tests in 1972, only between 10 and 15% were using the same tests in 1997. The one exception is TTD testing, which appears to have remained constant at 55 to 60% of the respondents. Most of the audiologists who use TTD employ a modified procedure that is faster to administer (Rosenberg or Olsen-Noffsinger).

Data from Chermak et al (1998) indicate that SCAN and SCAN-A are the most popular behavioral tests for auditory processing. All other auditory processing tests (Willeford, competing sentences, speech in noise, SSI with ipsilateral competing message [SSI-ICM] and contralateral competing message [SSI-CCM], staggered spondaic word [SSW], filtered speech, and performance intensity function for phonetically balanced words [PI-PB]) showed uniform declines in use from 1972 to 1997, and no more than half of the audiologists reported using auditory processing disorder tests at all.

Overall, available data clearly show that the procedures used in diagnostic audiology have changed significantly in the past 25 years. The behavioral diagnostic test battery for retrocochlear lesions has all but been abandoned, save for the TTD test. Many of the subsequent chapters in this book refer to the emerging potential use of auditory processing tests as a key to diagnostic audiology. In view of the low number of audiologists reporting their current use, if the optimism for their future application is to be realized, a major thrust must be made to develop and standardize effective and efficient diagnostic procedures that can be put into widespread use.

◆ Can Audiologists Diagnose Hearing Loss?

A question posed at times, especially in matters dealing with litigation, is whether audiologists can "diagnose" hearing loss. In the courtroom or in a deposition during the qualifying period, it is not uncommon for the opposing attorney to challenge the legality of an audiologist's rendering a "medical diagnosis" regarding the cause of hearing loss. Because the question posed includes the term *medical diagnosis,* the opposing attorney will attempt to disqualify the audiologist because giving a medical diagnosis requires medical training and licensing. The implication is that audiologists, because they are not physicians, are not qualified to "diagnose" hearing loss. As a result, the opinions of the audiologist regarding hearing loss cannot be entered into the proceedings.

One could go to several dictionaries and debate the meaning of the word *diagnose* and its use in various settings: in everyday language, in the clinic, in legal matters, and the like. For certain, to diagnose a condition, a need to administer and interpret diagnostic tests exists. In the case of hearing loss, diagnostic audiological tests would be administered and interpreted. This book testifies to the fact that many relatively simple and very complex diagnostic

protocols are used by audiologists on a regular basis and that audiologists in various settings are the ones interpreting the results.

However, the real question is whether the training and experience that audiologists receive qualify them to give an opinion about the possible cause or causes of a patient's hearing loss and its impact on the patient's ability to communicate. A corollary to this is that if the audiologist is not the professional who can render an opinion regarding the cause of a patient's hearing loss and its impact on communication ability, who is?

Controversial Point

- Some argue that audiologists cannot provide a diagnosis because they are not physicians, and only physicians have the credentials to give medical diagnoses.

Evidence suggests that audiologists are the primary professionals who are trained in hearing loss. As a result of the extensive training audiologists receive in the anatomy and physiology of the ear, pathophysiology of the auditory system, clinical experience, and professional skills, they are the most logical professionals to render an opinion regarding the effect of hearing loss on the communication function of patients. No other professional has the academic preparation. Otologists are the primary medical professionals who have expertise in diseases affecting the ear and auditory system. However, in most cases the otologist's expertise is limited to medical conditions of the ear, not hearing loss. In fact, in most medical schools audiologists are the faculty members who teach otology residents the curricula on hearing, hearing loss, and the impact of hearing loss on communication ability.

What about causation? Can audiologists render an opinion regarding causation? Certainly, by viewing audiometric results it is oftentimes possible to relate audiometric data to possible causation. For example, patients with conductive hearing loss cannot claim causation from continuous exposure to workplace noise of moderately high intensities. Audiologists, however, can confirm the causation of a patient's hearing loss with a history of noise exposure and the stereotypical 4000 to 6000 Hz sensorineural notch in the audiometric configuration to noise exposure. By examining other data, such as the intensity of workplace noise, the degree of threshold symmetry (or asymmetry), and social/medical history, including hobbies, sports, recreational activities, and medical conditions, an opinion can be given regarding the influence of each. These are clear examples of how the audiologist can, in fact, provide an opinion regarding the causation of hearing loss within the bounds of professional standards.

The *Scope of Practice in Audiology* by the ASHA states, "Audiologists provide comprehensive diagnostic and rehabilitative services for all areas of audiology, vestibular and related disorders" (American Speech-Language-Hearing Association, 1995). This statement gives audiologists national recognition that they can provide diagnostic testing and interpretation of results as they relate to hearing loss. However, care must be taken that audiologists keep within their recognized bounds. Performing diagnostic audiological tests properly is one thing, interpreting them properly and reporting them within acceptable limits is another. For example, audiologists cannot, on the basis of their test results, "recommend" surgery for a patient. Instead, referral of surgical candidates for possible treatment to be determined by the otologic surgeon is appropriate. Moreover, audiologists should not state that test findings are indicative of a specific otologic disease but rather suggest that test results are consistent with an otologic condition to be determined by the physician. In the ideal situation audiologists will collaborate closely with physicians, preferably otologists, in developing diagnostic information for each patient served.

Pearl

- Physicians provide medical diagnoses; audiologists provide audiological diagnoses.

It is unlikely that any audiologist who is not a physician would want to be perceived as a physician. The fact that audiologists function in the health care profession sometimes confuses patients, and every effort should be made to make it clear that the audiologist is not a medical practitioner. A way to prevent any misunderstanding about using the term *medical diagnosis* is to substitute the term *audiological diagnosis* to describe the contribution that audiologists make to the diagnostic process (D. Lipscomb, personal communication, October 1999). That is, "audiological diagnoses" can be made by audiologists, which clearly implies that "medical diagnoses" are in the exclusive purview of medical practitioners.

◆ Should Audiologists Use the Term *Patients* or *Clients*?

A question seldom posed formally, but having significant implications on how professionals perceive themselves and how they are perceived by others, is the terminology used to refer to those who receive audiology services. Put into a more specific framework, how should audiologists refer to those they serve? Are they "patients," "clients," or simply "customers?"

Controversial Point

- Some audiologists refer to those they serve as *clients*, and others use the term *patients*.

The noun *patient* is from the Latin *patiens*, the present participle of *pati*, which means "to suffer," and is used to denote an individual undergoing therapy or one who has or may have an affliction and is seeking therapy or a remedy. The word *patient* is associated with services provided by professions in health care (e.g., physicians, dentists, nurses, podiatrists). The word *client* is from the Latin *cliens*, meaning "dependent or follower," and refers to a customer or patron, one dependent on the patronage of another, or one for whom professional services are rendered. The word *client* is traditionally associated with professional services outside of health care, such as attorneys, accountants, and social workers.

In addressing the issue of what to call those served by audiologists, Harford (1995) asks the question,"Are audiologists hearing health care professionals?" He indicates that within the professions of speech-language pathology and audiology, organizations and segments within organizations promote the widespread use of the term *clients,* primarily because most of the members are providing services in the public schools where the use of the term *patients* would be questionable. He further states that audiologists are being influenced to use the term *clients* because of "lexical inbreeding," a process of exposing individuals to the use of terminology early in their careers as a result of the required exposure of audiologists-in-training to speech-language pathology instruction. Harford argues that many reasons exist why audiologists should use the term *patient,* including to be recognized as a viable part of the health care profession, to be recognized as the entry point into the health care system (the gatekeepers) for individuals with hearing impairment, to advance to a "doctoring profession," to be recognized by the health insurance industry, and to be favored in government health care regulations.

Practitioners will choose to call those they serve by the professional environment in which they work. Audiologists working in the public schools are unlikely to talk to teachers about the students in the school as their "patients." However, audiologists working in health care facilities, clinical settings, or private practices, providing diagnostic audiological services and rehabilitative programs, should carefully consider the professional implications, both internal and external, of how they refer to those they serve. For sure, all measures should be taken to avoid using the term *customers.*

The editors of all three volumes in this series have chosen to use the term *patients* when referring to those served by audiologists. Audiology is a health care profession, and using terminology identified with health care professionals will enhance the ability of audiologists to serve those with hearing loss by becoming a recognized and viable component of health care programs.

References

American Speech-Language-Hearing Association. (1995). Scope of practice in audiology. Rockville, MD: American Speech-Language Hearing Association.

Békésy, G. V. (1947). A new audiometer. Acta Oto-laryngologica (Stockholm), 35, 411–422.

Carhart, R. (1957). Clinical determination of abnormal auditory adaptation. Archives of Otolaryngology, 65, 32–39.

Chermak, G. D., Traynham, W. A., Seikel, J. A., & Musiek, F. E. (1998). Professional education and assessment practices in central auditory processing. Journal of the American Academy of Audiology, 9, 452–465.

Harford, E. (1995). Are audiologists hearing healthcare professionals? Audiology Today, 7(3), 10–11.

Hirsch, B. E., Durrant, J. D., Yetiser, S., Kamerer, D. B., & Martin, W. H. (1996). Localizing retrocochlear hearing loss. American Journal of Otology, 17, 537–546.

Jerger, J. (1960). Békésy audiometry in analysis of auditory disorders. Journal of Speech and Hearing Research, 3, 275–287.

Jerger, J., & Hayes, D. (1977). Diagnostic speech audiometry. Archives of Otolaryngology, 103, 216–222.

Jerger, J., & Herer, G. (1961). Unexpected dividend in Békésy audiometry. Journal of Speech and Hearing Disorders, 26, 390–391.

Jerger, J., & Musiek, F. (2000). Report of the Consensus Conference on the Diagnosis of Auditory Processing Disorders in School-aged Children. Journal of the American Academy of Audiology, 11, 467–474.

Jerger, J., Shedd, J., & Harford, E. (1959). On the detection of extremely small changes in sound intensity. Archives of Otolaryngology, 69, 200–211.

Jerger, S. (1983). Decision matrix and information theory analysis in the evaluation of neuroaudiologic tests. Seminars in Hearing, 4, 121–132.

Jerger, S., & Jerger, J. (1983). The evaluation of diagnostic audiometric tests. Audiology, 22, 144–161.

Martin, F. N., Champlin, C. A., & Chambers, J. A. (1998). Seventh Survey of Audiometric Practices in the United States. Journal of the American Academy of Audiology, 9(2), 95–104.

Musiek, F. E., Mueller, R. J., Kibbe, K. S., & Rackliffe, L. S. (1983). Audiological test selection in the detection of eighth nerve disorders. American Journal of Otology, 4, 281–287.

Olsen, W. O., & Noffsinger, D. (1974). Comparison of one new and three old tests of auditory adaptation. Archives of Otolaryngology, 99, 94–99.

Owens, E. (1964). Tone decay in eighth nerve and cochlear lesions. Journal of Speech and Hearing Disorders, 29, 14–22.

Rosenberg, P. E. (1958, November). Rapid clinical measurement of tone decay. Paper presented at the annual meeting of the American Speech and Hearing Association, New York.

Sanders, J. W. (1979). Recruitment. In W. F. Rintelmann (Ed.), Hearing assessment (pp. 261–280). Austin, TX: Pro-Ed.

Turner, R. G., & Nielsen, D. W. (1984). Application of clinical decision analysis to audiological tests. Ear and Hearing, 5, 125–133.

Wilson, D. F., Talbot, J. M., & Leigh, M. (1997). A critical appraisal of the role of auditory brain stem response and magnetic resonance imaging in acoustic neuroma diagnosis. American Journal of Otology, 18, 673–681.

Chapter 2

Anatomy and Physiology of the Peripheral Auditory System

Richard J. Salvi, Wei Sun, and Edward Lobarinas

- ♦ **Cochlear Anatomy**

  Ionic Composition of Endolymph and Perilymph Fluid
  Inner and Outer Hair Cells
  Prestin and Electromotility
  Afferent Innervation
  Efferent Innervation

- ♦ **Cochlear Mechanics**
- ♦ **Gross Cochlear Potentials**

  Endolymphatic Potential
  Cochlear Microphonic Potential

  Summating Potential
  Compound Action Potential

- ♦ **Hair Cell Physiology**
- ♦ **Outer Hair Cell Electromotility**
- ♦ **Otoacoustic Emissions**

  Spontaneous Otoacoustic Emissions
  Distortion Product Otoacoustic Emissions
  Transient Otoacoustic Emissions

- ♦ **Auditory Nerve Fiber Responses**
- ♦ **Summary**

The mammalian auditory system is remarkably sensitive and shows an extraordinary ability to extract signals of interest from a background of noise. In humans, it is able to detect changes in sound pressure that are slightly greater than the theoretical limit set by the Brownian motion of the air particles and is able to detect and process extremely high intensity sounds in excess of 130 dB sound pressure level (SPL). Thus, the dynamic range of the normal auditory system exceeds the range of most digital sound recordings, which have ranges on the order of 96 dB. The system is not only sensitive but also very selective. For example, in the midst of a noisy party, normal listeners can "tune in" to a particular conversation and quickly switch to processing another acoustic source that suddenly becomes more interesting or important. To determine the location of a sound in the environment, a listener must be able to detect small differences in the time of arrival of sounds reaching the two ears, time differences as small as 10 to 20 μs.

Elderly individuals or those exposed to loud sounds or ototoxic drugs have difficulty understanding speech in quiet or noisy rooms and in identifying the location of the speaker. These hearing deficits are invariably associated with damage to the sensory cells and neurons in the inner ear. To appreciate the biological bases underlying these hearing deficits, it is important to have a clear understanding of the basic anatomical elements in the inner ear and how the inner ear converts sound into neural activity that is transmitted from the inner ear to the central auditory pathway by way of the auditory nerve, the eighth cranial nerve.

♦ Cochlear Anatomy

Sounds in the environment are transmitted from the external ear and through the middle ear before entering the cochlea, which consists of three, coiled, fluid-filled membranous compartments surrounded by a bony shell. The external ear (pinna) and ear canal (external auditory meatus) are mainly responsible for funneling sound down to the tympanic membrane, causing the tympanic membrane (eardrum) to vibrate. The sound-induced vibrations of the tympanic membrane are subsequently transmitted to the inner ear through the three middle ear ossicles, first to the malleus, which is attached to the tympanic membrane,

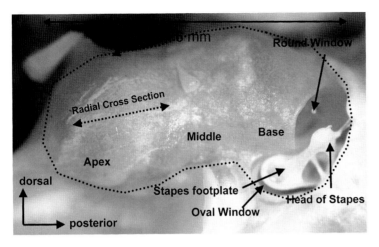

Figure 2–1 Photomicrograph of a chinchilla cochlea looking inward from the direction of the tympanic membrane. The enclosed dotted line shows the approximate boundaries of the cochlea. The stapes footplate inserts into the oval window in the base of the cochlea and is held in place by a membranous ring of tissue. The round window membrane in the base of the cochlea is oriented approximately perpendicular to the plane of the oval window. The location of the base, middle, and apex of the cochlea is indicated. The dotted line labeled Radial Cross Section shows the approximate plane of the radial section taken through the apex of the cochlea.

then to the incus, and finally to the stirrup-shaped stapes, the smallest bone in the body. **Figure 2–1** is a photomicrograph of the chinchilla cochlea showing the bony shell and the stapes. The footplate of the stapes inserts into the oval window, an opening in the base of the cochlea, behind which lies the scala vestibuli, a fluid-filled chamber. The stapes is loosely attached to the oval window by a ring of membranous tissue, allowing the stapes to move in and out in response to sound-induced vibrations transmitted through the middle ear. Two struts emerge from the footplate of the stapes and join together to form the head of the stapes; the head of the stapes attaches to the incus (not shown) by a cartilaginous joint. The round window membrane, also located at the base of the cochlea, is oriented at an angle of approximately 90 degrees relative to the oval window.

Figure 2–2A shows a schematic of a radial cross section (see black dotted arrow in **Fig. 2–1**) through one turn of the cochlea. The cross section reveals the location of the main components in each turn. The scala vestibuli, containing perilymph, is separated from the scala media by Reissner's membrane. The scala media, which is filled with endolymph, is bounded radially by the lateral wall containing the cells of the stria vascularis and spiral ligament. A large network of blood vessels course through the stria vascularis, and many of the cells lining the endolymphatic space contain numerous energy-dependent pumps for moving ions into and out of the scala media. These electrogenic pumps are responsible for generating the +80 mV potential in the scala media and the high concentration of potassium. The organ of Corti rests on the basilar membrane just below the scala media. The basilar membrane is attached laterally at the spiral ligament and medially at the osseous spiral lamina. The osseous spiral lamina projects out from the modiolus, a hollow bony canal through which the auditory nerve fibers pass as they exit the inner ear on their way to the cochlea nuclei in the brainstem. The scala tympani, also filled with perilymph, lies below the basilar membrane. Although the scala tympani and the scala vestibuli are separate compartments, they share a common fluid and communicate with one another through the helicotrema, a membranous opening

located in the apex of the cochlea. The basal end of the scala vestibuli ends at the footplate of the stapes, and the basal end of the scala tympani terminates at the round window membrane. Because the fluids in the scala tympani and scala vestibuli are connected at the helicotrema, a slow, inward movement of the stapes will result in outward displacement of the round window membrane. The sensory hair cells transduce sounds into neural activity. The spiral ganglion neurons are located near the entrance of the osseous spiral lamina. The peripheral processes of the spiral ganglion neurons extend out to the hair cells in the organ of Corti; their central axons extend medially into the modiolus, forming the auditory nerve. The auditory nerve passes through a small fenestra in the skull, the internal auditory meatus, where the fibers synapse on neurons in the cochlear nucleus.

Figure 2–2B is an expanded view of the organ of Corti showing the three rows of outer hair cells and one row of inner hair cells, plus several nonsensory cells collectively referred to as supporting cells. The inner hair cells are separated from the outer hair cells by the tunnel of Corti. The tunnel of Corti is formed by outer pillar cells and inner pillar cells; the feet of the pillar cells rest on the basilar membrane, and their heads join at the surface of the organ of Corti to create an arch. The inner hair cells are completely surrounded by supporting cells. The outer hair cells, by contrast, make contact with supporting cells only at their base, where they rest in a cuplike depression in the Deiters' cell, and at their apical pole. Importantly, the outer hair cell lateral wall is completely surrounded by fluid, allowing this portion of the cell to move freely. The inner hair cells are contacted by spiral ganglion neurons classified as type I, and the outer hair cells are contacted by type II spiral ganglion neurons. Hensen's cells are located lateral to the outer hair cells; the inner sulcus cells form a cavity medial to the inner hair cell. The tectorial membrane, a fibrous, acellular structure, sits above the hair cells. The lateral edge of the tectorial membrane is attached to the stereocilia, which protrude from the apical surface of the outer hair cell. The thin, medial edge of the tectorial membrane is attached to the cells of the inner sulcus; this thin attachment allows the tectorial

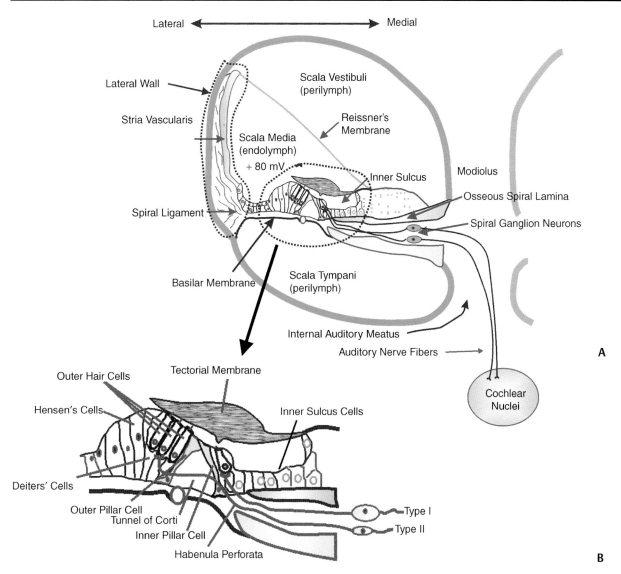

Figure 2–2 **(A)** Schematic showing radial cross section (see **Fig. 2–1**) through a turn of the cochlea. Each turn of the cochlea contains three fluid-filled compartments: the scala vestibuli and scala tympani, both filled with perilymph, and the scala media, filled with endolymph and with a +80 mV potential relative to the scala tympani and scala vestibuli. Reissner's membrane separates the scala vestibuli from the scala media. The lateral wall of the cochlea (enclosed dotted line) containing the stria vascularis and spiral ligament forms the lateral boundary of the scala media. The organ of Corti (enclosed dotted line and arrow pointing to panel B) contains the sensory hair cells that convert sounds into neural activity. The spiral ganglion neurons, which lie within the bony core of the modiolus (enclosed dotted line), have peripherally oriented neurites that make synaptic contact with the hair cells in the organ of Corti and centrally projecting axons that form the auditory nerve and which make synaptic contact with neurons in the cochlear nuclei that lie within the brainstem. The osseous spiral lamina projects out from the modiolus to form a bony shelf on which the medial edge of the organ of Corti attaches. The basilar membrane, on which the organ of Corti rests, projects medially from the osseous spiral lamina outward toward the spiral ligament in the lateral wall. (From Melloni, B. J. (1957). In: What's new, No. 199. North Chicago: Abbott Laboratories, with permission.) **(B)** Schematic showing enlargement of the organ of Corti region in panel A (enclosed dotted line at center). The outer hair cells rest on top of Deiters' cells; Hensen's cells lie lateral to the outer hair cells and Deiters' cells. The inner pillar cells and outer pillar cells form the arch of the organ of Corti. Inner hair cells lie medial to the inner pillar cells. The tectorial membrane lies above the hair cells and makes contact with the stereocilia projecting from the apical pole of the outer hair cells. The medial edge of the tectorial membrane attaches to the cells in the inner sulcus region. Type I and II spiral ganglion neurons with cell bodies in the modiolus send peripheral processes out to the inner hair cells and outer hair cells. (From Bess, F. H., & Hames, L. E. (1990). Audiology: The fundamentals. Baltimore: Williams & Wilkins, with permission.)

membrane to follow any vertical movement of the organ of Corti.

Ionic Composition of Endolymph and Perilymph

The ionic composition of perilymph in the scala tympani and scala vestibuli is similar to that of cerebrospinal fluid, that is, high in sodium (~150 mmol/L) and low in potassium (~3 mmol/L) (Bosher and Warren, 1968). The endolymph, in contrast, contains a high concentration of potassium (~160 mmol/L) and a low concentration of sodium (~1.5 mmol/L). The concentration of calcium in endolymph (~0.02 μm) is considerably lower than that in perilymph (~0.6–1.3 mmol/L). However, the concentration of chloride (~120–130 mmol/L) is similar in perilymph and endolymph. The boundaries of the endolymphatic space in the scala media are circumscribed by three structures: Reissner's membrane, the lateral wall of the cochlea, and the reticular lamina, the cells lining the apical surface of the organ of Corti. The intercellular junctions of the cell forming the reticular lamina at the apical surface of the organ of Corti are extremely tight, thereby preventing the flow of sodium and potassium ions down their respective concentration gradients. Thus, the apical surface of the organ of Corti is bathed by endolymph, whereas the fluid spaces below the reticular lamina (e.g., the tunnel of Corti) are filled with perilymph. The unique ionic composition of endolymph arises from energy-dependent adenosine triphosphate (ATP), electrogenic pumps located in the stria vascularis of the lateral wall. These pumps increase the concentration of potassium and the voltage in the scala media while reducing the concentration of sodium. For example, the sodium-potassium adenosinetriphosphatase (ATPase) electrogenic pumps bring two potassium ions into the scala media while removing three sodium ions on every cycle, resulting in a net increase in charge of +1 for every pump stroke (hence the term *electrogenic*). The +80 mV endolymphatic potentials act like a battery with its positive pole in the scala media and the negative pole inside the organ of Corti.

Inner and Outer Hair Cells

Figure 2–3A–C illustrates several of the important features of inner and outer hair cells, as well as the stereocilia bundles that emerge from the apical surface of the hair cells. The stereocilia, which are composed of rigid, polymerized actin filaments, taper near the rootlet region as each stereocilium enters the cuticular plate of the hair cell (not shown). Consequently, when the stereocilia are deflected, the rigid shaft of each stereocilium bends at the rootlet. The bundle consists of three parallel rows of stereocilia. When viewed from above (**Fig. 2–3A**), the stereocilia bundle on the inner hair cell is arranged in a gently curving arc located on the side of the hair cell closest to the lateral wall. The stereocilia bundle on the outer hair cells, in contrast, is arranged in a blunt W- or U-shaped configuration. When viewed from the side, the stereocilia bundle has a staircase arrangement, with the tallest stereocilia located on the side of the hair cell near the lateral wall (**Fig. 2–3B**). The individual stereocilia are attached to one another by side links near the base of the stereocilia. The side link attachments cause all the stereocilia in the bundle to move in unison when the bundle is deflected. Current models of hair cell transduction, whereby sound vibration is converted to neural activity, envision a mechanically gated ion channel near the tip of each

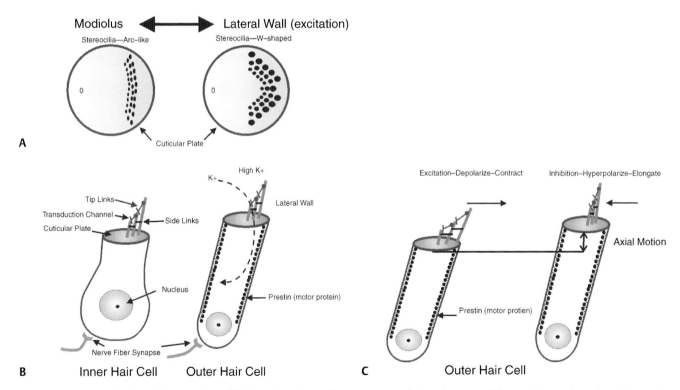

Figure 2–3 **(A)** Apical surface of an inner hair cell (left) and outer hair cell (right) showing the arrangement of a stereocilia bundle. The stereocilia bundle is arranged in a gently curving arc on the inner hair cell and in a W- or U-shaped pattern on the outer hair cell. **(B)** Radial view showing the pear-shaped cell body of an inner hair cell and the cylindrical shape of an outer hair cell. Numerous prestin motor protein molecules are arranged along the lateral wall of the outer hair cells. Stereocilia are arranged in a staircase pattern, with the tallest stereocilia oriented toward the lateral wall (excitatory direction) and the shortest stereocilia closest to the modiolus. Deflection of stereocilia toward the tallest stereocilia (lateral wall) leads to increased tension on tip links and opening of the transduction channel, resulting in the influx of potassium ions (K+). The side link connecting adjacent stereocilia causes all the stereocilia in the bundle to move in unison. **(C)** Deflection of stereocilia toward the tallest stereocilia results in depolarization of the outer hair cell and axial contraction (shortening) of the hair cell body. Deflection of stereocilia toward the shortest row of stereocilia results in hyperpolarization and slight elongation of the outer hair cell body. The vertical line in the rightmost outer hair cell shows the approximate direction of axial motion. (From Durrant, J., & Lovnnic, J. H. (1995). Bases of hearing science (3rd ed.) (p. 144). Baltimores: Williams & Wilkins, with permission.)

stereocilium (Hudspeth, 1992). Tip links, which apply tension to the mechanically gated channel, extend from the tip of the shorter stereocilia in one row of stereocilia to the side of another stereocilium in the adjacent taller row. The transduction channel, responsible for converting mechanical vibration (sound) into neural activity, is thought to be located near the tip of the stereocilia. Sound-induced deflection of the stereocilia toward the tallest stereocilia in the bundle (i.e., toward the lateral wall) causes tension to develop in the tip link, which leads to the opening of the mechanically gated ion channel at the tip of the stereocilia, resulting in the influx of potassium ions (K^+) into the hair cell.

Prestin and Electromotility

The inner hair cell soma is pear-shaped, whereas the outer hair cell soma is cylindrical. The nucleus of the hair cell is located near the basal end of the cell. The peripheral processes from the afferent spiral ganglion neuron extend out to the hair cells and make synaptic contact at the base of the inner and outer hair cells. Along the lateral wall of the outer hair cells lies the lateral cisternae (smooth endoplasmic reticulum) and a circumferential ring of filaments resembling a coiled spring; the circumferential filaments impart radial rigidity to the outer hair cell but allow it to move longitudinally (axial motion) (Holley and Ashmore, 1988). The membranes along the lateral wall are decorated with numerous proteins, dubbed prestin, that are linked to one another (**Fig. 2–3B**) (Dallos and Fakler, 2002). Prestin is a unique motor protein that can rapidly alter its shape (conformation) in response to changes in voltage across the outer hair cell membrane. The prestin motor proteins and the filamentous cytoskeletal spring in the lateral wall give the outer hair cell electromotile properties, causing the cell to elongate and contract in the axial direction at rates up to 20 kHz (Gale and Ashmore, 1997). When the stereocilia on the outer hair cell are deflected toward the tallest stereocilia, potassium ions flow in through the transduction channels, depolarizing the cell and causing the outer hair cell to contract in the axial direction (**Fig. 2–3C**, right). Conversely, when the stereocilia are deflected toward the shortest stereocilia, the influx of potassium ions is blocked; this leads to hyperpolarization of the outer hair cell and elongation in the axial direction (**Fig. 2–3C**, left). The axial movement of the outer hair cell is asymmetric, such that elongation is considerably less than contraction. The prevailing opinion is that the electromotile response of the outer hair cells serves as a "cochlear amplifier" that enhances the incoming sound vibration in a frequency-specific manner. Support for this hypothesis comes from lesion studies showing that when the outer hair cells are destroyed or prestin is eliminated from outer hair cells in genetically engineered mice, the threshold for hearing is elevated 40 to 50 dB, and frequency selectivity is impaired (Liberman et al, 2002; Ryan and Dallos, 1975). Because the electromotile response is asymmetric and nonlinear, it gives rise to distortion, which can be propagated in the reverse direction from the outer hair cells, into the cochlear fluids and back into the ear canal, a point that will be developed more fully in the section Otoacoustic Emissions.

Special Consideration

- Axial movement of the outer hair cells is facilitated by the fact that the lateral wall of an outer hair cell is surrounded by fluid rather than attached to surrounding supporting cells that would hinder the elongation and contraction of the outer hair cell.

Afferent Innervation

The human ear contains approximately 3000 inner hair cells aligned in a single row and roughly 12,000 outer hair cells aligned in three parallel rows; these orderly rows extend from the base of the cochlea to the apex over a distance of 34 mm. The 42,000 spiral ganglion neurons in the human cochlea provide the sole source of afferent innervation to the outer and inner hair cells. Approximately 90% of the spiral ganglion neurons, classified morphologically as type I neurons, make synaptic contact with inner hair cells (**Fig. 2–4A**). Each type I neuron contacts a single inner hair cell in a one-to-one manner; thus, the neural output from each type I neuron provides information from a single hair cell at a specific point along the basilar membrane. Each inner hair cell, however, is contacted by roughly 15 to 20 type I neurons; thus, the output from each inner hair cell is transmitted to the cochlear nucleus in a highly redundant manner. The remaining spiral ganglion neurons, classified morphologically as type II neurons, project out through the tunnel of Corti, bypassing the inner hair cells and extending across to the outer hair cells, where they spiral basalward for a few millimeters, contacting roughly 10 outer hair cells along the way (**Fig. 2–4A**) (Spoendlin, 1972). The axons of both type I and type II spiral ganglion neurons project centrally through the internal auditory meatus as the auditory nerve and then synapse on neurons in the cochlear nucleus located in the lateral portion of the brainstem.

Efferent Innervation

The cochlea not only receives acoustic information from the external environment but also receives feedback from neurons located around the superior olivary complex in the brainstem, referred to as the olivocochlear complex. The olivocochlear neurons arise from two major sources, one located near the lateral superior olivary complex, referred to as the lateral olivocochlear (LOC) neurons, and the other located near the medial superior olive, referred to as medial olivocochlear (MOC) neurons (**Fig. 2–4B**) (Warr and Guinan, 1979). The total number of olivocochlear neurons is roughly 1000. Approximately 65% of the olivocochlear efferent neurons in the cat are LOC neurons, and roughly 35% are MOC neurons. The MOC neurons give rise to thick, myelinated fibers that branch extensively after crossing the organ of Corti and then synapse on the base of many outer hair cells. The majority of the MOC efferents that project to the outer hair cells arise from neurons on the contralateral side of the brain (crossed) versus the ipsilateral side (uncrossed). The majority of the LOC neurons give rise to thin, unmyelinated fibers that

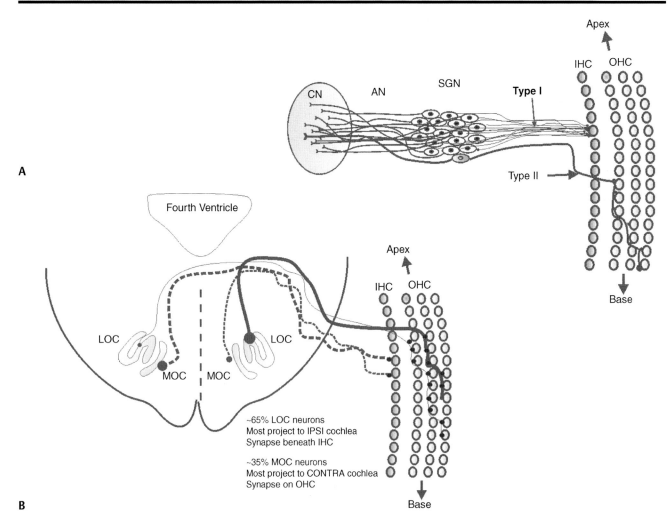

Figure 2–4 **(A)** Schematic illustrating afferent innervation of the mammalian inner ear. Three rows of outer hair cells and one row of inner hair cells form orderly rows that extend from the base of the cochlea to the apex. The spiral ganglion neurons (SGN) consist of type I and type II neurons, which constitute ~90% and 10% of the afferent population, respectively. The peripheral processes of type I neurons project to the inner hair cells; each type I neuron makes synaptic contact with a single inner hair cell. Approximately 20 type I neurons contact a single inner hair cell. The peripheral process of type II neurons cross the tunnel of Corti, ramify, and spiral basalward among the outer hair cells. Each type II neuron makes synaptic contact with ~20 outer hair cells. The axons of the SGN collect into the auditory nerve (AN), project centrally into the cochlear nuclei (CN), bifurcate, and make synaptic contact with many second-order neurons. (Reprinted from "The afferent innervation of the cochlea," Spoendlin, H. In *Evoked electrical activity in the auditory nervous system*, Naunton, R. F. & Fernandez, C.

(Eds.), p 35, copyright 1978, with permission from Elsevier.) **(B)** Schematic illustrating the olivocochlear efferent innervation of the inner ear. The cell bodies of the lateral olivocochlear (LOC) efferent neurons, which comprise ~65% of the efferent population, are located near the S-shaped lateral superior olivary nucleus. The axons of the thin, unmyelinated axons of LOC neurons synapse on afferent fibers located beneath the inner hair cells; most LOC neurons project to the ipsilateral (IPSI) cochlea, but some project to the contralateral cochlea. The cell bodies of the medial olivocochlear (MOC) efferent neurons, which comprise ~35% of the efferent population, are located near the medial superior olive. The axons of the thick, myelinated axons of MOC neurons synapse on outer hair cells; most LOC neurons project to the contralateral (CONTRA) cochlea, but some project to the ipsilateral cochlea. IHC, inner hair cell; OHC, outer hair cell. (From Liberman, M. C. (1990). Effects of chronic cochlear de-efferentiation on auditory-nerve response. Hearing Research 49, 209–224, with permission.)

synapse on the afferent type I fibers beneath the inner hair cells. Most of the LOC efferents project to the ipsilateral cochlea. The functional role of the olivocochlear system is not completely understood; however, there is a growing body of evidence suggesting that MOC neurons can influence outer hair cell function, alter outer hair cell electromotility, and enhance the detection of signal in noise (Winslow and Sachs, 1988). Because they make synaptic contact with the afferent dendrites beneath the inner hair cells, the LOC neurons are well positioned to influence the rate of neural activity transmitted through type I neurons (Puel et al, 2002).

♦ Cochlear Mechanics

Sound-induced motion of the stapes gives rise to pressure fluctuations in the cochlear fluids that cause the basilar membrane to vibrate; the location of the vibration pattern along the length of the cochlea varies with the intensity and spectral characteristics of the stimulus. The inward and outward motion of the stapes is opposed by the inertia of the fluid mass within the cochlea, the stiffness of the basilar membrane tissues, and the frictional resistance generated by fluid motion within the scalae. Because the fluids in the inner ear are incompressible, the pressure fluctuations in the fluids occur almost instantaneously along the entire length of the cochlea. Nevertheless, the entire basilar membrane does not move in unison because the mechanical impedance of the cochlear partition varies from base to apex. The stiffness of the basilar membrane gradually decreases from base to apex, while its mass increases from base to apex. Because the base of the cochlea is stiffer and the mass less than in the apex, the base responds sooner than the apex when pressure is applied to the basilar membrane. Consequently, the movement of the basilar membrane begins in the base and gradually shifts toward the apex with time, giving the appearance of a "traveling wave" displacement pattern.

Figure 2–5B shows the traveling wave displacement pattern along the length of the cochlea during stimulation with a high-frequency tone (8 kHz), a mid-frequency tone (2 kHz),

and a low-frequency tone (200 Hz). Each thin line represents a series of snapshot views of basilar membrane motion, showing how the peak response shifts from the base toward the apex of the cochlea. High-frequency sounds produce a traveling wave envelope (dotted line, **Fig. 2–5B**) that has a peak near the base of the cochlea; no activity occurs in the middle or the apex of the cochlea. The peak of the traveling wave for mid-frequency sounds is located near the middle of the cochlea. Low-frequency sounds produce a peak near the apex of the cochlea. However, low frequencies also activate the base and middle of the cochlea at high sound levels; that is, the mechanical vibration pattern spreads basalward with increasing intensity. The shift in the location of the peak results in a frequency-to-place transformation. That is, the basilar membrane acts as a frequency analyzer, segregating different frequencies according to the position of maximal excitation along the cochlear partition.

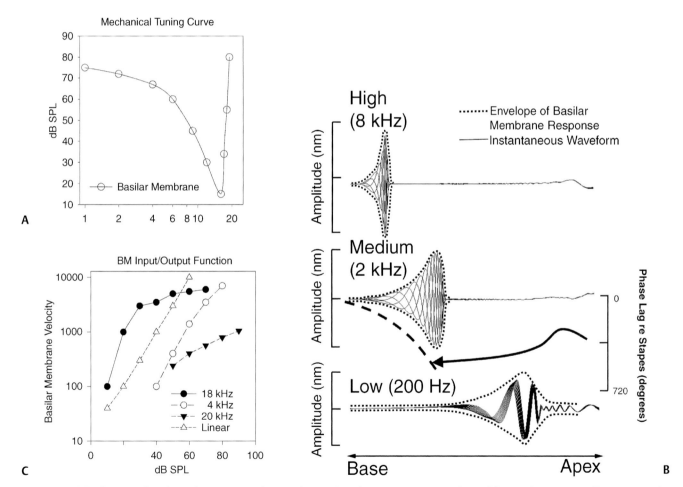

Figure 2–5 **(A)** Schematic of mechanical tuning curve showing the sound pressure level (SPL) in dB needed to produce a constant magnitude of basilar membrane velocity. (From Sellick, P. M., Patuzzi, R., & Johnstone, B. M. (1982). Measurement of basilar membrane motion in the guinea pig using the Mossbauer technique. Journal of the Acoustical Society of America, 72, 131–141, with permission.) **(B)** Schematics of traveling wave displacement along the basilar membrane (base to apex), for high-frequency tones (8 kHz), mid-frequency tones (2 kHz), and low-frequency tones (200 Hz). The dotted lines show the envelope of the basilar membrane response; note that the peak of the envelope is located near the base of the cochlea for high frequencies and near the apex for low frequencies. The thin lines show

the instantaneous waveform of the traveling wave at different times. The gray dashed line in the 2 kHz plot shows the phase lag of points along the basilar membrane relative to the stapes (ordinate shown on right). (From Sellick, P. M., Patuzzi, R., & Johnstone, B. M. (1982). Measurement of basilar membrane motion in the guinea pig using the Mossbauer technique. Journal of the Acoustical Society of America, 72, 131–141, with permission). **(C)** Schematic of basilar membrane input/output functions for the 18 kHz region of the cochlea. Basilar membrane (BM) velocity (logarithmic scale) plotted as a function of stimulus intensity (dB SPL) for stimulus frequencies of 4, 18 (characteristic frequency [CF]), and 20 kHz. White triangles show linear input/output function.

The mass and stiffness gradient of the cochlear partition also influences its temporal response. Because the base of the cochlea is stiffer and lighter than the apex, it responds more quickly to stimulation than more apical locations. Thus, although the pressure wave initiated by stapes motion is applied to the entire basilar membrane almost simultaneously, the basilar membrane near the base of the cochlea starts to move sooner than that in the apex. This results in a wave of motion that appears to move from base to apex over time. The time required for initiation of basilar membrane movement at any given point along the basilar membrane can be expressed in terms of phase lag. The phase lag can be compared with the phase of the stimulus or the phase of another point on the basilar membrane, such as the stapes. This is illustrated by the gray dashed line in **Fig. 2–5B** (2 kHz), which shows the phase lag (0–720 degrees, ordinate on right side of graph) of points along the basilar membrane (base to peak of the traveling wave) with respect to motion of the stapes. Note that the phase lag of the base relative to the stapes is small and that phase lag increases as the distance from the base increases.

The earliest traveling wave displacement patterns, measured by Békésy in ears from dead cadavers, were extremely broad due to the poor physiological condition of the tissues. Consequently, the results were difficult to reconcile with psychophysical measurements that suggested that the auditory system was extremely sharply tuned. More recent measurements from healthy cochleas have shown that the basilar membrane displacement patterns are extremely sharply tuned (Khanna and Leonard, 1982; Nuttall et al, 1991). The schematic in **Fig. 2–5A** shows a frequency-threshold-tuning curve for a point near the base of the cochlea. Threshold was defined as the minimum intensity required for producing a constant displacement of the basilar membrane. The frequency with the lowest threshold, referred to as the characteristic frequency (CF), was approximately 18 kHz. Threshold increased significantly at frequencies above and below CF. The mechanical tuning curve in a healthy ear consists of a low-threshold, narrowly tuned tip near CF and a high-threshold, broadly tuned tail below CF. The high-frequency side of the tuning curve has an extremely steep slope because the basilar membrane displacement envelope shifts farther toward the base of the cochlea as frequency increases (see **Fig. 2–5B**).

The schematic in **Fig. 2–5C** shows basilar membrane velocity (logarithmic ordinate) plotted as a function of the sound pressure level (SPL), that is, the basilar membrane input/output function. Input/output functions are shown for stimuli presented at CF (18 kHz), below CF (4 kHz), and above CF (20 kHz). For comparison, the solid line shows the response of a linear system with a slope of 1. Because the basilar membrane is most sensitive to frequencies near CF, the input/output function at CF is located farthest to the left (lower intensities). The input/output functions above and below CF are located farther to the right (higher intensities) to reflect the decreased sensitivity to off-CF frequencies. For frequencies below CF (4 kHz), the slope of the input/output function is close to 1, indicating that the

basilar membrane response is essentially linear. The input/output function above CF (20 kHz) is also linear, but the slope is less than 1. In contrast, the input/output function at CF shows a compressive nonlinearity. That is, the input/output function rises rapidly at low intensities but begins to saturate at high intensities, resulting in a slope that is less than 1 at high sound levels. Thus, the basilar membrane exhibits a frequency-dependent nonlinear response near CF and a linear response at frequencies far below and above CF. The sensitive, nonlinear response seen at frequencies near CF is believed to be linked to outer hair cell electromotile response, which is nonlinear and asymmetric (**Fig. 2–3C**).

Pearl

- The nonlinear response of the basilar membrane observed near the CF of the basilar membrane is believed to generate distortion products in the normal ear. The intrinsically generated distortion products are transmitted to the central auditory system, where they are heard as aural combination tones. The internally generated distortion is also propagated from the cochlea back into the ear canal (reverse transmission), where it can be recorded with a sensitive microphone.

◆ Gross Cochlear Potentials

The functional status of the cochlea can be assessed by measuring the electrical potentials from different locations within the inner ear in the presence of sound stimulation or in quiet. Low-impedance gross electrodes can be used to sample the electrical activity contributed by many cells. The electrical activity detected by the electrode is generally dominated by the cells closest to the electrode, and the contribution of more remote generators falls off with increasing distance from the electrode. As the electrode approaches the neural generator, the electrical potential increases, and as the electrode passes through the generator, the polarity of the electrical signal reverses polarity and then declines with increasing distance. The type of signal that is recorded depends on bandwidth of the measurement system and whether the electrode and amplifier are capable of recording alternating current (AC) or direct current (DC) signals. Because the voltages generated by the cells in the inner ear are relatively small, the neural activity picked up from the electrode must be amplified (1000–50,000 ×) and filtered to improve the signal-to-noise ratio. If the neural activity being recorded from the inner ear is time locked (synchronized), it can be averaged to further enhance the neural signal from the randomly occurring background noise. To accomplish this, every time the signal (e.g., tone burst) is presented, the output of the recording amplifier is digitized by a computer for a brief segment of time

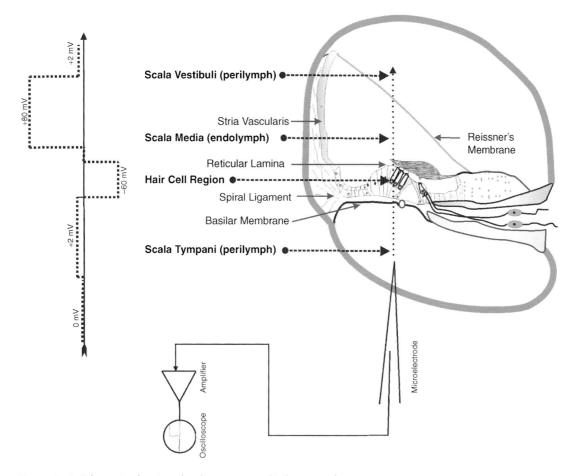

Figure 2–6 Schematic showing the direct current (DC) potential recorded from an electrode as it is gradually advanced through the scala tympani, basilar membrane, hair cell region, reticular lamina, scala media, Reissner's membrane, and finally scala vestibuli. Note the large −60 mV drop in voltage as the electrode passes through the hair cell region in the organ of Corti and then the large +80 mV increase as the electrode passes through the reticular lamina into the endolymph. The +80 mV endolymphatic potential disappears once the electrode passes through Reissner's membrane into the scala vestibuli.

following the onset of the stimulus (i.e., a sweep is a digital representation of the recorded waveform). Each sweep is added to previous ones so that the coherent (time locked) neural response increases in amplitude (i.e., the average waveform), and the random (incoherent) neural noise cancels out. Signal averaging is a powerful tool for enhancing weak biological signals that are often embedded in a noisy background.

Endolymphatic Potential

The endolymphatic potential is a standing potential that can be recorded from the endolymphatic space with any sound stimulation. To record this potential, a small hole must be drilled through the bony shell surrounding the cochlea to gain access to the tissues and fluids within. When a small, low-impedance glass microelectrode capable of measuring DC potentials is advanced through the hole into the fluid spaces in the cochlea and the organ of Corti in the absence of any sound stimulation, the magnitude and polarity of the DC potential (relative to ground) change dramatically as a function of electrode position, as

schematized in **Fig. 2–6**. As the electrode passes through the extracellular fluids into the scala tympani, the DC potential increases from 0 to +2 mV. As the electrode is advanced through the scala tympani, the potential remains near +2 mV until the electrode passes through the basilar membrane and enters the organ of Corti. At this point the potential abruptly drops to approximately −60 mV, presumably reflecting the intracellular potential (resting potential) of hair cells or supporting cells within the organ of Corti. As the electrode advances through the reticular lamina and enters the scala media, the potential abruptly jumps to +80 mV. As the electrode advances through the scala media, it remains at +80 mV until the tip of the electrode passes through Reissner's membrane and enters the scala vestibuli, at which point the potential abruptly drops to +2 mV, similar to the potential seen in the scala tympani. Importantly, the cuticular plate and stereocilia lie at the boundary of a large voltage gradient. Because the resting potential inside the hair cell is on the order of −60 mV and the endolymph fluid is at +80 mV, the voltage across the transduction channels at the apical pole of the hair cell is around 140 mV.

Pearl

• High doses of loop-inhibiting diuretics such as furosemide and ethacrynic acid temporarily abolish the endolymphatic potential, resulting in a temporary hearing loss. Some cases of age-related hearing loss arise from the degeneration of the vessels and cells in the lateral wall of the cochlea that are responsible for generating the endocochlear potential.

Cochlear Microphonic Potential

When a high-frequency tone burst is presented to the ear, an AC voltage fluctuation having the same frequency and duration can be recorded from a gross electrode in the inner ear (recording filter bandwidth ~100–20,000 Hz). Because the AC voltage fluctuation recorded from the cochlea resembles the acoustic input, the potential was termed the *cochlear microphonic*. The distribution of the cochlear microphonic potential as a function of sound frequency is shown in **Fig. 2–7A**. When a recording electrode is placed in the

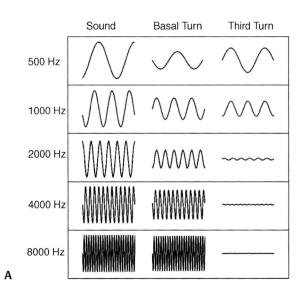

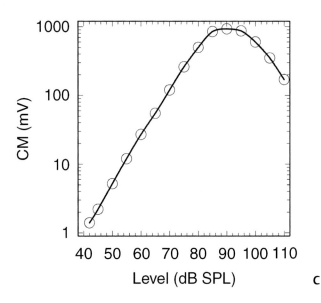

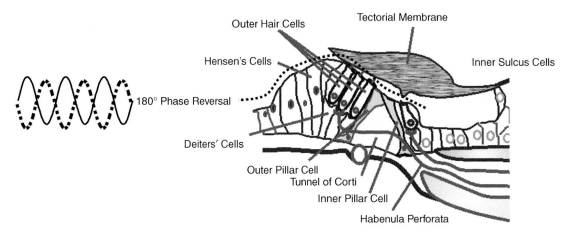

Figure 2–7 **(A)** Schematic showing the sound frequency (left column) and the cochlear microphonic waveform recorded from an electrode in the basal turn (middle column) and apical third turn (right column). (From Yost, W. A. (1994). Fundamentals of hearing: An introduction (3rd ed). San Diego: Academic Press, with permission.) The electrode in the apical third turn produces the largest cochlear microphonic voltage to the 500 Hz low-frequency tone; the cochlear microphonic amplitude decreases as stimulus frequency increases. The electrode in the high-frequency basal turn produces a large cochlear microphonic response to the 8000 Hz high-frequency tone. Low-frequency tones also activate the cochlear microphonic in the base, but at a slightly lower amplitude. **(B)** The polarity of the cochlear microphonic waveform reverses phase by 180 degrees (solid vs dotted sine wave) when the recording electrode moves from below the hair cells through the reticular lamina (dotted line) and into the scala media. **(C)** Schematic showing the plot of cochlear microphonic (CM) amplitude (logarithmic scale) versus sound pressure level (SPL). Cochlear microphonic amplitude initially increases with increasing level but saturates and rolls over at higher intensities.

apex of the cochlea, a prominent AC voltage oscillation can be recorded in response to a 500 Hz tone; however, as the frequency of the stimulus increases from 1000 to 8000 Hz, the amplitude of the AC response recorded from the apex decreases significantly. Thus, the apex of the cochlea is most sensitive to low frequencies consistent with the spatial distribution of a traveling wave envelope (**Fig. 2–7A**). The cochlear microphonic recorded from the basal end is largest for high-frequency sounds (e.g., 8000 Hz). As the frequency of the stimulus decreases, cochlear microphonic voltage decreases slightly. This is consistent with the fact that high-frequency sounds produce maximum vibration in the base; however, low-frequency sounds can also stimulate the base of the cochlea but at lower amplitude. If the cochlear microphonic waveform is monitored as the recording electrode is moved from below the hair cells into the scala media, the cochlear microphonic potential abruptly reverses phase at the reticular lamina (**Fig. 2–7B**). These results, along with others from lesion studies, suggest the cochlear microphonic is generated somewhere near the tips of the hair cells. The Davis model assumes that the transduction channels in the stereocilia bundles act like a variable resistor that modulates the potential between the endolymph ($+80$ mV) and the resting potential inside the hair cell (-60 mV) (Davis, 1965).

The cochlear microphonic potential is a graded potential that increases with sound intensity (**Fig. 2–7C**). When the amplitude of the cochlear microphonic potential is plotted on a logarithmic scale versus dB SPL, the amplitude initially increases approximately linearly but then saturates at higher intensities and rolls over. Because there are roughly 3 times as many outer hair cells as inner hair cells, the dominant source of the microphonic potential comes from the outer hair cells. Lesion studies involving selective destruction of either outer or inner hair cells confirm this view (Dallos et al, 1972; Wang et al, 1997).

Pitfall

- From a clinical perspective, the cochlear microphonic potential recorded by electrocochleography using an electrode on the promontory or electrodes located in the ear canal primarily reflect the response of outer hair cells. However, recordings made from the promontory primarily reflect the output of hair cells in the base of the cochlea. Therefore, it is difficult to use the cochlear microphonic potential recorded from the promontory to assess the condition of the outer hair cells in the middle or apex of the cochlea.

Summating Potential

The summating potential is a gross potential that is elicited by sound stimulation. The polarity of the summating potential can be both positive and negative, and the properties of this local field potential depend on whether the recordings are made with the differential electrode recording technique using electrodes in the scala tympani and scala vestibuli or simply

with a single active electrode on the round window. **Fig. 2–8A** is a schematic that illustrates how the polarity of the summating potential changes with frequency when recordings were made from the apical turn using the differential recording technique. The peak of the traveling wave envelope to a 500 Hz tone is located in the apex of the cochlea, the CF at this location in the cochlea. The polarity of the summating potential in the apex of the cochlea shows maximum negativity near 500 Hz, the CF, and the negativity of the response decreases at lower frequencies and higher frequencies. At around 1000 Hz, the summating potential becomes positive, increases to a maximum around 1200 Hz, and then gradually declines at higher frequencies. Thus, the summating potential recorded with the differential electrode technique shows relatively sharp spatial tuning and a marked polarity reversal.

Figure 2–8B is a schematic that shows the temporal features of the summating potential recorded (recording filter band width approximately 0.3 to 200 Hz) with a single electrode located on the round window membrane in response to 8000 Hz tone bursts. The summating potential consists of a positive DC shift during the duration of the tone burst; the DC response rapidly drops to zero at the offset of the stimulus. The summating potential is a graded response whose amplitude varies with stimulus intensity as schematized in **Fig. 2–8C**. When plotted on a logarithmic scale, the amplitude of the summating potential plotted initially increases approximately linearly with increasing sound intensity but gradually saturates at high intensities. The origins of the summating potential are not fully understood, but lesion studies with ototoxic drugs have shown that the amplitude of the summating potential is greatly reduced when the inner hair cells are destroyed; further loss of outer hair cells results in an additional but smaller decline (Durrant et al, 1998). These results suggest that the inner hair cells play a significant role in generating the summating potential.

Pearl

- The amplitude and polarity of the summating potential recorded by electrocochleography or ear canal electrodes are used clinically in the diagnosis of Meniere's disease.

Compound Action Potential

The compound action potential (CAP) is a local field potential of neural origin; that is, it originates from the spiral ganglion neurons that give rise to the auditory nerve. It is an onset response that arises from the simultaneous discharge of many auditory nerve fibers in response to a sound stimulus that has a rapid onset, for example, a click or tone burst with rapid rise time. **Figure 2–9A** is a schematic illustrating the waveform of the CAP (recording filter bandwidth: 30 to 3000 Hz) elicited by an 8 kHz tone burst with a short rise–fall time (1 msec). The CAP is characterized by two large negative peaks, one occurring around 1.5 msec after stimulus onset (N_1) and a second occurring around 2.3 msec (N_2). It is a graded potential that increases in amplitude with stimulus level. **Figure 2–9B**

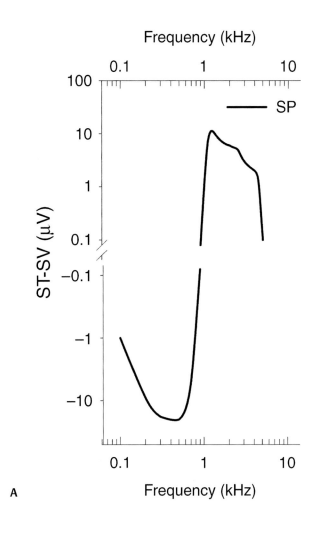

Frequency (kHz)

ST-SV (µV)

Frequency (kHz)

A

Summating Potential (8 kHz Tone Burst)

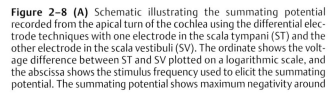

SP Amplitude (mV)

8 kHz Tone Burst

Time (ms)   B

8 kHz Tone Burst

SP Amplitude (mV)

dB SPL   C

Figure 2–8 (A) Schematic illustrating the summating potential recorded from the apical turn of the cochlea using the differential electrode techniques with one electrode in the scala tympani (ST) and the other electrode in the scala vestibuli (SV). The ordinate shows the voltage difference between ST and SV plotted on a logarithmic scale, and the abscissa shows the stimulus frequency used to elicit the summating potential. The summating potential shows maximum negativity around 500 Hz, the characteristic frequency of the apical turn of the cochlea. **(B)** Schematic illustrating the summating potential versus time waveform to 8 kHz tone burst recorded from the round window. Note the positive direct current–like response. **(C)** Schematic illustrating summating potential amplitude versus sound intensity (summating potential amplitude plotted on a logarithmic scale). SPL, sound pressure level.

is a schematic showing the typical input/output function for the CAP plotted on a linear amplitude scale. The amplitude of the N_1 potential initially increases with stimulus intensity and then saturates and rolls over at high intensities. The minimal SPL needed to produce a just noticeable response (e.g., 20 µV) is often used to define a neural threshold for the CAP. In the schematic shown in **Fig. 2–9B**, the threshold would be approximately 25 dB SPL using a 20 µV threshold criterion. If CAP input/output functions are measured over a range of frequencies and threshold is determined, then a plot of CAP threshold versus frequency can be used to obtain a so-called neural CAP audiogram, as schematized in **Fig. 2–9C**. The CAP audiogram can be useful for estimating hearing sensitivity of the cochlea.

Because 90% of the spiral ganglion neurons originate from type I neurons that innervate the inner hair cells, the amplitude of the CAP arises predominantly, if not exclusively, from the neural circuit involving inner hair cells, type I neurons, and the afferent synapse that connects them. However, the sensitivity and frequency selectivity of the inner hair cells and type I neurons are affected by the functional integrity of the outer hair cells, which enhance the sensitivity and frequency selectivity of the basilar membrane that provides the mechanical input to the inner hair cells. Consequently, when all the outer hair cells are destroyed, the CAP threshold will increase approximately 40 to 50 dB. When the inner hair cells are selectively destroyed, but the outer hair cells are intact, then the

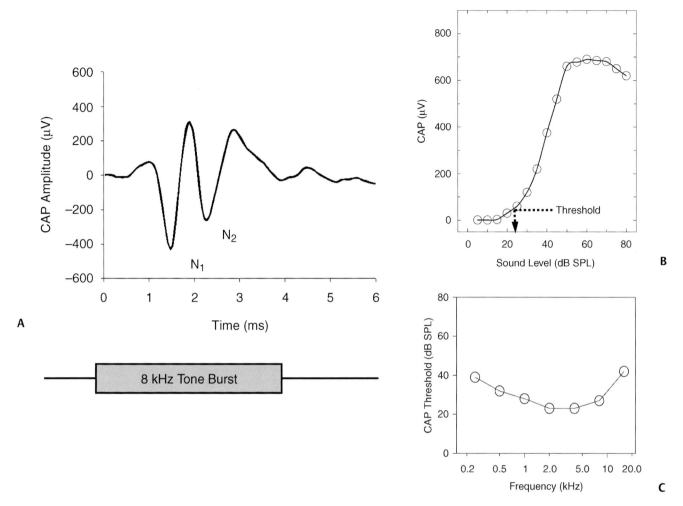

Figure 2–9 (A) Compound action potential (CAP) voltage versus time waveform showing the N_1 and N_2 components of the response. The envelope of the 8 kHz tone burst used to elicit the response is shown below. **(B)** Schematic showing typical compound action potential input/output function for N_1 amplitude plotted as a function of the sound intensity. Note the saturation of response at high intensities. The horizontal line depicts the threshold criterion used to define threshold; the arrow shows the sound pressure level needed to reach the threshold. **(C)** Schematic showing the compound action potential threshold across a range of frequencies, the so-called CAP neural audiogram. SPL, sound pressure level.

amplitude of the CAP will decrease in proportion to the amount of inner hair cell damage (Wang et al, 1997).

Controversial Point

• The clinical utility of the cochlear microphonic potential, summating potential, and CAP are described in more detail in Chapter 18. In patients with auditory neuropathy, the CAP is typically absent, whereas the cochlear microphonic potential is present. The mechanisms that lead to the loss of the CAP are still a subject of debate. The CAP could be absent due to impaired function of the inner hair cells, the type I auditory nerve fiber, the synapse connecting the inner hair cell or type I nerve fibers, or disturbance of the myelin sheath surrounding the afferent nerve fibers.

◆ Hair Cell Physiology

To record from individual hair cells or neurons, it is necessary to use electrodes with very small tip diameters ($< 1 \mu$m), so called microelectrodes or sharp electrodes with high electrical impedance (> 20 MΩ). Microelectrodes can be used to pick the extracellular response from individual cells or, if they penetrate the plasma membrane, the intracellular potentials. When an extremely fine microelectrode enters an inner hair cell, the potential drops abruptly to -35 to -45 mV DC, a potential that reflects the resting membrane potential of the cell (Sellick and Russell, 1978). When a tone burst is presented, the inner hair cells produce both an AC and a DC response. The AC response, which mirrors the frequency of the stimulus, is prominent at low frequencies but decreases in amplitude as frequency increases because the AC voltage is attenuated (i.e., filtered out) by the capacitance of the cell's membrane and the electrode. When low-intensity tone

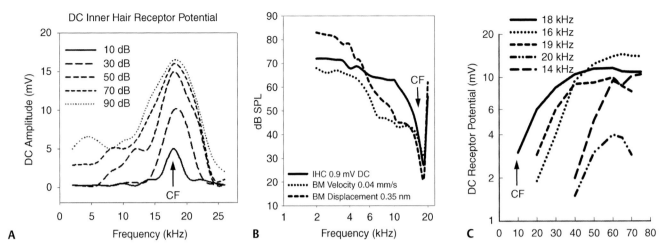

Figure 2–10 **(A)** Schematic showing the amplitude of the direct current (DC) receptor potential from an inner hair cell plotted as a function of frequency producing a response area map. Response area maps are shown for sound intensities ranging from 10 to 90 dB sound pressure level (SPL). Response area of inner hair cells is tuned to a characteristic frequency (CF) near 18 kHz. BM, basilar membrane; IHC, inner hair cell. **(B)** Schematic showing inner hair cell DC receptor potential tuning curve using a threshold criterion of 0.9 mV. Tuning curves are shown for a constant basilar membrane velocity (threshold criterion 0.04 mm/s) and a constant basilar membrane displacement (0.35 mm). Hair cell and mechanical responses are tuned to a CF near 18 kHz. **(C)** Schematic showing inner hair cell DC receptor potential input/output function. DC receptor potential amplitude is plotted on a logarithmic scale. The CF of the inner hair cell is located near 18 kHz. Note the saturation of the receptor potential for frequencies close to CF. (**A–C:** From Sellick, P. M., & Russell, I. J. (1978). Intracellular studies of cochlear hair cells: Filling the gap between basilar membrane mechanics and neural excitation. In: R. F. Naunton, & C. Fernandez (Eds.), Evoked electrical activity in the auditory nervous system (pp. 113–139). New York: Academic Press, with permission.)

bursts are presented to the ear, inner hair cells generate low-amplitude AC and DC responses over a narrow range of frequencies, the so-called characteristic frequency. When sound intensity increases, the amplitudes of the AC and the DC responses increase near the CF. In addition, AC and DC responses occur over a wider range of frequencies above and below the CF. **Figure 2–10A** shows the amplitude of the inner hair cell DC receptor potential plotted as a function of frequency, often referred to as the response area map. Note that at low sound levels, only a narrow range of frequencies produces a strong response around the cell's CF, 18 kHz. As the sound intensities increase, the DC receptor potential increases in amplitude at CF, and the response area becomes wider. At low-to-moderate sound levels, the broadening of the response area mainly occurs around CF. However, at moderate-to-high intensities, two changes occur in the growth pattern. First, the expansion of the response area occurs primarily below CF. Second, the amplitude of the DC response near CF increases very little with increasing intensity; that is, the response saturates near CF.

Another informative way to portray the response properties of an inner hair cell is to plot its threshold as a function of frequency, where threshold is defined as the SPL needed to produce a just noticeable increase in the DC receptor potential (e.g., 0.9 mV DC) (Sellick and Russell, 1978). The DC threshold versus frequency plot, or tuning curve, is schematized by the thin solid line in **Fig. 2–10B**. Threshold is lowest near 18 kHz, the cell's CF. The SPL needed to elicit a threshold response increases rapidly at frequencies above CF, resulting in a steep high-frequency edge to the tuning curve. Below CF, the threshold initially increases rapidly as frequency decreases, then rises more slowly, resulting in a

shallow, low-frequency tail to the tuning curve. **Figure 2–10B** also shows a schematic of basilar membrane tuning curves, one based on the sound level needed to produce a constant displacement of the basilar membrane (0.35 nm) and the other needed to produce a constant velocity (0.04 mm/s). The overall shape of the mechanical tuning curves is remarkably similar to the inner hair cell tuning curve, suggesting that the tuning curve of the hair cell is largely defined by the mechanical input from the basilar membrane.

The schematic in **Fig. 2–10C** shows the input/output function for the DC potential of an inner hair cell with a CF near 18 kHz. The input/output function at 18 kHz is shifted farthest to the left because this is the frequency to which the cell is most sensitive. The amplitude of the DC receptor potential rises rapidly over a 20 dB range and then saturates. The input/out functions near CF and 16 and 19 kHz, which are shifted slightly to the right of the 18 kHz function, rise steeply with increasing level and saturate. The saturation seen in the DC receptor potential of the inner hair cell is similar to the compressive nonlinearity seen in the basilar membrane mechanical response (**Fig. 2–5C**).

Outer hair cells in the apex of the cochlea produce AC potentials similar to those of apical turn inner hair cells. However, resting potentials of apical outer hair cells (−53 mV) tend to be somewhat larger than those of apical inner hair cells (−32 mV) (Dallos, 1985). Inner and outer hair cells in the apex also produce DC receptor potentials to tone bursts; those from inner hair cells are always depolarizing, whereas those from outer hair cells can be either hyperpolarizing or depolarizing. Outer hair cells in the base of the cochlea have large resting potentials (−71 mV) and produce AC receptor potentials of up to 15 mV in response to tone burst stimulation. However, their DC receptor potentials are quite small, particularly to tones near CF.

♦ Outer Hair Cell Electromotility

As noted earlier, outer hair cells contain the motor protein, prestin, and can elongate and contract in response to DC or AC electrical stimulation (Brownell et al, 1985; Dallos et al, 1991). AC stimulation results in a cycle-by-cycle change in cell length around a mean value. Outer hair cells contract when their membrane is depolarized and elongate when hyperpolarized. Electrical partitioning experiments have shown that the change in outer hair cell length is distributed along the length of the cell between the nucleus and the cuticular plate region. Electromotile responses have been observed at frequencies as high as 20 kHz (Gale and Ashmore, 1997). These results indicate that the outer hair cells are capable of moving in response to a change in the cell's membrane potential. Because acoustic stimulation can depolarize and hyperpolarize outer hair cells, the change in the cell's potential could induce AC or DC movements of the basilar membrane that in turn could provide positive or negative feedback and influence the movement of the basilar membrane in response to the incoming sound vibration.

The outer hair cells sit in a unique anatomical environment; the base of the outer hair cell is attached to a Deiters' cell, and the apex is attached at the reticular lamina. However, the lateral wall is surrounded by fluid spaces, allowing the outer hair cell to move unimpeded in this region. When an outer hair cell elongates or contracts along its main axis, the cell is able to exert an axial force that causes the organ of Corti to move (Mammano and Ashmore, 1993). Static DC movements could influence the stiffness of the cochlear partition and alter its vibration to sound. Because the outer hair cells are attached to the overlying tectorial membrane via their stereocilia, a change in the length of the outer hair cell could deflect the stereocilia bundle or alter the position of the overlying tectorial membrane. When electrical stimulation is applied to an isolated segment of the organ of Corti or the intact cochlea, the basilar membrane moves at the same frequency as the electrical stimulus (Nuttall and Ren, 1995). The electrically induced motion of the basilar membrane results in the production of traveling waves that propagate in the reverse direction out of the cochlea and into the ear canal. These electrically evoked sounds are referred to as electrically evoked otoacoustic emissions.

Pearl

- The remarkable sensitivity and frequency selectivity of the inner ear is believed to be derived in large part from the electromotile response of the outer hair cells that enhances the mechanical response of the basilar membrane in a frequency-specific manner, thereby increasing the mechanical input to the inner hair cells.

♦ Otoacoustic Emissions

The electromotile response of the outer hair cells provides a biological basis for understanding and interpreting a class of sounds that are generated in the inner ear and transmitted back through the middle ear ossicles and into the ear canal, where they can be recorded by a sensitive microphone. Otoacoustic emissions are generated in healthy ears but are reduced in amplitude or absent in ears with certain types of damage, such as loss of outer hair cells. Consequently, otoacoustic emissions provide a way of assessing the functional integrity of the circuit composed of the outer hair cell and the +80 mV potential generated by the stria vascularis. Although there are several types of otoacoustic emissions, as described in more detail in Chapter 22, the three most commonly studied are spontaneous otoacoustic emissions (SOAEs), transient otoacoustic emissions (TOAEs), and distortion product otoacoustic emissions (DPOAEs).

Spontaneous Otoacoustic Emissions

The ear can act as a robust sound generator, transmitting sounds, SOAEs, into the environment that, in some cases, are intense enough to be heard by individuals standing nearby (Powers et al, 1995). Approximately one third of all human subjects with normal hearing have been reported to have SOAEs (Probst et al, 1991). In most cases, human SOAEs are less than 20 dB SPL and generally occur in narrow frequency bands below 2 kHz. SOAEs generally remain stable within an ear, but the amplitude and spectrum of SOAEs vary from one ear to the next. SOAEs can be suppressed by external sounds; the frequency–intensity combinations needed to suppress the SOAEs by a fixed amount (e.g., 3 dB) define the SOAE suppression contour. **Figure 2–11A** shows an SOAE recorded from the ear of a chinchilla. The SOAE was located near 4.5 kHz, and its level was ~30 dB SPL, loud enough to be directly heard in a quiet sound booth. The emission, which was stable over time, could be temporarily abolished by sodium salicylate and suppressed by external tones. The SOAE suppression contour consisted of a low-intensity, narrowly tuned tip located slightly above 4500 Hz and a high-intensity, broadly tuned, low-frequency tail. The shape of the SOAE suppression contour was similar to basilar membrane tuning curves shown above (**Fig. 2–5B**).

Distortion Product Otoacoustic Emissions

As noted earlier, the basilar membrane motion and the outer hair cell electromotility respond to stimulation in a nonlinear manner and therefore can generate distortion. The distortion generated in the inner ear in response to sound can be demonstrated experimentally by presenting two primary tones, f_1 and f_2, and measuring the spectrum of the sound in the ear canal. If the cochlea were a linear system, then only sounds corresponding to f_1 and f_2 would be present in the ear canal. However, when two tones are presented to a healthy ear, additional frequencies are detected in the ear canal at

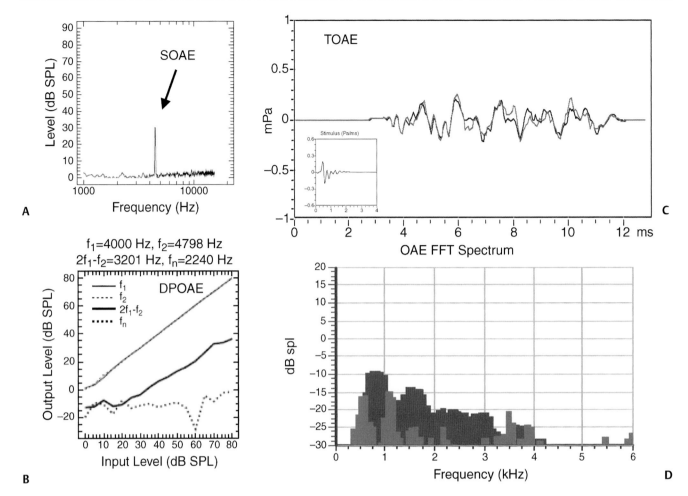

Figure 2–11 (A) Amplitude versus frequency spectrum recorded from the ear canal of a chinchilla using a sensitive microphone. Note the presence of 30 dB sound pressure level (SPL) spontaneous otoacoustic emission (SOAE) near 4.5 kHz. **(B)** Distortion product otoacoustic emission (DPOAE) input/output function recorded from the ear canal of a chinchilla. Primary tone $f_1 = 4000$ Hz and $f_2 = 4798$ Hz shown by thin solid line; $2f_1$-f_2 DPOAE at 3201 Hz shown by thick solid line. Primary tone level, $L_1 = L_2$, varied from 0 to 80 dB SPL. Dashed line shows the noise floor of the measurement system. DPOAE rises above the noise floor at levels greater than 20 dB SPL. **(C)** Transient otoacoustic emissions (TOAE) waveform recorded from human ear canal. Waveform of acoustic click is used to elicit the TOAE shown in inset. **(D)** Spectrum showing sound pressure level of the TOAE as a function of frequency (dark black area). FFT, fast Fourier transform.

intermodulation distortion frequencies, the most prominent of which are $2f_1$-f_2 and f_2-f_1. If primaries of 4000 Hz and 4800 Hz are presented to the ear, $2f_1$-f_2 and f_2-f_1 distortion products would be produced at 3200 Hz and 800 Hz, respectively. In a healthy ear, the largest distortion product, $2f_1$-f_2, is sometimes only 30 to 40 dB below the level of the primary tones.

Figure 2–11B shows the $2f_1$-f_2 DPOAE input/output function measured from the ear of a healthy chinchilla. The amplitude of $2f_1$-f_2 increased as the level of the primary tones, f_1 and f_2, increased. The two primary tones were presented at the same intensity, and the level increased from 0 to 80 dB SPL in 5 dB steps. At primary tone levels less than 25 dB, the $2f_1$-f_2 distortion product cannot be measured because its amplitude is equal to or below the noise floor of the measurement system. However, as stimulus level increased, the amplitude of $2f_1$-f_2 increased above the noise floor at a rate of ~1 dB of DPOAE amplitude per 1 dB increase in signal level. When the primary tones were at 80 dB SPL, the amplitude of $2f_1$-f_2 was roughly 40 dB SPL, that is, ~40 dB below the level of the primaries.

Lesion studies have shown that complete destruction of the inner hair cells has no effect on DPOAE amplitude; however, destruction of the outer hair cells leads to a significant reduction in DPOAE amplitude. In chinchillas, DPOAE amplitude decreased at the rate of 2 to 4 dB for every 10% loss of outer hair cells (Hofstetter et al, 1997). DPOAE amplitude is also altered by electrical or acoustic stimulation of the efferent neurons that synapse on the outer hair cells (Siegel and Kim, 1982). From a clinical perspective, it is clear that DPOAEs assess the functional integrity of the outer hair cells combined with the +80 mV endolymphatic potential generated by the stria vascularis. DPOAEs cannot be used to assess the functional integrity of the inner hair cells, which transmit virtually all of the input to the central nervous system by way of type I spiral ganglion neurons.

Transient Otoacoustic Emissions

TOAEs can be elicited by presenting a short duration acoustic signal, such as a click or tone burst, then recording the acoustic activity that occurs in the ear canal for a short period of time after the input signal has ended (Kemp, 1978). **Figure 2–11C** shows the time waveform of the TOAE recorded from a human ear in response to a click **(inset Fig. 2–11C)**. The amplitude of the acoustic click dropped down to the noise floor after 2 msec or more. However, beginning at 4 msec, an oscillatory response appears, increases to a maximum around 6 msec, then decays down into the background noise around 12 msec. **Fig. 2–11D** shows the spectrum (frequency domain representation) of the TOAE (time domain representation, **Fig. 2–11C**). The spectrum has a peak near 1 kHz (−8 dB SPL/half-octave band) and declines to approximately −25 dB/half-octave band near 4 kHz.

Because the TOAE appears after a short delay, it was originally referred to as an echo; however, this gives the misleading impression that it is a passive reflection. Passive acoustic echoes behave linearly, whereas TOAE amplitude increases nonlinearly when the stimulus level is raised. At high intensities, a 3 dB increase in the input signal may yield only a 1 dB increase in the level of the TOAE. The TOAE has a biological origin because conditions that damage the cochlea, such as acoustic trauma, metabolic inhibitors, and ototoxic drugs, reduce the amplitude of the TOAE (Kemp, 1978).

The instantaneous frequency spectrum of the click-evoked TOAE varies over the duration of the TOAE waveform, resulting in frequency dispersion. The initial portion of the TOAE contains mainly high-frequency energy, but the spectrum shifts to lower frequencies toward the end of the waveform. If tone bursts are used to elicit a TOAE, the spectrum of the TOAE is similar to the eliciting stimulus; however, the time delay between stimulus onset and the emergence of the TOAE is inversely related to frequency. Thus, low-frequency sounds take longer to emerge from the cochlea than high-frequency sounds. The time delays and frequency dispersion of the TOAE are related to the time delay imposed by the forward and reverse transmission of the frequency components of the click to their respective transduction sites along the cochlear partition. Because the base of the cochlea is stiffer and has less mass than the apex, the base of the cochlea begins to vibrate sooner than the apex; consequently, otoacoustic emissions generated from hair cells in the base of the cochlea appear in the ear canal before those produced in the apex of the cochlea.

Pearl

- DPOAE and TOAE are now widely used to screen for hearing loss in neonates and other difficult-to-test subjects. Because DPOAEs and TOAEs arise from the electromotile response of outer hair cells in conjunction with the +80 mV endolymphatic potential, these tests provide convenient methods for indirectly assessing the functional integrity of the outer hair cells and the cells in the lateral wall of the cochlea that generate the endocochlear potential. It is important to note that otoacoustic emissions do not assess the functional integrity of the inner hair cells and type I auditory nerve fibers, which are responsible for sending auditory information into the central auditory system.

♦ Auditory Nerve Fiber Responses

The only pathway by which sounds transduced in the cochlea can reach the central auditory system is by way of the spiral ganglion neurons that give rise to the auditory nerve. Since each type I spiral ganglion neuron contacts only one inner hair cell (**Fig. 2–4A**), the neural activity from each fiber reflects the output from a very small segment of the cochlea. Using extremely fine microelectrodes, it is possible to record the all-or-none spike discharges from individual nerve fibers (**Fig. 2–12A**) as they make their way to the cochlear nucleus, the first auditory relay station in the brain. Most auditory nerve fibers discharge spontaneously in the absence of controlled acoustic stimulation and their spontaneous discharge rates range from 0 to 120 spikes/s (**Fig. 2–12B**). A large proportion of fibers have spontaneous rates fewer than 18 or more than 30 spikes/s resulting in a bimodal distribution (Liberman, 1978).

When a tone burst with the appropriate frequency–intensity combination is presented to the ear, the discharge rate increases above the spontaneous rate. The stimulus intensity needed to produce a just detectable increase in the discharge rate defines the neuron's threshold. The frequency–threshold tuning curve is a plot that describes the neuron's thresholds as a function of frequency, as schematized in **Fig. 2–12C**. The frequency at which a response can be elicited at the lowest stimulus intensity is the unit's CF. Threshold increases significantly above and below the CF, resulting in a narrow, low-threshold tip around the CF. Responses can be elicited to a broad range of frequencies below the CF, but only at high SPLs. Thus, the auditory nerve fiber tuning curves are similar in shape to basilar membrane iso-response tuning curves (**Fig. 2–5B**) and inner hair cell receptor potential tuning curves (**Fig. 2–10B**).

The thresholds of neurons with similar CF can vary by as much as 50 to 60 dB. Neurons with the lowest thresholds at CF thresholds tend to have high spontaneous rates (> 18 spikes/s), whereas those with the highest thresholds at the CF have the lowest spontaneous rates (0–1 spike/s). Neurons with intermediate spontaneous rates have moderate thresholds at the CF. By injecting a dye tracer into a neuron, it has been possible to determine where the nerve fiber terminates in the organ of Corti. All of the labeled neurons that respond to sound have been found to synapse on inner hair cells (Liberman, 1982; Robertson, 1984). Thus, all of the acoustic information transmitted to the central auditory system appears to be conveyed by the type I auditory nerve fibers. There is no evidence that type II fibers, which contact outer hair cells, transmit spike activity to the central auditory system (Robertson, 1984).

Auditory nerve fibers respond to sound by increasing their discharge rate over the time when the stimulus is present; however, the amount of neural activity varies with stimulus level and as a function of time following stimulus onset. The change in discharge rate over the duration of a 200 msec tone burst is illustrated by the post-stimulus time (PST) histograms in **Fig. 2–13A**. PST histograms are constructed by counting the number of spikes that occur in a particular time bin following stimulus onset; responses are

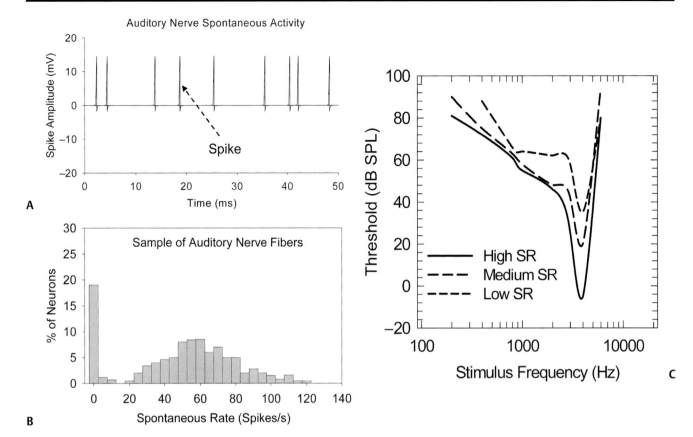

Figure 2–12 (A) Schematic showing spontaneous spike discharges from a single auditory nerve fiber. **(B)** Schematic showing the proportion of auditory nerve fibers with different spontaneous discharge rates. The spontaneous rate profile is bimodal, with a peak near one and a second mode near 40 to 60 spikes per second. **(C)** Schematic showing represen-tative frequency–threshold tuning curves from auditory nerve fibers with high, medium, or low spontaneous rates (SR). Tuning curves shown for neurons with characteristic frequency near 4 kHz. High spontaneous rate units have the lowest thresholds, and low spontaneous rate units have the highest thresholds. SPL, sound pressure level.

typically averaged over several hundred stimulus presentations to obtain an average temporal profile. At low sound intensities (18 dB SPL), the PST histograms tend to be nearly flat, reflecting the fact that the stimulus level is near or below threshold; thus, the spike counts mainly reflect the spontaneous discharge rate. As the sound intensity is increased above the threshold (e.g., 28 dB SPL), the PST histograms develop a profile that has a peak near stimulus onset followed by a gradual decay to a plateau discharge rate. Further increases in stimulus intensity lead to a more pronounced onset peak and a higher plateau firing rate in the PST histogram. The rapid decline in neural activity following stimulus onset presumably occurs because the pool of available neurotransmitters in the inner hair cell is partially depleted, a phenomenon referred to as neural adaptation.

Figure 2–13B is a schematic that shows the discharge rate–intensity function for a typical auditory nerve fiber. As the stimulus rises above the neuron's threshold, the discharge rate increases monotonically over a range of 30 to 50 dB, then remains fairly constant at higher stimulus levels. Because most auditory nerve fibers have a 30 to 50 dB dynamic range, they can only encode changes in sound level over a relatively narrow range of intensities. In contrast, normal listeners can scale the loudness of a stimulus over a range of 120 dB or more. How can this paradox be resolved? A solution to the discrepancy between the dynamic range

for loudness perception and single fiber dynamic range can be found in the large range of CF thresholds. Low-, medium-, and high-threshold neurons can process changes in intensity at low, medium, and high intensities, respectively, so that the total dynamic range of hearing can be approximated using the whole population of fibers.

As noted earlier, hair cells are depolarized when the stimulus deflects the stereocilia bundle toward the tallest stereocilia and are hyperpolarized when the bundle is deflected toward the shortest stereocilia. Hair cell depolarization leads to the release of a neurotransmitter, presumably glutamate, from the base of the inner hair cell on to the synapse of type I spiral ganglion neurons, which depolarizes the nerve fiber and increases its discharge rate. According to this scheme, auditory nerve fibers should produce phase-locked responses such that spike discharges occur during a preferred half-cycle of the stimulus that is associated with deflection of the bundle toward the tallest stereocilia. **Figure 2–13C** contains period histograms that show the phase-locked response of an auditory nerve fiber to a 1000 Hz tone presented at 40 and 70 dB SPL. The period histogram shows the number of spikes that occur at a particular time within one cycle of the 1000 Hz tone (1 msec period). At intensities above thresholds, spikes are clustered within a preferred half-cycle of the stimulus. Thus, the neural response pattern of an auditory nerve fiber resembles a half-wave rectified version of the stimulus. Neural

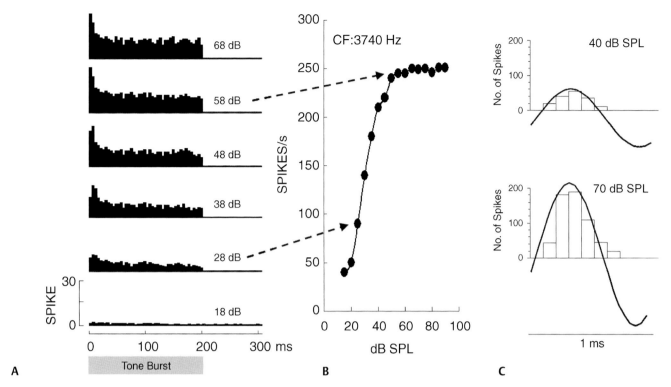

Figure 2–13 **(A)** Schematic showing representative post-stimulus time (PST) histogram of spike count versus time from an auditory nerve fiber stimulated with a 200 msec duration tone burst. Sound intensity increased from 18 to 68 dB sound pressure level (SPL). For intensities from 18 to 68 dB SPL, the PST histogram shows a high spike count near stimulus onset, followed by a gradual decay to a steady level over the duration of the stimulus. Little spike activity is evoked by an 18 dB SPL tone. **(B)** Schematic showing the spike rate (SR, spikes/s) versus stimulus level. The spike rate increases rapidly from 23 to 58 dB SPL, then plateaus at higher stimulus levels. CF, characteristic frequency. **(C)** Schematic of period histogram showing the distribution of spikes during one cycle of a 1000 Hz tone presented at 40 or 70 dB SPL. Spike discharges occur during one half of the stimulus cycle, indicating that neural activity is time locked to a preferred half-cycle of the tone. (From Rose, J. E., Hind, J. E., Anderson, D. J. & Brugge, J. F. (1971). Some effects of intensity on response of auditory nerve fibers in the squirrel monkey. Journal of Neurophysiology, 34, 685–699, with permission.)

phase locking is robust at the low frequencies (< 1500 Hz) where pitch perception is believed to be based on periodicity cues; however, phase locking deteriorates at higher frequencies and is absent at frequencies above 3 to 4 kHz.

♦ Summary

Many important aspects of hearing are determined by the biomechanical, anatomical, and physiological properties of the inner ear. The traveling wave displacement pattern provides a mechanism for segregating sounds of different frequencies into different locations along the basilar membrane. This provides a basis for place theories of pitch. From a clinical standpoint, damage at a specific place along the cochlea should result in a hearing loss in a specific frequency region. The morphological polarization of the hair cell and the phase-locking behavior observed in auditory nerve fibers provide the physiological basis for models of periodicity pitch at low frequencies. During the past 50 years, physiologists have gained a clearer understanding of the standing potentials and sound evoked potentials that originate in the cochlea, information that is essential for understanding and interpreting results from clinical electrocochleography made from electrodes placed near the round

window. The cochlear microphonic recording near the round window is generated mainly from outer hair cells in the base of the cochlea. The summating potential most likely reflects the neural activity originating from the inner hair cell near the base of the cochlea. The CAP reflects the neural activity emanating from the type I spiral ganglion neurons; selective damage to the inner hair cells reduces the amplitude of the CAP, whereas selective damage to the outer hair cells primarily increases the threshold of the CAP. The utility of otoacoustic emissions for infant hearing screening requires a thorough understanding of cochlear mechanics and cochlear anatomy. Selective damage to inner hair cells has no effect on sound evoked otoacoustic emissions; however, DPOAEs and TOAEs are reduced in amplitude or completely abolished by outer hair cell damage and loss of the endocochlear potential, which provides the +80 mV driving potential for the outer hair cells. Thus, otoacoustic emissions should be thought of as a test to assess the functional integrity of the outer hair cells and/or endocochlear potential generated by the stria vascularis.

Patients with sensorineural hearing loss are not only less sensitive to sound but are often unable to extract specific spectral features (e.g., consonants) from a complex signal. The ability to resolve the spectral components of a complex sound depends on the ear's sharp mechanical and neural tuning, which in turn depends on the functional integrity of the outer hair cells and the endolymphatic potential.

Because the cochlear microphonics and otoacoustic emissions are generated by the outer hair cells in conjunction with the endolymphatic potential, clinicians can use either or both of these measures to assess the functional condition of the outer hair cell system in hearing-impaired patients. For example, TOAEs and DPOAEs could be used to monitor the ototoxic effects of aminoglycoside antibiotics and anticancer drugs, such as cisplatin and carboplatin. The battery of physiological measures available to the clinician has proved useful in the diagnosis of subjects with auditory neuropathy (Starr et al, 1996). Patients with auditory neuropathy have normal otoacoustic emissions and cochlear microphonic potentials, suggesting that their outer hair cells are intact. However, the CAP (or wave I of the auditory brainstem response) is absent or greatly diminished in amplitude, suggesting that relatively little neural information is being transmitted to the central auditory system via the auditory nerve. Knowledge of the auditory periphery provides a scientific basis for understanding many facets of hearing and hearing loss.

Acknowledgments   The preparation of this chapter was supported in part by a grant from the Tinnitus Research Consortium and the National Institutes of Health (R01 DC00630).

References

Bosher, S. K., & Warren, R. L. (1968). Observations on the electrochemistry of the cochlear endolymph of the rat: A quantitative study of its electrical potential and ionic composition as determined by means of flame spectrophotometry. Proceedings of the Royal Society of London Series B, 171(23), 227–247.

Brownell, W. E., Bader, C. R., Bertrand, D., & de Ribaupierre, Y. (1985). Evoked mechanical responses of isolated cochlear outer hair cells. Science, 227, 194–196

Dallos, P. (1985). The role of outer hair cells in cochlear function. Progress in Clinical and Biological Research, 176, 207–230.

Dallos, P., Billone, M. C., Durrant, J. D., Wang, C. Y., & Raynor, S. (1972). Cochlear inner and outer hair cells: Functional differences. Science, 177, 356–358.

Dallos, P., Evans, B. N., & Hallworth, R. (1991). Nature of the motor element in electrokinetic shape changes of cochlear outer hair cells. Nature, 350 (6314), 155–157.

Dallos, P., & Fakler, B. (2002). Prestin, a new type of motor protein. Nature Reviews: Molecular Cell Biology, 3(2), 104–111.

Davis, H. (1965). A model for transducer action in the cochlea. Cold Spring Harbor Symposia on Quantitative Biology, 30, 181–189.

Durrant, J. D., Wang, J., Ding, D. L., & Salvi, R. J. (1998). Are inner or outer hair cells the source of summating potentials recorded from the round window? Journal of the Acoustical Society of America, 104(1), 370–377.

Gale, J. E., & Ashmore, J. F. (1997). An intrinsic frequency limit to the cochlear amplifier. Nature, 389(6646), 63–66.

Hofstetter, P., Ding, D., Powers, N., & Salvi, R. J. (1997). Quantitative relationship of carboplatin dose to magnitude of inner and outer hair cell loss and the reduction in distortion product otoacoustic emission amplitude in chinchillas. Hearing Research, 112(1–2), 199–215.

Holley, M. C., & Ashmore, J. F. (1988). A cytoskeletal spring in cochlear outer hair cells. Nature, 335(6191), 635–637.

Hudspeth, A. J. (1992). Hair-bundle mechanics and a model for mechano-electrical transduction by hair cells. Society of General Physiologists Series, 47, 357–370.

Kemp, D. T. (1978). Stimulated acoustic emissions from within the human auditory system. Journal of the Acoustical Society of America, 64, 1386–1391.

Khanna, S. M., & Leonard, D. G. B. (1982). Basilar membrane tuning in the cat cochlea. Science, 215, 305–306.

Liberman, M. C. (1978). Auditory-nerve response from cats raised in a low-noise chamber. Journal of the Acoustical Society of America, 63, 442–455.

Liberman, M. C. (1982). Single-neuron labeling in the cat auditory nerve. Science, 216, 1239–1241.

Liberman, M. C., Gao, J., He, D. Z., Wu, X., Jia, S., & Zuo, J. (2002). Prestin is required for electromotility of the outer hair cell and for the cochlear amplifier. Nature, 419(6904), 300–304.

Mammano, F., & Ashmore, J. F. (1993). Reverse transduction measured in the isolated cochlea by laser Michelson interferometry. Nature, 365(6449), 838–841.

Nuttall, A. L., Dolan, D. F., & Avinash, G. (1991). Laser Doppler velocimetry of basilar membrane vibration. Hearing Research, 51(2), 203–213.

Nuttall, A. L., & Ren, T. (1995). Electromotile hearing: evidence from basilar membrane motion and otoacoustic emissions. Hearing Research, 92(1–2), 170–177.

Powers, N. L., Salvi, R. J., Wang, J., Spongr, V., & Qiu, C. X. (1995). Elevation of auditory thresholds by spontaneous cochlear oscillations. Nature, 375(6532), 585–587.

Probst, R., Lonsbury-Martin, B. L., & Martin, G. K. (1991). A review of otoacoustic emissions. Journal of the Acoustical Society of America, 89, 2027–2067.

Puel, J. L., Ruel, J., Guitton, M., & Pujol, R. (2002). The inner hair cell afferent/efferent synapses revisited: A basis for new therapeutic strategies. Advances in Oto-rhino-laryngology, 59, 124–130.

Robertson, D. (1984). Horseradish peroxidase injection of physiologically characterized afferent and efferent neurons in the guinea pig spiral ganglion. Hearing Research, 15, 113–121.

Ryan, A., & Dallos, P. (1975). Effect of absence of cochlear outer hair cells on behavioural auditory threshold. Nature, 253(5486), 44–46.

Sellick, P. M., & Russell, I. J. (1978). Intracellular studies of cochlear hair cells: Filling the gap between basilar membrane mechanics and neural excitation. In R. F. Naunton & C. Fernandez (Eds.), Evoked electrical activity in the auditory nervous system (pp. 113–139). New York: Academic Press.

Siegel, J. H., & Kim, D. O. (1982). Cochlear biomechanics: Vulnerability to acoustic trauma and other alterations as seen in neural responses and ear-canal sound pressure. In R. P. Hamernik, D. Henderson, & R. J. Salvi (Eds.), New perspectives on noise-induced hearing loss (pp. 137–151). New York: Raven Press.

Spoendlin, H. (1972). Innervation densities of the cochlea. Acta Otolaryngologica, 73, 235–248.

Starr, A., Picton, T. W., Sininger, Y., Hood, L. J., & Berlin, C. I. (1996). Auditory neuropathy. Brain, 119(Part 3), 741–753.

Wang, J., Powers, N. L., Hofstetter, P., Trautwein, P., Ding, D., & Salvi, R. (1997). Effects of selective inner hair cell loss on auditory nerve fiber threshold, tuning and spontaneous and driven discharge rate. Hearing Research, 107(1–2), 67–82.

Warr, W. B., & Guinan, J. J. (1979). Efferent innervation of the organ of Corti: Two separate systems. Brain Research, 173, 152–155.

Winslow, R. L., & Sachs, M. B. (1988). Single-tone intensity discrimination based on auditory-nerve rate responses in backgrounds of quiet, noise, and with stimulation of the crossed olivocochlear bundle. Hearing Research, 35(2–3), 165–189.

Chapter 3

Anatomy and Physiology of the Central Auditory Nervous System: A Clinical Perspective

Frank E. Musiek, Jeffrey A. Weihing, and Victoria B. Oxholm

♦ Importance of the Anatomy and Physiology of the Central Auditory Nervous System to the Clinician

Knowledge of anatomy and physiology is important to the clinician for a variety of reasons. Certainly accurate and informed diagnosis of auditory disorders requires an understanding of the underlying structure and function of the auditory system, and it would be challenging to interpret test results without such knowledge. Additionally, a thorough knowledge of structure and function may benefit the clinician in the selection and fitting of hearing aids; only by understanding the normal auditory system can we understand how our treatments will modify the disordered system. There remain many other reasons for studying the anatomy and physiology of the auditory system, some of which follow.

♦ *Communication* Communication with medical personnel about clinical topics is easier and more relevant if audiologists are knowledgeable about the structure and function of the auditory system. Long-lasting opinions about our profession are often formed by these medical personnel on the basis of our knowledge of anatomy and physiology. Knowledge of anatomy and physiology is also helpful during the frequent communications with hearing scientists and other audiologists.

♦ *Test selection* Most audiological tests assess in some manner the function of the auditory system. Thus, in selecting tests to evaluate different parts of the auditory system, one should understand the relevant biology of a particular system. For example, because of anatomy and physiology research, it is known that certain tests are necessary to measure the integrity of interhemispheric transfer. Without this knowledge and the correct selection of tests, interhemispheric dysfunction may never be detected by the clinician.

♦ *Test interpretation* Perhaps the most critical need for anatomy and physiology is in the interpretation of audiological test results (especially diagnostic). Test results combined with the patient's history can provide valuable information if interpreted with a working familiarity of anatomy and physiology. For example, the acoustic reflex is of little value if one does not understand the anatomy of the reflex circuit. If one knows this circuit well, relevant clinical insight can be gained about the peripheral and part of the central auditory nervous system.

♦ *Radiology* Radiology is a medical specialty based on anatomy. The diagnostic audiologist must have at least a cursory knowledge of radiology to evaluate the audiological tests administered because imaging techniques are often the "gold standard" to which many diagnostic hearing test results are compared. In addition, radiologists look at brain images in a general sense and not for specifics, as would an auditory anatomist. Therefore, specific anatomical data on auditory structures often must be supplied by the clinician to optimize interpretation. Fundamental information on radiology should be included in courses of medical audiology, diagnostic audiology, and anatomy and physiology.

- *Hearing disorders*   An understanding of various hearing disorders, both peripheral and central, depends on a knowledge of anatomy and physiology. Hearing disorders can relate to dysfunction at a certain locus or loci. For example, we now know that kernicterus primarily affects the cochlear nucleus in the brainstem, and even though high-frequency pure-tone hearing loss is common, the cochlea is usually unaffected. This type of information is linked closely to anatomy and physiology; without this information, the clinician cannot fully understand the disorder and its consequences for hearing.

- *Patient counseling*   It is difficult to counsel patients if one does not have a good understanding of the condition's underlying anatomy and physiology. For example, if a patient asks why two hearing aids are recommended instead of one, part of the appropriate answer relates to the physiology of binaural hearing and even plasticity of the brain. Patient questions can often be best answered with the help of an anatomical model because a visual aid gives the patient something tangible with which to work.

At present in the field of audiology, many tests and clinical behaviors are associated with the central auditory nervous system. Most auditory-evoked potentials have a profound interaction with the central auditory nervous system, as do the various behavioral central auditory tests. The audiology–central auditory nervous system relationships go beyond these obvious procedures. For example, maturational factors in children, auditory deprivation influences, and auditory training procedures all are closely related to the central auditory nervous system. However, although modern audiology interacts increasingly with the central auditory nervous system, the education and training of audiologists about the central auditory nervous system have failed to keep pace. This is unfortunate, especially because current technology can help us learn more about the brain. The use of imaging techniques, such as positron emission tomography (PET), magnetic resonance imaging (MRI), and functional MRI (fMRI), allows knowledge of the human brain anatomy and physiology to be acquired. Before the availability of these techniques, neuroanatomists and physiologists depended on cadaver specimens and animal studies to learn about the central auditory nervous system.

It is difficult to use data from animal studies to generalize about the human anatomy and physiology of the central auditory nervous system (Moore, 1987). Fortunately, with the greater availability of imaging techniques, relevant human data can be acquired. In this chapter we refer to human data

as much as possible without compromising the critical knowledge gained from animal studies.

Pearl

- Many experts agree that the greater the knowledge of anatomy and physiology, the more effective the clinician. However, many audiologists receive little preparation in the anatomy and physiology of the central auditory nervous system. More than 70% of the 180 respondents in a survey of clinical audiologists had only one course or no courses in the anatomy and physiology of the central auditory nervous system at the graduate school level (Chermak et al, 1998). This finding emphasizes a need for training for students and professionals about the structure and function of the central auditory nervous system.

◆ Sequential and Parallel Processing in the Central Auditory Nervous System

In viewing the central auditory nervous system (or the entire auditory system) overall, it is important to consider the concepts of sequential and parallel processing (Ehret and Romand, 1997). Sequential processing could be seen as consistent with a hierarchical organization of the auditory system. This means that information is transferred from one center to another in a progressive manner, moving from lower nuclei in the brainstem to the key structures in the cortex. As the information progresses from one auditory center to the next, the different structures along the pathway influence impulses. These actions alter or preserve the pattern of information in ways that make it usable to more central centers. The sequence of processing in the central auditory nervous system implies that if certain sequences are skipped, optimal information flow is not achieved. This may be the case when nerves or nuclei are damaged and less than optimal auditory perception takes place.

Parallel processing depends on having at least two separate channels for information as it progresses through the system. At the auditory nerve level, type I and type II fibers could be viewed as two channels representing parallel processing. Further up in the system, much more parallel processing occurs as many channels come into play. Sequential and parallel processing are ways in which much information can be analyzed in abbreviated time periods, which is critical in the auditory system.

The auditory structures and their associated functions make up a system. Although there is some relationship between structure and function, it can be difficult to assign specific functions to each structure. This is because the structures work together as a system, with the interaction of different structures providing the end result of hearing.

◆ Central Auditory Nervous System: Anatomical Definition

The anatomical limits of the central auditory nervous system begin at the cochlear nucleus and end at the auditory cortex. However, the end point of the central auditory nervous system is unclear because it might be someplace in the efferent system or possibly in a nonauditory area of the cerebrum. The end point of the central auditory nervous system may also depend on the types of acoustic stimuli and the task to be completed. Thus, it may be physiologically rather than anatomically determined (**Fig. 3–1**).

The Brainstem

The Cochlear Nucleus

The cochlear nucleus is located in the cerebellopontine angle area, a lateral recess formed at the juncture of the pons, medulla, and cerebellum. It consists of three principal sections: the anterior ventral cochlear nucleus (AVCN), the posterior ventral cochlear nucleus (PVCN), and the dorsal cochlear nucleus. Auditory nerve fibers enter this complex at the junction of the AVCN and PVCN, where each fiber then divides and sends branches to the three individual nuclei (Schuknecht, 1974) (**Figs. 3–1** and **3–2**).

The cochlear nucleus is composed of multiple cell types. Among the most prominent of these are the pyramidal (fusiform), octopus, stellate, spherical (bushy), globular (bushy), and multipolar cells (Pfeiffer, 1966). The pyramidal cells in the cat are at the dorsal fringe of the dorsal cochlear nucleus, octopus cells are in the PVCN, and spherical cells are in the AVCN. Globular and multipolar cells are found between the AVCN and PVCN (Rouiller, 1997) (**Figs. 3–3** and **3–4**).

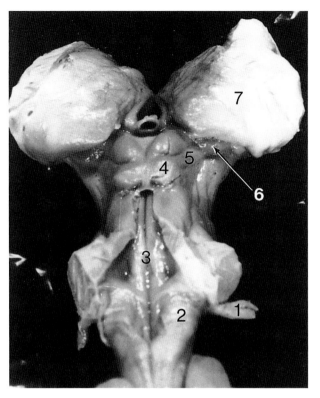

Figure 3–2 Posterior view of the human brainstem (cerebellum and vessels removed). 1, Eighth nerve (entering cochlear nucleus just below the cerebellar peduncle); 2, cochlear nucleus; 3, fourth ventricle; 4, inferior colliculus; 5, brachium of inferior colliculus; 6, medial geniculate body; 7, thalamus. (Courtesy of W. Mosenthal and F. Musiek, Anatomy Laboratory, Dartmouth Medical School, Hanover, NH.)

Incoming neural impulses can be modified by these cells in a characteristic manner that provides the basis for coding information by the type of neural activity within the

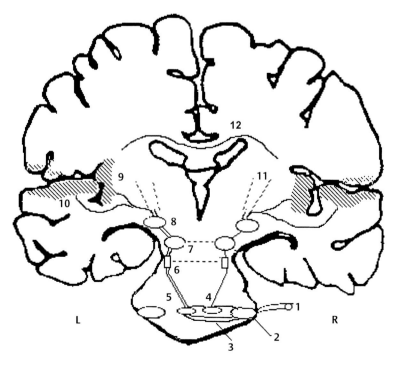

Figure 3–1 Coronal view of the brain with key auditory structures and areas defined. 1, auditory nerve; 2, cochlear nucleus; 3, stria (dorsal, intermediate, ventral); 4, superior olivary complex; 5, lateral lemniscus; 6, nuclei of lateral lemniscus; 7, inferior colliculus; 8, medial geniculate bodies; 9, insula (shaded); 10, primary auditory region in temporal and parietal lobes (shaded); 11, internal capsule; 12, corpus callosum.

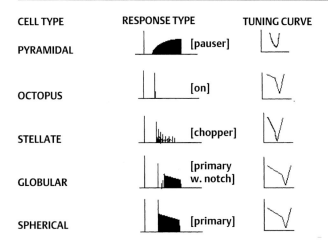

CELL TYPE	RESPONSE TYPE	TUNING CURVE
PYRAMIDAL	[pauser]	
OCTOPUS	[on]	
STELLATE	[chopper]	
GLOBULAR	[primary w. notch]	
SPHERICAL	[primary]	

Figure 3–3 Examples of five cell types found in the cochlear nucleus with associated post-stimulatory histogram types and tuning curve configurations.

cochlear nucleus. The average response of a particular neural unit over time to a series of short tones presented at the unit's characteristic frequency is shown in post-stimulatory histograms (Rhode, 1985). The principal response patterns include the following: (1) primary-like, an initial spike followed by a steady response until the stimuli ceases; (2) the chopper post-stimulatory response, an extremely rapid oscillatory neural response to the stimulus; (3) the onset response, a solitary initial spike at the onset of the stimulus; and (4) the pauser response, similar to the primary-like response, but it ends soon after the initial spike and resumes a graded response (Kiang, 1975). An additional pattern, the "buildup" response, is when the cell fires increasingly throughout the stimulus presentation (Kiang, 1975; Rhode, 1985). This correspondence between cell type and response pattern proposes a significant relationship between anatomy (structure) and physiology (function) of the cells within the cochlear nucleus. Post-stimulatory histograms

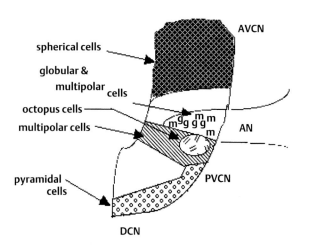

Figure 3–4 Location of cell types in the cochlear nucleus. AVCN, anterior ventral cochlear nucleus; AN, auditory nerve; PVCN, posterior ventral cochlear nucleus; DCN, dorsal cochlear nucleus. (Adapted from Osen, K. K. (1969). Cryoarchitecture of the cochlear nuclei in the cat. Journal of Comparative Neurolology 136, 453–484.)

from the cochlear nucleus supply details regarding the complex processing of auditory information at the cochlear nucleus, such as precise timing needed for localization and distinguishing interaural time differences (Rhode, 1991). The various cell types also have associated tuning curves; the main difference among the cell types is the shape of their tuning curve tails (**Figs. 3–3** and **3–4**).

The auditory nerve enters the brainstem on the lateral posterior aspect of the pontomedullary juncture and projects to the cochlear nuclear complex. Auditory nerve fibers entering each section of the cochlear nucleus are arranged in a systematic fashion that preserves the frequency organization from the cochlea (Sando, 1965). All three sections of the cochlear nucleus contain this tonotopic organization, with low frequencies represented ventrolaterally and high frequencies represented dorsomedially within each nucleus (Sando, 1965) (**Fig. 3–5A**). Some tuning curves derived from AVCN units using tone bursts have a similar shape to those of the auditory nerve (Rhode, 1991). However, some cochlear nuclear fibers produce wider tuning curves than do auditory nerve fibers (Moller, 1985). Frequency resolution of acoustic information coming from the auditory nerve may thus be maintained but not necessarily enhanced by cochlear nuclear units.

The tuberculoventral tract, a fiber pathway thought to be primarily inhibitory in nature, connects the dorsal and ventral portions of the cochlear nucleus (D. Ortel, personal communication, 1990). Three main neural tracts continue from the cochlear nuclear complex to the superior olivary complex (SOC) and higher levels of the central auditory nervous system.

A large fiber tract called the dorsal acoustic stria emanates from the dorsal cochlear nucleus and continues contralaterally to the SOC, lateral lemniscus (Whitfield, 1967), and inferior colliculus (Kiang, 1975). The intermediate acoustic stria originates in the PVCN and communicates with the contralateral lemniscus (ventral nucleus) as well as the central nucleus of the contralateral inferior colliculus (Kiang, 1975) (**Fig. 3–5B**). The ventral acoustic stria, the largest tract, arises from the AVCN and merges with the trapezoid body as it nears the midline of the brainstem (Whitfield, 1967). The ventral stria extends contralaterally along the lateral lemniscus to the SOC and other nuclear groups. Interestingly, in animal studies for simple detection tasks of tones or noise, performance was not affected by sectioning of the intermediate and dorsal acoustic stria. However, severe deficits were noted with sectioning of the ventral stria (Masterton and Granger, 1988).

In addition to these three primary tracts, other fibers project ipsilaterally from each division of the cochlear nucleus. Some of these fibers synapse at the SOC and nuclei of the lateral lemniscus within the pons. Other fibers synapse at the inferior colliculus only and completely bypass the SOC and the nuclei of the lateral lemniscus. The contralateral pathways carry the largest number of fibers even though many neural tracts project both ipsilaterally and contralaterally from the cochlear nucleus (Noback, 1985).

The cochlear nucleus is a unique brainstem auditory structure in that its only afferent input is ipsilateral, coming from the cochlea by way of the auditory nerve. Consequently,

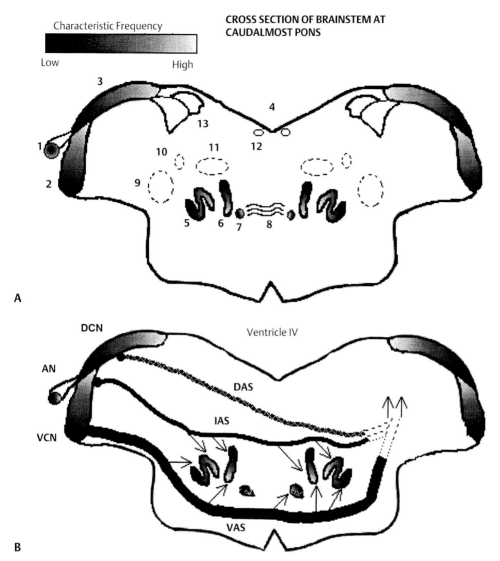

Figure 3–5 (A) Cross section of the lower pons focusing on the cochlear nucleus, superior olivary complex, and associated structures in this region of the brainstem. **(B)** The same cross section as in **(A)**, showing the three acoustic stria coursing from the left cochlear nucleus only. AN, auditory nerve; VCN, ventral cochlear nucleus; DCN, dorsal cochlear nucleus; DAS, dorsal acoustic stria; IAS, intermediate acoustic stria; VAS, ventral acoustic stria (arrows indicate fibers ascending through the lateral lemniscus).

damage to the nucleus can mimic auditory nerve dysfunction (Jerger and Jerger, 1974) because it may only produce ipsilateral pure-tone deficits (Dublin, 1976). Extra-axial tumors, such as acoustic neuromas, often affect the cochlear nucleus because of its posterolateral location on the brainstem surface (Dublin, 1976).

Tumors situated in this cerebellopontine region can often affect the cochlear nucleus and may produce central auditory deficits. Nevertheless, the cerebellopontine angle is large enough in some cases to accommodate lesions of sizable mass without compromising neural function (Musiek and Gollegly, 1985).

Other disorders that can influence the cochlear nucleus include kernicterus. Kernicterus is a pathological condition that results from severe cases of hyperbilirubinemia. It is caused by high bilirubin levels, which ultimately stain the brainstem nuclei. The cochlear nucleus is especially suscep-

tible to this damage (Moller, 2000). The root entry zone, or where the auditory nerve connects with the cochlear nucleus, is also frequently damaged in cases of kernicterus. Generally speaking, bilirubin levels that are greater than 15 mg/dL are considered high risk. Any damage to the cochlear nucleus as a result of kernicterus is likely to lead to a hearing loss.

Superior Olivary Complex

The SOC is positioned ventral and medial to the cochlear nucleus in the caudal portion of the pons (Noback, 1985) (**Fig. 3–5A**). It consists of numerous groups of nuclei, but this discussion will be limited to the following five: the lateral superior olivary complex (LSO), the medial superior olivary nucleus (MSO), the nucleus of the trapezoid body, and the lateral and medial preolivary nuclei. In humans, evidence suggests that the MSO is the largest of these nuclei (Brugge and Geisler, 1978). In some animal species, however, the largest and most prominent nucleus is the S-shaped LSO (Moore, 1987).

Similar to that of the cochlear nucleus, tonotopic organization in the SOC seems to be preserved in all groups of nuclei. The LSO and MSO have been studied most extensively. In the LSO, lower frequencies are represented laterally and the higher frequencies medially following the S-shaped contour of the nucleus, which gives it a unique tonotopic organization (Tsuchitani and Boudreau, 1966). The MSO has a primarily low-frequency representation, whereas the LSO responds to a broader range of frequencies (Noback, 1985). The nucleus of the trapezoid body has a tonotopic orientation, with the low frequencies represented laterally and the high frequencies medially.

The tuning curves for the trapezoid body, LSO, and MSO are mainly quite sharp, denoting good frequency selectivity (Rouiller, 1997). The trapezoid and MSO post-stimulatory responses are primary-like with a notch, whereas the LSO has shown chopper and primary-like responses (Keidel et al, 1983; Rouiller, 1997).

Within the SOC, the LSO is innervated bilaterally (Strominger and Hurwitz, 1976) and receives ipsilateral input from the AVCN and contralateral innervation from both the AVCN and PVCN (Warr, 1966). Both ipsilateral and contralateral input from the AVCN are also received in the MSO (Strominger and Strominger, 1971). Afferent input to the trapezoid body is not understood fully, but a significant contribution seems to arise from the contralateral cochlear nucleus (Strominger and Hurwitz, 1976). Innervation of the lateral and the medial preolivary nuclei may come primarily from the ipsilateral AVCN, but this is also unclear and appears to differ among species (Strominger and Hurwitz, 1976).

The SOC is a complex relay station in the auditory pathway. It is the first place where a variety of ipsilateral and contralateral inputs provide the system with the anatomical foundation for unique functions in binaural listening. Sound localization is determined mainly by interaural time (Masterton et al, 1975) and intensity (Boudreau and Tsuchitani, 1970) variations reflected in inputs to the SOC. The SOC has excitatory and/or inhibitory cells that are time (hence directionally) sensitive. These excitatory and inhibitory responses help clarify directional cues for the higher auditory system (Tsuchitani and Johnson, 1991). Tasks that necessitate the integration and interpretation of binaurally presented signals depend on the SOC and convergence of neural information from each ear. For example, audiological tests, such as rapidly alternating speech perception and the binaural fusion test (see Chapter 17), rely on binaural integration and the interaction of information in the SOC (Tobin, 1985). Abnormal results are often seen on these tests in cases with signal degradation before the SOC or SOC pathosis (Matzker, 1959). Binaural integration is also necessary for the measurement of masking level differences (MLDs), which are a sensitive index of brainstem integrity (Lynn et al, 1981). Changing the phase of the stimulus (tones or speech) in the presence of noise results in a change in the ability to detect the signal, which makes temporal cueing at

the SOC critical in MLDs. The importance of the SOC in the measurement of MLDs and the fusion of binaural signals is supported by several studies that show low brainstem lesions affect MLDs, whereas lesions in the upper brainstem or auditory cortex do not (Lynn et al, 1981).

The SOC also appears to be an important relay station in the acoustic stapedius muscle reflex arc (Borg, 1973). The reflex is thought to entail both direct and indirect neural pathways (Musiek and Baran, 1986), but the neurophysiology of the reflex arc is not entirely understood (Hall, 1985). The direct reflex arc appears to consist of a three- or four-neuron chain that is activated when a sufficiently intense acoustic stimulus is presented to one or both ears. Neural impulses are conveyed through the auditory nerve to the AVCN, then proceed to the ipsilateral MSO and/or facial nerve nucleus. Transverse input seems to arise from the AVCN and travels to the contralateral MSO by way of the trapezoid body. Neurons originating in the MSO region eventuate in the motor nucleus of the facial nerve area, where motor fibers then descend to innervate the stapedius muscle. Consequently, unilateral acoustic stimulation results in bilateral stapedius muscle contractions (Borg, 1973).

The existence of an indirect pathway for the acoustic reflex has also been postulated. A slower polysynaptic pathway, possibly including the extrapyramidal system of the reticular formation, has been contemplated by Borg (1973) as this indirect reflex arc. Although all the pathways involved in the neural arc are not specified, significant clinical acoustic reflex data support the existence of this neural pathway (Hall, 1985).

Lateral Lemniscus

The lateral lemniscus is the primary auditory pathway in the brainstem and is composed of both ascending and descending fibers. The ascending portion extends bilaterally from the cochlear nucleus to the inferior colliculus in the midbrain and contains both crossed and uncrossed fibers of the cochlear nucleus and SOC (Goldberg and Moore, 1967) (**Fig. 3–1**).

Within the lateral lemniscus are two main cell groups: the ventral and dorsal nuclei of the lateral lemniscus and a minor cell group called the intermediate nucleus of the lateral lemniscus. These nuclei are located posterolaterally in the upper portion of the pons, near the lateral surface of the brainstem (Ferraro and Minckler, 1977). Afferent input to the nuclei of the lateral lemniscus arises from the dorsal cochlear nucleus on the contralateral side and from the ventral cochlear nucleus from both sides of the brainstem (Jungert, 1958). The dorsal nuclei of the lateral lemniscus from either side of the brainstem are interconnected by a fiber tract called the commissure of Probst (Kudo, 1981). Lemniscal fibers may also cross from one side to the other through the pontine reticular formation (Ferraro and Minckler, 1977). Most neurons of the dorsal segment of the lateral lemniscus can be activated binaurally. However, most neurons from the ventral segment can be activated only by contralateral stimulation (Keidel et al, 1983).

Although a large number of afferent fibers originating from the cochlear nucleus and SOC actually bypass the lateral lemniscus altogether, there are several important connections between the lateral lemniscus and lower brainstem structures. The dorsal nuclei of the lateral lemniscus have more numerous afferent connections with structures lower in the brainstem than the ventral nuclei (Schwartz, 1992). Among these are bilateral inputs from the LSO, ipsilateral inputs from the MSO and ventral nuclei of the lateral lemniscus, and contralateral inputs from the ventral cochlear nucleus. Additionally, contralateral input is received from the other dorsal nuclei of the lateral lemniscus via the commissure of Probst. The ventral nuclei of the lateral lemniscus receive primarily contralateral input from the lower brainstem. These connections include the AVCN, PVCN, and SOC. Ipsilateral connections do exist between the medial nucleus of the trapezoid body and the ventral nuclei of the lateral lemniscus (Parent, 1996). There are no contralateral inputs between the ventral and the contralateral nuclei of the lateral lemniscus (Buser and Imbert, 1992).

In studies of nonhuman animals, a tonotopic arrangement of the dorsal nuclei of the lateral lemniscus has been identified such that neurons coding high frequencies are located in the ventral region and neurons coding low frequencies are in the dorsal region (Brugge and Geisler, 1978). The tonotopic arrangement of the ventral nuclei of the lateral lemniscus is not as well organized as the dorsal nuclei (Helfert et al, 1991) and may resemble a helicoid, or "corkscrew," pattern (Merchan and Berbel, 1996). For both the dorsal and ventral nuclei of the lateral lemniscus, frequency tuning is thought to be poorer than at lower levels in the auditory system.

The lateral lemniscus is a contributor to the auditory brainstem response (ABR). Specifically, neurons within the lateral lemniscus appear to contribute to the positive peak of wave V (Moller, 2000). Clinical evidence for the role of the lateral lemniscus in the ABR comes from patients with lesions of the central auditory pathway. In many cases, when lesions are confined to the lateral lemniscus, the characteristics of wave V are changed (Starr and Hamilton, 1976). It is unlikely, however, that the lateral lemniscus response makes up the entirety of wave V, since there is probably some contribution from lower brainstem structures.

Inferior Colliculus

The inferior colliculus is one of the largest and most identifiable auditory structures of the brainstem (Oliver and Morest, 1984). It is located on the dorsal surface of the midbrain, ~3.0 to 3.5 cm rostral to the pontomedullary junction (**Fig. 3–2**).

From the dorsal aspect of the midbrain, the inferior colliculus is clearly visible as two spherical mounds (Musiek and Baran, 1986). Two additional rounded projections, the superior colliculi, can be seen on the dorsal surface of the midbrain, slightly rostral and lateral to the inferior colliculus (Musiek and Baran, 1986).

There are three primary regions of the inferior colliculus (Rockel and Jones, 1973). The first of these is the central nucleus. The central nucleus is the core of the inferior colliculus and is composed of purely auditory fibers. This is a key

auditory region of the midbrain, connecting with many afferent fibers arising from the lower brainstem. This central nucleus, along with its inputs and thalamic projections, is a component in the main (e.g., classical) auditory pathway. The second and third regions of the inferior colliculus are the lateral and dorsal nuclei, or the pericentral nucleus. These regions are less well organized than the central nucleus. These latter two regions surround the central nucleus like a belt and are comprised of both auditory and somatosensory fibers (Keidel et al, 1983). The lateral region of the inferior colliculus also includes fibers that form the brachium (Geniec and Morest, 1971). Both the lateral and dorsal nuclei contribute to the nonclassical auditory pathway (Caird, 1991).

Other divisions for the inferior colliculus have been proposed. Geniec and Morest (1971) proposed a distinction between a caudal cortex and a dorsomedial nucleus within the inferior colliculus. Oliver and Morest (1984) found the need to divide the inferior colliculus into several additional regions. These included: the pars centralis, the pars medialis, and the pars lateralis (for a detailed review regarding these anatomical segments of the inferior colliculus, see Oliver and Shneiderman, 1991).

Most auditory fibers from the lateral lemniscus and the lower auditory centers synapse directly or indirectly at the inferior colliculus (Barnes et al, 1943). Van Noort (1969) found that the inferior colliculus receives input from the dorsal and ventral cochlear nuclei, lateral and medial superior olivary nuclei, dorsal and ventral nuclei of the lateral lemniscus, and contralateral inferior colliculus. Other reports (Keidel et al, 1983; Pickles, 1988; Whitfield, 1967) suggest that the lower nuclei provide both contralateral and ipsilateral input to the inferior colliculus. Many interneurons appear to exist in the inferior colliculus, suggesting the presence of strong neuronal interconnections (Oliver and Morest, 1984). The superior colliculi, generally associated with the visual system, also receive input from the auditory system, which is integrated into the reflexes involving the position of the head and eyes (Gordon, 1972).

Many of the functional properties of the inferior colliculus have been described. As with other brainstem auditory structures, the inferior colliculus has a high degree of tonotopic organization (Merzenich and Reid, 1974). In the inferior colliculus, the high frequencies are ventral and the low frequencies are dorsally positioned (Merzenich and Reid, 1974).

Moreover, the inferior colliculus contains a large number of fibers that yield extremely sharp tuning curves, suggesting a high level of frequency resolution (Aitkin et al, 1975). It contains many time and spatially sensitive neurons (Pickles, 1982) and neurons sensitive to binaural stimulation (Benevento and Coleman, 1970). This suggests a role in sound localization (Musiek and Baran, 1986). Finally, in considering its neural connections and its position astride the auditory pathways, the inferior colliculus has been referred to as the obligatory relay nuclear complex in transmitting auditory information to higher levels (Noback, 1985).

Similar to the lateral lemniscus, the inferior colliculus has a commissure that permits neural communication between the left and right inferior colliculus (Whitfield, 1967).

A unique feature of the inferior colliculus is its brachium, a large fiber tract that lies on the dorsolateral surface of the midbrain. This tract projects fibers ipsilaterally to the medial geniculate body (MGB), which is the principal auditory nucleus of the thalamus. Three cell types make up most neural elements in the inferior colliculus. Disk-shaped cells represent 75 to 85% of the cells in the central nucleus. Simple and complex stellate cells also exist in the inferior colliculus (Oliver and Shneiderman, 1991). In terms of response properties, the inferior colliculus has two main types of responses: transient onset and sustained. The transient onset has an increase in response that grows only at the beginning of the stimulus; the sustained response gradually increases for the duration of the stimulus (Moore and Irvine, 1980). It is important to know that in the inferior colliculus, all the response types described in the section on the cochlear nucleus are also present, although apparently to a lesser degree (Ehret and Merzenich, 1988). The temporal resolution of the inferior colliculus, as with the lateral lemniscus, is less efficient than at the lower brainstem auditory structures (Rouiller, 1997). Interestingly, intensity coding at the inferior colliculus reveals a large number of neurons with nonmonotonic functions (Ehret and Merzenich, 1988).

Medial Geniculate Body

The medial geniculate body is located on the inferior dorsolateral surface of the thalamus just anterior, lateral, and slightly rostral to the inferior colliculus (**Fig. 3–2**). Although the MGB sits in the thalamus and the inferior colliculus in the midbrain, these structures are located only ~1 cm apart. The MGB contains ventral, dorsal, and medial divisions (Morest, 1964). Cells in the ventral division respond primarily to acoustic stimuli, whereas the other divisions contain neurons that respond to both somatosensory and acoustic stimulation (Keidel et al, 1983; Pickles, 1988). The ventral division appears to be the portion of the MGB that transmits specific discrimination (speech) auditory information to the cerebral cortex (Winer, 1984). The dorsal division projects axons to association areas of the auditory cortex. This division may maintain and direct auditory attention (Winer, 1984). The medial division may function as a multisensory arousal system (Winer, 1984).

Besides the MGB, there are three areas of the thalamus that respond to acoustic stimulation. These include the posterior nucleus, the reticular nucleus, and the pulvinar. Viewing the thalamus from a lateroposterior, superior perspective, the posterior nucleus is located on the lateral side, the reticular nucleus is also located laterally bordering the internal capsule, and the pulvinar is located in the posterior section. These three areas effectively increase the amount of the thalamus that is responsive to auditory stimuli.

Afferent inputs to the MGB are primarily uncrossed, arriving from the inferior colliculus by way of the branchium. It is possible, however, that some input may come from the contralateral inferior colliculus and that some lower nuclei may input directly on the MGB (Pickles, 1982). In the cat, crossed inputs from the inferior colliculus connect to the medial division of the MGB (Morest, 1964; Winer, 1984). As with the inferior colliculus, the MGB has many neurons sensitive to binaural stimulation and interaural intensity differences (Aitkin and Webster, 1972; Pickles, 1988).

Tonotopic organization has been reported in the ventral segment of the MGB, with low frequencies represented laterally and high frequencies represented medially (Aitkin and Webster, 1972). Tuning curves range from broad to sharp, but MGB fibers in general are not as sharply tuned as are those of the inferior colliculus (Aitkin and Webster, 1972). As reviewed by Rouiller (1997), the MGB has neurons with response properties that include transient onset, sustained, offset, and inhibitory. The MGB also has sharp tuning curves that allow good frequency selectivity. Both monotonic and nonmonotonic neurons code the intensity. Temporal resolution varies across the three regions of the MGB, and the ventral division has the best fidelity (measured by phase locking or synchronization to individual clicks). In general, the temporal resolution of the ventral portion is similar to that of the inferior colliculus and much poorer than that of the cochlear nucleus.

In addition to the connections mentioned above, the MGB projects fibers to the amygdala (Russchen, 1982) and the posterior area of the caudate. These fibers primarily arise from the medial division of the MGB (LeDoux, 1986). Evidence for these connections comes from auditory fear conditioning research. In these studies, rats, which have been conditioned to a sound that created a fear response, showed no reduction in this response following ablation of the auditory cortex. However, when the MGB was ablated, the fear response could no longer be evoked. This speaks to the importance of the MGB in mediating emotional responses to auditory stimuli (LeDoux, 1986).

Reticular Formation

The auditory system, like other sensory and motor systems, is intricately connected to the reticular formation. The reticular formation can be viewed as having two subsystems: the sensory or ascending reticular activating system (ARAS) and the motor activating system. Our remarks pertain to the ARAS.

The reticular formation, which forms the central core of the brainstem, is a diffusely organized area with intricately connected nuclei and tracts (Sheperd, 1994). It is connected to the spinal cord by reticulospinal tracts and to the cerebrum by many (but poorly defined) tracts, such as the medial forebrain bundle, the mammillary peduncle, and the dorsal longitudinal fasciculus. The reticular formation also contains many brainstem nuclei and has both ascending and descending tracts on each side of the brainstem. These tracts extend from the caudal areas of the spinal cord through the medulla, pons, and midbrain, where diffuse tracts are sent throughout the cerebrum. Connections to the cerebellum also exist.

When the ARAS is stimulated, the cortex becomes more alert and aware. This increased alertness has been shown by changes in electroencephalogram patterns (French, 1957). Conversely, when the reticular formation is turned off, sleep or coma ensues (W. Mosenthal, personal communication, 1991). The ARAS is a general alarm that responds the same way to any sensory input. These responses prepare the entire brain to act appropriately to the incoming stimulus

(Carpenter and Sutin, 1983). Evidence suggests that the ARAS can become sensitive to specific stimuli (French, 1957). For example, this system has a greater reaction to important stimuli than to unimportant stimuli. This may be one of the mechanisms underlying selective attention and could be related to the ability to hear in the presence of noise. General listening skills may also be affected by the state of awareness. The profuse connections of sensory structures to the reticular formation and their extensive interactions may make it unnatural to try to separate attention from sensory or cognitive processing of information.

Vascular Anatomy of the Brainstem

Many auditory dysfunctions of the brainstem and periphery have a vascular basis. For example, vertebrobasilar disease, ministrokes, vascular spasms, aneurysms, and vascular loops have all been shown to affect the auditory system (Musiek and Gollegly, 1985).

The major blood supply of the brainstem is the basilar artery, which originates from the left and right vertebral arteries 1 to 2 mm below the pontomedullary junction on the ventral side of the brainstem (**Fig. 3–6**). At the low to midpons level, the anteroinferior cerebellar artery branches from the basilar artery to supply blood to the cochlear nucleus. The cochlear nucleus also may receive an indirect vascular supply from the posteroinferior cerebellar artery (Waddington, 1984). In many cases the anteroinferior cerebellar artery gives rise to the internal auditory artery, which supplies the eighth cranial nerve (CN VIII), then branches into three divisions to supply the cochlear and vestibular periphery. The internal auditory artery sometimes branches directly from the basilar artery (Portman et al, 1975).

At the midpons level, small pontine branches of the basilar artery, perhaps with the circumferential arteries, indirectly

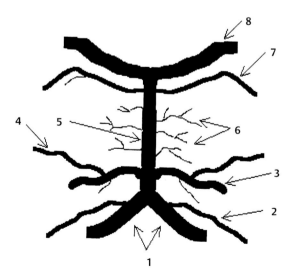

Figure 3–6 A drawing of the key vessels of the rostral medulla and pons segment of the brainstem. These vessels are located on the ventral side of the pons/medulla. 1, vertebral arteries; 2, posterior inferior cerebellar artery; 3, anterior inferior cerebellar artery (AICA); 4, internal auditory artery; 5, basilar artery; 6, pontine arteries; 7, superior cerebellar artery; 8, posterior cerebral artery.

supply the SOC and possibly the lateral lemniscus (Tsuchitani and Boudreau, 1996). In addition, a strong possibility exists that the paramedian branches of the artery supply the SOC and the lateral lemniscus. The superior cerebellar arteries are located at the rostral pons or midbrain level. Their branches supply the inferior colliculus and, in some cases, the nuclei of the lateral lemniscus (Carpenter and Sutin, 1983). At the midbrain level, the basilar artery forms the posterior cerebral arteries. Each posterior cerebral artery has circumferential branches that supply the MGB ipsilaterally (M. Waddington, personal communication, 1985).

Significant variability has been shown in the vasculature of the brainstem (Waddington, 1974, 1984). Because vascular patterns vary among specimens, no one description can encapsulate all vascular patterns. Additionally, most brainstem auditory structures are on the dorsal side of the brainstem, so they may receive secondary and tertiary branches of the key arteries mentioned previously.

Functional Concepts in Sound Processing

This section introduces concepts about general auditory anatomy and physiology and reviews them in reference to auditory brainstem structures.

Intensity Coding

As sound intensity increases, the firing rate of many of the auditory fibers in the brainstem increases; exceptions to this will be discussed later. Because the range between the threshold and saturation point of any given fiber is much smaller than the range of intensities audible to the human ear, large-intensity increases cannot be encoded by individual nerve fibers (Moller, 1983). Rather, at high intensities many neurons must interact to achieve accurate coding. The mechanisms of this interaction are poorly understood (Pickles, 1988) because most information on intensity coding is gained on the basis of the study of individual neurons.

Neurons of various brainstem nuclei respond to stimulus intensity in three principal ways (Pickles, 1988; Whitfield, 1967). One type of response is monotonic, meaning that as the stimulus intensity increases, the firing rate of the neuron(s) increases proportionally. The second type of intensity function is monotonic for low intensities, but as stimulus intensity increases, the firing rate levels off. The third type of intensity function is nonmonotonic. With this type of function, the neuronal firing rate reaches a plateau at a relatively low intensity and sometimes actually decreases as intensity increases, resulting in a rollover phenomenon. For example, some neurons in the inferior colliculus reach their maximum firing rate 5 dB above their threshold (Whitfield, 1967). These three types of intensity coding appear to be common throughout the auditory brainstem, although the extent of each type varies among nuclei groups. Most fibers in the cochlear nucleus, in contrast, have monotonic intensity function. The cochlear nuclear fibers have a 30 to 40 dB dynamic range and in this regard are similar to the auditory nerve fibers (Musiek and Baran, 2007; Rouiller, 1997).

One can hypothesize that a high-intensity signal would not be coded appropriately when damage to brainstem auditory neurons of the first type (monotonic) exists but not to the latter two types of neurons. This could result in higher intensities being coded incorrectly, which might result in what is known clinically as the rollover phenomenon (Jerger and Jerger, 1971).

Temporal Coding

> ### Pearl
>
> • The central auditory nervous system is an elegant time-keeper. Physiological measures of latency, phase locking, phase difference, and synchronicity are common ways of detailing temporal processing. The latency of brainstem neuronal responses varies, depending on the type of auditory stimulus and the neuron or neuron group analyzed (Pickles, 1988; Whitfield, 1967). Some neurons react quickly to stimulation, whereas others have lengthy latency periods. Some neurons respond only on termination of the stimulus.

Phase locking is another phenomenon related to timing in the auditory system (Keidel et al, 1983; Moller, 1985). Many auditory neurons appear to lock onto the stimulus according to phase and fire only when the stimulus waveform reaches a certain point in its cycle. This is particularly evident with low-frequency sounds. Moreover, at lower frequencies, certain neurons fire on every cycle, whereas at higher frequencies, they fire only at every third or fifth cycle. This phase relationship is especially apparent in lower brainstem auditory neurons and may have considerable relevance to the mechanisms underlying masking level differences (Jeffress and McFadden, 1971). Generally, the firing rates of brainstem auditory neurons are higher than those of cortical nerve fibers for steady-state signals or for periodic signals. The speed with which a neuron can respond to repeated stimuli depends on its refractory period. The refractory period is the time interval between two successive discharges (depolarization) of a nerve cell. The refractory period depends on the cell metabolism, and dysfunction of metabolic activity will lengthen it (Tasaki, 1954). Phase locking could be viewed as a form of synchronicity in that responses occur repeatedly in the same time domain. A good example of auditory synchronicity is the auditory brainstem response. In an ABR, the waves represent synchronous electrical activity.

In reviewing timing of the auditory system, it is necessary to discuss temporal processing. As Phillips (1995) conveys, this term may mean different things to different people. Clinicians often use the term *temporal processing* to indicate performance on an audiological test that requires some type of timing decision about the stimuli presented. Basic scientists look at various types of temporal processing and how these contribute to other auditory functions. Phillips (1995) provides several examples of how timing is key to certain auditory processes. Localization of a sound source requires relative timing of acoustic signal arriving at the two ears. The auditory system has a temporal sensitivity to

phase differences (of the signal) that may help us hear in noise. Masking level difference is a good example of phase differential sensitivity. The pitch percept of complex sounds depends on timing (and related coding) of rapidly repeating acoustic events. In addition, sequencing of successive stimuli, masking of signals (existing close in time), discrimination of element duration and time intervals, integration of acoustic energy, and pitch changes can all be considered aspects of temporal processing. Even detection, recognition, and discrimination processes operate over critical time periods and thus may be considered as having a temporal element.

Frequency Coding

The three concepts relevant to our discussion of frequency coding include tonotopicity, frequency discrimination, and physiological tuning curves. The central auditory system is tonotopically arranged, and certain neurons respond best to certain frequencies. This arrangement provides a "spatial array" of various frequencies to which the system responds. The characteristic frequency is the frequency at which a neuron has its lowest threshold to a pure-tone stimulus (the frequency that requires the least amount of intensity to raise a neuron's activity just above its spontaneous firing rate). A physiological tuning curve refers to a plot of the intensity level needed to reach the threshold of a nerve cell over a wide range of frequencies. This measure can convey much information about the frequency resolution of a neuron (or group of neurons). Frequency discrimination is the differential sensitivity to various frequencies. This differential measurement can be accomplished psychophysically and is often referred to as a difference limen, which is the smallest frequency difference that can be discerned between two acoustic stimuli. An electrophysiological correlate to the frequency difference limen can be accomplished using the evoked potential mismatched negativity. Differential sensitivity to intensity and duration of tones can be accomplished in the same way but is not used in physiological studies on audition as much as the frequency parameter is used.

The Auditory Brainstem Response

In concluding this section on the auditory pathways of the brainstem, it is important to discuss aspects of the auditory brainstem response (see Chapter 20). The ABR has gained most of its popularity because of its clinical applications, but it has also been a valuable addition to basic science. It has provided a physiological approach to the study of multiple neuron groups and the way they interact in the brainstem. This avenue of study is different from the single-neuron studies that have been common in auditory brainstem anatomy and physiology.

The exact origins of some elements of the ABR are uncertain, but research in humans has helped clarify the subject (Moller, 1985; Wada and Starr, 1983). Moller (1985) indicated that wave I of the ABR is generated from the lateral aspect of the auditory nerve, whereas wave II originates from the medial aspect. Wave III likely has more than one generator, as do other subsequent waves of the ABR, but the cochlear nucleus is probably the principal source of wave III

(Moller, 1985; Wada and Starr, 1983). In a study of patients with multiple sclerosis undergoing detailed MRIs and ABRs, observations indicated that waves I and II were generated peripheral to the rostral ventral acoustic stria (Levine et al, 1993). This same study indicated that wave III was generated by the AVCN and rostral ventral stria, with the IV/V complex generated rostrally to these structures. Clinical studies have shown that a midline lesion in the low pons that did not affect the cochlear nuclei preserved waves I, II, and III and delayed the waves IV/V complex. This lesion appeared to compromise the SOC (Musiek et al, 1994). Wave IV probably has multiple generator sites as well, but it arises predominantly from the SOC and has a contralateral influence that may be stronger than the ipsilateral contribution. According to Moller (1985) and Wada and Starr (1983), wave V is generated from the lateral lemniscus. Levine et al (1993) relate that the waves IV/V complex may be generated by the MSO system, perhaps where it projects contralaterally onto the lateral lemniscus or inferior colliculus. In a simplified view of the ABR origins, it is plausible that the first five ABR waves may be generated entirely within the auditory nerve and pons. However, the inferior colliculus may exert some influence on wave V, and this has been shown in detailed analyses of the ABR (Durrant et al, 1994).

Pitfall

- Certain nuclei in the brainstem may respond later in time than other nuclei at the same site. This creates difficulty in exact determination of the origin of waves—especially for the later waves of the ABR.

The typical clinical findings of ABR abnormalities on the ear ipsilateral to a brainstem lesion (Musiek and Geurkink, 1982) seem to be inconsistent with known neuroanatomy, which shows most of the auditory fibers crossing to the contralateral side at the level of the SOC. It is unclear what these ABR findings mean in reference to brainstem pathways and associated physiology. However, it is important to consider these clinical findings in the framework of how the brainstem pathways may function in the pathological situation.

Animal studies by Wada and Starr (1983) and our own observations with humans show that the first five waves of the ABR are not affected by specific lesions of the inferior colliculus, with the exceptions noted earlier. Unfortunately, the ABR may not be a useful tool in evaluating lesions at or above the inferior colliculus. Powerful clinical tests such as the ABR, MLDs, and acoustic reflexes appear to be restricted to detecting lesions below the midbrain level. In cases in which lesions of the inferior colliculus or the MGB (midbrain and thalamic levels) are suspected, other procedures are necessary to detect and define the abnormality.

The Cerebrum

Auditory Cortex and Subcortex

Neurons originating in the MGB and radiating outward to the auditory areas of the brain create the ascending auditory system that proceeds from the thalamic area to the cerebral cortex (**Fig. 3–7**).

The cerebral cortex, the gray matter overlay on the brain surface, consists of three principal types of cells: pyramidal, stellate, and fusiform. Six cell layers in the cortex can be distinguished by type, density, and arrangement of the nerve cells (Carpenter and Sutin, 1983). In the auditory region of the cortex, cells responsive to acoustic stimuli exist in all the layers, with the exception of the first layer (Phillips and Irvine, 1981).

Controversial Point

- Researchers disagree on which areas constitute the auditory cortex. This controversy results from adapting animal models to the human brain and from disagreement as to whether to include "association" areas as part of the auditory cortex (Musiek, 1986a). We believe these association areas are critical to understanding the system, although they also contain some fibers that are not sensitive to auditory stimuli.

The principal auditory area of the cortex is considered to be Heschl's gyrus, sometimes referred to as the transverse gyrus (**Fig. 3–8**). This gyrus is located in the sylvian fissure, approximately two-thirds posterior on the upper surface of the temporal lobe (supratemporal plane). It courses in a posterior and medial direction. Heschl's gyrus can be defined by the acoustic sulcus at its anterior and transverse sulcus at its posterior fringes. The temporal lobe must be displaced inferiorly or separated from the brain to expose the supratemporal plane to examine Heschl's gyrus (see Musiek and Baran, 2007).

Campain and Minckler (1976) analyzed numerous human brains and concluded that the configuration of Heschl's gyrus differed on the left side compared with the right. In some brains double gyri were present unilaterally, whereas in other brains double gyri were present on both sides. Musiek and Reeves (1990) studied 29 human brains and reported that several Heschl's gyri ranged from one to three per hemisphere, although no significant left-right asymmetry existed in the number of Heschl's gyri within individual brains. The mean length of Heschl's gyrus, however, was found to be greater in the left hemisphere (Musiek and Reeves, 1990).

The planum temporale is located on the cortical surface from the most posterior aspect of Heschl's gyrus, continuing posteriorly to the end point of the sylvian fissure. In the human brain, the planum temporale was shown to be significantly larger on the left side (3.6 cm) than on the right (2.7 cm) by Geschwind and Levitsky (1968). These researchers thought that the planum temporale may be an anatomical correlate to language (receptive) in humans because it is located in Wernicke's region and in the left hemisphere, which is dominant for speech. Musiek and Reeves (1990) supported these earlier findings on the differences in the length of the left and right planum temporale. Musiek and Reeves proposed, however, that asymmetries in higher

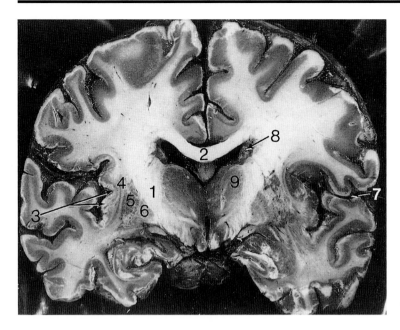

Figure 3–7 Coronal section through a human brain (gray matter stained), emphasizing the subcortical structures. 1, internal capsule; 2, corpus callosum; 3, insula; 4, external capsule with the claustrum (gray matter strip); 5, putamen; 6, globus pallidus; 7, sylvian fissure; 8, caudate; 9, thalamus. (Courtesy of W. Mosenthal and F. Musiek, Anatomy Laboratory, Dartmouth Medical School, Hanover, NH.)

auditory and language function may be related to anatomical differences of not only the planum temporale but also Heschl's gyrus.

Recently, the "belt-core" concept has been proposed as an alternative way to define the main auditory cortex areas (Hackett et al, 2001). Both the belt and core are located on the superior temporal plane and gyrus, with the belt comprising the posterior two thirds of the temporal plane and gyrus and the core being located between the posterior sulcus and the anterior temporal sulcus of Heschl's gyrus. The core is primarily divided into three sections: rostral temporal, which is anterior; rostral, which is in the middle, and the primary auditory region, which is posterior. Medial and lateral to the core are two belts. The medial belt is made up of three divisions: the rostral temporal medial, rostral medial, and caudal medial sections. The lateral belt is made up of four divisions: the rostral temporal lateral, anterior lateral, medial lateral, and caudal lateral sections. A third belt, the parabelt region, is located on the surface of the superior temporal gyrus. The parabelt region is made up of two sections: the rostral and caudal parabelt. Core and belt areas appear to receive different subcortical inputs. The main input from the ventral MGB is to the core, whereas the dorsal and ventral MGB connect to the belts. The core also has inputs into the belts and parabelt. The belt areas connect to other areas of the brain, including other regions of the temporal lobe, the parietal lobe, and the prefrontal cortex (Hackett et al, 2001).

The primary auditory area and a portion of the language area in humans are contained within the sylvian fissure. Rubens (1986) reviewed earlier anatomical work on the sylvian fissure, showing the left sylvian fissure to be larger

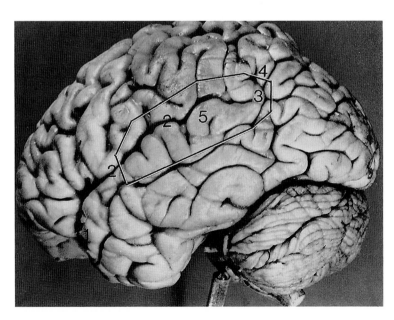

Figure 3–8 Lateral view of the left hemisphere of the brain with the auditory responsive area encircled. 1, temporal pole; 2, sylvian fissure; 3, supramarginal gyrus; 4, angular gyrus; 5, superoposterior temporal gyrus. (From Waddington, M. (1984). Atlas of human intracranial anatomy. Rutland, VT: Academy Books, with permission.)

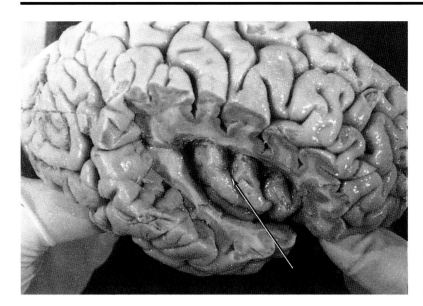

Figure 3–9 Right lateral view of the insula observed after removal of part of the parietal, frontal, and temporal lobes. (Courtesy of W. Mosenthal and F. Musiek, Anatomy Laboratory, Dartmouth Medical School, Hanover, NH.)

than the right. Others have corroborated this finding, including Musiek and Reeves (1990), who found that asymmetry of the sylvian fissure was correlated with the greater length of the planum temporale on the left side.

Curving around the end of the sylvian fissure is the supramarginal gyrus, an area responsive to acoustic stimulation (Celesia, 1976). It is located in the approximate Wernicke's area region, along with the angular gyrus, which is situated immediately posterior to the supramarginal gyrus (Geschwind and Levitsky, 1968). These constitute a portion of a complex association area that appears to integrate auditory, visual, and somesthetic information, making it vital to the visual and somesthetic aspects of language, such as reading and writing.

Also responsive to acoustical stimulation are the inferior portion of the parietal lobe and the inferior aspect of the frontal lobe (Celesia, 1976) (**Fig. 3–8**). The insula (a portion of the cortex located deep within the sylvian fissure medial to the middle segment of the temporal gyrus) is yet another acoustically responsive area. It appears that the most posterior aspect of the insula is contiguous with Heschl's gyrus. The only way to observe the insular cortex is by removing the temporal lobe or displacing it inferiorly (**Figs. 3–9** and **3–10**).

The insula contains fibers that respond to somatic, visual, and gustatory stimulation. Acoustic stimulation, however, causes the greatest neural activity (Sudakov et al, 1971). The posterior aspect of the insula, the section nearest to Heschl's gyrus, seems to possess the most acoustically sensitive fibers (Sudakov et al, 1971). Located just medial to the insula is a narrow strip of gray matter called the claustrum. The function of the claustrum is not well understood but seems to be highly responsive to acoustic stimulation (Noback, 1985; Sudakov et al, 1971).

The findings just mentioned are interesting for two reasons. First, the areas of symmetry versus asymmetry and microdysgenesias appear to involve areas that in humans are mostly considered auditory regions of the cerebrum. Second, the reason for the high incidence of cortical dys-

plasias in people with learning disorders is unknown. One might speculate that these morphological abnormalities have functional or perhaps dysfunctional correlates. For instance, people with dyslexia have been reported to have anatomical brain irregularities (Kaufmann and Galaburda, 1989). More studies are needed to relate these findings to behavioral consequences.

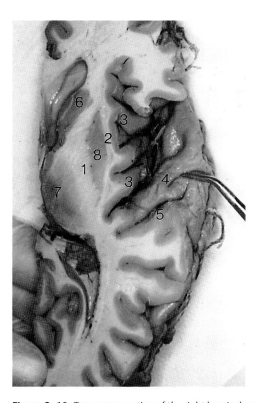

Figure 3–10 Transverse section of the right hemisphere cut along the sylvian fissure. 1, internal capsule; 2, external capsule with claustrum coursing through it; 3, insula; 4, Heschl's gyrus; 5, anterior part of the planum temporale (posterior part is cut away); 6, caudate; 7, thalamus; 8, lenticular process (putamen, globus pallidus).

Thalamocortical Connections

Pearl

- The planum temporale, normally significantly longer in the left hemisphere, was found to be symmetrical bilaterally in the brains of dyslexic patients, who also had an unusually large number of cell abnormalities called cerebrocortical microdysgenesias, which are nests of ectopic neurons and glia in the first layer of the cortex. These ectopic areas are often connected with dysplasia of cortical layers (including focal microgyria), sometimes with superficial growths known as brain warts. Up to 26% of normal brains may contain these focal anomalies, but they are usually found in small numbers, often in the right hemisphere. A greater number of anomalies occur in patients with developmental dyslexia, frequently in the left hemisphere in the area of the presylvian cortex (Kaufmann and Galaburda, 1989).

Auditory fiber tracts ascending from the MGB to the cortex and other areas of the brain follow multiple routes. One of these groups of fibers supplies input to the basal ganglia, which is the large subcortical gray matter structure consisting of the caudate nucleus, putamen, and global pallidus (**Figs. 3–7** and **3–10**). The lenticular process, or nucleus, lies between the internal and external capsules, the white matter neural pathways, and contains the putamen and globus pallidus. In animal studies the MGB has been shown to transmit fibers that connect with the putamen, the caudate nucleus, and the amygdaloid body, a small almond-shaped expansion located at the tail of the caudate nucleus (LeDoux et al, 1984).

Two main pathways link the MGB and the cortex, besides the aforementioned connections to the basal ganglia. The first pathway follows a sublenticular route through the internal capsule to the Heschl's gyrus and contains all auditory fibers emanating from the ventral MGB. The second pathway courses from the MGB through the inferior aspect of the internal capsule, ultimately under the putamen to the external capsule, and consists of auditory, somatic, and possibly visual fibers. Beyond the external capsule, fibers connect to the insula (Musiek and Gollegly, 1985; Streitfeld, 1980). Further connections proceed from the MGB to the auditory cortex and most likely overlap the two pathways discussed here. These pathways represent the varied and complex connections of the thalamocortical auditory anatomy.

Intrahemispheric Connections

Intrahemispheric and interhemispheric connections are both present within the primary auditory cortex. Primary auditory area lesions in primates have produced degeneration of the caudal (posterior) aspect of the superior temporal gyrus and the upper bank of the adjacent superior temporal sulcus (Seltzer and Pandya, 1978). This pattern of degeneration suggests the existence of multisynaptic pathways in the middle and posterior areas of the superior temporal gyrus (Jones and Powell, 1970). Fibers from the superior temporal gyrus also connect to the insula and frontal operculum.

Few connections exist between the auditory area and the temporal pole (i.e., the anteriormost aspect of the temporal lobe) (Noback, 1985). Some audiological studies have investigated the validity of several central auditory tests by evaluating patients whose temporal poles had been removed. One would not anticipate these patients having central auditory deficits considering the anatomy of this region.

The arcuate fasciculus, one of the "long" association pathways, adjoins the auditory cortical areas and other sections of the temporal lobe with areas in the frontal lobe. This large fiber tract passes from the temporal lobe, up and around the top of the sylvian fissure, and extends anteriorly to the frontal lobe (Streitfeld, 1980). The arcuate fasciculus is coupled with the longitudinal fasciculus, a larger tract that travels in the same direction by means of comparable anatomical regions. Wernicke's area in the temporal lobe and Broca's area in the frontal lobe are two important regions connected by way of the arcuate fasciculus (Carpenter and Sutin, 1983).

In animals, reciprocal connections exist between the posterior auditory cortex and the claustrum, which is located in the external capsule. Although the claustrum's function is uncertain, it is clear that it is acoustically responsive (Rouiller, 1997). Given its location and its neural connections, the claustrum may have functions related to insular and Heschl's gyrus interactions.

Connections also exist from auditory regions to occipital and hippocampal areas of the brain, although the pathways are not anatomically defined. These connections provide memory and visual associations necessary for such functions as reading.

Interhemispheric Connections

Located at the base of the longitudinal fissure, the corpus callosum is the primary connection between the left and right hemispheres (see Musiek and Baran, 2007) (**Figs. 3–1, 3–7,** and **3–11**).

The corpus callosum is covered by the cingulate gyri and forms most of the roof of the lateral ventricles (Selnes, 1974). It consists of long, heavily myelinated axons and is the largest fiber tract in the primate brain. In an adult the corpus callosum is ~6.5 cm long from the anterior genu to the posterior splenium and is ~0.5 to 1.0 cm thick (Musiek, 1986b). The corpus callosum seems to be larger in left-handed than in right-handed people, but it has significant morphological variability (Witelson, 1986).

The corpus callosum is not exclusively a midline structure (Musiek, 1986b) because it essentially connects the two cortices and thereby must span much of the intercortical space above the basal ganglia and lateral ventricles. It is probable that in many "cortical" lesions some region of the corpus callosum is involved because it encompasses such a large portion of the cerebrum.

Homolateral fibers (those that connect to the same locus in each hemisphere) are the primary fibers in the corpus callosum. The corpus callosum also contains heterolateral fibers, which are those connecting to different loci on each hemisphere (Mountcastle, 1962). Heterolateral fibers frequently have a longer and less direct route to the opposite

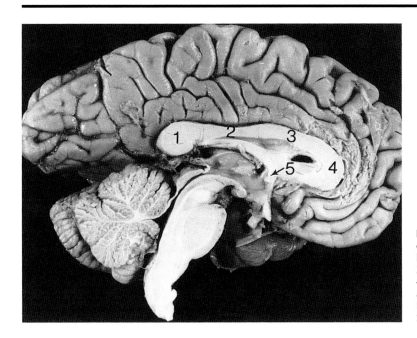

Figure 3–11 Sagittal cut separating the two hemispheres of the brain and sectioning the corpus callosum at its midline. Focus is the corpus callosum. 1, splenium (visual); 2, sulcus (auditory); 3, trunk or body (somatic and motor); 4, genu (olfactory frontal lobe fibers), rostrum (olfactory); 5, anterior commissure. (Courtesy of W. Mosenthal and F. Musiek, Anatomy Laboratory, Dartmouth Medical School, Hanover, NH.)

side, which may necessitate a longer transfer time than required by their homolateral counterparts. The latency of an evoked potential recorded from one point on the cortex after stimulation of the homolateral point on the other hemisphere is referred to as the transcallosal transfer time (TCTT). The TCTT in humans decreases with age, and minimum values are achieved during teenage years (Gazzaniga et al, 1962). These findings are consistent with increased myelination of the corpus callosum axons (Yakovlev and LeCours, 1967). The TCTT varies significantly, from a minimum of 3 to 6 msec to a maximum of 100 msec, in primates and humans (Salamy, 1978). The concept of inhibitory and excitatory neurons in the corpus callosum may be substantiated by this variability.

The anatomy of the corpus callosum subserves, and the neural connections correspond to, various regions of the cortex. The neural connections of the corpus callosum correspond to, and the anatomy subserves, various regions of the cortex. The genu, or anterior region of the corpus callosum, contains fibers leading from the anterior insula and the olfactory fibers (Pandya and Seltzer, 1986). The trunk comprises the middle section of the corpus callosum, where the frontal and temporal lobes are also represented. The posterior half of the trunk, called the sulcus, is thinner and contains most of the auditory fibers from the temporal lobe and insula. The splenium is the most posterior portion of the corpus callosum and contains mostly visual fibers that connect with the occipital cortex (Pandya and Seltzer, 1986).

Just anterior to the splenium in the posterior half of the corpus callosum is the auditory area of the corpus callosum at the midline. Although this information was obtained through primate research (Pandya and Seltzer, 1986), data on humans helped localize the auditory areas of the corpus callosum. Baran et al (1986) found little or no change in tasks requiring interhemispheric transfer (i.e., dichotic listening or pattern perception) after the sectioning of the

anterior half of the corpus callosum. However, markedly poorer performance on these auditory tasks was shown in patients with a complete section of the corpus callosum (Musiek et al, 1984).

Lesions along the transcallosal auditory pathway may bring about interhemispheric transfer degradation. Although we have much information about the anatomy of the corpus callosum at midline, we know little about the course of the transcallosal auditory pathway. It is thought to begin at the auditory cortex and course posteriorly and superiorly around the lateral ventricles. It then crosses a periventricular area known as the trigone and courses medially and inferiorly into the corpus callosum proper. This information about the transcallosal auditory pathway comes from anatomical and clinical studies (Damasio and Damasio, 1979).

A study by Hynd et al (1991) demonstrated size differences in the corpus callosum for children with attention deficits compared with control subjects. The auditory and the genu areas of the corpus callosum in the experimental group were smaller than those of the control group.

The vascular anatomy of the corpus callosum is simple. The splenium, or posterior fifth, is supplied by branches of the posterior cerebral artery (Carpenter and Sutin, 1983). The remainder of the corpus callosum is supplied by the pericallosal artery, a branch of the anterior cerebral artery (Carpenter and Sutin, 1983).

Tonotopic Organization in the Auditory Cortex

As in the brainstem, distinct tonotopic organization exists in the auditory cortex. Tonotopic organization exists in the primary auditory cortex of the primate, with low frequencies represented rostrolaterally and high frequencies represented caudomedially (Merzenich and Brugge, 1973). Using positron emission tomography (PET) to measure changes in cerebral blood flow, Lauter et al (1985) demonstrated a similar pattern in the human brain. Tones of 500 Hz evoked increased activity in the lateral part of Heschl's gyrus, whereas tones of 4000 Hz resulted in activity in the medial position. Most tonotopic information on the insular cortex has been obtained from studies of cats (Woolsey, 1960). In the cat insula, the high-frequency neurons appear to be located in the inferior segment (Woolsey, 1960).

In the primary auditory area where cells are sharply tuned, highly definable tonotopic organization and isofrequency strips (contours) can be found (Pickles, 1985). "Columns" within the cortex appear to have similar characteristic frequencies (Phillips and Irvine, 1981). A spatial component to frequency representation also seems to be present in the auditory cortex; ~2 mm is required to encompass the frequency range of one octave. For extremely high frequencies, less space is needed to represent an octave range (Mountcastle, 1968).

Special Consideration

- The tonotopicity of the auditory cortex has the plasticity to change if a lack of input is present at a given frequency range. Schwaber et al (1993) demonstrated in primates that if one frequency band of the auditory cortex was deprived of input, after ~3 months that frequency band shifted to the neighboring lower frequency for which there was input and stimulation; thus, the cortical tissue remains active and viable even though its tonotopic arrangement was different. This type of finding has important clinical implications.

Intensity Coding in the Auditory Cortex

The discharge or firing rate of cortical neurons in primates varies as a function of intensity and takes two forms: monotonic and nonmonotonic (Pfingst and O'Connor, 1981). Most neurons in the primary auditory cortex display rate–intensity functions similarly to the auditory nerve (i.e., the firing rate is monotonic for increments of ~10–40 dB). Intensities greater than 40 dB do not increase firing rates. Many neurons in the auditory cortex are sharply nonmonotonic. In some cases the firing rate may be reduced to a spontaneous level, with a 10 dB increase above the threshold intensity (Pickles, 1988).

Phillips (1990) reported similar results with cats, identifying both monotonic and nonmonotonic profiles. For some nonmonotonic neurons, firing rates decreased precipitously, often to zero, at stimulus levels slightly above threshold. Phillips (1990) also found that the introduction of wideband noise raised the threshold level of the cortical neurons. However, once threshold sensitivity was achieved in noise, the firing rate increased in a manner similar to the nonmasked condition, with the intensity profile remaining basically unchanged. With successive increments in the level of the masking noise, the tonal intensity profile is displaced toward progressively higher sound pressure levels. This phenomenon could be a way in which some cortical neurons can afford the auditory system an improvement in signal-to-noise ratio, perhaps permitting better hearing in noise. One may also hypothesize that if these cortical neurons are damaged, the signal-to-noise ratio is compromised and that hearing in noise may be more difficult.

Animal studies show some cortical neurons to be intensity selective. Certain cells respond only within a given intensity range, but collectively the neurons cover a wide range of intensities. For example, cortical cells may respond maximally, minimally, or not at all at a given intensity. When the intensity is changed, different cells may respond at a maximum level, and the previous neurons may respond minimally or not at all (Merzenich and Brugge, 1973).

Temporal Coding in the Auditory Cortex

Like the brainstem, the auditory cortex responds in various ways to the onset, presence, and offset of acoustic stimuli. Abeles and Goldstein (1972) found four types of responses of cortical neurons to a 100 msec tone. One type of neuron sustained a response for the duration of the stimulus, although the firing rate was considerably less at the offset of the tone. "On" neurons responded only to the onset, and "off" neurons responded only after the tone was terminated. The fourth type responded to both the onset and the offset of the tone but did not sustain a response during the tone.

Additional information on timing or temporal processing in the auditory cortex can be found in the work of Goldstein et al (1971). These investigators studied cells in the primary auditory area (A_1) of rats and found four categories of response to clicks presented at different rates. Approximately 40% of the A_1 cells responded to each click at rates of 10 to 1000 per second, whereas 25% of the A_1 cells did not respond at all. The third classification of A_1 cells showed varying response patterns as the click rate changed. The fourth group of cells responded only to low click rates. Eggermont (1991) reported that several studies found click rates of auditory cortex neurons to be ~50 to 100 per second or less. He also reported that recording methods may influence the quantification of the response rates of these neurons. However, it seems that cortical neurons have difficulty following high-rate periodic events.

The coding of transient events by the cortex is related to temporal resolution and is different from coding periodic events. Examples of transient events would be tasks such as click fusion and temporal ordering. For these kinds of tasks, the cortex is temporally sensitive (Phillips, 1995). Only 2 to 3 msec differences were needed between two clicks to determine in humans that two stimuli were present and not one (Lackner and Teuber, 1973).

Timing within the auditory cortex plays a critical role in localization abilities. Many neurons in the primary auditory cortex are sensitive to interaural phase and intensity differences (Benson and Teas, 1976). In a sound field, more cortical units fire to sound stimuli from a contralateral source than from an ipsilateral source (Evans, 1968). This finding provided the basis for the initial clinical work on sound localization.

In 1958, Sanchez-Longo and Forster reported that patients with temporal lobe damage had difficulty locating sound sources in the sound field contralateral to the damaged hemisphere. Moore et al (1990) studied the abilities of both normal and brain-damaged subjects to track a fused auditory image as it moved through auditory space. The perceived location of the auditory image, which varies according to the temporal relationship of paired clicks presented one each from matched speakers, is referred to as the precedence effect. Although the normal subjects were able to track the fused auditory image accurately, two subjects with unilateral temporal lobe lesions (one in the right hemisphere, one in the left) exhibited auditory field deficits opposite the damaged hemispheres. Results of these investigations are consistent with other localization and lateralization studies that show contralateral ear effects (Pinheiro and Tobin, 1969).

Electrical Stimulation of the Auditory Cortex

Various auditory stimulation experiments with humans during neurological procedures were performed by Penfield and Roberts (1959). These investigators electrically stimulated areas along the margin of the sylvian fissure while the patient, under local anesthesia, reported what he or she heard. Numerous patients reported experiencing no auditory sensation during the electrical stimulation. Some patients, however, reported hearing buzzing, ringing, chirping, knocking, humming, and rushing sounds when the superior gyrus of the temporal lobe was stimulated. These sounds were directed primarily to the contralateral ear but sometimes to both ears.

Patients in this study frequently reported the impression of hearing loss during the electrical stimulation, although they heard and understood spoken words. Furthermore, the patients claimed that the pitch and volume of the surgeon's voice varied during the electrical stimulation. In a later study, Penfield and Perot (1963) reported cases in which patients heard music and singing during electrical stimulation of the right auditory cortex. When the left posterosuperior temporal gyrus was stimulated, many patients who responded heard voices shouting and other acoustic phenomena.

Lateralization of Function in the Auditory Cortex

One important issue in central auditory assessment using behavioral tests relates to lateralization of the deficit. It is well known that behavioral testing often indicates deficiencies in the ear contralateral to the damaged hemisphere. The fact that each ear provides more contralateral than ipsilateral input to the cortex may explain this contralateral ear deficit. Solid physiological evidence upholds this theory. Mountcastle (1968) reported that contralateral stimulation of cortical neurons ordinarily had a 5 to 20 dB lower threshold for activation than did ipsilateral stimulation. Celesia (1976) also showed that near field potentials recorded from human auditory cortices during neurosurgery had larger amplitudes with contralateral ear stimulation than with ipsilateral stimulation. Studies of cats have also demonstrated comparable findings that indicate a stronger contralateral representation (Donchin et al, 1976).

Late auditory evoked potentials recorded with temporal/parietal region electrode placement in humans also revealed variances between contralateral and ipsilateral stimulation. The auditory evoked potentials recorded from contralateral stimulation were generally earlier and of greater amplitude than ipsilateral recordings (Utler et al, 1969). However, this may not always be the case, and these findings for far field evoked potentials are controversial (Donchin et al, 1976).

Behavioral Ablation Studies

Ablation experiments have served as the basis for the development of several auditory tests. By monitoring auditory behavior in animals, the effects of partial or total ablation of the auditory cortex have been measured and have been valuable in the localization of function.

Differences among animal species are shown in studies with opossums (Ravizza and Masterton, 1972) and ferrets (Kavanagh and Kelly, 1988), in which auditory threshold recovery is almost complete after bilateral lesions of the auditory cortex. The effects of auditory cortex ablation on frequency discrimination in animals remain unclear, even after many years of research. Early studies (Meyer and Woolsey, 1952) reported that frequency discrimination was lost after ablation of the auditory cortex, whereas later studies (Cranford et al, 1976) contradicted these early findings. These discrepancies may be related to the difficulty of the discrimination tasks because each study used a different test paradigm to measure pitch perception. The complexity of the tasks, rather than the differences in frequency discrimination, is likely responsible for the discrepant findings (Pickles, 1988).

Controversial Point

- Kryter and Ades (1943) found little or no effect on absolute thresholds or differential thresholds for intensity in the auditory cortex. These findings are consistent with data obtained from humans with brain damage or surgically removed auditory cortices (Hodgson, 1967). However, some investigators (Heffner and Heffner, 1986; Heffner et al, 1985) report that bilateral ablations of the primate auditory cortex result in severe hearing loss for pure tones. Bilaterally ablated animals demonstrated gradual recovery, but many retained some permanent pure-tone sensitivity loss, especially in the middle frequencies (Heffner and Heffner, 1986). Unilateral cortical ablations resulted in hearing loss in the ear contralateral to the lesion and normal hearing in the ipsilateral ear (Heffner et al, 1985). Permanent residual hearing loss also has been reported in humans with bilateral cortical lesions (Jerger et al, 1969).

Lesion effects on frequency discrimination in humans may differ from those in animals. Thompson and Abel (1992) showed that patients with temporal lobe lesions have significantly poorer frequency discrimination for tones than do normal control subjects. Patients with lesions of the left temporal lobe yielded a greater deficit than did patients

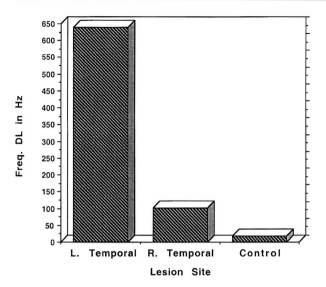

Figure 3–12 Column graph shows the mean difference limen (DL) in Hz obtained from subjects with left and right temporal lobe lesions compared with a control group. (Adapted from Thompson, M. E., & Abel, S. M. (1992). Indices of hearing in patients with central auditory pathology. Scandinavian Audiology Supplementum, 35, 3–22.)

with right temporal lobe lesions (**Fig. 3–12**). Similar results of poor frequency discrimination in patients with central auditory lesions have been noted on a more informal test basis by the authors of this chapter.

Because ablation of the auditory cortex has debatable effects on absolute or differential thresholds for intensity or frequency, more complex tasks were sought to examine the results of cortical ablation. Diamond and Neff (1957) used patterned acoustical stimuli to examine the ability of cats to detect differences in frequency patterns after various bilateral cortical ablations. After ablation of primary and association auditory cortices, the cats could no longer discriminate different acoustical patterns, and despite extensive retraining they could not relearn the pattern task. On the basis of subsequent studies, Neff (1961) reported that the auditory cortex ablations affected primarily temporal sequencing and not pattern detection or frequency discrimination of the tones composing patterns. Colavita (1972) demonstrated in cats that ablation of only the insular-temporal region resulted in the inability to discriminate temporal patterns. The early research of Diamond and Neff influenced Pinheiro in her development of the frequency (pitch) pattern test, a valuable clinical central auditory test in humans (Pinheiro and Musiek, 1985). Another pattern perception test, duration patterns, has emerged as a potentially valuable clinical tool (Musiek et al, 1990). Temporal ordering appears to be a critical part of pattern perception, which in turn is affected by lesions of the auditory cortex.

Other studies show that the temporal dimension of hearing is linked to the integrity of the auditory cortex. Gershuni et al (1967) demonstrated that a unilateral lesion of the dog's auditory cortex resulted in decreased pure-tone sensitivity for short but not long tones in the ear contralateral to the lesion.

In contrast, Cranford (1979) showed that cortical lesions had no effect on brief tone thresholds in cats. Cranford also demonstrated that auditory cortex lesions in cats markedly affected the frequency difference limen for short but not long duration tones presented to the contralateral ear. After the animal study, Cranford et al (1982) examined brief tone frequency difference limina in seven human subjects with unilateral temporal lobe lesions. Findings with human subjects were essentially the same as those with animals. Brief tone thresholds for subjects with temporal lobe lesions were the same as those of a normal control group, but the brief tone frequency difference limen was markedly poorer for subjects with lesions. The frequency difference limen was poorer for the contralateral ear for stimulus durations less than 200 msec.

Auditory Stimulation Influences on the Auditory Cortex

The auditory cortex appears to respond to acoustic stimulation and/or auditory training. This statement is associated with several important recent studies. One such study was conducted by Recanzone et al (1993) on owl monkeys. These animals were trained on a frequency discrimination task. After extensive training, each animal's auditory cortex was tonotopically mapped. The neural substrate matching the frequency of the training was 2 to 8 times larger than the same region in a control group of animals that did not receive training. In addition, these animals' behavioral frequency discrimination improved markedly after training. Other studies, although differently oriented, have also shown changes (reorganization) in the auditory cortex as a result of stimulation and/or training (Knudsen, 1988). This has changed our view on auditory training, especially its use with auditory processing disorders (for a review, see Chermak and Musiek, 1997).

Imaging Techniques

Advanced imaging technology has made anatomical and physiological inspection of the human brain possible. This is important because at the subcortical and cortical levels animal brains are structurally and functionally different from the human brain, and it has been with concern that inferences have been made from animal models to humans on brain function related to audition. With imaging techniques, it is possible to measure some functions of hearing in humans. Although it is too soon for these imaging techniques to replace animal studies, they have important potential.

Two types of imaging techniques will be discussed here: positron emission tomography and functional magnetic resonance imaging (Elliott, 1994) (**Fig. 3–13**). The basis of PET is the decay of radioactive tracers that have been introduced into the body and emit positrons. These positrons undergo transformations that result in the release of photons that are detected by the scanning equipment. The radioactive tracer becomes perfused in the brain, and brain activity results in photon emissions that are measured. Two types of PET exist: one based on regional blood flow and one based on glucose metabolism. The blood flow technique requires inhalation or injection of the radioactive tracer,

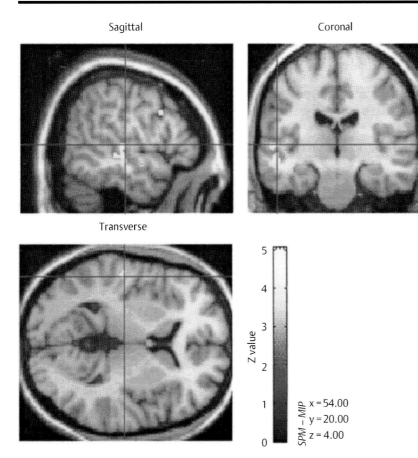

Sagittal   Coronal

Transverse

Figure 3–13 Functional magnetic resonance imaging of the brain of a subject who was required to discriminate nonsense words as being alike or different. Note activity in the midportion of Heschl's gyrus and extending inferiorly into the superoposterior midtemporal gyrus. Also note some frontal lobe activity on the sagittal view. All activity in these views seems to be limited to the left hemisphere. (Courtesy of Brain Imaging Laboratory, Dartmouth Medical School, Hanover, NH.) *(See Color Plate 3–13.)*

which has a short half-life of ∼2 minutes. Because the body clears the radioactive substance quickly, repeated tests are possible, but each test is obviously limited by time. The glucose metabolism technique uses fluoro-2-deoxy-D-glucose (FDG), which has a by-product linked to glucose, which in turn perfuses the brain differentially. The maximum perfusion is where the metabolism is greatest. The time window for measurement is 30 to 40 minutes after tracer injection, and multiple scans should not be performed because of risk to the patient.

The second imaging technique is fMRI. In fMRI, a strong magnetic field is used to align the body's protons, and a brief radio signal is then used to alter the tilt of the aligned protons. The energy released when the protons resume their original positions is measured. Because the blood acquires paramagnetic properties when the body is in a strong magnetic field, blood flow can be visualized by MRI. Blood flow is related to blood volume and oxygenation, which are increased when certain areas of the brain are active. Hence, magnetic susceptibility of the blood changes with increased neural activity, and these changes are reflected in the MRI measurements (Elliott, 1994). With fMRI, no radioactivity is involved, and its resolution is greater than that of PET. The noise present during fMRI testing is considerable, and this remains a factor in auditory studies.

Many contributions from imaging studies to auditory anatomy and physiology exist, but we will highlight only a few studies. As mentioned, one early PET study investigated the tonotopic arrangement of Heschl's gyrus (Lauter et al,

1985). This showed low frequencies (500 Hz) to be anterior and lateral, whereas the high frequencies (4000 Hz) were posteromedial. Similar tonotopic results have been reported using fMRI (Talavage et al, 1996).

An fMRI study (Millen et al, 1995) using speech (context, reading passages) and tonal stimuli showed primarily activation at the superior temporal gyrus, with more activity on the left side than on the right. Activity appeared to occur in the insula as well. The regions that were active along the superior temporal gyrus varied. Interestingly, different intensities of the stimuli seemed to have no effect on activation patterns. In an fMRI study on word presentation rates, greater activation was seen on the left side than on the right, with activity increasing from 10 to 90 words per minute and a drop in activity at 130 words per minute. The superior temporal gyrus areas, including Heschl's gyrus, planum temporale, and a small area immediately anterior to Heschl's gyrus, were activated at high rates of word presentation. The posterior insula also became involved at high rates (Dhankhar et al, 1997). In a PET study using words from a song for which pitch judgment of target words was required, the left cortex was more active than the right. Most activity was in the area of Heschl's gyrus but often extended both posteriorly and anteriorly beyond Heschl's gyrus. In this study the subjects were also asked to imagine performing the task. The auditory regions (though smaller and less intense) were activated for this type of task. This showed a way to activate the auditory cortex without external stimuli (Zatorre et al, 1996).

New Measures of the Sensitivity of Auditory Cortical Neurons

The auditory steady-state response (ASSR) is a measure of the sensitivity of the auditory cortex to amplitude modulated (AM) and frequency modulated (FM) signals. It has recently received interest clinically as a potential frequency-specific measure of the sensitivity of cortical auditory neurons. As initially demonstrated by Whitfield and Evans (1965), FM signals yield larger and more consistent cortical responses than steady-state tones of identical frequency. Cortical responses to FM signals are strongest when the modulation direction is toward the neuron characteristic frequency and when the signal stays within the response area of the cortex (Phillips et al, 1991). The modulation rates of FM signals to which the auditory cortex neurons are most responsive are in the 5 to 15 Hz range (Evans, 1974). Additionally, the greater frequency modulation range yields stronger neural responses (Moller, 2000). AM signals are similarly influenced by acoustic characteristics of the signal. The AM rates that the auditory cortex is most responsive to are in the 1 to 50 Hz range. Because the brainstem response surpasses the cortical response as the modulation rate exceeds 50 Hz (Phillips et al, 1991), slower modulation rates tend to yield better cortical responses.

Auditory Cortex Vascular Anatomy

The middle cerebral artery (MCA) branches directly from the internal capsule at the base of the brain and is the main artery supplying blood to the auditory cortex (Waddington, 1974). The length of the MCA varies. It can be only 2 cm long before its diffuse branching (Gershuni et al, 1967), or it can extend the full length of the sylvian fissure before becoming the angular artery and coursing posteriorly and laterally on the brain surface. Its route fluctuates greatly between species, but it courses primarily in an anterior-to-posterior direction within the sylvian fissure (Waddington, 1974).

Starting with an anterior view of the MCA, the fronto-opercular artery is the first major branch supplying an auditory region. This artery follows a superior route, supplying the anterior section of the insula. Just posterior to the fronto-opercular artery is the central sulcus artery that supplies the posterior insula and the anterior parietal lobe. Three arteries ascend from the MCA and course over the middle and posterior part of the temporal lobe (Waddington, 1974). These three are the anterior, middle, and posterior arteries, and they supply the middle and superior temporal gyri. A combination of the MCA and angular artery presumably supplies the primary auditory area along with the angular gyrus and a portion of the supramarginal gyrus. The posterior parietal artery supplies the remainder of the supramarginal gyrus.

Significant tissue damage to gray and white matter in the temporal-parietal regions of the brain may be caused by vascular insults involving the MCA. These lesions are devastating to both the structure and function of the auditory cortex and are among the most common anomalies affecting this region.

Pitfall

- The difference between the auditory cortex in animals and humans is a factor in interpreting animal studies pertaining to its physiology.

The Efferent Auditory System

The efferent auditory system likely functions as one unit, but the pathways are often viewed in two sections. The caudalmost part of the system, the olivocochlear bundle (OCB), has been studied, but little is known about the more rostral system. The rostral efferent pathway starts at the auditory cortex and descends to the medial geniculate and the midbrain regions, including the inferior colliculus. A loop system appears to exist between the cortex and these structures, and fibers descend from the cortex to neurons in the brainstem. The inferior colliculus also receives efferents from the medial geniculate (Pickles, 1988). The descending connections from the inferior colliculus to nuclei in the SOC have not been well established. Sahley et al (1997) reviewed these connections and stated that connections exist from the inferior colliculus to the ipsilateral trapezoid body nuclei and preolivary nuclei. Bilateral connections also appear to exist from the inferior colliculus that are widespread to different areas of the SOC. Some areas of the descending pathway are not well studied, but a system is known to exist that allows neural communication from the cortex to the cochlea. In this regard, it is known that electrical stimulation of the cortex results in the excitation or inhibition of single units in the lower auditory system (Ryugo and Weinberger, 1976). Physiological evidence exists for a descending train of impulses that eventually reach the cochlea from the cortex (Desmedt, 1975).

The OCB is the best known circuitry of the efferent system. It has two main tracts: the lateral and the medial (Sahley et al, 1997). The lateral tract originates from preolivary cells near the lateral superior olive and is composed mostly of uncrossed, unmyelinated fibers that terminate on the ipsilateral dendrites beneath the inner hair cells. These preolivary cells also send projections ipsilaterally to the cochlear nuclei by way of the ventral and dorsal acoustic stria. The medial tract of the OCB is composed of myelinated fibers that originate in preolivary nuclei in the area around the medial superior olive. Most fibers cross to the opposite cochlea, where they connect directly to the outer hair cells. Bilateral (mostly contralateral) connections to the cochlear nucleus also exist by way of both the dorsal and ventral acoustical stria. The lateral and medial OCB fibers after connecting to various divisions of the cochlear nucleus course along the vestibular nerves in the internal auditory meatus before terminating at the type I auditory nerve fibers below the inner hair cells and the base of the outer hair cells (for a review, see Sahley et al, 1997; see also Pickles, 1988).

Early physiological studies show that stimulation of the crossed (medial) OCB fibers results in reduced neural response from the cochlea and auditory nerve (Galambos,

1956). Since then, the suppressive effect of the medial system has been shown in humans. In 1962, Fex showed that acoustic stimulation of the contralateral ear will trigger the medial OCB function. By stimulating the contralateral ear in humans, the action potential is reduced in amplitude, as is the amplitude of the transient and distortion product otoacoustic emissions (Collet, 1993). It has also been shown that cutting the vestibular nerves in the internal auditory meatus (which is where the OCB fibers course) results in absent suppression of otoacoustic emissions (Williams et al, 1993). Hence, a procedure by which some facet of OCB function can be tested in humans exists by using otoacoustic emissions. This procedure is progressing toward clinical use.

Another important aspect related to function of the OCB is hearing in noise. Pickles and Comis (1973) showed that the application of atropine (a cholinergic blocker) in the region of the OCB resulted in poorer hearing in noise in animals. Other studies also show that the OCB has an important role for hearing in noise (Nieder and Nieder, 1970). The mechanism underlying this facilitation for hearing in noise may be related to the ability of the medial OCB to trigger outer hair cell expansion/contraction, thereby enhancing or damping basilar membrane activity. This, in turn, may limit auditory nerve activity to low levels for unimportant (e.g., noise) stimuli, resulting in a larger dynamic range for the auditory nerve neuron to respond to other acoustic stimuli (for a review, see Sahley et al, 1997). It is also important to consider that the OCB may sometimes enhance responses, even though data indicate many of its activities are related to suppression (see section Auditory Neurochemistry). Evidence shows that when an animal is surrounded by noise and the OCB is triggered (by electrical stimulation or by contralateral noise presented to the ear), a release of the auditory nerve from noise is accomplished, allowing better overall hearing in noise.

◆ Auditory Neurochemistry

Neurochemistry is reviewed as part of the discussion of auditory neuroanatomy and physiology because many known neurotransmitters are associated with the central auditory system. Neurotransmitters are neurochemical agents that convey information across the synapse between nerve cells. The type of synapse and particular neurotransmitters involved may influence many characteristics of auditory function and processing. Research findings on auditory neurotransmitters frequently have profound clinical implications.

The Anatomy of Neurotransmission

The synapse is the connecting link between nerve cells and the main structure in neurotransmission. It involves the synaptic button of the axon that communicates neurochemically with the dendrites, or in some cases the cell body, of another nerve cell. The neurotransmitters are released by vesicles and permeate the synaptic region to bind to proteins, called receptors, embedded in the adjacent cell membrane. Various events can take place as a result of this transmitter binding. One such event is a change in ions across the cell membrane, which may induce an alteration in a postsynaptic cell receptor potential. Several neurotransmitter interactions occurring in a restricted time period will cause the postsynaptic cell to depolarize and fire its own impulse or action potential. An excitatory neurotransmitter is associated with this response (Musiek and Hoffman, 1990).

Hyperpolarization of the postsynaptic cell membrane is caused by inhibitory neurotransmitters making the cells less likely to fire an impulse or more difficult to excite (Musiek and Hoffman, 1990). The synapse can also be influenced by other biochemical actions of the cell that are beyond the scope of this review.

Pearl

- Numerous therapeutic drugs are used to influence synaptic activity. Agonists can bind to and activate postsynaptic receptors, mimicking natural neurotransmitters. Antagonists can produce the opposite effect by binding to but not activating the receptor, thus blocking the natural neurotransmitter function.

Afferent Auditory Neurotransmission

If synaptic activity can be controlled by neurotransmitters, it may be feasible to control the functions that are based on these synaptic interactions. To accomplish this, neurotransmitters must first be localized and identified, keeping in mind that before a chemical can be considered as a neurotransmitter, it must meet strict criteria (Musiek and Hoffman, 1990). New information on function and dysfunction of a system may be obtained through the use of agonists and antagonists once these neurotransmitters are identified.

It is not known which neurotransmitter operates between the cochlear hair cells and auditory nerve fibers, but one possibility is glutamate (Bledsoe et al, 1988). Glutamate or aspartate is believed to be involved in auditory nerve-to-cochlear nucleus transmission (Bledsoe et al, 1988). Within the cochlear nucleus, it is likely that several excitatory neurotransmitters exist, such as aspartate, glutamate, and acetylcholine (Oliver et al, 1983). Inhibitory amino acids found at high levels within the cochlear nucleus are γ-aminobutyric acid (GABA) and glycine (Godfrey et al, 1977). Gamma-aminobutyric acid and glycine are also found in the SOC (Wenthold et al, 1987). Also located in the SOC are excitatory amino acids, including quisqualate, glutamate, and N-methyl-D-aspartate (NMDA) (Ottersen and Storm-Mathisen, 1984). Glycine and glutamate are likely neurotransmitters in the inferior colliculus (Adams and Wenthold, 1987). Increased activity at the level of the inferior colliculus has been shown from both NMDA and aspartate (Faingold et al, 1989).

Little information exists on auditory cortex transmitters. Evidence shows that acetylcholine and opiate drugs affect auditory cortex activity or evoked potentials, but further research is needed before the neurochemistry of this brain region is understood fully (Velasco et al, 1984).

Efferent Auditory Neurotransmission

More data are available about efferent neurotransmitters than with afferent neurotransmitters. Neurotransmission within the OCB, for example, has been studied extensively. The OCB can be viewed as two systems. One system is lateral and originates from the outlying lateral superior olive region. The second system is medial and ascends from the medial olive region. Both systems are cholinergic, and the lateral system also contains the opioid peptides enkephalin and dynorphin (Hoffman, 1986). These efferent neurotransmitters can be found in the perilymph of the cochlea. The results of electrical stimulation on the OCB can be mimicked by applying acetylcholine to this region (Bobbin and Konishi, 1971).

Auditory Function and Neurotransmitters

Several studies have examined neurotransmitter effects on auditory function that are measured electrophysiologically or behaviorally. Cousillas et al (1988) found that auditory nerve activity during sound stimulation was diminished when glutamatergic blockers were perfused through guinea pig cochleas. The application of aspartate, an excitatory amino acid, was also found to increase the spontaneous and acoustically stimulated firing rates of cochlear nuclear fibers. This effect was reversed when an antagonist drug was administered. Homogeneous neural modulating outcomes were shown in a similar study using antagonists and agonists such as glutamate, aspartate, and NMDA at the inferior colliculus level (Faingold et al, 1989).

The late auditory evoked potential (P_2) also showed an increased amplitude after administration of naloxone, an opioid antagonist, in humans. Fentanyl, an opioid agonist, was also found to reduce the P_2 amplitude in the same study (Velasco et al, 1984).

Auditory function of the OCB and neurotransmission also have been studied. The OCB plays a role in enhancing hearing in noise (Winslow and Sachs, 1987). The chemical interaction of the OCB and the hair cells of the cochlea may mediate this role. The fact that outer hair cells can expand and contract might show a link to the OCB because neurotransmitters may control this hair cell function. Regulation of this motor activity may in turn allow the OCB modulation of incoming impulses via the outer hair cells.

In studies on chinchillas, the auditory nerve action potential was enhanced significantly by injecting the opioid agonist pentazocine (Sahley et al, 1997). Because opioids are found in the lateral OCB system, this effect, only noted at intensity levels near threshold, assuredly involves the OCB system.

The pharmacological means to enhance hearing may be furnished ultimately through the study of auditory function and neurotransmission. Neurochemistry's intrinsic role in auditory physiology is underscored by research in this important area.

◆ Maturation of the Central Auditory System

Various segments of the brain and auditory system develop and mature at different rates. In a general sense, the auditory system matures in a caudal-to-rostral manner. Maturation of the auditory system evolves around several mechanisms, including cell differentiation and migration, myelination, arborization, and synaptogenesis. We discuss the last three mechanisms.

Myelination

Myelin is white matter of the nervous system. It covers and insulates the axons of a nerve fiber. Generally, the amount of myelin on a nerve fiber indicates how fast the impulses are conducted. A heavily myelinated nerve fiber will conduct impulses quickly (some large fibers up to 100 m/s), whereas nerve conduction is slow in unmyelinated fibers (< 2 m/s) (Mountcastle, 1968). Slow conduction limits the types of processing that take place. Examples come from the studies on the quaking mouse, a species that does not produce myelin because of a genetic disorder. Auditory brainstem response testing on these mice indicates that their interwave latencies are almost twice as long as in control mice (Shah and Salamy, 1980). In another study on myelination, the amount of myelin was measured in rats for 50 days postnatally. The study measured the amount of cerebroside (a lipid in the blood), which increases with the amount of myelin. As the rat pups grew older, the amount of myelin increased and the interwave latency of the ABRs decreased (Shah and Salamy, 1980).

Myelination of the brain occurs at different rates in different regions. It appears that the brainstem auditory tracts complete myelination before the subcortical regions of the brain. In humans, most of the ABR indices reach adult values at around 2 years of age. However, the middle latency and late auditory evoked potentials do not reach adult characteristics until a child is 10 to 12 years of age (McGee and Kraus, 1996). The P_1 component of the late potentials is thought by some investigators to be mature by 5 years of age (McPherson, 1996), but others believe full maturation of this potential occurs much later (Ponton et al, 1996). The P_2 response of the late potentials appears to mature around 5 years of age (McPherson, 1996). The P_{300} auditory potential does not mature until the early teenage years (Musiek and Gollegly, 1988). Although present at birth, the mismatched negativity does not reach adultlike characteristics until the early school-age years (Kraus and McGee, 1994). What characterizes the evoked potentials at all levels of the auditory system during maturation is great individual variability. We have noted absent middle and late potentials in some early school-aged children with no apparent problems of any sort, whereas in other school-aged children, these same potentials are well formed and easy to read. The development course of these evoked potentials is semiconsistent with the caudal-to-rostral myelination pattern in the brain.

Behavioral auditory tests also have an extended maturational course. Behavioral responses to sound involve more than the auditory system; therefore, maturation rates of the other systems involved may influence these measures. Auditory detection thresholds are 30 to 40 dB higher in 2- to 4-week-old infants than in adults. This difference decreases to 10 to 15 dB when the infant is 6 months old (Werner, 1996). These differences may be related to middle ear and auditory pathway influences. More central-type behavioral measures, such as masking level differences, are larger in preschoolers than in infants (Nozza et al, 1988). Jensen and Neff (1989) have shown that auditory frequency and duration discrimination is better in 6-year-old children than in 4-year-old children, but not as good as in adults. Dichotic listening and frequency pattern performance do not reach adult values until ~10 to 11 years of age. Although these behavioral measures do not depend only on the central auditory nervous system, the central system does play a significant role in these functions.

What is the myelin (maturational) time course to which we refer, and what is its foundation? Yakovlev and LeCours (1967) reported on years of study of human brains in regard to myelination at various ages and anatomical regions. Using a Loyez (silver) staining technique, they quantified the amount of myelin in a given region of the brain. Their large collection of brains covered a wide range of ages. Yakovlev and LeCours (1967) showed that the optic tracts myelinated before the auditory tracts. The prethalamic auditory tracts are essentially myelin complete at 5 to 6 months after birth. However, post-thalamic auditory tracts are not myelin mature until 5 to 6 years of age. The corpus callosum and certain auditory association areas may not have completed myelinogenesis until 10 to 12 years or older. The somatosensory-evoked potentials used to measure interhemispheric transfer time by comparing ipsilateral to contralateral stimulation latencies indicated that corpus callosum maturity ranges from ~10 to 20 years of age (Salamy et al, 1980). This was interpreted also as an index of myelination of the corpus callosum.

Another important factor of myelin maturation is the great variability in its rate (Yakovlev and LeCours, 1967). If the myelination rate varies, the processes it underlies may also vary. Therefore, if a certain amount of maturation is needed to complete a task but has not been achieved, the task cannot be completed. It is likely that the difference in children's performance on some auditory tests may be related to differences in the amount of myelination in critical regions of the brain.

Arborization and Synaptogenesis

The term *arborization* is used to mean axonal or dendritic branching. This is a maturational process of the nerve cell critical to the functioning of groups of neurons. Generally, as the cell matures, arborization is greater. However, increased arborization may also be a result of certain types of continued stimulation after the nerve cell is mature.

A nerve cell is composed of three main parts: soma (cell body), axon, and dendrites. The cell body and axons change with maturity. Axonic and dendritic branching is one of the most dynamic maturational actions of the cell. In the very early maturational course, growing axons make their way to specific areas of the immature brain. After reaching its destination, the axon develops branching (i.e., arborization), and each branch has a bulbous terminal. These bulbs in turn make synapses with dendrites (Kalil, 1989). In the first year of life, one cortical neuron may connect with as many as 10,000 other neurons through axonal/dendritic branching (Crelin, 1973). Arborization continues to increase for several years (Crelin, 1973). It is difficult to determine when arborization reaches its maturational peak because it is influenced by environmental experience (Kalil, 1989). Arborization provides an anatomical basis for more complex interactions among neurons in the brain. Appropriate connections are needed for appropriate function; thus, dendritic branching without connection to other cell bodies or axons is of little value. The course of dendritic maturation appears to show the greatest change in the first few years of life but then extends well into adulthood and even into old age.

Recent information about synaptic development suggests an important role of action potentials. When young axons are prevented from generating action potentials, the synaptic structures (i.e., terminal bulbs) do not develop (Kalil, 1989). Therefore, these electrical impulses (most of which come from external stimulation) of the axon are crucial to synaptogenesis.

The synapse is the communication between neurons that involves the transfer of a neurotransmitter. Earlier we discussed this aspect of neurochemistry. Because dendrites are necessary for synapses, their maturity influences the overall amount of synaptic development. Studies on kittens show an increase in synapses at the inferior colliculus until 14 days of age. Also, the number of synaptic terminals is considerably greater in an 8-day-old kitten than in a 3-day-old kitten (Reynolds, 1975).

Maturation is not the only influence on the synapse that can result in its change. Stimulation can alter the number of synapses and synaptic density after the system is mature. Conversely, a lack of stimulation (deprivation) may reduce the number of synaptic components.

♦ Summary

Knowledge of the structure and function of the central auditory nervous system is vital to the audiologist. Audiological procedures and related communication increasingly involve the central auditory nervous system, and without an understanding of the way this system works, potential clinical insights will not be realized. The central auditory nervous system is a complex system in which parallel and sequential processing takes place. Ipsilateral, contralateral, and commissural connections exist to various auditory nuclei in the brainstem. Auditory nerve cells in the brainstem are composed of a variety of different cell types. These cell types respond in certain ways (often according to their structure) to alter or preserve the impulse pattern coming into the cell. This same type of processing takes place in the cells of the auditory cortex, but fewer cell types are present in the cortex than in the brainstem. This type of processing may provide a basis for increased information pertaining to complex acoustical stimuli. The brainstem and the cortex are both highly tonotopic and present with a variety of tuning curves. In regard to intensity coding, most cells in the brainstem and cortex have a range of 30 to 40 dB; however, some have severely reduced dynamic ranges. Of interest is that in a listening situation with background noise, some cortical neurons will not respond until the target sound is above the noise floor, with apparently no restriction in their dynamic range. This relatively new information may provide an understanding of how we hear in noise that has not been considered previously.

In the cerebrum, the auditory regions have intrahemispheric and interhemispheric connections to other auditory areas and to sensory, cognitive, and motor regions. At the cortical level, seldom does a system function totally independently. This makes for an efficient processing of environmental input but also makes it difficult to design tests to isolate only auditory function. Much scientific study has been devoted to the afferent auditory system, and information on the efferent system is increasingly available. We have known for years that the efferent system—especially the OCB—can affect acoustical input. The OCB appears to play a role in allowing better hearing in noise. In a broader sense, the OCB (and likely the entire efferent system) may have a modulatory effect on peripheral function. Some influences of the OCB can be measured in humans by using otoacoustic emissions or evoked potentials.

Contributions to the anatomy and physiology of the central auditory nervous system have been, and will continue to be, made by careful study of patients with lesions of the auditory system. This kind of study often involves the clinician and clinical tests. The study of patients with structural abnormalities of the auditory system can now be enhanced by the use of PET or fMRI studies. These imaging techniques can provide insight about the locus and degree of function in normal and abnormal states. The use of new functional imaging techniques will help solve two major problems in the study of the central auditory nervous system. One is that now humans can be studied directly; the other is that more complex and relevant stimuli, such as speech, can be used to study associated physiology.

A new area of study of the central auditory nervous system is its neurochemistry or neuropharmacology. Surprisingly, the neurotransmitters of the OCB are better known than those of the afferent system. Neurotransmission takes place at the synapse of the nerve cell, and synaptic activity is governed largely by the type and amount of the neurotransmitter. Agonists are chemicals that can enhance the neural response and the synapse, whereas antagonists will shut down the response. Complex synaptic interactions among agonists and antagonists are the basis for complex auditory processing.

New information on the central auditory nervous system is increasing on all fronts. More data on audition are available from audiologists, pharmacologists, physiologists, anatomists, and psychologists. The basic scientists have provided much knowledge that will enhance the diagnosis and treatment of central auditory disorders. However, this basic knowledge can be used to its greatest potential only if the clinician is well versed in the structure and function of the central auditory nervous system.

References

Abeles, M., & Goldstein, M. (1972). Responses of a single unit in the primary auditory cortex of the cat to tones and to tone pairs. Brain Research, 42, 337–352.

Adams, J., & Wenthold, R. (1987). Immunostaining of GABA-ergic and glycinergic inputs to the anteroventral cochlear nucleus. Neuroscience Abstracts, 13, 1259.

Aitkin, L. M., & Webster, W. R. (1972). Medial geniculate body of the cat: Organization and response to tonal stimuli of neurons in the ventral division. Journal of Neurophysiology, 35, 365–380.

Aitkin, L. M., Webster, W. R., Veale, J. L., & Crosby, D. C. (1975). Inferior colliculus: I. Comparison of response properties of neurons in central, pericentral, and external nuclei of adult cat. Journal of Neurophysiology, 38, 1196–1207.

Baran, J. A., Musiek, F. E., & Reeves, A. G. (1986). Central auditory function following anterior sectioning of the corpus callosum. Ear and Hearing, 7(6), 359–362.

Barnes, W., Magoon, H., & Ranson, S. (1943). The ascending auditory pathway in the brain stem of the monkey. Journal of Comparative Neurology, 79, 129–152.

Benevento, L. A., & Coleman, P. D. (1970). Responses of single cells in cat inferior colliculus to binaural click stimuli: Combinations of intensity levels, time differences, and intensity differences. Brain Research, 17, 387–405.

Benson, D. A., & Teas, D. C. (1976). Single unit study of binaural interaction in the auditory cortex of the chinchilla. Brain Research, 103, 313–338.

Bledsoe, S., Bobbin, R., & Puel, J. (1988). Neurotransmission in the inner ear. In A. Jahn & J. Santo-Sacchi (Eds.), Physiology of the ear (pp. 385–406). New York: Raven Press.

Bobbin, R. P., & Konishi, T. (1971). Acetylcholine mimics crossed olivocochlear bundle stimulation. Nature: New Biology, 231, 222–224.

Borg, E. (1973). On the organization of the acoustic middle ear reflex: A physiologic and anatomic study. Brain Research, 49, 101–123.

Boudreau, J. C., & Tsuchitani, C. (1970). Cat superior olive S-segment cell discharge to tonal stimulation. In W. D. Neff (Ed.), Contributions to sensory physiology (Vol. 4, pp. 143–213). New York: Academic Press.

Brugge, J. F., & Geisler, C. D. (1978). Auditory mechanisms of the lower brain stem. Annual Review of Neuroscience, 1, 363–394.

Buser, P., & Imbert, M. (1992). Audition. Cambridge, MA: MIT Press.

Caird, D. (1991). Processing in the colliculi. In R. Altschuler, B. Bobbin, D. Clopton, & D. Hoffman (Eds.), Neurobiology of hearing: The central auditory system (pp. 253–291). New York: Raven Press.

Campain, R., & Minckler, J. (1976). A note in gross configurations of the human auditory cortex. Brain and Language, 3, 318–323.

Carpenter, M., & Sutin, J. (1983). Human neuroanatomy. Baltimore: Williams & Wilkins.

Celesia, G. G. (1976). Organization of auditory cortical areas in man. Brain, 99, 403–414.

Chermak, G. D., & Musiek, F. E. (1997). Central auditory processing disorders. San Diego, CA: Singular Publishing Group.

Chermak, G., Traynham, W., Siekei, A., & Musiek, F. (1998). Professional education and assessment in central auditory processing. Journal of the American Academy of Audiology, 9, 452–465.

Colavita, F. B. (1972). Auditory cortical lesions and visual patterns discrimination in cats. Brain Research, 39, 437–447.

Collet, L. (1993). Use of otoacoustic emissions to explore the medial olivocochlear system in humans. British Journal of Audiology, 27, 155–159.

Cousillas, H., Cole, K. S., & Johnstone, B. M. (1988). Effect of spider venom on cochlear nerve activity consistent with glutamatergic transmission at hair cell-afferent dendrite synapse. Hearing Research, 36, 213–220.

Cranford, J. L. (1979). Detection vs. discrimination of brief tones by cats with auditory cortex lesions. Journal of the Acoustical Society of America, 65, 1573–1575.

Cranford, J. L., Igarashi, M., & Stramler, J. H. (1976). Effect of auditory neocortical ablation on pitch perception in the cat. Journal of Neurophysiology, 39, 143–152.

Cranford, J. L., Stream, R. W., Rye, C. V., & Slade, T. L. (1982). Detection vs. discrimination of brief duration tones: Findings in patients with temporal lobe damage. Archives of Otolaryngology, 108, 350–356.

Crelin, E. (1973). Functional anatomy in the newborn. New Haven, CT: Yale University Press, pp. 22–24.

Damasio, H., & Damasio, A. (1979). Paradoxic ear extension in dichotic listening: Possible anatomic significance. Neurology, 29(4), 644–653.

Desmedt, J. (1975). Physiological studies of the efferent recurrent auditory system. In W. Keidel & W. Neff (Eds.), Handbook of sensory physiology (Vol. 2, pp. 219–246). Berlin: Springer-Verlag.

Dhankhar, A., Wexler, B. E., Fulbright, R. K., Halwes, T., Blamire, A. M., & Shulman, R. G. (1997). Functional magnetic resonance imaging assessment of the human brain auditory cortex response to increasing word presentation rates. Journal of Neurophysiology, 77(1), 476–483.

Diamond, I. T., & Neff, W. D. (1957). Ablation of temporal cortex and discrimination of auditory patterns. Journal of Neurophysiology, 20, 300–315.

Donchin, E., Kutas, M., & McCarthy, G. (1976). Electrocortical indices of hemispheric utilization. In S. Harnad, R. Doty; J. Jaynes, L. Goldstein, & G. Krauthamer (Eds.), Lateralization in the nervous system (pp. 339–384). New York: Academic Press.

Dublin, W. (1976). Fundamentals of sensorineural auditory pathology. Springfield, IL: Charles C. Thomas.

Dublin, W. B. (1985). The cochlear nuclei-pathology. Otolaryngology—Head and Neck Surgery, 93, 448–463.

Durrant, J. D., Martin, W. H., Hirsch, B., & Schwegler, J. (1994). ABR analysis in a human subject with unilateral extirpation of the inferior colliculus. Hearing Research, 72, 99–107.

Eggermont, J. J. (1991). Rate and synchronization measures of periodicity coding in cat primary cortex area. Hearing Research, 56, 153–167.

Ehret, G., & Merzenich, M. M. (1988). Complex sound analysis (frequency resolution, filtering and spectral integration) by single units of the inferior colliculus of the cat. Brain Research, 472, 139–163.

Ehret, G., & Romand, R. (1997). The central auditory system. New York: Oxford University Press.

Elliott, L. L. (1994). Functional brain imaging and hearing. Journal of the Acoustical Society of America, 96(3), 1397–1408.

Evans, E. (1968). Cortical representation. In J. Knight & A. de Reuck (Eds.), Hearing mechanisms in vertebrates (pp. 277–287). London: Churchill Livingstone.

Evans, E. (1974). Neural processes for the detection of acoustic patterns and for sound localization. In F. Schmitt & F. Worden (Eds.), Neurosciences: Third study program (pp. 134–145). Cambridge, MA: MIT Press.

Faingold, C. L., Hoffmann, W. E., & Caspary, D. M. (1989). Effects of excitant amino acids on acoustic responses of inferior colliculus neurons. Hearing Research, 40, 127–136.

Ferraro, J. A., & Minckler, J. (1977). The human lateral lemniscus and its nuclei: The human auditory pathways. Brain and Language, 4, 277–294.

French, J. (1957). The reticular formation. Scientific American, 66, 1–8.

Galambos, R. (1956). Suppression of auditory nerve activity by stimulation of efferent fibers to cochlea. Journal of Neurophysiology, 19, 424–437.

Gazzaniga, M. S., Bogen, J. E., & Sperry, R. W. (1962). Some functional effects of sectioning the cerebral commissure in man. Proceedings of the National Academy of Sciences of the United States of America, 48, 1765–1769.

Geniec, P., & Morest, K. (1971). The neuronal architecture of the human posterior colliculus. Acta Oto-laryngologica Supplementum, 295, 1–33.

Gershuni, G. V., Baru, A. V., & Karaseva, T. A. (1967). Role of auditory cortex and discrimination of acoustic stimuli. Zh. Vyssh. Nerv. Deiat. Im. I. P. Pavlova [Journal of Higher Nervous Activity named after I. P. Pavlov], 17, 932–946.

Geschwind, N., & Levitsky, W. (1968). Human brain: Left-right asymmetries in temporal speech region. Science, 161, 186–187.

Godfrey, D. A., Carter, J. A., Berger, S. J., Lowry, O. H., & Matschinsky, F. M. (1977). Quantitative histochemical mapping of candidate transmitter amino acids in the cat cochlear nucleus. Journal of Histochemistry and Cytochemistry, 25, 417–431.

Goldberg, J. M., & Moore, R. Y. (1967). Ascending projections of the lateral lemniscus in the cat and the monkey. Journal of Comparative Neurology, 129, 143–155.

Goldstein, M., DeRibaupierre, R., & Yeni-Komshian, G. (1971). Cortical coding of periodicity pitch. In M. Sachs (Ed.), Physiology of the auditory system. Baltimore, MD: National Education Consultants.

Gordon, B. (1972). The inferior colliculus of the brain. Scientific American, 227, 72–82.

Hackett, T. A., Preuss, T. M., & Kaas, J. H. (2001). Architectonic identification of the core region in auditory cortex of macaques, chimpanzees, and humans. Journal of Comparative Neurology, 441, 197–222.

Hall, J. W., III (1985). The acoustic reflex in central auditory dysfunction. In M. L. Pinheiro & F. E. Musiek (Eds.), Assessment of central auditory dysfunction: Foundations and clinical correlates (pp. 103–130). Baltimore, MD: Williams & Wilkins.

Heffner, H. E., & Heffner, R. S. (1986). Hearing loss in Japanese macaques following bilateral auditory cortex lesions. Journal of Neurophysiology, 55, 256–271.

Heffner, H., Heffner, R., & Porter, W. (November 1985). Effects of auditory cortex lesion on absolute thresholds in macaques. Paper presented at the annual meeting of the Society for Neuroscience, Dallas, TX.

Helfert, R., Sneed, C., & Altschuler, R. (1991). The ascending auditory pathways. In R. Altschuler, R. Bobbin, B. Clopton, & D. Hoffman (Eds.), Neurobiology of hearing: The central auditory system (pp. 1–26). New York: Raven Press.

Hodgson, W. R. (1967). Audiological report of a patient with left hemispherectomy. Journal of Speech and Hearing Disorders, 32, 39–45.

Hoffman, D. W. (1986). Opioid mechanisms in the inner ear. In R. A. Altschuler, D. W. Hoffman, & R. P. Bobbin (Eds.), Neurobiology of hearing: The cochlea (pp. 371–382). New York: Raven Press.

Hynd, G. W., Semrud-Clikeman, M., Lorys, A. R., Novey, E. S., Eliopulos, D., & Lyytinen, H. (1991). Corpus callosum morphology in attention deficithyperactivity disorder: Morphometric analysis of MRI. Journal of Learning Disabilities, 24, 141–146.

Jeffress, L. A., & McFadden, D. (1971). Differences of interaural phase and level of detection and lateralization. Journal of the Acoustical Society of America, 49, 1169–1179.

Jensen, J., & Neff, D. (April 1989). Discrimination of intensity, frequency and duration differences in preschool children: Age effects and longitudinal data. Paper presented at the biennial meeting of the SRCH, Kansas City, MO.

Jerger, J., & Jerger, S. (1971). Diagnostic significance of PB word functions. Archives of Otolaryngology, 93, 573–580.

Jerger, J., & Jerger, S. (1974). Auditory findings in brain stem disorders. Archives of Otolaryngology, 99, 342–350.

Jerger, J., Weikers, N. J., Sharbrough, F. W., III, & Jerger, S. (1969). Bilateral lesions of the temporal lobe: A case study. Acta Otolaryngologica, 258, 1–51.

Jones, E. G., & Powell, T. P. (1970). An anatomical study of converging sensory pathways within the cerebral cortex of the monkey. Brain, 93, 793–820.

Jungert, S. (1958). Auditory pathways in the brain stem: A neurophysiologic study. Acta Otolaryngologica Supplementum, 140, 183–185.

Kalil, R. E. (1989). Synapse formation in the developing brain. Scientific American, 261, 76–87.

Kaufmann, W. E., & Galaburda, A. M. (1989). Cerebrocortical microdysgenesias in neurologically normal subjects: A histopathological study. Neurology, 39, 238–243.

Kavanagh, G. L., & Kelly, J. B. (1988). Hearing in the ferret (*Mustela putorius*): Effects of primary auditory cortical lesions on thresholds for pure tone detection. Journal of Neurophysiology, 60, 879–888.

Keidel, W., Kallert, S., Korth, M., & Humes, L. (1983). The physiological basis of hearing. New York: Thieme-Stratton.

Kiang, N. Y. S. (1975). Stimulus representation in the discharge patterns of auditory neurons. In D. B. Tower (Ed.), The nervous system: Human communication and its disorders (Vol, 3. pp. 81–96). New York: Raven Press.

Knudsen, E. (1988). Experience shapes sound localization and auditory unit properties during development in the barn owl. In G. Edelman, W. Gall, & W. Kowan (Eds.), Auditory function: Neurobiological basis of hearing (pp. 137–152). New York: John Wiley & Sons.

Kraus, N., & McGee, T. (1994). Auditory event-related potentials. In J. Katz (Ed.), Handbook of clinical audiology (4th ed., pp. 406–423). Baltimore, MD: Williams & Wilkins.

Kryter, K., & Ades, H. (1943). Studies on the function of the higher acoustic centers in the cat. American Journal of Psychology, 56, 501–536.

Kudo, M. (1981). Projections of the nuclei of the lateral lemniscus in the cat: An autoradiographic study. Brain Research, 221, 57–69.

Lackner, J. R., & Teuber, H. L. (1973). Alterations in auditory fusion thresholds after cerebral injury in man. Neuropsychologia, 11, 409–415.

Lauter, J. L., Herscovitch, P., Formby, C., & Raichle, M. E. (1985). Tonotopic organization of human auditory cortex revealed by positron emission tomography. Hearing Research, 20, 199–205.

LeDoux, J. (1986). The neurobiology of emotion. In J. LeDoux & W. Hirst (Eds.), Mind and brain (pp. 342–346). Cambridge: Cambridge University Press.

LeDoux, J. E., Sakaguchi, A., & Reis, D. J. (1984). Subcortical efferent projections of the medial geniculate nucleus mediate emotional responses conditioned to acoustic stimuli. Journal of Neuroscience, 4, 683–698.

Levine, R. A., Gardner, J. C., Stufflebeam, S. M., Furst, M., & Rosen, B. (1993). Binaural auditory processing in multiple sclerosis subjects. Hearing Research, 68, 59–72.

Lynn, G. E., Gilroy, J., Taylor, P. C., & Leiser, R. P. (1981). Binaural masking level differences in neurological disorders. Archives of Otolaryngology, 107, 357–362.

Masterton, R. B., Thompson, G. C., Bechtold, J. K., & Robards, M. J. (1975). Neuroanatomical basis of binaural phase difference analysis for sound localization: A comparative study. Journal of Comparative and Physiological Psychology, 89, 379–386.

Masterton, R. B., & Granger, E. M. (1988). Role of acoustic striae in hearing contribution of dorsal and intermediate striae to detection of noises and tones. Journal of Neurophysiology, 60, 1841–1860.

Matzker, J. (1959). Two new methods for the assessment of central auditory functions in cases of brain disease. Annals of Otology, Rhinology, and Laryngology, 68, 1188–1197.

McGee, T., & Kraus, N. (1996). Auditory development reflected by the middle latency response. Ear and Hearing, 17(5), 419–429.

McPherson, D. L. (1996). Late potentials of the auditory system. San Diego, CA: Singular Publishing Group.

Merchan, M. A., & Berbel, P. (1996). Anatomy of the ventral nucleus of the lateral lemniscus in rats: A nucleus with a concentric laminar organization. Journal of Comparative Neurology, 372, 245–263.

Merzenich, M. M., & Brugge, J. F. (1973). Representation of the cochlear partition on the superior temporal plane of the macaque monkey. Brain Research, 50, 275–296.

Merzenich, M. M., & Reid, M. D. (1974). Representation of the cochlea within the inferior colliculus of the cat. Brain Research, 77, 397–415.

Meyer, D. R., & Woolsey, C. N. (1952). Effects of localized cortical destruction on auditory discriminative conditioning in the cat. Journal of Neurophysiology, 15, 149–162.

Millen, S. J., Haughton, V. M., & Yetkin, Z. (1995). Functional magnetic resonance imaging of the central auditory pathway following speech and pure tone stimuli. Laryngoscope, 105, 1305–1310.

Moller, A. R. (1983). Auditory physiology. New York: Academic Press.

Moller, A. R. (1985). Physiology of the ascending auditory pathway with special reference to the auditory brain stem response (ABR). In M. L. Pinheiro & F. E. Musiek (Eds.), Assessment of central auditory dysfunction: Foundations and clinical correlates (pp. 23–41). Baltimore, MD: Williams & Wilkins.

Moller, A. R. (2000). Hearing: Its physiology and pathophysiology. New York: Academic Press.

Moore, C. A., Cranford, J. L., & Rahn, A. E. (1990). Tracking for a "moving" fused auditory image under conditions that elicit the precedence effect. Journal of Speech and Hearing Research, 33, 141–148.

Moore, D. R., & Irvine, D. R. F. (1980). Development of binaural input, response patterns and discharge rate in single units of the cat inferior colliculus. Experimental Brain Research, 38, 103–108.

Moore, J. K. (1987). The human auditory brain stem: A comparative view. Hearing Research, 29, 1–32.

Morest, D. K. (1964). The neuronal architecture of medial geniculate body of the cat. Journal of Anatomy, 98, 611–630.

Mountcastle, V. (1962). Interhemispheric relations and cerebral dominance. Baltimore, MD: Johns Hopkins Press.

Mountcastle, V. (1968). Central neural mechanisms in hearing. In V. Mountcastle (Ed.), Medical physiology (Vol. 2). St. Louis: CV Mosby.

Musiek, F. E. (1986a). Neuroanatomy, neurophysiology and central auditory assessment: II. The cerebrum. Ear and Hearing, 7, 283–294.

Musiek, F. E. (1986b). Neuroanatomy, neurophysiology, and central auditory assessment: III. Corpus callosum and efferent pathways. Ear and Hearing, 7(6), 349–358.

Musiek, F. E., & Baran, J. A. (1986). Neuroanatomy, neurophysiology, and central auditory assessment: I. Brain stem. Ear and Hearing, 7, 207–219.

Musiek, F. E., & Baran, J. A. (2007). The auditory system: Anatomy, physiology, and clinical correlates. Boston: Allyn & Bacon.

Musiek, F. E., Baran, J. A., & Pinheiro, M. (1990). Duration pattern recognition in normal subjects and patients with cerebral and cochlear lesions. Audiology, 29, 304–313.

Musiek, F. E., Baran, J. A., & Pinheiro, M. (1994). Neuroaudiology: Case studies. San Diego, CA: Singular Publishing Group.

Musiek, F. E., & Geurkink, N. (1982). Auditory brain stem response and central auditory test findings for patients with brain stem lesions. Laryngoscope, 92, 891–900.

Musiek, F. E., & Gollegly, K. M. (1985). ABR in eighth nerve and low brain stem lesions. In J. T. Jacobson (Ed.), The auditory brain stem response (pp. 181–202). San Diego, CA: College-Hill Press.

Musiek, F. E., & Gollegly, K. M. (1998). Maturational considerations in the neuroauditory evaluation of children. In F. Bess (Ed.), Hearing impairment in children (pp. 231–250). Parkton, MD: York Press.

Musiek, F. E., & Hoffman, D. (1990). An introduction to the functional neurochemistry of the auditory system. Ear and Hearing, 11, 395–402.

Musiek, F. E., Kibbe, K., & Baran, J. (1984). Neuroaudiological results from split-brain patients. Seminars in Hearing, 5(3), 219–229.

Musiek, F. E., & Reeves, A. G. (1990). Asymmetries of the auditory areas of the cerebrum. Journal of the American Academy of Audiology, 1, 240–245.

Neff, W. (1961). Neuromechanisms of auditory discrimination. In W. Rosenblith (Ed.), Sensory communication (pp. 259–278). New York: John Wiley & Sons.

Nieder, P., & Nieder, I. (1970). Antimasking effect of crossed olivocochlear bundle stimulation with loud clicks in guinea pigs. Experimental Neurology, 28, 179–188.

Noback, C. R. (1985). Neuroanatomical correlates of central auditory function. In M. L. Pinheiro & F. E. Musiek (Eds.), Assessment of central auditory dysfunction: Foundations and clinical correlates (pp. 7–21). Baltimore, MD: Williams & Wilkins.

Nozza, R. J., Wagner, E. F., & Crandall, M. A. (1988). Binaural release for masking for speech sounds in infants, preschoolers and adults. Journal of Speech and Hearing Research, 31, 212–218.

Oliver, D. L., & Morest, D. K. (1984). The central nucleus of the inferior colliculus in the cat. Journal of Comparative Neurology, 222, 237–264.

Oliver, D. L., Potashner, S., Jones, D., & Morest, D. (1983). Selective labeling of spiroganglion and granule cells with D-aspartate in the auditory system of the cat and guinea pig. Journal of Neuroscience, 3, 455–472.

Oliver, D. L., & Shneiderman, A. (1991). The anatomy of the inferior colliculus: A cellular basis for integration of monaural and binaural information. In R. A. Altschuler, R. P. Bobbin, B. M. Clopton, & D. W. Hoffman (Eds.), Neurobiology of hearing: The central auditory system (pp. 195–222). New York: Raven Press.

Ottersen, O. P., & Storm-Mathisen, J. (1984). Glutamate- and GABA-containing neurons in the mouse and rat brain, as demonstrated with a new immunocytochemical technique. Journal of Comparative Neurology, 229, 374–392.

Pandya, D., & Seltzer, B. (1986). The topography of commissural fibers. In F. Lepore, M. Pitito, & H. Jasper (Eds.), Two hemispheres—One brain: Functions of the corpus callosum (pp. 47–74). New York: Alan R. Liss.

Parent, A. Carpenter's human neuroanatomy (9th ed.). Baltimore, MD: Williams & Wilkins.

Penfield, W., & Perot, P. (1963). The brain's record of auditory and visual experience: A final summary and discussion. Brain, 86, 596–695.

Penfield, W., & Roberts, L. (1959). Speech and brain mechanisms. Princeton, NJ: Princeton University Press.

Pfeiffer, R. R. (1966). Classification of response patterns of spike discharges for units in the cochlear nucleus: Tone burst stimulation. Experimental Brain Research, 1, 220–235.

Pfingst, B. E., & O'Connor, T. A. (1981). Characteristics of neurons in auditory cortex of monkeys performing a simple auditory task. Journal of Neurophysiology, 45, 16–34.

Phillips, D. (1990). Neural representation of sound amplitude in the auditory cortex: Effects of noise masking. Behavioural Brain Research, 37, 197–214.

Phillips, D. P. (1995). Central auditory processing: A view from auditory neuroscience. American Journal of Otology, 16, 338–350.

Phillips, D. P., & Irvine, D. R. (1981). Responses of single neurons in physiologically defined area AI of cat cerebral cortex: sensitivity to interaural intensity differences. Hearing Research, 4(9), 299–307.

Phillips, D. P., Reale, R. A., & Brugge, J. F. (1991). Stimulus processing in the auditory cortex. In R. Altschuler, R. Bobbin, B. Clopton, & D. Hoffman (Eds.), Neurobiology of hearing: The central auditory system (pp. 335–366). New York: Raven Press.

Pickles, J. O. (1982). An introduction to the physiology of hearing. New York: Academic Press.

Pickles, J. O. (1985). Physiology of the cerebral auditory system. In M. Pinheiro & F. Musiek (Eds.), Assessment of central auditory dysfunction: Foundations and clinical correlates. Baltimore, MD: Williams & Wilkins.

Pickles, J. O. (1988). An introduction to the physiology of hearing (2nd ed.). New York: Academic Press.

Pickles, J. O., & Comis, S. D. (1973). Role of centrifugal pathways to cochlear nucleus in detection of signals in noise. Journal of Neurophysiology, 36, 1131–1137.

Pinheiro, M., & Musiek, F. E. (1985). Sequencing and temporal ordering in the auditory system. In M. Pinheiro & F. Musiek (Eds.), Assessment of central auditory dysfunction: Foundations and clinical correlates (pp. 219–238). Baltimore, MD: Williams & Wilkins.

Pinheiro, M. L., & Tobin, H. (1969). Interaural intensity differences for intracranial lateralization. Journal of the Acoustical Society of America, 46, 1482–1487.

Ponton, C. W., Don, M., Eggermont, J. J., Waring, M. D., & Masuda, A. (1996). Maturation of human cortical auditory function: Differences between normal-hearing children and children with cochlear implants. Ear and Hearing, 17(5), 430–437.

Portman, M., Sterkers, J., Charachon, R., & Chouard, C. (1975). The internal auditory meatus: Anatomy, pathology, and surgery. New York: Churchill Livingstone.

Ravizza, R. J., & Masterton, B. (1972). Contribution of neocortex to sound localization in opossum (Didelphis virginiana). Journal of Neurophysiology, 35, 344–356.

Recanzone, G. H., Schreiner, C. E., & Merzenich, M. M. (1993). Plasticity in the frequency representation of primary auditory cortex following discrimination training in adult owl monkeys. Journal of Neuroscience, 13, 87–103.

Reynolds, A. (1975). Development of binaural responses of units in the intracolliculus of the neonate cat. Unpublished undergraduate paper, Department of Physiology, Monash University, Clayton Victoria, Australia.

Rhode, W. S. (1985). The use of intracellular techniques in the study of the cochlear nucleus. Journal of the Acoustical Society of America, 78, 320–327.

Rhode, W. (1991). Physiological-morphological properties of the cochlear nucleus. In R. Altschuler, R. Bobbin, B. Clopton, & D. Hoffman (Eds.), Neurobiology of hearing: The central auditory system (pp. 47–78). New York: Raven Press.

Rockel, A. J., & Jones, E. G. (1973). The neuronal organization of the inferior colliculus of the adult cat: I. The central nucleus. Journal of Comparative Neurology, 147, 11–60.

Rouiller, E. M. (1997). Functional organization of the auditory pathways. In G. Ehret & R. Romand (Eds.), The central auditory system (pp. 3–96). New York: Oxford University Press.

Rubens, A. (1986). Anatomical asymmetries of the human cerebral cortex. In S. Harnad, R. Doty; J. Jaynes, L. Goldstein, & G. Kranthamer (Eds.), Lateralization in the nervous system (pp. 503–517). New York: Academic Press.

Russchen, F. T. (1982). Amygdalopetal projections in the cat: II. Subcortical afferent connections: A study with retrograde tracing techniques. Journal of Comparative Neurology, 207, 157–176.

Ryugo, D. K., & Weinberger, N. M. (1976). Corticofugal modulation of the medial geniculate body. Experimental Neurology, 51, 377–391.

Sahley, T. L., Nodar, R. H., & Musiek, F. E. (1997). Efferent auditory system: Structure and function. San Diego, CA: Singular Publishing Group.

Salamy, A. (1978). Commissural transmission: Maturational changes in humans. Science, 200, 1409–1410.

Salamy, A., Mendelson, T., Tooley, W., & Chaplin, E. (1980). Differential development of brain stem potentials in healthy and high risk infants. Science, 210, 553–555.

Sando, I. (1965). The anatomical interrelationships of the cochlear nerve fibers. Acta Otolaryngologica, 59, 417–436.

Schuknecht, H. T. (1974). Pathology of the ear. Cambridge, MA: Harvard University Press.

Schwaber, M. K., Garraghty, P. E., & Kaas, J. H. (1993). Neuroplasticity of the adult primate auditory cortex following cochlear hearing loss. American Journal of Otology, 14(3), 252–258.

Schwartz, I. (1992). Superior olivary complex in the lateral lemniscal nuclei. In D. Webster, A. Popper, & F. Fay (Eds.), The mammalian auditory pathway: Neuroanatomy (pp. 117–167). New York: Springer-Verlag.

Selnes, O. A. (1974). The corpus callosum: Some anatomical and functional considerations with special reference to language. Brain and Language, 1, 111–139.

Seltzer, B., & Pandya, D. (1978). Afferent cortical connections and architectonics of the superior temporal sulcus and surrounding cortex in rhesus monkey. Brain Research, 149, 1–24.

Shah, S. N., & Salamy, A. (1980). Brain stem auditory potential in myelin deficient mice. Neuroscience, 5, 2321–2323.

Sheperd, G. (1994). Neurobiology (pp. 284–555). New York: Oxford University Press.

Starr, A., & Hamilton, A. (1976). Correlation between confirmed sites of neurological lesions and abnormalities of far-field auditory brain stem responses. Electroencephalography and Clinical Neurophysiology, 41, 595–608.

Streitfeld, B. D. (1980). The fiber connections of the temporal lobe with emphasis on the rhesus monkey. International Journal of Neuroscience, 11, 51–71.

Strominger, N. L., & Hurwitz, J. L. (1976). Anatomical aspects of the superior olivary complex. Journal of Comparative Neurology, 170, 485–497.

Strominger, N. L., & Strominger, A. L. (1971). Ascending brain stem projections of the anteroventral cochlear nucleus in the rhesus monkey. Journal of Comparative Neurology, 143, 217–232.

Sudakov, K., MacLean, P., Reeves, A., & Marino, R. (1971). Unit study of exteroceptive inputs to the claustrocortex in the awake sitting squirrel monkey. Brain Research, 28, 19–34.

Talavage, T. M., Ledden, P. J., Sereno, M. I., Benson, R. R., & Rosen, B. R. (1996). Preliminary fMRI evidence for tonotopicity in human auditory cortex. Paper presented at the Second International Conference on Functional Mapping of the Human Brain, Boston.

Tasaki, I. (1954). Nerve impulses in individual auditory nerve fibers of the guinea pig. Journal of Neurophysiology, 17, 97–122.

Thompson, M. E., & Abel, S. M. (1992). Indices of hearing in patients with central auditory pathology. Scandinavian Audiology Supplementum, 35, 3–22.

Tobin, H. (1985). Binaural interaction tasks. In M. Pinheiro & F. Musiek (Eds.), Assessment of central auditory dysfunction: Foundations and clinical correlates (pp. 151–171). Baltimore, MD: Williams & Wilkins.

Tsuchitani, C., & Boudreau, J. C. (1996). Single unit analysis of cat superior olive S-segment with tonal stimuli. Journal of Neurophysiology, 29, 684–697.

Tsuchitani, C., & Johnson, D. H. (1991). Binaural cues and signal processing in the superior olivary complex. In R. A. Altschuler, R. P. Bobbin, B. M. Clopton, & D. W. Hoffman (Eds.), Neurobiology of hearing: The central auditory system (pp. 163–193). New York: Raven Press.

Utler, R. A., Keidel, W. D., & Spreng, M. (1969). An investigation of the human cortical evoked potential under conditions of monaural and binaural stimulation. Acta Otolaryngologica, 68, 317–326.

Van Noort, J. (1969). The structure and connections of the inferior colliculus: An investigation of the lower auditory system. Leiden, Netherlands: Van Corcum.

Velasco, M., Velasco, F., Castaneda, R., & Sanchez, R. (1984). Effect of fentanyl and naloxone on human somatic and auditory-evoked potential components. Neuropharmacology, 23(3), 359–366.

Wada, S. I., & Starr, A. (1983). Generation of auditory brain stem responses: III. Effects of lesions of the superior olive, lateral lemniscus and inferior colliculus on the ABR in guinea pig. Electroencephalography and Clinical Neurophysiology, 56, 352–366.

Waddington, M. (1974). Atlas of cerebral angiography with anatomic correlation. Boston: Little, Brown.

Waddington, M. (1984). Atlas of human intracranial anatomy. Rutland, VT: Academy Books.

Warr, W. B. (1966). Fiber degeneration following lesions in the anterior ventral cochlear nucleus of the cat. Experimental Neurology, 14, 453–474.

Wenthold, R. J., Huie, D., Altschuler, R. A., & Reeks, K. A. (1987). Glycine immunoreactivity localized in the cochlear nucleus and superior olivary complex. Neuroscience, 22, 897–912.

Werner, L. A. (1996). The development of auditory behavior (or what the anatomists and physiologists have to explain). Ear and Hearing, 17(5), 438–446.

Whitfield, I. C. (1967). The auditory pathway. Baltimore, MD: Williams & Wilkins.

Whitfield, I. C., & Evans, E. F. (1965). Responses of auditory cortical neurons to stimuli of changing frequency. Journal of Neurophysiology, 28, 655–672.

Williams, E. A., Brookes, G. B., & Prasher, D. K. (1993). Effects of contralateral acoustic stimulation on otoacoustic emissions following vestibular neurectomy. Scandinavian Audiology, 22, 197–203.

Winer, J. A. (1984). The human medial geniculate body. Hearing Research, 15, 225–247.

Winslow, R. L., & Sachs, M. B. (1987). Effect of electrical stimulation of the crossed olivocochlear bundle on auditory nerve responses to tones in noise. Journal of Neurophysiology, 57, 1002–1021.

Witelson, S. (1986). Wires of the mind: Anatomical variation in the corpus callosum in relation to hemispheric specialization and integration. In F. Lepore, M. Ptito, & H. Jasper (Eds.), Two hemispheres—One brain: Functions of the corpus callosum (pp. 117–138). New York: Alan R. Liss.

Woolsey, C. (1960). Organization of cortical auditory system: A review and synthesis. In G. Rasmussen & W. Windell (Eds.), Neuromechanics of the auditory and visibility systems (pp. 3–236). Springfield, IL: Charles C Thomas.

Yakovlev, P., & LeCours, A. (1967). Myelogenetic cycles of regional maturation of the brain. In A. Minkowski (Ed.), Regional development of the brain in early life (pp. 3–70). Philadelphia: F. A. Davis.

Zatorre, R. J., Halpern, A. R., Perry, D. W., Meyer, E., & Evans, A. C. (1996). Hearing in the mind's ear: A PET investigation of musical imagery and perception. Journal of Cognitive Neuroscience, 8(1), 29–46.

Chapter 4

Anatomy and Physiology of the Vestibular System

Charles G. Wright and Nathan D. Schwade

- ◆ **The Vestibular Apparatus**
  - Structural and Functional Organization
  - Vestibular Neuroepithelia
- ◆ **The Vestibulo-ocular Reflex and Its Role in the Evaluation of Vestibular Function**

- ◆ **The Vestibular Nerve and the Central Vestibular System**

The vestibular sensory organs of the inner ear respond to physical stimuli related to movement and orientation of the head in three-dimensional space. In response to mechanical forces acting on the inner ear, neural messages regarding head motion and head position are generated by the vestibular apparatus and relayed to the brain. That information, along with visual and proprioceptive input, is used by the central nervous system (CNS) to help maintain clear vision during head movement, to control muscles responsible for maintaining body posture, and to provide a sense of orientation with respect to the surrounding environment.

Although the vestibular system is one of our major sensory modalities, it differs somewhat from other senses such as vision and hearing in that it operates largely in the service of motor reflexes outside the field of conscious perception. Thus, we are not ordinarily aware of vestibular sensory input, unless the system is subjected to unusually high levels of stimulation or is compromised by injury or disease, in which case the importance of vestibular function becomes acutely obvious. This chapter will present some fundamental aspects of vestibular anatomy and physiology with an emphasis on features of the system that provide the foundation for clinical testing of vestibular function.

◆ The Vestibular Apparatus

Structural and Functional Organization

As illustrated in **Fig. 4–1**, the petrous portion of the temporal bone contains a series of interconnected cavities known as the osseous (or bony) labyrinth. The central cavity of the osseous labyrinth, the vestibule, is situated medial to the oval window. Anterior to the vestibule is the cochlea, and posterior to it are the semicircular canals. The various sacs and ducts that make up the membranous labyrinth are enclosed within the osseous labyrinth. They are surrounded by a clear fluid, called perilymph, which is similar in composition to cerebrospinal fluid. The membranous labyrinth itself is filled with endolymph, which contains high potassium and low sodium concentrations, much like intracellular fluid (Correia and Dickman, 1991). It is within the membranous labyrinth that the sensory receptors of the auditory and vestibular systems are found. **Figure 4–2** depicts the membranous labyrinth isolated from the surrounding bone and provides some perspective regarding its actual size. As this illustration shows, the entire structure, including the cochlear duct and the vestibular apparatus, would easily fit within the circumference of a dime.

The position of the membranous labyrinth within the head is illustrated in **Fig. 4–3**. The vestibular portion of the inner ear includes five separate sensory organs (**Figs. 4–1, 4–3,** and **4–4**). These are the saccule and utricle, located in the vestibule, and the three semicircular ducts, which occupy the semicircular canals of the osseous labyrinth (Schuknecht and Gulya, 1995). The sensory receptors within the vestibular organs are oriented at different angles with respect to the vertical and horizontal planes; they are therefore differentially affected by head movements in different spatial planes. These receptors are all stimulated by forces associated with acceleration (i.e., change in velocity). However, the sensory organs of the vestibule are functionally distinct from those of the semicircular canals. The neuroepithelia of the saccule and utricle are sensitive to linear acceleration and to gravitational force (which in physical terms is indistinguishable from linear acceleration). They

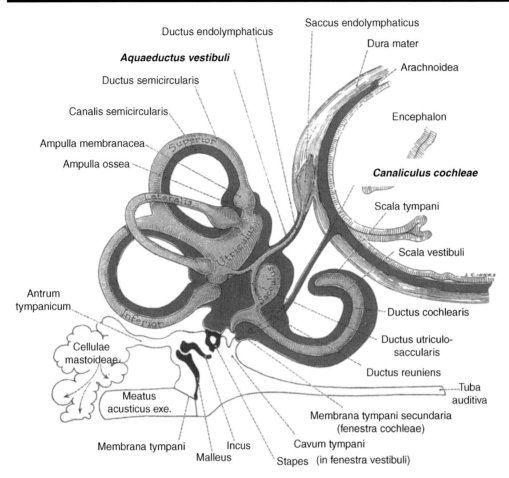

Ductus endolymphaticus
Saccus endolymphaticus
Aquaeductus vestibuli
Dura mater
Ductus semicircularis
Arachnoidea
Canalis semicircularis
Ampulla membranacea
Encephalon
Ampulla ossea
Canaliculus cochleae
Scala tympani
Scala vestibuli
Antrum tympanicum
Ductus cochlearis
Cellulae mastoideae
Ductus utriculo-saccularis
Ductus reuniens
Tuba auditiva
Meatus acusticus exe.
Membrana tympani secundaria (fenestra cochleae)
Membrana tympani
Incus
Cavum tympani
Malleus
Stapes (in fenestra vestibuli)

Figure 4–1 Schematic diagram of major components of the middle and inner ear. The organs of the membranous labyrinth are shown enclosed within the various cavities of the bony labyrinth. (From Anson, B. J., & Donaldson, J. A. (1973). Surgical anatomy of the temporal bone and ear (2nd ed.). Philadelphia: W. B. Saunders, with permission.) *(See Color Plate 4–1.)*

therefore provide information relating to linear motion and to head position within the earth's gravitational field. Because, on the earth's surface, these receptors are always acted upon by gravity, they continuously monitor the position of the head in space even when the head is not in motion. In contrast, the semicircular duct receptors are stimulated by angular acceleration (i.e., motion involving rotation); they are therefore influenced by head movements having a rotational component. Under normal conditions, the semicircular duct receptors do not respond to static head position because they are not stimulated by gravitational force.

The saccule is an ovoid membranous sac situated in a depression of the wall of the vestibule known as the spherical recess. It is located immediately adjacent to the basal portion of the cochlea and is connected with the cochlear duct by a narrow tube, the ductus reuniens (**Fig. 4–4**). The endolymphatic compartment of the cochlear duct is therefore in continuity with that of the saccule. The saccule does not communicate directly with the utricle; it does, however, give rise to the saccular duct, which joins a smaller duct from the utricle to form the endolymphatic duct, which leads to the endolymphatic sac (**Fig. 4–4**).

The sensory neuroepithelium of the saccule, the macula sacculi (**Fig. 4–4**), is a specialized area of the membranous saccular wall that lies against the bony wall of the spherical recess and is oriented predominantly in the vertical plane. The macula is an oblong, plate-like structure with a surface area of a little more than 2 mm^2; it contains ~16,000 sensory cells (Watanuki and Schuknecht, 1976). Its vertical orientation in the parasagittal plane makes it most sensitive to up-and-down translations of the head as well as to horizontal motion along the anteroposterior (front-to-back) axis.

The utricle is an irregularly shaped membranous tube that is considerably larger than the saccule (Igarashi et al, 1983). It has a superior-to-inferior orientation in the vestibule and lies behind (i.e., posterior to) the saccule.

The macula of the utricle is rounded in shape, has a surface area of roughly 4 mm^2, and contains ~31,000 receptor cells (Watanuki and Schuknecht, 1976). The utricular macula is situated in the superior portion of the utricle (**Fig. 4–4**) and lies in approximately the horizontal plane. This orientation makes it most sensitive to linear movements in the horizontal plane.

The three semicircular ducts are thin, curved tubes that are attached to the utricle and open into it, as shown in **Fig. 4–4**. Each of the ducts forms about two thirds of a circle, fact of importance for positioning the head during caloric testing.) Each of the semicircular ducts has a bulbous dilation at one end called the ampulla, which houses the sensory receptor. The nonampullated ends of the superior and posterior ducts unite to form the crus commune, which joins the posterior aspect of the utricle (**Fig. 4–4**). Thus, there are five (rather than six) openings into the utricle associated with the semicircular ducts. The sensory neuroepithelium of each of the ducts is located on a ridge of tissue called the crista ampullaris that extends transversely across the ampulla at right angles to the semicircular duct (**Fig. 4–5**). The neuroepithelium of each crista has a surface area of ~1 mm² and contains roughly 7000 sensory cells (Watanuki and Schuknecht, 1976).

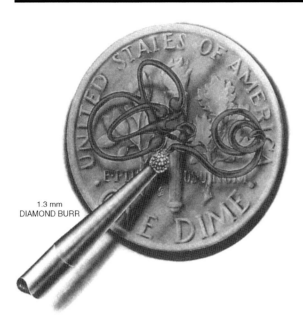

Figure 4–2 Drawing of the membranous labyrinth showing its size in relation to a dime and to a 1.3 mm dental burr. (From Anson, B. J., & Donaldson, J. A. (1973). Surgical anatomy of the temporal bone and ear (2nd ed.). Philadelphia: W. B. Saunders, with permission.)

Pearl

- All five sensory organs of the vestibular apparatus are stimulated by acceleratory forces. The maculae of the saccule and utricle respond to linear acceleration (linear motion and gravity). The cristae of the semicircular ducts respond to angular acceleration (rotational motion).

The Vestibular Neuroepithelia

Structure

Although the sensory receptors of the macular organs and the semicircular ducts are equipped with different types of accessory structures for stimulation of the vestibular sensory cells, the various neuroepithelia all have a similar structural organization (Lindeman, 1969). As shown in **Fig. 4–6**, which illustrates a cross section of the saccular

and each lies at right angles to the other two. As indicated in **Fig. 4–3**, the three semicircular canals and the membranous ducts they enclose are named according to their relative positions in the upright head: superior (or anterior vertical), inferior (or posterior vertical), and lateral (or horizontal). The superior and inferior ducts are oriented vertically, and the lateral duct lies in an approximately horizontal plane. (The lateral duct is actually tilted upward by ~30 degrees, a

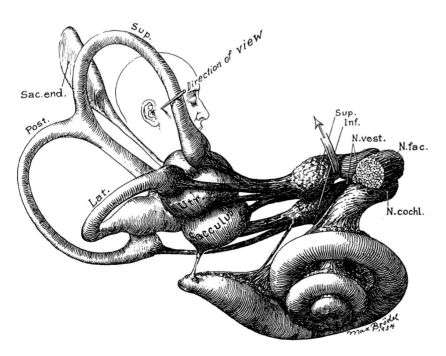

Figure 4–3 Orientation of the membranous labyrinth in the human head. The superior (sup.) and posterior (post.) semicircular ducts are vertically oriented, and the lateral duct (lat.) is tilted at ~30 degrees from the horizontal plane. Sac. end., endolymphatic sac; utr., utricle; Sup./Inf., superior and inferior components of the vestibular nerve (N. vest.). The arrow indicates that the superior division has been slightly elevated to make the two parts of the nerve more distinctly visible as separate elements. N. fac., facial nerve; N. cochl., cochlear nerve. (From Brödel M. (1946). Three unpublished drawings of the anatomy of the human ear. Philadelphia: W. B. Saunders, with permission.)

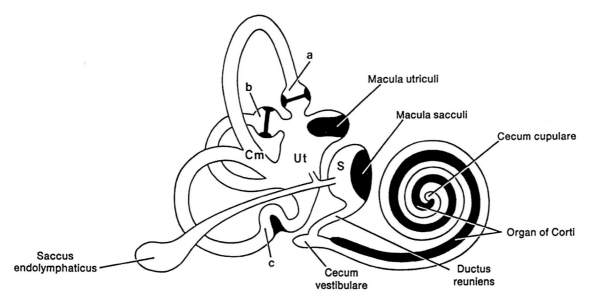

Figure 4–4 Diagram showing relationships between structures of the membranous labyrinth and location of the sensory epithelia within the vestibular apparatus. Labels a, b, and c indicate the superior, lateral, and posterior ampullae, respectively, with their sensory receptors (the cristae) shown in black. Cm, crus commune; Ut, utricle; S, saccule. (From Bloom, W., & Fawcett, D. W. (1962). A textbook of histology (8th ed.). Philadelphia: W. B. Saunders, with permission.)

macula, the vestibular neuroepithelia are composed of sensory and supporting cells together with the neural structures associated with the sensory epithelium. The sensory cells are arranged in a single layer and are separated from one another by supporting cells. The receptor cells have clusters of hair-like cilia at their apical ends and are therefore often called "hair cells." All vestibular hair cells have cilia of two types: stereocilia and kinocilia. The stereocilia are modified microvilli that are arranged in several rows that increase in height across the top of the cell. They are thus configured in a stairstep pattern in which short stereocilia are positioned on one side of the hair cell and long ones on the other (**Fig. 4–7**). Situated near the tallest row of stereocilia is a single, longer process known as the kinocilium, which has a more complex internal structure like that of true, motile cilia found in other parts of the body. The orderly arrangement of stereocilia and kinocilia across the top

of the vestibular sensory cell has important functional implications, as discussed below.

The stereocilia and kinocilia of the macular hair cells project into a sheet of gelatinous material that blankets the surface of the neuroepithelium (**Fig. 4–6**). Resting on the gelatinous sheet is a mass of tiny crystals called otoconia. The crystalline mass, together with the gelatinous layer, makes up the structure known as the otoconial membrane, which is responsible for stimulation of the macular hair cells in response to linear acceleration.

The otoconia are composed of calcium carbonate in the form of the mineral calcite, which has a density almost 3 times that of endolymph (Lim, 1984). As illustrated in **Fig. 4–8**, individual otoconial crystals are cylindrical in shape and have pointed ends, somewhat resembling miniature grains of rice. The otoconia range from less than 1 μm to ~20 μm in length, with crystals of differing size arranged in a definite pattern

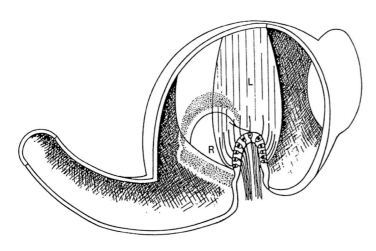

Figure 4–5 Schematic diagram of the sensory structures inside the ampulla of a semicircular duct. The crista (R), which extends across the ampulla, is covered by sensory epithelium. The cilia of the sensory cells project into the cupula (L), a gelatinous mass that fills the space between the surface of the crista and the opposite wall of the ampulla. (From Lindeman, H. H. (1969). Studies on the morphology of the sensory regions of the vestibular apparatus. Ergebnisse der Anatomie Entwicklungsgeschichte, 42(1), 1–113, with permission.)

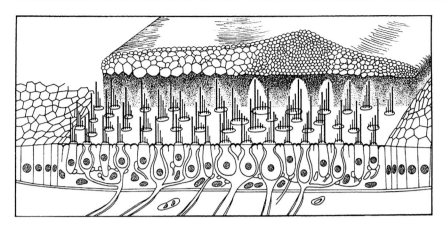

Figure 4–6 Drawing illustrating a cross section of the saccular macula. The stippled area above the macular surface represents the gelatinous layer of the otoconial membrane into which the stereocilia of the sensory cells project. Resting on the gelatinous layer are the otoconia. (From Lindeman, H. H. (1969). Studies on the morphology of the sensory regions of the vestibular apparatus. Ergebnisse der Anatomie Entwicklungsgeschichte, 42(1), 1–113, with permission.)

across the otoconial membrane. Under the influence of gravitational force or linear head movement, the otoconial membrane undergoes minute shifts in position on the macular surface, thereby deflecting the cilia on the underlying sensory cells. This changes the electrical polarization of the hair cells, which in turn alters the release of neurotransmitter so as to influence the activity of nerve fibers making contact with the sensory cells. It is in this way that the discharge rate of vestibular nerve fibers is modulated by stimulation of the macular receptor cells (Goldberg and Fernandez, 1984).

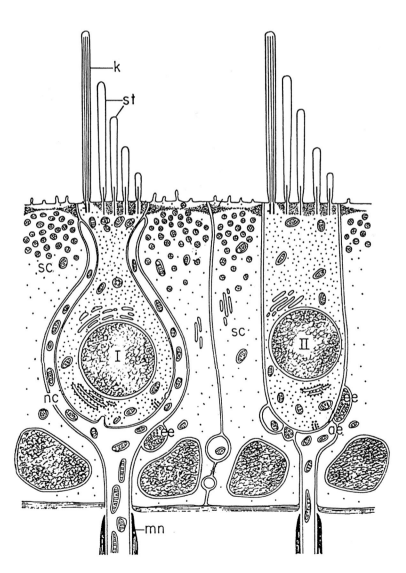

Figure 4–7 Diagrammatic cross section of the vestibular neuroepithelium illustrating type I and type II sensory cells surrounded by supporting cells (sc). The type I sensory cell is enclosed by an afferent nerve calyx (nc). Near its base, the type II cell receives small afferent (ae) and efferent (ee) nerve endings. Efferent endings are also found on the afferent nerve calyx. mn, myelinated vestibular nerve fiber approaching the sensory epithelium. Kinocilia (k) and stereocilia (st) are prominent features on the apical surfaces of both type I and type II receptor cells. Note that the kinocilium is located immediately adjacent to the tallest of the stereocilia. (From Lindeman, H. H. (1969). Studies on the morphology of the sensory regions of the vestibular apparatus. Ergebnisse der Anatomie Entwicklungsgeschichte, 42(1), 1–113, with permission.)

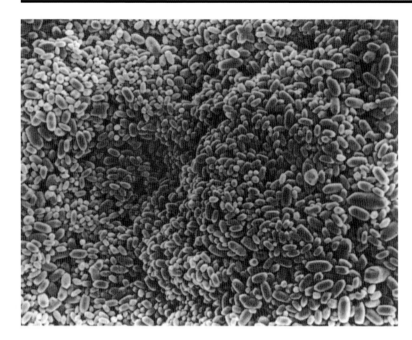

Figure 4–8 Scanning electron micrograph of the surface of the crystalline layer of the saccular otoconial membrane from a human infant. At this magnification (approximately × 1000), individual otoconial crystals are clearly seen.

In the ampullae of the semicircular ducts, the sensory cells are stimulated by the cupula, a gelatinous mass that rests on the crista and extends to the opposite wall of the ampulla, thereby closing off the opening between the semicircular duct and the utricle (**Fig. 4–5**). The cupula envelops the cilia of the hair cells and consists of material much like the gelatinous layer of the otoconial membrane, but it is without otoconia and therefore has the same density as endolymph. Very small fluid displacements occurring in the semicircular ducts during angular acceleration deflect the cupula, resulting in deflection of the cilia on the receptor cells.

All the vestibular neuroepithelia contain sensory cells of two different morphologic types (Lindeman, 1969), which are illustrated diagrammatically in **Fig. 4–7**. The type I receptor cell has a rather plump, goblet-like shape and is entirely surrounded by a single, large nerve ending, the so-called nerve calyx (or chalice). The calyceal endings are terminals of the large and medium-sized afferent fibers of the vestibular nerve (Correia and Dickman, 1991), which transmit information from the sensory cells to the CNS. The type II receptor cells are more slender and cylindrical in shape, and they have clusters of small nerve endings at their basal ends. Both afferent and efferent nerve fibers terminate on the type II sensory cells.

The efferent terminals are the peripheral endings of nerve fibers with cell bodies located in the brainstem in the vicinity of the vestibular nuclei. Thus, the efferent innervation projects from the CNS out to the periphery, where its fibers branch extensively and terminate in three locations: (1) on type II hair cells, (2) on afferent calyceal endings surrounding type I sensory cells, and (3) on afferent nerve fibers supplying both type I and type II hair cells (Correia and Dickman, 1991). Each labyrinth receives a total of 400 to 600 efferent fibers originating from neurons located on both the ipsilateral and contralateral sides of the brainstem (Gacek, 1980). The efferent innervation undoubtedly influences the flow of information transmitted from the vestibular neuroepithelia to the brain. However, the physiological significance of this innervation is not yet completely understood. Evidence exists that the efferent system may have both excitatory and inhibitory effects on afferent impulse transmission (Goldberg and Fernandez, 1984; Highstein, 1991; Marlinski et al, 2004).

Function

The afferent nerve fibers that supply the vestibular neuroepithelia are activated by release of neurotransmitter from the sensory cells. Because some release of transmitter apparently occurs even when the sensory cells are at rest, the afferent fibers transmit nerve impulses to the brain during periods when the neuroepithelia are not under active stimulation. As shown in **Fig. 4–9**, this "spontaneous" discharge may be increased or decreased by changes in transmitter release that occur when a stimulus is applied to the receptor cells (Goldberg and Fernandez, 1984; Leigh and Zee, 1991).

If the cupula or otoconial membrane moves so that the stereocilia on an underlying hair cell are deflected toward the kinocilium, the cell is depolarized. (Its membrane potential becomes less negative.) Depolarization increases the release of neurotransmitter onto the afferent nerve terminals, and the rate of neural discharge increases. If the stereocilia are deflected away from the kinocilium, the cell's membrane potential increases (becomes more negative or hyperpolarized), resulting in reduced transmitter release and a decrease in afferent discharge rate. Because the spontaneous discharge may be modulated either up or down, the system shows directional sensitivity; movement of the cupula or otoconial membrane in one direction increases afferent discharge, and movement in the opposite direction decreases the discharge (Correia and Dickman, 1991).

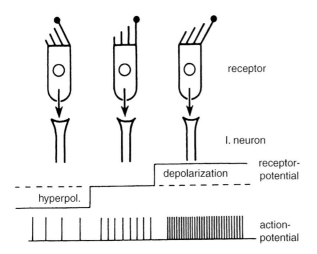

Figure 4–9 Effect of receptor cell stimulation on the activity of vestibular nerve fibers. In the absence of stimulation (center), vestibular neurons (I. neuron) show a continuous discharge of action potentials. Hair cell stimulation produces either depolarization (right) or hyperpolarization (left), depending on whether the stereocilia are deflected toward or away from the kinocilium (indicated here by the longest cilium with a beaded end). Hyperpolarization decreases the rate of action potential discharge, whereas depolarization increases the discharge rate. (From Leigh, R. J., & Zee, D. S. (1991). The neurology of eye movements (2nd ed.). Philadelphia: F. A. Davis, with permission.)

In each of the vestibular neuroepithelia, groups of sensory cells are oriented in such a way that all cells within a group are either depolarized or hyperpolarized by a given movement of the cupula or otoconial membrane (Lindeman, 1969). On the cristae of the semicircular ducts, all the receptor cells are oriented (or "polarized") in the same manner. In the case of the lateral crista, each hair cell is situated so that its kinocilium is on the side of the cell nearest the utricle. (The cells are said to be oriented in such a way that their kinocilia "face" the utricle.) Thus, if the head moves so as to displace the lateral cupula toward the utricle (i.e., utriculopetal deflection), the stereocilia will be deflected toward the kinocilia, depolarizing the sensory cells and producing increased neural discharge (excitation). Cupular deflection away from the utricle (utriculofugal displacement) will hyperpolarize the hair cells, resulting in reduction (inhibition) of neural discharge. The receptor cells of the superior and posterior cristae are polarized in a manner exactly opposite to those of the lateral crista. That is, they are oriented so that their kinocilia face away from the utricle. Therefore, cupular deflection toward the utricle produces inhibition of neural output, whereas deflection away from the utricle results in excitation.

The arrangement of sensory cells on the two maculae is somewhat more complex. That is, each macula is divided into two areas of roughly equal size in which the hair cells are oppositely oriented. Therefore, displacement of the otoconial membrane tends to excite cells on one half of the macula and inhibit those on the other half. The polarization patterns of sensory cells on the cristae and maculae are illustrated diagrammatically in **Fig. 4–10**.

◆ The Vestibulo-ocular Reflex and Its Role in the Evaluation of Vestibular Function

The reflex pathways connecting the vestibular system with the extraocular muscles of the eyes play an important role in clinical testing of vestibular function. Imagine an individual undergoing angular acceleration toward the right in the horizontal plane, as diagrammed in **Fig. 4–11**. As the head is rotated to the right, both lateral cupulae will be deflected toward the left. The lateral cupula on the right will therefore move toward the utricle, and the left cupula will move away from the utricle. Because the hair cells of the lateral cupulae are oriented with their kinocilia facing the utricle, this stimulus will increase the rate of neural discharge from the right ear and reduce the discharge rate on the left. The change in neural activity will be relayed via the vestibular nerves to the vestibular nuclei of the brainstem. From there, neural pathways lead to the nuclei that control the extraocular muscles (in this case, the medial and lateral rectus muscles that move the eyes in the horizontal plane). As **Fig. 4–11** shows, the increased discharge from the right ear will be transmitted to the abducens and oculomotor nerves that control the lateral rectus muscle of the left eye and medial rectus muscle of the right eye. These muscles will then draw the eyes toward the left. Thus, each labyrinth influences muscles that pull the eyes in a direction opposite to the direction of head rotation. When the head is rotated to the right, neural discharge from the right ear is increased, and the eyes move to the left with velocity and amplitude equal to the velocity and amplitude of the head movement (Barber, 1984). This response is known as the vestibulo-ocular reflex (VOR). The VOR functions to stabilize the visual field on the retina as the head moves, thereby reducing visual blurring during head motion, which helps to maintain clear vision as the body moves.

Pearl

- During head rotation, the extraocular muscles are stimulated so as to draw the eyes in a direction opposite to the direction of rotation. This reflex response (the VOR) is a result of vestibular stimulation, and it functions to stabilize the visual field on the retina as the head moves.

As the head moves to the right, the eyes move toward the left, but they can only move so far before they reach their limit of motion within the orbits. When that occurs, the eyes snap back to the midline position before moving left again. This repeated pattern of eye movement, in which the eyes move relatively slowly in one direction, then quickly return to the midline, is called nystagmus. The initial, slower phase of the nystagmic beat is controlled by the vestibular system. The quick return to midline is under the control of the brainstem reticular formation. Because the quick return is the more obvious part of the nystagmic beat, it is the direction of

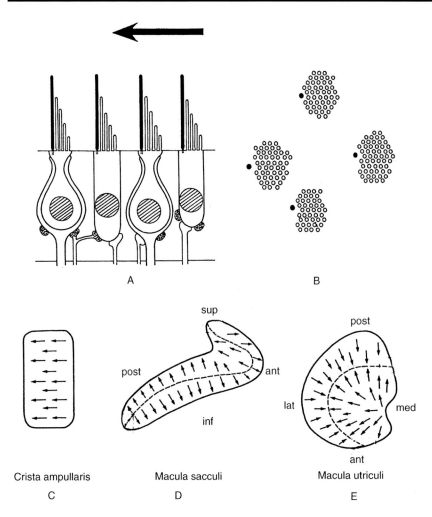

Figure 4–10 Diagram illustrating morphological polarization of the sensory cells and the polarization pattern of the vestibular sensory epithelia. The morphological polarization (arrow) of a sensory cell is determined by the position of the kinocilium in relation to the stereocilia. **(A)** Cross section of the neuroepithelium. Note the increasing length of stereocilia toward the kinocilium (shown in solid black). **(B)** Section through the stereociliary bundles parallel to the epithelial surface. The solid black dots indicate the kinocilia. **(C)** The sensory cells of the crista ampullaris are all polarized in the same direction. The saccular **(D)** and utricular **(E)** maculae are each divided into two areas in which the sensory cells are oppositely polarized; post (posterior), sup (superior), ant (anterior), inf (inferior), lat (lateral), and med (median) indicate the orientation of the maculae. (From Lindeman, H. H. (1969). Studies on the morphology of the sensory regions of the vestibular apparatus. Ergebnisse der Anatomie Entwicklungsgeschichte, 42(1), 1–113, with permission.)

eye movement during that phase that is said to be the direction of the nystagmus. Thus, angular acceleration of the head to the right induces a right-beating nystagmus. The assessment of nystagmus is an important tool for clinical evaluation of vestibular function. Nystagmus may occur spontaneously in various disorders, or it may occur when the head is placed in certain positions; it may also be induced in the clinic by rotational or caloric stimulation.

Pearl

- It is the fast component of the nystagmic beat that is used to designate the direction of nystagmus.

In some respects, caloric stimulation is more informative than rotational testing because with caloric tests, the two ears can be stimulated separately and their responses compared, thereby providing more diagnostically useful information. Caloric nystagmus is produced by irrigating the external ear canal with either warm or cool water or air, which changes the temperature of the middle ear cavity (Furman and Cass, 1996). The temperature change rather specifically affects the lateral semicircular duct because it lies in close proximity to the middle ear cavity. If the lateral duct is vertically oriented by appropriate tilting of the head, a warm stimulus to the right ear will increase the temperature of a portion of the endolymph in the lateral duct, causing it to rise and deflect the cupula toward the utricle. The resulting increase in neural discharge from the right side will then produce a right-beating nystagmus, as described above. A cool stimulus, in contrast, produces a response in the opposite direction. In that case, endolymph in the lateral semicircular duct is cooled, becomes more dense, and sinks, so that the cupula will be deflected away from the utricle. This will reduce the discharge rate from the right ear, making the left ear dominant so as to provoke a left-beating nystagmus. The mnemonic COWS (cold: opposite; warm: same) is a helpful aid for remembering the side of the head toward which the nystagmic beat is directed during caloric stimulation.

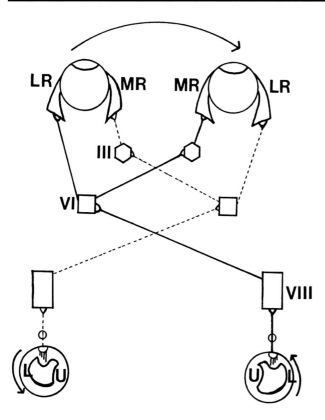

Figure 4–11 Simplified schematic illustrating the basic neurocircuits that mediate the horizontal vestibular ocular reflex. The circular figures at the bottom of the diagram represent the right and left vestibular labyrinths, with *L* indicating the lateral semicircular duct and *U* indicating the utricle. From the cristae of the lateral ducts, neural impulses are relayed via the vestibular nerve to the vestibular nuclei (VIII) and then to the nuclei of the abducens (VI) and oculomotor (III) nerves controlling the medial (MR) and lateral (LR) rectus muscles that move the eyes in the horizontal plane. These pathways involve relatively few neurons; the stimulus-to-response time (latency) of the vestibulo-ocular reflex is therefore short. When the head undergoes angular acceleration to the right (indicated by the large arrow at top), fluid displacement in the lateral duct deflects the stereocilia of the right crista toward the utricle and those of the left crista away from the utricle, as indicated by the small arrows. This results in increased neural discharge in the pathway drawn in solid lines and decreased activity in the pathway shown in dotted lines, producing a leftward shift of the eyes due to contraction of the medial and lateral rectus muscles on the left side of each eye. Thus, rotation of the head in one direction results in movement of the eyes in the opposite direction.

Pearl

- Under normal conditions, the vestibular receptors of the two ears operate in concert as they relay information to the CNS. The pattern of impulses flowing to the brain from the right and left ears changes with changes in head position and/or acceleration. It is the difference in neural activity between the two ears that provides the basis for the brain's interpretation of head motion and position. Lesions of the peripheral vestibular apparatus may severely upset the balanced flow of information from the two sides, resulting in disequilibrium, vertigo, and ataxia.

◆ The Vestibular Nerve and the Central Vestibular System

The sensory organs of the vestibular labyrinth are innervated by the vestibular component of the eighth cranial nerve (CN VIII), which carries both afferent and efferent fibers to the vestibular apparatus. Afferent fibers of the vestibular nerve have their cell bodies located in Scarpa's ganglion, which occupies the internal auditory canal of the temporal bone. The vestibular nerve (including Scarpa's ganglion) is divided into superior and inferior divisions; together the two divisions contain some 18,000 to 20,000 nerve fibers (Schuknecht, 1993). As indicated in **Fig. 4–12**, the peripheral portion of the superior division of the nerve innervates the utricular macula, the superior and lateral cristae, and the anterosuperior region of the saccular macula. Peripheral fibers of the inferior division supply the major portion of the saccular macula and the posterior crista. Central to Scarpa's ganglion, the vestibular nerve projects to the brainstem, where most of its fibers enter the vestibular nuclei (**Figs. 4–13** and **4–14**). A small contingent of fibers, however, bypasses the vestibular nuclear complex and projects directly to the cerebellum (Brugge, 1991; Goldberg and Fernandez, 1984).

The vestibular nuclei are located in the dorsolateral portion of the brainstem near the junction of the medulla and pons (**Fig. 4–13**). They consist of four major nuclei (superior, lateral, medial, and inferior or descending) together with several closely associated minor nuclear groups (Gacek, 1980). As the vestibular nerve fibers enter the brainstem, they bifurcate into ascending and descending branches, which distribute to the various nuclei in a highly organized fashion, with fibers from the cristae and maculae terminating in specific and, to some extent, independent areas of the vestibular nuclear complex.

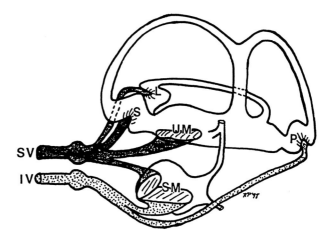

Figure 4–12 Drawing showing the peripheral distribution of the superior and inferior divisions of the vestibular nerve to the sensory organs of the inner ear. The superior division of the nerve (SV, shown shaded) supplies the cristae of the lateral (L) and superior (S) ampullae, as well as the macula of the utricle (UM) and a portion of the saccular macula (SM). The inferior division of the nerve (IV, stippled) innervates the main portion of the saccular macula and the crista of the posterior ampulla (P).

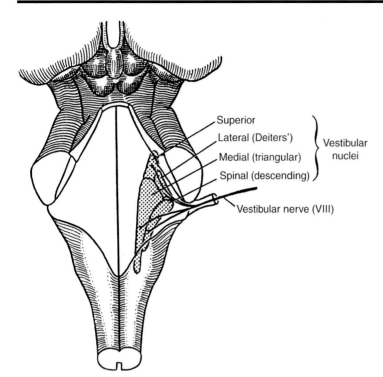

Figure 4–13 Drawing of the brainstem showing the location of the four major vestibular nuclei. For a detailed summary of the neuroanatomy of the vestibular nuclei and their connections with other brainstem centers, see Brugge (1991). (From House, E. L., & Pansky, B. P. (1967). A functional approach to neuroanatomy (2nd ed.). New York: McGraw-Hill, with permission.)

In addition to the vestibular nerve fibers, the vestibular nuclei receive input from various other sources, including the visual system, the cerebellum, the brainstem reticular formation, and the spinal cord. They therefore serve as more than simple relay stations for peripheral input; these nuclei play a significant role in the complex interaction between the vestibular system and other major centers of the CNS (Furman and Cass, 1996).

One of the most important central connections of the vestibular nuclei is with brainstem centers that control ocular motion (Barber, 1984; Goldberg and Fernandez, 1984; Leigh and Zee, 1991). As described previously, the vestibular

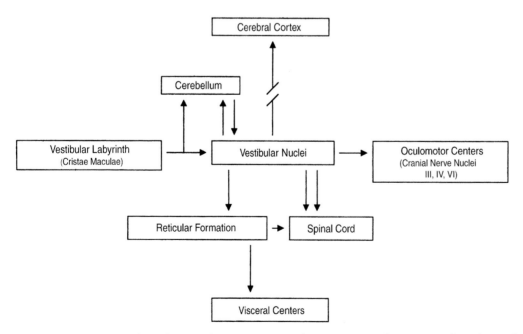

Figure 4–14 Highly simplified schematic showing major central nervous system connections of the vestibular system. The interrupted arrow from the vestibular nuclei to the cerebral cortex is to indicate that this is a multisynaptic pathway whose exact connections are still under investigation. The two arrows from the vestibular nuclei to the spinal cord represent the medial and lateral vestibulospinal tracts. See text for a discussion of central vestibular connections.

apparatus detects both static head position and head motion and through its central connections elicits compensatory eye movements that stabilize the visual image on the retina when the head moves or tilts (the VOR). The vestibulo-ocular pathways involved in horizontal eye movements have been outlined above. In addition to input from the lateral crista, signals from the superior and posterior cristae and the maculae are involved in reflex control of eye movement via connections through the vestibular nuclei to the oculomotor, trochlear, and abducens nuclei, which are the primary cranial nerve nuclei responsible for control of eye motion in all spatial planes.

As a major CNS center for motor coordination, the cerebellum plays a significant role in regulation of vestibulo-ocular and vestibulospinal reflexes (Brugge, 1991; Goldberg and Fernandez, 1984). The vestibular system has substantial reciprocal connections with the cerebellum. Vestibular input to the cerebellum includes a sizable projection from neurons in the vestibular nuclei, as well as a direct input from the peripheral vestibular apparatus (**Fig. 4–14**). (The direct vestibular fibers are the only afferents that reach the cerebellar cortex directly from a peripheral sensory organ without an intervening relay.) Vestibular signals reaching the cerebellum are integrated with information from visual, oculomotor, and proprioceptive pathways. The cerebellum, in turn, projects back to the vestibular nuclei and, after the vestibular nerve, supplies the second largest contingent of fibers to the vestibular nuclear complex. Although the cerebellum exerts both excitatory and inhibitory effects on the vestibular nuclei, its major influence on vestibular nuclear activity is inhibitory. Interaction between the vestibular nuclei and the cerebellum is of essential importance in coordination of eye and head movements and in control of balance and postural tone.

Vestibular influences on the spinal cord are mediated by two direct pathways from the vestibular nuclei and by indirect connections via the reticular formation of the brainstem (Brugge, 1991; Kevetter and Correia, 1997; Pompeiano, 1975). The first of the direct spinal pathways, which is of major importance with regard to postural control, is the lateral vestibulospinal tract that originates in the lateral vestibular nucleus, which receives sizable afferent input from the tilt-sensitive neurons innervating the utricular macula. The lateral vestibulospinal tract projects to all levels of the spinal cord and terminates in relation to motor neurons responsible for control of the antigravity muscles of the neck, trunk, and limbs. The second of the direct vestibulospinal pathways, the medial vestibulospinal tract, receives contributions from the medial, lateral, and inferior vestibular nuclei and descends to cervical (and probably upper thoracic) levels of the spinal cord. Reflexes mediated by the medial vestibulospinal tract operate to stabilize the head so as to provide a stable platform for the eyes during locomotion and also to maintain appropriate head position with respect to gravity.

In addition to the CNS regions just discussed, the vestibular nuclear complex makes functionally significant connections with other areas. These include the contralateral vestibular nuclei, brainstem centers controlling visceral reflexes, and the cerebral cortex.

The distressing symptoms produced by unphysiological vestibular stimulation or inner ear disease can be a major consideration in clinical management of patients with vestibular disorders. In addition to vertigo and disequilibrium, these patients may experience significant difficulty with autonomic/visceral upset due to high levels of vestibular system activity or markedly asymmetric vestibular input from the two ears. The neuroanatomical connections responsible for such symptoms are made via the reticular formation, which links the vestibular nuclei with various visceral reflex centers (**Fig. 4–14**), including the nuclei of origin of the vagus nerve, the phrenic nucleus, the salivatory nuclei, and the sympathetic chain ganglia (Crosby et al, 1962). These connections are responsible for the nausea, vomiting, sweating, and pallor that may result from intense vestibular stimulation or from diseases affecting the vestibular system.

It is now well established that the cerebral cortex receives vestibular input; however, the neuroanatomical pathways underlying vestibular representation at the cortical level are still the subject of active investigation. Evidence from neurophysiological and imaging studies indicates that multiple cortical areas are involved in processing vestibular information, and the neurons located in those areas tend to respond to multisensory neural input, especially optokinetic and somatosensory signals, in addition to vestibular input (Brandt and Dieterich, 1999). Vestibular impulses reaching the cortex are therefore integrated with incoming information from other systems so as to provide our sense of spatial orientation, including the perception of body position and body motion in three-dimensional space (Andersen et al, 1999; Guldin and Grusser, 1998).

Acknowledgment   We thank Karen S. Pawlowski for the artwork used in **Figs. 4–11** and **4–12**.

References

Andersen, R. A., Shenoy, K. V., Snyder, L. H., Bradley, D. C., & Crowell, J. A. (1999). The contributions of vestibular signals to the representations of space in the posterior parietal cortex. Annals of the New York Academy of Sciences, 871, 282–292.

Anson, B. J., & Donaldson, J. A. (1973). Surgical anatomy of the temporal bone and ear (2nd ed.). Philadelphia: W. B. Saunders.

Barber, H. O. (1984). Vestibular neurophysiology. Otolaryngology—Head and Neck Surgery, 92, 55–58.

Bloom, W., & Fawcett, D. W. (1962). A textbook of histology (8th ed.). Philadelphia: W. B. Saunders.

Brandt, T., & Dieterich, M. (1999). The vestibular cortex, its locations, functions, and disorders. Annals of the New York Academy of Sciences, 871, 293–312.

Brödel M. (1946). Three unpublished drawings of the anatomy of the human ear. Philadelphia: W. B. Saunders.

Brugge, J. F. (1991). Neurophysiology of the central auditory and vestibular systems. In M. M. Paparella, D. A. Shumrick, J. L. Gluckman, & W. L. Meyerhoff (Eds.), Otolaryngology: Basic sciences and related principles (Vol. 1, 3rd ed., pp. 281–314). Philadelphia: W. B. Saunders.

Correia, M. J., & Dickman, J. D. (1991). Peripheral vestibular system. In M. M. Paparella, D. A. Shumrick, J. L. Gluckman, & W. L. Meyerhoff (Eds.), Otolaryngology: Basic sciences and related principles (Vol. 1, 3rd ed., 269–279). Philadelphia: W. B. Saunders.

Crosby, E. C., Humphrey, T., & Lauer, W. L. (1962). Correlative anatomy of the nervous system. New York: Macmillan.

Furman, J. M., & Cass, S. P. (1996). Balance disorders: A case-study approach. Philadelphia: F. A. Davis.

Gacek, R. R. (1980). Neuroanatomical correlates of vestibular function. Annals of Otology, Rhinology, and Laryngology, 89, 2–5.

Goldberg, J. M., & Fernandez, C. (1984). The vestibular system. In J. M. Brookhart, V. B. Mountcastle, I. Darian-Smith, & S. R. Geiger (Eds.), Handbook of physiology: The nervous system (Vol. 3, Part 2, pp. 977–1021). Bethesda, MD: American Physiological Society.

Guldin, W. O., & Grusser, O.-J. (1998). Is there a vestibular cortex? Trends in Neurosciences, 21, 254–259.

Highstein, S. M. (1991). The central nervous system efferent control of the organs of balance and equilibrium. Neuroscience Research, 12, 13–30.

House, E. L., & Pansky, B. P. (1967). A functional approach to neuroanatomy (2nd ed.). New York: McGraw-Hill.

Igarashi, M., O-Uchi, T., Isago, H., & Wright, W. K. (1983). Utricular and saccular volumetry in human temporal bones. Acta Otolaryngologica (Stockholm), 95, 75–80.

Kevetter, G. A., & Correia, M. J. (1997). Vestibular system. In P. S. Roland, B. F. Marple, & W. L. Meyerhoff (Eds.), Hearing loss (pp. 54–70). New York: Thieme.

Leigh, R. J., & Zee, D. S. (1991). The neurology of eye movements (2nd ed.). Philadelphia: F. A. Davis.

Lim, D. J. (1984). The development and structure of the otoconia. In I. Friedman & J. Ballantyne (Eds.), Ultrastructural atlas of the inner ear (pp. 245–269). London: Butterworths.

Lindeman, H. H. (1969). Studies on the morphology of the sensory regions of the vestibular apparatus. Ergebnisse der Anatomie Entwicklungsgeschichte, 42(1), 1–113.

Marlinski, V., Plotnik, M., & Goldberg, J. M. (2004). Efferent actions in the chinchilla vestibular labyrinth. Journal of the Association for Research in Otolaryngology, 5, 126–143.

Pompeiano, O. (1975). Vestibulo-spinal relationships. In R. F. Naunton (Ed.), The vestibular system (pp. 147–180). New York: Academic Press.

Schuknecht, H. F. (1993). Pathology of the ear (2nd ed.). Philadelphia: Lea & Febiger.

Schuknecht, H. F., & Gulya, A. J. (1995). Anatomy of the temporal bone with surgical implications (2nd ed.). New York: Parthenon Publishing Group.

Watanuki, K., & Schuknecht, H. F. (1976). A morphological study of human vestibular sensory epithelia. Archives of Otolaryngology, 102(10), 853–858.

Chapter 5

Disorders of the Auditory System

Michael P. Castillo and Peter S. Roland

This chapter provides an overview of the most common diseases seen by otologists and audiologists. A general knowledge of the pathologic conditions of otology is necessary for the audiologist to do the testing necessary to help the physician properly diagnose and treat the patient. The chapter begins with a review of the otologic exam. Disorders of the ear canal; the tympanic membrane, middle ear, and mastoid bone; and the inner ear and internal auditory canal are then covered. Pertinent diagnostic information and treatment options are discussed for each disorder. Because the chapter reviews a wide range of disorders of the auditory system, material is covered that is presented in other portions of this textbook. This chapter is meant to be an overview and will complement other chapters.

◆ Otologic Examination

History

Patients seen by the otologist usually complain of one of several symptoms, which include tinnitus, vertigo, hearing loss, otalgia, and otorrhea. A complete history should include the following for each symptom:

- When was the symptom first noted?

- Is the symptom constant or intermittent?

- If intermittent, how often does it occur, and how long does it last with each occurrence? Do the symptoms come in clusters?

- How severe is the symptom?

- Is the symptom improving or worsening?

- Is the symptom bilateral or unilateral? If bilateral and intermittent, does it occur in each ear simultaneously or independently? If bilateral, did it begin simultaneously in both ears?

- If more than one symptom is troubling the patient, do the symptoms occur independently, or are they clustered together to form a symptom complex (syndrome)?

Tinnitus

Tinnitus refers to a sound that appears to be coming from one or both ears but is not related to an external stimulus. It is reported most frequently as a component of hearing loss. The perceived pitch is often close to the frequency at which hearing is worst: high-frequency hearing loss is often associated with high-pitched tinnitus, and low-pitched tinnitus is often related to low-frequency loss.

Millions of people experience varying degrees of tinnitus. At some time or another, almost everyone experiences brief episodes of tinnitus. Most individuals are not bothered by such brief episodes, but when tinnitus persists, they may experience substantial discomfort. Individuals with tinnitus report with some uniformity that tinnitus is exacerbated in quiet environments and in stressful situations. Whereas some merely regard the symptom as annoying, others are kept awake at night and may have difficulty concentrating. A few individuals find tinnitus disabling to the point that it prevents them from pursuing their usual daily activities. An occasional individual may find the experience so tortuous that suicide is contemplated.

It is important to determine if tinnitus is unilateral or bilateral, pulsatile or nonpulsatile, and constant or intermittent. Pulsatile tinnitus is often noted with vascular anomalies, such as vascular middle ear tumors (i.e., glomus tumors) or with carotid or temporal artery disease.

The same general considerations that apply to adults also apply to children. Children may have greater difficulty in expressing and describing their subjective sensations. On the whole, tinnitus seems to be less bothersome to children than to adults, but hearing loss still may be first identified during a workup for tinnitus in children.

There is evidence that tinnitus may be generated from more than one portion of the auditory or central nervous system (CNS). The tinnitus associated with aspirin intoxication appears to be generated in the cochlea and is associated with hearing loss. On the other hand, experience with eighth cranial nerve (CN VIII) section for control of tinnitus has variable efficacy and may even worsen it, suggesting a central origin. More recent neurophysiological and imaging evidence points to central auditory system changes as the source of some tinnitus (Eggermont and Roberts, 2004). Portions of the limbic and autonomic system also appear to be involved.

Although there currently are no drugs approved by the US Food and Drug Administration (FDA) for the treatment of tinnitus, multiple forms of therapies, including the use of benzodiazepines and antidepressants, amplification, maskers, and biofeedback, do exist. Antidepressants may be used for their neuroleptic (mood-stabilizing) and antidepressant effect. Medications such as amitriptyline are used for tinnitus and other chronic pain states. Benzodiazepines, typically used for control of anxiety, have a moderate efficacy in suppressing tinnitus but are potentially addictive.

Amplification partially remedies hearing loss and often has a beneficial effect on the underlying tinnitus. Relief from tinnitus may persist for hours after the hearing aid has been removed. Masking techniques use narrowband noise generators matched to the frequency of the patient's tinnitus. Noise is delivered at a sufficiently high intensity to "mask" the internally generated noise.

Habituation therapy (tinnitus retraining therapy) uses broadband, low-intensity noise generators to elevate the level of ambient background noise. This therapy does not seek to "mask" the tinnitus signal. It requires at least 12 to 18 months of treatment and includes supportive therapy. A variety of other alternative medical therapies have been advocated; however, there is no evidence of their effectiveness.

Hearing Loss

Formal audiometric testing is the most critical component in assessing hearing loss. However, it is useful to gain an understanding of how much difficulty the individual experiences due to the type and degree of hearing loss found. It is important to establish the circumstances in which difficulty arises and the degree to which the patient is affected. Such information can be helpful in determining the potential usefulness of amplification.

The time course of the hearing change is the most useful piece of historical information. Losses that have occurred many years before the current evaluation and are stable are not likely to require medical intervention. In making such determinations, it is very helpful to review old audiograms, and every effort should be made to obtain them. Inquiries should be made into the circumstances of chronic hearing losses, and any association with febrile illness, antibiotic therapy, noise exposure, trauma, or surgery must be noted. Each patient should be specifically asked about fluctuation of hearing loss. If present, it is important to determine the circumstances, frequency, and severity of these fluctuations.

Any association of the hearing loss with vertigo, tinnitus, otalgia, otorrhea, upper respiratory infection, nasal congestion, headache, dysarthria, dysphagia, visual changes, numbness or tingling in the extremities, or focal motor weakness should be established. The time and circumstance at which patients first noted the loss and its rate of progression should always be determined when possible. The patient's family history regarding hearing loss should be evaluated as well. If other family members have hearing loss, the nature of such losses should be explored and audiograms obtained, especially if this loss occurred early in life.

In evaluating children, consultation with family and teachers is critical. Parents are usually acute observers of their own child's hearing sensitivity and may be aware of fairly subtle changes. The parents' assessment should always be taken at face value initially, even though subsequent information may demonstrate inaccuracies.

Otalgia

Otalgia, or ear pain, is the chief complaint for many physician visits and can have a range of causes. In a high percentage of adults, otalgia is not otogenic. It is estimated that in the primary care setting, only one half of cases of otalgia in adults are caused by ear disease. Pain of otologic origin is usually dull, aching, and relatively constant. Pain that comes and goes frequently during the day is rarely otogenic.

Although nonotogenic otalgia is less common in children, the child, like the adult, may experience pain in the ear when it is actually referred from other embryologically related structures. Otalgia is commonly due to disorders affecting the larynx, pharynx, and tonsils. Tonsillitis and pharyngitis are the two common causes of referred otalgia in children.

Temporomandibular joint (TMJ) pain and myofascial pain dysfunction syndrome are important and common nonotogenic causes of otalgia. Most common is myofascial dysfunction syndrome involving the muscles of mastication. This disorder is characterized by inflammation, spasm, and tenderness of the muscles of mastication with pressure and pain transmitted to the TMJ. The joint itself is normal. In understanding this condition, it must be remembered that the glenoid fossa of the TMJ forms the anterior wall of the external auditory canal and portions of the anterior and lateral wall of the middle ear. Therefore, pain due to a cause in these areas will be localized to the ear and external canal. Myofascial pain dysfunction syndromes are often related to teeth grinding, clenching, or gritting (bruxism). It is more common in individuals with an overbite. It may follow changes in occlusion associated with orthodontic treatments or the fitting of dentures. Because these actions are related to stress, this disorder is frequently a manifestation of stress. As such, it is often associated with or accompanied by tension headaches and inflammatory conditions of the posterior and lateral cervical muscles. Diagnosis depends on identifying tenderness over the joint or within the muscles of mastication. The temporalis muscles are frequently tender, and frontal headaches may be present.

Occasionally, there may be degenerative or inflammatory processes arising from the TMJ itself. When the disease process is intrinsic to the joint, the condition is properly referred to as TMJ dysfunction. Popping, clicking, grinding, or crunching noises with mouth opening and mouth closure suggest intrinsic joint abnormalities. Definitive diagnosis usually depends on magnetic resonance imaging (MRI) or endoscopic evaluation of the TMJ.

The pain of both disorders is generally characterized as sharp or aching and described as either "deep in the ear" or centered around the tragus or TMJ. When asked to localize their pain, patients often point directly into the external ear canal, the tragus, or the joint. Pain commonly radiates inferiorly toward the hyoid bone along the ramus of the mandible. It generally lasts for several hours at a time. In patients who grind and clench their teeth at night, the pain may be worse in the morning and occasionally wake them at night. The pain will often disappear completely during the day in these cases. Although uncommon, the pain can escalate to be so severe as to be completely incapacitating, immobilizing or locking the jaw ("lockjaw").

Treatment of this pain is often successful with conservative approaches, such as application of heat and massage, patient education, and pain control with nonsteroidal anti-inflammatory drugs (NSAIDs). Such agents should be prescribed regularly for a period of 10 to 14 days. In individuals who grind or clench their teeth at night, the use of a nocturnal bite splint is frequently helpful.

Many important otologic conditions such as cholesteatoma, chronic otitis media, Meniere's disease, and acoustic tumors are not associated with pain. Otogenic ear pain may be due to cerumen impaction, acute infection, and, rarely, neoplasms. The most common cause of otogenic ear pain is infection. Both external otitis and acute otitis media may cause excruciating pain that precipitates a physician visit. Because most cases are treated in the primary care setting, the incidence of ear pain caused by otologic disease is actually lower in a referral otologic practice than it is in general practice.

Pearl

- Palpation (use of the hands and fingers to examine size, consistency, location, and tenderness) of the TMJ and muscles of mastication should be done when evaluating all patients with otalgia. Patients with joint or muscle tenderness should be treated with a 10 to 14 day course of nonsteroidal anti-inflammatory agents. If, despite treatment, pain persists, the patient should be referred to an oral surgeon.

Otorrhea

With the rare exception of cases in which spinal fluid drains through the ear, otorrhea, or drainage from the ear, is related to infection. The patient's history is especially important. Painless drainage is usually the result of chronic otitis media. This may be cholesteatoma, chronic mastoiditis caused by irreversible mucosal disease and tympanic membrane perforation, or chronic reflux through the eustachian tube. Otorrhea may occur episodically as the result of an otherwise asymptomatic tympanic membrane perforation, especially if water has inadvertently entered the middle ear space. Patients with a history of painless drainage for many months or years are highly suspect of harboring a temporal bone cholesteatoma. This is especially true if the drainage fails to resolve after vigorous treatment with systemic and topical antibiotics. Drainage associated with pain is more likely to be caused by an acute infectious process.

A perforation resulting from acute otitis media may be preceded by severe ear pain. Acute external otitis is frequently manifested by the simultaneous occurrence of aural drainage and acute ear pain. The prolonged use of antibiotic drops should alert the examiner to the possibility of fungal otitis, which occurs principally as a complication of broad-spectrum antibiotic treatment. Patients who routinely occlude the external auditory canal with hearing instruments or protective earplugs are more difficult to treat because occlusion of the canal interferes with the normal cleansing mechanism of the ear.

Vertigo

Vertigo—dizziness—has a myriad of causes, many of which are entirely unrelated to the temporal bone and ear. A detailed history is the most important piece of information in establishing a diagnosis. The following points should be clearly ascertained in every patient history:

- What exactly does the patient mean by "dizziness"?

- What does he or she experience?

- When did the symptoms first occur, how often do they occur, and how long do they last when they do occur?

- What is the shortest and longest time the dizziness has lasted?

- Is the dizziness associated with nausea, vomiting, or sweating?

- Is the patient aware of any change in hearing before, during, or after the dizzy spell?

- Do any activities reliably bring on the dizzy spell?

- Is the dizzy spell associated with any difficulty in swallowing or speaking or change in vision?

- Is consciousness ever completely lost during a dizzy spell?

- Is there associated tinnitus or a feeling of aural fullness?

- Can the patient tell when a dizzy episode is about to occur?

The answers to these questions vary dramatically. Vertigo arising from the vestibular system generally has as its principal component "the illusion of motion." This may be a sense of rotation or the sense of falling to one side or the other. When the patient uses such descriptors as *light-headed, giddy, confused, or faint*, the sensation is not likely to be of labyrinthine origin.

A special inquiry should be made into whether the patient has headaches before, during, or after each episode of vertigo or disequilibrium. It should be established whether a familial history of migraine exists. Migraine is a much more common cause of episodic vertigo in childhood than in adulthood and accounts for a substantial number of children with intermittent dizzy spells.

It is important to inquire about the patient's other medical problems, especially visual difficulties, history of diabetes, stroke, or hypertension. Additionally, obtain a list of the patient's medications. Elderly patients have a high incidence of balance complaints, many of which are exacerbated by medications. Antihypertensive medications can contribute to autonomic dysfunction, which may be attributed, in error, to the vestibular system. Careful evaluation of the history in light of basic audiometry will usually establish whether the vertigo is likely to be otogenic in origin and will probably suggest a diagnosis. Further diagnostic tests can then be ordered to confirm or deny these initial conclusions.

Physical Examination of the Ear Canal

Examination of the ear begins with examination of the auricle. The size and shape of the auricle and its position should be carefully noted. Some children will have no auricle as a result of congenital aural atresia; some will have one that is abnormally small or poorly formed (**Fig. 5–1**); other children may have an auricle placed either unusually low with respect to the remainder of the facial skeleton or unusually high.

The size and adequacy of the ear canal should be assessed. Some patients have collapsing ear canals with a slit-like opening, especially very young children. This should be noted before audiometry so that insert earphones can be used when hearing is tested to avoid prolapsing canals with supra-aural earphones. To assess the inner portion of the ear canal, the auricle should be drawn backward and upward. This opens the lateral portion of the cartilaginous

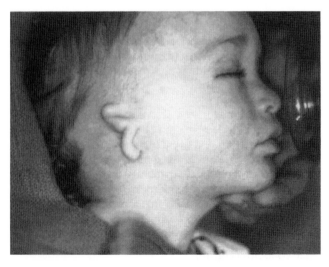

Figure 5–1 Young boy with unilateral microtia, or abnormal formation of the external ear.

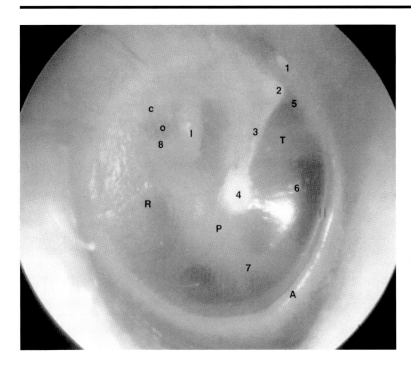

Figure 5–2 Normal tympanic membrane, right ear. 1, pars flaccida; 2, short process of the malleus; 3, handle of the malleus; 4, umbo; 5, supratubal recess; 6, tubal orifice; 7, hypotympanic air cells; 8, stapedius tendon; c, chorda tympani; I, incus; P, promontory; o, oval window; R, round window; T, tensor tympani; A, annulus. (From (2002) Color Atlas of Otoscopy: From Diagnosis to Surgery (2nd ed.). p. 22, Fig. 2.1, with permission.) *(See Color Plate 5–2.)*

canal and permits assessment of the bony canal. An otoscope may then be used to examine the external auditory canal and tympanic membrane.

Preliminary examination of the size of the canal will allow the appropriate-sized speculum to be selected. The largest speculum that can be comfortably inserted into the patient's ear canal should be chosen for maximum visualization. Specula for use in the ear canal are designed in such a way that they rarely protrude farther into the ear than the cartilaginous portion of the canal. This portion can be stretched and manipulated with minimal or no discomfort. Should the speculum reach the inner third of the ear canal, even the slightest pressure will be extraordinarily painful. The patient's head needs to be tilted toward the opposite shoulder to account for the normal upward direction of the ear canal.

It will often be necessary to remove cerumen from the external auditory canal to examine the tympanic membrane. Cerumen that is deep in the canal or is impacted may be very difficult to remove by untrained professionals. Such patients should be referred to an otolaryngologist, who can remove the cerumen by use of the operating microscope if other removal techniques are contraindicated or have failed. Occasionally, a general anesthetic will be required for cerumen removal in young children to reduce movement and to prevent harm to the ear canal and tympanic membrane.

Every attempt should be made to visualize the entire tympanic membrane. Otoscopic or microscopic examination of the ear cannot be considered complete until the entire tympanic membrane, including the pars flaccida, has been visualized. The anulus tympanicus should be followed anteriorly and posteriorly until it meets the anterior and posterior malleolar folds. The pars flaccida lies between these two folds (**Fig. 5–2**). Perforation or deep retraction of the pars flaccida is virtually diagnostic of a cholesteatoma. Both the long and short processes of the malleus can be seen

in the normal drum and their presence should be noted. The long process of the incus and the chorda tympani nerve can frequently, although not invariably, be seen through a normal tympanic membrane (**Fig. 5–3**). However, if the head of the malleus or body of the incus is seen, erosion of the superior auditory canal and lateral wall of the middle ear space has occurred. This is seen almost exclusively in cholesteatoma. Occasionally, a retracted drum lies directly on the incudostapedial

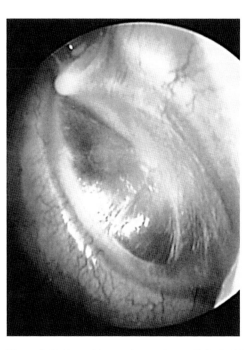

Figure 5–3 Normal tympanic membrane. Note that the short process of the incus and the malleus are well visualized. *(See Color Plate 5–3.)*

joint, forming a "myringostapediopexy." In such circumstances, long-term retraction probably caused by eustachian tube insufficiency can be assumed. Surprisingly, hearing can often be near normal in such situations.

A pneumatic otoscope is used to create positive or negative pressure on the tympanic membrane. Such pressure changes normally cause visible movement of the tympanic membrane. Using the pneumatic otoscope, the examiner can assess the degree of mobility of the tympanic membrane. Chronic middle ear effusion, for example, usually results in a sluggish or immobile tympanic membrane. In addition, brisk tympanic movements virtually exclude the possibility of tympanic membrane perforation. Often, a tympanic membrane perforation may heal without the middle fibrous layer of the eardrum, resulting in an extremely thin "secondary" membrane that is always translucent and often transparent. Such secondary membranes may be indistinguishable from perforations without the use of the operating microscope. Pneumatic otoscopy with the handheld otoscope can sometimes induce movement in healed secondary membranes, which makes it apparent that the drum is indeed intact although quite thin. Immittance testing can also confirm the presence of an intact membrane with a type A tympanogram.

Masses behind the tympanic membrane may be caused by a variety of pathological processes. Color is important and may be a clue to the cause. White masses suggest cholesteatoma, tympanosclerosis (**Fig. 5–4**), or, very rarely, middle ear osteoma. Dark blue masses suggest venous vascular structures, such as a high jugular bulb. Dark red masses suggest highly vascular tumors such as glomus tympanicum tumors or granulation tissue. The presence of pulsations within a mass strongly suggests that it is arterialized and vascular in origin. This can sometimes be confirmed by applying positive pressure to the tympanic membrane with the pneumatic otoscope. Positive pressure reduces blood flow within the mass and causes blanching of the drum overlying the middle ear mass. Such blanching is referred to as a positive Brown's sign and strongly suggests a vascular neoplasm. Occasionally, a red blotch will be seen in the area of the oval window. This may not be a mass but may represent the hypervascular bone characteristic of an active focus of otosclerosis.

No otologic examination is complete without evaluation of facial nerve function. The patient should be asked to frown, smile, wrinkle his nose, whistle, show his teeth, and shut his eyes. Any asymmetry between sides or the inability to perform any of these motions should be clearly noted. The earliest and most subtle sign of facial weakness is lagophthalmos. The eyelid closes a bit more slowly on the affected side than on the normal, contralateral side. This is clearly evident when the patient blinks spontaneously. The blink on the affected side appears to lag behind its normal contralateral partner.

> **Pitfall**
>
> • The examiner should be wary of the "dimeric membrane," which is the result of a tympanic membrane perforation healing without the middle fibrous layer of the eardrum. Dimeric membranes can be distinguished from tympanic membrane perforations by microscopy or pneumatic otoscopy.

◆ Disorders of the Ear Canal

Dermatitis

Seborrheic dermatitis is the most common type of dermatitis to affect the external auditory canal and is usually manifested by chronic itching and dry, flaky skin over the conchal bowl and within the lateral external auditory canal. Often there is a complete or near absence of cerumen. In addition to affecting the ear canal, there is often involvement of the scalp, eyebrows, nasal ala, and retroauricular creases with fine scale. The condition is important not only because the itching is subjectively distressing but also because the chronic irritation of the skin of the external canal reduces its effectiveness as a barrier to infection. Patients with chronic dermatitis are more susceptible to chronic bacterial external otitis than the normal population. In patients who present with recurrent episodes of external otitis, many will be discovered to have chronic, dry, flaking, and pruritic (itchy) external auditory canals. The condition is unpredictable, with some patients having little problem for years but with sporadic "flare-ups" lasting weeks to months. Often treatment of the ear canals with 2% hydrocortisone cream two or three times per week is sufficient. In more resistant cases, a more potent steroid may be needed. Some cases respond to the simple application of mineral oil or other emollient without the use of any medication whatsoever.

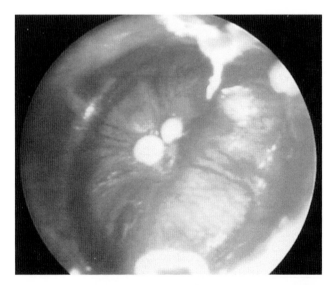

Figure 5–4 Two small white masses are visualized in the center of the tympanic membrane. These are cholesteatomas that have been implanted on the eardrum. *(See Color Plate 5–4.)*

Allergic dermatitis is another type of dermatitis that frequently occurs in response to exogenous materials placed in or around the ear canal. Many allergic reactions are seen in response to topical antibiotic drops, especially neomycin (Sood et al, 2002). Allergic reactions to neomycin and other topical antibiotics occur in two distinct forms. A fulminant (acute) form is occasionally seen that results in massive swelling of the canal, intense pain and tenderness, and skin color and texture changes involving the conchal bowl, lobule, and frequently the skin of the neck. This requires immediate discontinuation of the offending agent and the use of both topical and systemic steroid medications. A more indolent (chronic) form of hypersensitivity is manifested simply by the failure of a typical external otitis to resolve in response to what appears to be appropriate antibiotic therapy. Chronic drainage, edema of the external auditory canal, pain, and tenderness persist in the presence of both topical drops and mechanical cleansing. Discontinuing the offending agent and treating the external otitis with a nonantibiotic drop containing an antiseptic with or without a topical steroid can adequately treat such reactions. Allergic reactions of both the fulminant and indolent types can occur due to the materials from which both earmolds and earplugs are made. The mainstay of treatment is replacement of the offending agent with a more hypoallergenic material.

Acute Otitis Externa

Acute external bacterial otitis is an infection of the ear canal and portions of the pinna. The disorder is of relatively sudden onset and is characterized by severe pain localized to the affected external auditory canal. An important diagnostic feature is extreme sensitivity to any movement of the auricle or tissues surrounding the external auditory canal. Such tenderness is helpful in distinguishing external otitis from acute otitis media. The pain of acute otitis media is unaffected by even vigorous auricular movement. Erythema may be present, and severe cases may have sufficient subepithelial edema as to cause a pale blanching of the superficial tissues. Physical examination will show mucopurulent exudates, often thin or scant, accumulating in the external auditory canal, marked swelling of the tissues of the ear canal, and "weeping" (**Fig. 5–5**). In many cases it is not possible to examine the tympanic membrane fully because of the exquisite tenderness of the canal and a marked amount of canal swelling. There is rarely associated fever, malaise, or other sign of systemic infection.

Gram-positive bacteria commonly colonize normal ear canals and cerumen. Of the gram-positive organisms, staphylococci are most common, followed by coryneform bacteria, streptococci, enterococci, bacilli, and micrococci. Fungi can be cultured from normal ears as well, with *Candida* and *Penicillium* species found (Stroman et al, 2001). Bacterial organisms, generally gram-negative rods such as *Pseudomonas*, cause most external otitis. Staphylococci, followed by coryneform bacteria, are the next most common organisms to cause acute otitis externa. Fungi are only rarely cultured from ears with acute otitis externa (Roland and Stroman, 2002).

Pseudomonas is relatively ubiquitous in the environment, and in the appropriate circumstances may be pathogenic.

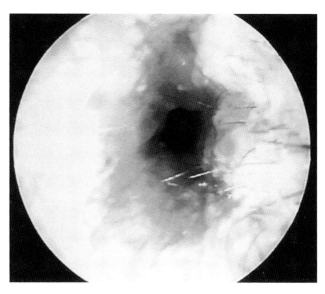

Figure 5–5   Bacterial otitis externa has led to a swollen ear canal with purulent debris. *(See Color Plate 5–5.)*

It is extremely sensitive to the local acidity of its environment and is incapable of growing or reproducing in low pH settings. Cerumen appears to maintain a slightly acidic environment, which prevents the growth of *Pseudomonas*. Introduction of water into the ear canal when swimming serves to wash out the normal acidity of the canal and may substitute a slightly alkali environment. In such circumstances, *Pseudomonas* may produce infection. This likely explains the finding that the incidence of acute bacterial otitis externa in summer is over 4 times the incidence in nonsummer months, as most swimming occurs during these months (Roland and Stroman, 2002).

Treatment of this disease process includes debridement (removal of infected tissue and purulent material), topical delivery of acidifying and antibacterial agents, and systemic antibacterial therapy. Preparations that combine antibiotics and corticosteroids, such as ciprofloxacin-dexamethasone, have been found in controlled studies to be more effective than topical antibiotics alone and should be considered first-line therapy in most cases (Roland et al, 2004). An external canal that is swollen closed can be addressed effectively by placing a small wick into the canal. The wick is made of an expandable material and draws the topical medication into the canal. When a large amount of mucopurulent debris has accumulated in the canal, mechanical removal of the debris using the operating microscope and suction is essential and crucial to successful management. In severe cases, such cleansing may need to be done on a daily or an every-other-day basis.

Pearl

- Avoid deliberately placing water in the ear of a diabetic patient, even for cerumen removal. This could lead to a medium favoring bacterial growth, which, in a diabetic patient who is prone to infections, could lead to necrotizing external otitis.

Fungal Otitis Externa (Otomycosis)

A wide variety of fungi colonize normal ear canals. Most often the fungal organisms grow on desquamated epithelium, cerumen, or the inspissated mucopurulent debris from a previous bacterial infection. True fungal external otitis with tissue invasion of fungal elements is uncommon and limited to those who are significantly immunocompromised. A recent review found only 1.7% of total isolates from ears diagnosed with acute otitis externa to be fungal organisms (Roland and Stroman, 2002). However, otomycosis can be a prevalent and troubling problem in the hot and humid areas of tropical climates, where the moisture and warmth fungi prefer predominate. In addition, healthy individuals subjected to long-term treatments with systemic antimicrobials or topical antibiotics may be at risk to develop fungal infections of the ear canal. This is of particular concern in children with tympanostomy tubes treated with multiple courses of ototopical antibiotics for post-tympanostomy tube otorrhea. Recent evidence shows they may be at risk to develop chronic otorrhea due to fungal infection (Schrader and Isaacson, 2003). Almost all clinically significant fungal otitis is caused by either *Candida* or *Aspergillus* species. Most often patients complain of chronic irritating itch, discharge, pain, hearing impairment, or a blocked sensation. Treatment involves discontinuation of antibiotic therapy, aural cleansing, removal of foreign bodies such as tympanostomy tubes, and the use of antiseptics, such as merbromin or gentian violet. Acidifying agents are also useful, as many fungi are sensitive to ambient pH. Occasionally, especially in immunocompromised individuals, the use of topical or even systemic antifungals may become necessary.

Malignant Otitis Externa

Malignant otitis externa (MOE)—osteomyelitis of the temporal bone and skull base—is a rare though life-threatening disease that begins in the ear canal and proceeds to invade the bone of the skull base. It is most often associated with elderly diabetic patients with poor glycemic control but can develop in patients with human immunodeficiency virus (HIV) and other immunocompromised states (Sreepada and Kwartler, 2003). *Pseudomonas* is the causative organism in nearly all cases of MOE associated with diabetes. Fungal infections may be the infecting organism in immunocompromised patients.

Radiological examination begins with computed tomography (CT) to evaluate the initial extent of soft tissue and skull base involvement. Technetium 99m scintigraphy is a rapid and inexpensive test used for evaluation of bony involvement and will show uptake early in the course of the disease. Gallium 67 citrate scans are more expensive and time consuming and will show uptake to areas of soft tissue involved in inflammation. These scans will show decreased uptake as the inflammation clears and are typically used to monitor for resolution of infection. Some authors suggest that the ease of administration of the technetium scan argues for its use as an initial monitor for response to treatment and would save gallium scanning for cases where the technetium scan remains positive nearing the end of treatment (Okpala et al, 2005).

Treatment of MOE may begin with oral quinolones and meticulous cleansing of the ear canal under the microscope. Treatment failures must be considered for inpatient intravenous antibiotic therapy. Ciprofloxacin is the drug of choice, although recent reports caution about the emergence of resistant strains (Berenholz et al, 2002).

Congenital Aural Atresia and Anotia/Microtia

Congenital aural atresias can involve the pinna, ear canal, middle ear space, or ossicles. Such malformations may occur alone or in association with other regional or distant malformations. A variety of different syndromes have been identified that are associated with malformations of the ear (**Table 5–1**). Malformations of the external and middle ear occur approximately once in every 10,000 to 20,000 births. The malformation occurs unilaterally 4 times more frequently than it does bilaterally. Because embryological development of the ear is finished by week 28 of gestation, injuries that occur in late pregnancy will not affect otologic development. Portions of the external auditory canal and middle ear develop from the same underlying embryological structures, so middle ear malformations are frequently associated with malformations of the ear canal. Fortunately, however, the cochlea, semicircular canals, and CN VIII are rarely affected. Most individuals with congenital aural atresia have a normally functioning sensorineural auditory system. The anatomical course of the facial nerve is frequently altered in malformations of the ear and temporal bone, but facial nerve function is rarely affected by the malformation. A bony plate frequently replaces the tympanic membrane, and a large variety of malformations and deformities to the ossicles may be present.

When gross malformation of the auricle occurs, the atresia is usually identified promptly, often on the day of birth. Malformation of the auricle is termed *anotia* when there is complete absence of an external ear and *microtia* when there is a vestige present. When the pinna is normal, identification of a stenotic or atretic ear canal may be delayed for several years. Physical examination should include a search for other anomalies, microscope evaluation of the contralateral ear, and assessment of facial nerve function. If an ear canal is present on the affected side, it is important

Table 5–1   Syndromes Associated with Congenital Aural Atresia

Alport's syndrome	Crouzon's disease
Marfan syndrome	Osteogenesis imperfecta
Treacher Collins syndrome	Pierre Robin syndrome
Goldenhar's syndrome	Franceschetti syndrome
Nager's acrofacial dysostosis	Wildervanck syndrome
Sprengel's deformity	Pyle's disease
Paget's disease	Möbius' syndrome
Levy-Hollister (LADD) syndrome	CHARGE syndrome
Alagille syndrome	Andersen's disease
Fraser's syndrome	Lenz's syndrome
Noonan's syndrome	

CHARGE, coloboma of the eye, heart anomaly, choanal atresia, retardation, and genital and ear anomalies; LADD, lacrimoauriculodentodigital syndrome.

to assess for medial canal stenosis or atresia. This may be difficult in young children, and radiographic assessment may be required.

On initial evaluation, more important than radiographic assessment is accurate determination of hearing thresholds. Auditory brainstem response (ABR) testing of both air and bone conduction is pivotal because hearing rehabilitation must occur long before these children are surgical candidates. Should a child have only unilateral involvement, further evaluation may be deferred until age 5 or 6. However, amplification must be provided immediately when a child is found to have bilateral involvement or if there is any question regarding hearing. The available options include the use of conventional amplification, externally applied bone-conducting hearing aids, and implantable bone-conducting hearing aids. As a general rule, when conventional amplification can be used, it is the treatment of choice. The use of an implantable bone-conducting aid, when appropriate, is preferred in patients with bilateral maximal conductive hearing losses and normal bone levels if they cannot be successfully fitted with conventional hearing aids.

Surgical repair of the external auditory canal, tympanic membrane, and middle ear space can be accomplished by a variety of different techniques. A grading scheme has been developed to assist in selection of those patients with the best potential for success and is based on anatomical variables found on high-resolution CT. Favorable outcomes are more likely in individuals with the least severe abnormalities. Successful surgery should be defined as a postoperative speech reception threshold of 15 to 25 dB hearing level (HL). Although repair of unilateral atresia has been controversial in the past, in children deemed good candidates and with parents who are realistic about postoperative results, surgical repair may be attempted (Trigg and Applebaum, 1988). Complications of surgery include injury to the facial nerve on rare occasions, high-frequency sensorineural hearing loss in 15% of cases, inability to close the air–bone gap to less than 30 dB, and restenosis of the ear canal (McKinnon and Jahrsdoerfer, 2002). Surgical repair of anotia or microtia is often handled earlier than atresia repair by a cosmetic facial surgeon once the patient reaches an age when his or her rib is of sufficient size for use as a graft material to create the scaffolding for a new external ear.

Controversial Point

- Whether surgical repair of unilateral atresia should be undertaken depends entirely on the patient and the parents. It is often useful to wait until the child is old enough to participate in the decision for surgical repair of the congenital atresia in unilateral cases. Surgical intervention is not without risks and complications.

Osteomas and Exostoses

Osteomas and exostoses are two distinct lesions of the ear canal that may develop and cause obstruction. These lesions are frequently confused but on histopathology are quite different. On clinical grounds there are several distinguishing features.

Exostoses are periosteal outgrowths that develop in the bony ear canal, usually in individuals who are often exposed to cold water. These lesions are often multiple and bilateral and only require removal in the case of severe conductive hearing loss or recurrent otitis externa (Tran et al, 1996). Osteomas, in contrast, are usually unilateral, pedunculated lesions that occur at the bony-cartilaginous junction of the ear canal. They are considered the most common bony neoplasm of the temporal bone. The indications for surgery for osteomas are similar to those for exostoses (Tran et al, 1996).

Keratosis Obturans

Keratosis obturans presents as an accumulation of keratin in the ear canal. Classically, these lesions are associated with acute conductive hearing loss, pain, a widened canal, thick tympanic membrane, and otorrhea. It occurs most commonly in younger individuals and is usually bilateral. It has been associated with systemic diseases such as bronchiectasis and sinusitis. Though not completely understood, the etiology of this disease is felt to be due to abnormal epithelial migration or excessive production of epithelial cells. Treatment involves regular aural cleaning and does not usually require surgery (Persaud et al, 2004).

Pitfall

- Keratosis obturans is often confused with external ear canal cholesteatoma. Cholesteatoma tends to affect older individuals, occurs in a discrete portion of the canal, and shows osteonecrosis (bone erosion) or bony sequestration (devascularized bone). Shallow canal cholesteatoma can be treated by marsupialization of the cholesteatoma sac. This involves incising the sac to create a pouch. Larger, deeper cholesteatomas require surgical excision.

◆ Neoplasms of the External Auditory Canal

Malignant cancer of the ear canal is rare. Histology most often shows squamous cell carcinoma; however, basal cell carcinoma, adenoid cystic carcinoma, adenocarcinoma, ceruminous carcinoma, and malignant fibrous histiocytoma have been reported. Most commonly, patients complain of otorrhea, aural fullness, pain, itching, and hearing loss (Nyrop and Grontved, 2002). Generally speaking, this disease is difficult to cure, as many patients present late in the course of disease, making complete resection difficult. Most patients undergo surgical resection of their lesion with postoperative radiation.

◆ Disorders of the Tympanic Membrane, Middle Ear, and Mastoid Process

Tympanic Membrane Perforations

Tympanic membrane perforations can arise as a consequence of either infection or trauma. Acute otitis media frequently results in perforation of the tympanic membrane. Such perforations often heal spontaneously, but occasionally the perforation fails to heal and becomes a permanent feature of the tympanic membrane. Severe, acute, necrotizing otitis media, almost always as a result of a streptococcal infection, has a much higher incidence of tympanic membrane perforation than the usual middle ear infections. Chronic infection with an unusual organism, such as tuberculosis, produces a much higher rate of permanent tympanic membrane perforation than occurs in the epidemic otitis media of schoolchildren.

Traumatic causes of perforation can include blasts, blunt and penetrating trauma, barotrauma, iatrogenic injury, and thermal and chemical burn. "Blast" trauma is much more common than penetrating injury. A slap to the side of the head, which completely occludes the external auditory canal, forcing a column of air down onto the tympanic membrane and rupturing it, is one form of blast trauma.

Most perforations heal spontaneously. When infection complicates an acute tympanic membrane perforation, the probability of spontaneous healing is significantly reduced. Increasing age (>30 years), malnutrition, and immunosuppression are felt to impair healing. In addition, large and central perforations or those in the posterosuperior quadrant are felt to have a diminished chance to heal spontaneously (Rizer, 1997).

Perforations of the tympanic membrane diagnosed on physical examination should be first categorized as to their location. They may occur in either the pars tensa or the pars flaccida. Perforations of the pars flaccida may be assumed to be cholesteatomas and should be managed as such. Perforations in the pars tensa can be divided into those that are central and those that are marginal. A central perforation has at least a small rim of intact tympanic membrane around it (**Fig. 5–6**). Marginal perforations extend all the way to the bony annulus of the external auditory canal. It is often difficult and sometimes impossible to determine whether an anterior perforation is marginal because the anterior canal wall makes it difficult to see the most anterior portion of the tympanic membrane. The distinction is important because marginal perforations have the potential to develop into cholesteatomas and should be considered dangerous. Central perforations are unlikely to develop into cholesteatomas and are sometimes referred to as "safe" perforations. Size can be recorded in terms of an estimate of diameter in millimeters or an estimate of the percentage of tympanic membrane involved in the perforation. The location should also be identified in terms of which quadrant or quadrants of the tympanic membrane are involved. Both location and size are important factors in determining the amount of conductive hearing loss expected with a particular perforation.

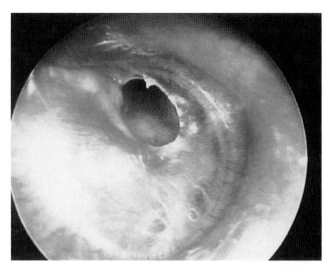

Figure 5–6 A small central perforation is seen involving the posterosuperior portion of the tympanic membrane. *(See Color Plate 5–6.)*

Perforations cause difficulties due to their potential to form cholesteatoma, as discussed above, significant conductive hearing loss, and recurrent infections. Hearing loss caused by tympanic membrane perforations is highly variable. Small pinpoint perforations may have no associated hearing loss, whereas larger perforations may produce losses up to 50 dB HL. Conductive hearing losses greater than 40 to 50 dB HL suggest associated ossicular discontinuity or fixation. Perforations may lead to infections by permitting bacterial entry into the middle ear space. If water is allowed into the ear canal, it is particularly likely to carry bacteria into this normally sterile space and increase the rate of infection. Protection of the middle ear space from water is an essential aspect of perforation management and should be advocated for swimming or bathing. Chronic obstruction of the external auditory canal also increases the likelihood of infections. Patients who use hearing aids or earplugs in an ear with a chronic perforation are much more likely to develop infections and chronic otorrhea.

The treatment of tympanic membrane perforations is surgical repair. In individuals with marginal perforations, the risk of developing cholesteatoma is sufficient to warrant surgical repair in most cases. Repair of central perforations, however, is entirely elective.

Pearl

- All apparent perforations in the pars flaccida are cholesteatomas.

Tympanic Membrane Retractions

Tympanic membrane retractions have been defined as any inward displacement of the tympanic membrane from its normal position. Retractions may be further classified as

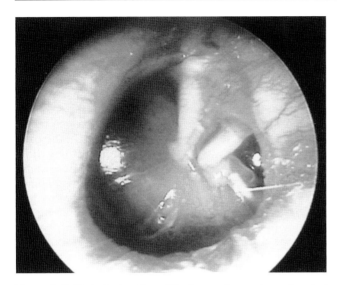

Figure 5–7 Marked retraction of the tympanic membrane is noted with a middle ear effusion. The incudostapedial joint is easily visualized. *(See Color Plate 5–3.)*

Special Consideration

- Patients with poor eustachian tube function and tympanic membrane perforation may need to have a permanent tympanostomy tube placed at the time of tympanic membrane repair.

Otitis Media

The eustachian tube serves to provide normal middle ear pressure when open and protect the middle ear from reflux and nasopharyngeal bacteria when closed. Abnormal eustachian tube function appears to be a common pathological feature in the development of otitis media. When chronically open (patulous), secretions from the nasopharynx may enter the middle ear and produce infection. When chronically closed, due to inflammation or tumors, consequences may include persistent or recurrent middle ear effusions with or without infection, tympanic membrane retractions or perforations, or further complications associated with the inner ear, mastoid process, or CNS. Infants and children are predisposed to otitis media because their eustachian tubes are more horizontal, shorter, and wider than those of adults. In addition, their palatal muscle function is less efficient, and therefore the active tubal opening is less reliable and vigorous.

Acute otitis media (AOM) is one of the most common diseases of early childhood. It affects more than 90% of children by the age of 7 and accounts for more than 25% of the prescriptions for oral antibiotics annually (Jung and Hanson, 1999). The peak incidence occurs between 6 and 24 months of age, and the disease is seen more frequently in the winter months. Exposure to secondhand smoke, male gender, and placement in day care facilities appear to increase the incidence of otitis media. AOM is caused by infection from one of several different relatively common bacteria and generally responds to prompt antibiotic therapy. Clinically, patients suffer from rapid onset of fever, pain, irritability, malaise, and elevated white blood cell count. The middle ear mucosa becomes edematous and hyperemic, and hemorrhage may occur. Local infiltration of white blood cells then follows and appears on physical exam as an accumulation of pus within the middle ear space (**Fig. 5–8**). The infection causes extreme pain to the patient, although there is no tenderness to the auricle or periauricular tissues as seen in otitis externa.

When untreated, AOM often resolves with spontaneous rupture of the tympanic membrane. The perforation in the tympanic membrane allows pus to drain from the middle ear and is often followed by rapid relief of pain and resolution of fever. In more than 90% of cases, the tympanic membrane heals spontaneously. When treated properly, most cases of AOM resolve without complication. However, despite the overall decrease in rates of complications compared with the preantibiotic era, life-threatening complications are still seen, often due to antibiotic-resistant bacteria. Complications include mastoiditis, facial nerve palsy, labyrinthitis with complete sensorineural hearing loss, meningitis, and brain abscess. Though currently most practitioners in the United States treat AOM with high-dose amoxicillin, it should be

simple retractions, when the diameter of the external opening is larger than that of the inner portion, or retraction pocket, when the diameter of the external opening is smaller. Retractions occur almost exclusively as a result of eustachian tube dysfunction. The normally functioning eustachian tube remains closed at rest but should open periodically to equalize middle ear pressure with ambient barometric pressure. The eustachian tubes are opened by active muscular contraction of small palatal muscles during swallowing or yawning. If the tube remains chronically shut, negative pressure will develop in the middle ear, which may result in a retracted tympanic membrane, middle ear effusion, or both (**Fig. 5–7**).

Development of deep retractions in the pars flaccida or pars tensa of the tympanic membrane leads to cholesteatoma. In addition, prolonged contact of the retracted tympanic membrane with the ossicles can cause ossicular erosion, ossicular discontinuity, and conductive hearing loss. Li et al (1999) reviewed a series of pediatric patients with otitis media with effusion who had developed retractions of the tympanic membrane. Although on average there was 5 dB hearing loss for pars tensa retractions and 6 dB for pars flaccida retractions, the researchers noted large intersubject variability, with some children having thresholds as poor as 30 dB HL. In addition, although they noted no significant relationship of severity of retraction with static admittance or tympanometric width, they did note significantly lower tympanometric peak pressures in children with retraction (Li et al, 1999).

Treatment of retractions is difficult, especially in the pars flaccida region. If even a partially ventilated middle ear space is present, a pressure-equalizing tube may be inserted into the region of the retraction. In cases of deep pars flaccida retraction that cannot be fully visualized, middle ear exploration to rule out the presence of cholesteatoma is warranted.

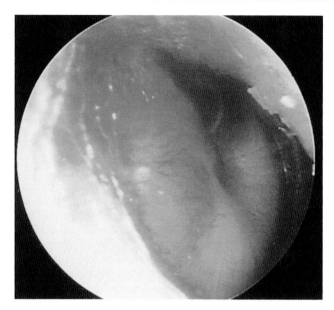

Figure 5–8 Purulent material is visualized behind a bulging tympanic membrane in acute otitis media. *(See Color Plate 5–8.)*

noted that watchful waiting is a valid strategy. The most recent evidence-based clinical practice guidelines for AOM published by the Agency for Healthcare Research and Quality (AHRQ) in 2004 allow for observation without antibiotics in otherwise healthy children (Kenna, 2005). Critical to this strategy of management is the presence of reliable follow-up and lack of signs of complications of otitis media.

A single episode of otitis media is generally followed by an effusion that clears within 3 months in 90% of cases. When the middle ear space harbors fluid for more than 3 months, the condition is termed *chronic middle ear effusion* (**Fig. 5–9**). Although culture of such fluid shows that it often does contain few bacteria, the condition is not properly referred to as an infection, as there is no pain, fever, or development of purulence. Many patients are completely asymptomatic. The persistence of fluid in and of itself is of no great consequence. The main concern with the presence of middle ear effusion is the presence of hearing loss or other symptoms. Such other symptoms in children may include disturbed sleep, imbalance, unexplained clumsiness, delayed speech or language, or recurrent AOM in addition to persistent effusion. In the past, recommendation was made for tympanostomy tube placement when middle ear effusion has lasted more than 4 to 6 months. However, the most recent guidelines by the AHRQ recommend surgery for persistent middle ear effusion when hearing loss is present to >20 dB HL, other symptoms remain present for a prolonged time, or when the patient is considered at risk for speech, language, or learning problems (Kenna, 2005). As with the case of AOM, it is essential to reexamine patients and assess hearing at appropriate intervals for those in whom observation of middle ear effusion is chosen. In addition, it is important to remember that conductive hearing loss associated with middle ear effusions is variable, and audiometric evaluation may occur when a child is hearing relatively well. Therefore, the input of parents or teachers should be given great credence. When a documented or even suspected problem with the acquisition of speech and language skills or difficulty in school exists, it is important to consider placement of tympanostomy tubes to eliminate the possibility of mild conductive hearing loss as an etiologic or confounding variable.

Tympanostomy tubes serve as prosthetic eustachian tubes, providing pressure regulation such that the external auditory canal and middle ear space equalize (**Fig. 5–10**). In addition, middle ear fluid may drain via the tube into the ear canal. For younger children, general anesthesia is necessary to perform this procedure. In older children and adults, it may be accomplished in the office with a topical

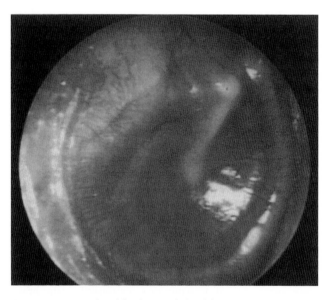

Figure 5–9 Tan-colored fluid is seen behind the tympanic membrane in chronic otitis media.

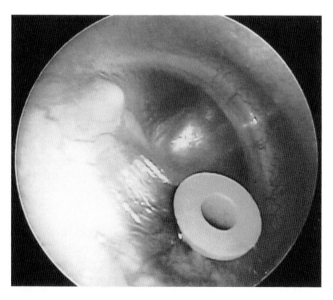

Figure 5–10 Otitis media with effusion has resolved with the placement of a tympanostomy tube. *(See Color Plate 5–10.)*

anesthetic. The tubes are spontaneously extruded from the tympanic membrane about 1 year after placement. Complications of tympanostomy tubes include recurrent or persistent otorrhea, retained tubes for longer than 2 years, foreign body reaction with granulation tissue formation, tympanic membrane perforation following extrusion, tympanosclerosis, and iatrogenic cholesteatoma (Derkay et al, 2000). It is useful to note that by far the most common complication is otorrhea and that the more serious complications occur infrequently. For example, one study estimated an incidence of post-tympanostomy tube otorrhea of 7.8%, whereas tympanic membrane perforation occurs on average only 1.7% of the time (Derkay et al, 2000). In most cases, tympanostomy tube otorrhea is treated with a course of topical antibiotic drops given over 5 to 7 days, which eliminates the drainage. Although tympanosclerosis of the tympanic membrane does appear related to placement of tubes, it is generally of no consequence, as no hearing loss develops.

Children with craniofacial abnormalities such as Down syndrome, cleft palate, Crouzon's syndrome, and Treacher Collins syndrome are predisposed to otitis media and frequently require multiple sets of tympanostomy tubes. These patients should be evaluated early in life for hearing difficulties and middle ear effusions. Almost all will benefit from tympanostomy tubes. In children with sensorineural hearing loss, the use of tympanostomy tubes is urgent. When the sensorineural component is severe to profound, elimination of the conductive component may be the difference between aidable and unaidable hearing. Other children who may benefit from tympanostomy tubes are those with a history of febrile seizures and those with drug allergies to common antibiotics. In children who develop recurrent symptoms of middle ear effusion after their first set of tympanostomy tubes have extruded, adenoidectomy should be considered concurrent with the second set of tympanostomy tubes.

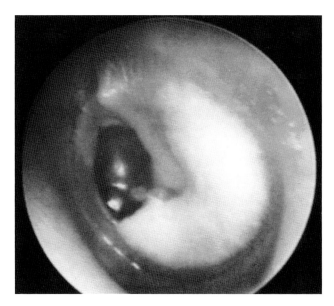

Figure 5–11 Tympanosclerosis is noted involving three fourths of the tympanic membrane. *(See Color Plate 5–11.)*

hearing loss. Tympanometry will often show type A_s tympanogram, indicating increased stiffness of the tympanic membrane. Most would agree that inflammatory processes in the middle ear incite development of tympanosclerosis. It appears that cytokines (inflammatory mediators), free radicals (by-products of metabolism that can alter proteins, deoxyribonucleic acid [DNA], and lipids), and nitric oxide (a molecule produced by inflammatory cells) may play a particular role in this disorder (Karlidag et al, 2004).

Pearl

- The audiologist can often serve to reinforce the recommendations of tympanostomy tubes in children when parents appear hesitant by reviewing the effects of mild hearing loss on speech and language development.

Pitfall

- Although it appears tempting to remove tympanosclerosis from the ossicles, it is usually unsuccessful. Hearing aids are the best option for hearing rehabilitation in this group of patients.

Tympanosclerosis and Myringosclerosis

Tympanosclerotic plaques are calcified (bone-like) portions of connective tissue that may form along the tympanic membrane or the heads of the ossicles within the middle ear space (**Fig. 5–11**). When limited to the tympanic membrane, this is termed *myringosclerosis*. Patients often have a history of acute or chronic otitis media. Myringosclerosis is more common and only rarely associated with hearing loss. Tympanosclerosis, however, will produce fixation of the ossicles and maximum conductive

Cholesteatoma

The lateral surface of the tympanic membrane is composed of stratified squamous epithelium, the same composition as skin, and like skin in other portions of the body, it sheds epithelial cells. Normally, the external auditory canal removes these desquamated products as they are produced. If a sufficient portion of the tympanic membrane is retracted far enough into the mastoid process, these products are unable to escape out of the canal and instead accumulate as a mass of dead skin within the temporal bone. Such collections of desquamated skin cells will erode bone slowly through a combination of pressure necrosis and enzymatic activity and is termed a *cholesteatoma*. The condition has also been

ACQUIRED CHOLESTEATOMA OF THE ATTIC

LATERAL ROUTE

MEDIAL ROUTE

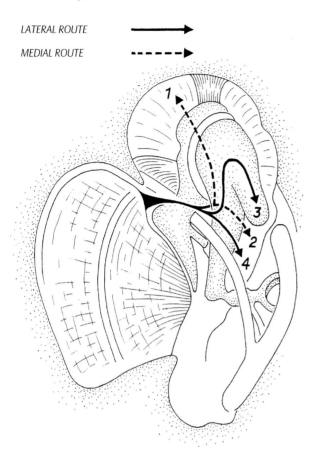

Figure 5–12 Routes of invasion of cholesteatoma of the attic. All routes usually result in ossicular erosion. The medial route (broken line) leads through a triangular space situated between the chorda tympani, malleus neck, and long process of the incus. The lateral route (solid line) follows the lateral surface of the incus and malleus. In extensive lesions, lateral and medial routes of invasion are combined. (From Fisch, U. (1994). Tympanoplasty, mastoidectomy and stapes surgery (p. 150). Stuttgart: Thieme, with permission.)

referred to as a *keratoma, epidermoid inclusion cyst,* or as was used in the older otologic literature, *pearly tumor*. The dead skin components at the center of such skin-filled cysts are an excellent medium for bacterial growth, and eventually infection will develop. Infection accelerates the process of bony destruction. Infections are particularly difficult to eradicate in cholesteatoma because of the difficulty antibiotics have in reaching such nonvascularized areas, and topical drops cannot penetrate to the core of the mass of dead skin.

As cholesteatomas expand, they do so only at the expense of surrounding normal structures (**Fig. 5–12**). Though uncommon, when an acute complication of cholesteatoma occurs, it can be very serious, with overall mortality rates between 14 and 32% (Osma et al, 2000). Conductive hearing loss can occur as one or all of the ossicles become destroyed. Labyrinthine fistula, which causes severe or profound sensorineural hearing loss and overwhelming vertigo, may result as the bone of the labyrinthine capsule is eroded and the membranous labyrinth is penetrated. Bacterial labyrinthitis

and total hearing loss are produced when the labyrinthine fluids become infected. Because these fluids are in direct contact with the brain and cerebrospinal fluid, bacterial meningitis may develop as a consequence of bacterial labyrinthitis. Of the intracranial complications of cholesteatoma, meningitis is the most common (Osma et al, 2000). Meningitis may be fatal within only a few hours when untreated. Erosion of the infected cholesteatoma matrix into the cranial cavity may produce brain abscess. Thrombosis or infection of the veins draining the brain may occur and can cause brain swelling, stroke, coma, and death. The major venous outflow tract of the mastoid, the sigmoid sinus, may become occluded and infected as well, and can lead to further sites of infection and death. Lastly, erosion into the facial nerve may result in paralysis of the face.

Surgical removal of cholesteatoma is the only reliable treatment and requires mastoidectomy in virtually all cases. Because the complications of cholesteatoma may be fatal, surgical therapy has as its goal complete removal of cholesteatoma and creation of a "safe" ear not subject to recurrent disease. Mastoidectomy itself has no effect on hearing. However, eradication of disease usually requires removal of one or more of the ossicles. Reconstruction of the disrupted middle ear transformer mechanism is of secondary importance. Even so, every effort is made to restore hearing when this is consistent with elimination of serious disease.

Pearl

- A second-look procedure is recommended in most cases of cholesteatoma 6 months after the initial surgery to check for residual disease that may have been missed at the initial operation. At this time, if no disease is found, ossicular reconstruction is usually performed.

Otosclerosis

Otosclerosis is a disease process in which vascular spongy bone replaces the normally hard bone of the otic capsule and ossicles. *Otospongiosis* is a more accurate term for ongoing disease; *otosclerosis* refers to the final inactive stage of the process when the bone becomes hardened. Otosclerotic changes have been found in 10% of the Caucasian population. In ~10% of these affected individuals, the otosclerotic process extends to involve the stapes footplate and annular ligament, causing decreased mobility of the footplate and a conductive hearing loss. Bilateral disease occurs in 75% of individuals. Although the cause of otosclerosis remains unknown, current theories include triggering by a viral infection such as measles, autoimmune disorders, or connective tissue disorders (Menger and Tange, 2003).

Otosclerosis is hereditary in many cases, with a form of inheritance that is most likely autosomal dominant; incomplete penetrance is estimated to be 40% (Menger and Tange, 2003). Definitive diagnosis depends on middle ear exploration with visualization of the otosclerotic focus and mechanical verification of stapes fixation. Presurgical diagnosis is based on the presence of slowly progressive conductive hearing loss in the absence of concurrent or preceding chronic ear disease.

The cardinal audiometric finding in otosclerosis is a progressively increasing air–bone gap. Early in the course of the disease, when only the anterior portion of the stapes is fixed, a marked low-frequency air–bone gap is seen. As footplate fixation becomes complete, high frequencies become involved, and the loss becomes a flat, conductive hearing loss. Depression of bone conduction scores isolated to the 2000 Hz range is characteristic of otosclerosis and referred to as "Carhart's notch." Tympanometry will often reveal a type A_s tympanogram despite a normal-appearing tympanic membrane.

Operative correction involves complete or partial removal of the fixed stapes and replacement with a prosthesis. The operation is a same-day surgical procedure and takes ~45 minutes. Regardless of the type of prosthesis used or the amount of stapes removed, most studies show correction of the air–bone gap to within 10 dB in over 80% of patients. A minority of patients will experience no improvement and will therefore continue to be good candidates for amplification. There is a 1 to 2% risk of complete and profound sensorineural hearing loss associated with this procedure, which does not necessarily seem to be related to technical intraoperative difficulties.

Ossicular Chain Discontinuity

Ossicular discontinuity may occur from a variety of causes. In children, the most frequent cause is necrosis (death and loss of tissue) of the long process of the incus because of recurrent or persistent middle ear infection or effusion. In such cases, the ossicular discontinuity is most often not complete, as a thin band of fibrous tissue replaces the necrotic distal segment of the long process of the incus. As the connection between the stapes and incus is then fibrous and not bony, it transmits sound inefficiently, and a significant conductive hearing loss is apparent. These children often have an air–bone gap that is larger in the high frequencies than in the lower frequencies. This high-frequency accentuated air–bone gap is thought to be characteristic of fibrous union of the incudostapedial joint. A type A_d tympanogram is seen in these cases.

In adults, trauma is one of the most common causes of ossicular dislocation. In general, trauma produces medial dislocation of the stapes and/or disruption of the incudo-malleolar joint. Less frequently, trauma produces complete subluxation of the stapes into the oval window, causing dizziness, sensorineural hearing loss, and conductive hearing loss. When suspected, immediate surgical intervention is recommended to limit the amount of sensorineural hearing loss and to close the perilymph fistula, which is an opening between the inner and middle ear space.

Previous surgical procedures can leave discontinuities in the ossicular chain. Oftentimes, surgery for cholesteatoma requires removal of part or all of one or more of the ossicles. Most frequently, the incus needs to be removed because of involvement with cholesteatoma. The head of the malleus and

capitulum of the stapes may also have to be removed. In many cases, bony destruction of the ossicles by the cholesteatomatous process has occurred before surgical intervention.

Treatment of ossicular discontinuity or dislocation is called *ossiculoplasty*. Repair of the ossicular chain is possible in most cases. Unfortunately, results are not as good with repair of defects involving the malleus and incus as stapes replacement is for otosclerosis. Closure of the air–bone gap to 10 dB occurs in less than three quarters of all patients, but it depends somewhat on the nature of the hearing deficit. When the malleus, incus, and stapes superstructure are gone and a total ossicular replacement prosthesis must be used, closure of the air–bone gap to within 25 dB is considered a good result. When the conductive hearing loss is caused by necrosis of the long process of the incus, complete closure of the air–bone gap can frequently be obtained.

Neoplasms of the Middle Ear

Glomus tumors are the most common benign neoplasm of the middle ear. They arise from paraganglionic tissue, which refers to cells that developed embryologically as nervous system cells, of the middle ear and may be more properly referred to as *paragangliomas* (**Fig. 5–13**). Although these

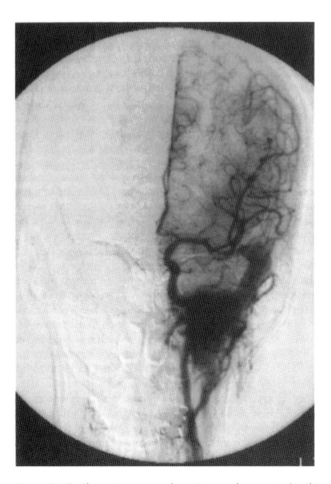

Figure 5–13 Glomus tumors can be quite vascular, as noted in this angiogram showing a large glomus jugulare tumor with multiple feeding vessels.

tumors can occur in all age groups, they are most common in middle-aged adults and may rarely show malignant potential (Manolidas et al, 1999). Symptoms of these tumors are related to its vascular nature and its tendency to erode surrounding structures. Most commonly, patients present with conductive hearing loss, pulsatile unilateral tinnitus, and a middle ear mass. Tympanometry will reveal a type A tympanogram with tiny sawtooth variations, which occur as a result of changes in tympanic membrane compliance related to blood flow in the middle ear mass. They may grow to a relatively large size prior to detection and may cause palsy of neighboring cranial nerves.

Treatment may include surgical resection, embolization, and radiation. Recently, stereotactic radiosurgery has been shown to have good results in controlling the progression of these tumors. This technique uses lower amounts of radiation and shorter overall treatment times than conventional radiation in an attempt to reduce post-treatment morbidity, such as brain necrosis, osteoradionecrosis of the temporal bone, and local tissue injury (Foote et al, 2002).

◆ Disorders of the Inner Ear and Internal Auditory Canal

Sensorineural Hearing Loss

Sensorineural hearing loss has many causes, which can be roughly divided into congenital and acquired causes. Both congenital and acquired causes can be further divided into genetic and nongenetic causes.

A large variety of congenital genetic etiologies for hearing loss exist. These etiologies may be even further subdivided into syndromic and nonsyndromic. There are over 400 syndromes that include hearing loss (Gurtler and Lalwani, 2002). Among the more frequently seen syndromes with hearing loss are Usher's syndrome, type II neurofibromatosis, Pendred's syndrome, and Waardenburg's syndrome. Nonsyndromic hearing loss is more common than syndromic causes and is frequently inherited in an autosomal recessive pattern. A mutation in the connexin 26 gene, which forms a protein that will combine into gap junctions that function in the cochlea to allow potassium recycling into the endolymph, has been found to cause over half of all cases of nonsyndromic hearing loss (Gurtler and Lalwani, 2002). This mutation can be detected via genetic screening of the patient.

Congenital nongenetic causes of sensorineural hearing loss include maternal infections, ototoxic drugs, prenatal developmental injuries, and birth trauma. Maternal rubella syndrome, although decreasing in frequency due to vaccination, is quite prevalent worldwide. Deafness from rubella is associated with congenital cataracts and congenital heart disease. Toxoplasmosis, cytomegalovirus, and syphilis are other infections that can involve the developing embryo and produce postnatal hearing loss. Each of these processes can cause progressive sensorineural hearing losses of childhood. Ototoxic drugs given to the mother during pregnancy

may result in congenital hearing loss. Hypoxia during intrauterine development can lead to significant injury to the auditory system. Prenatal injury to the vascular system of the branchial arches can produce either unilateral or bilateral hypoplasia of the membranous labyrinth. Perinatal injury, caused by birth trauma, may also result in sensorineural hearing loss, as may intracranial hemorrhage complicating delivery.

Acquired nongenetic causes of hearing loss are well known and consist most frequently of infection, neoplasm, ototoxic agents, noise, or trauma; they are discussed in other sections of this chapter. Meningitis, especially when caused by *Streptococcus pneumoniae*, is a frequent cause of hearing loss. A large variety of genetic causes for delayed sensorineural hearing loss exist, such as cochlear otosclerosis. Progressive sensorineural hearing loss can be attributed to a variety of syndromes that display musculoskeletal abnormalities. Among them are Paget's disease, van der Hoeve's syndrome, Alport's syndrome, and all of the mucopolysaccharidoses, such as Hunter's syndrome, Hurler's syndrome, Sanfilippo's syndrome, Morquio's syndrome, and Maroteaux-Lamy syndrome. However, the largest variety of delayed, genetically mediated sensorineural hearing losses occur sporadically as a consequence of a recessive inheritance pattern and are fortunately not associated with specific syndromes.

Sudden Sensorineural Hearing Loss

Sudden sensorineural hearing loss (SSNHL) is an uncommon condition, with onset of hearing loss within 72 hours. Most commonly, patients describe a unilateral hearing loss on awakening and may complain of fullness and tinnitus to the affected ear. Etiologies that cause sensorineural hearing loss may also cause SSNHL; however, most cases are felt to be due to a viral infection. Evaluation with audiometric testing and treatment should be instituted quickly, as most would consider this an otologic emergency. It is important to rule out other causes of hearing loss with appropriate laboratory studies and imaging, such as MRI. The only treatment option shown to improve outcome is steroids. Steroids may be delivered via an oral route or by direct injection into the middle ear. Despite the presumed viral etiology, treatment with antivirals has not been shown to improve hearing more effectively than steroids alone (Tucci et al, 2002).

Noise-Induced Hearing Loss

Noise-induced hearing loss has become recognized as a significant problem, especially in industrialized societies. Occupational noise exposure has been well studied, but nonoccupational noise exposure also accounts for a large amount of hearing loss in the general population. Noise-induced hearing loss begins with selective loss at 4000 Hz, which is seen as a notch on the audiogram (**Fig. 5–14**). With continued exposure, the notch widens and will affect all the high frequencies. Eventually, hearing loss can be seen in the middle and lower frequencies.

Initial exposure to loud noise causes a threshold shift, which is reversible within the first 24 hours. The threshold

PURE TONE AUDIOGRAM

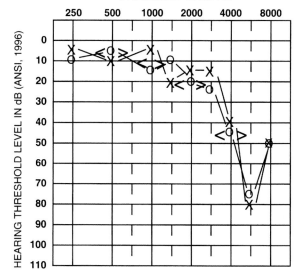

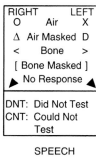

	RIGHT	LEFT
O	Air	X
△	Air Masked	D
<	Bone	>
[	Bone Masked	]
▲	No Response	◢

DNT: Did Not Test
CNT: Could Not Test

SPEECH

	RIGHT	LEFT
SRT	10 dB	10 dB
WRS	88 %	84 %

WRS Level 80 dB HL

PTA	13 dB	10 dB

Figure 5–14 Audiogram demonstrating noise-induced hearing loss. Note the notching present at 4000 Hz.

shift may be associated with tinnitus. Continued exposure can lead to permanent shifts. Temporary threshold shifts may occur with the discharge of a firearm without hearing protection or even after attendance at a rock concert. Permanent threshold shifts are often seen in persons with occupations requiring continued exposure to loud noises, such as airline mechanics and artillery experts. Children may also develop hearing loss from noise, which makes questions regarding such exposure important. In all patients with hearing loss, it is important to inquire whether any noise exposure occurred within the 24 hours prior to the onset of hearing loss because it may be a temporary threshold shift only.

Evidence suggests that a great individual variability exists in susceptibility to noise-induced hearing loss. Occupational noise limits are designed to eliminate noise-induced hearing loss in the average person and therefore may not protect the most sensitive individuals.

Aging and Hearing Loss

Hearing loss resulting from the physiologic process of aging alone is known as *presbycusis*. Current estimates place the incidence of hearing loss among geriatrics at between 25 and 50%. Most authorities believe that at least a portion of this hearing loss occurs solely because of the aging process and is not related to cumulative noise or other environmental exposures. However, identifying and studying presbycusis is difficult because of the multiple causes for hearing loss in elderly people and the effects of noise exposure, diet, hypertension, diabetes, or smoking on hearing thresholds.

Schuknecht, considered the founder of modern temporal bone histopathology, has classified presbycusis into four distinct types of clinical presentations, each associated with different pathologic alterations: sensory, neural, metabolic, and cochlear. Most patients have a combination of these types of presbycusis. Sensory presbycusis is characterized by the loss of hair cells in the organ of Corti, with audiograms revealing a high-frequency loss with a steep drop-off at 2000 Hz. Neural presbycusis occurs as a result of the loss of auditory neurons within the cochlea. This loss occurs evenly throughout the cochlear nerve and cochlea; however, pure-tone thresholds are not affected until ~90% of neurons are lost. Speech discrimination is often disproportionately worse than pure-tone audiometry would suggest. Metabolic presbycusis is characterized by atrophy of the stria vascularis, which provides nutritional support to the labyrinth. The audiogram is characterized by a flat or slightly descending audiogram with good preservation of speech discrimination. Cochlear conductive presbycusis is speculative but is thought to be caused by thickening of the basilar membrane, especially in the basal turn, leading to high-frequency hearing loss.

Pitfall

- Categorizing patients on the basis of audiograms is difficult because patients often have more than one pathological process occurring simultaneously.

Ototoxicity

A great number of medications are known to cause damage to the ear with associated auditory and vestibular dysfunction. In general, these drugs can be divided into distinct categories, including anti-inflammatory drugs, aminoglycoside antibiotics, loop diuretics, antimalarials, chemotherapeutic agents, and ototopical medications.

Ototoxicity as a result of aspirin use was first recognized in 1877. Aspirin ototoxicity is manifest as a flat mild-to-moderate reversible sensorineural hearing loss accompanied by pronounced tinnitus. The serum level required to produce symptoms is between 35 and 40 mg, which correlates to ~6 to 8 g/day or 18 to 24 regular-strength aspirin tablets. The mechanism of action of salicylate ototoxicity has not been identified, but it is believed to be due to reversible enzyme inhibition. Other NSAIDs, specifically ibuprofen and naproxen, have been associated with a very low incidence of associated hearing loss. However, the hearing loss associated with these medications is often permanent.

Aminoglycoside antibiotics have been an important treatment for a variety of infectious processes, but because of their known side effects of nephrotoxicity and ototoxicity, their use is decreasing. The ototoxic effects of aminoglycosides correlate directly with the amount of drug delivered to the perilymph. These drugs arrive in the inner ear from 30 minutes to 3 hours following intravenous administration and may remain in these tissues for months after treatment (Roland and Rutka, 2004). The ototoxic effects of the aminoglycosides are due to hair cell death from apoptosis following their uptake. The injury pattern seen is a high-frequency sensorineural hearing loss on the audiogram, which correlates with outer hair cell death at the basal turn of the cochlea. Inner hair cells may become damaged at high levels of toxicity.

Different types of aminoglycosides show different patterns of ototoxicity. Some are preferentially ototoxic, whereas others primarily affect the vestibular system. Streptomycin and gentamicin are primarily vestibulotoxic and have been used successfully to selectively destroy vestibular function as a part of the treatment of Meniere's disease. Dihydrostreptomycin, neomycin, amikacin, and tobramycin are primarily cochleotoxic. There does appear to be a genetic predisposition to aminoglycoside toxicity, with recent research showing a series of mitochondrial mutations account for ototoxicity in a significant portion of cases (Roland and Rutka, 2004). Prevention of ototoxic effects of aminoglycosides is difficult. Monitoring of serum peak and especially trough levels is helpful because toxicity is closely related to serum trough levels. Daily audiometric testing is usually not possible because of the gravity of illness typically present in patients receiving these drugs. When possible, extended high-frequency audiometry and otoacoustic emissions can be used to monitor for hearing loss during aminoglycoside treatment. Weekly or biweekly vestibular testing can detect vestibular injury before serious balance dysfunction becomes permanent.

Loop diuretics act by inhibiting reabsorption of electrolytes and water in the kidney. Toxicity is most likely in patients with preexisting renal dysfunction, patients receiving large boluses of loop diuretics over a short period, and patients receiving other potentially ototoxic medications such as aminoglycosides. The toxic effects are manifest by direct injury to hair cells and damage to the stria vascularis. Hearing loss is usually temporary, resolving after cessation of the drugs.

Both quinine and chloroquine, commonly used to treat malaria, have been associated with hearing loss even at very small doses. The hearing loss is usually temporary and primarily in the high frequencies because the basal turn of the cochlea is affected.

Many chemotherapeutic agents are known to have ototoxic effects. These include cisplatin, bleomycin, 5-flurouracil, and nitrogen mustard. The most studied drug is cisplatin, which is known to have its effects on the outer hair cells of the basal turn of the cochlea, causing a bilateral, symmetric, high-frequency hearing loss. The ototoxicity of cisplatin is dose dependent and permanent. Other risk factors include age extremes, previous or concurrent cranial irradiation, renal disease, use of other ototoxic medications, and prior hearing loss (Roland and Rutka, 2004).

Ototopical preparations have been shown to cause hair cell death and hearing loss when instilled into the middle ear of experimental animals. However, few reports of ototoxicity from topically applied antibiotics have been reported in humans (Roland and Rutka, 2004). Anatomical differences between humans and the animal models are most likely responsible for these differences. For example, the round window niche of experimental animals is highly exposed, whereas in humans it lies deep within a bony niche and often is partially or completely covered by a fold of mucous membrane. In addition, the round window membrane in humans is 6 to 10 times thicker than in experimental animals. Still, it is felt that caution is necessary with regards to these preparations, as vestibular toxicity has also been seen with their use. Newer ototopical agents such as the fluoroquinolones have been shown to be effective in treating otitis externa without ototoxic effects. Should potentially ototoxic topical medications be necessary, it is recommended to use short treatment durations to minimize toxic potential.

Vestibular Neuronitis

Vestibular neuronitis is an acute loss of unilateral peripheral vestibular function without associated auditory dysfunction. Four criteria can be used for the diagnosis of vestibular neuronitis: acute or subacute onset over minutes to hours, horizontal spontaneous nystagmus with fast-phase rotational component toward the unaffected ear, hyporesponsiveness on caloric irrigation of the affected ear, and perceived displacement of verticality with the eyes rotated toward the affected ear without showing vertical divergence of one eye above the other (Strupp et al, 2004). Through the course of this disease, prolonged severe rotational vertigo with nausea develops. Over time the vertigo typically improves, though the patient may experience mild positional vertigo for weeks to months. Symptoms most often resolve within 6 months. Audiometric testing is important to verify the lack of associated hearing loss. Recent study has shown the use of steroids improves recovery of peripheral vestibular function (Strupp et al, 2004). Treatment options also include antiemetics and vestibular suppressants during the acute stage; however, suppressants should be tapered once symptoms have subsided.

Benign Paroxysmal Positional Vertigo

Benign paroxysmal positional vertigo (BPPV) is a common disorder. Individuals with this disorder complain of brief rotational vertigo, from 15 to 30 seconds, associated with head movement and rapid position change. Brief vertigo after rolling onto one side in bed at night is virtually pathognomonic, but symptoms also commonly occur with neck hyperextension (e.g., reaching for something on a high shelf) and bending over. Symptoms can be provoked when the patient's head is moved rapidly into a supine position with the head turned such that the affected ear is 30 to 45 degrees below the horizontal. This position is known as the Dix-Hallpike maneuver, after the two individuals who fully defined the characteristics of BPPV. The vertigo has a brief latency (usually 1–5 seconds), limited duration, and is fatigable if the position is repeated. Characteristically, the nystagmus generated is predominantly rotatory, with the fast component directed toward the affected ear.

Two theories exist regarding the cause of BPPV. The first, known as "cupulolithiasis," proposes that debris or fragments of degenerating otoconia from the utricle become adherent to the cupula of the posterior semicircular canal. This converts the canal from an organ sensitive to angular rotation to a gravity-sensitive organ. When the canal is in a plane parallel to the force of gravity, the cupula is inappropriately deflected, producing vertigo. The "canalithiasis" theory is the more widely accepted theory and purports that debris is free floating in the posterior semicircular canal. When the head is moved into the provoking position, the debris moves to the most dependent position of the canal, which causes the endolymph to move away from the ampulla, provoking deflection of the cupula and vertigo. The etiology of otoconial detachment is unclear, although it is more common in older patients and those with a history of head trauma.

Treatment of BPPV focuses on repositioning maneuvers designed to deposit the semicircular debris into the vestibule. Epley's maneuver is based on the canalithiasis theory and has been shown by a large meta-analysis to improve symptoms in many patients. Seymont's maneuver is based on the cupulolithiasis theory and may be valuable in patients who do not respond initially to Epley's maneuver (Woodworth et al, 2004).

BPPV is a specific pathological and clinical entity. A large number of other causes for positional vertigo exist. The brief disequilibrium and vertigo that follow labyrinthitis and post-traumatic vertigo are two good examples. Such conditions and others are often referred to as benign positional vertigo and should not be confused with BPPV. Nomenclature is inconsistent, and care should be exercised to ascertain which condition is being discussed.

Perilymph Fistula

A perilymph fistula (PLF) occurs when disruption of the barrier between the perilymphatic space of the inner ear and the middle ear occurs with loss of perilymph. This can occur in a variety of clinical situations, including head trauma, barotrauma, congenital malformations of the inner ear, post-stapedectomy, or any situation that may increase cerebrospinal fluid pressure. Though considered rare, most experts do agree that spontaneous PLF may also occur (Friedland and Wackym, 1999). The clinical presentation is similar to Meniere's disease and may be indistinguishable

Table 5–2   Comparison of Meniere's Disease and Perilymph Fistula

Parameter	Meniere's disease	Perilymph fistula
Age at presentation	Third to sixth decade	Any age
History of trauma	No	Often
Abnormal electrocochleography	Yes	Yes
Hearing loss	Usually low-frequency fluctuating loss	Variable
Family history	Present in 20%	No
Vertigo	Episodic, rotational; lasts minutes to hours	Variable

(**Table 5–2**). Common complaints include episodic vertigo, disequilibrium, ataxia, and hearing loss (Friedland and Wackym, 1999).

No one test is diagnostic for PLF. Platform and electronystagmography fistula tests, when positive, strongly suggest fistula if Meniere's disease and syphilis can be excluded. Electrocochleography, which provides an electrophysiological measure of the cochlear microphonic summating potential (SP) and action potential (AP) of the cochlear nerve, has been shown to be sensitive in the diagnosis of PLF. Elevated SP/AP ratios can be seen with over half of patients with confirmed PLF. Even in the operating room, the diagnosis of PLF is difficult, because irrigation, blood, or injected anesthetic are often present in the middle ear and cannot be distinguished from escaping perilymph. In addition, PLFs may leak fluid only intermittently, adding to the diagnostic difficulty. Diagnosis of PLF often depends on history. When hearing loss, disequilibrium, or vertigo closely follows head trauma, rapid external pressure change (aircraft descent, scuba diving), or interval increase in cerebrospinal fluid pressure (straining, sneezing, coughing), PLF should be considered.

When hearing levels are stable, initial treatments are usually conservative and include bed rest, head elevation, and avoidance of situations that may increase intracranial pressure, such as sneezing and straining. Surgical treatment is considered in patients with deteriorating hearing levels or protracted vertigo. Treatment consists of oval and round window grafting. Vestibular symptoms often resolve promptly with repair, but recovery of hearing is uncommon.

Meniere's Disease

Meniere's disease is characterized by (1) spontaneous episodes of vertigo lasting several minutes to hours; (2) low-pitched, roaring tinnitus occurring or worsening during a vertiginous attack; (3) fluctuating low-frequency sensorineural hearing loss; and (4) aural fullness in the affected ear. For a diagnosis of Meniere's disease, in addition to the above symptoms, other sources of vertigo must be ruled out, most often by MRI. The vertigo is frequently violent and associated with nausea, vomiting, diaphoresis, and pallor. The onset of symptoms is typically between the third and sixth decades, with a slight female preponderance. Only ~3 to 4% of patients with Meniere's disease are seen in the pediatric age group. More

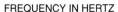

PURE TONE AUDIOGRAM
FREQUENCY IN HERTZ

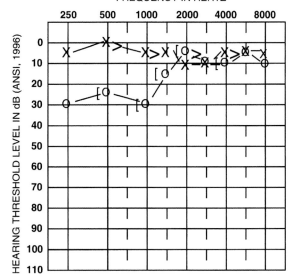

	RIGHT	LEFT
	O Air	X
	Δ Air Masked	D
	< Bone	>
	[Bone Masked]	
	▲ No Response	▲

DNT:	Did Not Test
CNT:	Could Not Test

SPEECH

	RIGHT	LEFT
SRT	NA	NA
WRS	92 %	100 %

WRS Level 80 dB HL

PTA	20 dB	5 dB

Figure 5–15 Audiogram demonstrating the typical findings in a patient with early Meniere's disease. Note the mild low-frequency sensorineural hearing loss.

than 40% of patients will eventually develop bilateral ear involvement, and 20% have a positive family history.

The proposed etiology of Meniere's disease is endolymphatic hydrops, a condition in which distension of the endolymphatic system occurs, which can only be confirmed on temporal bone examination. When suspected, the use of electrocochleography or vestibular testing may be helpful. Electrocochleography will often show an elevated SP/AP ratio to the affected ear. Although electrocochleography is helpful in establishing which ear is affected, it does not distinguish between Meniere's disease and perilymphatic fistula. ENG and sinusoidal harmonic acceleration can be useful in documenting unilateral labyrinthine dysfunction and confirming the diagnosis of Meniere's disease. The

definitive diagnosis is difficult and depends on the documentation of low-frequency sensorineural hearing loss and associated vestibular abnormalities.

The natural history of Meniere's disease is progressive; with fluctuating hearing that may be normal between attacks early in the course of disease but over years will often develop into permanent hearing loss. This can make early diagnosis difficult, as the patient may be seen for consultation at a time when symptoms have temporarily subsided. The hearing loss may follow any pattern, but low-frequency hearing losses are more common early in the course of disease. Patients with long-standing disease are more likely to have flat losses (**Figs. 5–15, 5–16,** and **5–17**). Some individuals will experience a relatively indolent variety of the disease

PURE TONE AUDIOGRAM
FREQUENCY IN HERTZ

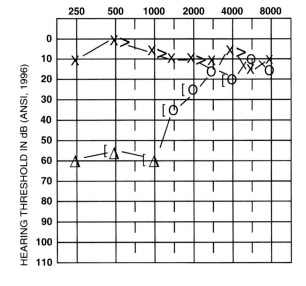

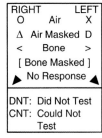

	RIGHT	LEFT
	O Air	X
	Δ Air Masked	D
	< Bone	>
	[Bone Masked]	
	▲ No Response	▲

DNT:	Did Not Test
CNT:	Could Not Test

SPEECH

	RIGHT	LEFT
SRT	45 dB	10 dB
WRS	80 %	96 %

WRS Level 80 dB HL

PTA	47 dB	5 dB

Figure 5–16 Audiogram demonstrating the typical findings in a patient with middle-stage Meniere's disease. Note the increasing low-frequency sensorineural hearing loss.

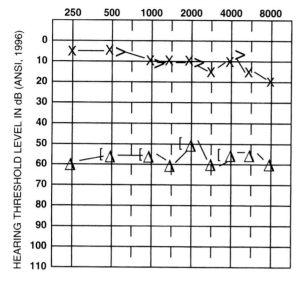
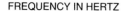
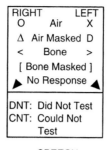

PURE TONE AUDIOGRAM

FREQUENCY IN HERTZ

	RIGHT	LEFT
O	Air	X
Δ	Air Masked	D
<	Bone	>
[	Bone Masked	]
▲	No Response	◄

DNT: Did Not Test
CNT: Could Not Test

SPEECH

	RIGHT	LEFT
SRT	NA	NA
WRS	64 %	100 %

WRS Level 80 dB HL

PTA	52 dB	8 dB

Figure 5–17 Audiogram demonstrating the typical findings in a patient with late Meniere's disease. Note the flat, moderate-to-severe sensorineural hearing loss.

with attacks separated by years, whereas others will lose all hearing and balance function over a period of several months. Most patients follow an intermediate course, with attacks coming in clusters lasting several weeks and separated by months or even years of symptom-free periods. Vertigo attacks continue to occur in some patients with Meniere's disease more than 20 years after diagnosis, with 75% still considering their attacks severe (Havia and Kentala, 2004). Although the development of complete bilateral anacusis is rare and reported to occur in only 1 to 6% of patients, it has been shown that cochlear implantation is beneficial in such patients (Lustig et al, 2003).

Most patients improve with medical management. Avoidance of caffeine and nicotine, which can exacerbate symptoms, is advised. The mainstay of treatment is the use of diuretic therapy and a rigorous salt-restricted diet. If the patient does not respond to medical therapy, selective vestibulotoxic aminoglycoside antibiotics can be infused into the middle ear to ablate the affected side. Surgical procedures for medically nonresponsive cases include endolymphatic shunt procedures, labyrinthectomy, and vestibular nerve section.

Autoimmune Inner Ear Disease

In 1979, McCabe first reported on a group of individuals with fluctuating sensorineural hearing loss responsive to immunosuppression, suggestive of an autoimmune cause. Although studies have shown that many of these patients do possess antibodies to inner ear antigens, many questions remain unanswered regarding the pathogenesis of this disease. Clinically, the diagnosis of autoimmune inner ear disease (AIED) is difficult. Patients are usually seen with bilateral, asymmetric, fluctuating sensorineural hearing loss. About 50% of patients will complain of vestibular abnormalities. Age at presentation is usually in the 40s to 50s, with a female preponderance. Approximately one third of patients will have evidence of a systemic autoimmune disorder such as lupus erythematosus, polyarteritis nodosa, rheumatoid arthritis, Behçet's disease, or Wegener's granulomatosis.

In addition to standard audiometry and vestibular testing, all suspected patients should be screened with an antinuclear antibody test, erythrocyte sedimentation rate, rheumatoid factor, syphilis serological studies, thyroid function tests, and a test for the 68 kD protein, which is the best available test for inner ear antibodies.

The treatment of choice for patients with autoimmune inner ear disease is high-dose steroids, 60 mg daily, for up to 4 weeks. A dramatic response is often noted in the presence of an accurate diagnosis. Chronic systemic steroid exposure does carry high risks of side effects. Other immunosuppressive medications that were developed for various rheumatological disorders have been attempted for AIED, with the hope that drugs with fewer systemic side effects, such as methotrexate, would show efficacy. The most recent large controlled clinical study has not shown methotrexate to be useful in AIED (Harris et al, 2003). At this point, should a patient not tolerate chronic steroid use, cochlear implantation appears to be the only alternative until novel immune modulators are developed for this disorder.

Tumors of the Internal Auditory Canal and Cerebellopontine Angle

Eighty percent of tumors arising in the cerebellopontine angle are acoustic neuromas (**Fig. 5–18**). The tumor arises from the Schwann's cells, which surround the sheath of the CN VIII, not from the nerve itself.

Most commonly, patients present with a progressive, unilateral, sensorineural hearing loss, which typically begins in the high frequencies and progresses to involve lower frequencies. Twenty percent of patients will

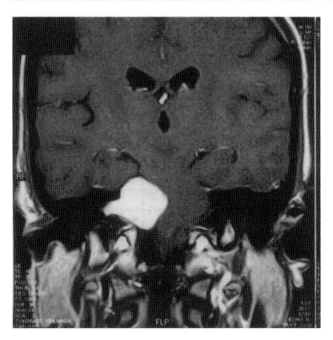

Figure 5–18 Coronal magnetic resonance imaging scan with gadolinium showing a large acoustic neuroma.

present with sudden sensorineural hearing loss (Sauvaget et al, 2005). Additionally, 20% will present with recurrent fluctuating hearing loss. Less common are vestibular complaints, which when present are usually vague complaints and tend to occur with smaller tumors (<1 cm). As the tumor enlarges, neurological changes may be evidenced as decreased function of CN VII and V. With continued growth, a patient may develop hydrocephalus from brainstem compression.

Several findings on audiometry should alert the examiner to the possibility of an acoustic neuroma. The patient will often have a speech discrimination score that is reduced out of proportion to the level of hearing loss. Often, "rollover" (decreased ability to understand words as the volume increases) is present. Most (95%) patients will have absent stapedial reflexes. ABR will demonstrate an increased wave I to V interpeak latency, usually greater than 0.2 msec. Up to 80% of patients will have abnormal results on ENG. Because the ENG tests the function of the horizontal semicircular canal, which is innervated by the superior vestibular nerve, a normal test suggests that the tumor originates from the inferior vestibular nerve. Because of the location of the cochlear nerve, in this situation, hearing preservation is less likely to be successful. MRI with gadolinium contrast is widely considered the gold standard for diagnosis of acoustic neuromas and can detect tumors as small as 2 mm. This imaging study should be ordered in patients with unilateral sensorineural hearing loss or bilateral asymmetric hearing loss.

Individuals with neurofibromatosis type 2 will develop multiple schwannomas of the CNS and often present with bilateral acoustic neuromas at a young age. Unlike patients with spontaneous acoustic neuromas, tumors in patients with neurofibromatosis type 2 may grow to a very large size before becoming symptomatic and tend to be more infiltrative into the nerve, making hearing preservation more difficult.

The usual treatment for acoustic neuroma is surgery. The surgical approach depends on tumor size and location, as well as the patient's audiometric results. In general, hearing conservation surgery is considered when the patient has a small tumor (<1.5 cm) and a pure-tone average of less than 50 dB HL with greater than 50% discrimination. Both the suboccipital and middle cranial fossa approaches allow for the possibility of hearing preservation. The most common approach to resection of acoustic neuromas is through the translabyrinth, which sacrifices hearing on the operated side. The risk of injury to the facial nerve increases with increasing tumor size and approaches 40% when tumor size increases beyond 3 cm.

Other treatment options include stereotactic radiation therapy (the "gamma knife") and observation. When tumors arise in elderly patients or patients who are poor candidates for surgery, a wait-and-see policy may be used. Serial MRI scans should be obtained every 6 months to detect changes in growth rate. Stereotactic radiosurgery has been shown to have excellent control over tumor growth; however, there has been some concern regarding incidence of continued hearing loss, facial nerve palsy, and trigeminal nerve dysfunction after this therapy. It appears that as the dosing of this modality has decreased, complications have decreased while tumor control still remains present in greater than 95% of patients (Wackym, 2005). In general, this modality is reserved for elderly patients, patients with medical problems that increase surgical risk, or individuals who refuse surgery.

Most other tumors that can occur in the cerebellopontine angle are meningiomas. Rarely, lipomas, cholesterol granulomas, cholesteatomas, or hemangiomas may present in the cerebellopontine angle. Meningiomas should be suspected when a patient presents with a large tumor and relatively normal hearing. In addition, meningiomas usually present eccentrically with respect to the internal auditory canal and fail to deform the bony auditory canal.

Pearl

- Because acoustic neuromas may present with symptoms similar to Meniere's diseases, all patients suspected of having Meniere's disease should have an MRI scan with gadolinium to look for the presence of an acoustic neuroma.

Vascular Compression Syndrome

Vascular compression of the cochleovestibular nerve in the internal auditory canal can cause vertigo and disequilibrium. Constant pulsations from a vessel lying on the nerve are believed to cause chronic irritation of the nerve and focal destruction of myelin. Usually the culprit vessel is a branch of the anteroinferior cerebellar artery. The vestibular complaints of patients with vascular compression of CN VIII often include constant, chronic vertigo with marked exacerbation by motion and chronic nausea. Audiometric testing shows a low-frequency hearing loss or a 15 dB notch at one octave. The most common finding is an increased wave I to III interpeak latency on ABR.

Relief of symptoms can be provided by either section of the vestibular nerve or vascular decompression. Symptoms seem to resolve more rapidly after nerve section.

References

Berenholz, L., Katzenell, U., & Harell, M. (2002). Evolving resistant *Pseudomonas* to ciprofloxacin in malignant otitis externa. Laryngoscope, 112, 1619–1622.

Derkay, D. S., Carron, J. D., Wiatrak, B. J., Choi, S. S., & Jones, J. E. (2000). Postsurgical follow-up of children with tympanostomy tubes: Results of the American Academy of Otolaryngology–Head and Neck Surgery Pediatric Otolaryngology Committee National Survey. Otolaryngology–Head and Neck Surgery, 122, 313–318.

Eggermont, J. J., & Roberts, L. E. (2004). The neuroscience of tinnitus. Trends in Neurosciences, 27, 676–682.

Foote, R. L., Pollock, B. E., Gorman, D. A., et al. (2002). Glomus jugulare tumor: Tumor control complications after stereotactic radiosurgery. Head and Neck, 24, 332–339.

Friedland, D. R., & Wackym, P. A. (1999). A critical appraisal of spontaneous perilymphatic fistulas of the inner ear. American Journal of Otology, 20, 261–279.

Gurtler, N. , & Lalwani, A. K. (2002). Etiology of syndromic and nonsyndromic sensorineural hearing loss. Otolaryngologic Clinics of North America, 35, 891–908.

Harris, J. P., Weisman, M. H., Dereber, J. M., et al. (2003). Treatment of corticosteroid-responsive autoimmune inner ear disease with methotrexate. Journal of the American Medical Association, 290, 1875–1883.

Havia, M., & Kentala, E. (2004). Progression of symptoms of dizziness in Meniere's disease. Archives of Otolaryngology–Head and Neck Surgery, 130, 431–435.

Jung, T. T. K., & Hanson, J. B. (1999). Otitis media: Surgical principles based on pathogenesis. Otolaryngologic Clinics of North America, 32, 369–383.

Karlidag, T., Ilhan, N., Kaygusuz, I., et al. (2004). Comparison of free radicals and antioxidant enzymes in chronic otitis media with and without tympanosclerosis. Laryngoscope, 114, 85–89.

Kenna, M. A. (2005). Otitis media and the new guidelines. Journal of Otolaryngology, 34, S24–S32.

Li, Y., Hunter, L. L., Margolis, R. H., Levine, S. C., Lindgren, B., Daly, K. & Gebink, G. S. (1999). Prospective study of tympanic membrane retraction, hearing loss, and multifrequency tympanometry. Otolaryngology–Head and Neck Surgery, 121, 514–522.

Lustig, L. R., Yeagle, J., Niparko, J. K., & Minor, L. B. (2003). Cochlear implantation in patients with bilateral Meniere's syndrome. Otology and Neurotology, 24, 397–403.

Manolidis, S., Shohet, J., Jackson, C. G., & Glasscock, M. E. (1999). Malignant glomus tumors. Laryngoscope, 109, 30–34.

McCabe, B. F. (1979). Autoimmune sensorineural hearing loss. Annals of Otology, Rhinology and Laryngology, 88, 585–589.

McKinnon, B. J., & Jahrsdoerfer, R. A. (2002). Congenital auricular atresia: Update on options for intervention and timing of repair. Otolaryngologic Clinics of North America, 35, 877–890.

Menger, D. J., & Tange, R. A. (2003). The aetiology of otosclerosis: A review of the literature. Clinical Otolaryngology, 28, 112–120.

Nyrop, M., & Grontved, A. (2002). Cancer of the external auditory canal. Archives of Otolaryngology–Head and Neck Surgery, 128, 834–837.

Okpala, N. C. E., Siraj, Q. H., Nilssen, E., & Pringle, M. (2005). Radiological and radionuclide investigation of malignant otitis externa. Journal of Laryngology and Otology, 119, 71–75.

Osma, U., Cureoglu, S., & Hosoglu, S. (2000). The complications of chronic otitis media: Report of 93 cases. Journal of Laryngology and Otology, 114, 97–100.

Persaud, R. A. P., Hajioff, D., Thevasagayam, M. S., Wareing, M. J., & Wright, A. (2004). Keratosis obturans and external ear canal cholesteatoma: How and why we should distinguish between these conditions. Clinical Otolaryngology, 29, 577–581.

Rizer, F. M. (1997). Overlay versus underlay tympanoplasty: 1. Historical review of the literature. Laryngoscope, 107(Suppl. 84), 1–25.

Roland, P. S., Pien, F. D., Schultz, C. C., et al. (2004). Efficacy and safety of topical ciprofloxacin/dexamethasone versus neomycin/polymyxin B/hydrocortisone for otitis externa. Current Medical Research and Opinion, 20, 1175–1183.

Roland, P. S., & Rutka, J. A. (2004). Ototoxity. Hamilton, Ontario, Canada: B. C. Decker.

Roland, P. S., & Stroman, D. W. (2002). Microbiology of acute otitis externa. Laryngoscope, 112, 1166–1177.

Sauvaget, E., Kici, S., Kania, R., Herman, P., & Tran Ba Huy, F. (2005). Sudden sensorineural hearing loss as a revealing symptom of vestibular schwannoma. Acta Otolaryngologica, 125, 592–595.

Schrader, N., & Isaacson, G. (2003). Fungal otitis externa–its association with fluoroquinolone eardrops. Pediatrics, 111, 1123.

Schuknecht, H. F. (1955). Presbycusis. Laryngoscope, 65, 402.

Sood, S., Strachan, D. R., Tsikoudas, A., & Stables, G. I. (2002). Allergic otitis externa. Clinical Otolaryngology, 27, 233–236.

Sreepada, G. S., & Kwartler, J. A. (2003). Skull base osteomyelitis secondary to malignant otitis externa. Current Opinion in Otolaryngology and Head and Neck Surgery, 11, 316–323.

Stroman, D. W., Roland, P. S., Dohar, J., & Burt, W. (2001). Microbiology of normal external auditory canal. Laryngoscope, 111, 2054–2059.

Strupp, M., Zingler, V. C., Arbusow, V., et al. (2004). Methylprednisolone, valacyclovir, or the combination for vestibular neuritis. New England Journal of Medicine, 351, 354–361.

Tran, L. P., Grundfast, K. M., & Selesnick, S. H. (1996). Benign lesions of the external auditory canal. Otolaryngologic Clinics of North America, 29, 807–825.

Trigg, D. J., & Applebaum, E. L. (1988). Indications for the surgical repair of unilateral aural atresia in children. American Journal of Otology, 19, 679–686.

Tucci, D. L., Farmer, J. C., Kitch, R. D., & Witsell, D. L. (2002). Treatment of sudden sensorineural hearing loss with systemic steroids and valacyclovir. Otology and Neurotology, 23, 301–308.

Wackym, P. A. (2005). Stereotactic radiosurgery, microsurgery, and expectant management of acoustic neuroma: Basis for informed consent. Otolaryngologic Clinics of North America, 38, 653–670.

Woodworth, B. A., Gillespie, M. B., & Lambert, P. R. (2004). The canalith repositioning procedure for benign positional vertigo: A meta-analysis. Laryngoscope, 114, 1143–1146.

Chapter 6

Genetics of Hearing Loss

Sonal S. Sheth and Richard K. McHugh

Hearing loss is the most common sensory deficit in developed countries. One in 1000 children is born profoundly deaf, and the prevalence of hearing impairment rises significantly with age to include 30% of people over 70 years old. With genetics playing a major role in hearing loss, it is critical to identify genes (definitions of terms are given in **Table 6–1**) involved in deafness. Our understanding of genetics has increased remarkably in the last century, especially in the last quarter of the 20th century (**Fig. 6–1**). Such advancements as the Human Genome Project are already leading to better diagnostic and treatment options. This chapter examines the genetics of hearing within the context of these advancements and their likely directions in the future.

A genetic basis accounts for approximately half of the cases of hearing impairment worldwide (**Fig. 6–2**). Although many forms of hearing loss are due to single genetic mutations, the more common forms are the result of complex interactions between genes and the environment. In common hearing disorders, for example, age-related hearing loss, the many genes that are involved in hearing control the susceptibility to the disease, with environmental influences, such as noise, further exacerbating the clinical manifestations. Because of environmental factors, there is a significant amount of variation in the severity of hearing loss. Recent advances provide ample evidence that genetics plays a fundamental role in the pathogenesis of hearing impairment.

Mapping and identification of genes involved in hereditary hearing loss began in the 1990s. As described in greater detail later in the chapter, gene identification requires several steps. Generally, a locus within chromosomal deoxyribonucleic acid (DNA) is found to include one gene that affects hearing among several other genes with functions that do not involve the hearing system. By analyzing the effects of each gene and refining the map to include the single causative gene, the hearing loss gene is eventually identified and confirmed by cloning.

Hereditary hearing loss is categorized into two major groups: syndromic forms, in which hearing loss is associated with other clinical disorders (SHL); and nonsyndromic forms, in which hearing loss is the sole disorder (NSHL). SHL accounts for 30% of all genetic forms of deafness. There are roughly 175 monogenic, or single gene, forms of SHL, of which 80 genes have been identified. The remaining 70% of hereditary hearing loss involves nonsyndromic hearing loss. Within the category of NSHL, ~90 genetic loci have been discovered, and more than 40 genes have been identified. The first locus contributing to hearing loss was mapped in a Costa Rican family exhibiting a dominant form of nonsyndromic hearing loss (DFNA1). Waardenburg's syndrome was the first syndromic form of hearing loss for which a causal gene, *PAX3*, was identified, although it was later determined that Waardenburg's syndrome was a heterogeneous disorder. A summary of the diagnostic criteria and examples of hereditary hearing loss are included in **Table 6–2**.

Table 6–1 Genetic Terms and Definitions

Term	Definition
Allele	The different forms or sequences that a gene may have in a population
Blastocyst	Embryo consisting of a spherical cell mass with a fluid-filled cavity and a cluster of cells called the inner cell mass (from which embryonic stem cells are derived)
Expressivity	The nature and severity of a trait as a result of a mutant allele
Gene	Fundamental unit of heredity
Genotype	An individual's specific DNA constitution at a particular locus
Heterogeneous disorder	A disorder that may be caused by any one of several gene mutations
Heterozygous	Possessing two different alleles for a given gene on a pair of chromosomes (individuals carry two homologous copies of each chromosome)
Homozygous	Possessing a pair of identical alleles for a given gene on a pair of chromosomes
Locus (pl loci)	The chromosome location of a specific gene
Missense mutation	A single DNA sequence change resulting in a different amino acid
Nonsense mutation	A single DNA sequence change resulting in a premature stop or termination of sequence
Nucleotide	The basic unit of DNA or RNA
Orthologous	Genes that exist between different species (*PAX3* is an orthologous gene existing in humans [*PAX3*] and in mice [*Pax3*])
Phenotype	The observable characteristics of an individual, produced by the interaction of genes and environment
Polymorphism	Any sequence variant present at a frequency > 1% in a population
Transgenic	Exchange of chromosomal material between two or more chromosomes
Translocation	An animal in which artificially introduced foreign DNA becomes stably incorporated into the animal's genome

Hearing loss is diagnosed by audiological testing that defines the functional loss, as it relates directly to the structure or structures affected. For example, conductive hearing loss may affect structures in the external or middle ear such that sound vibrations do not reach the inner ear. Sensorineural hearing loss involves lesions within the inner ear, brainstem, or cerebral cortex. In mixed hearing loss, the audiological profile of hearing loss may show components of both conductive and sensorineural types. Through genetics, one can understand the underlying reason for the functional and

470-320 BC – Hippocrates, Aristotle, Plato. Notes on inheritance of traits and semen as the hereditary agent.

1839 – Schleiden & Schwann. Cell theory including nuclei as fundamental units of life.

1858 – Darwin & Wallace. Theory of natural selection.

1866 – Mendel. Inheritance of "factors" in pea plants.

1902 – Sutton & Boveri. Chromosome theory of heredity.

1905 – Bateson. Coined term "genetics", 'to generate' in Greek.

1941 – Beadle & Tatum. Irradiation shows gene effects due to enzyme regulation.

1952 – Hershey & Chase. Labeling studies prove that DNA carries heredity.

1953 – Watson & Crick. DNA is a double helix.

1966 – Nirenberg & Khorana. Genetic code uses mRNA codons to specify 22 amino acids.

1986 – Mullis. Polymerase chain reaction.

2000 – Human Genome Project. Sequence of the human genome.

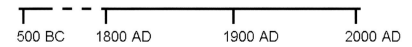

500 BC   1800 AD   1900 AD   2000 AD

Figure 6–1 Timeline of critical events in the field of genetics.

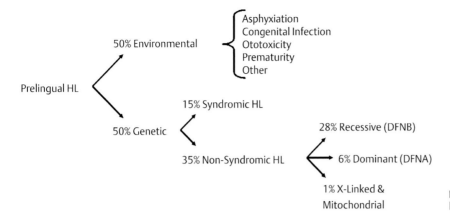

Figure 6–2 Tree diagram of the forms of hearing loss. HL, hearing level.

Table 6–2 Criteria Used in the Diagnosis of Hereditary Hearing Loss

Criteria	Category	Example
Clinical manifestation	Syndromic	30 to 40% of hereditary hearing loss
	Nonsyndromic	60 to 70% of hereditary hearing loss
Affected site	Sensorineural	Inner ear Acoustic nerve Brain
	Conductive	External auditory canal Middle ear
Onset	Prelingual	DFN3
	Postlingual	Usher's syndrome type II
	Fluctuating	DFNB1
Severity	Mild	21 to 40 dB
	Moderate	41 to 60 dB
	Moderately severe	61 to 80 dB
	Severe	81 to 100 dB
	Profound	>100 dB
Frequency in population	Low	DFNA1 DFNA6/14/38
	Medium	DFNA8/12 DFNA13
	High	DFNA3 DFNA5
Auditory neuropathy	Yes	DFNA2 DFNB9
Vestibular involvement	Yes	DFNA9 DFNA11
Radiology	Abnormal	DFNB4
Mutated genes	Nuclear	*SIX1*- BOR syndrome
	Mitochondrial	tRNALys: maternally inherited diabetes and deafness
	Structural	*CDH23*: DFNB12
	Transporter	*SLC26A4*: Pendred's syndrome
Mode of inheritance	Autosomal	Dominant Recessive
	X-linked	Dominant Recessive
	Mitochondrial	Maternal

Adapted from Finsterer, J., & Fellinger, J. (2005). Nuclear and mitochondrial genes mutated in nonsyndromic impaired hearing. *International Journal of Pediatric Otorhinolaryngology, 69*(5), 621–647, with permission.

anatomical dysfunctions leading to hearing loss (**Table 6–3**). Understanding the phenotype of hearing loss in terms of age of onset, progression, and functional-anatomical relationships is crucial. All of these phenotypic factors may involve genetics. We now have the ability to link genes to molecular mechanisms involved in hearing. As we continue to understand the influence of genetics in hearing, we will find better diagnostic and therapeutic modalities, thus improving many lives. The rapid pace of gene discovery and analysis will outpace our ability to fully describe any single gene in this chapter. We have chosen to discuss the methods used to find these genes and describe only a select few. Approaching the genetics of hearing with an understanding of the molecular biological methods and the systems of interaction within the hearing system enables the best preparation to further study the specifics of any gene.

Table 6–3 Functional and Anatomical Measures to Determine Cochlear Structures Affected by Hereditary Hearing Loss

Level	Measurement	Specific Structure(s)
Function	Otoacoustic emissions	Outer hair cell
	Cochlear microphonics	Outer hair cell
	Compound action potential	Inner hair cell (electrode on round window)
	Single unit recording	Spiral ganglion cell
	Endocochlear potential	Cochlear fluid
	Auditory brainstem response	Inner hair cell to cortex
Gross structure	CT	Bony structures
	MRI	Tissue structures
Microstructure	Light microscopy	Cells
	Immunohisto-chemistry	Proteins in cells
	Confocal microscopy	Subcellular localization of molecules
Ultrastructure	Transmission electron microscopy	Intracellular structure
	Scanning electron microscopy	Intracellular structure

CT, computed tomography; MRI, magnetic resonance imaging.

Pearl

- High-resolution computed tomography (CT) and magnetic resonance imaging (MRI) have provided valuable information for the diagnosis, counseling, and evaluation of hearing impairment. In addition to the study of anatomical dysfunctions, the identification of genetic loci and genetic defects involved in hearing loss, such as *GJB2*, has greatly facilitated the diagnosis of various forms of hearing loss.

◆ Mode of Inheritance in Genetic Disorders

Hereditary deafness can be the result of a single gene disorder (also known as Mendelian disorder) or the result of a complex disorder, in which multiple genes act in conjunction with environmental influences. Complex disorders have unparalleled genetic heterogeneity and affect all areas involved in hearing, including the external acoustic canal, middle ear, inner ear, acoustic nerve, and brain. Approximately 1% of the total number of human genes are necessary for hearing and contribute to syndromic and nonsyndromic hearing loss.

With each human having 3 billion nucleotide pairs encoding roughly 30,000 genes, mutations in these genes or various combinations of genes can lead to a large number of genetic disorders. These disorders can be classified based on the type of mutations or alterations and the pattern of inheritance. These include (1) Mendelian (or monogenic) disorders, in which a single gene is mutated, or chromosomal disorders, in which entire chromosomes or portions of them have been duplicated, deleted, or translocated; and (2) complex disorders, in which the convoluted interactions between environmental causes and multiple genes lead to variable clinical manifestations. Because of the differences in the genetic aspects of these disorders, each type of disease requires a specific genetic analysis for gene identification. However, Mendelian hearing loss is considered to be monogenic due to the significant effect of a single mutation. For instance, a deletion within one crucial gene may completely interrupt normal hearing function.

Pitfall

- Hearing loss of a specific type may be caused by many genetic defects. This is known as genetic heterogeneity. Likewise, a particular genetic defect may produce various symptoms including hearing loss. This is known as phenotypic heterogeneity and often is due to the effects of many other gene products acting with the primary genetic defect. Such genetic complexity complicates the ability of a clinical examination to yield a diagnosis. Genetic testing will be able to provide a correct diagnosis in such cases and therefore is becoming an indispensable adjunct to the clinical hearing evaluation.

Mendelian Disorders

Genetic analyses have been successful in identifying genes leading to monogenic disorders, with more than 5000 human characteristics attributed to Mendelian inheritance. The pattern of inheritance is generally deduced from observations of transmission patterns within families. Mendelian disorders are categorized based on the inheritance pattern and the chromosomal location of the genetic mutation.

A monogenic disorder is considered to be autosomal if the mutation arose on a gene encoded on one of the 22 pairs of autosomes (any chromosome other than the sex chromosomes X and Y). Autosomal inheritance is further subdivided such that a disorder can be dominant or recessive. In autosomal dominant disorders, the condition is expressed in heterozygous individuals (individuals with one mutant gene and one normal gene). Therefore, the individual will express the phenotype, which is the observable characteristic resulting from the genotype. Autosomal dominant disorders comprise 10 to 20% of all nonsyndromic hearing loss. On the contrary, autosomal recessive disorders make up the majority of nonsyndromic hearing loss, with 75 to 80% of all nonsyndromic disorders resulting from recessive traits (Finsterer and Fellinger, 2005). Autosomal recessive disorders are characterized by clinical manifestations that are expressed in individuals who carry two copies of the mutant allele. Individuals with two copies of an allele are said to be homozygous at that allele. If two individuals who are heterozygous for the mutant allele mate, then there is a 1 in 4 chance that each offspring will be affected by the autosomal recessive disorder.

Mendelian diseases can also be inherited maternally. In 1 to 5% of nonsyndromic hearing loss cases, the disorder is X-linked, or due to a genetic mutation on the X chromosome. X-linked genes are fully expressed in males because they carry only a single X chromosome. However, in females, two X chromosomes are present, but only one is active. Therefore, a disease encoded by a mutant X-linked gene may or may not be expressed clinically in heterozygous females. Another form of maternally inherited hearing loss is transmitted by the mitochondrial genome in the ovum but not in the sperm. The mitochondria carry their own set of cytoplasmic chromosomes separate from the cellular genome in the nucleus. Mutations in mitochondrial genes can account for up to 20% of nonsyndromic hearing loss.

Monogenic disorders can also be the result of other genetic anomalies. For example, uniparental disomy leads to several forms of hearing loss. Uniparental disomy occurs when one parent contributes two copies of a chromosome, and the other parent contributes none. It has been demonstrated that uniparental disomy of chromosome 13q leads to DFNB1 because of a mutation in connexin 26 (Alvarez et al, 2003). Another cause for monogenic hearing loss is genomic imprinting. Genomic imprinting is when only one copy of the gene is expressed, depending on the inheritance from the mother or father. Genomic imprinting of the mutant paternal allele of the *SDHD* gene has been shown to cause a form of sensorineural hearing loss (Badenhop et al, 2001). Lastly, the expansion of specific DNA sequences is another genetic cause for Mendelian forms of hearing loss.

In what is referred to as "repeat expansion," the number of repeated sequences commonly found in the genome increases with each generation; this is generally due to genetic instability at that specific locus. For example, the harmonin gene is susceptible to an expansion in the gene that underlies Usher's syndrome 1C (Verpy et al, 2000).

Complex Disorders

Genetics of hearing loss is further complicated by disorders exhibiting genetic heterogeneity, in which mutations in different genes cause an identical phenotype, or phenotypic variability, in which a spectrum of phenotypes result from mutations within one gene. Although the environment plays an important role in the clinical manifestation of the disease, it is the interplay between the environment and genes that significantly affects the etiology of the disease. Most common chronic diseases and common congenital defects are due to genetic predispositions. The two models for how a genotype may cause a phenotype are known as qualitative and quantitative genotype effects. The qualitative model states that multiple, small, genetically determined predispositions and environmental exposures work in concert to produce disease. However, in order for an individual to be considered affected by the disease, the confounding effects of predisposing genotypes and environmental effects must sum above a threshold. In the quantitative model, a specific genotype affects only a small percentage of a phenotype. For instance, a specific genotype involved in hearing loss may cause only a 1 to 5% loss in hearing. Multiple quantitative genetic effects work additively such that the severity of hearing loss is based on the summation of multiple genotypes and the interaction of their products with environmental stresses.

Two of the most common forms of hearing loss are complex disorders: presbycusis and noise-induced hearing loss. Within these disorders, genotypes have been found that follow the qualitative or quantitative models or both models.

Presbycusis

Presbycusis (or age-related hearing loss) is extremely common, with a prevalence of 40% of individuals older than the age of 65 years. This percentage increases to 80% of the population when older than 80 years. Presbycusis is characterized by reduced hearing sensitivity and speech understanding with slow central processing of acoustic information. Although the environment, in the form of acquired auditory stress, plays a role in presbycusis, there is a strong genetic component controlling the aging process. Presbycusis is further categorized based on the type of degeneration, such as metabolic and sensorineural forms.

Metabolic forms of presbycusis are the result of stria vascularis degeneration; sensorineural forms are the result of spiral ganglion and/or organ of Corti degeneration. Patients with metabolic presbycusis exhibit an elevated hearing threshold at all frequencies, primarily due to elevated high-frequency thresholds that progress to elevated lower frequency thresholds. The strial atrophy may be due to a decrease in the maintenance of ionic composition, which

affects both neural conductivity and cellular homeostasis. It has also been suggested that the metabolic changes are caused by oxidative damage and a decrease in superoxide dismutase levels in hair cells. This was determined by observing a decline in expression levels of this enzyme prior to hair cell degeneration (Keithley et al, 2005). Sensorineural presbycusis is primarily the result of progressive degeneration of sensory cells in the cochlea and spiral ganglion cells, with the outer hair cells affected the most.

Special Consideration

- Presbycusis is defined as age-related hearing loss in humans. However, it is difficult to separate the effects of age, genetics, and a lifetime of environmental exposures on the hearing apparatus in older humans. Further, the pathological description of presbycusis includes six types: sensory, neural, strial, cochlear conductive, mixed, and indeterminate. Therefore, presbycusis appears to be a heterogeneous collection of multiple disease processes, some of which involve heredity.

Pearl

- By convention, the shorthand names of human genes are in all capital letters and italicized. For example, the human gene that produces cadherin 23 is *CDH23*. Mouse gene names are also italicized, but only the first letter is capitalized. Using the same example, the orthologous mouse gene, which produces the mouse form of cadherin 23, is named *Cdh23*.

The study of model organisms, specifically mouse models, has contributed significantly to the field's progress. Several mouse strains exhibit age-related hearing loss (termed AHL in mice) and have been studied extensively to understand the genetic etiology of AHL. Based on these models, a susceptibility gene for AHL, cadherin 23 (*Cdh23*), was identified in mice (Johnson et al, 1997) and later discovered in humans (Di Palma et al, 2001; Noben-Trauth et al, 2003). *Cdh23* encodes a calcium-binding transmembrane protein that is involved in stereociliary structure and organization. Mutations in Cdh23 have been shown to cause susceptibility to both AHL and noise-induced hearing loss (NIHL). Since this finding, other genes, such as *Bcl-2* and *Sod1*, have been implicated in playing a role in AHL, and other loci contributing to the disorder, *Ahl2* and *Ahl3*, have been mapped. However, the molecular basis of AHL remains to be determined because of nongenetic factors, such as noise exposure and acoustic trauma, which interact with multiple genetic factors and affect the overall clinical manifestation of the disorder.

Noise-Induced Hearing Loss

Noise is the best known and most studied environmental factor to cause hearing loss. Noise causes hearing loss by two mechanisms, direct mechanical damage and secondary metabolic damage. Direct mechanical damage causes deafness due to very high energy noise. Metabolic damage to inner ear structures occurs from loud noises that overwork the hearing physiology without causing direct mechanical failure. Noise induces the release of free radicals, presenting one possible mechanism for cell death leading to hearing loss.

Presumably genetics plays a role in NIHL. Human heritability studies and gene association studies have not linked any hereditary factors to NIHL. However, several studies in mouse models demonstrate a genetic involvement. Targeted mutations in or deletions of several genes in mice lead to increased sensitivity to NIHL. Mutations in genes such as *Cdh23*, which codes for stereocilia linkages, and *Pmca2*, which codes for a calcium pump on the stereocilia, may inhibit reformation of normal stereocilia structures following noise exposure and thereby lead to hair cell dysfunction and death. Mutations in genes such as *Sod1* and *Gpx1*, which have antioxidant functions, also lead to increased sensitivity to noise exposure, probably because of increased cell damage by free radicals. However, the challenge now remains in determining the genetic link between the mouse models and human studies for NIHL.

Studies of hereditary hearing loss began with monogenic disorders that could be tracked through family inheritance patterns. Present technologies and animal models have advanced our abilities to study the complex forms of hereditary hearing loss, particularly in teasing apart genetic from environmental factors. Novel techniques, particularly in bioinformatics and genomics, will further facilitate gene discovery in monogenic and complex diseases.

◆ Approaches to Gene Identification

The mapping and identification of genes involved in common disorders, such as hereditary hearing loss, is critical both to increase the basic understanding of human genetics and to improve the diagnosis and preventive care of diseases. Until recently, there were very few successes in disease gene identification, and these resulted from knowledge of the biochemical basis of the gene product. Recently, advancements in recombinant DNA technology, the Human Genome Project, and bioinformatics have synergistically facilitated exponential growth in understanding the underlying genetic and molecular mechanisms conferring these phenotypes.

Identifying Chromosomal Disorders

Chromosomal disorders are caused by large alterations in chromosomal structure, such as duplications, deletions, and translocations. These alterations are responsible for a significant portion of genetic disorders in the population, with a frequency of 1 in 150 live births. They have a significant effect on mental retardation and spontaneous abortions. Some chromosomal aberrations, such as duplications within chromosomes X or 22, and deletions within chromosome 6, lead to forms of conductive and sensorineural hearing loss.

Cytogenetics involves the study of chromosomal structure. The first visualization of chromosomal structure was in peripheral blood lymphocytes. Later, researchers studied chromosomal replication by monitoring the incorporation of radioactively labeled thymidine into chromosomes. However, the most important advance in cytogenetics has been the development of fluorescence in situ hybridization (FISH), which utilizes fluorescently labeled markers to find chromosomal aberrations. Since the advent of FISH, several diseases that lead to hearing loss, such as Fanconi anemia, have been genetically characterized. The maximum resolution of FISH is several megabases, making it an ideal method for large chromosomal alterations. Although it is not a feasible technique for mapping mutations affecting single genes, it has been used successfully in mapping some loci for monogenic and polygenic disorders.

Identifying Mendelian Disorders

Polymorphisms are common variations in the DNA that occur in a particular population but do not cause disease. Polymorphisms have become important as a method to map disease genes. If a disease gene is near a polymorphism on a chromosome, then the polymorphism may act as a marker for the disease. There are several ways that polymorphisms have been measured, including microsatellites and single nucleotide polymorphisms (SNPs). Microsatellites are polymorphisms in the number of repeated segments that naturally occur as part of a chromosome. Microsatellite markers do not occur as frequently as single nucleotide changes but are easier to analyze. However, with the knowledge of the genomic sequence from the Human Genome Project, we are now able to be more specific and analyze single nucleotide changes, or SNPs. SNPs are the most frequent type of polymorphism in the genome and occur roughly every 1000 nucleotides. Sets of SNPs near one another on a chromosomal segment can be used to define specific DNA regions. Therefore, a specific DNA region, consisting of a series of SNPs that are linked, provides the most detailed DNA information for that particular region.

Linkage Analysis

Using these polymorphism-based markers, disease genes may be studied by linkage analysis. Linkage analysis is based on the premise that genes that reside near one another on a chromosome tend to travel together through meiosis and tend to be "linked," with the possibility that genes separated by a great distance on a chromosome may undergo recombination during meiosis. Shorter length of DNA between two chromosomal sites causes greater linkage, because a random recombination event is less likely to occur in a shorter sequence. The frequency of recombination between two genes provides an estimate of the genetic distance between them; therefore, the farther apart the genes, the higher the frequency of chromosomal breaks between the two. Generally, there are no clues about the chromosomal location of the disease gene, except in cases where the disease gene is X-linked or where there are large chromosomal aberrations. Therefore, to map a gene, markers must be systematically examined for linkage throughout the entire genome. This is referred to as a genome scan.

For Mendelian traits, the most common method for determining linkage is by the "logarithm of odds" (LOD) score. This method determines the likelihood of seeing the observed data in the presence or absence of linkage and depends on the rate of recombination between a marker and a disease gene. Therefore, making linkage comparisons by using an LOD score requires a model to explain the mode of inheritance (autosomal or sex-linked and recessive or dominant). Linkage analysis has been the first step to locate and identify the disease genes, particularly in monogenic diseases.

Special Consideration

- As the name suggests, the LOD is a base-10 logarithmic value. A threshold value for the LOD score must provide a certain level of statistical confidence. When using a genome scan involving multiple linkage comparisons and a statistical p value of .05, an LOD score of 3 or greater suggests significant linkage. An LOD of 3 may be represented in logarithmic form as $\log_{10}(1000) = \log_{10}(10^3) = 3$, indicating that the likelihood of linkage is 1000 times greater than the absence of linkage. However, the linkage represented by an LOD score is limited to ~20 megabase segments. When two loci are 20 megabases or greater apart, the likelihood of recombination is uniformly high.

Identifying Complex Disorders

For common complex diseases, such as AHL and NIHL, the genetic analyses become far more complicated. Because we do not have a concrete idea of the number of susceptibility genes involved, the gene frequencies, or the mode of inheritance, it becomes extremely difficult to apply a genetic model. Nevertheless, the identification of susceptibility genes in complex disorders is now a major part of human genetics research. To identify genes involved in complex disorders, there have been two major approaches to date. The first method, known as a position-independent strategy, does not require any knowledge of the chromosomal location or disease locus. This method is purely based on the functional analysis of genes. The second method is not dependent on functional knowledge and makes no assumptions on the gene product and its biochemical role. This method, known as a position-dependent strategy, is solely based on the position of the disease gene in relation to linkage markers.

Both of these methods have been combined, creating a dynamic process of gene identification. Most genes that contribute to complex diseases are first mapped to a small section of a chromosome using the position-dependent strategy. This yields a locus that may contain several putative genes. The position-independent strategy is then employed to analyze the functional properties of each candidate gene product in comparison to the disease process.

Position-Dependent Strategy

Positional cloning is a position-dependent strategy and has been effectively utilized to identify disease genes based solely on approximate chromosomal location. With the first success in 1986, several genes conferring hereditary hearing loss have been identified using this technique, including the branchio-oto-renal (BOR) syndrome gene (*EYA1*), the Treacher Collins gene (*TCOF1*), and the Waardenburg's syndrome gene (*PAX3*).

Fundamental positional cloning involves tracking a disease locus in families by linkage analysis. This is accomplished through the analysis of a genome-wide scan of known genetic markers and the segregation of these markers with the disease. Through the collection of many families, a dense set of markers can be created, and enough statistical power is established to determine the segregation

Table 6–4   Web Sites for Genomics, Bioinformatics, and Hearing Loss Databases

National Institute of Deafness and Other Communication Disorders	http://www.nidcd.nih.gov/
Information on hereditary hearing loss	http://hearing.harvard.edu http://dnalab-www.uia.ac.be/dnalab/hhh
Cochlear anatomy	http://www.iurc.montp.inserm.fr/cric/audition/english/start2.htm
Human Cochlear EST Database	http://hearing.bwh.harvard.edu/
Gene expression in the developing ear	http://www.ihr.mrc.ac.uk/Hereditary/genetable/index.shtml
Inner Ear Protein Database	http://oto.wustl.edu/thc/history.htm
Role of connexins in hearing loss	http://www.crg.es/deafness/
Genetic counseling	http://www.genetests.com
Gene therapy	http://www.nlm.nih.gov/medlineplus/genesandgenetherapy.html
Mouse genome	http://www.ncbi.nlm.nih.gov/Genomes/index.html http://www.informatics.jax.org
Mouse models for hearing loss	http://www.jax.org/hmr/index.html http://www.ihr.mrc.ac.uk/hereditary/MutantsTable.shtml
Bioinformatics/ genomics databases	http://www.ncbi.nlm.nih.gov/Database/ http://www.ensembl.org/index.html http://www.genome.ucsc.edu/ http://www.hapmap.org http://www.genome.jp/kegg/pathway.html http://www.genenetwork.org/home.html http://symatlas.gnf.org/SymAtlas/

EST, Expressed Sequence Tag.

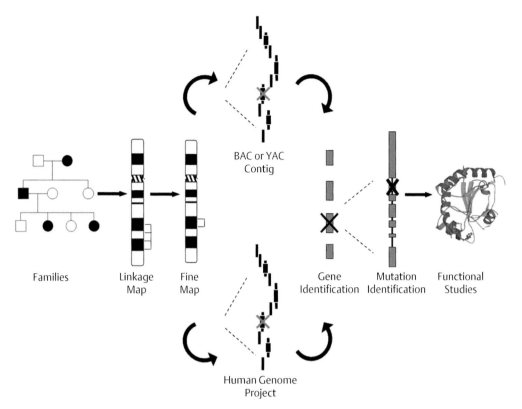

Figure 6–3   Positional cloning strategy as a position-dependent approach to gene identification. The disease locus is mapped through linkage analysis of affected families using a genome scan. A fine map is created through the analysis of polymorphic markers. Through the use of an overlapping set of human DNA, the candidate region is analyzed. With the completion of the Human Genome Project, the map location of the full human genome, including polymorphic markers, is now available for analysis. A survey of genes that are in the candidate region may yield a candidate gene. If not, the genes are sequenced or analyzed for expression differences to identify the gene involved in the disease. BAC, bacterial artificial chromosome; YAG, yeast artificial chromosome.

pattern. With the Human Genome Project, we are now able to locate and confirm the sequence of the polymorphic markers through the use of various databases (**Table 6–4**). Prior to the completion of the Human Genome Project, a long section of human chromosome would be broken into overlapping fragments of a feasible size and analyzed. The candidate regions could then be screened for sequence differences based on markers interspersed within the fragments. Today, genes within the candidate region are identified by searching databases for specific sequences. Through database searches, researchers now focus on genes in the region with a potential clinical significance. Through the determination of sequence or expression-level differences, the causative gene is then identified. The positional cloning strategy is summarized in **Fig. 6–3**.

The discovery of the gene leading to BOR syndrome is a great example of positional cloning leading to gene identification for hereditary hearing loss. BOR syndrome is an autosomal dominant disorder with patients exhibiting mixed hearing loss along with several other abnormalities. Based on the linkage analysis of affected families, BOR syndrome was mapped to human chromosome 8q13. Through the use of polymorphic markers whose map positions were known, the candidate region was then narrowed to ~500 kilobases. The critical region in genomic libraries was analyzed, and candidate genes were isolated. The various genes were se-quenced and confirmed against sequences in databases. With the ability to search the sequences of various organisms, a homology search was conducted, and sequence homology of one of the candidate genes to the *Drosophila* gene, *eyes absent (eya)*, was observed. The *eya* gene is a developmental gene and, when mutated, leads to reduced or absent compound eyes. The role of this gene was confirmed when seven mutations were identified in 42 unrelated BOR patients. This work unequivocally demonstrated that *EYA1*, the orthologous gene in humans, conferred the BOR phenotype (Abdelhak et al, 1997). However, further studies are warranted to determine the functional role of *EYA1* in BOR syndrome.

The discovery of the gene leading to Treacher Collins syndrome is an example of positional cloning in its absolute form. As an autosomal dominant disorder with variable expression, Treacher Collins syndrome leads to conductive deafness and atresia of the external ear canal and was linked to human chromosome 5q31-q34. To fine map the region, new markers were required because the region at the time was not well defined. This led to the refinement of the region and the ability to narrow the interval. By breaking the region into smaller fragments, a linkage and physical map were constructed. With further fine mapping, the region was narrowed to contain seven genes that were isolated and identified with no clinical role. Sequence analysis led to the discovery of the *TCOF1* gene ("Positional cloning of a gene involved in the pathogenesis of Treacher Collins syndrome: the Treacher Collins Syndrome Collaborative Group," 1996). Though this gene had no functional relevance, it was found to be mutated in patients with Treacher Collins syndrome. Different mutations were discovered in five unrelated families. Little is known of the function of the *TCOF1*; however, it has been demonstrated that the gene product has a role in ribosomal DNA gene transcription. Functional studies are being undertaken to further understand the molecular pathogenesis of Treacher Collins syndrome and how it involves *TCOF1*.

The last example of how positional cloning has led to the identification of genes involved in hereditary hearing loss is the identification of the Waardenburg's syndrome gene. Waardenburg's syndrome type 1 is another autosomal dominant disorder with variable expressivity. Analysis of affected families showed linkage on human chromosome 2q. Serendipitously, at the same time a mouse model with a similar phenotype emerged, which was studied to discover the orthologous gene leading to Waardenburg's syndrome. Linkage analysis of the mouse model showed mouse chromosome 1 segregated with the phenotype. The candidate region of mouse chromosome 1 was syntenic (when subchromosomal regions are conserved between two species) to human chromosome 2q, which provided the impetus to continue the positional cloning in both humans and mice. Based on the pathogenesis, it appeared that the same gene was causing the Waardenburg's syndrome phenotype. The candidate gene in the critical interval of the mouse was identified as *Pax3*, a transcription factor. It was further demonstrated that all families with Waardenburg's syndrome type 1 showed linkage to the *PAX3* region of chromosome 2 (Farrer et al, 1994). It has been suggested that the variable expressivity of the disorder may be the result of interactions between *PAX3* and other genes. With the mouse model, the molecular mechanisms involved in Waardenburg's syndrome are being studied extensively.

Position-Independent Strategy

In the position-independent strategy, specific gene products are studied for DNA variations based on their potential role in the manifestation of a target disease. Historically, this was the only approach utilized prior to mapping the sequence of various genomes. There are two ways to approach this strategy: identification of the gene through knowledge of its protein product, and identification of the gene through its function. If there is sufficient knowledge of the protein product, it is possible to identify and characterize the putative gene based on the biochemical basis of the inherited disease. The identification of a gene through function can be determined through cloning by a method called functional complementation. In this approach, if the cloning of potential target gene-containing DNA fragments into cell lines or model organisms leads to the desired change in phenotype, then the fragment of interest can be isolated and identified by sequence. Functional complementation has been successful in various cell lines and yeast to identify genes involved in DNA repair, transcriptional regulation,

and cell cycle regulation. It has also been successful in model organisms, such as transgenic mice. With this technique, DNA fragments from a candidate region found by position-dependent linkage are injected into normal mice. These transgenic mice are then crossed to mice expressing the disease of interest. If the offspring do not express the disease, the DNA fragment contains the gene responsible for the rescue of the disease phenotype. Further sequencing of the fragment will provide information about the gene and the mutation involved in the disorder. Often a disease mutation will produce the same phenotype in both an animal model and humans. Therefore, position-independent identification of a gene in an animal model may allow identification of the orthologous human disease gene. This technique was extremely successful in the identification of the DFNB3 gene, *Myo15* (**Fig. 6–4**).

Animal Models

Animal models, particularly mouse models, have been fundamental tools in understanding the genetics of hearing loss. In this chapter, we will focus on mouse models and the genetic manipulation possible in creating them. Mouse models, either through spontaneous mutations or through genetic engineering, are critical in learning about gene function and the pathogenesis of genetic diseases. With more efficient sequencing capabilities and the sequence of the mouse genome, it has become a goal to knock out or induce increased expression of every mouse gene sequentially and study the downstream effects. The major models to study gene modification are transgenic, gene-targeted, and spontaneously mutated mouse models.

Pearl

- As shown in the position-independent strategy section, mouse and other animal models may allow discovery of disease genes and thereby discovery of orthologous human disease genes. Animal models also have the advantage that environmental factors may be controlled in ways not possible in human populations.

Transgenic Mouse Models

Transgenic mouse technology, in which one or more genes are added to the mouse genome, provides a powerful way to overexpress genes to understand their function or to rescue mutant genes. Generally, genes are introduced into mouse oocytes just after fertilization. The oocyte is then reimplanted into a pseudopregnant female. The injected DNA, often in several copies, will be integrated into the DNA of the mouse progeny. With chromosomal integration, the developing animal will be fully transgenic, and all cells will contain the additional transgene. Often times, tissue or temporal specificity can be included with the transgene of interest to study the role of the gene in a certain tissue or to study the effects of the gene at a certain time in

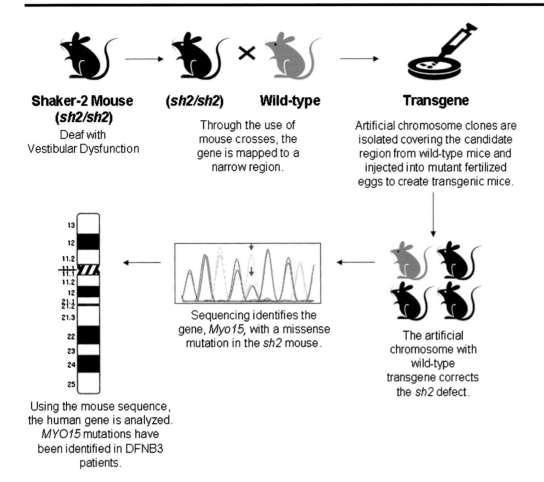

Shaker-2 Mouse (sh2/sh2)
Deaf with
Vestibular Dysfunction

(sh2/sh2)
Through the use of mouse crosses, the gene is mapped to a narrow region.

Wild-type

Transgene
Artificial chromosome clones are isolated covering the candidate region from wild-type mice and injected into mutant fertilized eggs to create transgenic mice.

Sequencing identifies the gene, *Myo15*, with a missense mutation in the *sh2* mouse.

The artificial chromosome with wild-type transgene corrects the *sh2* defect.

Using the mouse sequence, the human gene is analyzed. *MYO15* mutations have been identified in DFNB3 patients.

Figure 6–4 Functional complementation as a position-independent strategy to identify genes in hereditary hearing loss. The *Myo15* gene was identified as a causative gene for the *shaker-2* mouse, a model for DFNB3. Through the use of a transgene to rescue the disease phenotype, the gene was isolated, and the mutation was identified.

development. Transgenic mice are critical in understanding gene dosage effects. Furthermore, transgenic mice are important in confirming the identification of a disease gene. By inserting a wild-type transgene in the mutant model, one can determine if the disease gene, and subsequently the phenotype, is rescued. With the ability to regulate the time and location of gene expression, we have been successful in understanding the molecular mechanisms behind many genes. An example of this is the rescue of the *sh2* mutation leading to DFNB3, as shown in **Fig. 6–4**.

Gene-Targeted Mouse Models

In gene-targeted, or knockout, mouse models, in vivo mutagenesis is accomplished by introducing a mutation into a specific target gene. Using the sequence information of the gene, foreign DNA is introduced to displace the gene of interest. This introduction of a mutation is accomplished by homologous recombination. The intent is to insert the foreign DNA to disrupt the transcription of the target gene. To ensure proper insertion and to track the foreign DNA, a marker is also cloned in with the foreign DNA. The DNA containing the marker that will displace the endogenous gene is introduced into embryonic stem cells that are grown in vitro. The embryonic stem cells are injected into a mouse embryo at the blastocyst stage. The mouse embryo, which contain both wild-type and gene-targeted cells, are reimplanted into a female mouse uterus. The resulting progeny will display mixed expression because their somatic cells will have developed either with or without the targeted gene. In some progeny, the gene will be knocked out of the germline DNA, such that a stable, gene-targeted mouse line will be created. Both transgenic and gene-targeted models allow one to learn about gene expression and regulation.

Currently, large-scale projects are being conducted to investigate gene function. With complete access to sequence information, it is now feasible for universities and private companies to systematically knock out genes. For example, consortia are taking advantage of gene trapping, which is a gene-targeting technique in which a specific type of transgene is inserted into embryonic stem cells. This transgene contains a defective reporter or marker gene to displace a portion of the endogenous gene of interest. Once the reporter gene has inserted into the endogenous gene, it will be expressed, and this allows for confirmation of proper insertion. It is estimated that with this technique, there will be targeted disruption of ~2500 genes per year.

Spontaneous Mouse Models

Animal models may undergo spontaneous mutations that alter their genotype. A spontaneous animal genotype may produce a phenotype similar to the phenotype of a human disease. Such an animal may then be bred to maintain that phenotype, thus becoming a model to study human disease. Despite the difficulty in discovering spontaneous mouse models, various models, such as the *Splotch* mouse for Waardenburg's syndrome, have been characterized for hereditary hearing loss because of the close similarity in phenotypes. However, in other models, there is often considerable divergence with either the phenotype (when targeting the causative gene in humans and mice produces different disease manifestations) or genotype (when the phenotype in humans is due to a different gene than in the mouse model) because of species differences in biochemical and developmental pathways.

Modeling Complex Diseases

The focus of genetics is moving toward understanding the pathogenesis and networks involved in complex diseases, and the molecular basis of these complex traits is being studied with increasing interest. Although transgenic, gene-targeted, and spontaneous mouse models have been extremely valuable in understanding monogenic disorders, common disorders, which are due to many genes, require a more complex form of analysis, particularly because the clinical manifestations are different in humans from various populations. The different combinations of disease susceptibility genes on different combinations of backgrounds in mice are necessary to comprehend and appreciate the complexity of common disorders exhibited by humans.

Quantitative Trait Locus Analysis

Complex traits are the result of multiple genetic loci, either acting concertedly or independently to produce a phenotype with variable expressivity and time of onset. This results in a wide spectrum of severity and difficulty in clinical diagnosis. The chromosomal locus that contributes to the phenotype of the continuous characteristic is referred to as a quantitative trait locus (QTL). QTLs contain specific genetic variations that are responsible for the differences observed in a trait.

Mice are ideal models for QTL analysis in hearing loss because of two major reasons: (1) the ease of breeding allows for complex breeding programs that can be arranged to produce various types of strains; (2) the short generation time and life span allow for the effects of the transmission of specific genetic mutations through several generations to be monitored. The overall strategy in analyzing QTLs involves the intercrossing of inbred mouse strains that exhibit phenotypes on the opposite ends of the spectrum. For example, crossing a strain susceptible to a disease with a strain resistant to the disease will produce progeny that are theoretically identical, with 50% of their genome from the resistant strain and 50% of the susceptible strain. These progeny are then intercrossed to each other to produce mice that will exhibit the entire spectrum of phenotypes due to the shuffling of the genome during meiosis. The larger the number of individual genetic loci affecting the trait and/or the larger the number of polymorphisms at a given locus, the more likely an even distribution pattern will occur. With the advent of molecular biology and statistical techniques, one can study the intercross and correlate the disease trait with the contributing chromosomal loci.

Two inbred mouse strains have been studied extensively for AHL. To follow the segregation of hearing loss, these strains were crossed to each other, and the progeny were then intercrossed. Auditory brainstem response (ABR) thresholds at various ages have been applied to determine hearing in the intercrossed strains and analyzed as a quantitative trait for linkage association (**Fig. 6–5**). Utilizing this technique, researchers identified a major locus that contributes significantly to AHL (Johnson et al, 1997). Since this major discovery, the orthologous region in humans has been demonstrated to contribute to AHL. Upon fine mapping of the region, the gene was identified as *Cdh23*, the

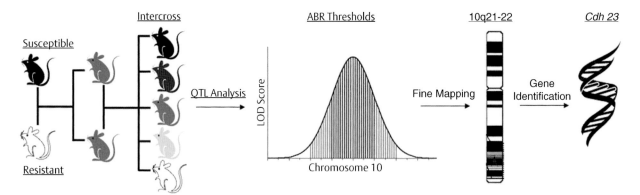

Figure 6–5 Quantitative trait locus (QTL) studies begin with a cross between two inbred strains that differ in their susceptibility to the trait of interest, in this case, age-related hearing loss (AHL). Statistical analysis of the correlation between phenotypes, such as auditory brainstem response (ABR) thresholds, and the genomic regions leads to the identification of QTL on chromosome 10. This is represented by a "logarithm of odds" (LOD) score, where the highest point of the curve is the most likely location of the underlying gene. Mapping techniques and further crossing then lead to gene identification of *Cdh23*.

same gene involved in AHL in humans (Noben-Trauth et al, 2003). Recent developments, especially in genomic resources and bioinformatics, may make this approach to identify more genes that underlie hearing loss QTLs more feasible.

Gene expression levels, like clinical traits such as ABR thresholds, can also serve as quantitative traits to identify genes, and differences in gene expression that trigger a disease phenotype can lead to contributing QTLs. With advances in microarrays, we now have the ability to investigate genome-wide expression profiles. Microarrays allow one to analyze gene transcript levels in an experimental sample simultaneously. Ribonucleic acid (RNA) that is isolated from the sample is quantitated based on fluorescence to provide the level of expression of all genes. This technique, in conjunction with genetics, has been successful in identifying polymorphisms that lead to natural changes in gene expression levels and thereby contribute to one's susceptibility to the disease. Combining QTL analysis and sequence information with microarray technology also identifies regulatory regions that control levels of expression and determines the amount of interaction of genes of interest in biochemical pathways and networks potentially involved in the pathogenesis of the disease.

Bioinformatics and Genomics Approaches

Hearing loss involves a large network of genes that interacts with risk factors, including noise, and involves many different cell types. In the past, these intertwined networks were studied through the perturbation of a single element, as in the case of transgenic or gene-targeted mouse models. With public accessibility and a worldwide collaborative effort to develop databases, the sequence information of many species, transcript information on all tissues, and QTL analyses and network data have made it possible to attack complex diseases using a multipronged approach.

Several databases have been established as a concerted effort to provide resources for sequence information, computational biology, and software tools to analyze genomes for various organisms (**Table 6–4**). Most databases are multidisciplinary with applied research in computational molecular biology. With the intersection of mathematical and computational methods with genetics and molecular biology techniques, several fields have come together to explore fundamental biomedical processes. Various fields have linked databases with sequencing, cloning, and mapping information and computational programs on several model organisms, including rodents, yeast, worm, fly, zebrafish, and plants. These sites not only provide access to data but also allow the ability to mine for data and upload data to contribute to the ongoing research. Web sites also serve to research molecular interaction networks for metabolic and regulatory pathways. Sites consists of interactive database resources that combine data on networks, sequences, expression levels, and phenotypes for complex disorders to access different reference populations of various organisms with extensive genetic and phenotypic information for each population. Currently, because of international efforts, researchers have compiled at least 30,000 pathways to

understand biological processes in several organisms. In this concerted approach, all databases are linked to each other, and each site in turn is specialized and caters to a specific field. This has led to a synergistic effect on the fast-paced field of genomics and bioinformatics.

In 2000, public and private efforts independently generated maps of the human genome. Since then, public and private groups have come together to annotate the sequence and identify genes. Although determining the human DNA sequence has been a large feat, the next great challenge will be to unravel the genome and understand it. With continuing advancements in the efficiency and cost-effectiveness of analyzing data, we hope to not only recognize the genetics behind hearing loss but also understand the biological mechanisms involved.

Human Studies for Complex Disorders

Through the discovery of genetic factors that lead to monogenic or complex diseases, the insights gained provide mechanistic clues to the biology of cells and organ systems. Whereas linkage analyses, as described above, have been successful in identifying genetic variants that cause rare, single-gene disorders, other techniques have been more fruitful in identifying genes in common human disorders.

The primary approach to studying common disorders in humans has been association studies, in which an association between a genetic variant, such as an SNP, and the disease is established based on a comparison between affected patients and unaffected controls. Because of the abundance of these variants in the genome, there is a broad spectrum in the frequency of polymorphisms throughout a population. In association studies, each putative variant is statistically tested for association with the disorder. With ~11 million SNPs in the human genome, this can be a very laborious and cost-intensive process. To narrow this approach, many studies have focused on specific candidate genes with a biochemical or physiological relevance to the disorder and have determined whether a sequence variant within these genes associates with the disease. These candidate genes are often selected based on either functional studies or animal models. This method was utilized in determining an association between a variant in *CDH23* and sensorineural hearing loss (Noben-Trauth et al, 2003).

Another method commonly used today is a genome-wide approach. Genome-wide association studies take advantage of the fact that common sequence variants in the genome are perfectly correlated with nearby variants. The genotype at one locus can predict the genotype at nearby locations. Therefore, one would only need to analyze a particular sequence variation in a region because it would serve as a representative or proxy marker for that specific locus. This is based on the idea that entire portions of chromosomes are inherited in blocks, and therefore, a few variants can be chosen to capture the entire block. By studying only the selected SNPs, one can acquire information or essentially the "fingerprint" of that specific region and test whether the region is associated with the disease. Like positional cloning, the genome-wide approach requires no prior knowledge and makes no assumptions of a functional role of the candidate gene.

Prior to the completion of the Human Genome Project, an association study was a daunting, if not impossible, task. Now, with the establishment of the International HapMap Project, one can identify common variations, their frequencies, and the correlation between them and surrounding variations in several different populations, including populations of African, Asian, and European ancestry. Started in 2002, the International HapMap Project is a partnership between the United States, Canada, China, Japan, the United Kingdom, and Nigeria. It is expected to be fully completed by 2010, although the data are readily available now. The International HapMap Project is an invaluable tool to study variations contributing to a disease through a whole genome approach or to study variations identified in a specific candidate gene. Whereas the Human Genome Project provided the sequence to the human genome, the International HapMap Project will provide the sequence variations that make populations so different. It is the next logical step proceeding from the success of the Human Genome Project. Because of the international collaborative efforts in this era of genomics and bioinformatics, studies that were once considered improbable are now on the forefront of producing the necessary information to understand the biology of humans and the pathogenesis of disease.

◆ Present Knowledge of Hereditary Hearing Loss

The functional genetics of hearing have been studied through hereditary hearing impairments. In particular, family studies have been essential in linking a genotype with a hearing loss phenotype. At present, DNA arrays and other technologies are allowing an unprecedented advance in the detection and understanding of hereditary hearing loss and the functions of genes involved in hearing (**Fig. 6–6**).

Various mutations within a single gene have been shown to produce both syndromic and nonsyndromic diseases. Modifier genes further broaden the phenotypic spectrum produced by a single gene mutation. Further, heterogeneity of gene mutations affects hearing such that several genes can produce the same type of hearing impairment. Therefore, classification by genotype is becoming as important as phenotypic description. Genotypic information may evolve into the primary classification system for hearing loss.

Here we review select genes and functional networks involved in hearing loss by functional or developmental anatomy. For a comprehensive review of syndromic hearing loss disorders, please refer to the comprehensive text by Toriello and colleagues (2005).

External Auditory Canal

Malformation of the external ear may be an isolated phenotype, or it may be found as part of a syndrome. Congenital malformation, specifically of the external auditory canal, can cause a conductive hearing loss due to direct obstruction of sound or indirect obstruction by predisposing a patient to otitis externa, cerumen impaction, or other potentially occluding factors.

Congenital aural atresia involves developmental obstruction due to lack of formation of the external auditory canal either with or without normal middle ear architecture. This disease usually occurs as part of a syndrome (e.g., Treacher Collins) and is rarely found in isolation.

Pearl

- The majority of syndromic hearing loss is due to conductive or mixed hearing impairment from malformation of the external auditory apparatus.

Middle Ear

Hereditary diseases involving the middle ear are relatively sparse. Otosclerosis is the major hereditary disease identified that affects function in this anatomical region. In addition, the X-linked DFN3 due to rare mutations in *POU3F4* may cause conductive and sensorineural hearing loss. The conductive hearing loss in this case is due to stapes fixation and is similar to otosclerosis.

Otosclerosis is a postlingual form of hearing loss generally described as a conductive hearing loss, although it may have components or be completely composed of sensorineural hearing loss. The prevalence of otosclerosis is 0.2 to 1.0% of the adult Caucasian population. Seven otosclerosis loci, labeled *OTSC1–7*, have been identified by linkage analysis. A mutation in *COL1A1*, which encodes type 1 collagen and is a major contributor to bone structure, has been identified within *OTSC1*.

Otosclerosis is a disease with associations to autoimmunity, infection, and heredity. It may involve any part of the petrous temporal bone, although there are some focal sites with higher prevalence. The most common site affected is the otosclerotic angle. Extension of the disease from this site to the footplate of the stapes can lead to conductive hearing loss. Otosclerotic sensorineural hearing loss is hypothesized to be due to lesions affecting the cochlea or cochlear nerve within the temporal bone.

Inner Ear

The inner ear presents the area of greatest structural and functional complexity within the hearing apparatus. This complexity creates a multitude of targets for hereditary and environmental hearing impairment. The vast majority of hereditary nonsyndromic hearing loss occurs due to genetic variation affecting inner ear cells and structures. This usually results in sensorineural hearing loss. We have categorized inner ear genes causing hearing loss by microanatomy or function, including hair cells and stereocilia, potassium recycling, acellular structures, mitochondria, and embryology.

COCHLEA CROSS SECTION

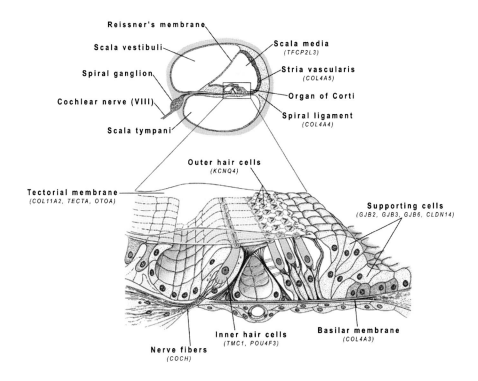

HAIR CELL

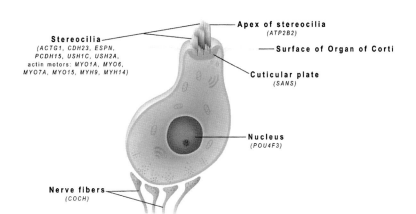

Figure 6–6 Anatomical locations of genes involved in hearing loss.

Hair Cells and Stereocilia

There are a multitude of gene products involved in hair cell function, particularly in stereocilia function. Genes expressed in hair cells that have also been found to be mutated in hearing loss may be classified by structure and function. These include actin (*ACTG1*), actin motors (*MYO1A, MYO7A, MYO15*), actin tertiary structure (*DIAPH1, ESPN*), stereociliary morphogenesis (*CDH23, MYO7A, PCDH15,*

SANS, USH1C), and hair cell morphogenesis (*DFNB9, WHRN*). Mutation in one of these genes often leads to hair cell death.

Allelism, in which specific kinds or locations of mutations occur within a single gene, has been found to correlate highly with phenotype in some genes such as *CDH23*. Cadherin 23, encoded by *CDH23*, is involved in linkages between stereocilia affecting both stereociliary development and function. For instance, missense mutations in

CDH23 allow translation of a less functional protein and result in presbycusis or DFNB12. However, nonsense mutations in *CDH23*, in which no cadherin 23 protein is present, result in Usher's syndrome type 1C. Decrease in cadherin 23 function may only inhibit tip link formation, whereas complete loss of cadherin 23 inhibits stereociliary morphogenesis and elongation. Many of the gene products expressed in hair cells are functionally interactive.

Usher's syndrome type 1, which is defined by blindness and profound deafness, has been associated with nonsense mutations in only five genes. The identified genes, which are usually affected by a null mutation, include *MYO7A* (Usher 1B), *USH1C* (Usher 1C), *CDH23* (Usher 1D), *PCDH15* (Usher 1F), and *SANS* (Usher 1G). Usher syndrome type 1 appears to be caused by dysfunction of a complex of proteins required for stereociliary development and function (Frolenkov et al, 2004). The loss of a component protein by a null mutation may inhibit formation of the entire protein complex, which then blocks the morphogenesis of stereocilia in the inner ear and retina.

Potassium Recycling

Potassium recycling within the cochlea involves a network of genes that produce gap junctions (*GJB2*, *GJB3*, and *GJB6*) and potassium channels (*KCNQ4* and *TMC1*).

Gap junctions are connecting tubes formed between cells that allow the passage and exchange of cytoplasmic components, including ions, metabolic intermediates, and second messengers, between cells. The gap junction tubes are formed by the assembly of subunit proteins called connexins. The connexins forming a gap junction differ between various tissues. These tissue-specific connexin isoform assemblies have differences in their gap junction function.

DFNB1 is a very common prelingual form of hearing loss and related to mutations in the connexin genes, *GJB2* and *GJB6*, located together on chromosome 13. Connexin 26 is encoded by *GJB2* and connexin 30 by *GJB6*. DFNB1 may be caused by mutations affecting these two genes in homozygous, compound heterozygous, or digenic heterozygous ways. Basically, two mutations among these two genes cause a critical reduction in the concentration of functional protein. It may be possible for mutated connexins to form gap junctions, but the function of such complexes would be retarded. Mouse knockout models of *Gjb6* and inner ear–specific knockout of *Gjb2* have shown deafness related to nonsensory cell and hair cell death.

Clouston's syndrome, also known as hidrotic ectodermal dysplasia, has been associated with autosomal dominant missense mutations in *GJB6* but not *GJB2*. The syndrome is marked by a skin disease including palmoplantar hyperkeratosis, hair defects, and nail hypoplasia with defects. Some individuals with Clouston's syndrome also experience hearing impairment. In contrast to the DFNB1-related mutations that produce a dysfunctional protein, the missense mutations in *GJB6* causing Clouston's syndrome result in impaired trafficking of the protein to the plasma membrane. Therefore, the skin disease is related to mutations that prevent the formation of the connexin 30–containing gap junction.

Pearl

- Mutations in *GJB2* account for up to 50% of human sensorineural hearing loss worldwide. Hearing loss due to *GJB2* mutations may respond better to cochlear implants than other prelingual hereditary forms of hearing loss (Green et al, 2002). Mutations in *GJB2* interrupt the potassium recycling from hair cells to supporting cells, possibly resulting in the death of these cells. However, the spiral ganglion neurons appear to be unaffected and remain able to interact with a cochlear implant. Many other forms of hereditary sensorineural hearing loss involve neuronal cell death such that a cochlear implant would not be as effective.

Acellular Structures

Cochlear function relies on several genes to produce acellular structures, including the various basement membrane structures formed by isoforms of type IV collagen (*COL4A3*, *COL4A4*, and *COL4A5*) and the tectorial membrane (*COL11A2*, *TECTA*, and *OTOA*). Type IV collagen is found in the basement membrane of the basilar membrane, spiral ligament, and vessels of the stria vascularis and renal glomeruli. Alport's syndrome is linked to mutations in type IV collagen and is defined by hereditary kidney disease (glomerulonephritis) that may be concurrent with several other symptoms, including sensorineural hearing loss.

Mutations in the three genes expressed within the tectorial membrane—*COL11A2*, *TECTA*, and *OTOA*—have been linked to hearing loss. Alpha-collagen XI type 2 is involved in collagen fibril structures within the tectorial membrane. Curiously, hearing loss linked to *COL11A2* mutations is postlingual, usually presenting after age 30. Collagen XI is also involved in formation of the eyeball, bone, and cartilage such that some mutations lead to Stickler's syndrome and affect these multiple organ systems in addition to the inner ear.

The *OTOA* gene encodes otoancorin, which appears to anchor the tectorial membrane to the apical surface of the cochlear sensory epithelium. It provides a similar function in the vestibular apparatus by anchoring the acellular gel to the apical surface of neurosensory cells. Otoancorin mutations presumably allow displacement of the tectorial membrane in relation to the hair cell stereocilia. This would interfere with the efficient transfer of vibrations in mechanotransduction.

Mitochondria

About 42 to 70% of individuals with mitochondrial disorders also experience sensorineural hearing loss. Approximately 3% of sensorineural hearing loss in a population is linked to mutations in mitochondrial DNA. Mitochondrial DNA mutations have been associated with both syndromic and nonsyndromic hearing loss, sensitivity to ototoxic agents, and presbycusis. Mutations affecting mitochondrial transfer

RNA (tRNA) cause MELAS (an acronym based on clinical symptoms including myopathy, encephalopathy, lactic acidosis, and stroke), MERRF (myoclonic epilepsy associated with ragged red fibers), and maternally inherited diabetes and deafness. Mutations in mitochondrial 12S ribosomal RNA (rRNA) have been linked to ototoxic sensitivity to aminoglycosides. Therefore, mitochondrial mutations may have a variety of phenotypic effects related to hearing loss. Recent work links acquired mutations in mitochondrial DNA with presbycusis.

Diseases linked to mitochondrial mutations often occur in cells with a high energy requirement, such as cochlear hair cells. It is hypothesized that mitochondrial dysfunction will reduce the available adenosine triphosphate (ATP) and lead to imbalances in ionic gradients. Such gradients are particularly active in muscle and nerve tissues.

Embryology

Genes directing embryological development are often active in multiple organs. Gene mutations that affect otocyst development generally cause syndromic hearing loss, including BOR syndrome (*EYA1* and *SIX1*), Treacher Collins syndrome (*TCOF1*), Waardenburg's syndrome (*MITF* and *PAX3*), and Wolfram syndrome (*WFS1*). Rarely, allelism of mutations in these genes will produce NSHL, such as DNFA6/14/38 (*WFS1*). Significant effort has been dedicated to study the timing of gene expression in embryological development.

◆ Clinical Aspects and Future Directions

Research into genetics ultimately seeks to reduce disease and improve health. The clinical application of genetics in hearing loss begins with genetic evaluation and counseling. Soon, this will lead to gene-based diagnosis and treatment modalities. The present capabilities and future directions of pharmacogenomics, stem cell, and gene-based therapies are reviewed.

Genetic Evaluation and Counseling

A genetic evaluation is usually conducted as part of the medical evaluation of a patient either presenting at birth with congenital malformations or presenting later in life with a related family history. In both cases, the geneticist's goal is a specific diagnosis to facilitate counseling regarding prognosis, treatment options, and related genetic issues. Note that any complete genetic evaluation will also include detailed information gathering of environmental exposures to ascertain the impact of both genetic and environmental factors. A genetic evaluation followed by appropriate genetic counseling is an important part of the medical evaluation in both syndromic and nonsyndromic forms of disease.

Genetic Evaluation for Hearing Loss

A specific diagnosis is the required, but often elusive, goal of genetic evaluation. Syndromic disease is generally recognized at birth or in the neonatal period. In the past, dysmor-

phologists would make a syndromic diagnosis based on patterns of malformation and related laboratory values. The American College of Medical Genetics has developed an algorithmic aid used in the evaluation of a child with congenital malformations (Reid and Robinson, 1999). Correct diagnoses of syndromes affecting the head and neck can benefit from a comprehensive listing of disease characteristics, as shown by Gorlin et al (2005). This encyclopedic text sorts craniofacial defects by known genetic causes, such as chromosomal, single gene, or multifactorial, or as unknown. At present, the genetic cause of most congenital malformations is unknown.

Syndromic classification by recognition of concurrent abnormalities in multiple organ systems is a phenotypic assessment. However, allelism within a single gene has been shown in multiple examples to lead to either syndromic or nonsyndromic hearing loss. Therefore, a nonsyndromic form of hearing loss may be diagnosed when related syndromic aspects are subtle or not expressed at birth. Future genetic diagnosis for the presence of specific mutations will greatly enhance early and accurate detection of both syndromic and nonsyndromic hearing loss.

For instance, early diagnosis of any hearing impairment is of great importance in neonates. However, genetic testing is of questionable value in the neonate except for diseases in which early intervention will significantly reduce morbidity or mortality. Universal newborn hearing screening is gaining support as a method to identify hearing loss prior to deficits in early language development. The present value of newborn genetic testing will only be achieved in several rare situations. Genetic testing should always be used in conjunction with the clinical assessment, including family history and physical exam, and the newborn hearing screening in the case of neonates.

Special Consideration

- A common ethical question in genetic diagnostics is whether one should test for a genetic disease if there are no available treatments. Recently, it was found that 85% of hearing and 62% of deaf or hearing-impaired people would desire genetic testing of hearing loss in their infant regardless of available treatments (Bauer et al, 2003).

- Some hereditary diseases manifest beyond congenital or childhood time periods. A familial disease may be first considered in the differential diagnosis of a parent when the child presents a similar phenotype. There are several nonsyndromic forms of progressive hearing loss that may present in later life, though most include measurable congenital hearing impairment.

Genetic Counseling

In 1947, the term *genetic counseling* was coined by Sheldon C. Reed and was considered to have three requirements: the knowledge of human genetics; the respect for sensitivities, attitudes, and reactions of clients; and the provision of genetic information to the fullest extent known (Veach and Leroy, 2003). Similar to the earlier standards, the goals of genetic counseling today include (1) an explanation of the diagnosis, pathophysiology, prognosis, and management options; (2) counseling support that takes into consideration ethnic, cultural, religious, and other aspects of family dynamics; and (3) an explanation of the risk of recurrence in future pregnancies and options in the case of recurrence for congenital diseases. It is important for a genetic counselor to meet these goals in a manner that takes into account the educational background of the patient and involved family. A genetic counselor may play a lifelong role in the care of patients with congenital malformations.

In recent years, genetic counseling has begun to include some form of specific genetic diagnosis, often for well-characterized monogenic disease linkages such as *BRCA1*. Due to continuing advances in both diagnostic abilities and the understanding of disease processes, genetic counseling requires continuous educational efforts. A geneticist is an important part of a multidisciplinary team and must be able to contribute the most up-to-date technical information and options.

Special Consideration

- Although disclosure of genetic information may lead to changes in health insurance and discrimination, situations may arise that will require disclosure. For example, during genetic counseling, it may prove necessary to warn at-risk relatives, and as a result, lead to the disclosure of a patient's genetic information. Present guidelines allow such disclosure only when there is a hereditary risk for a serious disease, along with early detection and therapy that may significantly reduce morbidity and mortality (Patenaude, 2005).

Gene-Specific and Stem Cell Therapies

Many potential gene-specific or stem cell therapies have been studied, though few have yielded clinical application. Here we review the major tenets of these approaches and focus on their progress and potential in hearing loss. The therapies reviewed include pharmacogenomics, stem cell therapies, and gene-specific therapies.

The majority of insults to the hearing apparatus, whether of genetic or environmental origin, affect the hair cells and the spiral ganglion neurons within the cochlea. Damage to these cells generally leads first to cell dysfunction and then to cell loss by apoptosis (programmed cell death). Therefore, these novel strategies have focused on preventing damage to or repopulating the hair cells and spiral ganglion neurons. For example, pharmacogenomics seeks to identify the interaction of drugs in relation to the genotype, which may lead to the creation and usage of more efficient and less toxic drugs. Stem cell therapies seek to regenerate tissues through the activation or transplantation of cells. Gene therapy attempts to alter the genotype of cells to correct a

genetic defect or to alter the phenotype of supporting cells, which could repopulate the sensory epithelium and spiral ganglion. Finally, some situations may require simultaneous usage of several of these modalities.

Pharmacogenomics in Hearing Loss   It has been shown in multiple examples that a patient's genotype may greatly affect the efficacy or toxicity of drug therapy. Pharmacogenomics involves alteration in the usage of medicines based on a patient's genotype. Pharmacogenomic principles were first used in highly penetrant monogenic diseases, in which clinicians sought to limit the number of adverse reactions due to a specific drug or dosage (Nebert and Vesell, 2004). It has been hypothesized that adverse drug reactions result in a fatality rate of more than 5% per year in hospitalized patients (Nebert and Vesell, 2004). In terms of hearing, pharmacogenomics has many potential avenues. These include recognition of either a potentially harmful drug or a particularly effective drug in relation to a genotype. Most of the work in this area has focused on how mitochondrial genotypes alter aminoglycoside sensitivity.

Initial studies in pharmacogenomics have involved linkage of genotypes to the specific activity of a drug in terms of efficacy or toxicity. For instance, as we find multiple genotypes that affect aminoglycoside sensitivity, then concurrent screening of these genotypes may enhance our ability to protect patients from toxic exposures. Though costly, DNA array technology is able to produce this kind of concurrent genetic screening.

Recently, DNA arrays have yielded unprecedented abilities to identify potential drug therapies without knowledge of gene function. The array uses genotypes and gene expression as markers for functional pathways. Diseased cells have expression profiles that are altered in very specific ways from normal cells of the same tissue. Arrays yield the potential to compare multiple linkages such that many different predisposing genotypes for a condition, such as sensitivity to aminoglycoside agents, could be simultaneously measured.

Cells and tissues involved in any process may be analyzed by a gene expression profile to extrapolate the effects of specific drugs. For example, expression profiling has been successful in identifying genes expressed in cancer cell lines that are associated with sensitivity to chemotherapeutic agents. Expression profiling may also identify drugs or functional groups on drugs as being particularly effective. This may lead to genomic-based drug design. Using expression profiles to tailor drug regimens will likely become more useful in the near future as a cost-effective and rational method. Widespread usage will require continuation of the efforts to expand our knowledge of expression profiles and their relation to physiological processes.

Stem Cells in Hearing Loss

It has been hypothesized that stem cells transplanted into the inner ear may be able to regenerate hearing. In contrast to most epithelia in the body, the hair cells in the human cochlea are both relatively few in number and do not regenerate. Furthermore, the cellular architecture responsible for hearing involves a complex interplay between hair cells, supporting cells, ionic contributions from local cells, and structural and neural connections. Stem cell therapy must be able to replace cells in both a gross fashion and in a way that reconstructs the complex microarchitecture required for hearing.

Stem cells have not been identified within the mammalian cochlea. Presently, stem cells transplanted into the cochlea may come from two main sources: embryonic and adult stem cells.

Embryonic Stem Cells   Embryonic stem cells are generated from the blastocyst stage. Due to collection at this extremely early stage of development, these cells are able to differentiate into any somatic cell type when given the appropriate induction signals. This multipotency, along with the ability to proliferate in vitro for an indefinite period, presents tremendous advantages to the usage of embryonic stem cells in transplantation procedures.

Embryonic stem cells require differentiation signals prior to transplantation, and naive embryonic stem cells spontaneously form multiple tissue types resembling teratomas upon in vivo transplantation. Such cells have been transplanted to the inner ear following in vitro differentiation into several cell types, including neurons, glia, hair cells, and supporting cells (Matsui and Okamura, 2005). Incorporation of transplanted cells into damaged sensory epithelium occurred in greater numbers than into undamaged epithelium. However, present studies have not shown functional hearing reconstitution following embryonic stem cell transplantation.

Somatic cell nuclear transfer (SCNT) is a subset of embryonic stem cells in which the blastocyst is enucleated and any desired nuclear material is added. These stem cells have earned the term *therapeutic cloning* due to the usage of cloning technology with stem cells for transplant purposes. SCNT technology is able to create an embryonic stem cell line specific for each patient; therefore, donor immunogenicity will not be a problem.

Adult Stem Cells   Initially, adult stem cells were thought to be significantly limited, being committed to the cell lineages in the tissue of origin. However, adult stem cells have now been shown capable of multipotential differentiation regardless of the originating tissue. Adult stem cells of various progenitor capabilities have been successfully harvested from human tissues, including dermis and skeletal muscle (Young et al, 2005). Autologous transplantation, which uses the patient's own cells, will avoid an immunogenic rejection. Epiblast-like stem cells are able to form any germ cell layer and represent the greatest multipotency of all adult-derived cells (Young et al, 2005). In contrast to embryonic stem cells, all forms of adult stem cells are quiescent unless receiving signals to differentiate or proliferate and, therefore, will not spontaneously form teratoma-like tissue in vivo. Interestingly, a gene therapy study to be discussed later points to local architectural cues from pillar cells (Izumikawa et al, 2005). These local signals may direct stem cells, particularly epiblast-like cells, to differentiate

into several different cell types with integration into the sensory epithelium. Furthermore, local cellular signals within the inner ear will likely be far superior to any culture media used to induce in vitro differentiation.

Epiblast-like stem cells have shown all of the multipotential advantages of embryonic stem cells. Additionally, epiblast-like stem cells may be a better substrate for direct transplantation, because they will receive local tissue differentiation signals. They have shown success in functional reconstitution of nigrostriatal neurons in a rat model of Parkinson's disease. Epiblast-like stem cells have also been incorporated into pancreatic, endothelial, and cardiac myocyte tissues (Young et al, 2005). However, they have not yet been transplanted into the cochlea of an animal model or human.

Ethics of Stem Cell Usage   Human embryonic stem cells are generated by harvesting a human blastocyst. This presently requires the sacrifice of an early human embryo. Many feel that this is the sacrifice of a living person and are opposed to such research. Debate in the United States has led to government funding for only a handful of approved embryonic stem cell lines. Research involving any other embryonic stem cells or cell lines is excluded from government funding but may be pursued with private funding. Adult stem cells, particularly when used in an autologous fashion, do not engender moral questions and therefore may be ethically superior to embryonic stem cells in transplantation.

Controversial Point

• Should embryonic stem cell research be an issue that requires government intervention? If so, should embryonic stem cell research on every level become legal in the United States? With a controversial issue such as stem cell research, should the government be responsible for providing funding for the research? And if investigators are to conduct stem cell research, do they need to consider any moral obligations involved? These are issues that perhaps should be addressed or considered, as there are moral and religious implications involved in stem cell research.

Gene Therapy in Hearing Loss

Gene therapy involves altering the genome of a cell, tissue, or organism. It relies on a vector to carry the desired genetic material to the target cells. Vectors may be applied in a systemic fashion, in which many cells in the body may be affected. The inner ear is a relatively closed, fluid-filled system, such that systemic application of vectors may not be effective. Vectors may also be applied in a local fashion directly to the organ or tissue. The small volume of endolymph and perilymph may be an advantageous local medium for the spread of locally applied vectors to inner ear structures. Similar to stem cell methods, local administration of vectors to the inner ear has the potential for surgical damage and ectopic transfection. Local administration and tissue-specific expression or targeting of the vector may yield greater specificity and limit ectopic transfection (Atar and Avraham, 2005).

Various anatomically based approaches for the administration of vectors directly to the inner ear have been studied. The majority involve surgical entry into inner ear structures with concomitant morbidity. Some studies have shown that various forms of vectors are able to pass through the round window membrane. Placement of vectors in the middle ear at the round window may be effective while minimizing surgical trauma to the inner ear. Not surprisingly, the method of vector administration and the type of vector affect many transfection variables.

Vectors come in several forms with important differences in their application to the inner ear (**Table 6–5**) (Atar and Avraham, 2005). Only adeno-associated virus (AAV) vectors and retroviral vectors are able to cause permanent transfection of a genome by incorporation into the chromosomal DNA. Unlike most vectors, retroviral vectors require cell division for transfection, which limits their usage. So far, only adenoviral vectors have produced effective transgene expression in the stria vascularis. The choice of vector must match the goals of the gene therapy.

Finally, the timing of administration of gene therapy must be considered. The majority of hereditary hearing loss is found postnatally and requires a disease correction form of gene therapy. Therefore, we will only consider gene therapy administration to postnatal inner ear structures.

The field of gene therapy has largely focused on the correction of single gene defects in autosomal recessive disease, though hereditary hearing loss has not been significantly included. Unfortunately, many of the hereditary diseases that affect the inner ear result in hair cell or neuron death. Therefore, gene therapy in the inner ear has largely focused on replacing the cells lost from the sensory epithelium. Gene therapy–based manipulation of the cell

cycle, differentiation status, or neurotrophin expression in the remaining cells of the inner ear may be able to reconstitute the lost hair cells and spiral ganglion neurons. Finally, we will review monogenic gene therapy and interference RNA methods.

Cell Cycle Manipulation

Cyclin-dependent kinases are proteins that function in cellular differentiation. They push differentiation toward a dedicated somatic cell state that will not reenter the cell cycle. Blocking one or more of the kinases involved in terminal differentiation may allow cells to reenter the cell cycle and proliferate. In damaged cochleas, the majority of cells remaining will be supporting cells following apoptosis of hair cells and spiral ganglion cells. This therapy will seek to cause proliferation of the remaining hair and spiral ganglion cells.

Supporting cells induced to reenter the cell cycle may potentially cause dedifferentiation to a progenitor cell type. Upon the second terminal differentiation, these progenitor cells may be able to form hair cells with cues from the local cellular milieu.

The cyclin-dependent kinase inhibitor, p27/Kip1, is the first expressed in the terminal mitosis pathway toward becoming a hair cell. Animal models with the p27/Kip1 gene knockout have shown transient prolongation of mitosis leading to overpopulation of hair cells and supporting cells. However, these cells soon undergo apoptosis. Our understanding of these differentiation pathways is presently too crude to control the multiple factors in a coherent manner. However, this is an important area for continued study, especially as DNA arrays and other technologies improve our understanding of the timing in gene expression.

Differentiation Control

Similar to manipulation of the cell cycle, alteration of the differentiation status of the supporting cells may reconstitute hair cells. Lower vertebrates provide models to better

Table 6–5   Gene Therapy Vectors

Vector	Genome	Insert (kB)	Site/expression	Efficiency	Cell division required?	Advantages	Disadvantages
AAV	ssDNA	4.5	Genome/permanent	Variable	No	No human disease	Difficult to produce
Retrovirus	RNA	6–7	Genome/permanent	Low	Yes	Suited for neoplasias	Insertional mutagenesis
Adenovirus	dsDNA	7.5	Episome/transient	Moderate	No	Ease of production	Inflammatory response
Herpesvirus	dsDNA	10–100	Episome/transient	Moderate	No	Neural tropism	Human disease
Plasmid	RNA/DNA	Infinite	Episome/transient	Very low	No	Safe, easy production	Low transfection
Liposome	RNA/DNA	Infinite	Episome/transient	Very low	No	Safe, easy production	Low transfection

AAV, adeno-associated virus; dsDNA, double-stranded DNA; ssDNA, single-stranded DNA.

understand the differentiation control of the sensory epithelium. These animals have shown spontaneous regeneration of damaged hair cells, which has not been found in mammals, however. Characterization of the regenerative pathways may lead to methods for mammalian hair cell regeneration. Regeneration in lower vertebrates appears to happen by two methods: mitotic proliferation and transdifferentiation (Matsui and Okamura, 2005). Transdifferentiation involves a somatic cell changing from one terminally differentiated state to another. Though lower vertebrate models present exciting potential, no gene therapy targets have yet been identified.

A mammalian model has provided the first functional restoration of damaged sensory epithelium utilizing differentiation-based gene therapy (Izumikawa et al, 2005). The gene, *Atoh1,* is a transcription factor that causes progenitor cells to differentiate into hair cells. Using an adenoviral vector, *Atoh1* has been delivered to deafened guinea pig cochleas via a cochleostomy. Histological studies showed cells with hair cell–like stereocilia and an increased number of cells within the cochlea. Functionally, hearing was regained up to near normal thresholds. The increased number of cells could be due to local migration of supporting cells or an unexpected proliferative response to the *Atoh1* gene therapy. Reconstitution of hearing function suggests that *Atoh1* not only induced transdifferentiation into hair cells, but these hair cells were able to make the appropriate mechanical and neuronal connections.

Because the guinea pigs had been deafened only days prior to the gene therapy, one can hypothesize that the spiral ganglion axons and the sensory cells still maintained the local signals to re-create the necessary cellular architecture. In humans, deafness and its related cellular death may have occurred years prior. In such long-term deafness, remodeling of the cellular microarchitecture may not maintain the local signals to rebuild the functional connections to produce hearing. However, the fact that *Atoh1* gene therapy was able to regenerate any functional hearing is a remarkable beginning toward differentiation-based gene therapy in humans.

Neurotrophins

Neurotrophins in the inner ear function to support the development of spiral ganglion neurons and their connections. Usage of neurotrophin therapy could assist the regrowth of neural connections and may be particularly beneficial in conjunction with cochlear implants.

Some factors, for instance brain-derived neurotrophic factor and neurotrophin-3, have been administered via a miniosmotic pump to adult guinea pigs several weeks after deafening. These neurotrophins reduced spiral ganglion neuron degeneration and promoted dendritic growth. Gene therapy may present a more permanent method to apply these factors to the inner ear with significantly less surgical morbidity. Many more factors remain to be found and studied in understanding the mechanisms regulating neuronal development.

Monogenic Gene Therapy and RNAi

Gene therapy protocols often seek to replace a gene lost due to an autosomal recessive disease. Certainly, when gene therapy comes of age, it will be able to replace dysfunctional genes in the inner ear. When used alone, this approach is limited because the cellular targets, hair cells and spiral ganglion neurons, usually undergo apoptosis. However, monogenic gene replacement may be advantageous if used with other novel methods that repopulate the sensory epithelium.

RNA interference (RNAi) is a naturally occurring biological process in multicellular organisms that causes gene suppression. Therapeutic RNAi may be able to suppress a multitude of unwanted genes, including viral, oncogenic, and autosomal dominant genes. It has been effective in animal models for several clinical conditions, including viral infections, neurodegenerative diseases, and inflammatory processes (Uprichard, 2005). RNAi and gene replacement therapy represent two sides of the monogenic gene therapy coin, able to, respectively, suppress or replace a targeted gene.

Combination Therapies

Using combinations of the above novel therapies may be required for some forms of hearing loss. Stem cell therapy or gene therapy for differentiation control may be able to repopulate some inner ear cells. Therefore, these methods will be effective for deafening due to acute or chronic exposures to ototoxic agents. Other forms of hearing loss may involve a dysfunctional gene product that will remain dysfunctional in its interaction with a regenerated sensory epithelium. Therefore, hereditary hearing losses that affect the cochlea and result in hair cell or neuronal death must be corrected by gene therapy concurrently with repopulation of the sensory epithelium.

Potentially, the first attempts to fix a gene defect in the inner ear will be for mutations in *GJB2* that cause DFNB1 because of its high prevalence in prelingual deafness. DFNB1 appears to cause both hair cell and supporting cell losses such that gene therapy may have only a small number of cochlear target cells. Usage of a vector containing a wild-type copy of *GJB2* could be combined with vectors containing *ATOH1* and perhaps a cell cycle regulator to induce proliferation of the remaining cells. In this case, all target cells would require successful transfection with the *GJB2* vector to allow normal gap junction transfer of potassium. This model would work for DFNB1 but perhaps not for the autosomal dominant and syndromic forms of hearing loss associated with *GJB2* mutations. RNAi technology could be applied to correct the autosomal dominant mutations in *GJB2*. Similarly, inner ear damage (e.g., presbycusis) that involves both hair cell and spiral ganglion neuron losses may be corrected by a combination of therapies. In such cases, neurotrophin gene therapy to repopulate the neurons may be combined with *ATOH1* gene therapy directed at repopulating the hair cells.

Ethics of Gene Therapy

Those nascent therapies with the greatest potential to advance medicine, gene therapy and stem cell therapy, include major ethical dilemmas. Gene manipulation in the morally unacceptable forms of eugenics, sterilization, specified human mating, and genocide has been occurring in rare instances over several centuries. Because technological advances now begin to allow unprecedented alteration of our genetics, the moral questions are more critical than ever and should be considered at every step.

In what ways will we be able to control our genes? Gene therapy, in which one or multiple selected genes are altered, will soon be able to cure monogenic diseases and affect several other disease processes. However, as our ability to manipulate specific genes grows, our cultural definition of what constitutes hereditary disease may change.

Historically, the most effective way to avoid ethical dilemma has been to maintain transparency in operation and access. Early applications of gene or stem cell therapies to patients may be limited due to resources. Perhaps a system similar to organ transplantation may be created to ensure that application of those limited resources is based on medical need and rigorously monitored. Unlike organ transplantation, these novel therapies should overcome their period of limited resources as the methods are refined and gain acceptance.

◆ Summary

Molecular genetic techniques have led to significant advances in the understanding of the genes involved in hearing loss. However, because of the rapid growth in this field, it is critical to proceed with caution and consider the ethical concerns of these applications. Moreover, as an integral component of diagnosis and treatment, conscientious genetic counseling is an important process to provide detailed information and to ensure that individuals are able to make informed choices regarding the use of genetic testing. Although carrier detection and reproductive risk counseling are currently used for a limited number of genes and disorders, the further identification of genes will greatly improve the field of genetic counseling.

The study of medical genetics in hearing loss translates directly into clinical genetics and the direct clinical care of persons with genetic disorders. One of the goals of genetic studies, including studies involved in hearing loss, is to identify and understand the causative genes in diseases. With the knowledge obtained from such research, we will have the ability to create precise diagnostic tests and to create preventive treatments for prenatal and postnatal care. The ultimate goal will be the application of this research in designing individualized therapy tailored to cure disorders based on a patient's distinct genetic background. However, an accurate diagnosis and consistent diagnostic criteria for genetic diseases will be the essential first step in utilizing genetics as a form of treatment.

The research in genetics of hearing loss is growing exponentially. To take full advantage of the vast amount of information and insight, it will be important to establish a strong network between biological, statistical, and computational principles, along with a strong system of bioinformatics. One of our aims in this chapter has been to demonstrate the accessibility of available genetic resources and the development of databases with comprehensive DNA information.

In this chapter, we have attempted to convey the fast-paced research, the concerted international effort, and the development of novel techniques to understand the genetics and etiology of hereditary hearing loss.

References

Abdelhak, S., Kalatzis, V., Heilig, R., et al. (1997). A human homologue of the *Drosophila* eyes absent gene underlies branchio-oto-renal (BOR) syndrome and identifies a novel gene family. Nature Genetics, 15(2), 157–164.

Alvarez, A., del Castillo, I., Pera, A., et al. (2003). Uniparental disomy of chromosome 13q causing homozygosity for the *35delg* mutation in the gene encoding connexin26 (*GJB2*) results in prelingual hearing impairment in two unrelated Spanish patients. Journal of Medical Genetics, 40(8), 636–639.

Atar, O., & Avraham, K. B. (2005). Therapeutics of hearing loss: Expectations vs reality. Drug Discovery Today, 10(19), 1323–1330.

Badenhop, R. F., Cherian, S., Lord, R. S., Baysal, B. E., Taschner, P. E., & Schofield, P. R. (2001). Novel mutations in the *SDHD* gene in pedigrees with familial carotid body paraganglioma and sensorineural hearing loss. Genes, Chromosomes and Cancer, 31(3), 255–263.

Bauer, P. W., Geers, A. E., Brenner, C., Moog, J. S., & Smith, R. J. (2003). The effect of *GJB2* allele variants on performance after cochlear implantation. Laryngoscope, 113(12), 2135–2140.

Di Palma, F., Pellegrino, R., & Noben-Trauth, K. (2001). Genomic structure, alternative splice forms and normal and mutant alleles of cadherin 23 (*CDH23*). Gene, 281(1–2), 31–41.

Farrer, L. A., Arnos, K. S., Asher, J. H., Jr., et al. (1994). Locus heterogeneity for Waardenburg syndrome is predictive of clinical subtypes. American Journal of Human Genetics, 55(4), 728–737.

Finsterer, J., & Fellinger, J. (2005). Nuclear and mitochondrial genes mutated in nonsyndromic impaired hearing. International Journal of Pediatric Otorhinolaryngology, 69(5), 621–647.

Frolenkov, G. I., Belyantseva, I. A., Friedman, T. B., & Griffith, A. J. (2004). Genetic insights into the morphogenesis of inner ear hair cells. Nature Reviews: Genetics, 5(7), 489–498.

Gorlin, R. J., Cohen, M. M., & Levin, L. S. (2005). Syndromes of the head and neck (3rd ed.). New York: Oxford University Press.

Green, G. E., Scott, D. A., McDonald, J. M., et al. (2002). Performance of cochlear implant recipients with *GJB2*-related deafness. American Journal of Medical Genetics, 109(3), 167–170.

Izumikawa, M., Minoda, R., Kawamoto, K., et al. (2005). Auditory hair cell replacement and hearing improvement by *Atoh1* gene therapy in deaf mammals. Nature Medicine, 11(3), 271–276.

Johnson, K. R., Erway, L. C., Cook, S. A., Willott, J. F., & Zheng, Q. Y. (1997). A major gene affecting age-related hearing loss in *C57bl/6j* mice. Hearing Research, 114(1–2), 83–92.

Keithley, E. M., Canto, C., Zheng, Q. Y., Wang, X., Fischel-Ghodsian, N., & Johnson, K. R. (2005). Cu/Zn superoxide dismutase and age-related hearing loss. Hearing Research, 209(1–2), 76–85.

Matsui, Y., & Okamura, D. (2005). Mechanisms of germ-cell specification in mouse embryos. Bioessays, 27(2), 136–143.

Nebert, D. W., & Vesell, E. S. (2004). Advances in pharmacogenomics and individualized drug therapy: Exciting challenges that lie ahead. European Journal of Pharmacology, 500(1–3), 267–280.

Noben-Trauth, K., Zheng, Q. Y., & Johnson, K. R. (2003). Association of cadherin 23 with polygenic inheritance and genetic modification of sensorineural hearing loss. Nature Genetics, 35(1), 21–23.

Patenaude, A. F. (2005). Genetic testing for cancer: Psychological approaches for helping patients and families. Washington, DC: American Psychological Association.

Positional cloning of a gene involved in the pathogenesis of Treacher Collins syndrome: the Treacher Collins Syndrome Collaborative Group. (1996). Nature Genetics, 12(2), 130–136.

Reid, C., & Robinson, L. (1999). Evaluation of the newborn with single or multiple congenital anomalies: Executive summary. New York, Oxford University Press.

Toriello, H. V., Reardon, W., & Gorlin, R. J. (2005). Hereditary hearing loss and its syndromes. New York: Oxford University Press.

Uprichard, S. L. (2005). The therapeutic potential of RNA interference. FEBS Letters, 579(26), 5996–6007.

Veach, P. M., & Leroy, B. S. (2003). Facilitating the genetic counseling process: A practice manual. New York: Springer-Verlag.

Verpy, E., Leibovici, M., Zwaenepoel, I., et al. (2000). A defect in harmonin, a PDZ domain-containing protein expressed in the inner ear sensory hair cells, underlies Usher syndrome type 1c. Nature Genetics, 26(1), 51–55.

Young, H. E., Duplaa, C., Katz, R., et al. (2005). Adult-derived stem cells and their potential for use in tissue repair and molecular medicine. Journal of Cellular and Molecular Medicine, 9(3), 753–769.

Chapter 7

Radiologic Imaging in Otologic Disease

Debara L. Tucci and Linda Gray

Modern neuroimaging capabilities have revolutionized the practice of otology. The use of a combination of computed tomography (CT) and magnetic resonance imaging (MRI) enables the otologist and neuroradiologist to define the nature and extent of most disease processes that affect the temporal bone and surrounding anatomical structures. With knowledge gained from interpretation of these images, the otologist can make an accurate diagnosis and plan an appropriate surgical procedure or other course of treatment. Proper use of neuroimaging can enhance patient care and reduce the risk of surgical or treatment-related complications.

This chapter describes basic imaging techniques, discusses the use of these techniques in the diagnosis of otologic disease processes, and presents a discussion of the specific uses of imaging in the evaluation of patients in an otologic practice. It is not meant to provide an exhaustive discussion of all otologic disease in which imaging could potentially be used. Rather, the chapter gives the reader a basic understanding of neuroimaging and of the most common uses of neuroimaging in the evaluation of the patient with otologic disease.

♦ Types of Radiologic Imaging

Conventional Radiology

Conventional radiologic techniques are rarely used for assessment of the temporal bone today. The ear is an extremely complex organ; many structures are located in a small space within the temporal bone. Conventional radiologic techniques do not permit the isolation of distinct anatomical structures because each point on the film is a summation of all the points crossed by the x-ray beam traveling through the skull and temporal bone. These techniques have been abandoned, for the most part, in favor of CT, which offers a much higher resolution and a precise reconstruction of the entire area of interest in a series of images. Current use in an otologic practice is probably limited to the transorbital, or frontal, projection, which shows the otic capsule and may be used to confirm the position of cochlear implant electrodes.

Pearl

- High-resolution temporal bone CT is typically used for preoperative assessment of a wide variety of otologic surgical problems, including cholesteatoma, tumors such as glomus tympanicum or glomus jugulare, cochlear implantation, and congenital atresia. CT may be helpful not only for diagnosis but also for the delineation of the surgical anatomy and for planning the operative procedure.

Computed Tomography

Computed tomography (Grossman and Yousem, 1994) was first developed in the early 1970s and has continued to evolve over the years. This technique uses a highly collimated (or focused) x-ray beam that is differentially absorbed by various tissues within the body. The beam is rotated over many different steps so as to get differential absorption patterns through a single section of a patient's body. By mathematical analysis, one can obtain an absorption value for each point in a CT slice. The scale for CT absorption ranges from 11,000 to 21,000, with 0 allocated to water and 21,000 to air. These units of absorption are termed Hounsfield units (HU) for the discoverer of CT. High-resolution CT techniques can provide slice thickness as narrow as 0.75 mm. Two or more projections are required for proper interpretation of a study. The most commonly used projections are the axial or horizontal and the coronal or frontal.

Special reconstruction algorithms can be used to highlight a particular tissue with CT. Bone algorithms are very useful for assessment of the anatomy of the temporal bone. Iodinated contrast may be used to opacify blood vessels or vascular tumors, such as paragangliomas. However, small vascular tumors will not take up enough contrast to produce opacification. In general, contrast is not administered for routine temporal bone studies.

In most cases, CT is the initial imaging study of choice for the evaluation of patients with suspected otologic disease. The major exception is the evaluation of acoustic neuroma, for which MRI is most useful, as discussed below.

Magnetic Resonance Imaging

Magnetic resonance is an imaging technique that does not expose the patient to ionizing radiation (Grossman and Yousem, 1994; Valvassori et al, 1995). Whereas CT is a technique that relies on differential attenuation of an x-ray beam, MRI relies on the unique response of various tissues to an applied magnetic field. For MRI, images are generated by the interaction of hydrogen nuclei or protons, high magnetic fields, and radiofrequency pulses. The intensity of the MR signal to be captured on the image depends on the density of hydrogen nuclei in the tissue and on two magnetic relaxation times, called T1 and T2, which are tissue-specific. The appearance of both normal and pathological tissue will vary, depending on the relative contribution of the T1 and T2 relaxation times in the image generated. Variation of relaxation times is obtained by changing the time between radiofrequency pulses, or repetition time (TR), and the time the emitted signal or echo is measured after the pulse, or echo time (TE).

The signal intensity of various tissues is directly proportional to the amount of free protons present within the tissue. Soft tissue and bodily fluids contain large amounts of free protons and emit a strong MR signal. In contrast, air and bone contain few free protons and emit a weak MR signal. Pathological processes are recognizable when the proton density and relaxation times of the abnormal tissue are different from those of normal tissue. Some pathological processes are definable on the basis of the appearance on T1-weighted versus T2-weighted images. The recognition and differentiation of pathological processes are enhanced by the use of a ferromagnetic contrast agent, such as gadolinium, which may be taken up by abnormal tissue. MRI is most useful for the detection of soft tissue tumors, such as acoustic neuroma and lesions of the petrous apex, and for the detection of intracranial involvement by pathological processes such as cholesteatoma.

Magnetic resonance angiography (MRA) depends on creating intensity differences between flowing matter and stationary tissue. By suppressing background stationary tissue and focusing on the high-signal flowing blood, it is possible to depict vascular structures in three-dimensional space. Although this technique is useful for detecting vascular abnormalities such as intracranial aneurysms, its usefulness in temporal bone evaluation is limited.

Pearl

- MRI cannot be used for patients with pacemakers or metallic implants, such as cochlear implants. Special non-ferromagnetic cochlear implants are available for use with patients who might be expected to need MRI in the future (Heller et al, 1996). Otologic prostheses, such as for stapedectomy or stapedotomy, are generally MRI compatible.

◆ Normal CT Temporal Bone Anatomy

A series of axial and coronal CT images showing normal temporal bone anatomy is given in **Figs. 7–1** and **7–2.** Some important structures and relationships to note include the following:

1. The internal auditory canal is located medial (or toward the middle of the head) to the external auditory canal

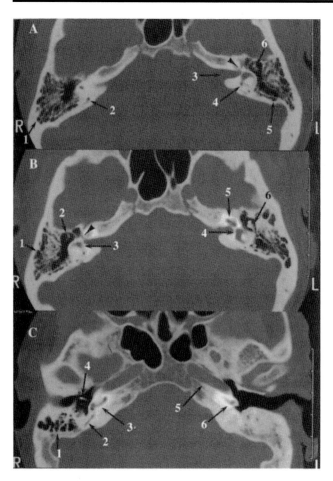

Figure 7–1 Series of axial computed tomography images through the normal temporal bone, from most superior to most inferior. **(A)** 1, mastoid air cells; 2, posterior semicircular canal; 3, internal auditory canal; 4, posterior semicircular canal ampulla; 5, mastoid air cells; 6, ossicles. **(B)** 1, mastoid air cells; 2, ossicles; 3, vestibule and horizontal semicircular canal; 4, vestibule; 5, cochlea (basal turn); 6, ossicles. **(C)** 1, mastoid air cells; 2, common crus (posterior and superior semicircular canals); 3, basal turn of cochlea; 4, manubrium of malleus; 5, canal of the internal carotid artery; 6, basal turn of cochlea. Arrowheads indicate the facial nerve, labyrinthine portion.

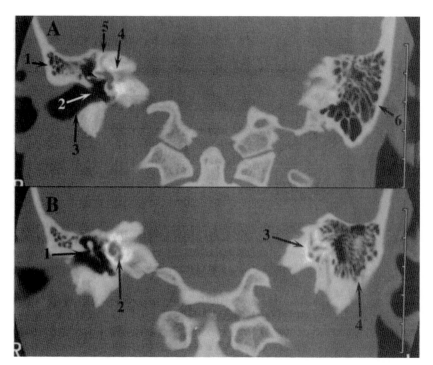

Figure 7–2 Series of coronal computed tomography images through a normal temporal bone. **(A)** At the level of the semicircular canals. 1, mastoid air cells; 2, tympanic membrane; 3, external auditory canal; 4, internal auditory canal; 5, superior semicircular canal; 6, mastoid air cells. **(B)** At the level of the cochlea, posterior to **(A)**. 1, scutum, or posterosuperior external auditory canal, and Prussak's space, which is the space between the pars flaccida of the tympanic membrane and the neck of the malleus in which cholesteatomas can form; 2, cochlea; 3, superior and horizontal semicircular canals; 4, mastoid air cells. Arrowhead, indicates the facial nerve seen above the oval window, inferior to the horizontal semicircular canal.

(which is lateral, or toward the outside of the head). The internal auditory canals should be uniform in size, within 2 mm. An enlarged internal auditory canal raises the suspicion of an acoustic neuroma, although an MRI is a better method of assessment. The internal auditory canal transmits the facial nerve, superior vestibular nerve, inferior vestibular nerve, and cochlear nerve. An internal auditory canal that is less than 2 mm in diameter is suspected of transmitting only a facial nerve, without a normal auditory-vestibular nerve (Jackler et al, 1987a; Shelton et al, 1989).

2. The middle ear space is noted, with attention to the size and degree of aeration and the presence of a mass, soft tissue, or fluid. The ossicles are noted in the middle ear space, particularly the head of the malleus and the body of the incus in the epitympanum.

3. The ossicles are noted, including the head of the malleus and body of the incus superiorly. Their configuration should resemble that of an ice cream cone, with the head of the malleus representing the "ice cream" in the "cone" of the incus. The stapes is most inferior and best visualized in the coronal plane, lateral to the vestibule. The patency of the oval window can be assessed in this plane as well.

4. The otic capsule is noted, particularly the patency and morphology of the cochlea and the vestibule and semicircular canals. The cochlea is located most anterior and medial, and semicircular canals are more posterior and lateral. The cochlea is in proximity to the carotid artery, seen best in the coronal image.

5. The major vascular structures of the temporal bone include the carotid artery and jugular bulb. The jugular bulb is in continuity with the sigmoid sinus in the mastoid and is posterior and lateral to the carotid artery.

6. The facial nerve takes a complicated path through the temporal bone and may be visualized in a series of axial and coronal images. Segments include an internal auditory canal segment, a labyrinthine segment that is in proximity to the semicircular canals ending in the geniculate ganglion, a tympanic segment that travels horizontally through the middle ear just superior to the oval window, and a mastoid or vertical portion that extends from the level of the horizontal semicircular canal and oval window to the stylomastoid foramen near the mastoid tip. The nerve makes two sharp turns, one at the geniculate ganglion, which is the first genu, and another at the juncture of the tympanic and mastoid segments, which is called the second genu.

7. The vestibular aqueduct is seen posterior to the posterior semicircular canal, extending to the endolymphatic sac on the posterior aspect of the temporal bone. The cochlear aqueduct extends from the region of the round window to the subarachnoid space, inferior to the internal auditory canal and medial to the jugular bulb at the level of the basal turn of the cochlea.

◆ Uses of Radiologic Imaging in Evaluation of Otologic Disease

Neuroimaging is of critical importance in diagnosis of otologic disease in the modern otolaryngology practice. Patient populations for whom neuroimaging plays an especially important role in assessment of the disease process are described below.

Pearl

- MRI is most useful for imaging soft tissue in contrast to CT, which is most useful for imaging bony detail.

Unilateral or Asymmetrical Sensorineural Hearing Loss

Because unilateral or asymmetrical sensorineural hearing loss (SNHL) and unilateral tinnitus are the most common presenting symptoms of acoustic neuroma, evaluation to rule out an eighth cranial nerve (CN VIII) tumor is indicated in patients with these symptoms (Tucci, 1997). Gadolinium-enhanced MRI (MRIg) is considered the gold standard for detection of an acoustic neuroma (National Institutes of Health Consensus Development Conference, 1991). Because the resolution of MRI is 500 mm, extremely small tumors (< 1 mm) may be detected. Auditory brainstem response (ABR) testing has been used in the past to screen for abnormalities that require follow-up imaging. However, recent studies of detection rates with ABR and MRI have raised the concern that ABR is not adequately sensitive to diagnose small tumors (Telian et al, 1989). Although ABR sensitivity is reported by most authors as ~90% for all size tumors, the sensitivity for diagnosis of small, intracanalicular tumors is significantly lower (Wilson et al, 1997). In one prospective study (Ruckenstein et al, 1996), all patients with significant asymmetrical SNHL (defined in this study as asymmetry of 15 dB at two frequencies or asymmetry in speech discrimination scores of 15%) were evaluated with both ABR and MRIg. Preliminary data from this study, based on 47 patients, indicate that ABR sensitivity and specificity are both ~60%, which supports the contention by some authors (Chandrasekhar et al, 1995; Welling et al, 1990; Wilson et al, 1997) that MRIg be used as the preferred screening test for assessment of all patients with unilateral auditory-vestibular symptoms. It may be argued that an exception to this recommendation be made in the case of elderly patients for whom a small slow-growing tumor is not likely to create a health risk within their expected lifetime. In certain circumstances, such as in rural areas, access to MRI may be limited. In these situations, ABR must be used for acoustic neuroma screening. In cases of asymmetrical hearing loss and a normal ABR, patient follow-up every 6 to 12 months is of critical importance. If hearing loss progresses or other symptoms such as tinnitus or vestibular dysfunction develop, repeated ABR is indicated (Tucci, 1997).

Appropriate MRI protocols will obtain adequately thin sections through the internal auditory canals (IACs) to rule out a small acoustic tumor. Gadolinium is used to increase the sensitivity of detection in the case of a small tumor. In the case of neuritis, the nerve may enhance with gadolinium in the

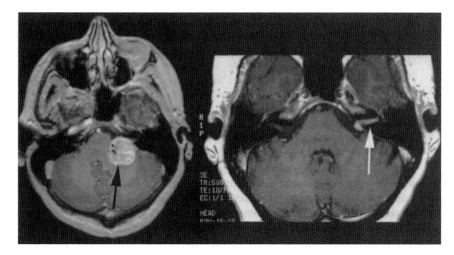

Figure 7–3 Axial magnetic resonance images showing large (left side) and small (right side) acoustic neuromas. On the left image, tumor fills the medial portion of the internal auditory canal (IAC) and expands the porus, or opening, of the canal. Tumor fills the cerebellopontine angle (CPA) and compresses the brainstem. The dark spaces within the tumor are indicative of small cysts. The small tumor on the right is seen to fill the entire IAC and extend minimally into the CPA.

absence of a tumor mass. In this situation, special MR techniques may facilitate the differential diagnosis (Syms et al, 1997). Some authors have advocated the use of abbreviated MRI techniques to screen for acoustic neuromas. These techniques have the advantage of reduced cost but the disadvantage of less comprehensive brain imaging, with the potential to miss other intracranial causes of auditory dysfunction, such as multiple sclerosis and small vessel disease (Wilson et al, 1997).

The typical radiologic appearance of an acoustic neuroma is that of a mass in the cerebellopontine angle (CPA) that extends into the IAC (**Fig. 7–3**). Tumor size may be described in terms of both an intracanalicular and an extracanalicular portion. The tumor tends to widen the most medial portion (or porus acusticus) of the IAC as it enlarges. However, small tumors may not erode the porus acusticus. This is why small tumors are not easily or reliably detected by conventional CT. Most tumors in the CPA are acoustic neuromas. Meningiomas may also occur in this region and usually have a somewhat different appearance on MRI (Valvassori et al, 1994, 1995). In general, hearing is less affected by a meningioma in this region than by an acoustic neuroma. Surgical resection that preserves the potential for hearing conservation may be indicated in these cases, as well as for patients with small acoustic neuromas (McKenna et al, 1992; Rosenberg et al, 1987; Shelton et al, 1990; Tucci et al, 1994).

Pitfall

- SNHL in children may be associated with malformations of the membranous cochlea. Examples include the Bing-Siebenmann deformity, which is characterized by underdevelopment of the membranous labyrinth, and the Scheibe deformity, in which the malformation is restricted to the organ of Corti and saccular neuroepithelium. These deformities cannot be detected with current CT imaging techniques.

Less common causes of unilateral hearing loss of adult onset include other skull base tumors, particularly those located in the petrous apex. The petrous apex is the portion of the

temporal bone that lies between the inner ear and the clivus, which is at the center of the skull base. The petrous apex is divided into two compartments by the IAC; the anterior compartment, which lies medial to the cochlea, is most frequently involved by disease processes. Patients may have unilateral hearing loss or other unilateral auditory-vestibular symptoms if lesions of the petrous apex involve either the inner ear or contents of the IAC. Although CT is very useful in delineating the extent of bony involvement of these lesions, MRI is most useful in defining the characteristics that help to make the

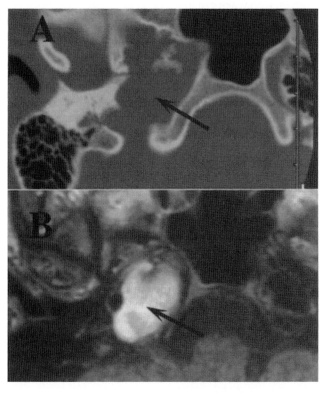

Figure 7–4 Lesion of the left petrous apex. **(A)** Axial computed tomography demonstrating an expansile lesion of the petrous apex with associated calcification. **(B)** Axial T1-weighted magnetic resonance scan demonstrating high signal intensity cholesterol cyst of the petrous apex.

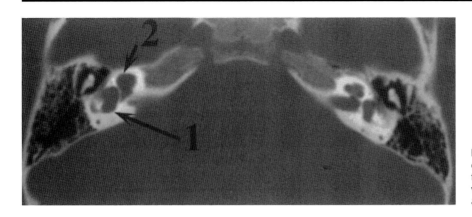

Figure 7–5 Cochlear malformation. Axial computed tomography image at the level of the otic capsule. 1, enlarged, malformed vestibule; 2, malformed cochlea. Normal anatomy is seen on the opposite side.

differential diagnosis. One common lesion of the petrous apex is the cholesterol granuloma (**Fig. 7–4**), which is an expansile cystic mass that is typically located in the anteromedial petrous apex. MRI is very characteristic and shows a markedly hyperintense lesion on both T1- and T2-weighted images, with no change after gadolinium administration. Cholesteatomas may arise in this location either from congenital squamous epithelial rests (a developmental anomaly) or, less typically, as a result of spread from cholesteatoma that occurred primarily in the mastoid. Cholesteatomas are much less common than cholesterol granulomas in this location and have a characteristic appearance on MRI, with low signal intensity on the T1-weighted images, high intensity on the T2-weighted images, and no enhancement with gadolinium. The T1-weighted images generally provide the information needed to make the diagnosis. Other, rarer tumors are also possible in this location (Jackler and Parker, 1992).

Pearl

• Although high-resolution CT is the gold standard for the evaluation of most aspects of temporal bone anatomy, it does have limitations, particularly in the assessment of cochlear patency (Jackler et al, 1987c; Seidman et al, 1994; Wiet et al, 1990). MRI can be a useful adjunct to CT for the assessment of implant candidates because it is possible to visualize the presence or absence of fluid within the cochlear turns, as well as the size of the cochleovestibular nerve within the IAC (Arriaga and Carrier, 1996; Tien et al, 1992). Many implant centers use both CT and MRI for the routine evaluation of implant candidates.

Sensorineural Hearing Loss in Children

In children, SNHL is less likely to be due to neoplasms or other pathological conditions as described for the adult and more likely to be the result of congenital anatomical or functional abnormalities. According to Jackler et al (1987b), ~20% of patients with congenital SNHL will have radiographic abnormalities that can be identified on temporal bone CT (**Fig. 7–5**). Jackler and colleagues developed a classification of cochlear malformation that is based on embryogenesis. Abnormalities include (1) complete aplasia of the inner ear—cochlea and labyrinth (Michel deformity); (2) cochlear aplasia; (3) cochlear hypoplasia, with a small cochlear bud; (4) incomplete partition, or a small cochlea with an incomplete interscalar septum (classic Mondini malformation); and (5) the common cavity malformation, in which the cochlea and vestibule form a common cavity without internal architecture. Malformations of the membranous portion of the cochlea are much more common than bony malformations; these are not detectable with currently available imaging techniques.

The radiographic finding of an enlarged vestibular aqueduct (**Fig. 7–6**) is known to be associated with SNHL, which can be progressive and profound (Jackler and De La Cruz, 1989). Enlargement of this structure may be due to the developmental arrest of the endolymphatic anlage, much like the arrest of cochlear development is thought to result in the malformations listed previously. This abnormality may also be associated with other malformations of the membranous cochlea.

Children who have SNHL often undergo radiologic imaging, particularly if the hearing loss is profound or progressive. Children with profound hearing loss are often

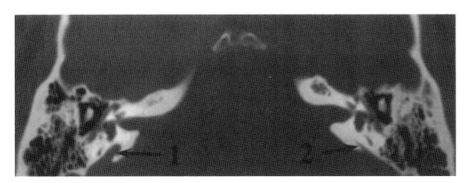

Figure 7–6 Axial computed tomography image showing an enlarged vestibular aqueduct (1) and a normal vestibular aqueduct (2).

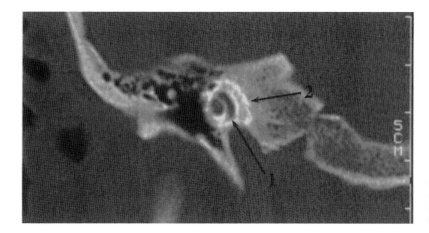

Figure 7–7 Coronal computed tomography image showing the cochlea in a patient with otosclerosis. Sclerosis of the cochlea is evident, with narrowing of the cochlear lumen. 1, cochlear lumen; 2, sclerotic bone.

imaged in the course of evaluation for cochlear implant candidacy (see the following discussion). Children with malformations of the temporal bone may be at greater risk of progression of hearing loss resulting from head trauma (Jackler and De La Cruz, 1989). Recurrent meningitis has been documented in children with cochlear malformations, particularly in association with cerebrospinal fluid (CSF) leak and an oval window fistula (Ohlms et al, 1990).

Cochlear Implant Evaluation

Imaging is an important part of the cochlear implant evaluation. A detailed temporal bone CT helps to define the surgical anatomy and alert the surgeon to potential abnormalities, such as cochlear ossification and malformation (**Figs. 7–7** and **7–8**). Modifications of conventional surgical techniques permit implantation of patients with a variety of cochlear anomalies; surgical planning and patient counseling are enhanced by preoperative identification of these abnormalities. Bony malformations of the cochlea have been associated with the absence of the oval and round windows and an aberrant course of the facial nerve. Free flow of CSF may occur into the cochlea from the IAC and may result in profuse flow of CSF on creation of the cochleostomy (Tucci et al, 1995). A narrow IAC may suggest absence of the auditory nerve, which is a contraindication to implantation in that ear (Jackler et al, 1987b; Shelton et al, 1989).

Pulsatile Tinnitus

The symptom of unilateral pulsatile tinnitus often warrants radiologic evaluation to rule out or diagnose abnormalities such as a vascular tumor of the temporal bone, vascular anomaly, or other rare disorders such as arteriovenous malformations or aneurysms. The two major blood vessels associated with the ear, the carotid artery and the jugular vein, both course along the floor of the middle ear, and either may demonstrate anomalous development. The carotid artery typically lies no farther laterally in the temporal bone than the lateral wall of the cochlea. Because of a developmental abnormality, the carotid artery can course over the cochlear promontory and turn anteriorly under the oval window. Patients with an aberrant carotid artery may have

pulsatile tinnitus and conductive hearing loss (**Fig. 7–9**). Otoscopic examination may reveal a red retrotympanic mass that does not blanch on pneumatoscopy.

In ~6% of temporal bones, the jugular bulb protrudes above the level of the floor of the external auditory canal. If the bony plate, which usually separates the jugular bulb and middle ear, is dehiscent, the bulb is exposed to the middle ear cavity. A "high-riding" jugular bulb may be visualized through the tympanic membrane as a bluish mass (**Fig. 7–10**); in severe cases, it may cause a conductive hearing loss by interfering with the normal movement of the ossicular chain. Pulsatile tinnitus may be produced by a variety of mechanisms, including turbulent blood flow in the high-riding jugular bulb, transmission of intratemporal carotid artery pulsations, or retrograde transmission of atrial pulsations (Sismanis, 1997).

Other abnormalities that may be commonly associated with pulsatile tinnitus are not diagnosed by conventional

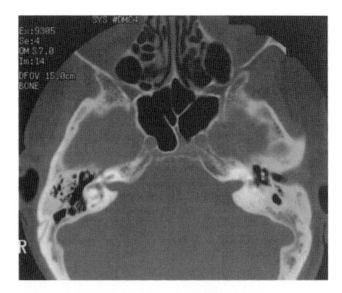

Figure 7–8 Axial computed tomography showing complete labyrinthine ossification, left ear (right side of figure). Right cochlea (left side of figure) is partially ossified, and the outline of a portion of the cochlea and semicircular canals is evident.

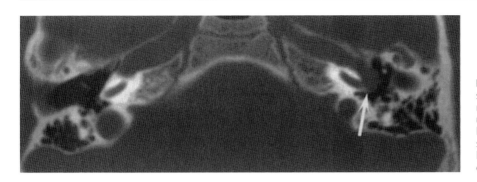

Figure 7–9 Axial computed tomography showing an internal carotid artery malformation (arrow). On the left side of the figure, the carotid artery is seen in its normal location medial to the cochlea. On the right side of the figure, the carotid artery courses lateral to the cochlea and extends over the cochlear promontory.

imaging techniques. Sismanis (1997) argues that many young women with this disorder have benign intracranial hypertension. Atherosclerotic carotid artery disease is thought to be a common cause of pulsatile tinnitus in patients older than 50, particularly when they have risk factors for atherosclerosis (hypertension, angina, hyperlipidemia, diabetes mellitus, and smoking).

The most common vascular tumor affecting the temporal bone is the paraganglioma or glomus tumor (**Fig. 7–11**). Temporal bone paragangliomas originate most frequently from the jugular bulb (glomus jugulare) and less commonly over the promontory of the cochlea (glomus tympanicum). Either can grow to involve a large portion of the temporal bone, and tumors may extend intracranially. Glomus jugulare tumors are typically much more extensive than tympanicum tumors, which can be quite small on diagnosis. Tympanicum tumors can be easily seen through a translucent tympanic membrane and appear as a circumscribed, often pulsatile, cherry red mass over the cochlear promontory. These patients may have conductive hearing loss, as a result of ossicular involvement, and pulsatile tinnitus.

Special Consideration

- The issue of whether to attempt elective surgical correction of a unilateral conductive hearing loss in a young child is controversial. Some surgeons advocate delaying intervention until the child is 18 or the age at which consent may legally be given. Others recommend early intervention to maximize development of speech perception and localization abilities that depend on binaural hearing (Hall et al, 1995; Pillsbury et al, 1991; Wilmington et al, 1994).

Pediatric Conductive Hearing Loss

Conductive hearing loss in the pediatric patient may be due to an obvious cause, such as congenital aural atresia or cholesteatoma. However, if the otomicroscopic examination is normal, the diagnosis may be more subtle. Imaging is frequently used for evaluation of the pediatric patient. In the case of congenital anomaly or cholesteatoma, the scan will

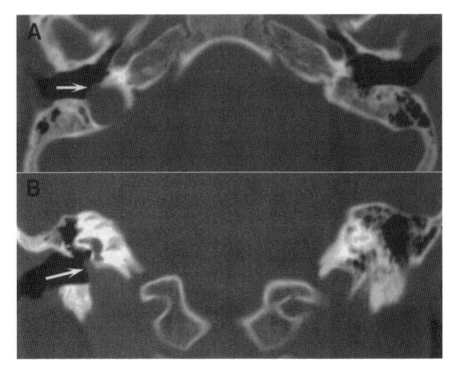

Figure 7–10 High-riding jugular bulb. **(A)** Axial image showing the jugular bulb at the level of the middle ear space, with dehiscence (lack of bone covering). **(B)** Coronal computed tomography image showing dehiscence and extension into the middle ear space. This could be visualized as a bluish mass behind the tympanic membrane on otoscopic examination. This patient also had a conductive hearing loss.

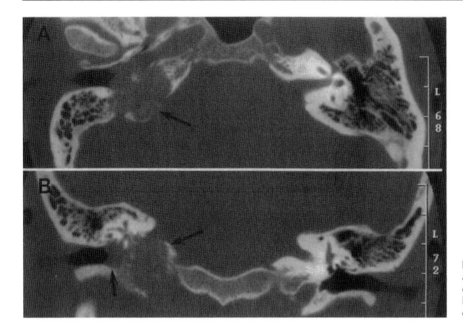

Figure 7–11 Glomus jugulare tumor. **(A)** Axial and **(B)** coronal computed tomography scans demonstrating an erosive lesion of the jugular bulb, with extension of tumor into the middle ear (**(B)**, vertical arrow).

help define the anatomy and help with surgical planning and family counseling. In the case of conductive hearing loss of unknown cause, a detailed temporal bone study will help to determine whether an indication exists for early surgical intervention. A cholesteatoma that is not evident on physical examination may be evident on an imaging study and would require treatment, whereas the absence of such a problem should reassure the physician and family that surgical treatment may be scheduled electively.

In cases of congenital aural atresia, it is essential to perform a careful preoperative assessment to determine whether the patient is a good candidate for reconstructive surgery. High-resolution CT of the temporal bone is used to assess the development of the temporal bone and anatomy of the middle ear space (**Fig. 7–12**). Jahrsdoerfer et al (1992) developed a guideline for assessment of the relevant anatomy and have made recommendations on the basis of surgical experience with a large number of patients with atresia. This grading system is based on the morphology of the ossicles, patency of the oval and round windows, size of the middle ear space, position of the facial nerve, degree of mastoid pneumatization, and appearance of the external ear. In general, surgery is not performed until a child reaches at least age 5, and canal reconstruction is preceded by auricular reconstruction if indicated (De la Cruz and Chandrasekhar, 1994; Jahrsdoerfer et al, 1992; Lambert, 1988). A CT scan may be performed long before the age at which surgery takes place to determine whether surgical intervention is appropriate and help with overall patient management decisions. In cases of bilateral atresia, surgical ear selection should be based both on middle ear and mastoid anatomy and, where possible, an assessment of cochlear integrity. This may be based on bony morphology of the cochlea as seen on CT and audiological assessment.

Several other congenital abnormalities of the middle ear are described (Sando et al, 1990). These abnormalities may be diagnosed in children with known syndromic disorders, nonsyndromic dysmorphic features, or, most commonly, in other-

wise normal children. In most cases, diagnosis of a specific ossicular problem cannot be made definitively on CT scan.

Chronic Ear Disease

The term *chronic middle ear* disease reflects a wide variety of pathological conditions, which can range in severity from

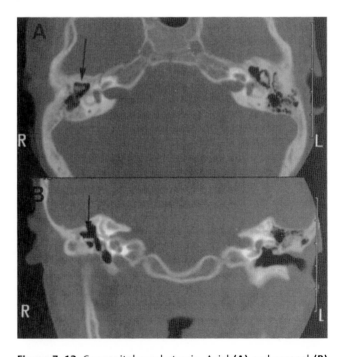

Figure 7–12 Congenital aural atresia. Axial **(A)** and coronal **(B)** computed tomography images showing right ear (left side of figure) congenital atresia. Arrows indicate globular ossicular mass with adherence to atretic plate. Normal ossicles are seen for the left ear. The size of the middle ear space is similar on the right and left sides. An external auditory canal is seen on the coronal **(B)** image for the left ear.

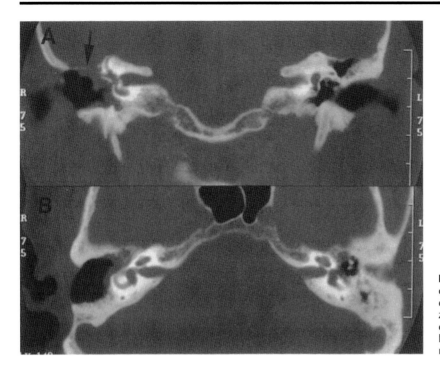

Figure 7–13 Cholesteatoma. **(A)** Coronal image demonstrates soft tissue in the middle ear space, a defect in the tegmen tympani (arrow), and a horizontal semicircular canal fistula. **(B)** Axial image also demonstrates soft tissue in the middle ear space and labyrinthine fistula. No ossicles are seen in the right middle ear space. (Right ear is on left side of figure.)

chronic otitis media with effusion to extensive cholesteatoma with associated aural and intracranial complications. It is not always possible on physical examination to determine the exact nature or extent of the disease process. For this reason, imaging studies, particularly temporal bone CT, are an important component of a patient evaluation (Glasscock et al, 1997; Hughes, 1997).

The most common reason to obtain an imaging study in a patient with chronic ear disease is to determine the absence or presence and extent of cholesteatoma (**Fig. 7–13**). Aural cholesteatoma is defined as keratinizing squamous epithelium that is present in the middle ear, mastoid, or petrous apex. Cholesteatoma can be termed primary acquired, secondary acquired, or congenital. Primary cholesteatoma is caused by severe retraction of the tympanic membrane as a result of chronic eustachian tube dysfunction and resultant negative middle ear pressure. In this case, the posterosuperior portion of the drum invaginates, forming an epithelial-lined cyst that accumulates keratin, enlarges, and destroys surrounding bone. This is commonly referred to as an "attic" cholesteatoma because it occurs in the most superior portion of the middle ear. Areas of bone destruction can include the ossicles; scutum or posterosuperior ear canal wall; tegmen or bone separating the ear from the intracranial cavity; semicircular canals, particularly the horizontal canal, which is closest to the middle ear; and the fallopian canal, which houses the facial nerve and is particularly vulnerable as it travels through the middle ear just above the oval window. Cholesteatoma may extend into the mastoid cavity or even into the intracranial cavity. Secondary acquired cholesteatoma occurs when squamous epithelium from the surface of the tympanic membrane enters the middle ear through a perforation. This may occur as a result of trauma or infection.

Congenital cholesteatoma occurs as a result of a developmental abnormality. The typical patient is a young child with a white mass visualized in the anterosuperior middle ear space, behind an intact, normal-appearing tympanic membrane. These patients have no history of tympanic membrane perforation, otorrhea, or otologic surgery to suggest a mechanism for acquired cholesteatoma. Disease can be extensive, regardless of the origin of the cholesteatoma.

Imaging is typically performed preoperatively for assessment of a known cholesteatoma only if clinically indicated (Blevins and Carter, 1998). Indications may include vertigo, a suspected labyrinthine fistula, facial paresis or paralysis, SNHL, cholesteatoma in unilateral hearing loss, and planned revision surgery. Other extracranial complications can include labyrinthitis, mastoiditis, petrositis, and soft tissue abscesses.

MRI may be indicated in cases of suspected intracranial extension or other complications. Intracranial complications include extradural/perisinus abscess, lateral (sigmoid) sinus thrombosis, subdural abscess, cerebral abscess, otitic meningitis, otitic hydrocephalus, and brain herniation.

Pearl

- CT may be useful in diagnosing conditions for which surgery is contraindicated. X-linked congenital mixed deafness is associated with a series of distinct morphologic features of the temporal bone that are evident on CT scan. Surgical treatment of the associated stapes fixation is likely to result in a CSF "gusher" during stapedectomy, with resultant profound SNHL (Talbot and Wilson, 1994). CT may also identify features such as an anomalous course of the facial nerve, which is important for surgical planning.

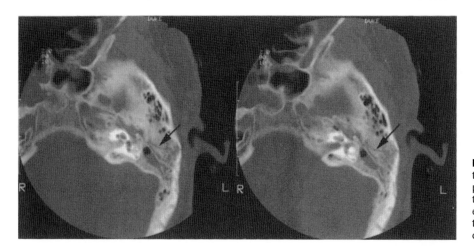

Figure 7–14 Longitudinal fracture through the temporal bone. Sequential axial computed tomography images demonstrate the fracture line (arrow) that parallels the external auditory canal. The fracture line extends toward the middle ear space and ossicles. The cochlea is not involved.

Temporal Bone Trauma

Temporal bone fractures (Swartz and Harnsberger, 1992) are described in terms of their predominant orientation with respect to the long axis of the petrous bone. Most fractures have either a longitudinal or transverse orientation. Complications associated with these fractures vary according to the orientation of the fracture and the temporal bone structures involved. Transverse fractures tend to be associated with more severe complications; fortunately, they are less common than longitudinal fractures.

About 70 to 90% of all temporal bone fractures are longitudinal (**Fig. 7–14**). These typically result from a blow to the temporal or parietal region. Fractures follow a path of least resistance, and because this fracture originates outside the dense bone of the otic capsule, it remains extralabyrinthine. The fracture line often involves the external auditory canal and middle ear. Involvement of the anulus tympanicus usually results in a tympanic membrane tear. Hemotympanum is often identified on examination, and these patients typically have a conductive hearing loss. In the absence of a perforation, the conductive hearing loss should resolve after several weeks. If it does not, ossicular discontinuity should be suspected. These fractures may result in facial paralysis or paresis. Cholesteatoma may form as a result of invaginating epithelium along the fracture line or through a perforation.

A transverse temporal bone fracture occurs less commonly (10–30% of the time) and usually results from a blow to the occiput. The fracture line typically begins in the vicinity of the jugular foramen or foramen magnum and extends to a foramen in the floor of the middle cranial fossa, often through the bony labyrinth (**Fig. 7–15**). When these fractures involve the otic capsule, deafness and severe vertigo usually result. Although the hearing loss is permanent, the vertigo can be transient. Hearing loss and vertigo can result from inner ear concussive injuries in the absence of fracture as well. In these cases, head trauma produces mechanical disruption of the membranous components of the inner ear.

Facial nerve paralysis or paresis is a common sequela of temporal bone trauma. Facial nerve injury is associated with transverse fractures in up to 50% of cases. Injury is less common with longitudinal fractures and occurs ~10 to 20% of the time. Patients with total paralysis and severely diminished responses on studies of facial nerve function (electroneuronography or electromyography) are candidates for facial nerve decompression surgery to reduce bony spicules or traction injuries and repair the nerve. CT imaging may be very useful in delineating areas of likely injury.

Imaging in the Diagnosis of Facial Paralysis

A partial or complete unilateral facial paralysis that occurs over a 24 to 48 hour period of time, with no associated abnormalities of hearing, vestibular function, other cranial nerves, or the head and neck exam, is likely to be due to Bell's palsy. This is a diagnosis of exclusion, so a thorough

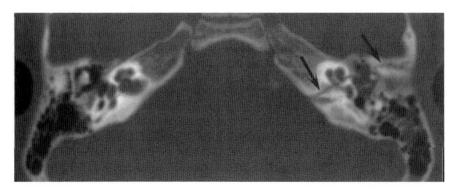

Figure 7–15 Transverse fracture of the temporal bone demonstrated on axial computed tomography. The fracture line (arrows) extends through the cochlea.

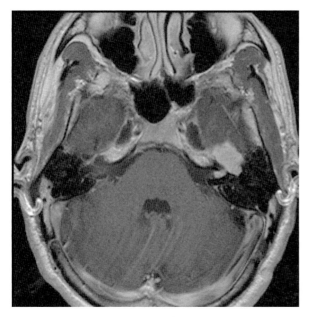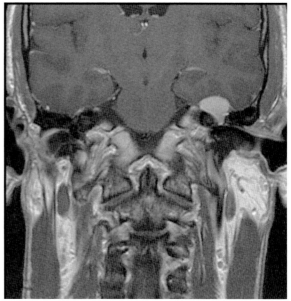

A   B

Figure 7–16 (A) Axial image showing enhancing tumor in the skull base with extension into the internal auditory canal (right side of figure, left side of patient). **(B)** Coronal image showing the same tumor.

history and physical examination are necessary to rule out other causes of facial paralysis, particularly skull base neoplasms, otitis media, and parotid tumors, all of which can present with facial weakness.

Tumors of the facial nerve, although rare, can present with facial paralysis or paresis. It is estimated that only 5% of peripheral facial paralysis is caused by tumors (Schaitkin and May, 2000); however, early diagnosis is important. In most cases, the facial paralysis related to neoplastic growths is slowly progressive rather than acute in onset, as for Bell's palsy. The most common intratemporal tumors causing facial paralysis include schwannomas and hemangiomas. Both are benign tumors but difficult to manage surgically because extirpation requires resection and grafting of the nerve. **Fig. 7–16** shows a schwannoma involving the geniculate ganglion portion of the facial nerve, in the base of the middle cranial fossa. This patient presented with near total facial paralysis, and so underwent resection of the tumor and nerve in this location with nerve grafting.

Parotid tumors can also cause facial paralysis either by compression of the nerve or by direct invasion. Early diagnosis and surgical resection are important for optimal management of these patients.

♦ Summary

This chapter discussed the basic imaging techniques, normal CT temporal bone anatomy, the use of techniques in diagnosing otologic disease processes, and the specific uses of imaging in the evaluation of patients in otologic practice.

References

Arriaga, M. A., & Carrier, D. (1996). MRI and clinical decisions in cochlear implantation. American Journal of Otology, 17, 547–553.

Blevins, N. H., & Carter, B. L. (1998). Clinical forum: Routine preoperative imaging in chronic ear surgery. American Journal of Otology, 19, 527–538.

Chandrasekhar, S. S., Brackmann, D. E., & Devgan. K. K. (1995). Utility of auditory brain stem audiometry in diagnosis of acoustic neuromas. American Journal of Otology, 16, 63–67.

De la Cruz, A., & Chandrasekhar, S. S. (1994). Congenital malformation of the temporal bone. In D. E. Brackmann, C. Shelton, & M. A. Arriaga (Eds.), Otologic surgery (pp. 69–84). Philadelphia: W. B. Saunders.

Glasscock, M. E. III, Haynes, D. S., Storper, I. S., & Bohrer, P. S.(1997). Surgery for chronic ear disease. In G. B. Hughes & M. L. Pensak (Eds.), Clinical otology (2nd ed., pp. 218–232). New York: Thieme Medical Publishers.

Grossman, R. I., & Yousem, D. M. (1994). Neuroradiology: The requisites (pp. 1–22). St. Louis: Mosby.

Hall, J. W. III, Grose, J. H., & Pillsbury, H. C. (1995). Long-term effects of chronic otitis media on binaural hearing in children. Archives of Otolaryngology—Head and Neck Surgery, 121, 847–852.

Heller, J. W., Brackmann, D. E., Tucci, D. L., Nyenhuis, J. A., & Chou, C. K. (1996). Evaluation of MRI compatibility of the modified nucleus multichannel auditory brainstem and cochlear implants. American Journal of Otology, 17, 724–729.

Hughes, G. B. (1997). Complications of otitis media. In G. B. Hughes & M. L. Pensak (Eds.), Clinical otology (2nd ed., pp. 233–240). New York: Thieme Medical Publishers.

Jackler, R. K., & De la Cruz, A. (1989). The large vestibular aqueduct syndrome. Laryngoscope, 99, 1238–1243.

Jackler, R. K., Luxford, W. M., & House, W. F. (1987a). Sound detection with the cochlear implant in five ears of four children with congenital malformation of the cochlea. Laryngoscope, 97(Suppl. 40), 15–17.

Jackler, R. K., Luxford, W. M., & House, W. F. (1987b). Congenital malformations of the inner ear: A classification based on embryogenesis. Laryngoscope, 97(Suppl. 40), 15–17.

Jackler, R. K., Luxford, W. M., Schindler, R. A., & McKerrow, W. S. (1987c). Cochlear patency problems in cochlear implantation. Laryngoscope, 97, 801–805.

Jackler, R. K., & Parker, D. A. (1992). Radiographic differential diagnosis of petrous apex lesions. American Journal of Otology, 13, 561–574.

Jahrsdoerfer, R. A., Yeakley, J. W., Aguilar, E. A., Cole, R. R., & Gray, L. C. (1992). Grading system for the selection of patients with congenital aural atresia. American Journal of Otology, 13, 6–12.

Lambert, P. R. (1988). Major congenital ear malformations: Surgical management and results. Annals of Otology, Rhinology, and Laryngology, 97, 641–649.

May, M., & Schaitkin, B. (Eds.). (2000). Tumors involving the facial nerve. New York: Thieme Medical Publishers.

McKenna, M. J., Halpin, C., Ojemann, R. G., Nadol, J. B., Jr., Montgomery, W. W., Levine, R. A., et al. (1992). Long-term hearing results in patients after surgical removal of acoustic tumors with hearing preservation. American Journal of Otology, 13, 134–136.

National Institutes of Health Consensus Development Conference. (1991). Consensus statement. Acoustic Neuroma, 9(4), 1–24.

Ohlms, L. A., Edwards, M. S., Mason, E. O., Igarashi, M., Alford, B. R., & Smith, R. J. (1990). Recurrent meningitis and Mondini dysplasia. Archives of Otolaryngology–Head and Neck Surgery, 116, 608–612.

Pillsbury, H. C., Grose, J. H., & Hall, J. W. III. (1991). Otitis media with effusion in children. Archives of Otolaryngology–Head and Neck Surgery, 117, 718–723.

Rosenberg, R. A., Cohen, N. L., & Ransohoff, J. (1987). Long-term hearing preservation after acoustic neuroma surgery. Otolaryngology–Head and Neck Surgery, 97, 270–274.

Ruckenstein, M. J., Cueva, R. A., Morrison, D. H., & Press, G. (1996). A prospective study of ABR and MRI in the screening for acoustic neuromas. American Journal of Otology, 17, 317–320.

Sando, I., Shibahara, Y., & Wood, R. P. II. (1990). Congenital anomalies of the external and middle ear. In C. D. Bluestone, S. E. Stool, & M. D. Scheetz (Eds.), Pediatric otolaryngology (2nd ed., pp. 271–304). Philadelphia: W. B. Saunders.

Seidman, D. A., Chute, P. M., & Parisier, S. (1994). Temporal bone imaging for cochlear implantation. Laryngoscope, 104, 562–565.

Shelton, C., Hitselberger, W. E., House, W. F., & Brackmann, D. E. (1990). Hearing preservation after acoustic tumor removal: l. Long term results. Laryngoscope, 100, 115–119.

Shelton, C., Luxford, W. M., Tonokawa, L. L., Lo, W. W. H., & House, W. F. (1989). The narrow internal auditory canal in children: A contraindication for cochlear implants. Otolaryngology–Head and Neck Surgery, 100, 227–231.

Sismanis, A. (1997). Pulsatile tinnitus. In G. B. Hughes & M. L. Pensak (Eds.), Clinical otology (2nd ed., pp. 445–459). New York: Thieme Medical Publishers.

Swartz, J. D., & Harnsberger, H. R. (1992). Imaging of the temporal bone (2nd ed., pp. 247–267). New York: Thieme Medical Publishers.

Syms, C. A. III, De la Cruz, A., & Lo, W. W. M. (1997). Radiologic findings in acoustic tumors. In W. F. House, C. M. Luetje, & K. J. Doyle (Eds.), Acoustic tumors: Diagnosis and management (pp. 105–133). San Diego, CA: Singular Publishing Group.

Talbot, J. M., & Wilson, D. F. (1994). Computed tomography diagnosis of X-linked congenital mixed deafness, fixation of the stapedial footplate, and perilymphatic gusher. American Journal of Otology, 15, 177–182.

Telian, S. A., Kileny, P. R., Niparko, J. K., Kemink, J. L., & Graham, M. D. (1989). Normal auditory brain stem response in patients with acoustic neuroma. Laryngoscope, 99, 10–14.

Tien, R. D., Felsberg, G. J., & Macfall, J. (1992). Fast spin-echo high-resolution MR imaging of the inner ear. AJR American Journal of Roentgenology, 159, 395–398.

Tucci, D. L. (1997). Audiological testing. In W. F. House, C. M. Luetje, & K. J. Doyle (Eds.), Acoustic tumors: Diagnosis and management. San Diego, CA: Singular Publishing Group.

Tucci, D. L., Telian, S. A., Kileny, P. R., Hoff, J. T., & Kemink, J. L. (1994). Stability of hearing preservation following acoustic neuroma surgery (pp. 93–104). American Journal of Otology, 15, 183–188.

Tucci, D. L., Telian, S. A., Zimmerman-Phillips, S., Zwolan, T. A., & Kileny, P. R. (1995). Cochlear implantation in patients with cochlear malformations. Archives of Otolaryngology–Head and Neck Surgery, 121, 833–838.

Valvassori, G. E. (1994). Update of computed tomography and magnetic resonance in otology. American Journal of Otology, 15, 203–206.

Valvassori, G. E., Mafee, M. F., & Carter, B. L. (1995). Imaging of the head and neck (pp. 31–35, 113–115). New York: Thieme Medical Publishers.

Welling, D. B., Glasscock, M. E., Woods, C. I., & Jackson, C. G. (1990). Acoustic neuroma: A cost-effective approach. Otolaryngology–Head and Neck Surgery, 103, 364–370.

Wiet, R. J., Pyle, F. M., O'Connor, C. A., Russell, E., & Schramm, D. R. (1990). Computed tomography: How accurate a predictor for cochlear implantation? Laryngoscope, 100, 687–692.

Wilmington, D., Gray, L., & Jahrsdoerfer, R. (1994). Binaural processing after corrected congenital unilateral conductive hearing loss. Hearing Research, 74, 99–114.

Wilson, D. F., Talbot, J. M., & Mills, L. (1997). Clinical forum: A critical appraisal of the role of auditory brain stem response and magnetic resonance imaging in acoustic neuroma diagnosis. American Journal of Otology, 18, 673–681.

Chapter 8

Functional Brain Imaging

Lynn S. Alvord, James N. Lee, Robert B. Burr, Cynthia McCormick Richburg, and Julie Martinez Verhoff

- ♦ **Functional Imaging Defined**
- ♦ **Functional Magnetic Resonance Imaging**

  General Principles
  BOLD Functional MRI
  Variability Factors
  Validity
  Resolution
  Determining Degree of Activation
  Other fMRI Techniques

- ♦ **Magnetoencephalography**

  General Principles
  Strengths and Limitations

- ♦ **Positron Emission Tomography**

  General Principles
  Strengths and Weaknesses

- ♦ **Single Photon Emission Computed Tomography**

  General Principles
  Strengths and Weaknesses
  Comparison of PET and SPECT

- ♦ **Auditory Findings from Functional Imaging Studies**

  Clinical Research
  Basic Research
  Clinical Application
  Role of Audiologists

- ♦ **Summary**

The recent advent of functional imaging has resulted in an explosion of information on the auditory system, often with surprising results. Instead of simple "brain maps" in which cortical areas are identified as having a single function, it has become increasingly apparent that a far greater degree of complexity is involved. For example, there is evidence that it may be important for some cortical areas to diminish instead of increase their activity during particular tasks (Zatorre et al, 1994). Because functional magnetic resonance imaging (fMRI) shows only areas of increased activation, such a decrease would only be apparent in standard techniques by comparing the activation of two separate stimulus presentations.

Controversial Point

- What is the meaning of decreased cortical activation in an area of the cortex in response to a stimulus? It is not fully understood whether areas of decreased activation represent reduced cognitive ability or are actually a sign of the brain's ability to focus function to another cortical area.

There is also evidence that, instead of the cortex processing sequentially at different cortical locations, parallel streams of information processing exist in which different cortical areas act simultaneously (Rauschecker, 1998; Rauschecker et al, 1997). These and other principles are emerging, the understanding of which lends relevance to both our clinical and research efforts as audiologists. Figuratively speaking, it is apparent that the line between "language" and "auditory" areas is blurring, not only anatomically but also professionally. That cortical areas may share auditory as well as language functions makes us realize that it is increasingly important for audiologists to have an understanding of language theory to best assess central auditory processing.

◆ Functional Imaging Defined

For many years, scientists interested in the brain have longed to see it functioning in vivo. Techniques collectively termed *functional imaging* allow this to be accomplished in a variety of modalities, including fMRI, positron emission tomography (PET), and magnetoencephalography (MEG). In functional imaging, areas of the brain that are active during mental processes, such as audition, may be visualized as computer-enhanced colored areas on the scan. This is made possible by advanced imaging techniques, whereby metabolic processes accompanying increased neuronal activation may be detected. Such changes are typically very small and must be determined by computer analysis post hoc.

Whereas previous attempts at "brain mapping" relied on injured, diseased, or indirect methods, functional imaging comes closer to direct determination of active cortical areas in normal and abnormal subjects. Descriptions such as "seeing the mind" depict the scope and future of this new technology that promises increased understanding of brain function.

Neuropsychologists, physicists, radiologists, and neurosurgeons are among those most often involved in the imaging team. In the clinical setting, a variety of stimulus types are used, including auditory and visual, to determine the location of critical language areas. This information helps the neurosurgeon predict the outcome of various surgical procedures. Because auditory stimuli are among the most often used, audiologists are becoming valuable members of the imaging team, bringing with them an in-depth knowledge of auditory neurophysiology and experience in stimulus design and delivery.

Special Consideration

- Because scanner time is expensive and competitively sought after, researchers and clinicians are organized into teams, thereby allowing more than one experiment to be performed on a given subject. For example, an auditory experiment may be performed during the same fMRI session in which another researcher is performing a visual or language experiment.

This chapter provides an overview of the principles, techniques, and recent findings using auditory stimuli for the various functional imaging modalities. Emphasis is given to

fMRI, including studies performed at the University of Utah. The chapter assumes a working knowledge of cortical anatomy. The reader is referred to Fitzgerald (1992) for an excellent review. A review of auditory cerebral anatomy and physiology may be found in Musiek (1986).

◆ Functional Magnetic Resonance Imaging

Since its inception in the early 1990s, fMRI has rapidly become the most widely used modality in functional imaging (Binder et al, 1994). With greater temporal and spatial resolution than previous methods, fMRI is producing an ever-increasing number of studies in the auditory modality. The purpose of this section is to (1) provide a brief overview of the principles, technique, and instrumentation involved in the acquisition of fMR images in the auditory mode; (2) describe general findings to date; and (3) discuss the role of audiologists in the future of fMRI.

General Principles

MRI Theory

Before discussing fMRI, a basic understanding of standard MRI is necessary. The reader is also referred to Sanders and Orrison (1995) for a more in-depth treatment of this subject. MRI differs from other imaging modalities such as x-ray imaging and computed tomography (CT) in that a magnetic field is used to produce images. MR images are formed using radiofrequency (RF) magnetic measures of water density within tissue. Along with these density measures, various "weightings" (T1, T2, etc) further affect the brightness of portions of the image and are chosen according to the desired goals of the scan.

Figure 8–1 shows a somewhat oversimplified explanation of how these weightings are achieved. A strong static magnetic field causes the magnetic moments (plus–minus orientations) of a majority of hydrogen atoms to align with the static field, creating a net magnetic vector (L). A strong RF signal is next applied transversely to these protons (90 degrees), which realigns the magnetic vectors into the transverse position (T). This realignment causes the longitudinal magnetic vector to lose strength while the transverse vector gains strength. When the RF signal is switched off, these vectors assume their original positions and strengths over a very short period, termed *relaxation time.*

Pearl

- In MRI, T1 is the time required for the longitudinal vector to regain strength, and T2 is the time required for the transverse vector to lose strength. Because time constants vary according to tissue type, the T1 and T2 information is used to enhance images into either T1- or T2-weighted images.

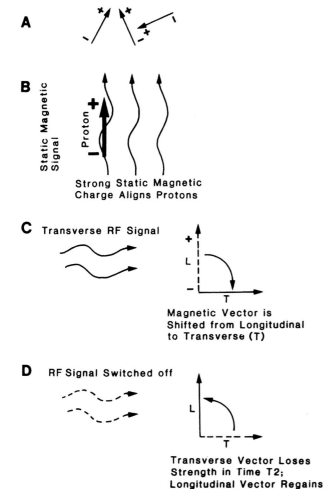

Figure 8–1 Derivation of T1 and T2 weightings of a magnetic resonance image. **(A)** Randomly aligned hydrogen protons. **(B)** Static magnetic signal aligns protons along the longitudinal axis of the body, creating a net magnetic vector (L) in this axis. **(C)** Transverse radiofrequency (RF) signal is applied, shifting the longitudinal vector (L), creating a magnetic vector (T) in the transverse direction. **(D)** When the RF signal is switched off, vectors return to their previous position. T2 is defined as the time in which vector T loses its strength. T1 is the time in which vector L regains its strength. Because T1 and T2 differ depending on tissue type, this information is used to produce T1- or T2-weighted images.

The time functions in which these vectors return to their original states are referred to as T1, the time in which the longitudinal vector regains strength, and T2, the time in which the transverse vector loses strength. Because these time constants vary according to tissue type, this information is used during image development to enhance the image into either a T1- or T2-weighted image. Various weightings are best for particular tissue combinations needing to be imaged. For example, a T1-weighted image is particularly good for differentiating normal anatomical tissue boundaries. T2-weighted images are sensitive to most abnormal tissue, including tumors, abscesses, and infected areas. A variation of T2, called T2*, is optimally suited for functional imaging in normal as well as abnormal individuals. Although a discussion of the difference between T2 and

T2* is beyond the scope of this chapter, T2* weighting is well suited for functional imaging because of its sensitivity to the status of deoxyhemoglobin concentration. This chemical affects MR signal intensity and forms the basis of the BOLD (blood oxygenation level–dependent) fMRI technique (Ogawa et al, 1990). BOLD fMRI is used in most current fMRI studies, including those described in this chapter. For a more in-depth treatment of general MRI theory, the reader is referred to Bronskill and Sprawls (1993). A simplified version of MRI theory is also published by Berlex Laboratories (1992).

Having metal in the body often contraindicates MRI or fMRI scanning. With the increasing number of cochlear implant recipients, the inability to scan these patients poses a problem. Strides have been made recently by cochlear implant manufacturers to make certain implant models compatible with MRI scanners. It is hoped that, in the future, most new implants will be MRI compatible.

Pitfall

- With the increasing number of cochlear implant recipients, care should be taken to identify such individuals, as MRI and fMRI scans may pose danger to the patient or damage to the implant.

BOLD Functional MRI

In BOLD fMRI, areas of the cortex that are active during mental tasks, such as listening, may be detected after computer analysis on the basis of the BOLD theory. According to this model (**Fig. 8–2**), increased neuronal activity in active cortical areas results in increased localized blood flow, bringing greater concentrations of oxygenated hemoglobin relative to deoxygenated hemoglobin (deoxyhemoglobin). Because deoxyhemoglobin is paramagnetic, this chemical interferes with the magnetic processes producing the image; therefore, lower concentrations of deoxyhemoglobin result in increases in the desired MR signal in the area. The above description is true particularly for T2*-weighted

BOLD Principle

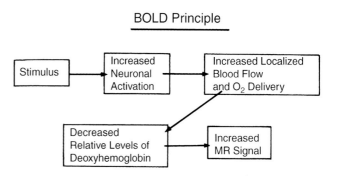

Figure 8–2 Sequence of events describing the blood oxygenation level-dependent (BOLD) theory on which BOLD fMRI is based. MR, magnetic resonance.

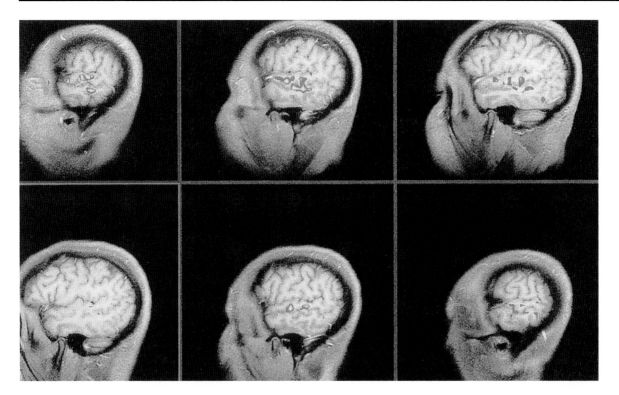

Figure 8–3 The functional magnetic resonance image of a normal 34-year-old right-handed man. Stimulus was a narrative story delivered auditorily at the upper level of comfortable loudness. The top three sagittal slices are of the right hemisphere. The bottom three slices are of the left hemisphere. *(See Color Plate 8–3.)*

images. A more detailed description of this theory may be found in Ogawa et al (1990). The increase in signal is not instantaneous but requires ~5 seconds to occur (Frahm et al, 1992). The small amount of increased brightness on the scan is not detectable to the naked eye but must be determined post hoc by computer analysis, which enhances active areas on the final version of the scan.

Stimulus Paradigm and Data Analysis

For analysis, the computer divides the cortical surface into tiny units (pixels if two dimensional, voxels if three dimensional). Analysis is made within each voxel to determine whether the MR signal (1) exceeds a certain threshold and (2) fluctuates in time with the on–off pattern of signal presentation (typically 30 seconds "on" alternated with 30 seconds "off").

An example fMRI scan performed in the University of Utah laboratory is shown in **Fig. 8–3**. The normal, right-handed male subject was asked to listen and remember details of a story switched on and off every 30 seconds. The figure shows sagittal images with the right hemisphere on top. Note that primary auditory areas and more posterior language areas are activated. Additional information regarding this figure will be presented in the following sections. **Figure 8–4** shows the on–off "boxcar" paradigm of signal delivery along with the change in MR signal for a particular voxel, termed the *time-intensity profile*. For auditory stimuli, words, tones, or sentences are presented to the patient

through nonmetallic earphones consisting of a length of polyethylene tubing terminating in foam ear inserts.

Pearl

- Besides correlation statistics, multiple *t*-tests and other statistical procedures are used in some software to determine the significance of the signal changes.

Post hoc computer analysis is made within each voxel to determine whether fluctuations in signal strength exceed random variations. To be considered significant, these fluctuations must exceed a certain amount, as well as "wax" and "wane" correspondingly with the "on–off" cycles of the stimulus. To determine this second criterion, a correlation statistic is run comparing the time course of the signal intensity in each voxel with an idealized curve created from the "on–off" pattern of task presentation and a model of the expected hemodynamic response function.

If this correlation is found, and if the signal changes also exceed a certain absolute value, the computer assigns a color depicting statistical significance (degree of activation) to the voxel being analyzed. Color schemes vary depending on the software.

Each voxel is analyzed independently in this manner to arrive at the final functional scan. Typically, correlation values of .35 or greater are necessary for significance. Although this

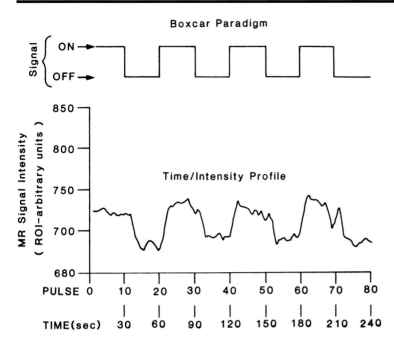

Boxcar Paradigm

Time/Intensity Profile

Figure 8–4 "Boxcar" stimulus delivery paradigm and "time/intensity profile" showing MR signal change in a single voxel, which fluctuates with the "on–off" pattern of the stimulus. MR, magnetic resonance; ROI, region of interest.

value seems low, according to the mathematical models used in the analysis software, this value corresponds to probability (*p*) values much lower than .001. Signal strength typically should increase by 2 to 6% (Rueckert et al, 1993). Signal changes greatly exceeding this amount (20–50% range) are likely caused by artifact, such as when scanning directly over a blood vessel. Besides correlation statistics, multiple *t*-tests and other statistical procedures are used in some software to determine the significance of the signal changes.

Alternative Boxcar Signal Paradigms

In a variation of the "boxcar" paradigm, instead of an "off" period, a second signal meant to activate a different area of the cortex (i.e., primary visual) is alternated with the auditory signal. By this "on–on" method (**Fig. 8–5**), two areas of the cortex may be analyzed in one session. The desired "off" period will still be achieved in the primary auditory cortex because visual stimuli, which do not activate primary auditory areas, will occur during the usual "off" cycle. For the primary visual area, the auditory stimulus serves as the "off" cycle. For example, the patient may receive auditory sentences for 30 seconds alternated with visually presented words for 30 seconds, thereby stimulating both the primary auditory and primary visual areas of the cortex. It should be remembered when using this method that any common areas activated by both stimuli will not be accurately assessed. Presumably such areas either would not activate due to the lack of an "off" period or would activate to a lesser extent, in which case it would not be clear which stimulus activated the area. A final consideration is that this method is employing a type of "alternating attention" task, which in itself may be a variable.

A third useful paradigm (**Fig. 8–6**) uses a type of subtraction technique to tease out a single feature within the same modality (e.g., semantic area vs primary auditory area). The

following example demonstrates this technique. In attempting to determine the cortical location of receptive language among other cortical areas activated by sound, it would be necessary to subtract the areas not involved in the specific language process. To achieve this, meaningless sentences could be alternated with meaningful sentences. In areas sensitive to sound but not meaning, the message would be meaningless during both the "on" and "off" cycles. Because no change is perceived, no activation would occur in this area. However, in the areas sensitive to meaning, "meaningful" words would be occurring every 30 seconds alternated with meaningless words. Thus, an "on–off" activation pattern would be achieved only in the semantic areas affected by the meaningful words.

Event-Related Paradigms

An alternative to the boxcar designs mentioned in the preceding paragraphs is the event-related (or single event) paradigm. An event-related paradigm uses the concept employed in such additive tests as auditory brainstem response (ABR), in which many small responses are added over a period of time. The event-related paradigm analyzes the response period at a point in time following a single short stimulus presentation. This response, however, will be very small and must be added to similar responses of many presentations. The resultant signal-to-noise ratio is therefore not as good as typically seen in the block design, which is a disadvantage to event-related paradigms. A disadvantage of the event-related paradigm is that sensitivity is somewhat less than in block designs. On the positive side, stimulus presentation can be randomized in event-related paradigms, thereby reducing expectation or habituation errors. The effects of scanner noise may also be reduced using event-related techniques (see discussion below).

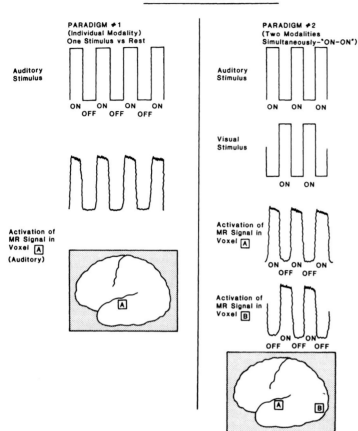

Figure 8–5 Standard stimulus paradigm (no. 1) and alternative stimulus paradigm (no. 2) in which two areas of the cortex are stimulated during the same experiment. MR, magnetic resonance.

For the most part, block paradigms are preferred when the goal is simple detection of activation in an area of the brain, whereas event-related paradigms are preferred when there is the need to study details of the hemodynamic response function. In short, for simple mapping studies, block paradigms are more sensitive in detecting activation. Newer versions of event-related paradigms, however, show promise in reducing the effects of scanner noise on auditory images, as explained in the following section.

Scanner Noise

Scanner noise is sometimes an obstacle when obtaining fMR images using auditory signals. Stimuli must be intense to be heard over the scanner noise. Although images are

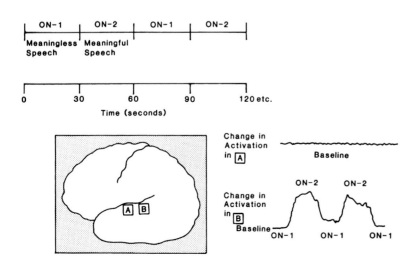

Figure 8–6 Subtraction paradigm used to tease out a subcategorical function (e.g., meaningful speech) within a broader category (e.g., "hearing" areas that include both meaningful and meaningless speech). Meaningful speech is alternated with meaningless speech. Because the software determines only those areas in which change occurs, only the areas activated by meaningful speech will be shown in the final scan.

successfully obtained in the block design by use of sound delivered through attenuating earphones, newer event-related paradigms are being tested to reduce or eliminate the effects of scanner noise by presenting the stimulus during periods of time when there is no scanner noise. For examples, see Belin et al (1999) and Talavage et al (1999). Talavage and Edmister (1998) proposed a method using "clustered volume acquisition" (CVA), in which the stimulus is presented during a period when there is no scanner noise. This results in a greater percentage of signal change and a higher statistical power per unit of imaging time. Attempts are also being made to reduce actual scanner noise during periods of signal acquisition (Seifritz et al, 2005). Although the 3 T (tesla) scanners with their greater sound intensity result in even greater noise problems, rapid strides are being made in the development of both hardware and paradigm design toward overcoming the challenges of scanner noise. Despite the challenges of scanner noise, we as well as others have been able to obtain good images at least in 2 T scanners using the block design by utilizing high-intensity stimuli, which are above the noise of the scanner.

Image Acquisition and Equipment

Functional MRI may be performed either on research scanners designed specifically for this purpose or on high-quality scanners designed primarily for clinical use. The field strength of the magnet should be at least 1.5 T (Moonen, 1995). Good images are certainly obtained with 1.5 T or 2 T using head coils, and there are now many 3 T scanners in use, although these produce somewhat greater acoustic scanner noise. To improve signal quality, a head coil (**Fig. 8–7**), which better detects the magnetic signal focused on the head, is highly beneficial. Custom-built encapped head coils are also available that further reduce noise. Studies reported in this article were performed at the University of Utah employing a General Electric (GE) Medical Systems (Milwaukee, WI) Signa "echo speed" Horizon Scanner (**Fig. 8–8**). Shown in **Fig. 8–7** is the quadrature (three-axis)

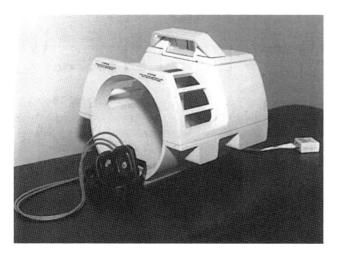

Figure 8–7 General Electric quadrature three-axis head coil used in functional magnetic resonance imaging scanning.

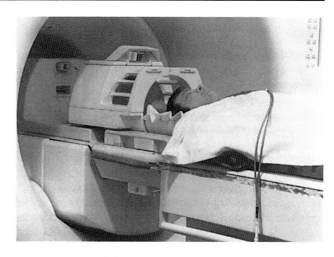

Figure 8–8 General Electric 1.5 T magnetic resonance imaging (MRI) high-speed "echo planar" scanner used in functional MRI. Note the quadrature head coil ready to be positioned over the head.

head coil ready to be positioned over the head. Pillows were then packed inside the coil around the head to reduce the chance of head motion during the scan.

Final fMR images are a composite of two sets of images. The statistical images computed from the functional images obtained during stimulus presentation are overlaid on separately acquired anatomical images. The following procedure outlines the methods used at the University of Utah to obtain six sagittal fMR images similar to those seen in **Fig. 8–3** (three images in the right and left hemispheres, respectively). A similar procedure may be used to obtain functional images in any other plane.

For the anatomical images, a three-axis T1 image is first acquired (axial, then coronal and sagittal). Both the functional and anatomical images are acquired at slices set at the same locations. **Figure 8–9** shows how these locations are chosen, using a different plane than the one in which the images are obtained. As seen in **Fig. 8–9**, locations are selected by first setting the sagittal slice locations in the coronal plane (19 vertical lines in **Fig. 8–9A**). Of these 19 slice locations, the outer three on each side were chosen (**Fig. 8–9B**) to obtain the final six sagittal images shown in **Fig. 8–3**. Scanning for the functional imaging occurs sequentially in the six chosen slices, with the scanner "seeing" each slice every 3 seconds.

From the computer analysis described previously, areas of functional activation (active voxels) are superimposed by the software onto the anatomical images to produce the final fMRI sagittal scans, an example of which is shown in **Fig. 8–3**. The three top images of **Fig. 8–3** represent increasingly deeper sagittal slices (**Fig. 8–9**) for the right hemisphere, whereas the bottom three slices show increasingly more lateral slices of the left hemisphere. Right and left hemispheres must always be identified because there is no standard orientation at this point for two separate scans showing right and left hemispheres. Additional techniques allow transposition of the functional data onto one of the other planes (axial or

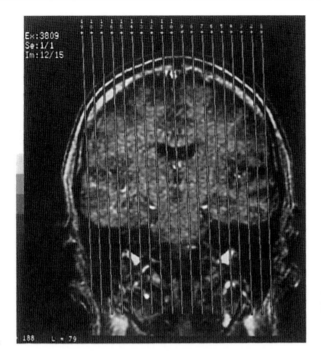

A

B

Figure 8–9 **(A)** Anatomical MRI locator scan (frontal radiologic view) with slice locator lines used to set slices for the sagittal plane for both the anatomical and functional magnetic resonance imaging acquisitions. **(B)** Six final slice locations chosen from the original 19 shown in **(A)**.

coronal). However, this requires an additional step during the anatomical imaging, termed a *whole head acquisition.*

Data Management

Images from both the anatomical and functional acquisitions represent a large amount of data, requiring substantial computer disk space. Typically, these data cannot remain in the scanner's computer but are transferred to another computer for analysis. Analysis requires commercially available software specifically written for this purpose. A typical analysis for a single patient requires ~1 to 2 hours, depending on user experience.

Variability Factors

Analysis Variables

Various analysis programs are available commercially, each resulting in slightly differing images, due to differences in underlying assumptions in the software. For example, software user variables may cause significant differences in the final image. During the analysis, a variety of options may be used, including various statistical significance threshold values. **Figure 8–10** shows the same scan given in **Fig. 8–3**, analyzed with the same software but using slightly higher statistical thresholds in the analysis. Note the result in a less "active"-looking scan. It would seem that a simple solution would be to use the same statistical values during analyses. However, clinical experience has shown that in cases of decreased patient motivation or alertness (discussed below), a slight lowering of the statistical threshold during analysis can result in a "normal"-looking scan,

whereas using the typical thresholds may show no activation. Appropriate statistical values for use during analysis, as well as interaction with patient state, are topics in need of further study.

Subject State or Effort

Initial fMRI studies demonstrate that the degree of activation is greatly affected by the conscious state of the subject. Similarly, the motivation or degree of effort used by the subject can affect scans. Sleeping subjects show little activation of cortical areas, which emphasizes the concept that areas of activity represent conscious thought processes. This is especially true when sensory stimuli are used or when the task involves memory or other cognitive abilities.

Pitfall

- The conscious state of the subject greatly affects the degree of activation. Sleeping or disinterested subjects may exhibit little or no activation.

Head Movement and Muscle Artifact

Head movement at any time during the scanning process produces significant location errors and other artifact. Because the final fMRI scan is a composite of functional images superimposed on detailed anatomical images, head motion of as little as a few millimeters in either scan can greatly reduce the accuracy of the final image. Surrounding the head with towels tightly packed in the coil housing is a

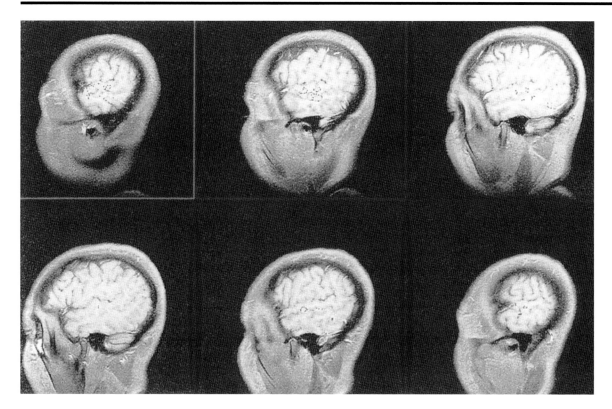

Figure 8–10 Functional magnetic resonance imaging scan using the same data from **Fig. 8–3** but a higher statistical cutoff during analysis. Note the apparent lesser degree of activation caused by the different statistical choice made during analysis. *(See Color Plate 8–10.)*

superior method to using a bite bar, which may also cause artifact because of active muscle clenching. Clenching of head or neck muscles may be particularly deceiving because this may occur in synchrony with "on" cycles. This timed head movement could conceivably cause areas on the cortex to appear active.

Pitfall

- Use of a bite bar may cause artifact because of muscle activation. Head motion, which is a great source of artifact, may be best eliminated by proper patient instruction and the use of firm pillows packed around the head.

Choice of Slice Location

Functional images are acquired at predetermined slice locations in a particular plane (sagittal, coronal, or axial). The location of the slice can affect the degree of activation seen on the final scan; therefore, it is best to observe activation at several different slice depths. In the sagittal plane, three slice depths on each side, such as those shown in **Figs. 8–3** and **8–10**, were utilized at the University of Utah. Having standard slice locations would aid in comparative studies; unfortunately, the choice of slice location is somewhat arbitrary between laboratories and between subjects within the same laboratory. Arriving at standard slice locations is com-

plicated by large variations in individual anatomy and head size. Until standardized methods can be achieved, small differences in slice location must be considered a possible source of error when comparing two datasets. However, the magnitude of this error may be quite small because studies of this issue report good correspondence between two such datasets having slight variations in slice location (DeYoe et al, 1994). Although of less significance clinically, it is likely that small variations in slice location could lead to erroneous research conclusions. It is likely that a system for choosing slice location based on an individual's own anatomical landmarks would have the greatest advantage for comparative studies.

Special Consideration

- Future efforts will be needed to improve the designation of slice locations within and between subjects.

Within and Between Subject Variability

Figure 8–11 shows test–retest results from a single subject evaluated at the University of Utah. The subject, a right-handed, 24-year-old normal woman, was given two scans in succession on the same day. She received an auditorily presented taped story about the city of Chicago. The stimulus was binaurally balanced for loudness by the subject

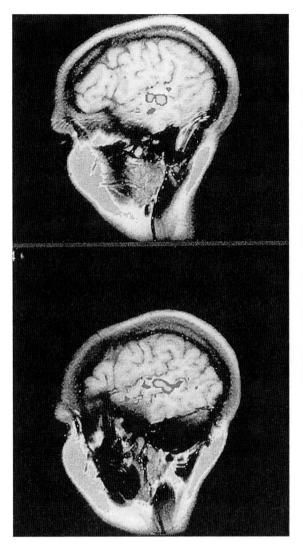

A

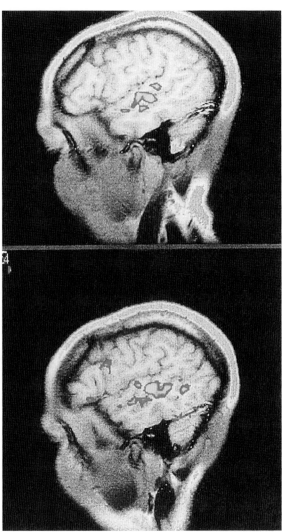

B

Figure 8–11 Two separate functional magnetic resonance imaging scans performed on the same subject 20 minutes apart using identical methodologies. **(A)** First scan performed. **(B)** Second scan performed 20 minutes later. Slice locations for the two scans were chosen to be as nearly the same as possible (right hemisphere is shown on top for both acquisitions). *(See Color Plate 8-11.)*

to her upper level of comfortable loudness prior to the test and was alternated "on–off" in 30-second periods. Resulting sound levels as measured at the foam tip with a sound level meter were 92 dB(A) in the right ear and 91 dB(A) in the left. The subject was asked to pay close attention to the details of the story. Before the second scan, the patient was removed from the scanner, repositioned on the table, and asked to readjust the volume of the stimulus, resulting in levels of 93 dB(A) in the right ear and 90 dB(A) in the left (levels within 1 dB of those used in the first scan). Analysis of the two scans used the same software with the same statistical values (Z thresholds 3–7). **Figure 8–11** shows the results of the first and second scans, respectively. As seen, similar but not identical results were obtained, with slightly more extensive activation occurring on the second scan. Although slices were chosen in the same manner for both scans (setting the outermost slice in the axial plane at the outer margin of the cortex), apparently some difference exists in slice

depth between the two scans, which may account for much of the difference between scans. This is possibly caused by slight differences in head orientation in the scanner because the technician noted the head being positioned slightly more forward (chin more downward) on the second scan (see earlier discussion "Choice of Slice Location"). DeYoe et al (1994) also found minor differences in scans performed on the same individuals 1 week apart. Subject alertness or slight differences in slice locations were possible causes. Other possible variables are differences in head orientation, movement of the head, and differences in motivation or attention.

Pearl

- It is well established that individual differences exist in cortical organization for language.

When performing the same task on different subjects, considerable variability of results occurs. Using visual stimuli, Rombouts et al (1997) noted large variability in the size and location of the cortical area activated between subjects. However, a high degree of overlap of at least some portion of the areas being activated was noted. The greatest portion of this intersubject variability presumably comes from actual differences in individual cortical organization. It is well established that individual differences exist in cortical organization for language (Ojemann, 1983).

Validity

The validity of fMRI relates to several issues. Functional MRI provides an indirect measure of neural activity by use of measures in or around microvasculature, which is very close to neurons being activated. Therefore, it is possible that areas of blood pooling in larger veins could pose as sites of activation. This artifact may usually be determined because an increase in MR signal strength in this case far exceeds the values typically achieved at true activation sites.

Another potential problem is encountered when scanning directly over a sulcus, because signals at various levels may add together. Attempts are being made through software design to virtually "blow up" the cortical surface like a balloon during analysis, thus avoiding this problem. However, this approach may introduce other forms of artifact.

MR activation by the BOLD technique does not occur instantaneously. A time lag of ~5 seconds occurs between neural activation and the beginning of the BOLD effect (DeYoe et al, 1994). Use of a 30-second stimulus period allows for this factor.

Resolution

It should be recognized that the BOLD theory is only an indirect measure of neural activity at a location slightly remote from the neurons, that is, in or around the microvasculature. As mentioned in the previous section, the possibility exists that scanning near larger vessels where blood pooling may occur could result in an area of inactivity being identified as an active area. Notwithstanding this possibility, agreement with other, more direct methods (MEG or intraoperative electrode stimulation) is good and on the order of a few millimeters (Elliott, 1994). However, the degree of spread of the image beyond the actual point of neural activation is not known.

Pearl

- The presence of activation on an fMRI scan provides evidence of some viable function in a particular area of the cortex.

Determining Degree of Activation

Another factor relating to validity is the unknown relationship between the degree of activation on the fMRI scan and the degree of neural activity present. For example, whether greater neural activity is best represented by a wider area of activation (number of voxels activated) or by a greater percent increase in signal strength in response to the stimulus (percent change of signal strength of individual voxels) is unknown. Realizing that fMRI activation relates to conscious thought, it is not clear exactly what a greater or lesser degree of response signifies. For example, it is possible that a greater degree of response may occur in a brain that has some loss of function because the subject is trying harder to comprehend the stimulus. Therefore, at present it is unclear whether greater amounts of activation represent greater cognitive ability, greater effort, tissue health, motivation, or a combination of the these and other factors. More studies are needed to clarify these issues. One thing that is clear is that the presence of activation on an fMRI scan provides evidence of some viable function in a particular area of the cortex.

Other fMRI Techniques

Other fMRI techniques are termed *perfusion fMRI*. These techniques, which measure cerebral blood flow, include bolus tracking, which requires the injection of a magnetic compound such as gadolinium, and spin labeling (Moseley et al, 1996). They are somewhat limited in that they are either invasive (bolus tracking), which limits the number of times an individual may be scanned without risk of kidney damage, or more time consuming (spin labeling). However, spin labeling can provide highly accurate results when only a specific area of the cortex is being examined.

Two other techniques, not technically considered functional imaging but utilizing MRI, will undoubtedly play an increasing role in studies of audition. These are diffusion tensor imaging and MR spectroscopy. In diffusion tensor imaging, white matter tracts may be followed and identified. Thus, auditory pathways below the cortex may be studied. In MR spectroscopy, analysis is made of the chemical composition of the brain tissue in the area being examined. The concentration of particular chemical compounds in an area of the brain gives an indication of the health of the tissue in that area. This technique may have potential for determining the effects of auditory deprivation or stimulation in auditory areas of the brain, including the cortex.

◆ Magnetoencephalography

General Principles

Of all the functional imaging techniques, MEG provides the most direct assessment of neural events, detecting the tiny magnetic signals generated directly from traveling current along activated neurons.

Controversial Point

- Some would argue that MEG is more valid than fMRI because it directly measures neural activity, whereas fMRI does this indirectly by assessing regions of increased blood flow.

During functional MEG, cortical regions involved in sensory, motor, or cognitive functions experience increased neuronal activity. Because a traveling electrical charge always produces an accompanying magnetic field, these small magnetic signals are detected by a magnetometer or gradiometer positioned around the patient's head. The headpiece contains several discrete sensing transducers, or SQUIDs (*superconducting quantum interference devices*), each sensing a small area of the cortex. The number of SQUIDs corresponds to the number of channels. Instruments are currently available having between 1 and 306 channels. **Fig. 8–12** shows a 306-channel device housed at the Center for Advanced Medical Imaging at the University of Utah.

The assorted analysis programs that produce the final image operate under a variety of assumptions. According to the often-used single equivalent current dipole (ECD) model, or single dipole model, the mathematics used by the program assumes that a discrete group of neurons is generating a "dipole-like" electrical field (Ganslandt et al, 1997). Alternative models are also used in some software and result in slightly different-looking images. A criticism of the single dipole model is that it tends to "see" areas of greatest neuronal activation while somewhat ignoring certain surrounding areas of lesser activation. Lewine and Orrison (1995) provide a more complete technical description of MEG technology and techniques.

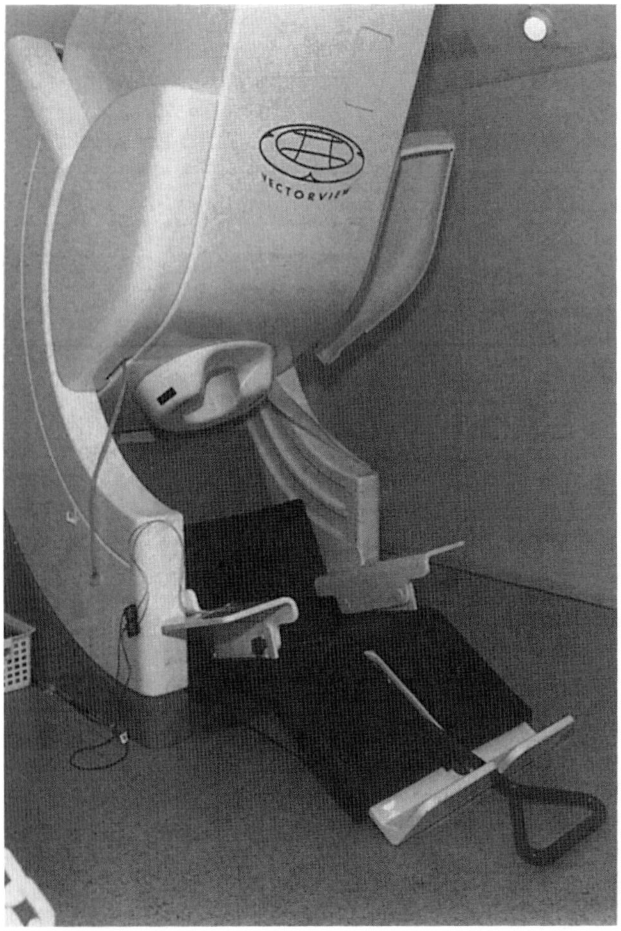

Superimposing Anatomical Images

Once the areas of magnetic activation have been identified, they are superimposed on anatomical MR images. These two acquisitions need to have the same precise orientation. During MEG, this orientation is accomplished by placing four small coils on the scalp: one on the front, back, and each side of the head. Additional infrared sensors are aimed below the nose and into each ear just superior to the tragus. The computer "marks" these locations, thereby determining head orientation. During the MRI anatomical scan, these locations are marked with small stickers placed on the head at the same locations so that the two final images may be aligned.

Pearl

- Evoked MEG, in which a stimulus is delivered and analysis is time-locked to the stimulus, is of great value in mapping cortical areas.

Figure 8–12 A 306-channel MEG scanner located at the Center for Advanced Medical Imaging, University of Utah.

Types of MEG Scans

MEG may be obtained in either spontaneous or evoked format. In spontaneous mode, the patient does nothing and receives no stimulus. Because effective spontaneous responses are obtainable only in the awake state, the patient is sometimes asked to read a passage from a book to maintain alertness, and a spontaneous sample is taken over a period of several minutes. Results of spontaneous MEG may be shown in a format similar to multielectrode electroencephalogram (EEG) tracings or may be "mapped" onto an anatomical grid, such as seen in **Fig. 8–13**. This figure shows results for a mildly autistic child having abnormal "epileptic" activity emanating from the location at the center of the left set of circles. Spontaneous MEG may be used to screen for abnormal cortical function, such as may occur in schizophrenia or after head trauma, in which case "slow" waves may be present. Other abnormal waveforms include altered alpha waves that are normally absent with the eyes open. Reading the raw data tracings of spontaneous multichannel MEG is a skill requiring highly specialized training. At present, only a few individuals are qualified to perform these analyses.

Of greater use in mapping cortical areas is evoked MEG, in which a stimulus is delivered and analysis is time-locked to the stimulus. For example, as a test of tonotopicity, a pure tone may be delivered multiple times with a separation of 3 seconds between each tone. The magnetic signal is sampled during a short time period surrounding each tone (beginning 50 msec before the tone and extending 2 seconds after). The sampling period before the tone is used to establish baseline values. The individual magnetic responses are then averaged and displayed as an image.

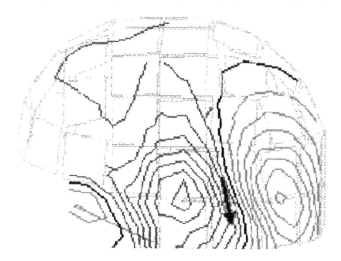

Figure 8–13 Posterolateral left view of spontaneous MEG scan of a mildly autistic child showing the focus of epileptiform activity in the left temporal lobe (at center of left circles). *(See Color Plate 8–13.)*

Pitfall

- A limitation of MEG is that any metal in the patient will greatly distort the signal, as with MRI.

Strengths and Limitations

As with MRI, a limitation of MEG is that metal existing in the patient will greatly distort the signal. Compared with fMRI, perhaps the greatest limitation is the short time frame (a few seconds) in which the data must be gathered. Therefore, single words or sounds rather than sentences lend themselves best to MEG. Sentences may be used for stimuli if careful timing of the target words is maintained. In addition, MEG has limited availability considering the paucity of centers possessing multichannel MEG devices. Finally, MEG only detects magnetic activity at or near the cortical surface, as opposed to analyzing deeper structures.

A great strength of MEG compared with all other functional techniques is its unique ability to determine the temporal order of events as they occur in various locations of the cortex. This feature will undoubtedly offer exciting insights into the function of the brain. Functional MEG results, in the form of scans, also agree favorably with those of fMRI and intraoperative electrocortical stimulation mapping.

◆ Positron Emission Tomography

Positron emission tomography, originally known as positron emission transverse tomography, has been used as a radiological imaging technique in biomedical research since the 1970s. It has been the pioneering technique of functional brain studies, including those in the auditory mode. The reader is referred to Engelien et al (1995), who used PET to study sound categorization in normal individuals and in a patient with auditory agnosia. This study contains many pertinent references.

General Principles

PET uses positron-emitting radionuclides ("tracers") to detect biochemical or physiological processes involved in cerebral metabolism. These specially selected radiolabeled compounds are bound with biochemical substances and intravenously injected or inhaled into the body. The isotopes begin to decay, producing positrons that interact with negative electrons. This process, termed *positron-electron annihilation,* produces two photons traveling colinearly (180 degrees) in opposite directions (annihilation radiation). In PET the positrons are then revealed in vivo by the detection of the annihilation radiation in a scanner encasing the head. The scanner reconstructs images on the basis of the distribution of the radioisotopes as they decay within tissue.

Pearl

- Physiological activity that is affected by a disorder or pathological condition can be seen as a departure from normal biochemical processes and can be detected with PET.

PET relies on the assumption that all physiological activities, including neural activation, are associated with biochemical processes. These biochemical processes can be assessed with PET techniques, allowing function to be indirectly localized. Likewise, physiological activity that is affected by a disorder or pathological condition can be seen as a departure from normal biochemical processes and, therefore, can be detected with PET (Ter-Pogossian, 1995).

Functional PET, properly termed *stimulation PET*, allows for localization of "functional" responses (detection of localized neuronal activity) on the basis of changes in metabolic activity associated with the delivery of the stimulus. These include changes in glucose metabolism and increased blood flow. PET was the first imaging modality by which successful functional studies were performed, and a large volume of PET data forms the basis of modern functional imaging.

PET data are often overlaid onto anatomical images obtained with MRI or CT, which have better resolution than the PET scan itself.

Radionuclides

PET techniques developed from the understanding that several radiopharmaceuticals have chemical properties that give them the ability to enter into, and therefore trace, physiological processes. Radioactive isotopes (radionuclides) produced in a cyclotron are used to (1) measure blood flow through the brain, (2) mark metabolic processes, or (3) bind to specific receptors (Ter-Pogossian, 1995). **Table 8–1** lists some commonly used radionuclides and indicates their half-lives (the amount of time required for half the atoms of the radioactive substance to undergo decay). The short half-life time (minutes) allows measurements to be repeated only at close intervals.

Table 8-1 Common Radionuclides Used in Positron Emission Tomography

Radionuclide	Symbol	Half-life (min)	Source
Oxygen 15	^{15}O	2.07	Cyclotron
Nitrogen 13	^{13}N	10.00	Cyclotron
Fluorine 18	^{18}F	109.70	Cyclotron
Gallium 68	^{68}Ga	68.00	^{68}GePE

This usually requires the cyclotron to be in the same building as the patient and scanner. A few radionuclides having longer half-lives have been used, eliminating the need for an on-site cyclotron (e.g., N4-methylthiosemicarbazone).

Instrumentation

For most PET applications, the detection of the annihilation radiation is accomplished with the use of a scintillator, an instrument that records flashes of light (scintillations) that occur when photons or high-energy particles bombard the transducer. Because the PET scanner must assess radiation at a particular region of the body, a collimator is also used. This device determines the location of the radioactive source in the body by detecting the presence and time of arrival of the photon emitted in the opposite direction. If no companion photon is found on the opposite side of the collimator, the signal is rejected as coming from a random source. Detection of the companion photon also allows for determination of the location of the generating source. This is done by comparing the time it takes the two photons to arrive at their respective transducers situated at opposing sides of the collimator (termed *time of flight*, [TOF]; see **Fig. 8–14**). Distance from the source (hence location) can then be easily calculated by the computer from the TOF.

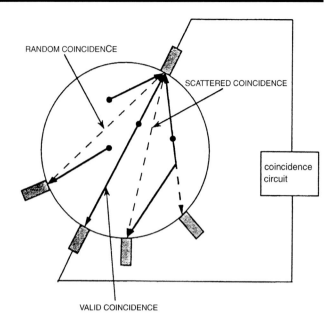

Figure 8–14 Function of a collimator in positron emission tomography scanning. Random photons are detected by the absence of a "companion" photon arriving at the opposite end of the collimator. True photons emitted by radioactive nuclides in the body are detected by the presence of a companion photon at the opposite end of the collimator. The location of the emitting source is determined by comparing the time of arrival of the two emitted photons.

Strengths and Weaknesses

A strength of PET is that scans may be obtained in patients having metal in their bodies, including cochlear implants. Limitations are poorer resolution, both spatially and temporally, (when compared with fMRI or MEG), the need for injection or inhalation of a radionuclide, and the paucity and high cost of available PET scanners. **Figure 8–15** shows a posterolateral left

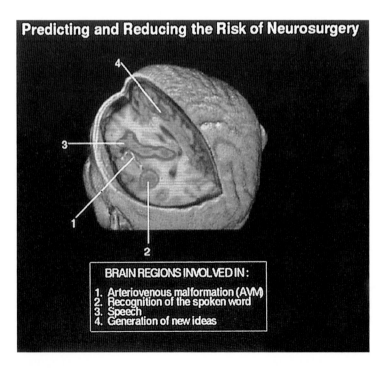

Figure 8–15 Posterolateral view of a three-dimensional positron emission tomography scan involving auditory, reading, and language areas. In this test, the patient is presented with the name of an animal on a screen and then required to read the word out loud, saying "yes" or "no" to signify whether the animal is dangerous or not. (Courtesy of The Banner Good Samaritan PET Center, Phoenix, Arizona.) *(See Color Plate 8–15.)*

view of a three-dimensional PET scan. The reader is also referred to Zatorre et al (1996) and Petersen and Fiez (1993) for examples of PET studies using auditory stimuli.

Pearl

- The goal of SPECT is to determine the relative or absolute concentration of radionuclides as a function of time.

◆ Single Photon Emission Computed Tomography

General Principles

Single photon emission computed tomography (SPECT), developed from emission CT (ECT), involves the detection of gamma rays emitted from radionuclides. SPECT is similar to PET in many ways. Both use radionuclides, which enter the body's metabolism and then emit radiation, which is detected to produce images. Janicek et al (1993) provide an example of how SPECT can be used for language analysis.

Radionuclides

As with PET procedures, radionuclides are necessary for producing SPECT images. SPECT uses radionuclides such as technetium 99m, xenon 133, and thallium 201. Several radionuclides used with SPECT are still in the experimental stage and are not approved by the U.S. Food and Drug Administration (Hartshorne, 1995; Jaszczak and Tsui, 1995).

Instrumentation

SPECT imaging requires the collimation (see the earlier discussion on PET) of gamma rays emitted from the radionuclide distribution within the body. A scintillation (gamma) camera, containing a lead collimator, is placed in front of a crystal (usually of sodium iodide containing a small amount of thallium), which acts as a lens in an optical imaging system. The collimator consists of multiple channels that allow rays traveling within a desired angle to pass through the channels and interact with the crystal. An array of photomultiplier tubes at the back of the crystal views the scintillations produced by the interaction of the radiation with the crystal. Determination is then made as to the location of each gamma ray interacting with the crystal (Jaszczak and Tsui, 1995). **Fig. 8–16** shows a clinical SPECT scanner.

SPECT systems reconstruct images in two basic planes, parallel and perpendicular to the axis of the body. The detector arrays come in a variety of configurations, including discrete scintillation detectors, one or more scintillation cameras, and hybrid systems that combine the arrays.

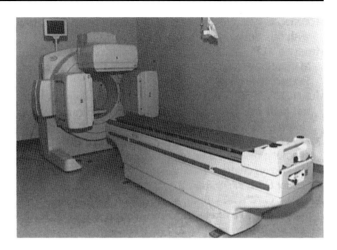

Figure 8–16 A single photon emission computed tomography scanner at the Center for Advanced Medical Imaging, University of Utah.

Pitfall

- Spatial resolution and noise are major factors that can affect the quality of SPECT images.

Strengths and Weaknesses

SPECT, like PET, has several weaknesses. The attenuation and scatter of gamma ray photons in the patient's body can affect image quality. The size and location of the structure being imaged and the stillness of the patient during imaging also affect quality and outcome.

Pearl

- Like PET and fMRI, SPECT has the ability to image deeper structures of the brain than MEG.

On the positive side, because SPECT systems are more widely available and less expensive to operate than PET, hospitals are more likely to have SPECT capabilities. Like PET and fMRI, SPECT has the ability to image deeper structures of the brain than MEG.

Comparison of PET and SPECT

SPECT scans look similar to PET, with colored areas indicating the degree of activation.

Both PET and SPECT systems produce three-dimensional images of anatomical structures from digitally stored data, which are then analyzed and displayed. Both procedures use radioactive isotopes injected into the body. PET uses two coincident annihilation photons from positron-emitting radionuclides, whereas SPECT uses gamma rays emitted from different types of radionuclides. Both procedures use the concepts of scintillation and collimation for imaging (Hartshorne, 1995).

PET is used in only ~100 centers around the world. Some of these systems are for clinical purposes, but most are used entirely for research. SPECT, in contrast, is much more common, less expensive to use, and primarily used for clinical purposes.

◆ Auditory Findings from Functional Imaging Studies

Studies using auditory stimuli began in the mid-1990s, using a variety of stimulus types, including pure tones and passive speech (Millen et al, 1995); nonspeech noise, single words, meaningless speech, or narrative text (Binder et al, 1994); and native versus foreign language comprehension (Schlosser et al, 1998). More recently, numerous studies have utilized auditory stimuli for topics as varied as language processing, schizophrenia, and musical perception. The principles learned to this point include the following:

1. Sound stimuli that require little or no linguistic analysis, such as noise, pure tones, and passive listening to uninteresting text, produce nearly symmetrical activity in or around the superior temporal gyrus of each hemisphere (Binder et al, 1994).

2. When the task requires listening for comprehension, significant lateralization to the language-dominant hemisphere is present (Schlosser et al, 1998).

Pearl

- When testing to determine the language-dominant hemisphere, use tasks that require linguistic analysis as opposed to passive listening tasks that tend to result in more symmetrical results.

---

3. Stimuli of higher presentation rates or greater difficulty produce greater activation. When words are presented too slowly, allowing time for the subject to daydream between stimuli, activation is greatly reduced. Tasks that are uninteresting, although "language rich," may produce activation of primary auditory areas but little activation of language areas.

Pearl

- Stimuli that are challenging or interesting produce greater activation.

---

4. There is evidence that certain cortical areas respond preferentially to a particular type of sound. For example, Obleser et al (2005) identified areas anterior to A1 as being specifically sensitive to vowels.

5. Recent studies have looked at a variety of other topics using auditory stimuli. Petacchi et al (2005) have noted several studies that report cerebellar activation in response to speech stimuli. The authors support a hypothesis that the cerebellum, among its other duties, plays a role that is purely sensory. Another recent study (Sokhi et al, 2005) has demonstrated that among male listeners, female voices activate different cortical areas than male voices. The results could not be accounted for by either pitch perception or behavioral response.

6. Cortical areas other than the primary auditory cortex are beginning to be better understood. Obleser et al (2005) observed that the anterosuperior temporal gyrus is involved in vowel recognition. Others have noted that more ventral areas, namely, the middle and inferior temporal gyri, are involved in semantic and lexical aspects of sound processing, especially on the left side, whereas other temporal lobe areas appear to be preferentially activated by speech sounds. The reader is referred to Zatorre and Binder (2000) for a review. Nontemporal areas are also activated by sound. For example, Griffiths et al (1998) reported that the right parietal cortex is involved in the analysis of sound stimulus movement.

When stimulating with meaningful speech, many additional areas of the cortex may be activated, the significance of which is not entirely understood. When the task is particularly difficult, such as listening in the presence of background noise, studies performed at the University of Utah as well as other sites have noted areas activated in the prefrontal cortex. This possibly represents decision-making processes for which the frontal lobe is particularly well suited. An alternative theory is that the frontal lobe, under difficult or noisy listening conditions, is playing its well-known role of selectively attending to the desired stimulus. Note the frontal lobe activation in the hearing-impaired subject in **Fig. 8–17**. This subject will be described more fully in the section "Clinical Research" below. Another theory to explain activation of the left frontal lobe regions is that these areas play a role in phonetic perceptual processing (Zatorre et al, 1992; Zatorre and Binder, 2000).

The number of functional imaging studies has grown exponentially in recent years, with new data frequently appearing in the literature. Auditory stimuli are among the most popular in functional imaging, which underscores the need and opportunity for audiologists to become more involved. The following section specifically reports studies involving audiologists as members of the functional imaging team. Audiologists are beginning to participate in functional imaging studies in both the clinical and basic research realms.

In the clinical realm, functional imaging has potential in at least three areas: determining the status of the auditory cortex in cochlear implant patients, assessment of central

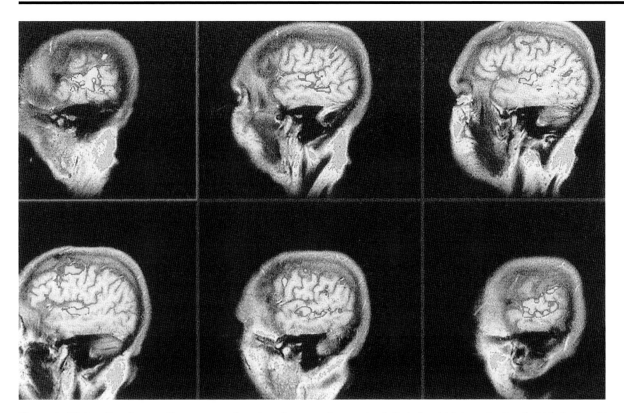

Figure 8–17 Functional magnetic resonance imaging of a severely hearing-impaired 73-year-old man (sagittal slices with right hemisphere on top). Note frontal lobe activation (middle bottom) in addition to normal areas of activation. *(See Color Plate 8–17.)*

auditory function in auditory processing disorders, and assessment for neurosurgical planning, such as in determining "language" areas to be avoided during surgery.

Clinical Research

Cochlear Implants

The potential use of functional imaging with cochlear implants is based on the concept that auditory areas of the brain may be assessed prior to implantation to ascertain their potential for future auditory stimulation. There is some evidence for the "use it or lose it" factor in that unused areas of the brain may become less capable of functioning after a certain period of disuse (auditory deprivation). Such a case could be due to simple inactivity or because the area has been recruited into another function. It is known, for example, that cortical visual areas in the blind can be "taken over" by other modalities.

Several technical issues make scanning the severely hearing impaired difficult, such as delivery of an intense stimulus. Also, several issues will have to be explored to assess the validity of such determinations, such as what degree of lessened activity is significant or nonrecoverable. Nevertheless, studies previously performed at the University of Utah, as well as other centers, have made some effort to begin such studies.

The study shown in **Fig. 8–17**, performed at the University of Utah, shows fMRI activation of a 73-year-old, severely hearing-impaired, right-handed male. The stimulus was the "Davy Crockett" story presented binaurally at the upper level of comfortable loudness (~115 dB hearing level). The patient had been postlingually deafened, presumably due to genetic factors, with the greater portion of the loss occurring at around age 35. Binaural amplification had been worn nearly constantly since the patient lost his hearing.

Hearing testing for the patient showed a nearly "corner audiogram" bilaterally. Pure-tone hearing thresholds were, right ear—55 dB at 250 Hz, 85 dB at 500 Hz, and no response at other frequencies; left ear—55 dB at 250 Hz, 50 dB at 500 Hz, 85 dB at 1000 Hz, and no response at other frequencies. Speech recognition thresholds were 95 dB, with 0% word recognition bilaterally.

As seen in **Fig. 8–17** (right hemisphere on top), there is strong, normal-appearing activation bilaterally in the temporal lobes. Also of interest is the lack of a strongly dominant hemisphere, a finding noted in many hearing-impaired subjects in our laboratory. The reason for this lack of dominance could be due to the stimulus sounding more like meaningless noise than a meaningful message. As noted earlier, meaningless sound often results in less hemispheric dominance in fMRI studies. Another explanation is that lack of strong hemispheric dominance is a "normal" characteristic of hearing-impaired subjects. Also of interest is the frontal lobe activation (middle bottom of **Fig. 8–17**). As noted in the previous section, this finding has sometimes been seen in normal individuals listening in difficult or noisy situations. The task for this subject would certainly be considered difficult because of the presence of the hearing loss. The subject shown in **Fig. 8–17** received a cochlear

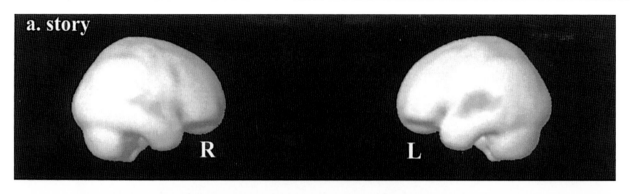

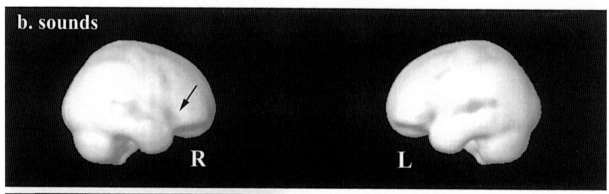

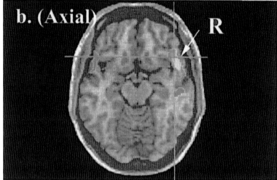

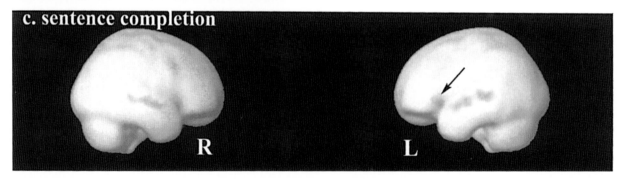

Figure 8–18 Composite functional magnetic resonance imaging scans of four normal subjects. In **(a)**, subjects were passively listening to a story ("Davy Crockett"). In **(b)**, subjects were attempting to mentally name sound effects. In **(c)**, subjects were mentally completing auditory sentences with the final word missing. Thus, trials **(b)** and **(c)** were both "naming" tasks in the auditory and visual modes, respectively. Note that sound effects also activate the right frontal cortex.

implant following the imaging study and is reportedly doing well.

In contrast to the above study, other investigators using SPECT as well as fMRI have found a general reduction in activation among postlingually deafened individuals (Roland et al, 2001; Truy, 1999; Wong et al, 1999). Depressed neural activity is generally observed bilaterally in primary and association cortices with long-term deafness (Truy, 1999). In addition, despite relatively similar hearing losses in each ear, significant differences in preoperative auditory cortex activation were observed between ears (Roland et al, 2001). In contrast, persons with residual hearing or deafness of short periods demonstrate more nearly normal resting cortical metabolism/perfusion in primary and secondary auditory cortices (Brodmann's areas 41, 42, 21, 22, and 38 for normal-hearing control subjects; Tobey et al, 2004).

In a study by Miyamoto and Wong (2001), cochlear implant subjects showed varying degrees of success in processing speech, which was reflected in their PET images. Individuals with functional speech processing also had activation in areas classically associated with speech processing for normal individuals (Miyamoto and Wong, 2001; Wong et al, 1999).

Tobey et al (2004), using SPECT, were able to show a relationship between activation of language areas and performance with the cochlear implant. Cochlear implant individuals with minimal open-set recognition demonstrated only minimal unilateral activation of auditory cortex in the hemisphere contralateral to the ear of implantation. In cochlear implant individuals who demonstrated high performance on open-set speech recognition tasks, bilateral activations were observed; however, activations were smaller in both amplitude and extent than those observed for normal-hearing individuals.

There is some evidence that cochlear implant users may utilize cortical areas differently than normal-hearing subjects. In a study by Wong and colleagues (1999), differing degrees of activation were seen among cochlear implant users and normal-hearing individuals in frontal and temporal areas when listening to multitalker babble. It was concluded that postlingually deaf cochlear implant users and normal-hearing subjects possibly use different perceptual processing strategies than normals under certain speech conditions.

Responsiveness of the auditory cortex in cochlear implant candidates has also been documented (Roland et al, 2001). In addition, research directly focusing on "repairing" neural architecture abnormalities in cochlear implant patients is also occurring (Tobey et al, 2005). Preliminary investigations have shown that the use of a pharmacologically enhanced treatment program resulted in a significant increase in activations in the primary and associative auditory cortex for adults with cochlear implants. Regional cerebral blood flow measures indicated an increase in both the extent and magnitude of primary and associative auditory cortex activations. In addition, auditory-only speech-tracking scores increased by 42% with the pharmacologically enhanced treatment program (Tobey et al, 2005).

Basic Research

In "brain mapping" studies, the goal is to identify cortical areas involved in a particular brain function. For example, in a recent review of the insular cortex (Bamiou et al, 2003), it is noted that tasks involving allocation of auditory attention, tuning into novel stimuli, temporal processing, and visual-auditory integration stimulate the insula.

Other examples of basic research studies are Moncrieff and Musiek (2002) and Moncrieff et al (2003), in which fMRI is used to study cortical activation during dichotic listening tasks.

At the University of Utah, we have performed fMRI studies of "naming" tasks using linguistic as well as nonlinguistic stimuli (sound effects). **Figure 8–18** shows composite fMRI scans using normal-hearing graduate students. For comparative purposes, part A shows the results of passive listening to a story ("Davy Crockett"). In part B, four normal-hearing subjects were mentally naming sound effects. In a similar study shown in part C, eight normal subjects were naming words described by an auditory sentence (i.e., "This is something that you use to cut your meat"). As shown in the passive listening task (part A), activation is almost exclusively limited to the superior temporal areas, possibly due to the fact that no language output (naming) is being required. In part C, in which the subjects are naming the auditorily described words, the left frontal cortex is also activated in an area roughly corresponding to Broca's area. In part B, naming sound effects, there is activation not only in Broca's area on the left but also in a similar area on the right, in addition to more superior areas. This result is evidence of a Broca's-like area in the right hemisphere possibly involved in the recognition or naming of environmental sounds. This is an example of a mapping study in which areas of the cortex are identified for a particular stimulus or task. This study used a block design, performed on a 1.5 T Marconi scanner, analyzed with the SPM99 statistical parametric mapping program (Wellcome Department of Imaging Neuroscience, University College London, London, UK).

Visual versus Auditory Naming

Another mapping study performed at our facility compared sentence completion (naming) in the visual and auditory modes. A single example normal subject is shown in **Figs. 8–19** and **8–20** performing both tasks. In **Fig. 8–19**, the subject is silently naming an auditorily described word (i.e., "This is something that you use to cut your meat"). As expected, auditory areas in the superior temporal lobe are activated, including more posterior areas possibly representing Wernicke's area, as well as areas in the frontal cortex. In the visual version of the task, **Fig. 8–20**, the subject is being shown sentences on a screen with the final word missing. As shown in **Fig. 8–20**, occipital visual areas are

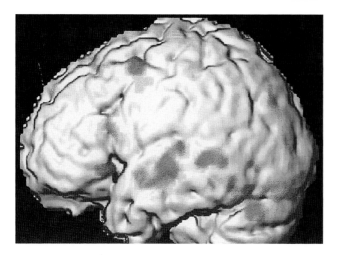

Figure 8–19 Single normal subject functional magnetic resonance imaging of an auditory naming task (i.e., "This is something that you use to cut your meat"). As expected, areas activated are in the superior and posterior temporal lobe, as well as in the frontal cortex. *(See Color Plate 8–19.)*

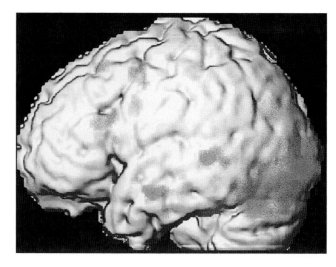

Figure 8–20 Single normal subject functional magnetic resonance imaging of a visual naming task (compare with Fig. 8–19). The subject was shown sentences on a screen with the final word missing. Note that occipital visual areas are being activated instead of auditory areas. Note also the common area activated by either the auditory or visual task located in the posterior temporal area, demonstrating that some language areas are modality independent. *(See Color Plate 8–20.)*

being activated instead of auditory areas. Interestingly, there is a common area activated by either task located in the posterior temporal area, demonstrating that some language areas are modality independent (activated by two different modalities).

Clinical Application

Neurosurgical Planning

In addition to the basic research studies just described, we have demonstrated that fMRI is a useful tool in neurosurgical planning (Heilbrun et al, 2001). Surgical candidates with space-occupying lesions are tested using stimuli similar to those described in the above studies to determine the location of language areas in relation to their lesion. Such images show the surgeon the location of important language areas in order that these may be avoided and that outcomes for language preservation may be better predicted. We have observed that tumors usually crowd out language areas, pushing them to one side as opposed to obliterating the language areas.

In summary, audiologists' involvement in functional imaging is needed for both research and clinical applications. Audiologists' expertise in the formulation of auditory stimuli, as well as our understanding of central auditory processes, provides important contributions to the functional imaging process.

◆ Summary

Functional imaging is an exciting technology, offering opportunities for audiologists to become involved in both clinical and research applications. Audiologists provide needed expertise to the imaging teams, which is necessary in performing such studies. Although PET and MEG are not widely available, fMRI and SPECT can be performed on standard high-quality scanners. Especially in the case of fMRI, data analysis requires additional software and training and computer hardware capable of storing large amounts of data. Such instrumentation may already be available in many larger hospitals and universities. Each of the imaging modalities described in this chapter has its own inherent strengths and weaknesses. MEG, for example, has the distinct advantage of being able to determine the order of events as they occur in the cortex. However, fMRI, PET, and SPECT can probe into deeper areas of the brain.

The information gained in functional imaging is currently useful in surgical planning and postsurgical evaluation of language function. Future research in functional imaging will provide new information on the basic mechanisms underlying central auditory and language function.

References

Bamiou, D. E., Musiek, F. E., & Luxon, L. M. (2003). The insula (island of Reil) and its role in auditory processing: Literature review. Brain Research: Brain Research Reviews, 42(2), 143–154.

Belin, P., Zatorre, R. J., Hoge, R., Evans, A. C., & Pike, B. (1999). Event-related fMRI of the auditory cortex. Neuroimage, 10(4), 417–429.

Berlex Laboratories. (1992). MRI made easy. Wayne, NJ: Author.

Binder, J. R., Frost, J. A., Hammeke, T. A., Cox, R. W., Rao, S. M., Prieto, T. (1997). Human brain language areas identified by functional magnetic resonance imaging. Journal of Neuroscience, 17, 353–362.

Binder, J. R., Rao, S. M., Hammeke, T. A., Yetkin, F. Z., Jesmanowicz, A., Bandettini, P. A., et al. (1994). Functional magnetic resonance imaging of human auditory cortex. Annals of Neurology, 35(6), 662–672.

Bronskill, M. J., & Sprawls, P. (Eds.). (1993). The physics of MRI. Woodbury, NY: American Institute of Physics.

DeYoe, E. A., Bandettini, P., Neitz, J., Miller, D., & Winans, P. (1994). Functional magnetic resonance imaging (fMRI) of the human brain. Journal of Neuroscience Methods, 54, 171–187.

Elliott, L. L. (1994). Functional brain imaging and hearing. Journal of the Acoustical Society of America, 96(3), 1397–1409.

Engelien, A. , Silbersweig, D., Stern, E., Huber, W., Doring, W., Frith, C., & Frackowiak, R. S. (1995). The functional anatomy of recovery from auditory agnosia. Brain, 118, 1395–1409.

Fitzgerald, M. J. T. (1992). Cerebral cortex. In M. J. T. Fitzgerald (Ed.), Neuroanatomy (2nd ed., pp. 197–210). London: Bailliere Tindall.

Frahm, J., Bruhn, H., Merboldt, K. D., & Hanicke, W. (1992). Dynamic MR imaging of human brain oxygenation during rest and photic stimulation. Journal of Magnetic Resonance Imaging, 2, 501–505.

Ganslandt, O., Steinmeier, R., Kober, H., et al. (1997). Magnetic source imaging combined with image-guided frameless stereotaxy: A new method in surgery around the motor strip. Neurosurgery, 41(3), 621–628.

Griffiths, T. D., Rees, G., Rees, A., et al. (1998). Right parietal cortex is involved in the perception of sound movement in humans. Nature Neuroscience, 1, 74–79.

Hartshorne, M. F. (1995). Single photon emission computed tomography. In W. W. Orrison, J. D. Lewine, J. A. Sanders, & M. R. Hartshorne (Eds.), Functional brain imaging (pp. 213–238). St. Louis: Mosby.

Heilbrun, M. P., Lee, J. N., & Alvord, L. (2001). Practical application of fMRI for surgical planning. Stereotactic and Functional Neurosurgery, 76, 168–174.

Janicek, M. J., Schwartz, R. B., Carvalho, P. A., Garada, B., & Holman, B. L. (1993). Tc-99m HMPAO brain perfusion SPECT in acute aphasia. Clinical Nuclear Medicine, 18(12), 1032–1038.

Jaszczak, R. J., & Tsui, B. M. W. (1995). Single photon emission computed tomography (SPECT): General principles. In H. N. Wagner, Z. Szaba, & J.W. Buchanan (Eds.), Principles of nuclear medicine (pp. 342–346). Philadelphia: W. B. Saunders.

Lewine, J. D., & Orrison, W. W. (1995). Magnetoencephalography and magnetic source imaging. In W. W. Orrison, J. D. Lewine, J. A. Sanders, & M. R. Hartshorne (Eds.), Functional brain imaging (pp. 369–417). St. Louis: Mosby.

Millen, S. J., Haughton, V. M., & Yetkin, Z. (1995). Functional magnetic resonance imaging of the central auditory pathway following speech and pure-tone stimuli. Laryngoscope, 105, 1305–1310.

Miyamoto, R. T., & Wong, D. (2001). Positron emission tomography in cochlear implant and auditory brainstem implant recipients. Journal of Communication Disorders, 34, 473–478.

Moncrieff, D., Briggs, R., Gopinath, K., et al. (June 2003). fMRI activation differences in children with dichotic words. Poster presented at the Organization for Human Brain Mapping Conference, New York.

Moncrieff, D. W., & Musiek, F. E. (April 2002). Functional MRI of children during dichotic listening. Research podium presented at the convention of the American Academy of Audiology, Philadelphia.

Moonen, C. T. W. (1995). Imaging of human brain activation with functional MRI. Biological Psychiatry, 37, 141–143.

Moseley, M. E., deCrespigny, A., & Spielman, D. M. (1996). Magnetic resonance imaging of human brain function. Surgical Neurology, 45, 385–391.

Musiek, F. E. (1986). Neuroanatomy, neurophysiology, and central auditory assessment: 2. The cerebrum. Ear and Hearing, 7(5), 283–294.

Obleser, J., Boecker, H., Drzezga, A., Haslinger, B., Hennenlotter, A., Roettinger M., et al. (2005). Vowel sound extraction in anterior superior temporal cortex. Human Brain Mapping, 27(7):562–571.

Ogawa, S., Lee, T. M., Ray, A. R., & Tank, D. W. (1990). Brain magnetic resonance imaging with contrast dependent on blood oxygenation. Proceedings of the National Academy of Sciences of the United States of America, 87, 9868–9872.

Ojemann, G. A. (1983). Brain organization for language from the perspective of electrical stimulation mapping. Behavioral and Brain Sciences, 6, 189–230.

Petersen, S. E., & Fiez, J. A. (1993). The processing of single words studied with positron emission tomography. Annual Review of Neuroscience, 16, 509–530.

Rauschecker, J. P. (1998). Cortical processing of complex sounds. Current Opinion in Neurobiology, 8, 516–521.

Rauschecker, J. P., Tian, B., Pons, T., & Mishkin, M. (1997). Serial and parallel processing in rhesus monkey auditory cortex. Journal of Comparative Neurology, 382, 89–103.

Roland, P. S., Tobey, E. A., & Devous, M. D.S. (2001). Preoperative functional assessment of auditory cortex in adult cochlear implant users. Laryngoscope, 111, 77–83.

Rombouts, S. A. R. B., Barkhof, F., Hoogenraad, F. G. C., Sprenger, M., Valk, J., & Scheltens, P. (1997). Test–retest analysis with functional MR of the activated area in the human visual cortex. AJNR American Journal of Neuroradiology, 18, 1317–1322.

Rueckert, L., Appollonio, I., Grafman, J., et al. (1993). Functional activation of left frontal cortex during covert word production. Abstracts of the 12th Meeting of the Society of Magnetic Resonance in Medicine, New York, 1, 60.

Sanders, J. A., & Orrison, W. W. (1995). Functional magnetic resonance imaging. In W. W. Orrison, J. D. Lewine, J. A. Sanders, & M. F. Hartshorne (Eds.), Functional brain imaging (pp. 239–326). St. Louis: Mosby.

Schlosser, M. J., Aoyagi, N., Fulbright, R. K., Gore, J. C., & McCarthy, G. (1998). Functional MRI studies of auditory comprehension. Human Brain Mapping, 6, 1–13.

Seifritz, E., Di Salle, F., Esposito, F., Herdener, M., Neuhoff, J. G., Scheffler, K. (2005). Enhancing BOLD response in the auditory system by neurophysiologically tuned fMRI sequence. Neuroimage, 29, 1013–1022.

Sokhi, D. S., Hunter, M. D., Wilkinson, I. D., & Woodruff, P. W. (2005). Male and female voices activate distinct regions in the male brain. Neuroimage, 27(3), 572–578.

Talavage, J. M., Edmister, W. B., Ledden, P. J., & Weisskoff, R. M. (1999). Quantitative assessment of auditory cortex responses induced by imager acquisition noise. Human Brain Mapping, 7, 79–88.

Talvage, J. M., & Edmister, W. B. (February 1998). Measuring and reducing the impact of imaging noise on echo-planar functional magnetic resonance imaging (fMRI) of the auditory cortex. Abstracts of the 21st Midwinter Research Meeting, Association of Research in Otolaryngology, 138, 35.

Ter-Pogossian, M. M. (1995). Positron emission tomography (PET): General principles. In H. N. Wagner, Z. Szabo, & J. W. Buchanan (Eds.), Principles of nuclear medicine (pp. 342–346). Philadelphia: W. B. Sanders.

Tobey, E. A., Devous, M. D. Sr., Buckley, K., Cooper, W. B., Harris, T. S., Ringe, W., & Roland, P. S. (2004). Functional brain imaging as an objective measure of speech perception performance in adult cochlear implant users. International Journal of Audiology, 43, S52–S56.

Tobey, E. A., Devous, M. D., Buckley, K., Overson, G., Harris, T., Ringe, W., & Martinez-Verhoff, J. (2005). Pharmacological enhancement of aural habilitation in adult cochlear implant users. *Ear and Hearing, 26,* 45S–56S.

Truy, E. (1999). Neuro-functional imaging and profound deafness. *International Journal of Pediatric Otorhinolaryngology, 47,* 131–136.

Wong, D., Miyamoto, R. T., Pisoni, D. B., Sehgal, M., & Hutchins, G. D. (1999). PET imaging of cochlear-implant and normal-hearing subjects listening to speech and nonspeech. *Hearing Research, 132,* 34–42.

Zatorre, R. J., & Binder, J. R. (2000). Functional and structural imaging of the human auditory system. In A. W. Toga & J. C. Mazziotta (Eds.), *Brain mapping: The systems* (pp. 365–402). San Diego, CA: Academic Press.

Zatorre, R. J., Evans, A. C., Meyer, E., & Gjedde, A. (1992). Lateralization of phonetic and pitch processing in speech perception. *Science, 256,* 846–849.

Zatorre, R. J., Evans, A. C., & Meyer, E. (1994). Neural mechanisms underlying melodic perception and memory for pitch. *Journal of Neuroscience, 14*(4), 1908–1919.

Chapter 9

Pharmacology in Audiology

Kathleen C. M. Campbell

Although audiologists in the United States do not prescribe medications to patients, every audiologist should have a basic understanding of pharmacology, drugs that can commonly affect the auditory system, classes of medications that are frequently used by physicians, and the approval process of the U.S. Food and Drug Administration (FDA). We can better manage our patients if we can fully communicate with pharmacists and otolaryngologists about a specific patient's medical care, understand some of the drugs our patients may be taking, and be aware of how these drugs can impact audiologic test results. We also want to be able to be full collaborators in clinical trials of new drugs that may be either ototoxic or otoprotective. Some audiologists may wish to pursue further study in chemistry and pharmacology, as I have, and participate in the exciting drug discovery process of identifying, patenting, and developing new therapeutic agents for the auditory system.

Pearl

- To communicate fully with other professionals about a patient's clinical care and to recognize the impact that drugs may have on hearing, each audiologist needs a basic understanding of pharmacology and ototoxicity.

♦ Definition of Pharmacology and Drugs

In a sense, humans have studied pharmacology since the earliest of times. Even primitive civilizations used plant or animal substances to ward off disease, to treat disease, to induce religious or meditative states, or to kill animals or human enemies. Sometimes the same substance would be used at a low dose for therapeutic effect and at a high dose for lethal effects. Thus, even early humans knew some of the basic principles of pharmacology.

Pharmacology is broadly defined as the study of the interaction of chemicals, both toxic and therapeutic, with living systems. This broad definition includes all natural and synthetic compounds. Thus, pharmacology can include the study of how the caffeine in our coffee affects us and how the nitrogen content in soil affects plants. However, in patient care and most medical research, we generally define *pharmacology* as the study of how drugs and the body interact.

Given that every time we eat or drink we are taking in chemicals, when does one of these substances become a "drug"? Technically, a drug is any natural or synthetic substance that has a physiologic action on a living body. That action may be beneficial or toxic depending not only on the substance but also on the dosage, the body's endogenous state, other concomitant drugs, the body's genetic profile, and a host of other factors. For example, acetaminophen may be beneficial at lower doses in relieving a headache, but at high doses it can permanently damage the liver. For most of us, peanuts are a healthy snack, but to a person with a peanut allergy, they may be lethal. Similarly, dairy products are a part of most nutritious diets, but for those with lactose intolerance, determined by genetics, dairy products can cause gastrointestinal disturbance.

In medicine, the term *drug* refers to any substance that is used in the diagnosis, treatment, or prevention of disease. Therefore, a nutritional supplement may be considered a drug if it is recommended or used to prevent or treat disease rather than to promote general health. Nutraceuticals are foodstuffs, such as supplements or fortified food products, that are designed to provide specific health benefits over and above the general nutritional value of the food product. Whether the nutraceutical is also considered a drug generally depends on the health claims made, although dosing and safety may also be factors. However, because nutritional supplements are not regulated by the FDA, the packaging may or may not note exactly what is in the nutraceutical.

Pearl

- Any time a substance is specifically recommended or used to diagnose, treat, or prevent a disease, it is considered a drug.

Sometimes the intended therapeutic effect of a drug also includes deliberate toxicity. For example, an overdose of an anesthetic may be used to euthanize an animal. A chemotherapy drug may be therapeutic to the patient but deliberately toxic to the cancer cells. Similarly, an antibiotic is intended to be beneficial to the patient but toxic to the targeted bacteria.

Most drugs have unintended side effects or toxicities, particularly at high dosage levels. When a drug is administered systemically, such as orally or by injection, it is distributed throughout the body and not just to the intended cells or organ system. Although drugs are developed to try to preferentially affect certain cell types or organ systems, usually the distribution and effects are more widespread. Side effects are unwanted effects that are not deleterious (i.e., truly harmful). For example, many drugs may cause slight nausea or indigestion, and the patient may tolerate these side effects to obtain the more important therapeutic effect, such as pain relief. A toxic effect is an unwanted effect that is deleterious, such as permanent liver damage, hearing loss, or peripheral neuropathy. Sometimes a drug is used even when it has known toxicities, such as a chemotherapeutic agent for a patient with a life-threatening cancer.

Most drugs have at least two names. All drugs will have a generic name, but most will also have trademarks, which are assigned by the pharmaceutical companies for marketing rather than scientific purposes. The *Physicians' Desk Ref-*

erence (*PDR*) lists both trademarks and generic names for each drug. For example, the loop diuretic furosemide is sold under the trademark Lasix. Some drugs will have several trademarks, usually for different marketing venues, particularly after the drug is out of patent. For example, the drug ibuprofen is marketed under the brand names Motrin, Advil, and Midol, as well as its generic name.

Branches of Pharmacology

There are five different disciplines of pharmacology: pharmacokinetics, pharmacodynamics, toxicology, pharmacogenetics, and pharmacogenomics. Pharmacokinetics is the study of how the body acts on the drug, and pharmacodynamics is the study of how the drug acts on the body. Toxicology is the study of the unwanted effects of drugs on physiologic systems, including both side effects and toxic effects. Pharmacogenetics is the study of how drugs impact the body's genetic response. Pharmacogenomics is the study of how we may use genetic information to guide the choice of drug therapy for each individual patient. Of course, it is clear that all of these areas overlap and cannot truly be studied independently.

Pitfall

- Drugs can have high intersubject variability. Drug safety and efficacy levels derive from studies of thousands of patients and will protect most but not all of them. Patients vary in their pharmacokinetics, pharmacodynamics, toxicity profiles, and genetic makeup. Further, each patient's diet, age, obesity level, disease states, genetic structures, exercise habits, use of other drugs and supplements, and health habits, such as smoking, may all affect how a drug works in his or her particular body.

Pharmacokinetics

Every audiologist should have a basic understanding of the principles of pharmacokinetics to understand why different drugs act differently from each other or why the same drug may act differently in different patients. Drugs may differ in their distribution throughout the body, the time course of that distribution, rate of absorption, manner of metabolism, how quickly and effectively they are excreted or eliminated from the body, how they interact with other substances in the body such as food or other drugs, and how they are affected by the method and timing of administration.

One of the major ways drugs may vary in their distribution throughout the body is whether or not they cross the blood–brain barrier. The blood–brain barrier comprises a series of tight endothelial cell junctions, which prevent many drugs, particularly large-molecule drugs, from reaching the brain. Sometimes that is a desirable result, for example, in avoiding the sedating effects of antihistamines.

Older antihistamines, as well as many of those sold over the counter, do have a sedating effect because they cross the blood–brain barrier. Some of the newer antihistamines avoid the side effect of sedation by not crossing that barrier. However, sometimes the inability of certain drugs to cross the blood–brain barrier can inhibit the intended therapeutic effect. For example, carboplatin, a chemotherapeutic agent, generally cannot cross the blood–brain barrier, which is desirable when the cancer is located outside the brain but is problematic for brain cancers. For this reason, in some current clinical studies, researchers first disrupt the blood–brain barrier with a drug called mannitol, which opens the tight endothelial cell junctions for a period of time so that the carboplatin can be delivered. As the mannitol wears off, the blood–brain barrier once again becomes intact.

Similarly, there is a cochlea–blood barrier that affects the distribution of systemic drugs to the cochlea. For example, when the blood–brain barrier and presumably the blood–Cochlea barrier are disrupted, carboplatin, which usually has a relatively low incidence of ototoxicity, has a very high incidence of ototoxicity. Consequently, researchers are attempting to use otoprotective agents to offset the ototoxicity.

The cochlear–blood barrier also can affect the distribution of otoprotective agents. For example, some agents that may protect the kidneys and peripheral neural system from the effects of cisplatin chemotherapy may not protect hearing, possibly because the molecule does not effectively cross the blood–cochlea barrier. Other otoprotective agents comprising smaller molecules may more readily cross the blood–cochlea barrier and thus be able to protect hearing.

The route of administration is also an important aspect of pharmacokinetics. Routes of administration include inhalation through the lungs, nasal sprays, oral administration, administration to other mucous membranes, as in the use of suppositories or injections into the vein (intravenous), the artery (intra-arterial), the muscle (intramuscular), and the sheath of membranes surrounding the spinal cord (intrathecal), or under the skin (subcutaneous), under the tongue (sublingual), or on the skin (topical). Sometimes drugs are delivered to the cochlea by direct administration to the round window membrane, either in basic science studies or for therapeutic intervention. For example, in Meniere's disease, gentamicin, a known ototoxin, is sometimes delivered to the round window of patients with intractable vertigo in the hope that it will deactivate the vestibular system without causing hearing loss.

Not all drugs can be safely, quickly, and effectively administered through all routes. For example, most patients would prefer to take an oral medication as opposed to an injection. However, aminoglycoside antibiotics, such as gentamicin, amikacin, and tobramycin, cannot be effectively delivered through the oral route and thus must be delivered by injection, whereas other antibiotics can be effectively delivered as a pill or oral suspension. Other drugs, such as the aminoglycoside neomycin, can be administered topically for skin infections, but it can cause severe hearing loss if given systemically. However, if the skin is seriously compromised, as in some burn patients, the transmission of neomycin through the skin can increase, resulting in ototoxic hearing loss. That increased transmission of the drug is only one example of how absorption may affect drug dose.

Absorption must be considered for each drug and for each route of delivery. Many characteristics of the drug itself may affect its absorption into the system. For example, a drug may be hydrophilic or lipophilic. Hydrophilic drugs dissolve preferentially in water, and lipophilic drugs dissolve preferentially in fats or oils. Drugs may vary by ionization state or molecular weight. As previously mentioned, drugs with a high molecular weight are less likely to cross the blood–brain and cochlea–brain barriers. In some cases, a delayed- or slow-release formula is used to slow absorption. Bioavailability is primarily an issue for oral medications, as nearly all of an injected drug enters the bloodstream. It is usually described as the fraction of the dose administered that actually reaches the bloodstream. Therefore, if the oral version of a drug has 50% bioavailability, the drug's oral dose may have to be doubled relative to the injected dose to have the same serum level and equal efficacy.

Different drugs may also be metabolized differently. The body has many natural defense mechanisms to detoxify and eliminate foreign substances or sometimes even high levels of natural substances. Most drug metabolism occurs in the liver. The most common forms of metabolism are (1) reactions that modify the structure of the drug itself, often by hepatic (i.e., liver) enzymes, and (2) reactions that conjugate the drug to other molecules that render it more water soluble so it can be excreted via the kidneys. Sometimes drugs are designed to avoid this problem. For example, if we really want to administer drug Y, but the liver changes the structure of the drug or binds it to other molecules for elimination, it may be more effective to administer a drug X that the liver converts to drug Y in its attempt to detoxify drug X.

Many patients, particularly the elderly, are on multiple medications. Additionally, many people take herbal or nutritional supplements. Drug-to-drug interactions, including interactions with herbal and nutritional supplements, may occur, and the most common site for those interactions is at the liver. One drug may affect how another drug is converted or its rate of excretion. Thus, it is easy to see why patients with impaired liver or kidney function are at higher risk of drug toxicities, such as ototoxicity. Unfortunately, drug interactions—or precisely how or to what degree liver or kidney dysfunction will affect a given drug in the body—is not always predictable.

Pitfall

- Patients with kidney or liver problems may not process drugs normally. They may not be able to take some medications at all and are frequently at higher risk for side effects and toxicities from the drugs they take. For most ototoxic drugs, the risk of ototoxicity is higher in patients with liver or kidney problems.

The status of the liver and kidney is always important to consider when developing drug therapies. Oral administration means not only that a given drug could potentially be digested or poorly absorbed but also that it must go through the liver as the first-pass effect and survive that process to be effective. Parenteral administration, meaning that the drug is delivered in one of the routes not involving the gut, avoids the first-pass effect. Because the liver is the body's major detoxification system, if the liver is not functioning properly, drug selection and dosage may need to be adjusted accordingly.

One important measure of drug pharmacokinetics is the serum half-life of the drug. The half-life is how long it takes the drug to drop to half of its original level. Generally, it is desirable to maintain a steady-state serum level of the drug rather than having marked swings in the peak and trough serum levels. Sometimes maintaining a relatively constant serum level requires a steady infusion of the drug or multiple administrations. Other drugs that are more slowly metabolized or cleared (longer half-life) may be administered less frequently. As previously mentioned, sometimes a drug's serum half-life is deliberately slowed with a time release formula or altered by liver or kidney dysfunction (see **Fig. 9–1**).

Drug clearance is also an important issue that may vary by both drug and patient. Clearance is a particular issue for people on long-term drug administration, not only to avoid markedly fluctuating peak and trough levels of the drug but also to ensure that the drug does not build up as it can in patients with poor renal clearance (i.e., kidney failure) or poor hepatic function. For example, the risk of ototoxicity is generally greatly increased if cisplatin or aminoglycosides are given to patients with poor kidney function, which is more frequent in the elderly. However, because these drugs may be considered part of life-saving measures, the treatment options available to the physician and patient are often limited. Thus, the audiologist needs to be particularly assiduous in monitoring the hearing of these patients and helping them if ototoxicity develops.

It is not always desirable to maintain a constant serum level. Certain drugs, such as cisplatin, are usually administered every 3 to 4 weeks. Aminoglycoside antibiotics have been reported to have less nephrotoxicity and equal antimicrobial efficacy if they are administered once a day rather than at more frequent intervals. Sometimes it is desirable to have a "washout" period, that is, a period after drug administration when the drug can no longer be detected in the system, before another dose of that drug or a different drug is administered to the patient.

Pharmacodynamics

Pharmacodynamics is the study of how drugs act on the body, particularly at their intended sites of action. Although the intended clinical action is always beneficial, the drug may produce adverse reactions, either side effects or toxicities, at the target site or other sites in the body. Frequently, but not always, drugs act on receptors within the surface of the cell's membrane and attach to them. Conceptually, the attachment can be thought of as a key fitting into a lock, but the "fit" may not just be mechanical. The fit may also be bioelectric or chemical. Furthermore, the attachment does not necessarily trigger the desired result directly but may trigger a series of reactions to obtain the desired (or undesired) effect. Sometimes a drug will help another drug to attach to a receptor; such a drug is called an agonist. Conversely, a drug may inhibit another drug from attaching; such a drug is called an antagonist. Therefore, the response of a drug is frequently deliberately or inadvertently modified by administering agonists or antagonists in conjunction with that particular drug. Sometimes agonists or antagonists are administered to alter the response of a chemical the body produces naturally, such as a neurotransmitter or histamine.

In some cases, a drug is designed to alter enzymes. For example, ibuprofen is considered an analgesic (i.e., painkiller), but it works by inhibiting enzymes that are needed to produce inflammatory prostaglandins, caused by muscular injury or cramping. By reducing the inflammation, which can both signal and promote pain, pain is reduced, but that is not the initial or direct action of the drug.

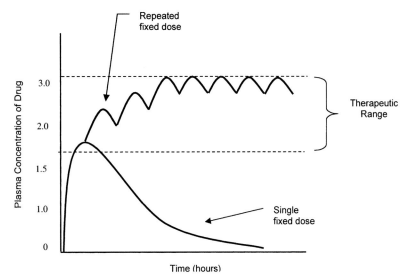

Figure 9–1 Graph of plasma concentration over time for a hypothetical drug showing the difference between repeated periodic dosing and single dosing. The drug's therapeutic range is also indicated. (From Schwade, N. D. (2000). Pharmacology in audiology practice. In R. Roeser, M. Valente, & H. Hosford-Dunn (Eds.), Audiology: Diagnosis (pp. 139–152). New York: Thieme Medical Publishers, with permission.)

> **Pitfall**
>
> • Nutritional and herbal supplements are not regulated by the FDA. However, they may interact with other drugs and have side effects and toxicities, particularly at high doses. Furthermore, the contents of the packages for herbal and nutritional supplements are not regulated; therefore, the package may or may not contain the substance and concentration indicated on the labeling.

Keep in mind that the primary purpose of the FDA approval process is to ensure that a drug is safe and effective. Many drugs, such as aspirin, have been used for decades, but we are still discovering more about their mechanisms of action and possible new applications for their use. Sometimes, even after a drug is on the market for a while, new side effects or toxicities are discovered that may not be evident until the drug is in long-term use or used in specific populations that are particularly and unexpectedly vulnerable. In the initial approval process, studies are designed to determine not only if the drug is safe and effective but also the lowest dose that is safe and effective as well as the lowest dose that causes toxicity. These levels are reflected in the therapeutic index of the drug.

The therapeutic index, also called the therapeutic range or therapeutic window, describes a particular drug's desirable dosing range. For example, for drug X, an over-the-counter analgesic, the minimum effective dose is 10 mg per kilogram (mg/kg) every 4 hours. Therefore, a 220 pound (100 kg) man should take 1000 mg every 4 hours. For convenience, the drug may be made available in tablets containing 500 mg, so adults may be advised to take two tablets every 4 hours. However, some adults may be only 45 kg, and others may be 200 kg. Thus, if all adults take two tablets every 4 hours, the actual mg/kg dose varies depending on the patients' weights. It may be preferable from a dosing standpoint to have each person compute the dose relative to his or her individual weight, but most patients won't do this accurately. Furthermore, the absorption of the drug may vary by when and what the patient just ate. The drug may also interact with other drugs or supplements the patient is taking. For example, some fiber supplements limit or slow a drug's absorption or bioavailability. There also may be a lot of intersubject variability in how various patients metabolize a given drug. Even a patient's body composition (fat vs muscle) can affect the way a given drug acts in his or her system. A safe and effective dose for one patient may be toxic or ineffective for another. Patients may also assume that "more is better" for a drug and deliberately exceed the recommended dose, although for most drugs the efficacy does not continue to increase above a certain level. Therefore, the drug must be safe and effective over as wide a dosing range as possible to account for all these common variables.

Consequently, it is desirable for each drug, particularly an over-the-counter drug, to have as wide a therapeutic index, or dosing range between the lowest effective level and the toxicity level, as possible. If the therapeutic window is narrow, the risks of both lack of efficacy and toxicity increase. Drugs with a narrow therapeutic index are frequently restricted to prescription-only availability, and others may not be approved at all, particularly if other drugs with a wide therapeutic index can treat the same disorder. However, it cannot be assumed that over-the-counter drugs are safe at any dose. For example, aspirin can cause gastrointestinal bleeding, tinnitus, and hearing loss at high and chronic dosages. Even the upper limit of the therapeutic index may not be safe for all patients, as up to 5 to 10% of all patients may still experience a toxic effect at that level.

> **Pearl**
>
> • The therapeutic index, range, and window of a drug all refer to the drug dosing levels from the lowest effective dosing level to the toxicity, not side effect, level. Even if the upper level of that range is not exceeded, 5 to 10% of patients may experience toxicity. Therefore, dosing is generally kept well below that level.

The therapeutic index is usually derived from several measures, including dose–response curves. Dose–response curves are generated by administering the study drug at dosing levels ranging from low to high levels, then measuring the desired biological effect. Any toxicities and side effects noted during generation of the dose–response curves are generally noted but are not the focus of these studies. Separate studies are usually performed to determine toxicities and the upper limit of the therapeutic index.

In the dose–response curves in **Fig. 9–2,** the dosing levels of three different drugs—A, B, and C—are on the abscissa (horizontal axis), and the biological effect of each drug at each dosing level is on the ordinate (vertical axis).

As seen in **Fig. 9–2,** it takes less of drug A than drug B to obtain a 50% biological effect. A drug's potency indicates the dosage that produces a 50% level of the desired biological effect. Thus, drug A is more potent than drug B. However, drug A and drug B have equal efficacy because they are equally effective in producing the desired biological effect. Efficacy is measured at 100% or maximal biological response level. It just takes more of drug B to produce that effect. Potency is not usually the critical issue unless there are problems either reducing the level of drug A to a suitable dose (i.e., for infants) in a reasonable volume or delivering adequate volumes of drug B to obtain the required effect. For example, if one needs to give only half a drop of an oral formulation of drug A to an infant, and he tends to spit it out, it may be difficult to measure dosing accurately, particularly in the home environment. Conversely, if a patient had to take 10 large pills per dose of drug B every 4 hours, patient compliance would probably decrease. Also, if drug A and drug B have the same cost per gram, than drug A may be cheaper to administer than drug B. Aside from these practical issues, however, efficacy, and not potency, of a

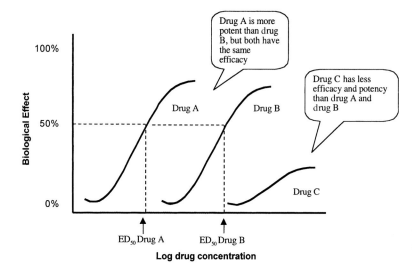

Figure 9–2 Dose–response curves showing the dosing levels of three different drugs, A, B, and C, on the abscissa (horizontal axis) and the biological effect of each drug at each dosing level on the ordinate (vertical axis). (From Schwade, N. D. (2000). Pharmacology in audiology practice. In R. Roeser, M. Valente, & H. Hosford-Dunn (Eds.), Audiology: Diagnosis (pp. 139–152). New York: Thieme Medical Publishers, with permission.)

given drug is generally the critical issue. Note that no level of drug C provides the biological effect of either drug A or drug B. Thus, drug C is neither potent nor effective.

Also note that all three drugs reach asymptotic levels, meaning that above a certain dosing level, increased dosing does not increase the biological effect, although the increased dosing may still greatly enhance side effects or toxicities.

Pharmacogenetics and Pharmacogenomics

Pharmacogenetics, which analyzes the body's genetic response to a drug, and pharmacogenomics, which is using each patient's genetic information to individualize drug therapies, will play increasingly larger roles in health care over the next decades.

For example, for many patients, low-dose or short-term aminoglycosides carry a relatively low risk of hearing loss, but in patients with the A1555G mitochondrial genetic mutation, a single dose of aminoglycosides can result in deafness. Although this genetic predisposition was initially discovered in Asian populations, this mutation has also subsequently been found in individuals in Spain, Italy, Germany, the United States, and New Zealand. The mechanisms of how this mutation renders individuals susceptible not only to aminoglycoside-induced hearing loss but also to hearing loss even in the absence of aminoglycosides are being carefully investigated. Thus, the A1555G mutation is an example of pharmacogenetics in audiologic practice.

The discovery of the A1555G mutation in pharmacogenetics has resulted in some major medical centers now recommending screening for the A1555G mutation before administering aminoglycoside antibiotics. Thus, pharmacogenetics has led to pharmacogenomics in the A1555G mutation, individualizing patient care based on each patient's genetic profile. Currently, there may not always be sufficient time for genetic testing to be completed before aminoglycosides are administered to treat a life-threatening infection. However, as genetic tools improve and

become faster, and as new alternative drug therapies become available, pharmacogenomics will undoubtedly play a larger role in patient care in optimizing the choice of drug therapies.

For further information on pharmacology, the FDA process, and nutraceuticals, the reader is referred to Meldrum (2007), Rey (2007), Bhattaram et al (2007), and Seidman and Moneysmith (2007).

◆ Ototoxicity

General Considerations

Audiologists need to be aware of ototoxic agents for several reasons. Some drugs, such as cisplatin and long-term aminoglycoside antibiotics, have a fairly high incidence of ototoxicity. Therefore, careful audiologic monitoring should be routinely scheduled for these patients. Other drugs, for example, loop diuretics in adults, difluoromethylornithine (DFMO), vincristine, vinblastine, low-dose quinine, high-dose aspirin, and erythromycin, can cause hearing loss and tinnitus that is reversible, usually returning to normal, if the drug is discontinued. In those cases, the audiologist may be the first to recognize the possible connection between the drug and the hearing loss. The alert audiologist should then contact the patient's treating physician so that the physician can consider changing the patient's medication to see if hearing returns. In the case of aspirin and some herbal medications, the patient may be self-medicating and not sharing that information with his or her physician, yet reveal it to their audiologist.

Audiologists should use the *PDR* with reservation when determining if a drug is ototoxic. Although the *PDR* lists drugs that are clearly ototoxic, others may be listed as having hearing loss, tinnitus, or dizziness as a possible side effect, although ototoxicity has not been clearly established.

For example, if drug X is in clinical trials, and a small percentage of patients experiences hearing loss, tinnitus, or dizziness while on drug X, the pharmaceutical company may simply decide to list ototoxicity as a possible side effect rather than spend the time and money to determine if it is actually ototoxic. In some cases, the hearing loss, tinnitus, or dizziness may have been secondary to factors other than the drug, as these disorders occur in the population at large irrespective of drug use. Consequently, the lists of drugs derived from the *PDR* indicating ototoxicity as a possible side effect should be interpreted accordingly. It is always advisable to consult the patient's treating physician if there is a concern about the auditory or vestibular effects of any medication the patient is taking. Contacting the patient's physician whenever there is a concern also improves patient care by encouraging interdisciplinary communication and management.

Pitfall

- Do not assume that every side effect listed for a drug in the *PDR* has been necessarily proven or occurs in a significant number of patients at therapeutic doses. If hearing loss, tinnitus, or dizziness is listed as a side effect, do not assume that the drug is necessarily ototoxic. It may be that symptoms occurred in a few patients in the clinical trials, but these symptoms may or may not have been drug related.

Even for drugs that are clearly ototoxic, the intersubject variability among patients can be high. For the exact same drug and dosing protocol, some patients may have marked bilateral hearing loss, whereas others experience no hearing changes even with continued administration. The factors underlying the high intersubject variability are largely unknown. Knowing that many otoprotective agents, which are often antioxidants, are also micronutrients found in common foods leads us to suspect that a person's diet and other health habits may influence their susceptibility to drug- and noise-induced hearing loss. The patient's endogenous oxidative state, which can be adversely affected by smoking, poor diet, and lack of exercise, may play a role in his or her vulnerability to these cochlear insults.

Other factors can exacerbate a patient's risk of ototoxicity. For many ototoxins, noise exposure can increase the risk of ototoxicity during, and often for several months after, ototoxic drug exposure. Therefore, the audiologist should question patients on each visit about noise exposure and counsel them accordingly. Other factors, such as liver and kidney dysfunction, may change the pharmacokinetics and pharmacodynamics of a drug and thus may increase its ototoxic risk. In those cases, the audiologist may choose to increase the frequency of the monitoring schedule.

Chemotherapeutic Agents

Some, but not all, chemotherapeutic agents carry a risk of ototoxicity. Although the ototoxic risk of some of these agents is well known, and the incidence of ototoxicity is high, often physicians have no other effective treatment option for these patients. In some cases, if the audiologist notes an ototoxic change in hearing, the patient may be switched to a less ototoxic drug. However, in some cases, the treatment for a life-threatening illness cannot be changed without compromising the potential for survival. In those cases, the audiologist's role is to assist the patient and family in maintaining communication if hearing loss develops.

Cisplatin is the most ototoxic agent in common clinical use. It also is effective in treating a variety of cancers, including testicular, ovarian, head and neck, bladder, lung, and cervical tumors. Therefore, cisplatin will continue to be used because of its excellent tumor kill for these types of cancers. Ototoxicity is not the only side effect of cisplatin. Other side effects include nephrotoxicity, peripheral sensory and autonomic neuropathy, and severe nausea and vomiting. The degree and incidence of these side effects, including ototoxicity, vary according to the cumulative dose of cisplatin, but the relationship is not perfect. As previously mentioned, intersubject variability of side effects is high. However, for cancers that require a high dose of cisplatin, such as ovarian cancer, which is generally discovered in a late stage after the cancer has spread, the incidence of ototoxic hearing loss can exceed 50% (Blakley and Myers, 1993).

Carboplatin is another platinum-based chemotherapeutic drug. The incidence of carboplatin-induced hearing loss is less than cisplatin, but carboplatin can cause ototoxic hearing loss and can exacerbate the risk of cisplatin-induced hearing loss for those patients receiving both drugs. However, there is high intersubject variability in the incidence of hearing loss for most ototoxic drugs, including both cisplatin and carboplatin. Consequently, the degree of ototoxicity cannot be predicted for an individual patient simply on the basis of the drug and dose. Audiologic monitoring for these patients is required.

Most ototoxic hearing loss, including cisplatin- and carboplatin-induced hearing loss, is bilateral, sensorineural, and starts at the high frequencies. With continued treatment, and sometimes even if the drug is discontinued, the hearing loss progresses into lower frequency regions, thus causing increasingly greater impact on communication. If testing is conducted above 8000 Hz (i.e., high-frequency audiometry), changes will first be observed in that frequency range (Fausti et al, 1984a,b; Jacobson et al, 1969; see also reviews by Campbell, 2004; Fausti et al, 2007).

Clinically, the patient may first notice only some difficulty communicating in groups or background noise. Mild tinnitus may develop. Without systematic audiologic monitoring, the patient's early symptoms of ototoxicity may be attributed to malaise or the distress of dealing with a life-threatening illness. By the time ototoxicity symptoms have clearly developed, the hearing loss has almost invariably progressed into the communication frequency range. Unfortunately, platinum-induced hearing loss is almost always irreversible. Thus, prospective audiologic monitoring is always advisable for these patients. Hearing loss may develop at any point during the course of platinum-based chemotherapy and may be particularly pronounced in pediatric patients (Helson et al, 1978, Li et al, 2004).

As is consistent with hearing loss, cisplatin-induced cochlear damage first affects the outer hair cells in the basal turn, then progresses into the middle and apical turns with further drug administration (Schweitzer et al, 1984, Van Ruijven et al, 2004). Damage to the stria vascularis can also be extensive (Campbell et al, 1999; Meech et al, 1998). For most species, carboplatin follows the same pattern of outer hair cell loss. Selective inner hair cell loss, secondary to carboplatin, has been reported only in the chinchilla (Wake et al, 1993) and not in other species (Saito et al, 1989).

Although other platinum-based chemotherapeutics are in use in the United States, only cisplatin and carboplatin have been reported to be ototoxic. For cisplatin, several other factors can increase the risk of ototoxicity, including noise exposure, concomitant aminoglycoside antibiotics, prior irradiation, and possibly loop diuretics. The audiologist should counsel patients to avoid noise exposure during and for several months after cisplatin treatment. If the audiologist notes that a patient is receiving concomitant drugs that could exacerbate the risk of ototoxicity, this increased risk should be discussed with the patient's treating physician.

Other chemotherapeutic agents, including nitrogen mustard, the vinca alkaloids (vincristine and vinblastine sulfate), and DFMO, can be ototoxic. However, the incidence of ototoxic hearing loss with those drugs is less than with cisplatin. Audiologists may not routinely see patients on these medications for ototoxicity monitoring. If a patient is referred for hearing loss and has been taking one of these drugs, the audiologist should be aware that these agents are potentially ototoxic and explore a possible relationship between the drug and the patient's hearing loss. Currently, nitrogen mustard is rarely used in the United States, but when it is, cochlear toxicity can result (Cummings, 1968). The audiologist may see patients being treated with DFMO, which is used in various antineoplastic (i.e., anticancer) and antiparasitic treatments. In cancer treatment, it is generally used for colon cancers and recurrent malignant melanomas, but it may also be used in metastatic liver disease and sometimes in brain cancer in combination with other drugs (Croghan et al, 1991; Levin et al, 2003). In parasitic illnesses, the audiologist is most likely to see it used with acquired immune deficiency syndrome (AIDS) patients being treated for *Pneumocystis carinii* pneumonia; it may also be used in the treatment of African trypanosomiasis, or sleeping sickness (Legros et al, 2002; Sahai and Berry, 1989; Sjoerdsma et al, 1984; see also the review by McCann and Pegg, 1992). Most patients receiving DFMO will not be referred for prospective audiologic monitoring, but the audiologist should recognize DFMO as an ototoxin if a patient presents with hearing loss and is taking that drug. If DFMO ototoxicity is recognized early and administration is discontinued, hearing may return in ~4 to 6 weeks (Croghan et al, 1988, 1991; Meyskens et al, 1986). DFMO ototoxicity is different from cisplatin-induced ototoxicity, as DFMO-induced hearing loss generally takes at least 4 weeks of treatment before

developing (Jansen et al, 1989; Lipton et al, 1989; Meyskens et al, 1994; Pasic et al, 1997). If a hearing loss secondary to DFMO does develop, it may progress from high to low frequencies in some but not all cases (Abeloff et al, 1986; Creaven et al, 1993; Lipton et al, 1989). Several audiometric configurations have been reported secondary to DFMO ototoxicity, including low-frequency (Croghan et al, 1991; Pasic et al, 1997) and flat (Meyskens et al, 1986) hearing losses.

Pearl

- Audiologists must consider the possibility of ototoxicity for a variety of audiometric configurations.

In most cases, the vinca alkaloids, including vincristine and vinblastine sulfate, will not cause hearing loss. Therefore, patients on these regimens will generally not be referred to the audiologist unless hearing loss develops. Because these drugs are used for a variety of cancers, generally as part of combination drug therapies, most patients will never be referred to the audiology clinic. However, if a patient develops a hearing loss and is taking one of these drugs, the possible link of the hearing loss to the vinca alkaloid should be considered. For vincristine, the incidence of ototoxicity is very low, but when it does occur, it can range from fairly flat, moderate bilateral sensorineural hearing loss to sudden, severe hearing loss. Hearing may or may not fully recover if the drug is identified as the cause and discontinued (see the review by Rybak et al, 2007). For vinblastine, only one case report is in the literature with an incident of mild, high-frequency hearing loss, but the patient had been reporting tinnitus after each cycle (Moss et al, 1999).

Aminoglycoside Antibiotics

Most antibiotics do not cause hearing loss. However, aminoglycoside antibiotics, which are used primarily to treat gram-negative bacterial infections, can cause hearing loss, particularly with high-dose or long-term treatment. Because the peak and trough levels of these drugs are now carefully monitored in patients in the United States, sometimes physicians assume that ototoxicity is no longer an issue. For those patients on aminoglycosides whose hearing is monitored, changes in hearing can be observed. In 1999, Fausti et al reported ototoxic hearing changes in about one third of Veterans Affairs patients. Incidence of aminoglycoside-induced hearing loss in developing countries has been reported to be substantially higher because the dosing and availability are less controlled.

Like cisplatin, aminoglycoside-induced ototoxicity almost invariably starts in the very high frequencies and then progresses into lower frequencies. Thus, high-frequency audiometry above 8 kHz can frequently detect aminoglycoside-induced ototoxicity before it progresses into the frequency range critical for understanding speech. Unlike cisplatin-induced hearing loss, aminoglycoside-induced hearing loss may reverse if the drug is discontinued but does not always do so. Like cisplatin-induced hearing loss, amino-glycoside-induced hearing loss may progress after the drug is discontinued and can be exacerbated by noise exposure. Generally, aminoglycoside-induced hearing loss, if permanent, is less severe than cisplatin-induced hearing loss. Simultaneous treatment with loop diuretics can markedly increase the risk of aminoglycoside-induced ototoxicity.

As is consistent with the high-frequency hearing loss, cochlear outer hair cell loss generally starts in the basal turn and progresses into the more apical regions, particularly if treatment is continued. Following the outer hair cell loss, inner hair cell loss and then spiral ganglion cell loss can occur. Aminoglycosides can also damage the stria vascularis.

Aminoglycoside antibiotics vary in their propensity for causing cochleotoxicity, vestibulotoxicity, or both. For example, gentamicin and streptomycin can cause hearing loss but are more likely to cause vestibular disturbance. Kanamycin, amikacin, and tobramycin are more likely to cause hearing loss than vestibular problems. Kanamycin is highly ototoxic and thus rarely used systemically except for very short periods of time. However, when kanamycin has been used at high doses for long periods of time, complete deafness has sometimes resulted. Neomycin is also highly ototoxic and so is not used systemically. Neomycin is used in some eardrops and in some topical antibiotics. Neomycin is generally only used in the presence of an intact tympanic membrane to avoid the possibility of its seeping through a perforated tympanic membrane, permeating the round window, and causing ototoxic hearing loss.

Vancomycin, another antibiotic, sounds like an aminoglycoside antibiotic, but it is actually a glycopeptide antibiotic and a different drug class. It is generally reserved for resistant strain infections that are severe and potentially life-threatening. Whether or not vancomycin is ototoxic is a subject of some debate. If it is ototoxic, the incidence appears to be less than 1%, although it is possible that it may exacerbate the ototoxicity of aminoglycosides (Campbell et al, 2003). Because vancomycin is often used after aminoglycoside therapy has failed to cure the infection and because aminoglycosides can cause delayed hearing loss, it is sometimes difficult to determine if a hearing loss is secondary to the vancomycin or to the previous aminoglycoside treatment in a given patient.

Another antibiotic that can cause hearing loss but is not an aminoglycoside is erythromycin. Erythromycin is a macrolide antibiotic that is widely used. The risk of ototoxicity with this drug is very low. However, hearing loss can be sudden and severe. If the drug is discontinued, the hearing loss may reverse. Thus, it is important for the audiologist to recognize this type of ototoxicity when it occurs.

Pearl

- As for most other ototoxins, the risk of aminoglycoside ototoxicity increases with increased length of treatment, cumulative dose, and daily dose. Patients with liver or kidney dysfunction are also at increased risk of ototoxicity.

Loop Diuretics

Loop diuretics are very potent and generally are used for cases of systemic fluid retention, such as congestive heart failure with pulmonary edema and other serious medical conditions. Most types of diuretics do not cause hearing loss, but loop diuretics can be ototoxic and can greatly exacerbate the ototoxicity of aminoglycoside antibiotics and possibly cisplatin.

The three most commonly used loop diuretics are furosemide, which is known by the trademark Lasix; bumetanide, which is known by the trademark Bumex; and the less commonly used ethacrynic acid. Furosemide is the most commonly used loop diuretic in children and neonates. Bumetanide is 40 to 60 times as potent as furosemide and thus generally used only in adults. In adults, loop diuretics occasionally exhibit reversible ototoxicity, unless they are used in combination with aminoglycoside antibiotics, which can result in permanent and sometimes severe hearing loss. Neonates may be at higher risk of permanent hearing loss from loop diuretics even in the absence of aminoglycosides. Further research is warranted to determine the risk to neonates. Fausti et al (1978) reported that low-dose bumetanide treatment did not alter even high-frequency hearing thresholds from 8000 to 20,000 Hz in adults.

Loop diuretics can affect both cochlear outer hair cells and the stria vascularis. The primary histologic change, noted in animal studies, appears to be extracellular edema in the stria vascularis, with consequent changes in the endocochlear potential (see the review by Rybak et al, 2007). These changes in the stria vascularis may underlie the variability in the audiometric configurations seen in patients experiencing loop diuretic–induced ototoxicity. Unlike the progressive high-frequency hearing losses associated with cisplatin- and aminoglycoside-induced hearing loss, loop diuretic ototoxicity may yield a variety of hearing loss patterns.

Other Ototoxic Drugs: Aspirin and Quinine

Aspirin, a salicylate, is perhaps the most commonly used ototoxic drug but is generally ototoxic only at high dosing levels. The high dosing levels may be seen when aspirin is used as an anti-inflammatory, but they usually occur as a result of a patient's self-medicating. Many times patients do not understand that even over-the-counter drugs can have side effects, particularly when they exceed the recommended daily dose.

When aspirin-induced ototoxicity occurs, it generally causes a flat sensorineural hearing loss of a mild or moderate degree. The hearing loss usually reverses over time after the aspirin is discontinued. Tinnitus commonly occurs and may precede the hearing loss. Tinnitus usually, but not always, disappears after the aspirin is discontinued. Therefore, patients should always be queried about their aspirin use as well as their use of prescription drugs (see the review by Lonsbury et al, 2007).

Quinine is rarely used in the United States at high dosages. Historically, it was used at high dosages as an antimalarial drug in many countries. In some developing countries, it may still be used for that purpose. Hearing loss and tinnitus often resulted. It is still used to control leg cramps at low dosages. However, anecdotal reports of reversible hearing loss secondary to low-dose quinine treatment for leg cramps is reducing the frequency of its use for that application (see the review by Lonsbury et al, 2007).

Environmental Ototoxins

A full discussion of environmental ototoxins is outside the scope of this chapter. However, audiologists should be aware that several chemicals, other than drugs, can either cause hearing loss or exacerbate noise-induced hearing loss (see the review by Pouyatos and Fechter, 2007). The exposure may occur secondary to organic solvents, asphyxiants and gases, or heavy metals in the work or even home environment. Usually the exposure is by inhalation, but some toxins, such as toluene in paint thinners, can be absorbed directly through the skin. Other exposures include deliberate recreational use, as in glue sniffing. The different chemicals have various effects on the peripheral, central auditory, and vestibular systems (Morioka et al, 1999; Pouyatos and Fechter, 2007; Rybak, 1992; Sulkowski et al, 2002). Therefore, the audiologist may also wish to include questions about these types of exposures when obtaining a case history.

◆ Audiologic Monitoring for Ototoxicity

Audiologic monitoring for ototoxicity is generally performed for patients receiving long-term and/or high-dose cisplatin and/or carboplatin chemotherapy treatment and for patients receiving aminoglycoside antibiotics. Prospective audiologic monitoring is also conducted as a part of clinical trials in which the study drug may be either ototoxic or otoprotective.

A baseline hearing assessment is always essential. Without a baseline evaluation, it will be difficult if not impossible to determine to what extent the patient's hearing changed during drug treatment, because any possible preexistent hearing loss cannot be parceled out. Similarly, at baseline, the patient should be questioned about any balance or vestibular problems and any tinnitus. If these symptoms change in the future, they can then be differentiated from preexistent problems. There are currently no nationally accepted standard procedures or formal guidelines for monitoring vestibulotoxicity or ototoxin-induced tinnitus. However, recommendations for vestibular testing can be found in Black and Pesznecker (2007) and Handelsman (2007).

Clinically, the audiologic monitoring schedule will vary by ototoxic agent. For cisplatin, the tests are generally scheduled just before each round of chemotherapy, usually every 3 to 4 weeks, when the patient is feeling well enough to cooperate and before he or she is connected to intravenous or other equipment. Any threshold shifts noted just prior to the next round of chemotherapy will probably reflect permanent rather than transient changes. For aminoglycosides, monitoring is generally scheduled once or twice per week, depending on the degree of risk from that particular agent and the dosing protocol. For both agents, follow-up testing at least once or twice in the 6 months after drug discontinuation is recommended to check for any possible progression of hearing loss.

A variety of audiologic tests may be part of the test battery, depending on the purpose of the testing. For adults and older children, pure-tone air conduction thresholds from 250 to 8000 Hz will generally be standard procedure. High-frequency audiometry above 8000 Hz will also be a standard procedure for most ototoxicity monitoring. However, if the drug treatment protocol cannot be changed, even if ototoxic hearing loss develops, such as in the treatment of some life-threatening cancers, high-frequency audiometry may not be needed. Instead, the focus of testing may be on assisting the patient with amplification or communication strategies if and when ototoxic hearing loss develops. Some investigators are determining if only monitoring the upper frequency range of the patient's hearing is adequate for ototoxicity monitoring (Dreschler et al, 1989, Fausti et al, 1992, 2007), but most centers now test in both the conventional and high-frequency ranges.

At baseline and if a significant change in hearing occurs, word recognition, bone conduction thresholds, and tympanometry should also be included. Both chemotherapy patients and patients on aminoglycosides may be particularly vulnerable to otitis media—chemotherapy patients because of the immunosuppression caused by the chemotherapy, and aminoglycoside patients because of the infectious disease for which they are being treated. Therefore, if a change in hearing occurs, the audiologist must determine if the change is secondary to conductive hearing loss or ototoxic sensorineural hearing loss. Word recognition, using 50-word lists and significant change criteria, as given in Thornton and Raffin (1978), should also be tested when a significant change in hearing thresholds occurs to help determine the impact on the patient's communication abilities.

Controversial Point

- Currently, no national guidelines exist for monitoring environmental toxins that may cause hearing loss, increase the risk of noise-induced hearing loss, or cause vestibular disturbance, including in work environments that routinely involve exposure to these chemicals. Ongoing discussion exists regarding how to monitor and regulate these substances and their potential effects on hearing.

Special Consideration

- Because patients on ototoxic medications are frequently quite ill, they may have difficulty tolerating extended testing. They also may have difficulty concentrating because of their illness or related stress. Audiologic tests, therefore, must be carefully selected and prioritized to obtain the most information in the shortest period of time.

Several criteria have been suggested for determining significant ototoxic threshold shifts. In the United States, the most widely used criteria are (1) a threshold shift of 20 dB or greater at any one test frequency, (2) threshold shifts of 10 dB or greater at any two adjacent frequencies, and (3) loss of response at any three consecutive frequencies where thresholds were previously obtained (American Speech-Language-Hearing Association, 1994). It is also critical that the noted changes be replicated within 24 hours (frequently, the replication occurs on the same test appointment). Patients on ototoxic medications can be quite ill or preoccupied, and the audiologist must ensure that the change is a true change in threshold and not just variability in the patient's responses before notifying the patient and his or her physician of a significant change in hearing. These criteria have excellent sensitivity and specificity (Campbell et al, 2003; Fausti et al, 1999; Frank, 2001) and may be used for either the conventional or high-frequency threshold ranges (Campbell et al, 2003).

For research applications and for pediatric testing, several other measures may be used for monitoring, including otoacoustic emissions and electrophysiologic measures. A full discussion of all monitoring techniques is outside the scope of this chapter, but fuller reviews are available (Campbell, 2004; Fausti et al, 2007).

Patients on ototoxic medications sometimes need special considerations. Frequently, they are ill and may have difficulty concentrating on the testing. Their scheduling may be complex because of the multiple services they need. If the medication cannot be changed, they and their families may need particular assistance in communication strategies and sometimes amplification that does not exacerbate the ototoxic hearing loss with noise exposure. Helping the patient in maintaining communication with his or her friends and family during a sometimes life-threatening illness is one of the most important roles audiologists can play. Patients frequently endure the misery of chemotherapy not just to prolong their life but to put their affairs in order and to communicate with loved ones, who may only be available by telephone. Hearing is a major factor in their quality of life.

♦ Future Directions

In the future, it is hoped that more non-ototoxic drugs will be developed that can replace some of the ototoxic drugs in clinical use. Several researchers are currently developing otoprotective agents to reduce the ototoxicity and other side effects of cisplatin, carboplatin, and aminoglycosides. Agents are also being developed to protect against noise-induced hearing loss. Several drugs are already in clinical trials. Within the next decade, several FDA-approved drugs should be available to prevent permanent hearing loss from ototoxic drugs or noise exposure. For example, one of the drugs that I have been developing in my laboratory, D-methionine, protects against cisplatin-, carboplatin-, aminoglycoside-, and noise-induced hearing loss in animal studies (Campbell et al, 1996, 1999; Campbell and Rybak, 2007; Kopke et al, 2002; Sha and Schacht, 2000). We are in clinical trials for some of these applications and approaching clinical trials for the others. However, it is only through the clinical trials process that we will know the safety and efficacy of this and other promising agents. Otoprotective agents will eventually reduce the incidence of ototoxicity. However, the audiologist will play a continuing role in monitoring for ototoxic hearing loss, recognizing ototoxic hearing loss when it occurs, counseling patients, and, perhaps in the future, working with physicians to determine when an otoprotective agent is appropriate for a given patient.

References

Abeloff, M. D., Rosen, S. T., Luk, G. D., Baylin, S. B., Zeltzman, M., & Sjoerdsma, A. (1986). Phase II trials of alpha-difluoromethylornithine, an inhibitor of polyamine synthesis in advanced small cell lung cancer. Cancer Treatment Reports, 70, 843–845.

American Speech-Language-Hearing Association (1994). Guidelines for the audiologic management of individuals receiving cochleotoxic drug therapy. ASHA, 36(Suppl. 12), 11–19.

Bhattaram, V. A., Madabushi, R., & Derendorf, H. (2007). Role of Food and Drug Administration in drug development. In K. C. Campbell (Ed.), Pharmacology and ototoxicity for audiologists (pp. 33–43). Clifton Park, NY: Thomson Delmar Learning.

Black, O., & Pesznecker, S. (2007). Vestibular toxicity. In K. C. Campbell (Ed.), Pharmacology and ototoxicity for audiologists (pp. 252–267). Clifton Park, NY: Thomson Delmar Learning.

Blakley, B. W., & Myers, S. F. (1993). Pattern of hearing loss resulting from cisplatinum therapy. Otolaryngology—Head and Neck Surgery, 109, 385–391.

Campbell, K. C. M. (2004). Audiologic monitoring for ototoxicity. In P. Roland & J. Rutka (Eds.), Ototoxicity (pp. 153–160). Hamilton, Ontario, Canada: B. C. Decker.

Campbell, K. C. M., Kelly, E., Targovnik, N., et al. (2003). Audiologic monitoring for potential ototoxicity in a phase I clinical trial of a new glycopeptide antibiotic. Journal of the American Academy of Audiology, 14(3), 157–169.

Campbell, K. C. M., Meech, R. P., Rybak, L. P., & Hughes, L. P. (1999). D-methionine protects against cisplatin damage to the stria vascularis. Hearing Research, 138, 13–28.

Campbell, K. C., & Rybak, L. P. (2007). Otoprotective agents. In K. C. Campbell (Ed.), Pharmacology and ototoxicity for audiologists (pp. 287–296). Clifton Park, NY: Thomson Delmar Learning.

Campbell, K. C. M., Rybak, L. P., Meech, R. P., & Hughes, L. (1996). D-methionine provides excellent protection from cisplatin ototoxicity in the rat. Hearing Research, 102, 90–98.

Creaven, P. J., Pendyala, L., & Petrelli, N. (1993). Evaluation of alpha-difluoromethylornithine as a potential chemopreventive agent: Tolerance to daily oral administration in humans. Cancer Epidemiology, Biomarkers and Prevention, 2, 243–247.

Croghan, M. K., Aickin, M. G., & Meyskens, F. L. (1991). Dose-related alpha-difluoromethylornithine ototoxicity. American Journal of Clinical Oncology, 14, 331–335.

Croghan, M. K., Booth, A., & Meyskens, F. L., Jr. (1988). A phase I trial recombinant interferon-alpha and alpha-difluoromethylornithine in metastatic melanoma. Journal of Biological Response Modifiers, 7(4), 409–415.

Cummings, C. W. (1968). Experimental observations on the ototoxicity of nitrogen mustard. Laryngoscope, 78(4), 530–538.

Dreschler, W. A., van der Hulst, R. J., Tange, R. A., & Urbanus, N. A. (1989). Role of high frequency audiometry in the early detection of ototoxicity: 2. Clinical aspects. Audiology, 28(4), 211–220.

Fausti, S. A., Frey, R. H., Henry, J. A., Olson, D. J., & Schaffer, H. I. (1992). Early detection of ototoxicity using high frequency, tone-burst evoked auditory brainstem responses. Journal of the American Academy of Audiology, 3, 397–404.

Fausti, S. A., Frey, R. H., Rappaport, B. Z., & Erickson, D. A. (1978). An investigation of the effect of bumetanide on high frequency (8–20 kHz) hearing in humans. Journal of Audiology Research, 18(4), 243–250.

Fausti, S. A., Helt, W. J., Gordon, J. S., Reavis, K. M., Phillips, D. S., & Konrad-Martin, D. L. (2007). Audiologic monitoring for ototoxicity and patient management. In K. C. Campbell (Ed.), Pharmacology and ototoxicity for audiologists (pp. 230–248). Clifton Park, NY: Thomson Delmar Learning.

Fausti, S. A., Henry, J. A., Helt, W. J., et al. (1999). An individualized, sensitive frequency range for early detection of ototoxicity. Ear and Hearing, 20(6), 497–505.

Fausti, S. A., Rappaport, B. Z., Schechter, M. A., Frey, R. H., Ward, T. T., & Brummettt, R. E. (1984a). Detection of aminoglycoside ototoxicity by high frequency auditory evaluation: Selected case studies. American Journal of Otolaryngology, 5, 177–182.

Fausti, S. A., Schechter, M. A., Rappaport, B. Z., Frey, R. H., & Mass, R. E. (1984b). Early detection cisplatin ototoxicity: Selected case reports. Cancer, 53, 224–231.

Frank, T. (2001). High frequency (8 to 16 kHz) reference thresholds and intrasubject threshold variability relative to ototoxicity criteria using a Sennheiser HAD 200 earphone. Ear and Hearing, 22(2), 161–168.

Handelsman, J. (2007). Audiologic findings in vestibular toxicity. In K. C. Campbell (Ed.), Pharmacology and ototoxicity for audiologists (pp. 272–286). Clifton Park, NY: Thomson Delmar Learning.

Helson, L., Okonkwo, E., Anton, L., & Cvitkovic, E. (1978). Cis-platinum ototoxicity. Clinical Toxicology, 13(4), 469–478.

Jacobson, E. J., Downs, M. P., & Fletcher, J. L. (1969). Clinical findings in high frequency thresholds during known ototoxic drug usage. Journal of Audiology Research, 9, 379–385.

Jansen, C., Mattox, D. E., Miller, K. D., & Brownell, W. E. (1989). An animal model of hearing loss from alpha-difluoromethylornithine. Archives of Otolaryngology—Head and Neck Surgery, 115, 1234–1237.

Kopke, R. D., Coleman, J. K. M., Liu, J., Campbell, K. C. M., & Riffenburgh, R. H. (2002). Enhancing intrinsic cochlear stress defenses to reduce noise-induced hearing loss. Laryngoscope, 112, 1515–1532.

Legros, D., Ollivier, G., Gastellu-Etchaegorry, M., Paquet, C., Burri, C., & Jannin, J. (2002). Treatment of human African tympanosomiasis—present situation and need for research and development. Lancet Infectious Diseases, 2, 437–440.

Levin, V. A., Hess, K. R., Choucair, A., et al. (2003). Phase III randomized study of postradiotherapy chemotherapy with combination alpha-difluoromethylornithine: PCV versus PCV for anaplastic gliomas. Clinical Cancer Research, 9, 981–990.

Li, Y., Womer, R. B., & Silber, J. H. (2004). Predicting cisplatin ototoxicity in children: The influence of age and the cumulative dose. European Journal of Cancer, 40, 2445–2451.

Lipton, A., Harvey, H. A., Glenn, J., et al. (1989). A phase I study of hepatic arterial infusion using difluoromethylornithine. Cancer, 63, 433–437.

Lonsbury Martin, B., & Martin, GK. (2007). Other ototoxins: Aspirin, quinine, non-steroidal anti-inflammatory drugs, and the macrolides. In K. C. Campbell (Ed.), Pharmacology and ototoxicity for audiologists (pp. 187–194). Clifton Park, NY: Thomson Delmar Learning.

McCann, P. P., & Pegg, A. E. (1992). Ornithine ecarboxylase as an enzyme target for therapy. Pharmacology and Therapeutics, 54, 195–215.

Meech, R. P., Campbell, K. C., Hughes, L. P., & Rybak, L. P. (1998). A semiquantitative analysis of the effects of CDDP on the rat stria vascularis. Hearing Research, 124, 44–59.

Meldrum, M. (2007). Introduction to pharmacology. In K. C. Campbell (Ed.), Pharmacology and ototoxicity for audiologists (pp. 1–9). Clifton Park, NY: Thomson Delmar Learning.

Meyskens, F. L., Emerson, S. S., Pelot, D., Mehkinpour, H., Shassetz, L. R., & Einsphahr, J. (1994). Dose de-escalation chemoprevention trail of alpha-difluoromethylornithine in patients with colon polyps. Journal of the National Cancer Institute, 86, 1122–1130.

Meyskens, F. L., Kingsley, E. M., Glattke, T., Loescher, L., & Booth, A. (1986). A phase II study of alpha-difluoromethylornithine (DMFO) for the treatment of metastatic melanoma. Investigational New Drugs, 4(3), 527–562.

Morioka, I., Kuroda, M., Miyashita, K., & Takeda, S. (1999). Evaluation of organic solvent ototoxicity by the upper limit of hearing. Archives of Environmental Health, 54(5), 341–346.

Moss, P. E., Hickman, S., & Harrison, B. R. (1999). Ototoxicity associated with vinblastine. Annals of Pharmacotherapy, 33, 423–425.

Pasic, T. R., Heisey, D., & Love, R. R. (1997). Alpha-difluoromethylornithine ototoxicity. Archives of Otolaryngology—Head and Neck Surgery, 123, 1281–1286.

Pouyatos, B., & Fechter, L. (2007). Industrial chemicals and solvents affecting the auditory system. In K. C. Campbell (Ed.), Pharmacology and ototoxicity for audiologists (pp. 197–210). Clifton Park, NY: Thomson Delmar Learning.

Rey, J. (2007). Pharmacokinetics and pharmacodynamics. In K. C. Campbell (Ed.), Pharmacology and ototoxicity for audiologists (pp. 10–18). Clifton Park, NY: Thomson Delmar Learning.

Rybak, L. P. (1992). Hearing: The effects of chemicals. Otolaryngology—Head and Neck Surgery, 106(6), 677–686.

Rybak, L. P. (2007). Renal function and ototoxicity of loop diuretics. In K. C. Campbell (Ed.), Pharmacology and ototoxicity for audiologists (pp. 177–183). Clifton Park, NY: Thomson Delmar Learning.

Rybak, L. P., Huang, X., & Campbell, K. C. (2007). Cancer and ototoxicity of chemotherapeutics. In K. C. Campbell (Ed.), Pharmacology and ototoxicity for audiologists (pp. 138–155). Clifton Park, NY: Thomson Delmar Learning.

Sahai, J., & Berry, A. J. (1989). Eflornithine for the treatment of Pneumocystis carinii pneumonia in patients with the acquired immunodeficiency syndrome: A preliminary review. Pharmacotherapy, 9, 29–33.

Saito, T., Saito, H., Saito, K., Wakui, S., Manabe, Y., & Tsuda, G. (1989). Ototoxicity of carboplatin in guinea pigs. Auris, Nasus, Larynx, 16, 13–21.

Schwade, N. D. (2000). Pharmacology in audiology practice. In R. Roeser, M. Valente, & H. Hosford-Dunn (Eds.), Audiology: Diagnosis (pp. 139–152). New York: Thieme Medical Publishers.

Schweitzer, V. G., Hawkins, J. E., Lilly, D. J., Litterst, C. J., Abrams, G., & Davis, J. A. (1984). Ototoxic and nephrotoxic effects of combined treatment with cis-diamminedichloroplatinum and kanamycin in the guinea pig. Otolaryngology—Head and Neck Surgery, 92, 38–49.

Seidman, M., & Moneysmith, M. (2007). Nutraceuticals and herbal supplements. In K. C. Campbell (Ed.), Pharmacology and ototoxicity for audiologists (pp. 57–69). Clifton Park, NY: Thomson Delmar Learning.

Sha, S. H., & Schacht, J. (2000). Antioxidants attenuate gentamicin-induced free radical formation in vitro and ototoxicity in vivo: D-methionine is a potential protectant. Hearing Research, 142, 34–40.

Sjoerdsma, A., Golden, J. A., Schechter, P. J., Barlow, J. L., & Santi, D. V. (1984). Successful treatment of lethal protozoal infections with the ornithine decarboxylase inhibitors, alpha-difluoromethylornithine. Transactions of the Association of American Physicians, 97, 70–79.

Sulkowski, W. J., Kowalska, S., Matyja, W., Guzek, W., Wesolowski, W., Szymczak, W., & Kostrzewski, P. (2002). Effects of occupational exposure to a mixture of solvents on the inner ear: A field study. International Journal of Occupational Medicine and Environmental Health, 15(3), 247–256.

Thornton, A. R., & Raffin, M. J. (1978). Speech discrimination scores modeled as a binomial variable. Journal of Speech and Hearing Research, 21, 507–518.

Van Ruijven, M. W. M., De Groot, J. C. M. J., & Smoorenburg, G. F. (2004). Time sequence of degeneration pattern in the guinea pig cochlea during cisplatin administration: A quantitative histological study. Hearing Research, 197, 44–54.

Wake, M., Takeno, S., Ibrahim, D., Harrison, R., & Mount, R. (1993). Carboplatin ototoxicity: An animal model. Journal of Laryngology and Otology, 107, 585–589.

Chapter 10

An Introduction to Acoustics and Psychoacoustics

Prudence Allen

Psychoacoustics links the physical parameters of sounds with the sensations and perceptions that they evoke. Psychoacoustic findings have provided the foundation for behavioral testing in audiology and likewise hold the promise for future improvements and expansions in that testing. The breadth of areas that have been studied using behavioral techniques is wide and more than can be considered, however briefly, in a single chapter. The focus of this chapter will therefore be on the psychoacoustic findings that provide the basis for current audiological practices as well as those that hold promise for assessment and rehabilitation of hearing and hearing disorders in the future. Without clear and complete understanding of normal hearing processes and how those processes change throughout life, the evaluation of hearing disorders and their impact on communicative behavior will be limited.

♦ Basic Acoustics

The physical basis of sound is a large topic, complete discussion of which would exceed the bounds of this chapter. This section will therefore be limited to providing a definition of some basic terms and mathematical relationships. This should enable the reader to understand the essential elements of sound production and measurement. (For more detailed information, see Hartmann, 1998.)

Signal Magnitude

Instantaneous Magnitude

Sound is acoustic energy produced by a moving object. The movement of the object is transmitted through the medium in which the object lies, producing a pressure wave that varies over time and is propagated in all directions. When a sound is described in the time domain, $x(t)$ denotes the instantaneous pressure of the signal at time t, and the sound is presumed to begin at $t = 0$.

Figure 10–1 shows a time domain representation of some simple signals. The x-axis shows time, and the y-axis shows instantaneous magnitude, both displayed in arbitrary units. When these signals are sounds traveling through air, there are three-dimensional condensations of air particles at the positive values and rarefactions at the negative values. Condensations and rarefactions are increases and decreases, respectively, in the density of air particles relative to that measured when the medium is in a state of rest. It is through this motion of particles in the air medium that sound is transmitted through space to arrive at and propagate through the external auditory meatus to a listener's tympanic membrane.

The magnitude of an acoustic waveform at any given moment will be determined not only by the instantaneous pressure created by the moving force that is driving the disturbance but also by the characteristics of the medium in which the pressure wave is expected to travel. For example, a sound wave traveling through air will be very different from one traveling through water, even if they were created with the same force. The magnitude of the wave in a medium is the waveform intensity, $I(t)$, and it is determined by the instantaneous pressure and the particle velocity, $u(t)$, of the medium. Wave velocity is equal to the instantaneous pressure, $x(t)$, divided by the specific impedance, ρc, of the medium in which the signal is transmitted; ρ refers to the density of the medium, measured in kg/meter², and c is the speed of sound (343.2 m/sec at 20°C). The unit of measurement for intensity is watts/meter². The relation between pressure and intensity is monotonic but nonlinear.

$$I(t) = x(t) * u(t) = x(t) * x(t) / \rho c = x^2(t) / \rho c$$

Note that sound intensity values will be positive for all time values, even though the pressure measurements from which they may be derived are both positive and negative.

Average Magnitude

It is often of interest to know not only the instantaneous magnitude of a signal (pressure or intensity) but also the average magnitude. This is calculated by averaging the instantaneous magnitudes over the duration of the signal, T_D, or some briefer time interval if the signal duration is very long.[1]

The equation for computing average pressure is

$$\bar{P} = \frac{1}{T_D} \int_0^{T_D} dt P(t).$$

The typical measure of average pressure is the root-mean-square value, denoted as X_{RMS} and calculated as follows:

$$X_{RMS} = \sqrt{\frac{1}{T_D} \int_0^{T_D} dt x^2(t)}.$$

The instantaneous pressures are squared, averaged over the time interval T_D, and the square root of the average is taken.

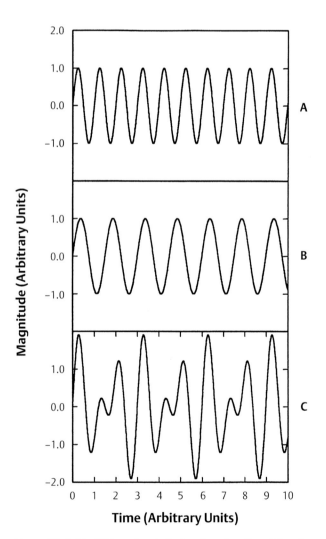

Figure 10–1 (A–C) Three signals displayed as a function of time, in arbitrary units. **(A)** and **(B)** show signals that are periodic within the time displayed. These signals are combined and displayed in **(C)**.

---

[1] To obtain an adequate representation of signal magnitude, the average must be taken over a time interval that is greater than the duration over which typical moment-to-moment variations occur. For very brief signals, the average should be made over the duration of the entire signal, but for longer signals, a time period less than the total duration could be sampled so long as the interval is longer than the minor moment-to-moment fluctuations.

Absolute and Relative Sound Levels

To this point, the discussion has been on the absolute values of sounds. But dealing with absolute values, particularly for acoustic signals, may easily become unruly. For example, the smallest pressure that can be detected by the human ear under ideal situations is $2*10^{-12}$ N/m^2, where N is the abbreviation for newtons.[2] Intensity is related to pressure (squared) divided by the specific impedance of air, which is commonly 415 rayls, although it may vary with atmospheric pressure and temperature. Thus, the smallest detectable intensity is $(2*10^{-5}$ N/m$^2)^2/415 = 0.964*10^{-12}$ W/m^2, where W is the abbreviation for watts. For convenience, this is approximated by 10^{-12} W/m^2. Listeners can also perceive, although perhaps painfully, intensities of 1 W/m^2 or greater. This is a very large range, and discussion of magnitudes within that range requires the use of very large numbers. Signal magnitudes are therefore more commonly reported as relative levels, computed with the log transformation. Signal level is equal to the log of a measured magnitude relative to a reference magnitude. The unit of measurement is the bel, or decibel (dB). (One bel is equal to 10 dB.)

$$\text{Level (dB)} = 10\log\left(\frac{\text{Measured magnitude}}{\text{Reference magnitude}}\right)$$

When level (in dB) is equal to 0, it does not suggest there is no signal but that the magnitude of the measured signal is equal to the magnitude of the reference signal, $10\log(1) = 0.0$. Although any reference value may be used in the measurement of sound levels, there is a standard reference agreed upon by the community of users (in audiology, hearing research, and engineering). The absolute reference for intensity is the minimum detectable, 10^{-12} W/m^2.[3]

The actual measurement of sound is most often made with pressure-sensitive microphones and sound level meters even though it is signal intensity that is the more relevant measure in practice, as it reflects both waveform magnitude and the influence of the medium in which the waveform is transmitted. Because intensity is proportional to the square of the pressure, the computation for intensity levels, computed from measured and reference pressure values, is

$$L(\text{dB}) = 10\log\left(\frac{\text{Measured pressure}}{\text{Reference pressure}}\right)^2.$$

By simple algebra [$\log(a/b)^x$ is equal to $x\log(a/b)$], the exponent can be moved to precede the log such that the computation of sound intensity from pressure values is

$$L(\text{dB}) = 20\log\left(\frac{\text{Measured pressure}}{\text{Reference pressure}}\right).$$

The absolute reference for sound pressures is the smallest pressure detectable, or $2*10^{-5}$ N/m^2, or 20 μPa. When this absolute reference value is used, the level is noted as dB sound pressure level (SPL).

Electrical Calibration

Sometimes sound measurement is performed electrically rather than acoustically. Knowing the sound pressure level that is produced when a given electrical magnitude is passed through a transducer enables the electrical calibration of acoustic signals. The unit of measurement is the volt. Likewise, because electric signals must also be transmitted through a medium, their magnitude can be noted as power, which is similar to sound intensity. Power is equal to the instantaneous magnitude multiplied by the current flow, $i(t)$. Current is equal to the instantaneous voltage, $x(t)$ divided by the resistance of the medium, R. Thus, power $= x(t)^* x(t)/R$. When signal levels are computed in dB from voltage measurements, they are noted as dBV. It is common for transducer outputs in SPLs to be calibrated according to the output achieved with a 1 V root-mean-square (RMS) signal passed across it.

Adding Signals

When signals are added in the time domain, their instantaneous pressures add linearly; thus, $x_{1+2}(t) = x_1(t) + x_2(t)$. The instantaneous pressure of the combined waveform is a sum of the instantaneous pressures of the components. **Figure 10–1C** shows the result of adding the signals shown in **Figs. 10–1A and 10–1B.** Note that the magnitude of the waveform in **Fig. 10–1C** is produced by a linear addition of the magnitudes in **Figs. 10–1A and 10–1B** at each moment in time.

Unlike pressures, intensities do not add linearly. Intensity is related to pressure by squaring. Thus, the intensity of a combined signal, I_{1+2}, is

$$I_{1+2} = \left[x_1(t) + x_2(t)\right]^2.$$

This expands algebraically to

$$I_{1+2} = x_1^2(t) + x_2^2(t) + 2x_1(t)x_2(t).$$

Because x_1^2 is the intensity of signal 1, and x_2^2 is the intensity of signal 2, the equation for computing the average intensity of the combined signal will be

$$I_{1+2} = I_1 + I_2 + 2\frac{1}{T_D}\int_0^{T_D} dt\, x_1(t)x_2(t).$$

Therefore, the combined intensity of two waveforms is equal to the sum of their individual intensities plus a sum that is related to the correlation between, or the cross-product of, the two waveforms. If x_1 and x_2 are uncorrelated, the integral is equal to 0, so that the intensity of the combined waveform reduces to the simple combination of the intensities

---

[2]Pressure is a force (measured in newtons, N) applied over an area (square meters, m^2). Thus, the standard unit of pressure in the MKS (meter-kilogram-second) system is the newton/meter^2, or N/m^2. Pressure may also be measured in pascals (Pa): 1 Pa = 1 N/m^2.

[3]Using this equation, it can be seen that the range of human hearing (in dB) is large, $10^*\log(1$ W/m$^2/10^{-12}$ W/m$^2) = 120$ dB.

in the two signals themselves. (This is the general assumption.) However, if the two waveforms are identical, then their combined intensity is simply 4 times greater than that of one component because the integral would be equal to 1.0. However, if the correlation between the two is equal to −1.0, that is, they are exact opposites, 180 degrees out of phase with one another, their combined intensity would be 0, as the two signals would cancel one another out. If the correlation is other than 1, 0, or –1, as described in these examples, the computation is less simple.

Adding Sound Levels (Decibels)

The preceding examples show how to combine intensities when they are in absolute terms. However, it is more customary to add intensities that have been measured in decibels. The overall level of a combined signal, in dB, will be

$$L = 10\log\left(\frac{\text{Intensity}_1}{\text{reference level}}\right) + 10\log\left(\frac{\text{Intensity}_2}{\text{reference level}}\right).$$

Because the two signals have a common reference level, for example, 10^{-12} W/m², the intensities of the individual waveforms can be computed from their dB values, $I(dB) = 10\log(I/10^{-12})$; solving for $I = 10^{I(dB)/10} \cdot 10^{-12}$. The several values of I obtained for each signal to be added can then be combined. The overall level will be equal to

$$10\log\left[\left(\sum_1^n I_n\right)/10^{-12}\right].$$

Periodic and Aperiodic Signals

When a signal repeats its pattern of vibration infinitely over time, it is said to be periodic. The time interval over which it repeats is the period. One of the simplest of periodic signals is the sinusoid, or in acoustics, the pure tone. (A gated pure tone, that is, one that is turned on and off and therefore not truly continuous in time, is the most common signal used in audiometric testing.) The pure tone or sinusoid is produced by a pattern of activity (voltage or pressure changes with time) that is defined according to the sine function such that

$$x(t) = A\sin(2\pi t/T + \phi),$$

where A is the maximum amplitude of the signal, T is the period (usually in seconds), and ϕ is the starting phase (in radians). The amplitude can take on any positive value. Because the sine function varies between 1 and −1, the signal magnitude will vary between A and −A. As can be seen in the definition of the sine wave, the magnitude will repeat with every cycle of the wave, that is, every 360 degrees or $2p$ radians. Assuming a starting phase of 0, (i.e., $\phi = 0$), $x(t)$ will be equal to 0 whenever $2pt/T$ is equal to 0 or p because the sine of both are equal to 0.0. $X(t)$ will reach a maximum, or peak amplitude, A, when the argument to the sine function is $p/2$ radians, or 90 degrees, and a minimum, −A,

when the argument is $3p/2$ radians (or 270 degrees). As time, t, progresses, the pattern repeats. The frequency of the signal is $1/T$, noted in cycles per second, or Hertz (Hz). The equation for the sinusoid can also be written as $x(t) = A\sin(2\pi ft + \phi)$, where f is the frequency. If the starting phase is not zero, the function is identical in shape to one starting at zero phase but shifted in time by an amount corresponding to the phase shift. Note that a time shift corresponding to a given phase shift will be different as the frequency varies. That is, for a signal of 1000 Hz frequency, a phase shift of 2π corresponds to a time shift of 500 μs, yet for a signal of 500 Hz, a shift of 2π corresponds to a time shift of 1000 μs. Signals are sometimes said to have phase lags or leads. This refers to the relative position of the first peak in amplitude. Thus, a signal with a starting phase of 90 degrees is said to have a phase lag relative to another signal with a starting phase of at 0 degree.

The signals shown in **Figs. 10–1A** and **10–1B** are sine waves with starting phase of 0 degree and are periodic over the time interval shown. If the time units were milliseconds, the period of the waveform in the upper panel would be 1 msec, and zero crossings would occur at $t = 0.0, 0.5$, and 1.0 msec, corresponding to phases of 0, π, and 2π. The positive and negative maxima occur at 0.25 and 0.75, corresponding to $\pi/2$ and $3\pi/2$ radians. This pattern repeats for all successive replications of the period. (Note that the absolute magnitude shown in **Figs. 10–1A** and **10–1B** varies between + and −1.0. If this were a real signal, the magnitudes shown here would be multiplied by the peak amplitude, A.)

When sinusoids are added together, perceptible fluctuations may result in the amplitude, or envelope, particularly if the components are different frequencies. The envelope of the combined signal will be modulated at a frequency that coincides with the difference in the frequencies of the two constituent tones. This modulation frequency is often called the beat frequency. When one listens to the combined tones, the amplitude modulates at a rate corresponding to the beat frequency, which corresponds to the slow variations in the envelope of the combined signal that resulted from the orderly addition of instantaneous pressures. The effect on the envelope of signals produced by the addition of individual signals with other relations may be more complex. Note that the signal in **Fig. 10–1B** is slightly different from that in **Fig. 10–1A**. The addition of these two signals produces the waveform shown in **Fig. 10–1C**. Note the slower variations in the overall amplitude of the envelope, which contrast with the constant envelope of the signals in **Figs. 10–1A** and **10–1B**.

Noise

Sounds that do not repeat in time are said to be aperiodic. A class of aperiodic sounds that are common in audiometry and hearing research are noises. A noise signal consists of frequency components that are not discrete but continuous. That is, they contain energy at every frequency over a specific range, and therefore, energy is represented as a continuous function of frequency. The noise is defined by the manner in which the amplitudes of the individual components are represented and by the bandwidth of frequencies represented. Gaussian noise, the most common type of noise used in hearing applications, is noise for which the amplitudes of the individual components are distributed normally. In contrast, uniform noise is that for which the amplitudes of the individual components are all the same.

The frequency composition of a noise is most often defined by its bandwidth. Band limited noise refers to a noise consisting of components only over a range of frequencies. The bandwidth (BW) of the noise is defined as the difference between the upper (f_u) and lower (f_l) cutoff frequencies ($BW = f_u - f_l$). White noise is gaussian, with energy present as a continuous function of frequency. The bandwidth is limited only by the output characteristics of the transducer. Pink noise contains energy as a continuous function of frequency, but the relative amplitude of components decreases at a rate of 3 dB/octave as frequency increases, thus biasing toward the lower frequencies. Other common noise types used in audiometric and hearing research are third-octave noise bands. These noises are defined by their center frequency and contain energy at frequencies only in the one-third octave wide region surrounding this center frequency. Other types of noise are also common in hearing research. For example, band stop noise refers to noise for which components are presented at all frequencies except those defined by the band stop region. This is also called notched noise.

Power Spectra of Signals

The overall power in a signal can be expressed as a function of the spectrum level of the individual components:

$$\bar{P} = \int_{f_l}^{f_u} df N_0(f).$$

The energy in each 1 Hz wide band of noise, N_0, is summed for each frequency component, f, over the entire bandwidth, noted by the integral with f_u and f_l representing the upper and lower cutoff frequencies, respectively. This measure is most often referred to as the power spectrum. When the power spectrum is noted in absolute units, dB relative to 10^{-12} W/Hz, the spectrum level, or level of individual components, can be calculated from the overall level, L_0: $L_0 = 10 \log(N_0/10^{-12})$. When the power spectrum is constant with frequency, the spectrum level in dB, N_0, can be calculated from the total level, L: $N_0 = L - 10 \log(BW)$, where BW is the bandwidth of the noise.

Fourier Analysis

Most natural sounds are complex and consist of energy at multiple frequencies, although the energy distribution may not be as easily defined as in the preceding examples of pure tones and noises. A frequency domain representation, or spectral representation, is most useful for displaying the relative amplitudes of individual components. To obtain spectral information, signals are analyzed mathematically using the Fourier transform. The Fourier transform and the inverse Fourier transform enable movement back and forth between time and frequency domain representations of signals. There are two types of Fourier transformations: the

Fourier series, which is applicable only to periodic signals, and the Fourier integral, which can be applied to all signals. (Although full treatment of this transform is not possible here, a brief introduction of the basic concepts will be provided. An excellent reference is Ramirez, 1985.)

Fourier Series

The Fourier series is used to evaluate signals that are infinite, a requirement to be truly periodic. As periodic signals, all of the components must have a period that will fit exactly into the period of the waveform, T. The lowest frequency for which this is true is the fundamental frequency, f_0, which is equal to $1/T$. Other components will be integer multiples of the fundamental and thus harmonics of it. The general form of the Fourier series states that a waveform, $x(t)$, can be written as a sum of sine and cosine functions, each of which is weighted by a magnitude:

$$x(t) = A_0 + \sum_{n=1}^{\infty} A_n \cos(\omega_n t) + B_n \sin(\omega_n t),$$

where A_0 is a constant representing the average magnitude, such as the direct current (DC) offset in an electrical signal, A_n and B_n are Fourier coefficients that weight each sine and cosine component; and ω_n is the frequency of each component. Note that ω is equal to $2\pi n/T$.

To solve for the Fourier coefficients, which are the magnitudes associated with each frequency component, two equations are needed, one to solve for the cosine components and one for the sine components:

$$A_n = \frac{2}{T} \int_{-T/2}^{T/2} dt \, x(t) \cos(\omega_n t)$$

and

$$B_n = \frac{2}{T} \int_{-T/2}^{T/2} dt \, x(t) \sin(\omega_n t), \text{ for } n > 0.$$

To solve for the constant:

$$A_0 = \frac{1}{T} \int_{-T/2}^{T/2} dt \, x(t).^4$$

When signals are analyzed using the Fourier transform, a spectral representation of a signal can be visualized by plotting the Fourier coefficients (or frequency component magnitudes) and the starting phases as a function of frequency.

---

[4]The equation for the series can also be represented in polar form such that

$$x(t) = A_0 + \sum_{n=1}^{n} C_n \cos(\omega_n t - \phi_n),$$

where C_n represents the amplitude and ϕ_n is the phase of each component. By expansion using trigonometric identities:

$$x(t) = A_0 + \sum_{n=1}^{N} \left[C_n \cos(\omega_n t) \cos(\phi_n) + C_n \sin(\omega_n t) \sin(\phi_n) \right].$$

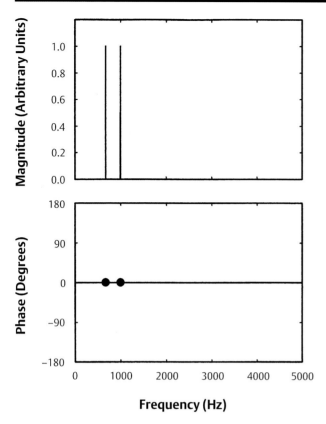

Figure 10–2 Amplitude and phase spectra, in the upper and lower panels, respectively, of the signal shown in the upper panel of **Figure 10–1**.

Figure 10–2 shows the amplitude and phase spectra of the signal shown in **Fig. 10–1C** (assuming, of course, that the signals in **Fig. 10–1** continue past the minimum and maximum time intervals shown).

Fourier Integral

The Fourier integral is more general than the Fourier series and can be used with signals that are not periodic. The rule states that from the frequency domain representation of a waveform, $X(\omega)$, a time domain representation, $x(t)$, can be written as

$$X(\omega) = \int_{-\infty}^{\infty} dt e^{-i\omega t} x(t).$$

The inverse integral, to move from the frequency domain to the time domain, is

$$x(t) = \frac{1}{2\pi} \int_{\infty}^{\infty} d\omega \, e^{i\omega t} X(\omega).$$

Discrete versus Continuous Fourier Transforms

Many signals used in hearing research laboratories and audiology clinics are not continuous analog signals but are produced digitally. As such, their instantaneous magnitudes do not occur as a continuous function of time but at discrete time intervals, the spacing of which is defined by the sampling rate (e.g., for a signal produced with a sampling rate of 10,000 points/second, an instantaneous magnitude will be available every 100 μs). To perform a spectral analysis on a discrete signal, the discrete Fourier transform (DFT) is often used, as is the fast Fourier transform (FFT). Because brief duration signals can never be truly periodic, as they will not be continuous in time, it is often assumed that the period is equal to the duration of the signal itself. Another difference between the DFT and the Fourier series is that, in the Fourier series, the number of frequencies and coefficients extends infinitely, whereas in the DFT, the components are limited by the Nyquist frequency, which is equal to half of the sampling frequency. (For a frequency to be represented, there must be at least two samples for the period.) Thus, for a sampling rate of 10 kHz suggested above, only frequencies up to 5 kHz will be represented accurately.

Wave Propagation in Space

Acoustic signals are transmitted over space as well as time. A periodic signal will therefore repeat itself not only over the period but also over a distance in space. This distance is the wavelength, λ, and it is related to the period, $\lambda = cT$, and to the frequency $\lambda = c/f$, where c is the speed of sound. In general, sounds will move around objects if their size is smaller than the wavelength. Thus, lower frequency sounds, with larger wavelengths, are less affected by objects in space as they are more likely to move around them. In contrast, higher frequencies with smaller wavelengths are more likely to bounce off objects in their path, thus producing differences in magnitudes on the two sides of the object, higher on the side facing the sound and lower on the opposite side.

Although sounds propagate through a space, they lose intensity as the distance they travel increases, particularly if there is low room reverberation. Signal intensity varies inversely with the square of the distance traveled. Because sound intensity is a function of force per unit area, as area increases with the space in which the sound is dispersed, the intensity decreases. The exact magnitude of the decrease will be proportional to the characteristics of the room itself. In a highly reverberant room, the intensity may not be reduced at all because reflected sounds will add with direct sounds. In a dead room, with little or no reverberation, sound intensity may be reduced quite rapidly with distance traveled. In general, sound waves propagate in all directions. However, some transducers and rooms cause sound to radiate in specific directions. This is a called a directional sound, and the levels recorded will vary with the location of the recording microphone relative to the direction in which the source transmits.

♦ Psychometric Methods

Measurement of sound perception requires not only a working knowledge of the physical basis of sounds but also reliable methods for measuring a listener's responses to those sounds.

Thresholds and Psychometric Functions

As audiologists, much of our focus is on thresholds. The measurement of absolute thresholds (or thresholds of audibility) is the most basic and agreed upon audiometric measure. In more general terms, threshold indicates the physical value of a stimulus at which a predetermined level of performance is obtained. It may apply to detection of, or discrimination between, events. It may be assumed that performance changes instantaneously from very poor to very good at the stimulus value corresponding to threshold. In reality, though, a single value at which this change occurs does not exist. Instead, perceptions change relatively gradually over a range of stimulus values.

The function used to describe this gradual change in perception is the psychometric function. It relates performance, such as percent correct detection or discrimination, to measurable parameters of the stimuli. Therefore, in a task for which a listener is asked to detect a signal presented in quiet, the psychometric function would relate performance, possibly in terms of percent correct detections, to signal intensity. If threshold were a single value below which detection was not possible and above which the signal would be detected with 100% accuracy, the psychometric function would be a step function moving abruptly from 0 to 100% correct at a single value of the stimulus. Detection, however, is probabilistic, changing gradually from 0 to 100% over a range of ~10 to 15 dB with adult listeners. (With young children, the range may be somewhat larger, and the functions may reach an asymptote at a performance level below 100% correct; see Allen and Wightman, 1994.) The shape of the function is nonlinear, often approximated by a logistic function. Because the rate of change in detection (or the slope of the psychometric function) is fairly constant for listeners under similar circumstances, in the clinic performance it is seldom measured over a wide range of levels as would be needed to fit a psychometric function. Instead, performance is estimated at predetermined levels, generally corresponding to performance at the inflection point on the psychometric function. That performance level is taken as threshold. When the psychometric function ranges from 0 to 100% correct, as in standard clinical testing procedures, threshold corresponds to the 50% correct level.

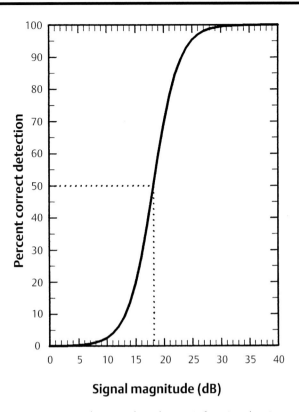

Figure 10–3 A theoretical psychometric function showing percent correct detections as a function of signal magnitude. The dotted line indicates the threshold magnitude corresponding to the 50% correct level.

Figure 10–3 shows a sample psychometric function. The solid line shows a function that would best fit observed performance data.

Note that predicted performance (detection accuracy) increases gradually as signal level increases from 10 to 25 dB. In this example, threshold, taken as the 50% correct level, corresponds to a signal intensity of slightly greater than 18 dB.

Signal Detection Theory

In general, individuals try to make informed decisions when asked to do so. This concept extends to the detection and discrimination of auditory signals. When an individual is asked to listen to two sounds and decide which is louder, which is a tone plus noise versus a noise alone, or which of a set of sounds is higher in pitch, and so on, the listener will try to make the decision based on the available sensory information and do so in a way that will maximize the probability of making a correct decision, weighted, of course, by the costs and values associated with incorrect and correct decisions. Statistical decision theory, and, from that, signal detection theory, assist in explaining how these decisions are likely made (see Green and Swets, 1988).

In a simple detection task, a listener has some sensory activity that he or she must judge as representing either the presence of a signal or simply random background activity.

Pearl

- Often, when measuring an audiometric threshold there may be uncertainty about whether a threshold value has actually been obtained. In those instances, we sometimes present a signal at a level 5 dB above the suspected threshold. If the response to the signal is clear, it can be assumed that the level measured probably did correspond to the 50% correct threshold. If, however, the response at this 5 dB higher level is unclear, the threshold estimate is questioned, and threshold seeking procedures should continue. This is because an individual's psychometric function ranges from 50 to 100% accuracy in ~5 dB as the whole function ranges over only 10 dB; thus, performance 5 dB above a threshold value, if it represents the intercept in the function, should produce near-perfect detection.

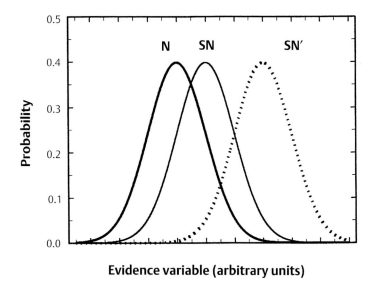

Figure 10–4 Three sample probability distributions of a hypothetical evidence variable used to make a decision in a signal detection or discrimination task. The heavy solid curve labeled *N* shows the probability of each value of the evidence variable associated with a noise alone, or no signal state. The lighter solid curve labeled *SN* shows the distribution of values associated with the introduction of a low level signal. The dotted line labeled SN′ shows the distribution of values associated with the addition of a higher level signal.

The evidence variable with which the listener must make that judgment, *x*, is, in this case, the amount of sensory activity in the system at the time of the observation. As signal intensity increases, so does the associated sensory activity. Because there is always some spontaneous activity in the system (noise), the listener must decide at what point the sensory activity is sufficiently high to warrant changing his or her description of it from that of "no signal" (or "noise") to "signal" (or "signal plus noise"). Where the listener sets this criterion will vary with costs and values associated with the mistakes he or she is willing to make and correct responses, respectively.

Assume that the random amount of activity that the listener experiences in the absence of a signal is normally distributed. **Figure 10–4** shows a hypothetical distribution of this "evidence variable." The distribution representing the values of sensory activity present when there is noise alone, or no signal, and the probability of each of those values occurring is labeled *N*. When a signal is added to this background activity, the mean of the distribution will increase, but the variance will remain the same. The signal simply adds a constant value to the probable values of sensory activity present in general. This new distribution is labeled *SN*, indicating that it is a signal plus noise distribution. On a given trial, a listener is asked whether or not he or she believes a signal was present. The listener will make this decision by examining the amount of sensory activity, *x*, that is present at the time of the trial. He or she must decide if the value of *x* sampled at that time is more consistent with the existence of no signal, *N* (i.e., that it is just random activity) or signal plus noise, *SN*. The only information the listener has to go on is the amount of activity sampled at that moment. For a particular value of *x*, there will be two probabilities: one that it came from the *N* distribution and another that it came from the *SN* distribution. Whenever *N* and *SN* overlap, as they will unless the signal level is very high, there is bound to be some error in the decision. All that the listener can do, according to statistical decision theory, is calculate the relative probabilities that the sensory experience was drawn form each of these two sensory states and compare them. This comparison is done by means of the likelihood ratio (*L*). It compares the probability that the activity came from a signal state divided by the probability that the activity came from a noise alone state: $L = P(x/SN)/P(x/N)$. If the value of *x* is such that it is equally likely to have been drawn from either of the two distributions (i.e., if it is equally probable to obtain this value of *x* in either state), the value of *L* is 1.0. In **Fig. 10–4**, this would occur for values of *x* for which the *N* and *SN* distributions intersect. Higher values of *L* will occur for values of *x* that exceed this value and therefore indicate that it is more likely that the activity was produced by the presence of a signal, and lower values of *L* indicate the opposite. The listener's task is to determine a critical value of the likelihood ratio above which he or she will say that a signal is present and below which he or she will say that none is present. This value of the likelihood ratio at which the decision changes from no signal to signal is the listener's criterion. When the signal is very intense, it will drive the level of the activity above that which is ever associated with simple, spontaneous activity; because the likelihood ratio will be large for nearly all of the expressed values of *x*, the decision will be easily made. A change in activity resulting from the addition of such a signal to random background activity is suggested by the dotted line in **Fig. 10–4** labeled SN′. When the signal is weak (e.g., SN in **Fig. 10–4**), it may only increase the background activity slightly, making the decision much harder and much more prone to error.

There are two ways in which a correct response can be made: first, the listener may judge that a signal is present when it in fact is (hit) and, second, the listener can judge that no signal is present when it is not (correct rejection). Similarly, there are two types of errors. One is that the listener will judge that a signal is present when it is not (false alarm), and the other, that the listener will judge that no signal is present when it is (miss). Obviously, for a block of trials, the proportion of hits and misses can be calculated if only one of the two is known, as they sum to 1.0. (Measuring both, therefore, provides no more information than measuring only one of the two.) Similarly, if the rate of correct rejections is known, so also is the rate of false alarms; again, these must sum to 1.0. To summarize, if the listener says there is a signal, he or she is either right (hit) or wrong (false alarm); if the listener says there is no signal, he or she is either right (correct rejection) or wrong (miss). The key for understanding sensitivity is to know not only the rates at which correct and incorrect responses are made on signal trials but also the rates of correct and incorrect responses on no signal trials. It is only by measuring performance on both signal and no signal trials that true sensitivity can be estimated.

For example, assume two listeners with equal sensitivity; for a particular stimulus level, the amount of sensory activity received would be indicated by the *SN* distribution of **Fig. 10–4**, and sensory activity with no signal would be indicated by *N*. Suppose the first listener wants us to think he or she has excellent hearing. That listener decides that no matter what he or she hears, he or she will claim to have heard a signal. The listener wants to be sure to say "yes" to every signal you present and miss none of them, regardless of what he or she can actually hear. Nearly every time the listener is presented with a trial, or asked if a sound was heard, he or she will respond in the affirmative. That would give the first listener a hit rate near 1.0 and a miss rate near 0.0. To achieve this level of performance would require that the listener set the criterion at a very low value of *x*. This listener would be described as having an extremely liberal response criterion. Suppose, in contrast, the second listener is much more conservative. This listener is very worried about his or her hearing. The second listener decides that he or she will only acknowledge hearing a sound when he or she is absolutely sure, that is, when the sound is fairly loud. He or she would set the criterion at a very high value of *x*. The second listener's hit rate would be much lower than that of the first listener. Without knowing anything else, one would be led to assume that the second listener has poorer hearing than the first listener. The only difference between these two listeners, however, is the bias in their response patterns, not their actual sensitivity. Only by also measuring their responses on no signal trials would the difference become apparent. If the rate at which they make mistakes is examined, it will be seen that the first listener, because of the low criterion value, will often say there is a signal present when there is not, that is, when merely experiencing a sample drawn from the *N* distribution. The false alarm would be quite high, and the correct rejection rate would be very low. This would suggest that the first listener's sensitivity may be much poorer than his or her very high hit rate had suggested. Conversely, the second listener would have far fewer false alarms and many correct rejections, suggesting that perhaps his or her sensitivity was better than the relatively low hit rate had indicated initially. Thus, only by examining responses on signal and no signal trials can an individual's true sensitivity be determined in a manner that is free of bias in his or her criterion.

Clearly, these extremes are rare in most settings. A listener is free to vary response criterion throughout the range of possible values of the likelihood ratio. Where a listener sets the criterion will vary with the costs and values associated with both forms of incorrect and correct responses. If the value in a hit is high and the cost of a false alarm is low, the listener may set a more liberal criterion, but if the value of hits decreases and the cost of false alarms increases, he or she may choose to become more conservative. To evaluate true sensitivity requires an estimate of performance that includes responses on both signal and no signal trials, so that both hit and false alarm rates can be estimated.

Special Consideration

- In the clinic, we seldom measure false alarm rates. When unsolicited responses occur, we reinstruct our client, encouraging them to be more conservative ("Press the button only if you are sure that there is a sound"). Our goal is to keep the false alarm rate as low as possible so that it will not bias the estimates of performance that are based solely on hit rates.

D-Prime and Forced Choice Procedures

Many experimental measures of performance are reported as d-prime (d') values, not percent correct; d' is a bias free estimate of performance that incorporates both hit and false alarm information. What is of interest in the measurement of performance is the relative detectability or discriminability of a particular stimulus and how that may change with changes in stimulus values. That is, how far does the distribution of *SN* values lie above the noise alone distribution? Does it lie only slightly above the *SN* distribution, suggesting that sensitivity for this sound was quite low (*SN*), or does it lie substantially above it, suggesting that sensitivity must be quite high (*SN'*)? To determine how far from the *N* distribution the *SN* distribution lies at each stimulus value, the mean of the *SN* distribution must be calculated relative to a normalized *N* distribution with a mean and $s = 1.0$. In simple terms, the mean of the *SN* distribution is calculated in standard deviation units relative to the mean and standard deviation of the *N* distribution: $d' = \text{Mean} ((SN) - \text{Mean} (N))/s(N)$. Because the mean and standard deviation of the noise alone distribution are 1.0, d' is actually the mean of the signal plus noise distribution in units normalized to the distribution of noise alone values. So, for a $d' = 0$, the signal should not be discriminable better than chance levels because the *N* and *SN* distributions must overlap completely. When $d' = 1.0$, it is assumed that the signal produced a mean value of *x* that lies 1 second above the mean of the *N* distribution. Once d' values reach ~3.0, discriminability should be near perfect, as the *N* and *SN* distributions will have little or no overlap.

In an experimental setting, it is customary to measure performance in forced-choice procedures. Trials, usually consisting of multiple listening intervals, are well defined. Signals are presented in only one of the intervals of each trial. In this way, performance is measured for both signal and no-signal options, simultaneously evaluating a combination of hit and false alarm rates. The listener's task is to choose which of the intervals presented on each trial has the greatest likelihood of containing a signal (or being different from the rest). The listener must respond on every trial, even if he or she is unsure. In such a task, performance can range from chance to a maximum that may or may not be associated with 100% correct levels.

Pitfall

- Best performance will often, but not always, be associated with 100% correct, depending on the task and the ability of the listener, and the performance associated with chance performance will vary with the number of listening intervals. If two intervals are presented, chance performance will be 50% correct. If three intervals are presented, chance will be 33% correct. Yet in both cases, chance indicates a $d' = 0.0$. This makes it difficult to compare performance across several conditions using percent correct measures if the task was not identical. For a quick reference, refer to tables presented in Swets (1964), that show d' values corresponding to a full range of percent correct values obtained in multiple-alternative forced-choice tasks.

Psychophysical Methods

There are many psychophysical methods that can be used to collect detection and/or discrimination data. Each has its own advantages and disadvantages, and selection of an appropriate procedure must be made based on consideration of speed and efficiency in data collection, the nature of the experimental/clinical question being asked, and the capabilities of the listener. A few examples will be discussed.

Method of Limits

In the method of limits, the listener is presented with a series of trials for which the physical value being tested is varied in an orderly and predetermined manner. For example, when the task is to determine an individual's threshold for the audibility of a signal, the signal level is presented in both ascending and descending series. In the ascending series, the stimuli are initially presented at a very low intensity, and as trials proceed, the stimulus level is increased. In the descending series, the level begins high and is gradually reduced. The listener simply responds if he or she does or does not hear the signals or, in a forced-choice task, which of the intervals is most likely to contain the signal. The lower and upper stimulus values tested are determined prior to the initiation of a trial block, usually requiring prior knowledge of the listener's overall response capabilities so that performance at stimulus values both above and below threshold levels can be measured. Thresholds are determined by averaging the stimulus values associated with changes in the listener's responses (e.g., from signal to no signal) obtained in both ascending and descending series.

An advantage of this procedure is that a full range of performance levels can be estimated. However, a disadvantage, if only threshold estimates are of interest, is that many trials may be presented at stimulus values quite remote from threshold levels. This makes the procedure somewhat inefficient for threshold determinations.

Variations on the methods of limits are adaptive procedures that use algorithms to select stimulus values for each trial based on the listener's responses on the preceding trial(s). These are also called *staircase procedures*. Rules are applied to the way stimulus values are chosen with the goal of concentrating trials at near the desired percent correct (threshold) signal values. For example, in a one-down, one-up procedure, the stimulus value is decreased every time a correct response is made and increased every time an incorrect response is made. The resulting threshold value tracked is that corresponding to 50% correct performance. This performance level is extrapolated from the midpoint between stimulus values for which a change in stimulus direction is noted (a reversal). If two correct responses are required before the stimulus value is decreased but the one-up rule is kept (i.e., two-down, one-up rule), the threshold level that is estimated will correspond to a higher level of performance than that estimated from a one-down, one-up rule, ~70.7% correct (Levitt, 1971).

Pearl

- On average, more trials will be presented at higher stimulus values, with a rule requiring a greater number of correct responses before the stimulus value is decreased. Thus, performance averaged across stimuli will be higher than when fewer sequential correct responses are required for a decrease in stimulus value. The performance level tracked in a one-down, one-up procedure will be equal to $\sqrt[n]{0.5}$. In the audiology clinic, a one-down, one-up rule is generally applied to a task for which chance is 0% correct, thus tracking 50% correct performance levels.

Adaptive procedures have the advantage of placing nearly all trials in and around the region of the threshold, avoiding stimulus values that lie distant from the threshold value in either direction. The starting values in an adaptive procedure are usually set relatively high to ensure that the listener knows what to listen for. The stimulus values are then reduced, usually with a slightly larger step size than will be used for the remainder of the trial block. Once the direction has changed from going down to going up (a reversal has occurred), the step size may be reduced. Generally, the first or second reversal values are not included in the calculation of the threshold estimate. (Stimulus levels at reversal points can be averaged, or the stimulus levels midway between successive reversals can be calculated and averaged for the final threshold estimate.) The rule for stopping an adaptive track is that either a fixed number of trials have been completed, or a predetermined number of reversals have occurred.

Method of Adjustment

In the method of adjustment, the stimulus values are under the control of the listener, not the experimenter. For example, in the measurement of detection thresholds, the level of the signal may gradually increase and decrease automatically, with the direction of change under the control of the listener. The listener is instructed to keep the signal level at a value that is just barely detectable by responding when he or she does and does not hear the sound. Signal intensity may gradually increase until the listener presses a response button to indicate that the signal is audible. At that point, the intensity begins to decrease gradually. When the sound is no longer audible, the listener releases the response button, signaling the system to now increase signal intensity. Threshold levels are determined from the average level falling between successive responses, indicating audible and inaudible signal values.

Method of Constant Stimuli

The experimenter may also select a variety of stimulus values that are both above and below the individual's threshold, rather than estimate only a single threshold value. Several trials are presented at each of many stimulus values, often chosen randomly across a block of trials, and performance is calculated for each stimulus value. A psychometric function may then be fitted to those performance data. Threshold values can be extrapolated from these fitted functions, if desired. This procedure is similar to the method of limits, in that a wide range of signal values are tested, but differs in the order in which those values are presented and perhaps in the interval between values.

Scaling

Often it is of interest to know how the magnitude of a psychological percept changes as a physical parameter of a sound varies, rather than simply measure an individual's ability to detect and/or discriminate between sounds. This information may be obtained by presenting listeners with a stimulus and asking them to rate the perceived stimulus magnitude (magnitude estimation) or by asking listeners to adjust a stimulus magnitude to match a number that is presented to them (magnitude production). Listeners may also be presented with a signal and asked to adjust the magnitude of another signal to be a fraction or integer multiple of that first signal. Each of these procedures may be used alone or in combination with others to develop sensory scales. Developing a scale relating perception to sensory magnitude must be done with care, as there are many potential sources of bias in these tasks (e.g., Gravetter and Lockhead, 1973; Pradhan and Hoffman, 1963). For example, when performing matching tasks (matching stimulus values, numbers, etc.), listeners often tend to limit or shorten the range of the parameter that is under their control. This is called the *regression effect*. Thus, when listeners are asked to estimate the loudness of a sound, they may avoid using very small or very large numbers; when listeners are asked to adjust a stimulus magnitude to correspond to numbers

they are given, they may avoid the extremely high and low signal values. One way to limit the expression of this bias is to begin the task by presenting a listener with the full range of stimuli (or magnitude values) that will be presented during the task. This allows the listener to calibrate his or her internal scale prior to the start of the task. Another bias that is common in scaling procedures is the sequential effect. Listeners try to respond on each trial in a manner that is consistent with their previous responses. The effect of this bias can be observed over five to seven previous trials and occurs even if listeners are told to judge each stimulus independently of all others.

Pitfall

- Some rating procedures present stimuli to listeners in ascending or descending series rather than randomly. This can exacerbate the sequential effect. The listener's responses may appear to be more consistent (internal reliability will be high), but the judgments may be less valid, as each judgment is not independent, but linked to previous judgments.

Lastly, as with detection and discrimination procedures, listeners may be biased by costs and values associated with their responses or by their concerns about the subsequent use that will be made of the judgments they provide. One way to limit the biases commonly associated with scaling tasks is to use matching tasks for which there is a very strong correlation between the items to be matched. For example, in a task for which loudness is rated numerically, the biases will be strong because there is not a perfect match between loudness levels and numbers. If loudness scales are created by matching similar stimuli, such as pure tones of slightly different frequencies (as is used in the measurement of equal loudness contours), the biases will be much smaller.

◆ Level, Spectral, and Temporal Encoding

Armed with a basic knowledge of the physical parameters of a sound and of the procedures used to measure a listener's responses to those sounds, the limits and abilities of humans to encode and use auditory information can be explored. As a first step toward understanding the perception of natural sounds, which are inherently complex, this chapter begins with an attempt to describe the perception of acoustically simple sounds.

Intensity Encoding

Absolute Detection of Sounds in Quiet

Data describing detectability as a function of stimulus frequency provides the foundation of audiometric threshold

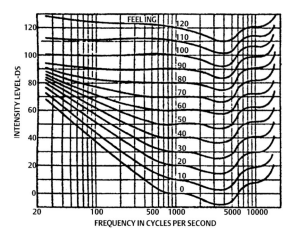

Figure 10–5 Equal loudness contours. The lowest curve, labeled *0*, reflects thresholds of audibility. (From Fletcher, H., & Munson, W. A. (1933). Loudness, its definition, measurement and calculation. Journal of the Acoustical Society of America, 5, 82–108, with permission.)

testing. Absolute threshold data shown by the lower curve in **Fig. 10–5** indicate the average SPL required by young, healthy adult listeners to detect a signal of known frequency presented in quiet. Audiometric measures of hearing level (dB HL) are referenced to these types of threshold values noted in dB SPL (American National Standards Institute, 2004). Specific reference equivalent threshold SPL levels for a variety of transducer types are stated in these standards. Note that the human ear is most sensitive to frequencies in the 1 to 5 kHz range and that higher signal levels are required for the detection of signal frequencies above and below this range.

Loudness

The psychological correlate of intensity is loudness. Near-threshold level sounds are perceived as very soft, and loudness increases with increases in stimulus intensity. Through a combination of loudness estimation procedures, it has been suggested that loudness grows exponentially with increases in signal intensity, $L = k\,I^{0.3}$, where L is loudness, k is a constant, and I is the signal intensity (Stevens, 1955). Thus, loudness increases more slowly with increasing intensity at lower intensities and more rapidly at higher intensities. Loudness also grows most slowly in midfrequencies and more rapidly at higher and lower frequencies. This is most clearly shown in the equal loudness contours, which were constructed by asking listeners to balance the loudness of sounds at several frequencies to that of a reference tone of predetermined frequency and level (Fletcher and Munson, 1933). Generally, the reference signal is a 1000 Hz tone whose level is systematically varied, so that matches to different frequencies can be made at many intensities. Data from Fletcher and Munson (1933) are shown in **Fig. 10–5**. Note that loudness growth is slowest for frequencies in the region of greatest sensitivity. That is, smaller increments in intensity are required at very high or very low frequencies to match the loudness growth of much larger increments in

the midfrequencies. Note also that at threshold levels, sounds of different frequencies must be set at very different overall SPLs to achieve equal loudness, but at high signal levels, sounds of different frequencies are perceived as equally loud at very similar SPLs. The equal loudness curves become flatter with changes in frequency at very high levels, suggesting that dynamic range is narrower at frequency extremes than at midfrequencies and that sound frequency is less of a determiner of loudness at high levels than at low. Small increments in intensity at extreme frequencies may be perceived as equivalent.

Dynamic Range

The human ear is capable of detecting and discriminating sounds across a very wide range of intensities. A listener's dynamic range is defined at the lower limit by detection thresholds and at the upper limit by thresholds of discomfort, feeling, and/or pain. For a normal-hearing listener, dynamic range may easily exceed 100 dB, but for a listener with a sensorineural hearing impairment, elevated thresholds and/or reduced thresholds of discomfort can combine to produce a reduced dynamic range.

Pearl

- Listeners with cochlear hearing impairments typically perceive very high sound levels in much the same way as do normal-hearing listeners. This, combined with their elevated detection thresholds, produces reduced dynamic ranges and faster than normal loudness growth functions, or "recruitment." Conversely, neural hearing losses are sometimes not associated with the normal perception of loudness at high intensities, regardless of whether thresholds are elevated or not. Conductive hearing impairments, though associated with elevated thresholds, are typically not associated with reduced thresholds of discomfort, and so these listeners retain a relatively wide dynamic range.

Loudness and detection thresholds are affected not only by signal frequency and intensity but also by signal complexity and duration. Detection of a signal (d') has been shown to vary approximately with the square root of the number of components (Green and Swets, 1988). When the bandwidth of the signal is less than a critical band, the loudness of the complex will be similar to that of a pure tone of equal intensity, centered at the center frequency. However, when the bandwidth exceeds a critical band, the loudness of the complex will increase (Zwicker et al, 1957). As with bandwidth, both detection and perceived loudness also vary with signal duration as signal energy is integrated over the ~200 msec (temporal integration). Beyond 200 msec, energy is not fully integrated, and loudness growth and detection thresholds remain stable.

In many modalities, the magnitude of a percept may decrease over time. A decrease in the perceived loudness of a continuous sound is referred to as *loudness adaptation*. Simple adaptation is that which is attributable solely to the duration of the stimulation. Few studies have successfully demonstrated the presence of simple adaptation to signals that are presented at moderate to high intensities (i.e., ≥ 30 dB SL [sensation level]). At these higher sensation levels, loudness adaptation is likely to occur only if the measurement procedures involve matching the loudness of a continuous tone with that of an intermittent tone. Adaptation is measured for the loudness of the continuous tone; the intermittent tone is used only to indicate the perceived loudness of that tone. The reference (intermittent) tone can be presented to either the ipsilateral or the contralateral ear. Often in these procedures the loudness of the continuous tone will appear to decrease. But this form of adaptation is most commonly referred to as induced and appears to be linked to the interaction between the two tones. The effect is largest at higher sound levels and at higher frequencies. It is greater for tones than for noise bands and for sounds that are steady-state rather than modulated. When an intermittent tone is not used, little loudness adaptation has been observed at higher levels. However, at relatively low intensities, a form of loudness adaptation may be measurable in which the loudness of a signal may decrease such that the signal is no longer audible. This phenomenon is termed *threshold fatigue*. In a normal-hearing listener, threshold fatigue is usually minimal (often < 10–15 dB).

Pearl

- In an individual suffering from a retrocochlear hearing loss, threshold fatigue may be much higher than in a normal-hearing listener or a listener with a cochlear hearing loss. It is this observation that gave rise to the many tests of tone decay that became common in audiological practice beginning in the 1950s.

A fairly thorough evaluation of loudness adaptation and threshold fatigue was given by Scharf (1983).

Intensity Discrimination

An important aspect of how the auditory system processes acoustic information is related to the ability to discriminate changes and/or differences in intensity. This ability can be evaluated by measuring the smallest intensity difference required for a listener to judge which of two sounds is more intense or the minimum intensity increment that can be detected when added to a continuous sound.

The ability of a listener to detect small changes in intensity is most often reported as a normalized value in the Weber fraction. This measure relates the minimum discriminable change in a stimulus parameter to the base value of that parameter. For intensity, the minimum detectable difference, or difference limen (DL), is equal to $10 \log_{10}((I + DI)/I)$, where I is the intensity of the sound and DI is the minimum detectable intensity increment.

Special Consideration

- Weber's law holds that the just discriminable difference of a stimulus value will be a constant proportion of the base magnitude. For intensity processing, Weber's law holds true only if the signals are broadband. For narrower sounds, such as pure tones, discrimination of intensity increments/changes is better at higher levels than the law predicts, thus constituting the "near miss" to Weber's law.

As with detection thresholds and loudness, the discrimination of intensity also varies with frequency. Sensitivity to intensity differences is greatest for the midfrequencies (1–4 kHz), where the ear is most sensitive, and poorest for frequencies both above and below the region. Discrimination accuracy also improves with increases in signal level and reaches values of less than 1 dB as the base level reaches 40 dB HL.

Pearl

- The short increment sensitivity index (SISI) was developed because it was observed that listeners with sensorineural impairments may be able to detect smaller intensity increments than listeners with normal hearing. However, this observation is confounded by the sensation level at which individuals are tested. The SISI is typically administered at 20 dB SL. For a normal-hearing listener, this equates to hearing levels < 30 dB, regions where intensity discrimination may be reduced. Yet for an individual with significant sensorineural hearing loss, 20 dB SL could easily be well above the 40 dB level at which performance reaches asymptotic levels. It is for this reason that high-level SISIs were developed. Only individuals with retrocochlear hearing losses would fail to discriminate intensity increments of at least 1 dB when presented at fairly high levels, in dB HL (or SPL).

The ability to detect an intensity difference in a signal will also vary with signal duration. Progressively larger increments are required for intensity discrimination if the signal duration decreases below 250 msec (Florentine et al, 1987).

Mechanisms of Intensity Encoding

Description of how processing of information changes with changes in stimulus level is important for better understanding of differences in the processing abilities of normal-hearing and hearing-impaired listeners. Whereas normal-hearing listeners have a broad range of signal levels that are audible, listeners with cochlear hearing impairments must operate largely at mid to high stimulus levels. One way that intensity is encoded is by changes in the average firing rate of neurons. As level increases, so does average firing rate, but the dynamic range of the auditory system can be well over 100 dB in the normal-hearing listener, and the average intensity range over which an individual auditory nerve fiber can increase its firing rate is typically $\leq$ 30 dB. Two other mechanisms that may contribute to intensity encoding have been proposed: spread of excitation and the existence of high threshold nerve fibers (see Delgutte, 1996, for a review).

At low intensities, the movement of the basilar membrane is restricted to the regions representing the frequency composition of the signal, and displacement increases with signal level. Basilar membrane motion is nonlinear with respect to stimulus level. At high levels, intensity increments do not produce proportional increases in basilar membrane displacement as are observed at lower levels. Similarly, displacement may saturate. Associated with this saturation is a spread of excitation to adjacent areas. This spread of activity and the concomitant recruitment of more auditory nerve fibers that results may contribute to auditory processing at higher levels. Thus, basilar membrane displacement and the firing rate of individual fibers may saturate at relatively low intensities. However, a wider population of fibers is stimulated as intensity increases, and the spread of excitation becomes less focal. Yet these two findings alone cannot fully account for processing at high levels. Other mechanisms must be involved. These may include differences in the spontaneous discharge rates of different nerve fiber populations as well as differences in their dynamic ranges. It has been suggested that many fibers in the eighth cranial nerve (CN VIII) have higher thresholds of excitation. The recruitment of these fibers may play a role in the encoding of intensity, especially at higher levels. The role of the olivo-cochlear system, the role of temporal processing in the form of coincidence detectors at higher levels of the auditory system, and the impact of external noise may also contribute (Delgutte, 1996).

Pearl

- We often observe clinically that individuals with damage to the cochlea perform poorest at low intensities, but that as intensity is increased, performance is generally better. This may be because, at low signal levels, the place mechanisms are damaged, but that at higher levels, they are able to rely more on the available temporal information. In contrast, individuals with damage to the auditory nerve often show reduced function predominantly at higher levels. For example, speech discrimination scores may be poor at high levels (rollover), listeners may be unable to detect intensity increments at high levels (reduced high-level SISI scores), and tone decay may be worst at the highest levels (e.g., suprathreshold adaptation test). This may result because, at very low levels, listeners can utilize place mechanisms, but at higher intensities, where they should rely on temporal mechanisms, neural damage prevents this.

Frequency Encoding

Frequency Discrimination and Pitch Perception

Discrimination   One of the simplest ways to think of how the auditory system processes frequency information is to examine how well a listener can discriminate between sounds of different frequencies. There are several methods for measuring frequency discrimination. A listener may be presented with a sequence of two sounds and asked to judge which is higher or lower in frequency; a listener may be presented with a steady tone of a given frequency and asked to discriminate between it and a similar signal whose frequency is modulated; or a listener may be asked to detect a small and transient change in the frequency of a continuous tone. The smallest difference that is discriminable at a predetermined level of accuracy is taken as the differential threshold, again most often expressed as a proportion of the base frequency (DF/F). In general, difference limens for frequency are smallest for the midfrequencies, where the listener is most sensitive, and tend to improve with increases in signal level (Sek and Moore, 1995). For midfrequency sounds (around 1000 Hz) presented at moderate sound levels (e.g., 60 dB), differences of as little as 2 to 3 Hz are discriminable. When sound duration is reduced below ~200 msec, performance worsens.

Pitch   The psychological correlate of frequency is pitch. The function describing the relation between frequency and pitch is nonlinear. Frequencies below 1000 Hz are perceived as higher in pitch than their absolute frequency would suggest, and frequencies above 1000 Hz are perceived as slightly lower than their absolute frequency, thus compressing the range (Stevens and Volkman, 1940). Similarly, pitch may not change linearly with changes in signal level. Higher level sounds are often perceived to be exaggerated in pitch such that at high intensities, sounds below 2 kHz are perceived to be lower in pitch than they are at lower levels, and sounds above 4 kHz appear to be higher in pitch (Verschuure and van Meeteren, 1975).

Periodicity Pitch and the Missing Fundamental   The pitch of a signal is not always related only to the frequency of its components. The pitch of a complex sound may be related to the interval between the harmonics, or the fundamental frequency of the signal, even if no energy is present at the fundamental (i.e., missing fundamental). The specific harmonics that are present give the signal its characteristic timbre, but the pitch is a function of the fundamental frequency. Also, when a signal is repeated at a relatively slow repetition rate, the pitch of the signal may correspond to the rate of the repetition more than to the specific spectral components of the signal. This phenomenon is termed *periodicity pitch*.

Frequency Resolution   The ability of the ear to resolve the individual frequency components of a complex sound has a significant impact on a listener's ability to perceive the important subtleties of spectral shape in nearly all sound discriminations and identifications. When frequency resolution is very good, all or most frequency components can be detected, and the internal spectral representation of the signal will be faithful to the spectral characteristics of the sound itself, sharp and full of detail. But when resolution is poor, as is often the case in sensorineural hearing impairment, the internal spectrum of the signal may lack clarity and detail, making discrimination of similar signals difficult.

The encoding of spectral information is commonly modeled as though the periphery were composed of a bank of overlapping, band-pass filters. Each hypothetical filter corresponds to the highly frequency-specific movement of the basilar membrane. The narrower these filters, the finer will be the internal spectral representation of sounds. Frequency-resolving abilities, or estimates of the widths and shapes of the theoretical auditory filters, are most often studied behaviorally in humans through masking experiments. One sound, usually a pure tone, is presented in the presence of another sound, usually a noise masker, and the degree of interference from the masker on detection of the signal is measured.

Recent studies and knowledge of basilar membrane mechanics suggest that the auditory filter is neither rectangular nor symmetrical as critical band data may lead one to believe. The shape of the auditory filter at low signal levels is more likened to a rounded exponential with very steep slopes above the signal and more shallow slopes below it. At higher intensities, it becomes much more symmetrical and more broadly tuned (Patterson, 1976).

There are several methods by which the frequency-resolving ability of the auditory system and the shape of the auditory filter can be measured behaviorally. Two procedures, the measurement of psychoacoustic tuning curves and notched-noise masking procedures, will be discussed here. Though not all-inclusive, they provide an example of ways in which frequency resolution can be measured with relative ease.

Psychoacoustic Tuning Curves

The psychoacoustic tuning curve (Zwicker, 1977) is measured by asking listeners to detect a low-level signal, usually a pure tone at 10 to 20 dB SL, in the presence of maskers. The maskers are usually very narrow bands of noise that vary in both frequency and intensity.

Special Consideration

- Masking occurs when one sound interferes with a sensation evoked by another sound, rendering it less audible. This can be effected through a variety of mechanisms. One sound may not evoke a perception because another sound, with similar spectral and temporal characteristics, is already stimulating the system. This is the most common way in which we think of masking, but there are others. Masking can occur through suppressive mechanisms that operate when the signal and masker occupy different frequency regions, but the presence of one necessitates that higher levels are needed to excite other regions (i.e., the level of a signal must be increased to be detected) than would be required were the masker not present. Masking can also occur through adaptation, which occurs when the masker is of relatively long duration and the signal is either a transient or, at least, is much shorter than the masker. This would occur with a continuous masker and a briefer duration signal.

Pitfall

- Usually the maskers are no more than 50 Hz wide, much narrower than the one-third octave narrowband noises available on an audiometer. Therefore, to evaluate psychoacoustic tuning curves clinically would require specialized equipment and/or an external filter that could provide these very narrow spectra. Pure-tone maskers, although significantly narrow, are poor choices as maskers because their temporal structure, when combined with the tonal signal, will produce audible beats that could be a useful cue to the listener that both a signal and masker are present.

In a series of masking studies published first many years ago (Fletcher, 1940), it was noted that detection of a tonal signal decreases as the bandwidth of a noise masker, centered at the signal frequency, increases. This decrease in detectability continues until a critical masker bandwidth is reached, at which point, although masker loudness continues to grow, the masker has no additional effect on the detection of the tone. The bandwidth at which masking effects reach an asymptote is termed the *critical band*. Estimates of the critical band show that it increases with increases in signal frequency and is ~160 Hz at 1000 Hz (Scharf, 1970).

Maskers frequencies will be at, above, and below the signal frequency, with level varied to determine the minimum masker level needed to render the signal inaudible. Results consistently show that maskers falling at or near the signal are most effective at masking the signal and do so at very low levels (**Fig. 10–6**). As the frequency of the masker moves away from the signal, increasingly higher levels of masker are needed to obscure the signal. The relative increase in masker level required for masker frequencies higher than the signal frequency is greater than that for frequencies below the signal. This results in very steep high-frequency slopes and shallower low-frequency functions. Data obtained with this procedure are evaluated in terms of the bandwidth of the masking function, usually at an intensity 10 dB from the tip of the function, and in terms of efficiency, which reflects the overall level of the masked thresholds independent of the shape of the masking function. Narrower bandwidths and lower overall thresholds

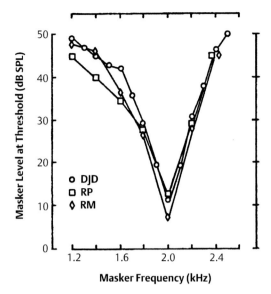

Figure 10–6 Psychoacoustic tuning curves obtained from three listeners. The signal was a 2000 Hz sinusoid. The masker was a 100 Hz wide band of noise. Data points show thresholds in dB spectrum level of the masker. (From Johnson-Davies, D., & Patterson, R. D. (1979). Psychophysical tuning curve: Restricting the listening band to the signal region. Journal of the Acoustical Society of America, 65, 765–770, with permission.)

imply better resolution and efficiency than do wider bandwidths and higher thresholds.

Controversial Point

- *Efficiency* is a term that is often used to describe higher than normal thresholds and/or reduced performance levels. There is no well-accepted definition of efficiency nor of the elements that may contribute to it. However, it is generally agreed that efficiency is a result of processing beyond the cochlea itself, perhaps in the auditory nerve or higher centers of the brain.

Notched-Noise Masking

Another procedure for measuring the width and shape of the auditory filter is the notched-noise masking technique (e.g., Patterson, 1976). A listener is asked to detect a tonal signal in the presence of a noise masker with either a flat or notched amplitude spectrum. The masker level is fixed at a fairly moderate intensity, for example, 30 to 40 dB sensation level, and signal level is varied in a search for a detection threshold. Thresholds are obtained under several masker conditions representing a variety of widths in the spectral notch. Sample data, shown in **Fig. 10–7**, suggest that thresholds are highest when the masker spectrum is flat, with no spectral notch, and decrease as a notch in the masker is widened.

Thresholds should approach quiet detection levels when the notch is wide enough so that it no longer interferes with

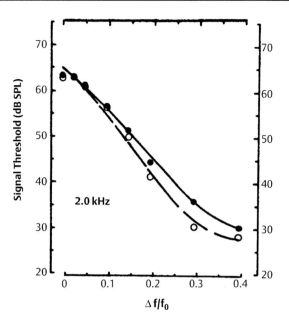

Figure 10–7 Threshold curves for a young adult listener plotted as a function of notch width in the masker. Open and filled symbols show right and left ears, respectively. The signal was a 2000 Hz sinusoid, and the masker was a noise with a spectral notch at the signal frequency. (From Patterson, R. D., Nimmo-Smith, I., Weber, D. L., & Milroy, R. (1982). The deterioration of hearing with age: Frequency selectivity, the critical ratio, the audiogram, and speech thresholds. Journal of the Acoustical Society of America, 72, 1788–1803, with permission.)

the detection of the tone, that is, when the excitation pattern of the masker and the signal no longer interfere with one another. Results are analyzed in terms of the slope of the function relating threshold to notch width. If the function drops quickly as the notch is widened, it is assumed that the frequency resolution of the listener is quite good. If instead the function is shallow with little change in threshold as notch width is increased, it is assumed that frequency-resolving abilities are poor (or that the hypothetical filters are wide). Efficiency, as with the psychoacoustic tuning curve, is indicated by the overall threshold levels (intercept of the function) and is independent of the slope of the function.

When notched-noise masking procedures are used with the noise bands and spectral notches placed asymmetrically around the signal frequency, not only the width of the auditory filter but also its shape can be mapped. When this is done, it can be seen that the shape of the auditory filter is best approximated by a rounded exponential with steeper high-frequency sides and shallower low-frequency tails, consistent with data obtained using other masking procedures and with neural tuning curve data (Patterson, 1976).

Time Course of the Auditory Filter

There has been much speculation regarding the time course of the auditory filter. The question is whether frequency-resolving ability is instantaneously as sharp as possible, or if there is a time, however brief, over which frequency resolution reaches its maximum sharpness. Moore and colleagues (1987) examined this question by asking listeners to detect very brief (e.g., 20 msec) signals that were placed at the beginning, middle, and end of a slightly longer (400 msec) masker. Their results showed that thresholds did not vary with position of the signal relative to that of the masker and therefore concluded that auditory filters do not require very much time to develop to their maximum sharpness.

Mechanisms of Frequency Encoding

Analysis of the frequency composition of a sound is largely accomplished by basilar membrane mechanics and temporal firing patterns of auditory nerve fibers. The basilar membrane performs an initial spectral analysis of incoming sounds because of its unique structural properties. High-frequency sounds cause the membrane to vibrate at the base, and lower frequency sounds cause vibration to localize at the more apical regions. The sharpness of the vibration pattern is facilitated through the active mechanisms of the outer hair cells. Because the auditory nerve is attached to the basilar membrane in an organized manner, the area of maximal vibration corresponds to a specific tonotopic map within the auditory nerve. Thus, place of excitation contributes frequency information to higher level centers of the brain. Additionally, as the basilar membrane vibrates, the pattern of auditory nerve responses also reflects temporal phase locking to signals that may be remote from the auditory nerve's characteristic frequency. Thus, auditory nerve fibers respond in a manner that reflects both the place of excitation on the basilar membrane and the temporal fine structure of the basilar membrane movement. This temporal information contributes useful frequency information to the central nervous system even though it often arises from regions adjacent to and/or remote from the place associated with the signal frequency. Thus, frequency-specific information is encoded both by spatial place mechanisms and by temporal mechanisms. The existence of both mechanisms of encoding frequency information may facilitate frequency processing across a wide range of absolute levels and signal-to-noise ratios.

Special Consideration

- This information may be useful for understanding the effect of hearing impairment on processing. For example, it could be hypothesized that listeners with cochlear damage are able to process frequency information at higher levels through the use of temporal cues in the auditory nerve's firing patterns. However, individuals with neural lesions typically have difficulty with high-level signals, potentially because of an inaccessibility of these temporal cues because of the auditory nerve damage.

Temporal Encoding

A primary source of information in every auditory signal lies in its temporal structure. Perhaps more than any other of the human senses, temporal information is critical to the discrimination and identification of signals.

Temporal Fine Structure: The Encoding of Periodicity

The auditory nerve will respond best to frequencies that vibrate maximally in the region of the basilar membrane to which the fiber is connected. However, remote frequency regions may be stimulated particularly at higher stimulus levels. The neural activity in these neurons may at first appear to be random. However, upon closer inspection, it can be seen that these neurons respond only at certain phases of the stimulus. They may not respond to every cycle, but when they do respond, their activity will be phase locked to the signal frequency, thereby providing information that encodes signal frequency, particularly when the activity of many fibers is summed. The phase-locked activity of neurons, both at and remote from the signal frequency, provides listeners with information that enables them to discriminate periodic from aperiodic signals, likely important in the perception of complex sounds (Allen and Bond, 1997), and for the detection of periodic signals in noise maskers (Allen et al, 1998; Hartmann and Pumplin, 1988). Binaural phase information plays a key role in the ability to localize sounds in the free field.

Temporal Resolution: The Detection and Discrimination of the Temporal Envelope

Gap Detection Important temporal information is also provided by the shape of a signal's envelope, which reflects the slower fluctuations in a signal. The ability of a listener to encode temporal envelope is proportional to his or her temporal resolving ability. One very basic measure of temporal resolution is provided by gap detection thresholds. To measure these thresholds, a listener is presented with a signal in which a temporal gap, or silent period, has been inserted. The listener's ability to detect the presence of the gap is measured as a function of gap size. The minimum detectable gap is used to indicate temporal resolving ability. Generally, adult listeners can detect gaps of 2 to 3 msec if the signals containing the gaps are bands of noise. With sinusoidal signals, the estimates of gap detection thresholds are slightly higher, ~4 to 5 msec (e.g., Shailer and Moore, 1983).

Pitfall

- Care must be taken when measuring gap detection thresholds in stimuli with very narrow spectral distributions, such as narrow bands of noise or pure tones. The introduction of a gap may produce spectral splatter in remote frequency regions, thus providing an additional cue to the listener that the gap is present. This cue can be masked by the use of a broad-spectrum masker with a spectral gap at the signal frequency.

Temporal Modulation Transfer Functions Another method for evaluating the temporal resolving capability of the auditory system is the temporal modulation transfer function. A listener is provided with a steady-state signal, usually a noise, and asked to discriminate it from one for which the amplitude is sinusoidally modulated. Both the rate (modulation frequency) and the depth of modulation can be varied. Generally, the minimum detectable depth of modulation is measured as a function of modulation frequency. The function that relates threshold modulation depth to modulation frequency is the temporal modulation transfer function. Using this technique, it has been suggested that listeners are very good at perceiving modulation at relative slow rates (e.g., < 50 Hz), but as the rate of modulation increases (i.e., the changes in amplitude occur more quickly over time), a greater depth of modulation is required for detection. Thresholds fall off slowly at first until ~100 Hz, at which point threshold modulation depth increases (e.g., Bacon and Viemeister, 1985). Very slow rates of modulation, below 20 Hz, are perceptible largely as rhythm and often correspond to the rate at which words are spoken in continuous speech. Slightly faster rates of modulation (20–100 Hz) correspond to a sense of roughness or unpleasantness in a sound. These modulation rates often occur when two or more frequencies are combined in a complex signal if the two frequencies fall within a critical band (~10–15% of the center frequency), so that they are not fully resolved (Pickles, 1988). The perception will be of roughness associated with the slower amplitude fluctuations produced by the combination of the components. Faster rates of modulation are more often associated with rates of vocal fold vibration and the perception of periodicity or voicing (Langner, 1992).

Duration Discrimination   Judgments about absolute duration, especially for speech sounds, are often used by listeners to infer something about speaker intent or emotion. Often when speakers wish to emphasize a word or token, they may increase its overall duration, usually by increasing the duration of the steady-state portions of the sounds, or the vowels. Yet information derived from absolute duration is seldom useful, at least in the English language, for discrimination between tokens. Small and Campbell (1962) showed that duration discrimination is good for very low frequency signals but that performance may worsen for higher frequencies (e.g., 5000 Hz). In general, listeners require proportionally larger changes to discriminate duration differences as the base duration of the signal increases (Abel, 1972). Thus, for durations around 100 msec, a change of ~15 msec is required for discrimination, but for longer stimuli, 1000 msec, ~60 msec change is required. Discrimination of the duration of a silent interval is slightly better, ~15 msec for 320 msec base silences (Divenyi and Danner, 1977). These findings are roughly independent of the spectral content of the signals but may vary with overall intensity, being slightly poorer at lower levels than at high.

Detection of Onset/Offset Asynchronies   For multiple component signals, the onset/offset characteristics of the components may provide useful information to the listener. Listeners are good at detecting onset asynchronies,

being able to discriminate onset disparities of 1 msec if the components are harmonically related (e.g., Zera and Green, 1993). If the components are not harmonically related, discrimination accuracy may be much poorer by factors as large as 50 times. The detection of offset asynchronies is somewhat poorer. Even with harmonically related components, 3 to 10 msec may be required. Sensitivity to onset/offset asynchronies may be important to listeners, as it often indicates whether component frequencies arise from a single or multiple sources. Sounds arising from a single source often have simultaneous onsets and offsets.

Judgments of Temporal Order   Individuals are usually good at discriminating the temporal order of sounds, particularly if the sounds presented in a particular order have meaning. For example, the order of sounds in some sequences of speech elements (e.g., morphemes or simple words) is important such that if the order of elements were to be changed, the item would no longer have the same meaning. In those instances, listeners can discriminate order changes for sounds 7 msec or shorter (e.g., Divenyi and Hirsh, 1974). However, if the sounds are unrelated, the listener may require slightly longer durations (10–20 msec) for the same level of discrimination accuracy (Hirsh, 1988; Warren, 1974).

♦ The Perception of Complex Sounds

Much of what has been discussed so far has focused on the processing of discrete features of acoustically relatively simple sounds. This approach fails to capture the full range and intricacy of auditory processing. It is only when we examine how more complex sounds are processed that the amazing capabilities of the human auditory system are evident. The topics selected for inclusion in this section are by no means exhaustive, but it is hoped that they will provide the reader with an introduction to the range of abilities and processes that contribute to the processing of complex auditory signals.

Profile Analysis

Many natural sounds have similar frequency content, but the relative distribution of energy within their bandwidth is different. Such differences in the shape of the amplitude spectra are useful in discrimination and identification tasks. Classic examples of listeners' use of spectral shape information can be found in the importance of formant ratios for the identification of vowels (Peterson and Barney, 1952) and the importance of frequency contours in the onset spectra of stop consonants (Stevens and Blumstein, 1978). To perceive spectral shape requires resolution of the primary frequency components and assessment of the relative amplitudes of those components, thus necessitating good frequency resolution and cross-channel level processing. The ability to perceive differences in spectral shape is termed *profile analysis* (Green, 1988).

In a standard intensity discrimination task, traditional models of intensity processing assumed that the listener evaluated the relative energy levels arriving from the auditory filter centered at the signal frequency. Comparison is made between levels of sounds, and the listener decides which of the sounds is more or less intense than the other. This task is thus affected by the listener's ability to hold a representation of the sound intensity in memory. If the time between stimulus presentations is increased from 250 to 8000 msec, intensity discrimination thresholds can decrease by as much as 10 dB (Green et al, 1983), reflecting these memory limitations. However, if the listener is provided with a background sound, such as a noise or other tones, performance may improve relative to that obtained with no background sound and will be unaffected by changes in the interstimulus interval. Furthermore, a listener's ability to judge intensity changes remains high, even if the overall level of the background sound is varied randomly from presentation to presentation (thereby removing absolute level information), so long as the signal-to-background ratio is kept constant. This suggests that listeners make simultaneous, within-signal comparisons of levels at different frequency regions, rather than between signals at a fixed frequency in performing intensity discrimination tasks for which a background sound is present. Thus, the overall shape of the signal spectrum is the important factor.

Models of Encoding Spectral Shape Information

At least two models of auditory processing have been suggested to explain listeners' discrimination of spectral shape. When the component frequencies lie within a critical band, it is likely that they compute an overall estimate of average frequency, or pitch. Feth and colleagues (1982) have shown that if a listener is presented with two tonal complexes, each of which is composed of two identical frequency components but for which one component is more intense than the other, a listener can discriminate when the relative levels are reversed. For example, a listener is presented with two complexes, one consisting of frequencies f and $f + Df$, such that f is more intense than $f + Df$, and another, such that $f + Df$ is more intense than f. If both f and $f + Df$ fall within one critical band, the two complexes will have the same overall RMS value and the same frequency components, yet they are discriminable from one another. The listener likely evaluates the complexes by computing a mean frequency that is weighted by the amplitude of each component. The overall average frequency and the corresponding pitch value will be higher when $f + Df$ is more intense than f and lower when their relative amplitudes are reversed. Thus, this spectral shape discrimination is made based on an extracted feature of the complex that corresponds to its overall pitch, which is computed from weighting the energy levels in the relative frequency components.

To explain spectral shape discrimination for components that are widely spaced in frequency may require some other model of auditory processing. Durlach et al (1986) proposed an excitation model in which peripheral processing occurs in multiple parallel filters. As a sound is heard, the listener performs a spectral decomposition of the sound, thus analyzing the relative energy levels in a range of frequencies. These theoretical filter outputs, each of which may contain some noise due to inaccuracies, for example, in peripheral resolution, are combined at a more central level where a rough estimate of spectral shape is formed. This central representation may also have some error associated with it (often modeled as a form of central internal noise), but the error is in the way in which cross-frequency information is combined rather than in the quality of the analysis at each frequency. Internal correlation between the outputs of the independent frequencies is performed, and the listener uses this information to compute the likelihood that it may or may not contain a signal.

Comodulation Masking Release

Another interesting phenomenon in auditory processing that reflects cross-channel processing is observed in comodulation masking release (CMR; Hall et al, 1984). The listener is asked to detect a masked signal. Usually the signal is a tone, and the masker is a narrow band of noise centered at the signal frequency. Thresholds increase as the noise band is increased until the bandwidth of the masker exceeds the critical band, as expected. Yet, if the masker is amplitude modulated very slowly, thresholds will improve as the bandwidth of the masker is increased beyond the critical band, contrary to critical band theory and inconsistent with our understanding of the mechanisms of masking. These results are obtained even though no energy in the masker surrounding the signal is removed and the overall level of the masker, because of its broader bandwidth, is much higher. In similar experiments, detection is evaluated for conditions in which the masker is a narrow band of noise placed at the signal frequency, and there is a flanking noise masker added at a remote frequency. When the flanking (off-frequency) masker is comodulated with the on-frequency masker, detection of the signal improves. However, if the flanking masker has an independent temporal structure from that at the signal frequency, detection thresholds show no change. These findings suggest that the auditory system is able to compare the temporal similarities in the masker at regions at, and remote from, the signal frequency in a manner similar to profile analysis. The amount of unmasking that occurs in the presence of temporally similar maskers at remote frequencies varies from 5 to 20 dB, depending on the specific stimulus and masker conditions. The theoretical explanations for CMR are many and outside the scope of this chapter, but its existence is a challenge to our understanding of how the auditory system processes complex sounds. A good review of CMR is provided by Green (1993).

Pearl

- Detection of similarities in modulation patterns across frequencies may provide a useful cue to the perception of sound sources. A single vibrating source may produce many frequency components, but their temporal modulation patterns will be similar and will reflect the vibration of the source. Thus, sounds that are not modulated with those produced by the source will not be perceived as part of it but as a separate source. Modulation similarities and differences across frequencies may provide an essential cue for the separation of sound sources in space and may aid in the discrimination of signals in noise.

Classification of Complex Sounds

One of the primary goals of auditory processing is to assign meaning to sounds. Among the ways in which meaning is assigned to sounds is classification, which requires the perception of similarities in individual features and/or patterns of features. One method that has been used successfully to study the processing of complex sounds and reveal the acoustic features and feature patterns that listeners attend to when recognizing sounds is a multidimensional scaling (MDS) analysis of paired comparisons data. Listeners are asked to rate the relative similarity (or dissimilarity) of all possible pairs of a set of stimuli. The similarity ratings are used to place the stimuli in a multidimensional space (generally euclidean) of few dimensions. Stimuli that are rated as very similar are placed closer together in that space than are stimuli that are rated as dissimilar. The axes or dimensions in the space are assumed to represent the perceptual attributes of the sounds that were used in making the judgments. Each attribute may correspond to a single auditory feature or to a combination of features. Howard and Silverman (1976) used an MDS analysis to evaluate listeners' processing of unfamiliar complex sounds. Their results suggested that encoding included both spectral and temporal characteristics of the sounds but that the relative weighting given to features varied with the previous experiences and training of the listener. (Listeners with musical training were more likely to place greater weight on temporal cues than did listeners with no musical training who weighted spectral cues more heavily.) Christensen and Humes (1996) showed that individual differences in dimension weightings can be useful for predicting classification and categorization responses. In their study, dimensions that were weighted most heavily by a listener in the paired comparisons task tended to be those used by that listener to form categories in a subsequent classification task. MDS analyses of similarity data are therefore a useful tool for discovering the underlying structure of listeners' perceptions of complex sounds and can be used successfully with young children as well as adults (Allen and Bond, 1997).

Information Processing

Masking

The way that acoustic features are combined to form categories, particularly when there is variability in those features or in the context in which they are presented, has received much attention in psychoacoustics. Watson and colleagues (Watson and Foyle, 1985; Watson and Kelley, 1981) were among the earliest investigators to study listeners' ability to detect subtle changes in acoustically well-controlled complex sounds. Their work showed that the perception of changes in the components of a complex sound is not easily predicted by a listener's ability to detect similar changes in an isolated sound. The presence of other sounds (context), even when they are irrelevant to the task, can reduce detection and discrimination accuracy, especially if they are similar to or more salient than the relevant features. For example, using word length sequences consisting of ~10 brief duration tone pips (~40 msec), Watson and Kelley (1981) found that listeners' ability to discriminate changes to the frequency, duration, or level of a target component in the sequence were ~10 to 20 Hz, 6 to 8 msec, and 2 to 3 dB, respectively. These measures are quite good and perhaps only slightly poorer than for sounds in isolation. Yet if the acoustic features of the nontarget components, the context tones, are varied from trial to trial, performance became much worse. This variation in the context tones is termed *informational masking*. Because the auditory periphery is likely processing simple and complex sounds in a similar manner, changes in performance associated with context effects are most likely attributable to more central auditory processing abilities (Watson and Foyle, 1985). Similar effects of uncertainty associated with stimulus and context variance also extend to the processing of components that are presented simultaneously (Green, 1988; Neff and Callaghan, 1988; Neff and Jesteadt, 1996).

Information Integration

Although variance can create uncertainty that is detrimental to the processing of complex sounds, it can also contribute to their encoding. Consider the task of learning a new word. If every time the word is heard it is exactly the same, as though it were a recorded signal, it would be difficult to recognize that same word if spoken by a different speaker, perhaps with a different accent or intonation pattern. It is only by hearing the word many times, in many contexts, and spoken by many speakers that the critical features of the item can be determined, enabling recognition in different contexts. Through the normal variability associated with a sound's repetition, the critical features are encoded. Thus, variability or uncertainty can be equated to information. As another example, consider a task in which a set of items are to be organized. If the items are very similar, this task will be very difficult, as there will be no features along which the items vary to provide dimensions along which the items can be grouped. Variability in the features of the items provides information that can be used to discriminate between them.

To resolve and make use of the uncertainty that naturally accompanies variability, listeners must attend to patterns in and relationships between features. This requires fine discriminations along each acoustic dimension, an ability that is related to peripheral resolving abilities, and integration of information from each feature into a meaningful whole, a process that is likely performed more centrally in the system. Both levels of processing can be tested auditorily using a sample discrimination paradigm (Berg and Robinson, 1987; Lutfi, 1989, 1990, 1992) in which a listener is asked to discriminate between two complex sounds. The components for each of the sounds are drawn from overlapping distributions of features such that some feature values may be equally likely to be drawn from either distribution, whereas other values have a higher probability of being drawn from one or the other. If only one sample of a feature is available, performance will be limited by the amount of overlap in the two distributions from which the features are selected. As greater numbers of features or components are sampled, the listener's performance will improve. Results have shown that performance in a sample discrimination task will be limited by two factors: the listener's ability to discriminate between feature values (or components) sampled and the ability to combine, or integrate, information obtained from the total number of features sampled. If the components sampled are not discriminably different from one another, then drawing more of them will provide no additional information. This limitation is related directly to peripheral resolving abilities. In contrast, limits to the individual's ability to integrate multiple bits of information is likely a more central process. It is the limits to integration ability that prevents performance from increasing linearly as the number of sampled components increases. Performance will improve at a rate consistent with the individual's integration ability and will reach an asymptote that reflects his or her capacity for information processing. In general, d′ in a sample discrimination task increases with the cubed root of the number of components sampled and will reach an asymptote at ∼2 to 3 bits of information, with each bit representing a dimension along which a stimulus can vary (see Lutfi, 1989). The sample discrimination technique holds promise for elucidating the nature and magnitude of changes in complex sound processing that occur with maturation (Allen and Nelles, 1996) or hearing impairment (Doherty and Lutfi, 1996).

Weighting Functions and Attention

It is important to know what information was used when a listener makes a decision about a complex sound. One way to perform such an analysis is through the use of COSS functions (Berg, 1989). With this technique, a listener's decision about a stimulus is analyzed according to the values of the individual components within the complex signal. Correlation functions are derived between the acoustic parameters of each component and the listener's response. In this way, the relative weight the listener gives to each component in making his or her decision can be determined. Using this technique, it has been shown that listeners make comparisons of acoustic features across components within

a stimulus, that they weight reliable information more heavily than unreliable information, and that when the intensity of a feature is increased, it may be weighted more heavily than lower intensity features, even if it is a less reliable parameter (Berg and Green, 1990). This form of analysis has the potential of being extremely useful in facilitating our understanding of what responses a listener makes when asked to perform a task involving complex signals and can provide useful information as to why those specific responses are made. It can tell far more about the features an individual listens to when performing a discrimination task than can be determined from a single estimate of performance, such as percent correct or d′.

The weighting of various acoustic features of a complex sound, derived either from MDS analyses of dissimilarity data or from COSS analyses of discrimination data, is in many ways an indication of the salience of that feature and/or the attention given to it by the listener. An extension of research in feature salience is to evaluate the extent to which a listener can intentionally focus on a sound or on specific acoustic features of that sound, particularly in the presence of other sometimes irrelevant and often interfering and distracting features or sounds.

One example of the role of auditory research in selective attention can be found in the study of auditory attention bands. This work asks questions about the extent to which listeners can focus attention on a single frequency region and how narrowly can that auditory attention be focused. The dominant technique used to study auditory attention is a probe-signal method (Greenberg and Larkin, 1968) in which a listener is led to expect a signal of a certain frequency. On an infrequent and randomly distributed percentage of the trials, the signal is of a slightly different frequency, but it is presented at a level such that if the listener were expecting the signal, it would be detected with a high degree of accuracy. Using this technique, it has been shown that many listeners do not detect the off-frequency probes as well as the on-frequency expected signals. In fact, detection accuracy appears to decrease for the probes in a way that mirrors that derived in studies of frequency resolution, suggesting that listeners are able to focus attention on a very narrowly tuned region of the basilar membrane. Performance is highly contingent upon the stimulus (and masker) parameters. When the signals are presented with noise maskers, the attention bands appear to stay relatively focused so long as the noise is not gated simultaneously with the signal. If the maskers are continuous, the measured attention bands are usually quite sharp (Scharf et al, 1987). If, however, the signals and maskers are gated on and off together, there is much more individual variability, and only some listeners show very sharply tuned functions (Dai and Buus, 1991). This suggests that with brief duration signals with similarly gated maskers, listeners may not be able to focus frequency-specific attention as sharply as possible. Similarly, attention bands may vary with signal duration in spite of the gating characteristics of the masker. When the signals are of a very short duration (e.g., 5 msec), attention bands are wider than those measured in response to longer duration signals (e.g., 295 msec) even though auditory filter widths, as measured with notched-noise maskers, are equivalent at the two durations (Wright and Dai, 1994). Collectively, these results suggest that a listener is less likely to use a highly frequency-specific listening strategy for the detection and identification of very brief duration tones, that as signal duration exceeds the temporal integration limits of the ear and as long as the signal and masker are temporally discrete from one another, listeners are capable of a very highly tuned, frequency-specific analysis.

In summary, there are many ways to study a listener's ability to process complex auditory signals that go beyond those used in traditional audiometry. Furthermore, there is strong evidence to suggest that many of these information-processing abilities, including detection and discrimination in instances of uncertainty, information integration, and auditory attention, can be evaluated in children and do show strong age-related trends (Allen and Nelles, 1996; Allen and Wightman, 1995; Bargones and Werner, 1994). These tasks may therefore be useful in evaluating the auditory-processing abilities of children, as well as adults, and may ultimately shed light on the nature of auditory-processing disorders.

Binaural Hearing and Sound Localization

How the auditory system combines information arriving at the two ears and the manner in which sounds are localized in space are areas of psychoacoustics for which tremendous advancements have been made very recently. In addition to the importance of understanding binaural hearing for completing our appreciation of the richness and complexity of auditory processing, binaural hearing research has important technological applications relevant to the design and fitting of assistive listening devices and the creation of virtual spaces.

Much of what is known about binaural hearing comes from studies in which listeners are presented with stimuli under headphones. In this way, the signals arriving at each ear can be well controlled acoustically, and the effects of interaural disparities on sound perceptions can be studied. Binaural images produced by presenting dichotic sounds under headphones remain perceptually inside the listener's head and are not perceived as originating from sources external to the listener. It is only when sounds are perceived outside the head that localization, rather than lateralization, may be studied. This section will begin with an introduction to binaural hearing as observed in headphone studies and proceed to a discussion of listening in real (and virtual) three-dimensional auditory environments.

Discrimination of Interaural Time and Intensity Differences Presented under Headphones

The human auditory system is very sensitive to even small interaural time and intensity disparities. When a signal is presented to the two ears at equal intensities, the image will be perceived in the center of the head. If the intensity at one ear is increased slightly, the image will shift toward the ear with the more intense signal (Blauert, 1983a). As little as a 1 dB difference is sufficient to move the image off the center. When the interaural intensity differences are larger (on the order of 10 dB), the image will be fully lateralized to the ear receiving the more intense signal, and the listener will be unaware that a signal is even being presented to the other ear.

> ### Pearl
>
> - A useful technique for the biologic calibration of earphones is to listen to a sound presented binaurally at equal levels. If the sound appears lateralized away from the center of the head, it is possible that the output from the two earphones may not be perfectly matched and should be calibrated.

Similarly, the time of arrival of sounds at the two ears will also exert a strong influence on the perceived lateralization of the sound (Blauert, 1983a). When the sounds are presented simultaneously, the perception will be of a sound located in the center of the head, but when one ear leads the other ear by as little as 10 μs, the image will be shifted toward the leading ear. With a 1 msec interaural time difference, the image will be fully lateralized to the leading ear. Thus, the binaural auditory system is highly sensitive to both interaural time and intensity differences.

Interaural Disparities in the Free Field

When a sound is presented in the free field, the image arrives at both ears, but each receives a slightly different image in accordance with intensity and phase differences at the two ears. Intensity differences result as some sounds are diffracted when they reach the head, such that the ear on the side opposite the sound source will receive a slightly less intense image. Sounds are most likely to be reflected off the head if their wavelength is small relative to the diameter of the head, producing a lower intensity representation at the far ear relative to that arriving at the near ear. This is termed the *head shadow effect*. Assuming that the diameter of the adult head is roughly 18 cm, sounds with frequencies above ~2000 Hz will be subjected to the head shadow and produce interaural intensity differences. (A wavelength (λ) of 18 cm corresponds to a frequency (f) of ~1907 Hz, given that the speed of sound (c) is 343.2 M/s ($f = c/\lambda$)). The magnitude of the head shadow will vary not only with the frequency of the sound but also with the position of the sound source. The greatest interaural intensity difference will be achieved when the sound source is located directly opposite to one ear, and the signal is greater than 2000 Hz. It may be as much as 20 dB for the higher frequencies. When the sound source is located directly in front of, above, or behind the listener, no interaural intensity differences will be observed. Interaural intensity differences are therefore useful for localizing a sound in space if the sound is high frequency and located sufficiently off the midline (Wightman and Kistler, 1993).

Lower frequency sounds, with wavelengths that are larger than the human head, will arrive at each ear with little or no interaural intensity differences. At these frequencies, the dominant cue for localization is provided by interaural time disparities. Sounds will arrive first at the leading ear and later at the lagging ear. This interaural time difference is, on average, slightly more than 650 µs in the adult when the sound is directly opposite one ear (Wightman and Kistler, 1993). For lower frequency sounds, this will be perceived as a phase lag. Higher frequencies will also be delayed in time of arrival at the lagging ear relative to the leading ear, but the differences are less likely to be discriminable to the listener, as phase coding is strongest at lower frequencies. At higher frequencies, the interaural time delay is more likely to be perceived as a delay in the envelope of the sound rather than as a phase delay of the individual components.

In the free field, interaural time and intensity differences are available as cues to a sound's location. Studies examining the relative salience of these cues suggest that interaural time differences are generally the dominant cue used by listeners in determining the source of a sound (Wightman and Kistler, 1997), unless the cues are not plausible. If an unreasonably large interaural difference is presented to a listener (e.g., one that is greater than that possible in the space), and that cue is made to conflict with a plausible interaural intensity difference, the listener will ignore the time cue and bias his or her judgments toward the intensity cue even though intensity is generally a weaker cue (Hartmann, 1997).

However, interaural time and intensity cues are often ambiguous. For example, when a sound is presented in the median sagittal plane, it will arrive simultaneously at the two ears with equal intensity. No interaural disparities will be present. The ambiguity produced is similar to that obtained for many other sound locations. Imagine an axis running through the two ears. As concentric circles are drawn around that axis, parallel to the direction in which the listener is facing, it can be seen that sound sources placed anywhere on one of those circles will provide equal interaural time cues, in spite of the fact that these points on the circle may be above, below, in front of, and behind the listener. This is commonly called the "cone of confusion," a region for which the binaural cues are ambiguous and could potentially lead to localization errors. However, listeners seldom make such confusions in the real world because most sounds are broadband. Thus, ambiguities for individual components will not be as strong when considered within the context of the entire stimulus. Also, position-dependent, monaural spectral cues are available.

Monaural Cues to Sound Localization

The ability to correctly localize sounds is likely facilitated through the use of broadband, monaural cues provided by the filtering characteristics of the pinna. For example, when a sound is in front of a listener, the spectral representation arriving at the tympanic membrane will be different from that of a sound arriving from behind the listener, even if the interaural cues are the same (Wightman and Kistler, 1989). The filtering characteristics of the pinna are position dependent; this filtering likely provides strong

information for localizing sounds in the free field. Many researchers (e.g., Wightman and Kistler, 1989) have suggested that these spectral cues play an important role in the determination of elevation and in the resolution of front-back confusions arising from ambiguous interaural time and intensity differences.

It must be noted that although interaural time and intensity disparities and spectral filtering by the pinna are the dominant cues used to position sounds in space, other, nonauditory factors, including vision, memory, and listener expectations, also play a role. For example, the well-known ventriloquism effect is a strong example of how visual cues can override auditory cues in sound localization (Warren et al, 1981). Even though a listener may be well aware that a puppet, or a figure on a movie or television screen, is not actually speaking, the sound is perceived as coming from those sources. There is a strong bias toward perceiving sounds as originating from a likely source. It is for this reason that many studies of sound localization are conducted in chambers where listeners' eyes are covered, so that they will not see speaker locations and thus be biased to those locations in the localization of auditory signals with which they are presented.

The Precedence Effect

The free field condition is also complicated by the acoustics of the room, or space, in which the sound is presented. Most rooms are reverberant; that is, sounds will be reflected off hard surfaces in the room and back to the listener as secondary and delayed sources. The listener is thus faced with several waveforms from which to extract source localization information. There will be the direct sound coming from the source and the reflected waveforms that are highly correlated with the direct source but come from locations that may be disparate from the source. If the reflected sounds arrive at the listener's ear with very little delay relative to the direct source, they may be integrated into the direct waveform and increase the sound level of the signal. However, if they arrive somewhat later and are significantly out of phase with the direct sound, they may produce an interference that degrades the quality of the signal. Furthermore, if the reflected sounds arrive late relative to the direct sound, they may be perceived as an echo. To localize a sound source, a listener must determine which of the many waveforms being received is the direct waveform and arising from the source and which are reflected and arising from the surfaces of the room, thereby providing misleading localization information. It is the functioning of the binaural auditory system that tells the listener which waveform arises from the source and where that source is located. Potentially interfering reflections are suppressed (dereverberation).

The precedence effect holds that a sound source location will be determined by the waveform that reaches the listener first, even if later arriving reflected waveforms are more intense. Consider a signal presented to a listener in a reverberant room. If the reflected waveform arrives after a very short delay (1 msec for a click) relative to the direct waveform, perception of the source location will be determined from an average of the acoustic cues provided by each waveform. However, the relative weight given to the lagging waveform will decrease as the magnitude of the delay increases. This is called *summing localization*.

When the reflected sound arrives slightly later (1–4 msec for a click stimulus) relative to the direct waveform, the perception of the source location will be affected only slightly by the reflected source, largely in terms of increasing error around the true location (localization blur), but not altering the location in the direction of the origin of the reflected source. The reflected sound will add with the direct source in such a way as to give the perception of the room acoustics, or spaciousness. If the reflected sound arrives with a greater delay (5–10 msec for a click), it may be perceived as an additional sound, or an echo. When signals are longer in duration than a click, such as would be the case for speech and music, much longer reverberation times produce integrated, single images than for clicks. The upper limit for reverberation before the reflected waves cause destructive rather than constructive interference is 10, 50, and 80 msec, for clicks, speech, and music, respectively (Blauert, 1983b).

A Note on Room Acoustics

Rooms with no reverberation, such as an anechoic chamber, are dead, and sounds appear dull and flat in them. However, rooms with very long reverberation times may also sound poor, with reflected sounds adding to the direct sounds in an interfering and destructive manner. This is often the case in very large rooms with poor acoustics, such as school gymnasiums. A room with good acoustics is one in which the reverberation time is sufficient to give a feeling of spaciousness but not so long as to produce destructive interference. That only one image is perceived even though several waveforms are received at the listener's ear is attributable to the binaural hearing capabilities of the listener. These effects are not observed in the absence of binaural hearing. For example, when a recording is made in a room through a single microphone, the quality of the sound will be poor. The reflected waves will interfere with the direct source, making the sound appear distorted and possibly difficult to understand. It is only because of the "dereverberation" provided by the precedence effect in the free field that clarity of sound is maintained in highly reverberant rooms. Thus, binaural hearing plays an important role in sound source separation, location, and discrimination in noise.

◆ Summary

Audiology has drawn much from psychoacoustics and will likely continue to do so in the future. Much of our methodology in behavioral assessment was refined by psychophysicists, enabling us to evaluate the hearing abilities of individual listeners with efficiency and rigor. As well, our understanding of normal hearing abilities and how those abilities may be impaired when there is damage or dysfunction in the auditory system comes largely from psychoacoustic study. There have been, particularly in the past, limitations to extending psychoacoustic findings to the clinic.

One of those limitations was that most earlier research in psychoacoustics focused on understanding how humans, in general, processed sounds. The aim was to define group, or average, trends. Although for many tasks this is reasonable because between-subject variability is relatively low (e.g., quiet detection thresholds), for others, the individual differences, and hence the between-subject variability, may be large. This is unfortunate because clinically we do not typically face a group of individuals but rather a single individual, and we must decide if his or her ability to perform an auditory task is within the range acceptable for normal-hearing listeners or whether it reflects an impairment of some sort. Thus, we must be cognizant of individual variability and the extent to which data from an individual can be compared with that averaged across a group of listeners. More recently, psychoacoustic studies have addressed issues of individual variance, particularly as they relate to the processing of more complex sounds where individual differences appear to be largest (Neff et al, 1993) and to the auditory processing ability of children (e.g., Allen and Wightman, 1994, 1995). Thus, we are learning not only how people should perform on average, but also what is the acceptable range of variability and how this variability changes with the task and with listener age.

Another limitation in the direct application of psychoacoustic research to clinical practice is that the psychoacoustic procedures are often lengthy and tedious, certainly not what is acceptable in a clinical practice. In many psychoacoustic studies, the participants are trained listeners with hours and thousands of trials of practice and experience. Given that practice and training effects may sometimes be large, it is difficult to extrapolate from these highly practiced listeners what performance should be expected from a relatively naive patient whom you are seeing for the first time. Similarly, it is unrealistic to expect that your client should perform thousands of trials before you can begin to assess his or her hearing abilities. Fortunately, some more recent studies have presented data from more naive listeners and have attempted to develop procedures that enable quicker estimates of performance.

Many of our clients are either children or elderly individuals, and much less is known about these populations than about the performance of young, healthy adult listeners. Until recently, relatively little was known about age-related changes in psychoacoustic abilities, often because few methods were available with which to test young children or very elderly listeners. Again, this pattern is changing, and very recently there has been an increase in interest and available data examining the psychoacoustic performance of a wide age range of listeners. Most notable is an interest in psychoacoustic performance in the assessment of (central) auditory processing disorders for which extensive measures of temporal and spectral resolution, the processing of complex auditory patterns, and sound localization and lateralization are recommended (e.g., American Speech-Language-Hearing Association, 2005).

Lastly, psychoacoustic studies have typically relied on advanced and often complicated equipment and computer software. The stimuli and techniques often required facilities, software, and equipment that were not available in the clinic. Audiologists have been, and sometimes continue to be, limited by what their clinical audiometer can do. However, the future is bright for bringing advanced psychoa-

coustic assessment into the clinic. The availability of small personal computers and highly sophisticated software that is now commercially available hold promise for the growth of behavioral testing and the further integration of psychoacoustics and audiology.

References

Abel, S. M. (1972). Duration discrimination of noise and tone bursts. Journal of the Acoustical Society of America, 51, 1219–1223.

Allen, P., & Bond, C. (1997). Multidimensional scaling of complex sounds by school-aged children and adults. Journal of the Acoustical Society of America, 102, 2255–2263.

Allen, P., Jones, R., & Slaney, P. (1998). The role of level, spectral, and temporal cues in children's detection of masked signals. Journal of the Acoustical Society of America, 104, 2997–3005.

Allen, P., & Nelles, J. (1996). Development of auditory information integration abilities. Journal of the Acoustical Society of America, 100, 1043–1051.

Allen, P., & Wightman, F. (1994). Psychometric functions for children's detection of tones in noise. Journal of Speech and Hearing Research, 37, 205–215.

Allen, P., & Wightman, F. (1995). Effects of signal and masker uncertainty on children's detection. Journal of Speech and Hearing Research, 38, 503–511.

American National Standards Institute. (2004). Specification for audiometers (ANSI S3.6–2004). New York: Author.

American Speech-Language-Hearing Association. (2005). (Central) auditory processing disorders. Retrieved from http://www.asha.org/members/deskref-journals/deskref/default

Bacon, S. P., & Viemeister, N. F. (1985). Temporal modulation transfer functions in normal- and hearing-impaired ears. Audiology, 24, 117–134.

Bargones, J. Y., & Werner, L. A. (1994). Adults listen selectively, infants do not. Psychological Science, 5, 170–174.

Berg, B. G. (1989). Analysis of weights in multiple observation tasks. Journal of the Acoustical Society of America, 86, 1743–1746.

Berg, B. G., & Green, D. M. (1990). Spectral weights in profile listening. Journal of the Acoustical Society of America, 88, 758–766.

Berg, B., & Robinson, D. (1987). Multiple observations and internal noise. Journal of the Acoustical Society of America, 81(Suppl. 1), S33.

Blauert, J. (1983a). Spatial hearing. Cambridge, MA: MIT Press.

Blauert, J. (1983b). Review paper: Psychoacoustic binaural phenomena. In R. Klinke & R. Hartmann (Eds.), Hearing—Physiological bases and psychophysics. Berlin: Springer-Verlag.

Christensen, L. A., & Humes, L. E. (1996). Identification of multidimensional complex sounds having parallel dimension structure. Journal of the Acoustical Society of America, 99, 2307–2315.

Dai, H. P., & Buus, S. (1991). Effect of gating the masker on frequency-selective listening. Journal of the Acoustical Society of America, 89, 1816–1818.

Delgutte, B. (1996). Physiological models for basic auditory perceptions. In H. L. Hawkins, T. N. McMullen, A. N. Popper, & R. R. Fay (Eds.), Auditory computation. New York: Springer-Verlag.

Divenyi, P. L., & Danner, W. F. (1977). Discrimination of time intervals marked by brief acoustic pulses of various intensities and spectra. Perception & Psychophysics, 21, 124–142.

Divenyi, P. L., & Hirsh, I. J. (1974). Identification of temporal order in three tone sequences. Journal of the Acoustical Society of America, 56, 144–151.

Doherty, K. A., & Lutfi, R. A. (1996). Spectral weights for overall level discrimination in listeners with sensorineural hearing loss. Journal of the Acoustical Society of America, 99, 1053–1058.

Durlach, N. I., Braida, L. D., & Ito, Y. (1986). Toward a model for discrimination of broadband signals. Journal of the Acoustical Society of America, 80, 63–72.

Feth, L. L., O'Malley, H., & Ramsey, J., Jr. (1982). Pitch of unresolved, two-component complex tones. Journal of the Acoustical Society of America, 72(5), 1408–1412.

Fletcher, H. (1940). Auditory patterns. Reviews of Modern Physics, 12, 47–65.

Fletcher, H., & Munson, W. A. (1933). Loudness: Its definition, measurement and calculation. Journal of the Acoustical Society of America, 5, 82–108.

Florentine, M., Buus, S., & Mason, C. R. (1987). Level discrimination as a function of level for tones from 0.25 to 16 kHz. Journal of the Acoustical Society of America, 81, 1528–1541.

Gravetter, F., & Lockhead, G. R. (1973). Criterial range as a frame of reference for stimulus judgment. Psychological Review, 80, 203–216.

Green, D. M. (1988). Profile analysis: Auditory intensity discrimination. New York: Oxford University Press.

Green, D. M. (1993). Auditory intensity discrimination, In W. N. Yost, A. Popper, & R. R. Fay (Eds.), Human psychophysics. New York: Springer-Verlag.

Green, D. M., Kidd, G. Jr., & Picardi, M. C. (1983). Successive versus simultaneous comparison in auditory intensity discrimination. Journal of the Acoustical Society of America, 73, 639–643.

Green, D. M., & Swets, J. A. (1988). Signal detection theory and psychophysics. New York: John Wiley & Sons.

Greenberg, G. Z., & Larkin, W. D. (1968). Frequency-response characteristics of auditory observers detection signals of a single frequency in noise: The probe signal method. Journal of the Acoustical Society of America, 44(6), 1513–1523.

Hall, J. W., Haggard, M. P., & Fernendes, M. A. (1984). Detection in noise by spectro-temporal pattern analysis. Journal of the Acoustical Society of America, 76, 50–56.

Hartmann, W. M. (1997). Listening in a room and the precedence effect. In R. H. Gilkey & T. R. Anderson (Eds.), Binaural and spatial hearing in real and virtual environments. Mahwah, NJ: Lawrence Erlbaum Associates.

Hartmann, W. M. (1998). Signals, sounds, and sensations. New York: Springer-Verlag.

Hartmann, W. M., & Pumplin, J. (1988). Noise power fluctuations and the masking of sine signals. Journal of the Acoustical Society of America, 83, 2277–2289.

Hirsh, I. J. (1988). Auditory perception of temporal order. Journal of the Acoustical Society of America, 31, 759–767.

Howard, J. H., & Silverman, E. B. (1976). A multidimensional scaling analysis of 16 complex sounds. Perception & Psychophysics, 19, 193–200.

Johnson-Davies, D., & Patterson, R. D. (1979). Psychophysical tuning curve: Restricting the listening band to the signal region. Journal of the Acoustical Society of America, 65, 765–770.

Langner, G. (1992). Periodicity coding in the auditory system. Hearing Research, 60, 115–142.

Levitt, H. (1971). Transformed up-down methods in psychoacoustics. Journal of the Acoustical Society of America, 49, 467–477.

Lutfi, R. A. (1989). Informational processing of complex sounds: 1. Intensity discrimination. Journal of the Acoustical Society of America, 86, 934–944.

Lutfi, R. A. (1990). Informational processing of complex sounds: 2. Cross-dimensional analysis. Journal of the Acoustical Society of America, 87, 2141–2148.

Lutfi, R. A. (1992). Informational processing of complex sounds: 3. Interference. Journal of the Acoustical Society of America, 91, 3391–3401.

Moore, B. C. J., Poon, P. W. F., Bacon, S. P., & Glasberg, B. R. (1987). The temporal course of masking and the auditory filter shape. Journal of the Acoustical Society of America, 81, 1873–1880.

Neff, D. L., & Callaghan, B. P. (1988). Effective properties of multicomponent simultaneous maskers under conditions of uncertainty. Journal of the Acoustical Society of America, 83, 1833–1838.

Neff, D. L., Dethlefs, T. M., & Jesteadt, W. (1993). Informational masking for multicomponent maskers and spectral gaps. Journal of the Acoustical Society of America, 94, 3112–3126.

Neff, D. L., & Jesteadt, W. (1996). Intensity discrimination in the presence of random-frequency, multicomponent maskers and broadband noise. Journal of the Acoustical Society of America, 100, 2289–2298.

Patterson, R. D. (1976). Auditory filter shapes derived with noise stimuli. Journal of the Acoustical Society of America, 59, 640–654.

Patterson, R. D, Nimmo-Smith, I., Weber, D. L., & Milroy, R. (1982). The deterioration of hearing with age: Frequency selectivity, the critical ratio, the audiogram, and speech thresholds. Journal of the Acoustical Society of America, 72, 1788–1803.

Peterson, G. E., & Barney, H. L. (1952). Control methods used in a study of the vowels. Journal of the Acoustical Society of America, 24, 175–184.

Pickles, J. O. (1988). An introduction to the physiology of hearing. New York: Academic Press.

Pradhan, P. L., & Hoffman, P. J. (1963). Effect of spacing and range of stimuli on magnitude estimation judgments. Journal of Experimental Psychology, 66, 533–541.

Ramirez, R. W. (1985). The FFT: Fundamentals and concepts. Englewood Cliffs, NJ: Prentice-Hall.

Scharf, B. (1970). Critical bands. In J. V. Tobias (Ed.), Foundations of modern auditory theory (Vol. 1). New York: Academic Press.

Scharf, B. (1983). Loudness adaptation. In J. V. Tobias & E. D. Schubert (Eds.), Hearing research and theory (Vol. 2). New York: Academic Press.

Scharf, B., Quigley, C., Aoki, N., Peachey, N., & Reeves, A. (1987). Focused auditory attention and frequency selectivity. Perception & Psychophysics, 42, 215–223.

Sek, A., & Moore, B. C. (1995). Frequency discrimination as a function of frequency, measured in several ways. Journal of the Acoustical Society of America, 97, 2479–2486.

Shailer, M. J., & Moore, B. C. (1983). Gap detection as a function of frequency, bandwidth, and level. Journal of the Acoustical Society of America, 74, 467–473.

Small, A. M., & Campbell, R. A. (1962). Temporal differential sensitivity for auditory stimuli. American Journal of Psychology, 75, 401–410.

Stevens, K. N., & Blumstein, S. E. (1978). Invariant cues for place of articulation in stop consonants. Journal of the Acoustical Society of America, 64, 836–842.

Stevens, S. S. (1955). The measurement of loudness. Journal of the Acoustical Society of America, 27, 815–829.

Stevens, S. S., & Volkman J. (1940). The relation of pitch to frequency: A revised scale. American Journal of Psychology, 53, 329–353.

Swets, J. A. (1964). Signal detection and recognition by human observers. New York: John Wiley & Sons.

Verschuure, J., & van Meeteren, A. A. (1975). The effect of intensity on pitch. Acustica, 32, 33–44.

Warren, R. M. (1974). Auditory temporal discrimination by trained listeners. Cognitive Psychology, 6, 717.

Warren, D. H., Welch, R. B., & McCarthy. T. J. (1981). The role of visual-auditory "compellingness" in the ventriloquism effect: Implications for transivity among the spatial senses. Perception & Psychophysics, 30, 557–564.

Watson, C. S., & Foyle, D. C. (1985). Central factors in the discrimination and identification of complex sounds. Journal of the Acoustical Society of America, 78, 375–380.

Watson, C. S., & Kelley, W. J. (1981). The role of stimulus uncertainty in the discrimination of auditory patterns. In D. G. Getty & J. H. Howard (Eds.), Auditory and visual pattern recognition. Hillsdale, NJ: Lawrence Erlbaum Associates.

Wightman, F. L., & Kistler, D. (1989). Headphone simulation of free-field listening: 2. Psychophysical validation. Journal of the Acoustical Society of America, 85, 868–878.

Wightman, F. L., & Kistler, D. (1993). Sound localization. In W. A. Yost, A. N. Popper, & R. R. Fay, (Eds.), Human psychophysics. New York: Springer-Verlag.

Wightman, F. L., & Kistler, D. (1997). Factors affecting the relative salience of sound localization cues. In R. H. Gilkey & T. R. Anderson, T.R. (Eds.), Binaural and spatial hearing in real and virtual environments. Mahwah, NJ: Lawrence Erlbaum Associates.

Wright, B. A., & Dai, H. (1994). Detection of unexpected tones in gated and continuous maskers. Journal of the Acoustical Society of America, 95, 939–948.

Zera, J., & Green, D. M. (1993). Detecting temporal onset and offset asynchrony in multicomponent complexes. Journal of the Acoustical Society of America, 93, 1038–1052.

Zwicker, E. (1977). On a psychoacoustic equivalent of tuning curves. In E. Zwicker & E. Terhardt (Eds.), Facts and models in hearing. New York: Springer-Verlag.

Zwicker, E., Flottorp, G., & Stevens, S. S. (1957). Critical bandwidth in loudness summation. Journal of the Acoustical Society of America, 29, 548–557.

Chapter 11

Basic Instrumentation and Calibration

Tom Frank and Allyson D. Rosen

The practice of audiology requires that audiometers and acoustic immittance instruments produce accurate and controlled signals and that testing be conducted in an acoustically controlled environment. This is needed for making reliable and valid interpretations regarding a patient's hearing sensitivity, speech-processing ability, and middle ear status. Thus, the extent to which audiometers and acoustic immittance instruments conform to standardized performance characteristics, and that testing is performed in an appropriate environment, is a major concern to audiologists. Manufacturers are responsible for designing accurate and reliable instruments; however, audiologists are responsible for maintaining the accuracy of these instruments by conducting routine calibration measurements and daily inspection and listening checks.

The goal of this chapter is to provide an overview concerning the performance characteristics of audiometers and acoustic immittance instruments and the requirements for audiometric test rooms. To achieve this goal, the chapter has been divided into sections devoted to standards, audiometers, calibration instrumentation, performance characteristics of pure-tone audiometers, automatic audiometers, speech audiometers, inspection and listening checks, acoustic immittance instruments, and audiometric test rooms. The sections concerning audiometers and acoustic immittance instruments contain information regarding the classification of instruments, transducers, calibration procedures, and standardized values. The audiometric test room section contains information regarding the measurement of ambient noise, standardized ambient noise levels, and sources and ways to reduce ambient noise. Appendix A provides a list of the national and international standards referenced in this chapter, as well as other standards having application to audiology. Appendix B provides forms that can be used for recording calibration.

◆ Standards

Purpose

A standard is a written document developed by a committee of experts based on scientific evidence and accepted practices. Standards contain terms and definitions, as well as specifications concerning the measurement and performance characteristics of various instruments. They are developed as a public service for consumers, industry, and governmental agencies having the primary purpose of providing uniformity among their users. For example, if all audiometers are calibrated to the same standard, intraclinic and interclinic hearing tests conducted for the same individual will result in equivalent results under comparable test conditions. Even though compliance with a standard is voluntary, audiologists should use audiometers, acoustic immittance instruments, and audiometric test rooms that meet specifications issued by the American National Standards Institute (ANSI). Only when standards are written into a law do they become mandatory. However, accreditation by professional associations and other accrediting agencies typically require that audiometric instrumentation and test rooms comply with ANSI standards.

Development of an ANSI Standard

In the United States, standards dealing with acoustics are the responsibility of four accredited standards committees of the Acoustical Society of America (ASA), known as S1-Acoustics, S2-Mechanical Vibration and Shock, S3-Bioacoustics, and S12-Noise. Standards dealing with audiometers, acoustic immittance instruments, audiometric test rooms, and calibration couplers fall under the jurisdiction of the S3-Bioacoustics committee. Each accredited committee is composed of working groups having an appointed chair and expert members. The purpose of each group is to develop, maintain, and revise a standard. Once a working group has drafted a standard, it is reviewed and balloted by members of the accredited committee, individuals representing professional organization members, and individual experts. After the draft standard has been approved by the chair of the ASA accredited committee and ANSI, it is recognized as an American National Standard, called an ANSI standard, given a number, published, and distributed by the ASA.

Pearl

- S1, S2, S3, and S12 ANSI standards can be obtained from the ASA Standards Secretariat, 35 Pinelawn Road, Suite 114E, Melville, NY 11747 or via the Internet at http://asa.aip.org.

ANSI requires that each standard be reviewed every 5 years so that any new scientific information, procedures, and equipment can be incorporated into the standard. When an ANSI standard is reviewed, the working group can recommend that the standard be revised, reaffirmed, or withdrawn. If a standard is revised, it retains its number and name, but the year changes to the year in which the revision was completed. For example, the ANSI standard S3.6–1996, *American National Standard Specification for Audiometers*, was revised in 2004. The standard has kept its title but is now designated as ANSI S3.6–2004. If a standard is reaffirmed, the year in which the reaffirmation occurred preceded by an *R* appears in parentheses after the number and year that the standard was originally completed. For example, ANSI S3.39–1987 was reaffirmed in 2002 and is now designated as ANSI S3.39–1987 (R2002), *American National Standard Specifications for Instruments to Measure Aural Acoustic Impedance and Admittance (Aural Acoustic Immittance)*.

International Standards

International standards have also been developed by the International Organization for Standardization (ISO) and the International Electrotechnical Commission (IEC). Since the early 1990s, ASA and ANSI have attempted to make all new standards and revisions of existing standards compatible and consistent with comparable ISO and IEC standards to promote international uniformity. For example, ANSI S3.6–2004, *Specification of Audiometers*, is consistent with several ISO and IEC standards to ensure that all audiometers would meet the same specifications, regardless of where in the world they were manufactured or used.

♦ Audiometers

The standard governing audiometers is ANSI S3.6–2004, *American National Standard Specification for Audiometers*, which was developed in 1969, revised in 1989, 1996, and 2004; it includes terms and definitions, specifications for audiometers and transducers, signal sources, reference threshold levels, and calibration procedures. Frank (1997) provides a history of the development of ANSI S3.6 from 1969 to 1996.

Types of Audiometers

Historically, audiometers have been given names in reference to (1) the type of signal they produce (pure tone or speech), (2) the frequency range over which they operate (limited, normal, or high frequency), (3) the method in which hearing is measured (manual, automatic, or computer-controlled), (4) the purpose for which they are being used (clinical, diagnostic, industrial, or screening), (5) the number of independent audiometers contained in one unit (one channel, two channel, or channel and a half), and (6) whether they are portable. ANSI S3.6–2004 classifies audiometers by the type of signal generated, mode of operation, and range of auditory functions tested on the basis of minimum required features, frequencies, and maximum hearing levels (HLs) they contain.

Pure-Tone Audiometers

In its simplest form, a pure-tone audiometer consists of a pure-tone generator, interrupter switch, amplifier, attenuator, output selector switch, and earphones. The generator produces pure tones at discrete frequencies selected with a frequency control. The interrupter switch is used to turn the tone on and off before it is routed to the amplifier. Each pure tone is amplified to its maximum by the amplifier and directed to the attenuator. The tones are attenuated with the HL control, which is numbered in decibels relative to normal hearing. Turning the HL control from minimum to maximum decreases the amount of attenuation but increases the level of the tone delivered to the output selector switch. The output selector switch is used to direct the tone to either the right or left earphone.

ANSI S3.6–2004 classifies pure-tone audiometers as types 1, 2, 3, and 4, where the minimum required features, frequencies, and maximum HLs decrease as the type number increases, as shown in **Tables 11–1** and **11–2**. For example, the minimum required features for a type 1 audiometer include four transducer types, frequencies from 125 to 8000 Hz for air conduction and 250 to 6000 Hz for bone conduction, and maximum HLs. A type 4 audiometer, in contrast, is only required to have supra-aural earphones and frequencies from 500 to 6000 Hz, with a maximum output of 70 dB HL at each frequency. For types 1 to 4, the minimum HL is −10 dB. If insert or circumaural earphones are used with a type 1 audiometer, the maximum HLs can be reduced by 10 dB. If a type 4 audiometer is used for hearing conservation purposes, the maximum HLs must be extended to 90 dB at each frequency.

Pearl

• Careful planning is needed before the purchase of an audiometer. Among other things, audiologists must consider the audiometer's size, record of stability, computer interface capabilities, warranties, the use of a loaner, and, most importantly, user-friendliness. Typically, instrument suppliers will provide a complete demonstration and allow a trial period with an audiometer before its purchase.

Automatic Audiometers

Historically, automatic audiometers were used for diagnostic purposes (Brunt, 1985; Jerger, 1960); however, in current practice, they are typically used to obtain air-conduction thresholds in industrial hearing testing programs. Automatic audiometers are also called Békésy, computer-controlled, or self-recording audiometers because they allow listeners to record their own hearing thresholds by controlling the level of a pure tone by means of a hand switch. When the listener hears a tone, the hand switch is depressed and the audiometer automatically lowers the level of the tone. When the tone is no longer audible, the listener releases the hand switch, and the audiometer automatically increases the level of the tone. Over a period of time, the listener has traced or bracketed his or her hearing threshold, which is recorded on an audiogram, on a form, or in a computer. ANSI S3.6–2004 types automatic audiometers using the same features, frequencies, and maximum HLs as specified for pure-tone audiometers.

Speech Audiometers

A speech audiometer has many of the same components as a pure-tone audiometer except the pure-tone generator is replaced by a microphone and external inputs, and a monitoring meter is located between the amplifier and the attenuator (i.e., HL control). The microphone allows for live-voice speech testing, and external inputs allow for playback devices (e.g., cassette tape or CD player) to be connected into the audiometer for recorded speech testing. Historically, speech audiometers were stand-alone instruments; however, in current practice, speech and pure-tone audiometers are typically combined into one unit called a clinical or diagnostic audiometer.

ANSI S3.6–2004 classifies speech audiometers as type A, B, or C, where type A has the most and type C has the fewest required features (**Table 11–1**). All types are required to have a speech replay device or an input for a playback device, but only types A and B are required to have a microphone input. Types A and B are required to have outputs for a supra-aural earphone and loudspeaker, whereas type C is only required to have an output for a supra-aural earphone.

Extended High-Frequency Audiometers

ANSI S3.6–2004 classifies extended high-frequency audiometers as type HF and defines these audiometers as

Table 11–1   Minimum Required Features for Pure-Tone and Speech Audiometers

Pure-Tone Speech Minimum Required Features	1	2	3	4	HF*	A	B	C
Transducers								
Supra-aural earphones	Yes	Yes	Yes	Yes	Yes	Yes†	Yes†	Yes†
Insert earphones	Yes	No	No	No	No	No	No	No
Loudspeakers or electrical output‡	Yes	Yes	No	No	No	Yes	Yes	No
Bone vibrator	Yes	Yes	Yes	No	No	Yes	No	No
Hearing Levels, Test Frequencies								
(see Table 11–2)	Yes	Yes	Yes	Yes	No	Yes	No	No
Test Signal Switching								
Presentation interruption	Yes	Yes	Yes	Yes	Yes	Yes	Yes	Yes
Pulsed tone	Yes	Yes	No	Yes§	Yes	No	No	No
Frequency modulation (FM)	Yes	Yes	No	No	No	No	No	No
Reference Tone								
Alternate presentation	Yes	Yes‖	No	No	No	No	No	No
Simultaneous presentation	Yes	No	No	No	No	No	No	No
Speech Input								
Replay device¶ or electrical input for recorded material‖	Yes	Yes	No	No	No	Yes	Yes	Yes
Microphone	No	No	No	No	No	Yes	Yes	No
Masking								
Narrowband noise	Yes	Yes	Yes	No	Yes	No	No	No
White noise	Yes	Yes	No	No	No	No	No	No
Speech spectrum noise	No	No	No	No	No	Yes	Yes	Yes
Routing of Masking								
Contralateral earphone	Yes	Yes	Yes	No	Yes	Yes	Yes	Yes
Ipsilateral earphone	Yes	No	No	No	No	Yes	No	No
Loudspeaker	Yes	Yes	No	No	No	Yes	Yes	No
Bone vibrator	Yes	No	No	No	No	No	No	No
Subject Response	Yes	Yes	Yes	Yes§	Yes	Yes	No	No
Signal Indicator	Yes	Yes	No	No	Yes	Yes	Yes	Yes
Audible Monitoring	Yes	No	No	No	No	Yes	Yes	No
Operator-to-Subject Communication	Yes	No	No	No	No	Yes	No	No
Talk-Back System	No	No	No	No	No	Yes	Yes	No

Source: Adapted from ANSI S3.6–2004, American National Standard Specification for Audiometers, © 2004 with permission of the Acoustical Society of America, 35 Pinelawn Road, Suite 114E, Melville, NY 11747.

*Audiometers used for testing high-frequency (HF) pure tones from 8000 to 16,000 Hz.

†Free field equivalent recommended; when provided the designation is type E.

‡If loudspeakers are not supplied, manufacturer must specify how conformity will be achieved.

§Not required for manual audiometers.

¶Replay device not always supplied by the manufacturer.

‖Not required for automatic recording audiometers.

instruments for measuring pure-tone thresholds from 8000 to 16,000 Hz. An extended high-frequency audiometer contains the same components as a pure-tone audiometer, except that the generator is capable of producing tones from 8000 to 16,000 Hz, and typically, circumaural rather than supra-aural earphones are used. The standard specifies the minimum HL as –20 dB and the maximum HL as 90 dB from 8000 to 11,200 Hz and 50 dB from 12,000 to 16,000 Hz. Some commercially available stand-alone high-frequency audiometers exist; however, high-frequency testing capabilities are included in several audiometers typically used for testing from 125 to 8000 Hz.

Free Field Equivalent Audiometers

ANSI S3.6–2004 classifies a free field equivalent audiometer as type E. It was included in the standard to be compatible with ISO and IEC audiometer standards. A free field

Table 11–2   Minimum Required Frequencies and Maximum Hearing Levels for Pure-Tone Audiometers

	Maximum Hearing Levels (dB HL) *							
	Type 1§		Type 2†		Type 3†		Type 4‡
Frequency (Hz)	Air	Bone	Air	Bone	Air	Bone	Air
125	70	—	60	—	—	—	—
250	90	45	80	45	70	35	—
500	120	60	110	60	100	50	70
750	120	60	—	—	—	—	—
1000	120	70	110	70	100	60	70
1500	120	70	110	70	—	—	—
2000	120	70	110	70	100	60	70
3000	120	70	110	70	100	60	70
4000	120	60	110	60	100	50	70
6000	110	50	100	—	90	—	70
8000	100	—	90	—	80	—	—
Speech	100	60	60	55	—	—	—

*Minimum HL is ≤ −10 dB for types 1 to 4.

†Sound field loudspeaker output within 250 to 6000 Hz is within 20 dB of the air tabled values for type 1, 2, and 3 for pure tones, warble tones, or speech.

‡Maximum HL is extended to 90 dB HL for type 4 if used for hearing conservation purposes.

§Maximum HL may be 10 dB less than tabled values for type 1 using circumaural or insert earphones.

Note: Maximum HL for type HF is 90 dB HL from 8000 to 11,200 Hz and 50 dB HL from 12,000 to 16,000 Hz; minimum HL is −20 dB HL at all frequencies above 8000 Hz.

Source: Reprinted from ANSI S3.6–2004, *American National Standard Specification for Audiometers,* © 2004 Acoustical Society of America, 35 Pinelawn Road, Suite 114E, Melville, NY 11747, with permission.

equivalent audiometer is a pure-tone and/or speech audiometer, whose transducer output levels are calibrated to be equivalent to sound field reference threshold levels. As such, hearing test results with an earphone or bone vibrator are equivalent to hearing tests performed in a sound field at 0 degree azimuth. Interested readers are referred to ANSI S3.6–2004, Annex A.

Supra-Aural Earphones

A supra-aural earphone consists of an earphone mounted in a circular cushion attached to a headband. The most common supra-aural earphones are Telephonics Corporation (Huntington, NY) Telephonics Dynamic Headphone (TDH) 39, 49, and 50. **Figure 11–1** shows Telephonics TDH

Controversial Point

- Several members of the ANSI working group were reluctant to include the specifications for a free field equivalent audiometer in ANSI S3.6–2004 because they questioned the need, and several manufacturers indicated that the circuitry for this type of audiometer would be very difficult to develop.

Types of Transducers

The function of a transducer is to convert one form of energy to another. A supra-aural, insert, or circumaural earphone and a loudspeaker convert the electrical output from the audiometer to acoustic energy, whereas a bone vibrator converts the electrical output to mechanical energy.

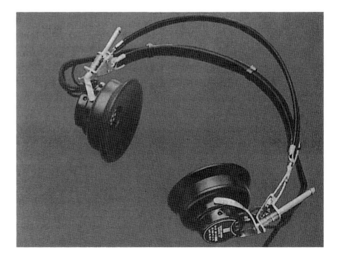

Figure 11–1 Telephonics Dynamic Headphones Model 51 cushions and headband. (From Telephonics Corporation, Huntington, NY, with permission.)

earphones mounted in Model 51 cushions and connected to a headband. These earphones have high sensitivity, low distortion, and the TDH 49 and 50 earphones have a relatively flat frequency response with limited output above 8000 Hz. Thus, TDH-type earphones are only used for testing from 125 to 8000 Hz. ANSI S3.6–2004 specifies the characteristics of earphone cushions (ANSI S3.6–2004, Annex F), which are met by a Telephonics Model 51 and MX-41/AR. Both cushions are made of molded rubber; however, the Model 51 is a one-piece cushion, and the MX-41/AR is constructed from two pieces glued together. Headbands are produced by several manufacturers. Typically, the earphones are attached to the headband by a device consisting of a Y-shaped yoke. The Y-shaped ends of the yoke insert into the sides of the earphone to allow it to swivel vertically, and the other end of the yoke extends through a holding or spring-loaded clip on the headband to allow horizontal adjustments of the earphones.

When fitted, the cushion rests on and presses against the surface of the pinna. ANSI S3.6–2004 specifies that the static headband force should be 4.5 ± 0.5 N. The procedure for measuring static headband force requires that the supra-aural earphones be mounted on a test fixture, with the earphone diaphragms aligned and separated horizontally by 145 mm and positioned 129 mm from the top center of the headband. Once positioned on the test fixture, the static headband force can be measured with a calibrated strain gauge or with an electromechanical force transducer built into the test fixture.

Pitfall

- Static headband force is rarely measured because very specialized instrumentation is required. Unfortunately, it is not unusual to find new headbands with a static force ranging from 2 to 12 N. Audiologists should purchase headbands only from suppliers who can guarantee that the static headband force is within 4.5 ± 0.5 N.

The most common insert earphones for audiometry are manufactured by Etymotic Research Inc. (ER; Elk Grove Village, IL). The original model is called the ER-3A (Killion, 1984), and the latest model is the ER-5A. These insert earphones are also distributed by Aearo Corporation (Indianapolis, IN) E-A-R Auditory Systems under the names E-A-RTone 3A and E-A-RTone 5A. The ER-3A and E-A-RTone 3A, as well as the ER-5A and E-A-RTone 5A, are functionally equivalent because they are built to the same specifications. The ER-3A and ER-5A are shown in **Fig. 11–2**. The 3A consists of a shoulder-mounted transducer coupled to the ear canal by means of a sound tube (240 mm long, 1.37 mm [inside diameter] ID) attached to a connecting nipple (11 mm long, 1.37 mm ID) and then to an eartip tube (26 mm long, 1.93 mm ID), which runs through a foam eartip. The eartips are disposable and available in three sizes. Each size has the same length (12 mm) but different outside diameters to accommodate individuals with very large ear canals (17.8 mm), normal ear canals (13.7 mm), or small ear canals (9.7 mm). When fitted, the foam eartip is rolled and compressed and inserted into the ear canal so that its outer end is flush or just inside the bowl of the concha and then held in place for at least 30 seconds to allow it to expand. The 5A consists of a smaller ear-level transducer than the 3A, and the foam eartip directly attaches to the transducer, thereby eliminating the sound tube used with the 3A.

The frequency response of the 3A (Frank and Richards, 1991) and the 5A is relatively flat from 100 to 4000 Hz and then decreases. Even though the 3A or 5A can be used for testing from 125 to 8000 Hz, the available maximum output at 6000 and especially at 8000 Hz is reduced compared with the output at 1000 Hz. Lilly and Prudy (1993) have reported the advantages and disadvantages of using an insert earphone.

Circumaural Earphones

Circumaural earphones consist of an earphone, cushion, and headband. The earphone is typically attached or suspended to the inside of a plastic dome. The cushion on the plastic dome may be round or oval, depending on the

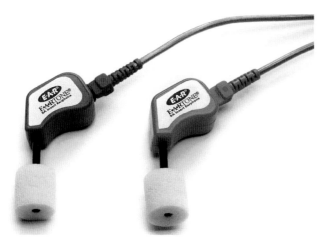
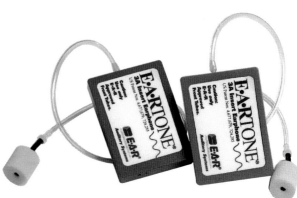

Figure 11–2 Etymotic ER-5A (left) and ER-3A (right) insert earphones. (From Etymotic Research Inc., Elk Grove Village, IL, with permission.)

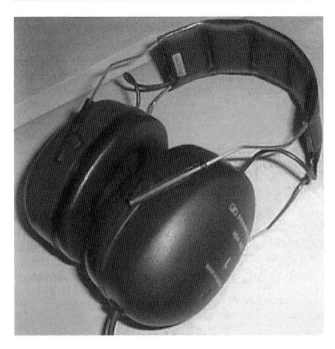

Figure 11–3 Sennheiser HDA 200 circumaural earphones. (From Sennheiser Electronic Corporation, Old Lyme, CT. Used with permission.)

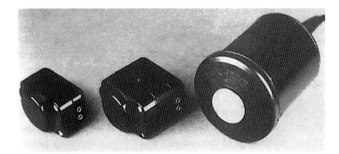

Figure 11–4 Left to right, Radioear B-71 and B-72 and Pracitronic KH 70 bone vibrators. (From American Speech-Language-Hearing Association, Rockville, MD. Used with permission.)

opening of the dome, and may be detachable or glued to the dome. Examples of a circumaural earphone include the Sennheiser Electronic Corporation (Old Lyme, CT) HDA200 and Koss Corporation (Milwaukee, WI) HV/1A. Sennheiser HDA 200 circumaural earphones are shown in **Fig. 11–3**. When fitted, the cushion of a circumaural earphone fits over and around the pinna similar to an earmuff used for personal hearing protection. ANSI S3.6–2004 specifies that the static headband force should be 9 to 10 N, measured with the same test fixture and procedures used for supra-aural earphones. Circumaural earphones are most commonly used for testing hearing above 8000 Hz.

Loudspeakers

Loudspeakers should have a bandwidth between 100 and 10,000 Hz, a smooth frequency response, and be housed in an enclosure. To meet these requirements, typically two or more limited-range, frequency-response speakers are contained in the same enclosure. The output is controlled by an electrical crossover network that minimizes overlap between the frequency response of each speaker to obtain an overall smooth frequency response. A loudspeaker should be capable of producing a sound pressure level (SPL) from 0 to 120 dB at a reference point in the sound field, be electrically isolated so that circuit or line noise is not amplified, and have very low distortion, especially at very high output levels.

Bone Vibrators

A bone vibrator consists of an electromagnetic transducer having a plane circular tip area of 175 ± 25 mm². However,

bone vibrators differ in size, shape, weight, input impedance, encapsulation, and frequency response. **Figure 11–4** shows a Radioear Corporation (New Eagle, PA) B-71 and B-72 and a Pracitronic KH-70 bone vibrator. The most common bone vibrator used in the United States is a Radioear B-71. The B-71 weighs 20 g and is encapsulated in a plastic case. The electromagnetic transducer in the B-71 (and B-72) is connected to the inside back of its plastic case so that the entire case vibrates when the transducer is activated. The frequency response of a B-71 is characterized by three resonant peaks at 450, 1500, and 3800 Hz that decrease in amplitude as frequency increases followed by a sharp drop in output above 4000 Hz (Richards and Frank, 1982). Thus, bone-conduction testing with the B-71 is typically conducted from 250 to 4000 Hz. Another Radioear bone vibrator, called a B-72, also has a frequency response characterized by three resonant peaks; however, the peaks occur at lower frequencies (250, 1350, and 3400 Hz) because the B-72 has an added dynamic mass of 28 g compared with the B-71 (Frank et al, 1988). The B-72 presents several clinical problems because it tends to slip off the mastoid process as a result of its weight, especially with small children. Another bone vibrator, manufactured in Germany but no longer available, is called a Pracitronic KH-70, but because of its size and weight (96 g) its clinical usefulness is limited. The frequency response of a KH-70 is characterized by one major resonance at 200 Hz followed by a gradual decline in output. For the same input voltage, the overall output of the KH-70 is less than the B-71 and B-72 from 100 to 8000 Hz (Frank et al, 1988), but it has a relatively flat frequency response from 8000 to 16,000 Hz so that it can be used for testing high-frequency (8000–16,000 Hz) bone-conduction thresholds (Richter and Frank, 1985).

When fitted, a bone vibrator can be placed on the mastoid or forehead using a headband. ANSI S3.6–2004 specifies the static headband force as 5.4 6 ± 0.5 N for either mastoid or forehead placement. The headband force can be measured with the same test fixture used for supra-aural earphones, except the horizontal separation for forehead placement is 190 mm.

General Requirements

ANSI S3.6–2004 specifies that audiometers are required to have a stable output for temperatures ranging from 15° to

35°C (59°–95°F) and for humidities from 30 to 90%. Furthermore, all audiometers must meet several safety requirements so that an electrical shock and external electrostatic or electromagnetic interference will not endanger the patient or audiologist or invalidate the test results. For battery-powered audiometers, manufacturers must provide an indicator showing if the battery is providing the appropriate voltage.

All audiometers are required to have several markings or labels and an instruction manual. If an audiometer is calibrated to ANSI S3.6–2004 specifications, the marking *ANSI/ISO Hearing Level* must appear on the front panel or hearing level control, and the audiometer type must be displayed on the front panel. It should be noted that one audiometer may meet several type designations. For example, the designation 1A would mean the audiometer meets the minimum requirements for a type 1 pure tone and type A speech audiometer. If the audiometer also meets the minimum requirements for an extended high-frequency audiometer, the type designation would be 1HFA. ANSI S3.6–2004 also requires that the maximum HL at each frequency be marked on the frequency control if the audiometer does not automatically limit the HL output at each frequency. In addition, the name of the manufacturer, model number, serial number, transducers to be used with the audiometer, country of origin, and safety standards must be marked on the audiometer. An instruction manual must be provided with each audiometer, and it is required that manufacturers include information as to how the audiometer and/or transducers meet several ANSI S3.6–2004 specifications. Interested readers should review ANSI S3.6–2004, Clause 10.2.

Pearl

• Audiologists should read the instruction manual before using the audiometer, then reread the instruction manual as they are learning to use all the audiometer's features.

♦ Calibration Instrumentation

An electroacoustic calibration is conducted by measuring performance characteristics of an audiometer and each transducer with couplers and electronic instrumentation. If the measured values agree with the standardized values specified in ANSI S3.6–2004, the audiometer is said to be calibrated or operating within ANSI specifications. An electroacoustic calibration involves measuring output levels, attenuator linearity, frequency accuracy, distortion, tone switching, masking levels, frequency response, and other performance characteristics.

All audiometers should (1) undergo an exhaustive calibration before they are used and thereafter at least once a year or sooner if there is reason to believe the output has changed, (2) be calibrated when the audiometer and transducers are in their customary locations, (3) be placed on a routine calibration schedule, (4) be calibrated quarterly for output level, and (5) be evaluated daily using inspection and listening checks. All of the calibration measurements, history of repair, and inspection and listening checks should be documented. This will assist in determining how well an audiometer remains in calibration and if a continual problem is occurring. Older audiometers, portable audiometers, and audiometers moved from one site to another (e.g., audiometers in a mobile testing unit) should be calibrated with more regularity because they are more susceptible to being damaged. Audiology clinics accredited by professional organizations or doing work regulated by law should check the time intervals for audiometer calibration required by these organizations or in the law.

The basic calibration instrumentation includes (1) couplers, (2) a sound level meter (SLM) having one-third octave band filters, (3) a voltmeter, (4) an electronic counter/timer, and (5) an oscilloscope. Other instrumentation such as a spectrum analyzer, distortion meter, and overshoot, rise/fall, and envelope detectors can also be used. Several manufacturers have developed audiometer calibration kits that include individual instruments or instruments packaged into an integrated unit. Unfortunately, the cost of calibration instruments may be prohibitive for some audiology clinics so that calibration services would have to be purchased from an outside source. However, an SLM having one-third octave band filters for measuring the output of loudspeakers, acoustic couplers used for measuring the output of supra-aural or insert earphones, and ambient noise levels should be considered standard instrumentation for all audiology clinics. The following provides a discussion of couplers and calibration instruments. For a more in-depth discussion, the reader is referred to Curtis and Schultz (1986) and Decker (1990).

Types of Couplers

Couplers are standardized devices used for measuring the output of transducers. Acoustic couplers are used for earphone measurements, have a standardized shape and volume, contain a calibrated microphone, and include the National Bureau of Standards (NBS) 9-A, IEC 60318–3, Hearing Aid (HA) type 1 and 2, and an occluded ear simulator. A mechanical coupler has a standardized mechanical impedance and contains an electromechanical transducer for measuring the force-level output of a bone vibrator.

NBS 9-A Coupler

The NBS 9-A coupler (ANSI S3.7–1995 (R2003)) shown in **Fig. 11–5** is used to measure the output of a supra-aural earphone. Placing a supra-aural earphone on the top of the coupler creates an enclosed volume of air that couples the earphone to a calibrated microphone at the bottom of the coupler. The enclosed volume of air is 6 cc and was chosen to approximate the volume of air between the diaphragm of a supra-aural earphone and the tympanic membrane (Corliss and Burkhard, 1953). Thus, the NBS 9-A coupler has been called a 6 cc coupler or an artificial ear. However, the NBS 9-A coupler does not simulate the acoustic impedance of a human ear over the entire

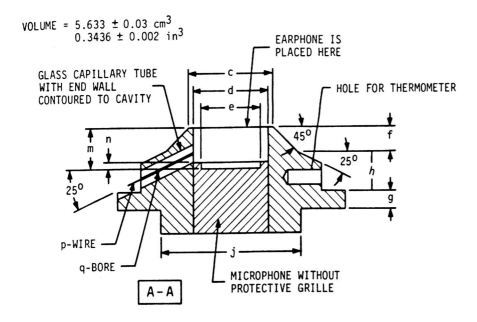

VOLUME = 5.633 ± 0.03 cm³
          0.3436 ± 0.002 in³

GLASS CAPILLARY TUBE WITH END WALL CONTOURED TO CAVITY

EARPHONE IS PLACED HERE

HOLE FOR THERMOMETER

p-WIRE

q-BORE

A-A

MICROPHONE WITHOUT PROTECTIVE GRILLE

Dimensions					
	in	cm		in	cm
a	2.874	7.30	g	0.187	0.475
b	2.252	5.72	h	0.490	1.245
c	1.00	2.54	j	1.750	4.445
	+0	+0	m	0.528	1.3410
	−0.1	−0.025		± 0.001	± 0.0025
d	0.938	2.3825	n	0.077	0.195
	± 0.0006	± 0.0015			
e	0.728	1.85	p (dia)	0.016	0.041
f	0.295	0.75	q (dia)	0.024	0.061

Figure 11–5 National Bureau of Standards 9-A coupler used for the calibration of supra-aural earphones. (Adapted from ANSI S3.7–1995 (R2003), *American National Standard Method for Coupler Calibration of Earphones,* © 1995 Acoustical Society of America, 35 Pinelawn Road, Suite 114E, Melville, NY 11747, with permission.)

frequency range (Corliss and Burkhard, 1953) and should not be considered as a true artificial ear. Several studies have demonstrated that the SPL developed in an NBS 9-A coupler is different than that measured in real ears (Hawkins et al, 1990; Killion, 1978; Zwislocki, 1970, 1971). Furthermore, because of its size, shape, and hard walls, the NBS 9-A coupler has a natural resonance around 6000 Hz, and standing waves may occur within the coupler at frequencies higher than 6000 Hz (Rudmose, 1964). Despite its shortcomings, the NBA 9-A coupler is the accepted device for measuring the output of supra-aural earphones because it produces highly repeatable results. When measurements are obtained, a supra-aural earphone is positioned on the top of the coupler, and a 500 g weight is placed on top of the earphone to simulate the static headband force.

Pearl

- Placing a small circular level on top of a 500 g weight used to load a supra-aural earphone will help position the diaphragm of the earphone parallel to the diaphragm of the microphone in an NBS 9-A coupler.

IEC 60318–3 Coupler

To promote international uniformity, ANSI S3.6–2004 recognizes that the output of a supra-aural earphone can also be measured with an IEC 60318–3 coupler (IEC 60318–3:1998–08). The IEC 60318–3 (formerly called a 318) coupler contains three acoustically coupled cavities and a calibrated microphone that simulates the average human ear from 20 to 10,000 Hz and can be used for measuring the output of physically dissimilar supra-aural earphones. When measurements are obtained, a supra-aural earphone is positioned on the top of the coupler and loaded with a 500 g weight.

The IEC 60318–3 coupler can be adapted to become an IEC 60318–2 coupler (IEC 60138–2:1998–08) to measure the output of a circumaural earphone by mounting either a type 1 or 2 flat plate adapter on the top of the coupler as described in ANSI S3.6–2004, Annex C. When measurements are obtained, the circumaural earphone is positioned on the flat plate and loaded with a 900 to 1000 g weight. To differentiate between an NBS 9-A and IEC 60318–3 coupler, ANSI S3.6–2004 refers to the NBS 9-A as an acoustic coupler and to the IEC 60318–3 as an artificial ear.

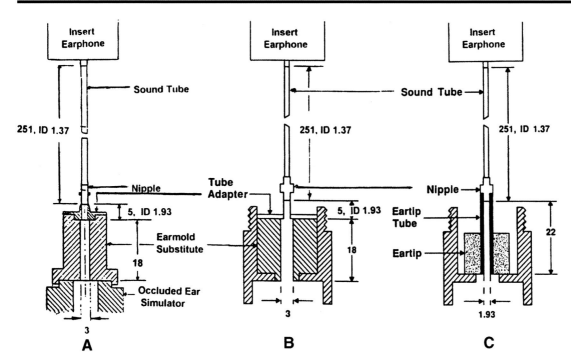

Figure 11–6 Couplers used for the calibration of insert earphones: **(A)** occluded ear simulator, **(B)** hearing aid type 2 coupler with rigid tube attachment, and **(C)** hearing aid type 1 coupler. (From ANSI S3.6–2004, *American National Standard Specification for Audiometers,* © 2004 Acoustical Society of America, 35 Pinelawn Road, Suite 114E, Melville, NY 11747, with permission.)

Hearing Aid Couplers and Occluded Ear Simulator

A hearing aid type 1 coupler (HA-1) or a hearing aid type 2 coupler (HA-2) with rigid tube attachment (ANSI S3.7–1995 (R2003)) or an occluded ear simulator (ANSI S3.25–1989 (R2003), IEC 60711, 1981–01) can be used for measuring the output of an insert earphone. Both the HA-1 and HA-2 couplers contain an effective volume of air of 2 cc and a calibrated microphone; however, the HA-2 also contains an earmold substitute and tube adapter. Thus, these couplers are also called 2 cc couplers. An occluded ear simulator contains acoustically coupled cavities and a calibrated microphone. **Figure 11–6** shows how an insert earphone is connected to these couplers. For the occluded ear simulator or the HA-2 with entrance through a rigid tube, the insert earphone eartip is removed, and the nipple is connected to the tube adapter of the coupler through a 5 mm piece of no. 13 tubing so that the nipple outlet will be held tightly and flush against the inlet of the tube adapter. For the HA-1 coupler, the end of the eartip is sealed to the top of the HA-1 cavity so that the eartip opening is centered over the cavity inlet hole.

Pearl

- The easiest and perhaps most efficient way to measure the performance characteristics of an insert earphone is to use an HA-2 coupler with rigid tube attachment.

A mechanical coupler is used for measuring the output of a bone vibrator. Because a bone vibrator is typically placed on the mastoid, a mechanical coupler is often called an artificial mastoid. However, a mechanical coupler is also called an artificial headbone because a bone vibrator can also be placed on the forehead. ANSI S3.13–1987 (R2002) and IEC 60373 (1990–01) specify the design characteristics of a mechanical coupler that are met by a Brüel & Kjaer (B&K; Nærum Denmark) 4930 artificial mastoid. The standards also specify the mechanical impedance of the coupler that should be presented to a bone vibrator and a device for measuring the alternating force level produced by the bone vibrator. **Figure 11–7** shows a schematic diagram of a B&K 4930 mechanical coupler. Unfortunately, the impedance of the coupler's rubber pad has higher mechanical impedance values than specified in ANSI S3.13–1987 (R2002) and IEC 60373 (1990–01) (Dirks et al, 1979). Another problem with the B&K 4930 is that its output is temperature dependent, especially in the higher frequencies (Frank and Richter, 1985). Thus, ANSI and IEC standards specify that the temperature of the mechanical coupler should be 23° ± 1°C (71.6–75.2°F) when it is used to calibrate the output of a bone vibrator. Even though the mechanical impedance of the B&K 4930 does not conform to ANSI and IEC standards, it is still the most common device for measuring the output of a bone vibrator. When measurements are obtained, a circular-tipped bone vibrator is positioned on the top of the coupler and loaded with a 550 g weight.

Sound Level Meter

A sound level meter (SLM) combines a microphone, amplifying and filtering circuits, and a meter into one unit and is used

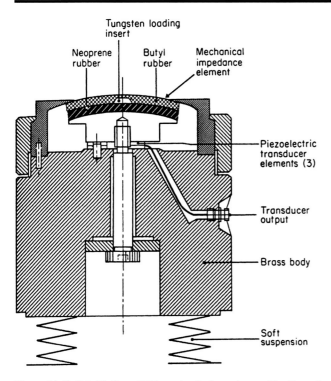

Figure 11–7 Brüel & Kjaer 4930 mechanical coupler used for the calibration of bone vibrators. (From ANSI S3.13–1987 (R2002), *American National Standard Mechanical Coupler for Measurements of Bone Vibrators,* © 1987 Acoustical Society of America, 35 Pinelawn Road, Suite 114E, Melville, NY 11747, with permission.)

to measure the SPL developed in an acoustic coupler by earphones or in a sound field by a loudspeaker. ANSI S1.4–1983 (R2001) specifies several types of SLMs on the basis of features they contain.

Pitfall

- It cannot be assumed that the output of a mechanical coupler will remain stable from year to year. Like all measurement instrumentation, a mechanical coupler needs to be recalibrated to ensure that its output is stable.

For audiometer calibration, a type 1 SLM having one-third octave band filters (ANSI S1.11–2004) and a condenser microphone should be used. A type 1 SLM has two response integration times called slow and fast. The slow response is useful for measuring signals that have level fluctuations typically greater than 4 dB, as would be the case for masking signals or ambient noise. The fast response is used to measure signals having slight or no level fluctuations, such as pure tones. One-third octave band filtering is used because the filtering allows for measuring only the sounds contained within a very narrow frequency range and excludes the contribution of other sounds having frequencies outside the bandwidth of the filter. A condenser microphone has low noise levels and a flat frequency response

over a wide range of frequencies, and operates in a linear manner over a wide intensity range. A pressure condenser microphone should be used for all coupler measurements, whereas a sound field condenser microphone should be used for all loudspeaker measurements. Condenser microphones are sensitive to temperature and humidity, which must be taken into account when an SLM is calibrated. An SLM is calibrated by placing a pistonphone, sound level calibrator, or acoustic calibrator over the microphone. These devices generate a known SPL output at one or more frequencies (ANSI S1.40–1984 (R2001)). The SLM reading should be adjusted to the output of the calibrator. Calibrating an SLM with a multiple-frequency and multiple SPL acoustic calibrator is a very good idea. This provides a quick check of the frequency response and linearity, which could change over time because of aging and variables associated with the microphone.

Pearl

- When not in use, microphones should be stored in a low-humidity environment. This can be performed by placing microphones in a sealed jar containing materials that act to reduce the humidity and eliminate condensation, which could influence the performance of the microphone.

Voltmeter

A voltmeter is used to measure the output of an electronic device. Because the acoustic output of a transducer follows the waveform and is directly proportional to the input voltage, except in nonlinear ranges, voltmeters can be used to determine whether a problem exists with a transducer, a cord, or the audiometer. For audiometer calibration, a voltmeter should have a very high impedance (e.g., megohm [MΩ] range) so that it will not influence the circuit load it is measuring, read the output in true root-mean-square, have a decibel scale, and have a sensitivity between 0.01 mV and 120 V. Some SLMs can also function as voltmeters.

When a voltmeter is used, the voltage is typically measured between the audiometer and transducer so that the audiometer continues to be loaded by the transducer. This can be completed using a Y-patch cord, where each end of the Y has a receptacle called a phone jack and the other end has a phone plug. In use, the patch cord phone plug is inserted into the appropriate audiometer output, the phone plug of the transducer is inserted into one of the patch cord phone jacks, and the voltmeter is inserted into the other phone jack. Whenever an electrical measurement is conducted, it is assumed that the transducer cord and transducer are functioning normally.

Electronic Counter/Timer

An electronic counter/timer is used to provide measurements of frequency and time. These devices typically measure frequency to within 1 Hz and time intervals to within hundredths of a second.

Oscilloscope

An oscilloscope can be used for several purposes (e.g., as a voltmeter, timer, and frequency monitor); however, its primary use is for measuring tone-switching performance characteristics, including rise/fall times, overshoot, and pulse durations. Because an oscilloscope is capable of measuring very low level voltages, it can also be used for measuring whether a signal directed to one output crosses over to another output. However, this could also be performed with a voltmeter using low-sensitivity settings. The most desirable oscilloscope would be one that has two channels capable of storing signals, a bandwidth from direct current (DC) to 100 kHz, voltage sensitivity ranging from 0.5 mV to 10 V, time base from 1 msec to 1 second, and internal and external triggers. Unfortunately, an adequate oscilloscope is somewhat expensive. As an alternative, rise/fall time, overshoot, and/or envelope detectors are available from several manufacturers at a relatively low price. If these devices are used, they must be sensitive enough to measure the rise/fall times and overshoot specified in ANSI S3.6–2004.

Special Consideration

- The instruments used for calibration must be calibrated to ensure that they have significantly less measurement error than the standardized tolerances for each performance characteristic.

◆ Performance Characteristics of Pure-Tone Audiometers

Output Levels

The output levels of audiometer transducers must be calibrated to standardized reference threshold levels shown in **Table 11–3**. For air-conduction transducers, the reference threshold levels are called reference equivalent threshold sound pressure levels (RETSPLs), and for bone-conduction transducers, reference equivalent threshold force levels (RETFLs). RETSPLs are the SPLs measured in an acoustic coupler, and RETFLs are the force levels measured on a mechanical coupler that equal the mean hearing thresholds of otologically normal individuals of both genders from 18 to 30 years old. Stated another way, RETSPLs are the SPLs and RETFLs are the force levels that are equal to normal-hearing or 0 dB HL. However, during calibration, RETSPLs and RETFLs are not measured at 0 dB HL. This occurs because air- and bone-conduction transducers have very low output levels at 0 dB HL, which may exceed the lower limits of the measurement instrumentation, and ambient noise might influence the measurements for air-conduction transducers. RETSPLs are typically measured at 70 dB HL, so that the transducer output level will be within the range of the measurement instrumentation and well above the ambient noise level. RETFLs are typically measured at 20 dB HL at 250 Hz and 50 dB HL from 500 to 4000 Hz.

Because it is impossible and impractical for all transducers and measurement instruments to perform exactly the same,

---

Table 11–3 Reference Threshold Levels for Different Transducer Types

Transducer, coupler	Frequency (Hz)											
	125	250	500	750	1000	1500	2000	3000	4000	6000	8000	Speech
TDH type, IEC 60318–3[*]	45.0	27.0	13.5	9.0	7.5	7.5	9.0	11.5	12.0	16.0	15.5	20.0
TDH 39, NBS 9-A[*]	45.0	25.5	11.5	8.0	7.0	6.5	9.0	10.0	9.5	15.5	13.0	19.5
TDH 49/50, NBS 9-A[*]	47.5	26.6	13.5	8.5	7.5	7.5	11.0	9.5	10.5	13.5	13.0	20.0
3A/5A Insert, OES[*†]	28.0	17.5	9.5	6.0	5.5	9.5	11.5	13.0	15.0	16.0	15.5	18.0
3A/5A Insert, HA-1[*]	26.5	14.5	6.0	2.0	0.0	0.0	2.5	2.5	0.0	−2.5	−3.5	12.5
3A/5A Insert, HA-2[*]	26.0	14.0	5.5	2.0	0.0	2.0	3.0	3.5	5.5	2.0	0.0	12.5
Loudspeaker Bin at 0[‡]	22.0	11.0	4.0	2.0	2.0	0.5	−1.5	−6.0	−6.5	2.5	11.5	14.5
Loudspeaker Mon at 0[‡]	24.0	13.0	6.0	4.0	4.0	2.5	0.5	−4.0	−4.5	4.5	13.5	16.5
Loudspeaker Mon at 45[‡]	23.5	12.0	3.0	0.5	0.0	−1.0	−2.5	−9.0	−8.5	−3.0	8.0	12.5
Loudspeaker Mon 90[‡]	23.0	11.0	1.5	−1.0	−1.5	−2.5	−1.5	−6.5	−4.0	−5.0	5.5	11.0
Bone Vib, Mastoid[§]	—	67.0	58.0	48.5	42.5	36.5	31.0	30.0	35.5	40.0	40.0	55.0
Bone Vib, Forehead[§]	—	79.0	72.0	61.5	51.0	47.5	42.5	42.0	43.5	51.0	50.0	63.5

Source: From ANSI S3.6–2004, *American National Standard Specification for Audiometers,* © 2004 Acoustical Society of America, 35 Pinelawn Road, Suite 114E, Melville, NY 11747, with permission.

[*]In dB re: 20 μPa.

[†]Occluded ear simulator.

[‡]In dB re: 20μPa at reference point at least 1 m from loudspeaker.

[§]In dB re: 1 μN using Brüel & Kjaer 4930 mechanical coupler.

an acceptable variation or error, called a tolerance, is allowed for each performance characteristic. The tolerance for all reference threshold levels is ± 3 dB from 125 to 5000 Hz and ± 5 dB at 6000 Hz and higher. In theory, it would be possible to have an output level difference between earphones of 6 dB from 125 to 5000 Hz and 10 dB at 6000 Hz and above and still be within tolerance. However, this might be detrimental to interpreting differences between ears and for determining a change in hearing sensitivity from one test to another. If this extreme situation occurs, or if the transducer output is higher or lower than the tolerance, the output of the audiometer is too strong or too weak and has to be corrected. All microprocessor-based audiometers have a calibration mode for easily changing transducer output levels. Older audiometers have adjustable potentiometers, or it may be necessary to replace some internal resistors to obtain the desired output level.

As a general rule, if the transducer output, regardless of frequency, is not within ± 2.5 dB compared with the reference threshold level and cannot be corrected during the calibration process, audiologists should develop a correction card as shown in **Fig. 11–8**. This occurs even though the tolerance is ± 3 from 125 to 5000 Hz and ± 5 dB at 6000 Hz and higher. The correction card indicates adjustments, rounded to the nearest 5 dB at each frequency, that must be made to the HL setting when a patient is tested. If the transducer output is lower than the reference threshold level, the amount of deviation is subtracted from the HL setting. For example, the RETSPL at 1000 Hz for a TDH 49/50 earphone is 7.5 dB SPL (**Table 11–3**). If the HL control is set at 70 dB, the earphone output should be 77.5 dB SPL. If the measured output was 72.5 dB, the audiometer output is 5 dB too low. Testing a patient with a true threshold of 60 dB HL would have resulted in a threshold of 65 dB HL. To eliminate this inaccuracy, a correction of –5 dB is applied to the patient's threshold of 65 dB HL, so that the patient's true threshold of 60 dB HL is recorded on the audiogram. If the transducer output level is higher than the reference threshold level, the amount of the deviation is added to the HL setting. Using the previous example, if the measured output was 82.5 dB SPL instead of 77.5 dB SPL, the output is 5 dB too high. Testing the patient with a true threshold of 60 dB HL would have resulted in a threshold of 55 dB HL. Thus, a correction of +5 dB is applied so that the patient's true threshold of

Penn State University, Speech and Hearing Clinic, 110 Moore Building, University Park, PA 16802
Audiometer Output Level Correction Card

Audiometer: _____   Serial No: _____   Channel: _____   Date: _____

Frequency	Transducer Type					
	Right Earphone	Left Earphone	Right Insert Earphone	Left Insert Earphone	Bone Vib Mastoid	Bone Vib Forehead
125						
250						
500						
750						
1000						
1500						
2000						
3000						
4000						
6000						
8000						
Speech						

NEGATIVE table value means audiometer output is too weak; make threshold better/Hearing Level setting lowered by table value.

POSITIVE table value means audiometer output is too strong; make threshold worse/Hearing Level setting increased by table value.

Figure 11–8 Audiometer output level correction card.

60 dB HL will be recorded on the audiogram. If a correction of more than 10 dB is needed, the audiometer should be repaired and recalibrated.

Pitfall

- The danger of using a correction card is that it may get lost, or the correction may not be applied to a patient's threshold. If a correction card is used, it should be tightly secured to the audiometer.

Supra-Aural Earphones

The output levels of a supra-aural earphone are measured by placing the earphone on either an NBS 9-A or an IEC 60318–3 coupler loaded with a 500 g weight. The coupler microphone is connected to an SLM. If the SLM has one-third octave band filters, the filter is adjusted to the frequency of the pure tone being measured. The position of the earphone is checked by directing a continuous 125 or 250 Hz tone at 70 dB HL to the earphone while it is adjusted to a position that produces the highest SPL. After this, the SPL is measured at each frequency for each earphone and recorded on a calibration form (see Appendix B, Form 1). If the audiometer has two channels, the measurements are repeated using the other channel. After each individual measurement, the measured SPL is checked against the RETSPL (**Table 11–3**) + 70 dB HL for the earphone type and coupler used during the measurements to determine if the earphone output level is in calibration. For example, at 2000 Hz, the RETSPL for a TDH 49/50 earphone measured in a NBS 9A coupler is 11.0 dB SPL. Because the HL was set at 70 dB, the measured SPL should be 81.0 dB SPL.

If the measured SPL is not within ± 2.5 dB of the RETSPL + 70 dB HL, the earphone output level should be changed to the desired level using the audiometer's internal calibration mode. If this is not possible, a correction card (**Fig. 11–8**) should be developed.

Insert Earphones

The output levels of an insert earphone (Etymotic ER-3A or ER-5A or E-A-RTone 3A or 5A) are measured by connecting the insert earphone to an occluded ear simulator, HA-1, or HA-2 coupler with rigid tube attachment, as shown in **Fig. 11–6**. The procedures used for measuring insert earphone output levels are the same as those for a supra-aural earphone, and the coupler output SPLs should be recorded on a calibration form (see Appendix B, Form 1). For example, at 1000 Hz, the output level of an insert earphone measured in an HA-2 coupler with rigid tube attachment should be 70.0 dB SPL because the RETSPL is 0.0 dB SPL and the audiometer was set at 70 dB HL.

The insert earphone RETSPLs specified in ANSI S3.6–2004 (**Table 11–3**) were taken directly from the insert earphone RETSPLs specified in ISO 389–2:1994 based on the mean insert earphone threshold levels reported from three studies

(Brinkman and Richter, 1990). The ANSI 2004 RETSPLs are somewhat lower than those reported by Wilber et al (1988) and Frank and Vavrek (1992), especially from 500 to 4000 Hz.

Controversial Point

- Even though the ANSI S3.6–2004 insert earphone RETSPLs are somewhat lower and are not supported by the findings of Wilber et al (1988) and Frank and Vavrek (1992), they were included in ANSI S3.6–2004 to promote international uniformity.

Type 1 pure-tone audiometers are required to have insert earphones (**Table 11–1**). For other types of pure-tone audiometers, insert earphones are typically connected to the audiometer's output jacks normally used for supra-aural earphones. If this is the case, the manufacturer has recommended plug-in correction values because the audiometer thinks that supra-aural earphones are still being used. However, to be precise, audiologists should measure the coupler output of each insert earphone at each frequency and determine their own correction values, which should be listed on a correction card (**Fig. 11–8**) attached to the audiometer. Recall that, if the measured output level is lower than the reference level, the amount of deviation is rounded to the nearest 5 dB and subtracted from the patient's threshold. If the measured level is higher than the reference level, the amount of the deviation is rounded to the nearest 5 dB and added to the patient's threshold.

Circumaural Earphones

The output levels of a circumaural earphone are measured by placing the earphone on an IEC 60318–2 coupler equipped with the appropriate flat plate coupler loaded with a 900 to 1000 g weight. The coupler microphone is connected to an SLM. At each frequency, the HL is set so that the measurements will not be influenced by environmental ambient noise. ANSI has not officially standardized hearing testing with circumaural earphones. However, ANSI S3.6–2004 Annex C provides RETSPLs for a Sennheiser HDA200 from 125 to 16,000 Hz and for a Koss HV/1A at 1000 and 4000 Hz and from 8000 to 16,000 Hz. The measured SPL for each frequency and earphone is checked against the RETSPL plus the HL setting to determine whether the earphone output is in calibration. If the measured SPL is not within ± 2.5 dB of the desired level (i.e., RETSPL plus HL setting), the earphone output level should be adjusted using the audiometer's internal calibration mode. If this is not possible, a correction card should be developed.

Bone Vibrators

The output levels of a bone vibrator are measured by placing the bone vibrator on a mechanical coupler loaded with a weight or spring-tension device that will produce a force of

5.4 N. The output of the mechanical coupler is connected to a voltmeter having a decibel scale calibrated in μN. Typically, bone vibrators are calibrated for mastoid placement, and a correction (dB difference between forehead minus mastoid RETFLs, **Table 11–3**) is applied if testing is performed using forehead placement. Furthermore, the audiometer HL is set to 20 dB HL at 250 Hz and 50 dB HL at higher frequencies. The force level is measured at each frequency and recorded on a calibration form (see Appendix B, Form 1). After each individual measurement, the measured level is checked against the RETFL plus the HL setting. For example, at 1000 Hz with the audiometer set to 50 dB HL, the measured force level for mastoid placement should be 92.5 dB re: 1 μN because the RETFL at 1000 Hz is 42.5 dB and the audiometer was set at 50 dB HL. If the measured force level is not within ± 2.5 dB of the desired output level (RETFL plus HL setting), the bone vibrator output should be adjusted using the audiometer's internal calibration mode or a correction card should be developed. The ANSI S3.6–2004 RETFLs are the same as those specified in ISO 389:3:1994. This occurred even though Frank et al (1988) reported that thresholds with a Radioear B-72 and Practronic KH 70 were ~10 dB higher at 250 Hz and ~5 dB lower at 500 Hz than a Radioear B-71 bone vibrator.

Controversial Point

• Audiologists commonly report that bone-conduction thresholds are not equal to air-conduction thresholds for normally hearing listeners or patients with a sensorineural hearing loss. In part, this occurs because the RETFLs are for any bone vibrator having a plane circular tip with a nominal area of 175 ± 25 mm² applied with a static headband force of 5.4 ± 0.5 N, were not adjusted to equal air conduction thresholds, and were obtained with 30 to 40 dB of effective masking directed to the contralateral ear. Interested readers are referred to Hood (1979), Frank (1982), and Frank et al (1988) for more information.

Loudspeakers

Before measuring the output levels of a loudspeaker, a decision has to be made as to whether to calibrate the loudspeaker output to RETSPLs for monaural or binaural listening. Historically, audiologists have used reference thresholds for monaural listening. In part, this is completed so that sound field thresholds can be compared with monaural air-conduction thresholds. If the decision is made for monaural listening, then a decision is needed concerning the placement of a loudspeaker relative to the patient specified in degrees and commonly referred to as the incidence or azimuth. For example, if a loudspeaker is directly in front of a listener, the listener is said to be seated at 0 degree azimuth. Typically, if one loudspeaker is used, it should be located at 0 degree azimuth. If two loudspeakers are used, the location for each loudspeaker should be 45 degrees azimuth

on either side of the patient; however, some audiologists use a position of 90 degrees on either side of the patient.

ANSI S3.6–2004 specifies that the loudspeaker should be positioned to the head height of a seated patient and that output level measurements should be completed at a reference point at least 1 m from the loudspeaker. Typically, the reference point is permanently marked with a dot on the ceiling or floor or by hanging a plumb bob from the ceiling. The reference point is where the middle of the patient's head would normally be located during testing. If two loudspeakers are used, they should have the same reference point. Loudspeaker output levels are measured by substituting an SLM at the reference point so that sound from the loudspeaker will pass across the top of the SLM microphone. Furthermore, the audiometer is set to produce a test signal at 70 dB HL so that ambient noise will not influence the measurements. The SPL or one-third octave band SPL is measured at each frequency for each loudspeaker, and each signal type to be used during testing is recorded on a calibration form (see Appendix B, Form 2). After each individual measurement, the measured level is checked against the RETSPL + 70 dB. For example, at 1000 Hz for monaural listening at 45 degrees, the measured level should be 70 dB SPL because the RETSPL is 0.0 dB SPL, and the hearing level was set at 70 dB. If the measured output level is not within ± 2.5 dB of the RETSPL + 70 dB, the loudspeaker output level should be adjusted using the audiometer's internal calibration mode or a correction card should be developed.

The ANSI S3.6–2004 RETSPLs for sound field testing (**Table 11–3**) were taken directly from ISO 389–7:1996. Because ANSI did not specify RETSPLs for sound field testing until 1996, many audiologists have calibrated their sound field using the reference threshold levels reported by Morgan et al (1979), Walker et al (1984), or the levels recommended in a 1991 American Speech-Language-Hearing Association (ASHA) tutorial. **Table 11–4** lists the ANSI S3.6–2004 monaural sound field RETSPLs, the reference threshold levels recommended by ASHA in 1991, and the differences. The ANSI S3.6–2006 RETSPLs tend to be lower than the ASHA 1991 reference threshold levels, especially for a 90 degree azimuth. The cause of the ANSI minus ASHA reference threshold level differences is difficult to determine. However, it is probably related to the size, absorption characteristics, and other physical differences of the sound field.

Controversial Point

• To promote international uniformity, the ANSI S3.6–2004 sound field thresholds were taken directly from ISO 389–7:1996 even though they are lower than reported in the literature and recommended in a 1991 ASHA tutorial. It would seem that more research is needed to determine the cause of the ANSI minus ASHA differences.

ANSI S3.6–2004 also specifies that measurements for each frequency, loudspeaker, and signal type must be completed at several locations around the reference point to ensure that the

Table 11–4   Monaural Sound Field RETSPLs Reported in ANSI S3.6–2004, ASHA-1991, and the Threshold Differences

	Frequency (Hz)											
	125	250	500	750	1000	1500	2000	3000	4000	6000	8000	Speech
Monaural at 0 degree												
ANSI S3.6–2004	24.0	13.0	6.0	4.0	4.0	2.5	0.5	−4.0	−4.5	4.5	13.5	16.5
ASHA (1991)	32.0	16.0	9.5	7.5	5.5	4.5	2.5	.05	1.5	7.5	13.0	16.5
Differences	−8.0	−3.0	−3.5	−3.5	−1.5	−2.0	−2.0	4.5	6.0	−3.0	0.5	0.0
Monaural at 45 degrees												
ANSI S3.6–2004	23.5	12.0	3.0	.5	0.0	−1.0	−2.5	−9.0	−8.5	−3.0	8.0	12.5
ASHA (1991)	—	20.5	9.0	0.5	0.9	2.0	−0.5	−4.1	−3.1	3.8	—	12.5
Differences	—	−8.5	−6.0	0.0	−0.9	−3.0	−2.0	−4.9	−5.4	−6.8	—	0.0
Monaural at 90 degrees												
ANSI S3.6–2004	23.0	11.0	1.5	−1.0	−1.5	−2.5	−1.5	−6.5	−4.0	−5.0	5.5	11.0
ASHA (1991)	32.0	16.0	7.5	—	3.5	2.0	4.0	0.5	1.0	1.5	9.0	15.0
Differences	−9.0	−5.0	−6.0	—	−5.0	−4.5	−5.5	−7.0	−5.0	−6.5	−3.5	−4.0

ANSI, American National Standards Institute; ASHA, American Speech-Language-Hearing Association; RETSPLs, reference equivalent threshold sound pressure levels.

SPL around the patient's head is stable. Measurements must be performed at 0.15 m (6 inches) from the reference point on a left-right and up-down axis and must be within ± 2 dB of the SPL at the reference point for any test signal and at 0.1 m (4 inches) in front of and behind the reference point. The decibel difference between the front and behind measurements can deviate from the theoretical value given by the inverse square law by no more than ± 1 dB for any test signal.

Attenuator Linearity

Measuring attenuator linearity is performed to be sure that changes in the HL control result in the same changes in the audiometer's output level and can be measured acoustically or electrically. For two-channel audiometers, the linearity of the attenuator in each channel must be measured. If attenuator linearity is measured acoustically, a supra-aural earphone is placed and loaded with a 500 g weight on an NBS-9A coupler connected to an SLM having a one-third octave band filter. The SPL is measured and recorded (see Appendix B, Form 3) using a 1000 Hz tone and with the filter set to 1000 Hz, when the HL control is at maximum and for each 5 dB decrement or at 70 dB HL as a reference for each 5 dB step in both directions. At lower HLs, accurate measurements might not be obtained because the coupler SPLs might approach the noise floor of the SLM, or the measurement may be influenced by the ambient noise in the room. However, switching to a 125 or 250 Hz test tone and filter setting typically allows for measurements to be completed over the entire HL range.

If attenuator linearity is measured electrically, it is necessary to connect a voltmeter between the output of the audiometer and earphone with a Y-patch cord so that the audiometer is loaded with an earphone. Using a 1000 Hz tone, the voltage is measured over the entire HL range in 5 dB steps. This procedure assumes that measuring voltages will provide an accurate indication of the SPL output of an earphone. Thus a transducer having a nonlinear output will not be detected.

ANSI S3.6–2004 specifies that the output level difference between two successive HL settings should be no more than 5 dB apart, cannot deviate by more than three tenths of the indicated difference or more than 1 dB, whichever is smaller, and the maximum linearity deviation at any HL setting cannot exceed ± 2 dB. If the attenuator linearity does not meet the ANSI specifications, the cause of the problem should be determined, and the audiometer should be repaired and recalibrated.

Pearl

- Our experience has shown that the output of some audiometers may not be linear at 4000, 6000, and 8000 Hz even though the output at 1000 Hz was linear. Thus, checking attenuator linearity at multiple frequencies is a good idea.

Frequency

Accuracy

Pure-tone audiometers must accurately produce the frequencies indicated on the frequency control. If this does not occur, the patient would be responding to pure tones having different frequencies than those that the audiologist thought were being presented. In addition to the required

Special Consideration

- Once a sound field is calibrated, if additional furniture, instrumentation, or other objects are moved within or placed in the audiometric test room, the sound field should be recalibrated.

test frequencies for the different audiometer types (**Table 11–2**), audiometers can have additional frequencies located at half, one-third, and one-sixth octave bands. Frequency is measured by connecting an electronic counter/timer between the output of the audiometer and earphone using a Y-patch cord so that the audiometer is loaded with an earphone and then setting the HL so that the audiometer's output activates the electronic counter/timer. Frequency accuracy is measured for each frequency control setting and is recorded on a calibration form (see Appendix B, Form 3). ANSI S3.6–2004 specifies that the measured frequency compared with the frequency indicated on the audiometer must be within ± 1% for type 1, 2, and HF and ± 2% for type 3 and 4 audiometers. For example, the measured frequency at 1000 Hz for a type 1 audiometer should be between 990 and 1010 Hz.

Frequency Modulated Signals

Type 1 and 2 audiometers are required to have frequency modulated (FM) signals (**Table 11–1**). FM signals that are most commonly used for sound field testing to avoid standing waves. FM signals have three definable characteristics known as the carrier (i.e., center or nominal) frequency, modulation rate, and frequency deviation. ANSI S3.6–2004 specifies that the carrier may be modulated with either a sinusoidal or triangular waveform. The modulation or repetition rate is the number of times the FM signal changes per second and can range from 4 to 20 Hz, with a tolerance of ± 10% of the value stated by the manufacturer. Frequency deviation refers to the frequency range over which a change occurs for each modulation. ANSI S3.6–2004 specifies frequency deviation in percent around the carrier frequency, which can range from 5 to 25%, with a tolerance of ± 10% of the value stated by the manufacturer. Most type 1 and 2 audiometers allow the audiologist to select the frequency deviation, which typically ranges from 1 to 5%. Measuring the characteristics of an FM signal is typically not performed during a routine calibration. Interested readers are directed to Walker et al (1984) and ASHA (1991) for more information.

Harmonic Distortion

Pure-tone audiometers must present a pure signal that does not contain other frequencies so that the patient will only respond to hearing the frequency of the test tone and not its harmonics. For example, if a 500 Hz tone had excessive harmonics, the patient with an upward sloping audiogram might respond to the 1000 or 1500 Hz harmonic at a lower HL than responding to a 500 Hz tone that did not have excessive harmonics.

Harmonic distortion for each earphone type is measured by mounting the earphone on an appropriate coupler, with the coupler microphone connected to an SLM having one-third octave band filters. ANSI S3.6–2004 specifies that harmonic distortion be measured at 75 dB HL at 125 Hz, 90 dB HL at 250 Hz and 6000 to 16,000 Hz, and 110 dB HL at 500 to 4000 Hz or the maximum hearing level, whichever is lower. With the audiometer adjusted to the appropriate HL and the SLM one-third octave band filter adjusted to the test frequency, the earphone SPL is measured and recorded. Then, without changing the audiometer settings, the SLM filter is changed to the second harmonic of the test frequency, and the earphone SPL is measured and recorded. If the SLM filter center frequency does not correspond to the frequency of the harmonic, the next higher filter center frequency setting is used. This procedure is repeated until all of the higher frequency harmonics are measured. After this, measurements are obtained for the next frequency, and all harmonics and the measurements continue until harmonic distortion has been measured at every audiometer test frequency for each earphone. For bone vibrators, harmonic distortion is measured using similar procedures, except the bone vibrator is mounted on a mechanical coupler, the mechanical coupler output is directed to an analyzing instrument (which could be an SLM having one-third octave band filters), and the HL is set at 20 dB at 250 Hz, 50 dB at 500 and 750 Hz, and at 60 dB at 1000 to 5000 Hz. The ANSI S3.6–2004 recognizes that measurements of harmonics greater than 5000 Hz might be inaccurate because of limitations of acoustic and mechanical couplers and allows for electrical measurements greater than 5000 Hz. Form 4 in Appendix B can be used for recording the results of total harmonic distortion (THD). Harmonic distortion for loudspeakers is reported in the "Speech Audiometer" section.

> **Pitfall**
>
> - Octave band filters are not suitable for measuring harmonic distortion because they do not have rejection rates sufficient to measure distortion products lower than 24 to 28 dB below the level of the test tone.

ANSI S3.6–2004 specifies the maximum THD for earphones as ≤ 2.5% from 125 to 16,000, ≤ 2% from 125 to 16,000 Hz for the second harmonic and from 125 to 4000 Hz for the third harmonic, ≤ 0.3% from 125 to 4000 Hz for the fourth and higher harmonics, and ≤ 0.3% from 250 to 16,000 Hz for all of the subharmonics. The maximum THD for bone vibrators is ≤ 5.5% from 250 to 5000 Hz, ≤ 5% for the second harmonic, and ≤ 2% for third and higher level harmonics. The percentage of THD can be computed with the formula: $\% \text{THD} = 100 \sqrt{(p_2^2 + p_3^2 + p_4^2 + \ldots / p_1^2}$, where p_1 is the sound pressure of the test frequency and $p_2, p_3, p_4, \ldots$ are the sound pressures of the second, third, fourth, and so on, harmonics. It is important to note that the p's in the formula are sound pressure, not SPLs. Sound pressure and SPL are related by the formula $\text{SPL} = 20 \log_{10} (p/p_o)$, where p_o is the reference sound pressure of 20 µPa; conversely, $p = p_o \text{antilog}_{10} (\text{SPL}/20)$. The following is an approximation of the percent of distortion corresponding to the decibel difference between the level of the test frequency minus the level of a harmonic: 5.5% = 25 dB, 5.0% = 26 dB, 2.5% = 32 dB, 2.0% = 34 dB, and 0.3% = 50 dB.

Special Consideration

- Although ANSI S3.6–2004 requires measurements at fourth and higher harmonics and at all subharmonics, it is unlikely to have excessive distortion at these harmonics if the distortion for the second and third harmonics is acceptable. Measurements of distortion at all subharmonics are difficult and require extremely sensitive measurement instrumentation.

Excessive harmonic distortion is typically due to a problem with the transducer and not the input signal coming from the audiometer. The first step to solve a problem with excessive harmonic distortion should be to replace the transducer with one of the same type and repeat the measurements. If the problem was due to the transducer, the audiometer should be completely recalibrated with the new transducer.

Signal Switching

For manual audiometers, the pure tone is normally off and turned on by pressing an interrupter or tone switch. Most audiometers also have another switch that turns the tone on continuously, so that pressing the interrupter switch turns off the tone. To ensure that a patient is responding only to a pure tone and not other sounds, ANSI S3.6–2004 specifies performance characteristics for on/off ratio, crosstalk, rise/fall times, and overshoot.

On/Off Ratio

Checking the on/off ratio is performed to ensure that a tone will not be audible when it is turned off. ANSI S3.6–2004 requires that the earphone output must be 10 dB less than the RETSPL when the tone is off at HL settings ≤ 60 dB or increased by no more than 10 dB for each 10 dB increase in HL above 60 dB. The on/off ratio can be checked acoustically or electrically. If checked acoustically, the HL could be set to maximum, and the coupler output should be measured with and without a tone directed to the earphone. If the measurements are completed electrically, a Y-patch cord, voltmeter, and dummy resistive load would be required. A dummy resistive load can be made by soldering a resistor equal to the impedance of the transducer at 1000 Hz across the terminals of a phone plug. The phone plug of the Y-patch cord would be inserted into the audiometer's earphone output jack, a voltmeter would be connected into one jack of the patch cord, and the dummy load would be connected to the other patch cord jack. The tone on minus the tone off measured with one-third octave band SLM readings or voltmeter readings at each frequency, should be ≥ 70 dB and recorded on a calibration form (see Appendix B, Form 3).

Crosstalk

Crosstalk, or crossover, is another form of unwanted noise and occurs when a signal is directed to one earphone but is audible in the other earphone. Crosstalk can be measured acoustically or electrically, as done to determine the on/off ratios. The measure is performed by turning the HL to ≥ 70 dB and measuring the acoustical or electrical output in the other or nontest earphone. The measured signal must be at least 70 dB below the level of the signal directed to the test earphone.

Rise/Fall Times and Overshoot

Rise time is the time required for a tone to increase from a turned off to steady-state level. Fall time is the time required for a tone to decrease from a steady state to a turned off level. Overshoot occurs when a tone is turned on or off and temporarily exceeds its steady-state level. ANSI S3.6–2004 requires that the level of a tone that is off should be at least 60 dB less than the level when the tone is on. When the tone is turned on, the rise time from −60 to −1 dB of the steady-state level cannot exceed 200 msec and from −20 to −1 dB cannot be less than 20 msec. When the tone is turned off, the fall time from 0 to −60 dB of the steady-state level cannot exceed 200 msec and from −1 to −20 dB cannot be less than 20 msec. Only 1 dB of overshoot above the steady-state value is allowed when the tone is turned on or off. Verification of rise/fall times and overshoot can be completed electrically by connecting the audiometer output to an oscilloscope (or a rise/fall or overshoot detector) with a Y-patch cord so that the audiometer is loaded with an earphone. Typically, testing is performed with a 1000 Hz tone. However, it is good practice to also do the measurements at 250 and 6000 Hz, especially for older audiometers having switching mechanisms that might produce different rise/fall times as a function of frequency. ANSI S3.6–2004 requires that overshoot should be measured acoustically, but if overshoot is not observed during the electrical measurements, it is doubtful that it will occur acoustically. To be in compliance, an acoustic measurement of overshoot should be considered by placing each transducer on an appropriate coupler and connecting the coupler output to an SLM. The output of an SLM is connected to an oscilloscope to measure overshoot and possibly rise/fall times. The measurements for rise/fall time and overshoot should be recorded on a calibration form (see Appendix B, Form 3).

Pitfall

- It cannot be assumed that signal switching characteristics will be the same at each frequency. This occurs because some audiometers use a nonoptical keying circuit to turn the tone on and off.

Pulsed Tones

Type 1, 2, and HF audiometers are required to have a pulsed-tone feature that might be used to obtain threshold or for suprathreshold measures. Typically, a pulsed tone is activated by means of a switch that will automatically pulse a tone that is normally continuously on. For pulsed tones, ANSI S3.6–2004 specifies that the rise time from −20 to −1 dB and the fall time from −1 to −20 dB of the steady-state level must be 20 to 50 msec. The plateau of the pulsed tone must be ≥ 150 msec, and the time that a pulsed tone is on and off (duty cycle) must be 225 ± 35 msec measured 5 dB below the steady-state level. Furthermore, the signal level during the off phase must be 20 dB lower than during the on phase. These measurements are typically performed electrically with an oscilloscope; some can be completed with an electronic counter/timer.

Masking

Narrowband and white noise signals are used to eliminate the possibility that a tone presented to one ear is heard in the other ear and are adjusted by a masking level control marked in at least 5 dB steps. ANSI S3.6–2004 specifies that the masking output level must be sufficient to mask a tone of 60 dB HL at 250 Hz, 75 dB HL at 500 Hz, and 80 dB HL from 1000 to 8000 Hz.

Narrowband Noise

Narrowband noise (NBN) is required for all audiometers equipped with a bone vibrator (types 1, 2, and 3) and for HF audiometers (**Table 11–1**). This occurs because the RETFLs were standardized with 40 dB of effective masking (EM) presented to the nontest ear (Frank, 1982). ANSI S3.6–2004 specifies the bandwidth of each NBN from 125 to 16,000 Hz and requires that the output level be calibrated in EM level. A 0 dB EM level is the SPL of a masking signal that masks a pure tone presented at 0 dB HL 50% of the time when the masking signal and pure tone are presented to the same ear. The standard specifies the SPL of each NBN equal to 0 dB EM using a correction factor added to the RETSPL of any earphone type from 125 to 8000 Hz. The correction factors were taken directly from ISO 389–4:1994 and were derived on the assumption that an NBN having a critical bandwidth (Zwicker and Terhardt, 1980) will just mask a tone having the same frequency as the NBN at a signal-to-noise ratio of −4 dB.

The NBN output levels are measured the same way as pure-tone output levels are measured with an SLM with one-third octave band filters. For each NBN, the measured SPL should be equal to the correction factor plus the earphone RETSPL plus the EM level control setting. For example, at an EM control level setting of 70 dB, the SPL of a 1000 Hz NBN for a TDH 49 earphone measured in a NBS 9A coupler should be 83.5 dB SPL. This occurs because the 1000 Hz NBN correction factor is 6 dB, the TDH 49 RETSPL at 1000 Hz is 7.5 dB, and the EM control was set at 70 dB. Form 5 in Appendix B can be used for recording the measurements of masking signals and includes the NBN correction factors when the SPL of the NBN is measured with an SLM having one-third octave band filters. If the measured NBN SPLs are not within −3 to +5 dB of the desired SPL (correction factor plus earphone RETSPL plus EM control level setting) at any frequency, the NBN output level should be adjusted with the audiometer's internal calibration mode to the desired SPLs. If this is not possible, a correction card should be developed showing the adjustments that

will have to be applied to the EM level control when masked thresholds are obtained using NBN.

ANSI S3.6–2004 specifies that the NBN masking level control must range from 0 dB EML to the maximum air-conduction HL (**Table 11–2**) at each frequency but cannot exceed 115 dB SPL at any frequency. The linearity of the NBN masking level control is measured the same way as conducted for a pure tone.

White Noise

White noise (WN), also called broadband noise, is required for type 1 and 2 audiometers. The sound pressure spectrum level for WN must be within ± 5 dB of the level at 1000 Hz from 250 to 5000 Hz when measured in an acoustic coupler. The output of WN noise is typically calibrated in SPL; however, it can be calibrated in EM. If the WN is calibrated in SPL, the measured unfiltered SPL of the WN should be the same as the number on the EM level control within −3 to +5 dB and recorded on a calibration form (see Appendix B, Form 5).

Reference Signals

Some audiometric tests require the use of a reference signal that is independently controlled by the use of a second channel on the audiometer. Type 1 and 2 audiometers are required to have a reference tone that can be alternately presented with the test tone, and type 1 audiometers are required to have a reference tone that can be simultaneously presented with the test tone (i.e., tone from the other channel) (**Table 11–1**).

ANSI S3.6–2004 specifies that the performance characteristics of a reference signal generated from the second channel must meet the same requirements as those previously described for a single-channel audiometer, except for frequency range, HL range, increments, output level, and operation. The required reference signal frequencies must range from 250 to 6000 Hz, and the HL must range from 0 to 80 dB HL at 250 Hz and to 100 dB HL at 500 to 6000 Hz, with increments of 2.5 dB steps or less for a type 1 and 2 audiometer and in 5 dB steps for a type 3 audiometer. The reference tone output level must be calibrated to the same RETSPLs as the test tone and must be within ± 3 dB of the output level of the test tone from 500 to 4000 Hz and within ± 5 dB at 250 and 6000 Hz; with the reference signal on (second channel is operating), the output level of the test signal cannot change by more than ± 1 dB.

◆ Performance Characteristics of Automatic Audiometers

Automatic audiometers are required to meet the same performance characteristics as pure-tone audiometers plus additional performance characteristics related to the rate of signal level change, recording period, and frequency accuracy. The rate of signal level change is 2.5 dB/s for types 1 to 3 and 2.5 or 5 dB/s for types 4 and HF with a ± 20% tolerance. The rate of signal level change can be measured with a stopwatch by starting the audiometer and measuring the time it takes to change the signal level. The decibels per second rate can be determined by dividing the time into the decibel change. For example, a change in signal level of 40 dB should take 16 seconds for a 2.5 dB/s or 8 seconds for a 5 dB/s rate of signal level change. The rate of change should be measured for both increasing and decreasing signal levels.

If an automatic audiometer uses fixed frequencies, ANSI S3.6–2004 requires a minimum recording period of 30 seconds at each frequency before the next fixed frequency begins. The frequency accuracy is the same as for a pure-tone audiometer. If an audiometer uses a continuously variable or sweep frequency, the rate of frequency change is one octave per minute, and the frequency accuracy must be within ± 5% of the frequency indicated on the recording audiogram.

◆ Performance Characteristics of Speech Audiometers

Even though many of the performance characteristics for a speech audiometer are similar to those for a pure-tone audiometer, additional measurements are needed. This occurs because speech signals cover a wider range of frequencies and have more amplitude and temporal fluctuations than a pure tone. The additional measurements for speech audiometers include the performance characteristics of the monitoring meter, speech RETSPLs for each transducer, the frequency response of each transducer, playback device, and the microphone, harmonic distortion, and masking signal.

Monitoring Meter

Speech audiometers have a meter to monitor the input level of the speech signal presented live voice using a microphone (required for types A and B) or by presenting recorded material from a playback device (required for types A, B, and C). The monitoring meter (traditionally called a volume units or VU meter) is calibrated in decibels having a minimum value of −20 dB, maximum value of +3 dB, and a 0 dB reference position located between two thirds and three quarters of the full scale. Within the circuitry of a speech audiometer, the monitoring meter is located after the amplifier and before the attenuator (i.e., HL control). This is so that a speech signal input can be monitored while the HL is increased or decreased when a patient is tested. The amplifier preceding the monitoring meter must have a gain control of at least 20 dB for adjusting the input speech level. It is important to note that the speech signal input level must be adjusted to 0 dB on the monitoring meter using the gain control so that the speech signal output level will be equal to the level indicated on the HL control. For example, if the 1000 Hz calibration tone preceding a recorded speech test is adjusted to 0 dB on the monitoring meter, the recorded speech test will be presented to the patient at the level indicated on the HL control. If the level of the 1000 Hz calibration tone was adjusted

to −10 dB on the monitoring meter, the test will be presented 10 dB lower than indicated on the HL control.

The monitoring meter must be accurate and stable so that undershoot and overshoot are at a minimum. The accuracy of a monitoring meter can be checked by directing a 1000 Hz tone from an external oscillator to a 1 dB step attenuator and then to the audiometer's microphone or playback input, making sure that all impedances are matched. With the monitoring meter adjusted to +3 dB, increasing the attenuator output (more attenuation) in 1 dB steps should result in 1 dB decreases on the monitoring meter through its entire range. ANSI S3.6–2004 specifies the stability of a monitoring meter in reference to response time, defined as the time that it takes the monitoring meter to reach 99% of the 0 dB reference point, as 350 ± 10 msec with an allowable overshoot of 1.0 but not more than 1.5%. Furthermore, the response time for frequencies from 250 to 8000 Hz can differ by no more than 0.5 dB compared with the response time for a 1000 Hz tone. One way to measure response time is to develop a calibration tape (or CD) containing pure tones from 250 to 8000 Hz in octave intervals. At each frequency, a 10 second tone should be recorded for adjusting the monitoring meter to 0 dB, followed by the same frequency tone having durations of 350 (standard time) and 315 and 385 msec (± 10% of 350 msec). The test tape is directed into the audiometer through a playback device. After the adjustment of the monitoring meter to 0 dB for the 10 second tone, the level of the monitoring meter is visually observed for the 350 msec tone and for the tones of shorter and longer duration to ensure that the meter accurately deflects to 0 dB.

Reference Equivalent Threshold Sound Pressure Levels for Speech

ANSI S3.6–2004 specifies the RETSPLs for speech as 12.5 dB above the 1000 Hz RETSPL for any transducer when the monitoring meter and HL control are adjusted to 0 dB. Thus, a 1000 Hz tone is the test signal used for measuring the RETSPL for speech. For measuring the RETSPL using the microphone, an external source can be used to generate a 1000 Hz test signal. For example, a calibrated pure-tone audiometer could be set to produce a 1000 Hz tone through an earphone to deliver the test signal to the microphone. The level of the 1000 Hz tone should be at least 40 dB higher than the ambient room noise. For measuring the RETSPL using each playback device, a recording containing a 1000 Hz calibration tone at least 40 dB above the background noise of the recording can be used. With the monitoring meter adjusted to 0 dB for the 1000 Hz test signal and the HL control set at 70 dB, the coupler output level for each earphone should be 12.5 dB plus the RETSPL at 1000 Hz for the earphone being tested plus 70 dB. For a loudspeaker, the SPL at the reference test position should be 12.5 dB above the RETSPL at 1000 Hz for the listening condition (e.g., binaural or monaural at 0, 45, or 90 degrees azimuth) that will be used for sound field speech audiometry. The output levels for each transducer using the microphone and each playback device should be recorded on a calibration form (see Appendix B, Forms 1 and 2). The tolerance is ± 3 dB; however, as done with pure-tone audiometer output calibration, the transducer output should be adjusted using the audiometer's internal calibration mode so that the measured SPL is within ± 2.5 dB of the desired level. If this is not possible, a correction card should be developed.

Frequency Response

Because a speech signal covers a wide range of frequencies, ANSI S3.6–2004 has specified the frequency response characteristics to ensure that each transducer, playback device, and microphone has an acceptably flat response.

Output Transducers

For measuring the frequency response of each output transducer, ANSI S3.6–2004 specifies that the test signal should be WN directed to an input for an external signal (e.g., input normally used for a playback device). The source of the WN can be an external WN generator, where the output of the generator would be directed to an input for an external signal through a patch cord (making sure the impedances match). Another source would be the audiometer's internal WN generator directed to a nontest earphone. The nontest earphone phone plug should be removed and replaced by one end of a patch cord, and the other end of the patch cord would be plugged into an input for external signals. Regardless of the source, once the WN has been directed into an input for external signals, the monitoring meter should be adjusted to 0 dB and the HL control set to 70 dB. The monitoring meter should not be readjusted during the measurements. For earphone measurements, each earphone is positioned on an appropriate coupler; for loudspeaker measurements, the SLM is positioned at the reference test position. One-third octave band coupler or sound field SPLs for each band from 125 to 8000 Hz are then recorded on a calibration form for each transducer and loudspeaker (see Appendix B, Form 6). ANSI S3.6–2004 requires that the one-third octave band SPL for each band between 250 and 4000 Hz must be within ± 3 dB of the average SPL for all the bands; from 125 to 250 Hz, within +0 to −10 dB; and from 4000 to 6000 Hz, within ± 5 dB of the average SPL for all the bands.

Controversial Point

- A one-third octave band analysis of the frequency response of a transducer may indicate a smooth frequency response. However, significant output level deviations may occur between the one-third octave bands. Thus, a $^1/_{10}$, $^1/_{16}$, or $^1/_{32}$ octave band analysis of the frequency response of a transducer, especially a loudspeaker, may be needed to sufficiently describe its frequency response.

Playback Devices

The frequency response of each playback device is also measured acoustically using the transducer normally employed during the presentation of speech from a playback device. The recommended test signals are one-third octave bands of WN centered at one-third octave intervals from 125 to 8000 Hz (ANSI S3.6–2004, Annex B). This requires that a test signal tape or CD recording has to be developed or purchased. Each test signal should have a duration longer than 15 seconds, and any background noise in the recording should be at least 40 dB less than the level of the test signals. The same measurement procedures are performed for each output transducer as previously reported, except the test signals are one-third octave bands of noise rather than WN. The frequency response requirements for playback devices are increased by ± 1 dB from 250 to 4000 Hz and by ± 2 dB for frequencies outside 250 to 4000 Hz but within 125 to 8000 Hz compared with those for the output transducers. Form 6 in Appendix B can be used for recording the frequency response of each transducer using playback devices.

Microphone

ANSI S3.6–2004 requires that the output voltage level of the microphone has to be within ± 3 dB of the average level for all of the test signals from 125 to 8000 Hz when the signals are presented at 80 dB SPL under free field or equivalent conditions. The recommended test signals are the same as those used for measuring the frequency response of a playback device (i.e., one-third octave bands of WN centered at one-third octave intervals from 125 to 8000 Hz). These requirements create several problems in reference to delivering and acoustically measuring the test signals and the testing environment.

One method is to play the recorded test signals from a tape player to an external amplifier and then to an output transducer (e.g., loudspeaker or earphone). The audiometer microphone is positioned at the approximate distance and orientation from the output transducer as would normally occur during speech audiometry. The microphone of an SLM is placed into the sound field between the output transducer and as close as possible to the audiometer microphone without obstructing the sound pathway. The output of the microphone can be connected to a voltmeter using a Y-patch cord, where the microphone phone plug is inserted into one phone jack, the voltmeter into the other phone jack, and the patch cord phone plug into the audiometer microphone input. During the measurement, the output voltage level of the microphone is recorded in decibels after each test signal has been adjusted to 80 dB SPL, as monitored with the SLM. If the audiometer has two channels, another method to deliver the test signals to the microphone is to route the tape player output to one channel and then to a supra-aural earphone. To obtain a constant 80 dB SPL at the audiometer microphone, the earphone output level could be adjusted using the HL control and/or adjusting the gain control of the monitoring meter to a level less than 0 dB.

The problem with each method is that the audiometer microphone may not be in a free field or may be picking up ambient noise during the measurements. One way to avoid these problems is to place the test signal transducer and the microphone in a hearing aid test box using the reference microphone normally used during hearing aid measurements to monitor the SPL at the audiometer microphone. The ambient noise problem can also be addressed by measuring the ambient noise in the test environment before the measurements. This can be completed with the SLM placed in the position used for monitoring the test signals and with all of the instrumentation for delivering the test signals turned on. If the one-third octave band ambient noise SPL measurements from 125 to 8000 Hz are ≤ 40 dB SPL, it can be assumed that the ambient noise will not influence the microphone measurements because the input to the microphone is a constant 80 dB SPL. Form 6 in Appendix B can be used for recording the microphone frequency response.

Harmonic Distortion

THD for speech audiometers is tested with pure tones and measured acoustically for each transducer. For this measurement, a 250, 500, and 1000 Hz pure tone from an external source is directed into the audiometer's microphone or playback device input, and the monitoring meter is adjusted to +9 dB. It is important that the pure-tone test signals do not have excess distortion (i.e., ≥ 1%) at each individual harmonic. If a calibrated portable pure-tone audiometer is used as an external source, the monitoring meter can be adjusted to –1 dB. Then, increasing the portable audiometer's HL by 10 dB will drive the monitoring meter to +9 dB. For earphone measurements, the earphone is placed on an appropriate coupler, and the HL control is adjusted to produce 110 dB SPL for each test frequency. After this, the coupler SPL is determined with one-third octave band filtering at each harmonic of the test tone frequency. ANSI S3.6–2004 requires that the THD should not exceed 2.5% for each test tone.

For loudspeaker measurements, the same test tones and procedures are used, except the SLM is positioned at the reference test position in the sound field, and the output of each test tone is adjusted by the HL control to 80 dB SPL. The THD for each test tone frequency cannot exceed 3%. The procedure is then repeated with a loudspeaker output level of 100 dB SPL. At this level, the THD cannot exceed 10% for each test tone. Form 4 in Appendix B can be used for recording the harmonic distortion of each loudspeaker.

Unwanted Noise

It is important to note that the internal background noise of transducers should be significantly lower than the speech signal. This can be measured acoustically for each transducer by turning the HL control to a relatively high level and turning on the speech circuit. Without an input into the speech circuit, the background noise level should be at least 45 dB less than the HL setting with the earphone mounted on the appropriate coupler and the SLM set to the A-weighting frequency response. This measure should also be completed for each loudspeaker because they are known to produce more amplifier hum, static, or internal noise than earphones. The background noise of a loud-speaker should be 45 dB less than the HL setting when measured at the reference test position using the A-weighting response of an SLM. However, a more precise measure of background noise from each earphone and loudspeaker would be to measure the one-third octave band SPLs from 125 to 8000 Hz in the appropriate coupler or at the reference test position when the HL control is set at 80 dB HL. With no signal directed to the earphones or loudspeakers, the SPL in each one-third octave band should be at least 45 dB below the HL control. If this does not occur, the source of the problem should be determined and corrected. For loudspeakers, a common cause of excessive background noise occurs because the amplifier is not properly grounded.

Masking

All speech audiometers are required to have a masking signal (**Table 11–1**) called weighted random noise, or speech noise, having a sound pressure spectrum level shaped to approximate the long-term pressure spectrum level of speech. ANSI S3.6–2004 specifies that the pressure spectrum level should be constant from 100 to 1000 Hz and decrease at a rate of 12 dB/octave from 1000 to 6000 Hz within 5 dB. Furthermore, ANSI S3.6–2004 specifies that the speech noise output must be calibrated in EM level, where the SPL of the speech noise when the EM level control is set to 0 dB equals the RETSPL for speech. The EM level for speech noise is measured for each transducer using the same procedures and tolerance (−3 to +5 dB) used for NBN, except the SLM is adjusted to a linear frequency response. Form 5 in Appendix B can be used for recording the level of speech noise. If the SPL of the speech noise is not within −3 to +5 dB of the desired value, the earphone output level should be adjusted using the audiometer's internal calibration mode. If this is not possible, a correction card should be developed showing the adjustments in the EM level control that will have to be applied when speech noise masking is used.

♦ Inspection and Listening Checks

The operational status of an audiometer should be checked on a daily basis by completing several inspection and listening checks. These checks are not a substitute for the electroacoustic performance measurements; rather, they are performed to help ensure that the audiometer is functioning properly and to detect any problems that might require an immediate electroacoustic check. Inspection and listening checks are especially important for portable audiometers and audiometers transported to different testing sites (e.g., audiometers in a mobile van) because they are more susceptible to internal and transducer damage. The following are some daily inspection and listening checks. **Figure 11–9** shows a form for recording inspection and listening checks.

Penn State University, Speech and Hearing Clinic, 110 Moore Building, University Park, PA 16802
Audiometer Inspection and Listening Checks

Audiometer Name/Model No: _____   Serial No.: _____   Location: _____

Inspection Checks		Date & Tester Initials (If Inspection and Listening Check are okay check box; if not report problem immediately)												
Power Cord														
Earphone Cords														
Insert Earphone Tubing														
Bone Vibrator Cord														
Headband and Cushions														
Controls and Switches														
Listening Checks														
Frequency	Right													
	Left													
Attenuator Linearity	Right													
	Left													
Tone Switch, Hum, Static	Right													
	Left													
Crosstalk	Right													
	Left													
Known Threshold	Right													
	Left													
Acoustic Radiation														

Figure 11–9 Audiometer inspection and listening checks.

> **Pearl**
>
> • To save time, inspection and listening checks can be performed at the same time using the procedure reported by Frank (1980) or Martin (1998).

Inspection Checks

Power Cord and Light

For audiometers that are consistently being plugged in and out of electrical outlets, the entire length of the power cord should be checked before it is plugged in, especially at each end. If signs of wearing, cracking, or exposed wires are visible, the power cord should not be plugged in and should be replaced immediately. Almost every audiometer has a power light (or a lighted control window) that comes on when the audiometer is turned on. There could be several reasons that the power light is not on once the power cord has been plugged in and the audiometer power switch has been turned on. One could be that the light is loose or burned out. If this is the case, the audiometer should still function normally, but the light should be checked and replaced. If the audiometer is powered by batteries, the

battery indicator should be checked to see whether the batteries need to be replaced. Another reason could be that power to the electrical wall outlet has to be turned on (common in day care centers) by a wall switch or a circuit breaker. Yet another reason could be a burned-out fuse contained in some older audiometers as a protection from an excessive electrical input. Typically, the fuse is located next to the entrance of the power cord into the audiometer. To check a fuse, the audiometer must be unplugged and turned off. The fuse should be removed from its holder and inspected to see whether the filaments running through the fuse are intact. If the fuse is burned out, it must be replaced with one having the same size and ampere rating. The final, most likely reason is that the audiometer power switch has become defective and needs to be replaced.

Transducer Cords

Visual inspection should be made of each transducer cord along the entire length to look for signs of wearing and cracking, especially where the cord enters the transducer and the phone plug. A worn or cracked cord should be replaced with one of the same type and length. Although it is not a cord, the plastic tube of each 3A insert earphone should be checked to be sure that it is tightly connected to the transducer and nipple and that there are no cracks along the entire length. Also, the inside of the tube and nipple for a 3A and nipple for a 5A insert earphone should be checked to be sure that it is clear of moisture and debris.

Cushions and Headband

The cushion of a supra-aural earphone should be tightly connected to the earphone or the plastic housing covering the earphone. This can be checked by holding the earphone or plastic housing and rotating the cushion. If the cushion can be easily rotated, it should be replaced. If a two-piece cushion (e.g., Telephonics Corporation [Farmingedale, NY] MX-41/AR) is being used, the connection between the two pieces should be inspected to be sure that the pieces are tightly glued together. A defective cushion should be replaced. Audiometer recalibration is not necessary. The earphone headband should have a certain tension to hold the earphones tightly against the pinna. This can be checked by positioning each post that connects the earphone to the headband to a midpoint position. When holding the top of the headband, the inside of the cushions should mate. If this does not occur, the headband should be bent (twisted) to restore its tension or be replaced.

Controls and Switches

All the dials, switches, and pushbuttons must be tightly connected, move through their entire function, and be in proper alignment. If a defect is found, the audiometer should be repaired and, depending on the problem, recalibrated, especially if an alignment problem was detected.

Listening Checks

Listening checks are done for many of the performance characteristics measured during an electroacoustic calibration. All listening checks should be completed with a normally hearing listener and the audiometer and transducers in their customary locations. If an audiometer and transducers are located in separate rooms, two people are required to do listening checks, and a talk-over and talk-back system is typically required. However, in this situation many audiologists who work alone unplug the transducers from the audiometric test room jack box and plug them directly into the audiometer after unplugging the patch cords that go from the audiometer to the control room jack box. The danger with this procedure is that all the phone plugs that were removed have to be fully reinserted into the appropriate jacks, and it is assumed that the connections from the audiometer through the audiometric test room side of the jack box are functioning normally. If this procedure is used, the final check should be listening to a 1000 Hz tone at 60 dB HL through each transducer after they were reinserted into the audiometric test room jack box. An alternative procedure is to use a patch cord having a phone plug at each end, as suggested by Martin (1998). The phone plug of the transducer to be checked is unplugged from the test room jack box and replaced by one end of the patch cord. The other end of the patch cord is inserted into an open jack

on the jack box, which leads to an open jack on the control room jack box. The phone plug of the transducer to be checked is then inserted into the open jack on the control room jack box.

Pearl

- Always be sure that a transducer phone plug is fully inserted into the output jack. If this does not occur, the transducer may have no or a reduced output, which could influence test results.

Audiometer Noise

If an audiometer is operated in the same room as the patient, the audiometer should not produce unwanted sounds that could invalidate the test results. That is, any sound that results from the operation of any control or sound radiated from the audiometer should not be audible; this does not apply to sound created by the movement of the frequency control or output selector when the patient is not actually being tested. This can be checked by disconnecting the earphones from the audiometer and terminating the earphone outputs with a dummy resistive load (i.e., a resistor equal to the impedance of the transducer soldered across the terminals of a phone plug). The listener wears the earphones, disconnected from the audiometer, while all of the controls on the audiometer that would normally be used during a test (e.g., interrupter switch, HL control) are manipulated. If the audiometer has a bone vibrator, the bone vibrator cord is disconnected and replaced by a dummy load. The listener wears the bone vibrator on one ear and an earphone occluding the other ear while the controls are manipulated. If unwanted sounds are detected, the audiometer needs to be checked to determine the source and repaired.

Frequency

Checking frequency is completed by setting the frequency control to its lowest setting and directing a continuous 70 dB HL tone to one earphone. The frequency control is slowly moved through its entire range and repeated for the other earphone. A nonwavering tone should be heard at each frequency in each earphone. If this does not occur, the audiometer needs to be checked for frequency accuracy.

Attenuator Linearity

Checking linearity is performed by setting the HL control to its lowest level and directing a continuous 1000 Hz tone to one earphone, then moving the HL control through the entire range and repeating for the other earphone. The result should be hearing a tone that increases in loudness without any other noises at or between the HL steps. If this does not occur, the audiometer needs to be checked for linearity.

Transducer Cords

Transducer cords can be checked by directing a continuous 1000 Hz tone at 70 dB HL into each transducer. The cord should be twisted and flexed along its entire length, especially where it inserts into the transducer and the phone plug. The result should be hearing a steady-state 1000 Hz tone in each transducer. A defective cord will usually produce static or cause the tone to be intermittent. If a problem occurs at the transducer connection, tightening the screws that hold the cord into the earphone might solve the problem. If a problem occurs at the phone plug end, a wire within the cord may be broken, or the solder joint connecting a wire to the phone plug may have broken loose and may need to be resoldered. However, many earphone cords have a plastic casing around the phone plug that cannot be removed. If a cord is defective, it should be replaced by one of the same type and length, and a quick output level calibration should be considered.

Interrupter Switch and Static/Hum

This check can be done by directing a tone at 70 dB HL into one earphone at each frequency from 125 to 8000 Hz and pressing the interrupter switch, then repeating for the other earphone. The result should be hearing a smooth tone on-set and off-set. When the tone is off, static, hum, or other noises should not be present. If turning the tone on and off does not produce a smooth tone on-set or off-set or when the tone is off, if static, hum, or other noises are present, the audiometer should be checked electroacoustically.

Crosstalk

Recall that crosstalk, or crossover, is a form of unwanted noise that occurs when a signal is directed to one earphone but is audible in the other earphone. Checking for crosstalk is completed by wearing each earphone, but one earphone is disconnected from the audiometer and replaced with a dummy resistance load. With the audiometer set at 70 dB HL, a tone is directed to the disconnected earphone while the frequency is changed over its entire range. The listener should not hear a tone in the earphone connected to the audiometer. The check is repeated in the same manner for the other earphone. If crosstalk occurs, the audiometer needs to be checked electroacoustically.

Acoustic Radiation

Unwanted sound from a bone vibrator can occur from sound leaking or radiating from the enclosure housing the electromagnetic transducer. This type of unwanted sound is termed *acoustic radiation* and may cause an invalid high-frequency air–bone gap in patients who do not have a conductive pathological condition or collapsing ear canals. This occurs because the patients are responding by means of air conduction to the acoustic radiation at a lower HL than their true bone-conduction threshold (Shipton et al, 1980). Typically, acoustic radiation occurs in the higher frequencies, especially at 4000 Hz, and is greater for a Radioear B-72

than a B-71 bone vibrator (Frank and Crandell, 1986; Frank and Holmes, 1981). ANSI S3.6–2004 specifies an objective test for acoustic radiation that manufacturers must conduct to determine whether their bone vibrators produce acoustic radiation. The manufacturer must state the frequencies at which acoustic radiation may occur that would invalidate unoccluded bone-conduction thresholds. Acoustic radiation can be checked by obtaining bone-conduction thresholds at 2000 and 4000 Hz using mastoid placement. Next, a foam earplug is placed between the surface of the bone vibrator and the mastoid to isolate the bone vibrator from the mastoid. The 2000 and 4000 Hz tones are then turned on individually at the HL that corresponded to the bone-conduction threshold. If acoustic radiation is present, the 2000 and/or 4000 Hz tone will be audible. If this occurs, the screws holding the bone vibrator together should be tightened and the test repeated. If acoustic radiation is still present, the bone vibrator should be replaced, and bone-conduction calibrations must be completed.

Known Threshold

This check is performed by obtaining air-conduction thresholds for each transducer on a listener (i.e., audiologist) and comparing them to previous thresholds. If the thresholds are not within ± 5 dB of the previous thresholds, the output levels should be measured electroacoustically.

◆ Acoustic Immittance Instruments

The term *acoustic immittance* does not have a physical reference. Rather, it refers to the reciprocal quantities of acoustic impedance or acoustic admittance, or to both quantities. Historically, instruments referenced to acoustic impedance were used to measure the ear's opposition to the flow of energy. However, all modern-day instruments are referenced to acoustic admittance and are used to measure the ease in which energy flows through the ear. As such, the following discussion only describes the performance characteristics of acoustic admittance instruments. All acoustic admittance instruments require a method to deliver a sound, measure the resultant SPL, and control the air pressure in the ear canal. This is done by coupling the instrument to the ear canal using a probe having a soft rubber tip so that an airtight seal is created when the probe tip is fitted in the ear canal. The probe contains several openings that are connected to different systems within the instrument. These systems typically include (1) a miniature loudspeaker that produces a probe tone (e.g., 226 Hz) in the ear canal and activating signals for measuring the ipsilateral acoustic reflex, (2) a microphone that measures the ear canal SPL of the probe tone, and (3) an air pump for changing the air pressure in the ear canal. To learn more about the principles underlying acoustic admittance measurements, interested readers are directed to Margolis (1981), Popelka (1984), and Wiley and Fowler (1997).

Acoustic admittance instruments are most commonly used to obtain a tympanogram and to measure the threshold or the presence of an acoustic reflex. A tympanogram is a measure of the acoustic admittance at the end of the probe tip (measurement plane) or at the eardrum (compensated) as a function of air pressure in the ear canal. The acoustic reflex is a measurement of stapedius muscle contraction to an activating stimulus (e.g., pure tones or noise) presented ipsilaterally through the probe or contralaterally using a supra-aural or insert earphone.

Terminology regarding acoustic admittance and the performance characteristics of acoustic admittance instruments using a 226 Hz probe tone have been specified in ANSI S3.39–1987 (R2002), *Specifications for Instruments to Measure Aural Acoustic Impedance and Admittance (Aural Acoustic Immittance)*, and IEC 60645-5 (2004–11), *Instruments for the Measurement of Aural Acoustic Impedance/ Admittance*. Form 7 in Appendix B can be used for recording the results of an electroacoustic calibration of an acoustic admittance instrument.

Terminology, Plotting, and Symbols

Terminology used to describe acoustic admittance instruments and, more importantly, the test measurements has been inconsistent, confusing, and sometimes misleading (Popelka, 1984). In an effort to eliminate this problem and promote uniformity, ANSI S3.39–1987 (R2002) provides standardized terms and their definitions and abbreviations for measured quantities. These terms have been accepted and are currently used throughout the literature.

ANSI S3.39–1987 (R2002) has also standardized the tympanogram by defining labels and scale proportions because the morphological aspects of a tympanogram (height and width) are influenced by the aspect ratio. The standard specifies that the vertical axis of a tympanogram must have a linear scale labeled "Acoustic Admittance $[10^{-8}\ m^3/Pa \times s$ (acoustic mmho)]," or "Acoustic Admittance of Equivalent Volume of Air (cm^3)," or both. The horizontal axis must be labeled "Air Pressure (daPa) [1 daPa = 1.02 mm H_2O]," where 0 daPa (dekapascal) represents the ambient air pressure at the test site. The scale proportions (aspect ratio) for a 226 Hz tympanogram is defined as 300 daPa on the horizontal scale equals the length of 1 acoustic mmho (1 cm^3) on the vertical axis. The standard also specifies symbols for plotting the threshold levels of ipsilateral and contralateral acoustic reflexes on an audiogram.

Controversial Point

• ANSI S3.39–1987 (R2002) only specifies performance characteristics for acoustic admittance instruments having a 226 Hz probe tone. The 2007 revision of ANSI S3.39 will probably incorporate IEC specifications and specifications for acoustic admittance instruments having multiple frequency probe tone frequencies.

Types

ANSI S3.39–1987 (R2002) classifies acoustic admittance instruments into types based on the features they contain and measurement capabilities, shown in **Table 11–5**, where types 1 and 2, typically used for diagnostic testing, have more features, functions, and capabilities compared with type 3, typically used for screening purposes. Type 4, not shown in **Table 11–5**, has no minimum requirements and are instruments usually having the capability for just tympanometry or acoustic reflex testing.

Range and Accuracy

All of the types of acoustic admittance instruments have a range of measurement capabilities referenced to $m^3/Pa \times s$ or in acoustic mmho, or in an equivalent volume of air with units in cm^3. If the instrument provides an assessment of the admittance at the frontal surface of the probe (i.e., measurement plane), the minimum range for all types is 0.2 to 5.0 acoustic mmho. If the instrument corrects for the acoustic admittance in the ear canal (i.e., compensated measurement), the minimum range for types 1 and 2 is 0.0 to 2.0 acoustic mmho and for type 3, 0.0 to 1.2 acoustic mmho with an accuracy of ± 5% of the indicated value.

Calibration Cavities

An enclosed volume of air can be used to calibrate acoustic admittance instruments. This occurs because the acoustic admittance of a cavity is proportional to its volume for a 226 Hz probe tone if certain constraints regarding the dimensions of the cavity are met. ANSI S3.39–1987 (R2002) requires that type 1, 2, and 3 instruments have three calibration cavities having volumes of 0.5, 2.0, and 5.0 cm^3 with a tolerance of ± 2% or 0.05 cm^3, whichever is greater. Additional cavities having volumes of 1.0, 1.5, 2.5, 3.0, 3.5, 4.0, and 4.5 cm^3 are optional. For a 226 Hz probe tone, the admittance magnitude reading on the instrument in mmho should be the same as the volume of each cavity. Many instruments perform an automatic calibration once the probe is sealed in a cavity, whereas others require an internal or external adjustment to obtain the desired value.

Special Consideration

• It is important to note that acoustic admittance measures are influenced by atmospheric pressure and might require an adjustment. Shanks (1987) has provided correction factors for atmospheric pressure at different altitudes above sea level.

Probe Tone

All acoustic admittance instruments use a probe tone that must be calibrated for frequency, SPL, and distortion. ANSI S3.39–1987 (R2002) requires that types 1 to 3 instruments have a 226 Hz probe tone. If the instrument has additional

Table 11–5 Characteristic, Function, or Capability of Acoustic Immittance Instruments per Instrument Type

Characteristic, Function, or Capability	Instrument Type		
	1	2	3
Probe signal			
Sinusoidal, 226 Hz	Yes	Yes	Yes
Pneumatic System			
Manual control of air pressure	Yes	No	No
Automatic control of air pressure	Yes	No	No
Manual or automatic control of air pressure	No	Yes	Yes
Analog or digital output proportional to air pressure	Yes	No	No
Graphic display or indicator	Yes	Yes	Yes
Static Acoustic Immittance			
Measurement plane	Yes	No	No
Compensated	Yes	Yes	No
Proportional analog or digital output	Yes	No	No
Graphic display or indicator	Yes	Yes	Yes
Tympanometry			
Measurement plane	Yes	No	No
Compensated	Yes	Yes	No
Proportional analog or digital output	Yes	No	No
Graphic display or indicator	Yes	Yes	Yes
Acoustic-Reflex Activating System			
Noise-activating signal (stimulus)	Yes	No	No
Pure-tone activating signals (stimuli)	Yes	Yes	No
Pure-tone or noise-activating signal	No	No	Yes
Contralateral presentation of stimulus	Yes	No	No
Ipsilateral presentation of stimulus	Yes	No	No
Contralateral and ipsilateral stimulus	No	Yes	Yes
Manual control of stimulus level	Yes	No	No

Source: Adapted from ANSI S3.39–1987 (R2002), *American National Standard Specification for Instruments to Measure Aural Acoustic Impedance and Admittance (Aural Acoustic Immittance),* © 1987 Acoustical Society of America, 35 Pinelawn Road, Suite 114E, Melville, NY 11747, with permission.

probe tones, the manufacturer has to describe their acoustic characteristics. The SPL of a probe tone is below the threshold of the acoustic reflex but high enough to obtain a favorable signal-to-noise ratio. The manufacturer has to specify the SPL of the probe tone, which cannot exceed 90 dB SPL. The SPL of the probe tone is measured using an HA-1 coupler by sealing the end of the probe flush with the opening of the coupler cavity, being careful to avoid any leaks between the end of the probe and the opening of the coupler cavity. The coupler SPL is measured with an SLM. If the SLM has a one-third octave band filter, the filter is set at 250 Hz. The measured SPL should be equal to the SPL stated by the manufacturer within ± 3 dB. Typically, an internal or external calibration control changes the level of the probe tone level if the measured SPL is not within tolerance.

The frequency accuracy of any probe tone has to be within ± 3% of the indicated value and can be measured with an electronic counter/timer. Harmonic distortion measurements of any probe-tone frequency are conducted with the probe coupled to an HA-1 coupler in the same manner as done for measuring the output level. Then the coupler SPL is measured in one-third octave bands with a filter setting corresponding to the frequency and harmonics of the probe tone. The THD cannot exceed 5%.

Air Pressure

Type 1 to 3 instruments must have the capability of changing air pressure in the ear canal and in the calibration cavities. The maximum limits are –800/+600 daPa measured in a 0.5 cm^3 cavity; however, each type has a minimum air pressure range. For type 1 and 2 instruments, the minimum range is –600/+200 daPa, for type 3 it is –300/+100 daPa, and for type 4 the range has to be stated by the manufacturer if provided. The tolerance in the calibration cavities from 0.5 to 2.0 cm^3 for type 1 and 2 instruments cannot differ from the indicated reading on the instrument by ± 10 daPa or ± 10%, whichever is greater, and for type 3 and 4 instruments by ± 10 daPa or ± 15%, whichever is greater. The air pressure and the linearity of the air pressure scale can be measured by sealing the probe to a calibrated manometer or U tube water displacement device. Many instruments have the means to change the air pressure by an internal calibration mode or external control. For some instruments, air pressure can be changed manually or automatically; however, most instruments automatically change air pressure once a seal is obtained. For these instruments, the manufacturer has to state the rate (daPa/s) and direction (positive to negative, negative to positive, or both) of the change.

Activating Signals for the Acoustic Reflex

Pure-tone and noise signals can be used as reflex activating signals (RASs) for determining the threshold or the presence of the acoustic reflex when presented contralaterally through a supra-aural or insert earphone and ipsilaterally through the probe.

Pure-Tone RASs

ANSI S3.39–1987 (R2002) specifies that type 1 instruments must have 500, 1000, 2000, and 4000 Hz pure tones for both contralateral and ipsilateral stimulation, and type 2 instruments must have at least 500, 1000, and 2000 Hz pure tones for contralateral or ipsilateral stimulation. The output levels for the RAS tones presented through a supra-aural earphone are referenced to HL using the RETSPLs listed in ANSI S3.6–2004, shown in **Table 11–3**, and must range from 50 to 90 dB at 250 Hz, 50 to 120dB from 500 to 4000 Hz, and from 50 to 100 dB at 6000 Hz. For an insert earphone, the output of the RAS pure tones can be calibrated in SPL or HL using the RETSPLs specified in ANSI S3.6–2004, shown in **Table 11–3**. The output level for RAS pure tones presented through the probe can also be calibrated in SPL or HL; however, the manufacturer has to provide the RETSPLs if the output level is calibrated in HL using the procedure outlined in Annex D of ANSI S3.6–2004. The insert earphone and probe output levels must range from 60 to 110 dB SPL from 500 to 2000 Hz and from 60 to 90 dB SPL at 4000 Hz.

Pitfall

- Some manufacturers report that the output level of different frequency ipsilateral RASs are calibrated in HL when in fact all the frequencies have the same SPLs at 0 dB HL.

Noise RASs

A broadband noise RAS is required for type 1 admittance instruments and may be used instead of pure-tone signals for type 3 instruments. When broadband noise is presented through a supra-aural earphone, the acoustic pressure spectrum level must be within ± 5 dB relative to the level at 1000 Hz from 250 to 6000 Hz and must range from 50 to 115 dB SPL. For an insert earphone or the probe, the acoustic pressure spectrum level must be within ± 5 dB relative to the level at 1000 Hz from 400 to 4000 Hz and must range from 50 to 100 dB SPL. Some acoustic admittance

instruments also have low-pass, high-pass, band-pass noise RASs. If this is the case, the manufacturer has to specify the acoustic pressure spectrum level of the noise, all other characteristics, and tolerances.

Measurement of RASs

The performance characteristics of RASs presented through a supra-aural or insert earphone are measured in the same manner using the same couplers used for a pure-tone audiometer. For RASs presented through the probe, the probe is sealed to an HA-1 coupler as previously described for measuring the characteristics of the probe tone. The required measures include output levels, attenuator linearity, frequency accuracy, total harmonic distortion, and rise/fall times. The coupler output levels for pure-tone RASs from 250 to 4000 Hz have a tolerance of ± 3 dB and ± 5 dB for 6000 Hz and higher, as well as for any noise RAS. The attenuator linearity cannot differ from the indicated difference between intervals of 5 dB on the instrument or less by more than three tenths or 1 dB, whichever is smaller, and the cumulative error cannot be more than the output level tolerance. Frequency accuracy is ± 3% of the indicated value. THD cannot exceed 3% for tone RASs presented through a supra-aural earphone when the output is set at 90 dB HL at 250 and 8000 Hz and at 110 dB HL from 500 to 6000 Hz. For insert earphones and the probe, the THD cannot exceed 5% when the output is 85 dB HL or 95 dB SPL at 500 Hz, 100 dB HL or SPL from 1000 to 3000 Hz, and at 75 dB HL or SPL at 4000 Hz. The rise/fall time of a RAS cannot exceed 50 msec or be less than 5 msec with 1 dB of overshoot.

Temporal Characteristics

The temporal characteristics of acoustic admittance instruments must be known if the instrument is going to be used for latency measurements of the acoustic reflex. For accurate measurements, the response time must be faster than the response of the acoustic reflex. ANSI S3.39–1987 (R2002) requires that manufacturers specify the response time, which cannot exceed 50 msec. Interested readers are referred to a procedure for measuring the temporal characteristics of an acoustic admittance instrument provided in Appendix B of ANSI S3.39–1987 (R2002) reported by Popelka and Dubno (1978) and Shanks et al (1985), who have suggested an alternative procedure. Briefly, the procedures involve a technique to simulate an instantaneous change in the acoustic admittance at the probe tip while measuring the temporal characteristics of the instrument to define initial latency, rise time, terminal latency, and fall time (Lilly, 1984). Initial latency is the time from the beginning of the instantaneous change in admittance to 10% of the measured change in the steady-state admittance. Rise time is the time from 10 to 90% of the change in the measured steady-state admittance. Terminal latency is the time from the end of the instantaneous change to 90% of the measured steady-state admittance change. Fall time is the time from 90 to 10% of the measured steady-state admittance change from the end of the instantaneous change.

Artifacts

ANSI S3.39–1987 (R2002) does not address the need to be concerned about artifacts caused by a possible interaction of the RAS and the probe tone during the measurement of the ipsilateral acoustic reflex. The presence of an artifact can be easily determined by placing the probe in the 0.5 cm^3 cavity and presenting each activating stimulus at increasingly higher levels. If no artifact is present, the method of displaying the acoustic reflex on an acoustic admittance instrument should remain stationary for each RAS at each output level. If an artifact is present, the display will change when the RAS is presented. The frequency and level at which each RAS creates an artifact should be recorded and placed on the acoustic admittance device, and ipsilateral acoustic reflex measurements should not be measured at that frequency or above that level.

Inspection and Listening Checks

Daily inspection and listening checks of an acoustic admittance instrument are performed in the same manner as for a pure-tone audiometer. In addition, the probe should be checked to be sure that each opening is free of wax and debris. Furthermore, the instrument should be calibrated before its daily use by placing the probe in each calibration cavity, and the audiologist should obtain a tympanogram and ipsilateral and contralateral acoustic reflexes. These measures can then be compared with previous measures to be sure that the instrument is operating correctly.

◆ Audiometric Test Rooms

Audiometric test rooms are also called audiometric test booths or sound-treated rooms. The purpose of an audiometric test room is to provide an acceptably quiet listening environment so that external or internal ambient noise will not elevate hearing thresholds caused by masking. Typically, audiometric test rooms are prefabricated with single-walled or double-walled construction. A double-walled room provides ~20 to 30 dB more attenuation of external ambient noise than a single-walled room, especially in the higher frequencies. Audiometric test rooms can range in size to accommodate a single person for just earphone testing or be large enough to allow for sound field testing. Before purchasing an audiometric test room, several variables have to be considered. Information concerning these variables can be found in ANSI S3.1–1999 (R2003), Annex G.

ANSI Ambient Noise Levels

Because it is impossible to eliminate all ambient noise, ANSI has developed a standard (ANSI S3.1–1999 (R2003)) specifying maximum permissible ambient noise levels (MPANLs) allowed in an audiometric test room for testing hearing down to 0 dB HL. Frank et al (1993) and Frank (2000) have provided an overview of all of the previous ANSI standards regarding the specification of MPANLs allowed in audiometric test rooms. The ANSI S3.1–1999 (R2003) MPANLs are specified in octave and one-third octave band intervals for two test conditions and three test frequency ranges. The one-third octave band MPANLs are shown in **Table 11–6**

Table 11–6 One-third Octave Band Maximum Permissible Ambient Noise Levels for Three Test Frequency Ranges for Ears Covered with a TDH or Insert Earphone and for Ears Not Covered

Test Frequency Range One-Third Octave Band (Hz)	Ears Covered						Ears Not Covered		
	125–8000 Hz		250–8000 Hz		500–8000 Hz		125–8000 Hz	250–8000 Hz	500–8000 Hz
	TDH	Insert	TDH	Insert	TDH	Insert			
125	30.0*	54.0	34.0	62.0	44.0	73.0	24.0	30.0	39.0
250	20.0	48.0	20.0	48.0	30.0	59.0	16.0	16.0	25.0
500	16.0	45.0	16.0	45.0	16.0	45.0	11.0	11.0	11.0
800	19.0	44.0	19.0	44.0	19.0	44.0	10.0	10.0	10.0
1000	21.0	42.0	21.0	42.0	21.0	42.0	8.0	8.0	8.0
1600	25.0	43.0	25.0	43.0	25.0	43.0	9.0	9.0	9.0
2000	29.0	44.0	29.0	44.0	29.0	44.0	9.0	9.0	9.0
3150	33.0	46.0	33.0	46.0	33.0	46.0	8.0	8.0	8.0
4000	32.0	45.0	32.0	45.0	32.0	45.0	6.0	6.0	6.0
6300	32.0	48.0	32.0	48.0	32.0	48.0	8.0	8.0	8.0
8000	32.0	51.0	32.0	51.0	32.0	51.0	9.0	9.0	9.0

*Figures given are in decibels.

Note: Octave band MPANLs are 5 dB higher than each tabled level.

Source: From ANSI S3.1–1999 (R2003), *American National Standard Maximum Permissible Ambient Noise Levels for Audiometric Test Rooms,* © 1999 Acoustical Society of America, 35 Pinelawn Road, Suite 114E, Melville, NY 11747, with permission.

(octave band MPANLs are 5 dB higher for each tabled value). One test condition is called ears not covered and applies when either one or both ears are not covered by an earphone, as would typically occur during bone-conduction or sound field audiometry. The other test condition is called ears covered and applies when both ears are covered simultaneously by a supra-aural or insert earphone, as would typically occur during air-conduction audiometry. The ears covered MPANLs exceed the ears not covered MPANLs by the attenuation provided by a supra-aural earphone derived using the mean attenuation values averaged across three studies (Arlinger, 1986; Berger and Killion, 1989; Frank and Wright, 1990) and by an insert earphone derived using the mean attenuation values averaged across three studies (Berger and Killion, 1989; Frank and Wright, 1990; Wright and Frank, 1992). The three frequency ranges are 125 to 8000 Hz, 250 to 8000 Hz, and 500 to 8000 Hz. The frequency ranges 125 to 8000 Hz and 250 to 8000 Hz are typically used for clinical testing, and the frequency range 500 to 8000 Hz is typically used for industrial testing and hearing screening.

The MPANLs take into account the upward spread of masking because it is well known that excessive low-frequency noise can mask higher frequency thresholds. For the purpose of specifying MPANLs, the upward spread of masking was defined to have a slope of 14 dB/octave below the lowest test frequency. Thus, the MPANL one octave below the lowest test frequency (125 Hz for the 250–8000 Hz range and 250 Hz for the 500–8000 Hz range) is equal to the lowest test frequency MPANL + 14 dB, and the MPANL two octaves below the lowest test frequency (125 Hz for the 500–8000 Hz range) is equal to the lowest test frequency MPANL + 28 dB.

ANSI S3.1–1999 (R2003) assumes that if the ambient noise levels in a test room are equal to or less than the MPANLs, hearing thresholds measured at 0 dB HL will not be elevated. However, when the level of a noise is near the level of a patient's unmasked threshold, the patient's thresholds might be elevated by as much as 2 dB. Thus, the MPANLs have an uncertainty or negligible masking of 2 dB. That is, a maximum threshold shift of 2 dB may occur when thresholds are obtained at 0 dB HL in an audiometric test room having ambient noise levels equal to the MPANLs. Research by Berger and Killion (1989) and Frank and Williams (1993a) has verified this assumption.

Measurement and Verification

Ambient noise levels are measured using an SLM having an octave or one-third octave band filter. Because some of the ears not covered MPANLs are very low, it is important that the noise floor of the SLM-filter combination does not interfere with the measurements. ANSI S3.1–1999 (R2003) specifies that the SLM-filter combination must have an internal noise at least 3 dB below the MPANLs and describes ways (Annex E) that this can be measured. If this condition is not met, an SLM having lower internal noise must be used. During the measurements, the SLM microphone should be placed at the location of the patient's head, and all possible sources of noise should be operating. This would include the ventilation system, lights, and all instrumentation inside and outside the test room. Octave or one-third octave band SPL measurements are obtained within the inclusive range of 125 to 8000 Hz, regardless of the test condition, earphone type, or frequency range to be used in the test room, and should be recorded. Form 8 in Appendix B can be used for recording MPANLs. The measured SPLs are then compared with the MPANLs for the test condition, earphone type, and frequency range to be used in the test room. The test room is acceptable if the measured SPLs do not exceed the MPANLs at each octave or one-third octave band from 125 to 8000 Hz for the test condition, earphone type, and frequency range to be used in the test room. If the measured SPLs are equal to or less than the ears not covered MPANLs for the 125 to 8000 Hz range, the test room is acceptable for all test conditions, earphone types, and frequency ranges. Ambient noise should be measured annually and whenever a new noise source is operating inside or outside the test room.

If testing is going to be performed at hearing levels other than 0 dB, the MPANLs can be adjusted using an equal trade-off between the hearing level to be used and the MPANLs. For example, if an air-conduction screening using supra-aural earphones is going to be conducted at 25 dB HL from 500 to 6000 Hz, then 25 dB can be added to each of the MPANLs for the ears covered, supra-aural earphone, and 500 to 8000 Hz range. To verify compliance, the ambient noise in the test room is measured from 125 to 8000 Hz in octave or one-third octave band intervals. The measured SPLs are compared with each MPANLs + 25 dB for the ears covered supra-aural earphone test condition and 500 to 8000 Hz range. If measured SPLs are equal to or less than the MPANLs + 25 dB, the test room is acceptable for screening at 25 dB HL with a supra-aural earphone from 500 to 6000 Hz.

Frank and Williams (1993b) reported the ambient noise levels for 136 audiometric test rooms used for clinical audiometry. Unfortunately, only ~50% had acceptable ears covered supra-aural earphone MPANLs for the 125 to 8000 Hz and 250 to 8000 Hz range and 82% for the 250 to 8000 Hz range. More unfortunately, only ~14% had acceptable ears not covered MPANLs for the 125 to 8000 Hz and 250 to 8000 Hz range and 37% for the 500 to 8000 Hz range. These results indicate that clinical audiometry is being conducted in many test rooms having excessive levels of ambient noise for obtaining thresholds down to 0 dB HL.

OSHA Ambient Noise Levels

MPANLs have also been specified by the Occupational Safety and Health Administration (OSHA, 1983) for the purposes of industrial hearing testing. The OSHA MPANLs assume that ambient noise will be measured with an SLM in octave bands from 500 to 6000 Hz and that testing will be performed with a supra-aural earphone. **Table 11–7** shows the OSHA MPANLs and the ANSI 1999 (R2003) octave band ears covered with a supra-aural earphone MPANLs for the 500 to 8000 Hz test frequency range for comparison. The OSHA are much higher than the ANSI MPANLs and do not take into account the upward spread of masking. For industrial testing,

Table 11–7 Octave Band Maximum Permissible Ambient Noise Levels Specified by OSHA and ANSI S3.1–1999 (R2003) for Ears Covered for the Test Frequency Range 500 to 8000 Hz

Octave Band (Hz)	OSHA	ANSI	Differences
125	—	49.0*	—
250	—	35.0	—
500	40.0	21.0	19.0
1000	40.0	26.0	14.0
2000	47.0	34.0	13.0
4000	57.0	37.0	20.0
8000	62.0	37.0	25.0

ANSI, American National Standards Institute; OSHA, Occupational Safety and Health Administration.

*Figures given are in decibels.

ANSI S3.1–1999 (R2003) recommends using the ears covered MPANLs for the 500 to 8000 Hz range.

Frank and Williams (1994) reported ambient noise levels for 490 single-walled prefabricated audiometric test rooms used for industrial testing. All 490 of the test rooms met the OSHA MPANLs, but only 162 (33%) also met the ANSI MPANLs for ears covered testing with a supra-aural earphone from 500 to 8000 Hz. They recommended that the OSHA MPANLs be revised to the more stringent ANSI MPANLs so that hearing thresholds for baseline and annual audiograms could be measured down to 0 dB HL.

Controversial Point

• Several studies (Berger and Killion, 1989; Frank and Williams, 1993a; Franks et al, 1992) have reported that accurate hearing thresholds cannot be obtained down to 0 dB HL when testing is conducted in a room with ambient noise levels equivalent to the OSHA MPANLs using a supra-aural earphone or when a supra-aural earphone is mounted in a passive noise-reducing earphone enclosure. Yet OSHA has not lowered its maximum permissible ambient noise levels.

Sources and Reduction of Ambient Noise

There are many sources of ambient noise; however, the primary source within a test room can be attributed to low-frequency (125–500 Hz) noise created by the ventilation system (Frank and Williams, 1993b, 1994). To determine whether the ventilation system is producing excessive noise, ambient noise levels within the test room can be measured with the ventilation system on and off. If the test room meets the MPANLs with the ventilation system off but not on, steps should be taken to reduce the noise. This might include replacing worn-out fan parts, replacing the

fan mounting gaskets, balancing or replacing the fan blade(s), or cleaning the air ducts. If the test room does not meet the MPANLs with the ventilation system off, measures should be taken to increase the noise reduction of the test room. This would include replacing faulty door seals, truing the door, tightening the door latch, and installing acoustic insulation in and around the jack panel.

Passive Noise-Reducing Earphone Enclosures

The use of a passive noise-reducing earphone enclosure has been suggested as an alternative to a supra-aural earphone when hearing tests are conducted in excessive ambient noise. A passive noise-reducing earphone enclosure contains a supra-aural earphone mounted in a plastic dome that fits over and around the pinna like an earmuff used for hearing protection. The theory is that the enclosure will attenuate more excessive ambient noise than just a supra-aural earphone at the patient's ear so that hearing thresholds will not be elevated as a result of ambient noise masking. However, the use of passive noise-reducing earphone enclosures has been strongly criticized for three reasons. The first reason concerns the calibration of the earphone output because ANSI S3.6–2004 does not have a provision or procedure specifying the output of a supra-aural earphone mounted in a passive noise-reducing enclosure. The second reason concerns hearing thresholds and threshold repeatability. Several studies (Billings, 1978; Cozad and Goetzinger, 1970) have demonstrated significant threshold differences between a supra-aural earphone and when the same earphone was mounted in an enclosure. Frank et al (1997) reported that when a supra-aural earphone cushion is recessed within the enclosure or flush with the enclosure's circumaural cushion, hearing thresholds are elevated and are less repeatable compared with a supra-aural earphone. The third reason concerns the amount of attenuation produced by a passive noise-reducing enclosure. Typically, enclosures having an oval cushion with a small opening supply more attenuation because they have a more consistent and efficient enclosure-to-ear coupling than those having a round cushion with a large opening. Because ambient noise is primarily contained in the low frequencies, the important aspect concerns the amount of low rather than high frequency attenuation supplied by the enclosure. Frank et al (1997) reported that some enclosures supply less low-frequency attenuation than a supra-aural earphone. If the ambient noise in a test room is too high to use a supra-aural earphone, an insert earphone rather than a supra-ear-phone mounted in a passive noise-reducing enclosure level is the best alternative.

Pitfall

• Even though the theory of using passive noise-reducing earphone enclosures sounds very good, ample research indicates that passive noise-reducing earphone enclosures should not be used for testing hearing in excessive levels of ambient noise or, for that matter, even in quiet.

♦ Summary

Audiometers and acoustic admittance instruments must produce accurate and controlled signals so that audiologists can make reliable and valid interpretations regarding a patient's peripheral hearing sensitivity, speech processing ability, and middle ear status. Consequently, audiometers, acoustic admittance instruments, and audiometric test rooms must conform to standardized performance characteristics. Audiologists are responsible for maintaining the accuracy of the instruments they use by doing routine calibration measurements and daily inspection and listening checks. It is hoped that the information in this chapter will provide audiologists with a better insight into the development and usefulness of standards, calibration instrumentation and measurement of audiometer, acoustic admittance, and audiometric test room performance characteristics, as well as a greater appreciation of basic instrumentation and calibration.

Appendix A

♦ ANSI, ISO, and IEC Standards Used for the Calibration of Audiometers and Acoustic Immittance Instruments and Other Standards Having Application to Audiology

The following ANSI standards can be purchased from the Standards Secretariat, Acoustical Society of America, 35 Pinelawn Road, Suite 114E, Melville, NY 11747 or via the Internet (http://asastore.aip.org). ANSI standards referenced in this chapter are designated by an asterisk.

S1.1–1994 (R2004) Acoustical Terminology

*S1.4–1983 (R2001) Specification for Sound Level Meters

S1.9–1996 (R2001) Instruments for the Measurement of Sound Intensity

*S1.11–2004 Specification for Octave-Band and Fractional-Octave-Band Analog and Digital Filters

S1.13–2005 Measurement of Sound Pressure Levels in Air

*S1.40–1984 (R2001) Specification for Acoustic Calibrators

S1.42–2001 Design Response of Weighting Networks for Acoustical Measurements

S1.43–1997 (R2002) Specifications for Integrating-Averaging Sound Level Meters

*S3.1–1999 (R2003) Maximum Permissible Ambient Noise Levels for Audiometric Test Rooms

S3.2–1989 (R1999) Method for Measuring the Intelligibility of Speech over Communication Systems

S3.4–2005 Procedure for the Computation of Loudness of Noise

S3.5–1997 (R2002) Methods for Calculation of Speech Intelligibility Index

*S3.6–2004 Specification for Audiometers

*S3.7–1995 (R2003) Method for Coupler Calibration of Earphones

*S3.13–1987 (R2002) Mechanical Coupler for Measurement of Bone Vibrators

S3.20–1995 (R2003) Bioacoustical Terminology

S3.21–2004 Method of Manual Pure Tone Threshold Audiometry

*S3.25–1989 (R2003) Occluded Ear Simulator

*S3.39–1987 (R2002) Specifications for Instruments to Measure Aural Acoustic Impedance and Admittance (Aural Acoustic Immittance)

The following ISO standards can be purchased from the Central Secretariat, International Organization for Standardization (ISO), 1 rue de Varembe, Case Postale 56, CH-1211 Geneva 20, Switzerland or via the Internet (http://asastore.aip.org/shop.do?cID=11). ISO standards referenced in this chapter are designated by an asterisk.

ISO 389–1:1998 Acoustics—Reference zero for the calibration of audiometric equipment. Part 1: Reference equivalent threshold sound pressure levels for pure tones and supra-aural earphones

*ISO 389–2:1994 Acoustics—Reference zero for the calibration of audiometric equipment. Part 2: Reference equivalent threshold sound pressure levels for pure tones and insert earphones

*ISO 389–3:1994 Acoustics—Reference zero for the calibration of audiometric equipment. Part 3: Reference equivalent threshold force levels for pure tones and bone vibrators

*ISO 389–4:1994 Acoustics—Reference zero for the calibration of audiometric equipment. Part 4: Reference levels for narrow band masking noise

ISO/TR 389–5:1998 Acoustics—Reference zero for the calibration of audiometric equipment. Part 5: Reference equivalent threshold sound pressure levels for pure tones in the frequency range 8 kHz to 16 kHz

*ISO 389–7:1996 Acoustics—Reference zero for the calibration of audiometric equipment. Part 7: Reference threshold of hearing under free-field and diffuse-field listening conditions

ISO 389–8:2004 Acoustics—Reference zero for the calibration of audiometric equipment. Part 8: Reference equivalent threshold sound pressure levels for pure tones and circumaural earphones

The following IEC standards can be purchased from the International Electrotechnical Commission (IEC) Central Office, 1 rue de Varembe, CP-131 Geneva 20, Switzerland or via the Internet (http://www.iec.ch/searchpub/cur_fut.htm (key word: electroacoustics)). IEC standards referenced in this chapter are designated by an asterisk.

IEC 60318–1 (1998–07) Electroacoustics—Simulators of human head and ear. Part 1: Ear simulator for the calibration of supra-aural earphones

*IEC 60318–2 (1998–08) Electroacoustics—Simulators of human head and ear. Part 2: An interim acoustic coupler for the calibration of audiometric earphones in the extended high-frequency range

*IEC 60318–3 (1998–08) Electroacoustics—Simulators of human head and ear. Part 3: Acoustic coupler for the calibration of supra-aural earphones used in audiometry

*IEC 60373 (1990–01) Mechanical coupler for measurements on bone vibrators

IEC 60645 (2001–06) Electroacoustics—Audiological equipment. Part 1: Pure-tone audiometers

*IEC 60645 (2004–11) Electroacoustics—Audiological equipment. Part 5: Instruments for the measurement of aural acoustic impedance/admittance

*IEC 60711 (1981–01) Occluded-ear simulator for the measurement of earphones coupled to the ear by ear inserts

Appendix B

◆ Calibration Forms

Form 1: Calibration form for earphone and bone vibrator output levels.

Penn State University, Speech and Hearing Clinic, 110 Moore Building, University Park, PA 16802
Calibration Form for Earphone and Bone Vibrator Output Levels (re: ANSI S3.6-2004)

Audiometer: _____ Serial No.: _____ Channel: _____ Date: _____ Calibrated by: _____

Transducer Type	Frequency in Hertz (Hz)											
	125	250	500	750	1000	1500	2000	3000	4000	6000	8000	Speech
1. Right TDH 49/50, SPL*												
2. Left TDH 49/50, SPL*												
3. RETSPL + 70 dB HL	117.5	96.5	83.5	78.5	77.5	77.5	81.0	79.5	80.5	83.5	83.5	89.5
Rt TDH 49/50, Error (1-3)†												
Lt TDH 49/50, Error (2-3)†												
4. Right ER-3A, SPL‡												
5. Left ER-3A, SPL‡												
6. RETSPL + 70 dB HL	96.0	84.0	75.5	72.0	70.0	72.0	73.0	73.5	75.5	72.0	70.0	82.5
Right ER-3A, Error (4-6)†												
Left ER-3A, Error (5-6)†												
7. Bone Vib, Mastoid, FL§												
8. RETFL		67.0	58.0	48.5	42.5	36.5	31.0	30.0	35.5			
9. Hearing Level Setting		20	50	50	50	50	50	50	50			
Bone Vib, Error (7-(8+9))†												

*One-third octave band SPL in NBS 9A coupler with an HL setting of 70 dB.
†Error equals measured output level minus RETSPL/RETFL plus HL setting; tolerance is ±3 dB from 125-5000 Hz and ±5 dB at 6000 Hz and above.
‡One-third octave band SPL in HA-2 coupler with rigid tube attachment with a HL setting of 70 dB.
§Force level using B&K 4930 mechanical coupler.

Form 2: Calibration form for loudspeaker output levels.

Penn State University, Speech and Hearing Clinic, 110 Moore Building, University Park, PA 16802
Calibration Form for Loudspeaker Output Levels (re: ANSI S3.6-2004)

Audiometer: _____ Serial No.: _____ Channel: _____ Date: _____ Calibrated by: _____

Transducer Type	Frequency in Hertz (Hz)											
	125	250	500	750	1000	1500	2000	3000	4000	6000	8000	Speech
1. Right Speaker, SPL*												
2. Left Speaker, SPL*												
3. RETSPL[†] + 70 dB HL	93.5	82.0	73.0	70.5	70.0	69.0	67.5	61.0	61.5	67.0	78.0	82.5
Right Speaker, Error (1-3)[‡]												
Left Speaker, Error (2-3)[‡]												
Rt Sp: Rt/Lt Error (±2 dB)	—	—	—	—	—	—	—	—	—	—	—	
Rt Sp: Up/Down Error (±2 dB)	—	—	—	—	—	—	—	—	—	—	—	
Rt Sp: Ft/Back Error (±1 dB)	—	—	—	—	—	—	—	—	—	—	—	
Lt Sp: Rt/Lt Error (±2 dB)	—	—	—	—	—	—	—	—	—	—	—	
Lt Sp: Up/Down Error (±2 dB)	—	—	—	—	—	—	—	—	—	—	—	
Lt Sp: Ft/Back Error (±1 dB)	—	—	—	—	—	—	—	—	—	—	—	

*One-third octave band SPL at reference point with an HL setting of 70 dB.
[†]Monaural listening at 45 degrees azimuth.
[‡]Error equals measured output level minus RETSPL plus HL setting; tolerance is ±3 dB from 125-5000 Hz and ±5 dB at 6000 Hz and above.

Form 3: Calibration form for attenuator linearity, frequency accuracy, tone switching, and on/off ratio.

Penn State University, Speech and Hearing Clinic, 110 Moore Building, University Park, PA 16802
Calibration Form for Attenuator Linearity, Frequency Accuracy, Tone Switching, and On/Off Ratio

Audiometer: _____ Serial No.: _____ Channel: ___ Date: _____ Cal by: _____

Attenuator Linearity			Frequency Accuracy			Tone Switching	
HL	Output	Error*	Freq.	Measured	Error[†]	Rise/fall[‡]	Overshoot[§]
120			125			/	
115			250			/	
110			500			/	
105			750			/	
100			1000			/	
95			1500			/	
90			2000			/	
85			3000			/	
80			4000			/	
75			6000			/	
70			8000			/	
65							
60							

On/Off Ratio[ǁ]				
	SA Phones TDH _____		Insert Phones _____	
Freq.	Right	Left	Right	Left

Attenuator Linearity			On/Off Ratio				
55			125				
50			250				
45			500				
40			750				
35			1000				
30			1500				
25			2000				
20			3000				
15			4000				
10			6000				
5			8000				
0							
Total							

*Error between 5 dB intervals is ≤1 dB, total error is ±3 dB from 125 to 5000 Hz and ±5 dB at 6000 Hz and above.
[†]Error is ±1% for type 1, ±2% for type 2, ±3% for types 3 to 5 of indicated frequency.
[‡]Error is <20 or >200 ms.
[§]Error is >+1 dB.
[ǁ]SPL output with tone switch off must be ≥70 dB less than with tone switch on.

Form 4: Calibration form for total harmonic distortion.

Penn State University, Speech and Hearing Clinic, 110 Moore Building, University Park, PA 16802
Calibration Form for Total Harmonic Distortion (re: ANSI S3.6-2004)

Audiometer: _____ Serial No.: _____ Channel: _____ Date: _____ Calibrated by: _____

Freq.	Supra-aural Earphone, TDH 49/50				Insert Earphone, ER-3A				Bone Vibrator, B-71		
	dB HL*	Allowed†	Right	Left	dB HL*	Allowed†	Right	Left	dB HL*	Allowed‡	Measured
125	75	≤2.5%			75	≤2.5%					
250	90	≤2.5%			90	≤2.5%			20	≤5.5%	
500	110	≤2.5%			110	≤2.5%			50	≤5.5%	
750	110	≤2.5%			110	≤2.5%			50	≤5.5%	
1000	110	≤2.5%			110	≤2.5%			60	≤5.5%	
1500	110	≤2.5%			110	≤2.5%			60	≤5.5%	
2000	110	≤2.5%			110	≤2.5%			60	≤5.5%	
3000	110	≤2.5%			110	≤2.5%			60	≤5.5%	
4000	110	≤2.5%			110	≤2.5%			60	≤5.5%	
6000	90	≤2.5%			90	≤2.5%					
8000	90	≤2.5%			90	≤2.5%					

Loudspeakers	Allowed§	250 Hz	500 Hz	1000 Hz	Loudspeakers	Allowed§				250 Hz	500 Hz	1000 Hz
Right, at 80 dB SPL	≤3%				Right, at 100 dB SPL	≤10%						
Left, at 80 dB SPL	≤3%				Left, at 100 dB SPL	≤10%						

*Or maximum HL, whichever is lower.
†Allowed percent for total harmonic distortion; ≤2% for second and third harmonic; ≤0.3% for fourth and higher harmonics; ≤0.03% for all subharmonics.
‡Allowed percent for total harmonic distortion; ≤5% for second harmonic; ≤2% for third and higher harmonics.
§Allowed percent for total harmonic distortion.

Form 5: Calibration form for masking output levels.

Penn State University, Speech and Hearing Clinic, 110 Moore Building, University Park, PA 16802
Calibration Form for Masking Output Levels (re: ANSI S3.6-2004)

Audiometer: _____ Serial No.: _____ Channel: _____ Date: _____ Calibrated by: _____

Narrow Band Noise	125	250	500	750	1000	1500	2000	3000	4000	6000	8000
1. Right TDH 49/50, SPL*											
2. Left TDH 49/50, SPL*											
3. CF† +RETSPL+70 dBEML	121.5	100.5	87.5	83.5	83.5	83.5	87.0	85.5	85.5	88.5	88.0
Rt TDH 49/50, Error (1-3)‡											
Lt TDH 49/50, Error (2-3)‡											
4. Right ER-3A, SPL§											
5. Left ER-3A, SPL§											
6. CF† +RETSPL+70 dBEML	100.0	88.0	79.5	77.0	76.0	78.0	79.0	79.5	80.5	77.0	77.5
Right ER 3A, Error (4-6)‡											
Left ER-3A, Error (5-6)‡											

	White Noise Setting	White Noise Error‡	Speech Noise Setting	Speech Noise CF‖	Speech Noise Error‡
Right TDH 49/50, SPL*	70		70		
Left TDH 49/50, SPL*	70		70		
Right ER-3A, SPL†	70		70		
Left ER-3A, SPL†	70		70		

*One-third octave band SPL in NBS 9A coupler with a setting of 70 dB EML.

†Correction factor for narrow band noise measured with one-third octave band filter.

‡Error equals measured output level minus CR plus RETSPL plus EML setting; tolerance is +5/-3 dB of indicated value.

§One-third octave band SPL in HA-2 coupler with rigid tube attachment with a setting of 70 dB EML.

‖Correction factor supplied by the manufacturer.

Form 6: Calibration form for frequency response.

Penn State University, Speech and Hearing Clinic, 110 Moore Building, University Park, PA 16802
Calibration Form for Frequency Response (re: ANSI S3.6-2004)

Audiometer: _____ Serial No.: _____ Channel: _____ Date: _____ Calibrated by: _____

Freq.	Supra-aural phones; TDH Earphones* Rt	Supra-aural phones; TDH Earphones* Lt	Tape† Rt	Tape† Lt	CD† Rt	CD† Lt	Insert phones; Earphones* Rt	Insert phones; Earphones* Lt	Tape† Rt	Tape† Lt	- CD† Rt	- CD† Lt	Loudspeakers Speakers* Rt	Loudspeakers Speakers* - Lt	Tape† Rt	Tape† Lt	CD† Rt	CD† Lt	Mic‡
125																			
160																			
200																			
250																			
315																			
400																			
500																			
630																			
800																			
1000																			
1025																			
1600																			
2000																			
2500																			
3150																			
4000																			
5000																			
6300																			
8000																			

*One-third octave band SPL of WN; compared with average from 250 to 4000 Hz, tolerance is ±3 dB from 250 to 4000 Hz, 0/-10 from 125 to 250 Hz, ±5 dB from 4000-6300 Hz.

†One-third octave band SPL of one-third octave band test signals; compared with average from 250 to 4000 Hz, tolerance is ±4 dB from 250 to 4000 Hz, +2/-12 from 125 to 250 Hz, +7 dB from 4000 to 8000 Hz.

‡Output voltage level for constant 80 dB SPL of one-third octave band test signals; tolerance is ±3 dB from 125 to 8000 Hz.

Form 7: Calibration form for acoustic immittance instrument.

Penn State University, Speech and Hearing Clinic, 110 Moore Building, University Park, PA 16802
Calibration Form for Acoustic Immittance Instrument (re: ANSI S3.39-1987 (R 2002))

Instrument: _____ Serial No.: _____ Date: _____ Calibrated 2002)

Source	Freq.	Frequency Accuracy		SPL Output*			Harmonic Distortion*	
		Measured	Error†	Measured	Expected‡	Error§	SPL‖	Percent¶
Probe Tone	226							
Ipsilateral Reflex Activating Signal	500						95	
	1000						100	
	2000						100	
	4000						75	
	Noise							
Contralateral Reflex Activating Signal	500				83.5		90	
	1000				77.5		110	
	2000				81.0		110	
	4000				80.5		110	
	Noise							

Attenuator Linearity

Setting	Output	Error#
120		
110		
105		
100		
95		
90		
85		
80		
75		
70		
65		
60		
55		
50		

Linearity of Air Pressure System: _____   Rise/Fall Time: _____

On/Off Ratio	500	1000	2000	4000	Noise
Ipsilateral					
Contralateral					

*Measured in HA-1 or NBS 9A coupler.

†Error is ±3%.

‡SPL of probe tone, ipsi activating signal, and noise from manufacturer; SPL of contra activating signal equals RETSPL + 70 dB HL for TDH 49/50.

§Error is ±3 dB for tones, ±5 dB for noise.

‖SPL in HA-1 or NBS 9A coupler.

¶Percent of total harmonic distortion must be is ≤5% for probe tone and ipsi signals, ≤3% for contra signals from TDH 49/50.

#Error between 5 dB intervals is ≤1 dB.

Form 8: Calibration form for maximum permissible ambient noise levels.

Penn State, Speech and Hearing Clinic, 110 Moore Building, University Park, PA 16802
Calibration Form for Maximum Permissible Ambient Noise Levels (re: ANSI S3.1–1999 [R2003])

Test Room Number: _____ Date: _____ Measured by: _____

Source	One-third Octave Band Center Frequency in Hertz (Hz)										
	125	250	500	800	1000	1600	2000	3150	4000	6300	8000
1. One-third octave band SPLs											
2. ENC: 250–8000 Hz	30.0	16.0	11.0	10.0	8.0	9.0	9.0	8.0	6.0	8.0	9.0
Difference (1 minus 2)											
3. ENC: 500–8000 Hz	39.0	25.0	11.0	10.0	8.0	9.0	9.0	8.0	6.0	8.0	9.0
Difference (1 minus 3)											
4. EC: Supra-aural, 250–8000 Hz	34.0	20.0	16.0	19.0	21.0	25.0	29.0	33.0	32.0	32.0	32.0
Difference (1 minus 4)											
5. EC: Supra-aural, 500–8000 Hz	44.0	30.0	16.0	19.0	21.0	25.0	29.0	33.0	32.0	32.0	32.0
Difference (1 minus 5)											
6. EC: Insert, 250–8000 Hz	62.0	48.0	45.0	44.0	42.0	43.0	44.0	46.0	45.0	48.0	51.0
Difference (1 minus 6)											
7. EC: Insert, 500–8000 Hz	73.0	59.0	45.0	44.0	42.0	43.0	44.0	46.0	45.0	48.0	51.0
Difference (1 minus 7)											

EC, ears covered; ENC, ears not covered; MPANL, maximum permissible ambient noise level; SPL, sound pressure level.
Note: If the difference is positive (i.e., measured SPL higher than MPANL), the test room should not be used for testing down to 0 dB HL for that test condition, earphone type, and frequency range.

References

American Speech-Language-Hearing Association. (1991). Sound field measurement tutorial. ASHA, 33(Suppl. 3), 25–37

Arlinger, S. D. (1986). Sound attenuation of TDH 39 earphones in a diffuse field of narrow band noise. Journal of the Acoustical Society of America, 79, 189–191.

Berger, E. H., & Killion, M. C. (1989). Comparison of the noise attenuation of three audiometric earphones, with additional data on masking near threshold. Journal of the Acoustical Society of America, 86, 1392–1403.

Billings, B. L. (1978). Performance characteristics of two noise-excluding audiometric headsets. Sound Vibrations, 13, 20–22.

Brinkman, K., & Richter, U. (1990). Reference zero for the calibration of pure tone audiometers equipped with insert earphones. Acoustica, 70, 202–207.

Brunt, M. A. (1985). Békésy audiometry and loudness balancing testing. In J. Katz (Ed.), Handbook of clinical audiology (3rd ed., pp. 273–291). New York: Williams & Wilkins.

Corliss, E. L. R, & Burkhard, M. D. (1953). A probe tube method for the transfer of threshold standard between audiometer earphones. Journal of the Acoustical Society of America, 25, 990–993.

Cozad, R. L., & Goetzinger, C. P. (1970). Audiometric and acoustic coupler comparisons between two circumaural earphone and earphone-cushion combinations vs a standard unit. Journal of Audiology Research, 10, 62–64.

Curtis, J. F., & Schultz, M. C.. (1986). Basic laboratory instrumentation for speech and hearing. Boston: Little, Brown.

Decker, T. N. (1990). Instrumentation: An introduction for students in speech and hearing sciences. New York: Longman, Addison-Wesley.

Dirks, D. D., Lybarger, S. F., Olsen, W. O., & Billings, B. L. (1979). Bone conduction calibration status. Journal of Speech and Hearing Disorders, 44, 143–155.

Frank, T. (1980). Pure-tone audiometer inspection and listening checks. Journal of National Studies of the Speech-Language-Hearing Association, 10, 33–41.

Frank, T. (1982). Influence of contralateral masking on bone-conduction thresholds. Ear and Hearing, 3, 314–319.

Frank, T. (1997). ANSI update: Specification of audiometers. American Journal of Audiology, 6, 29–32.

Frank, T. (2000). ANSI update: Maximum permissible ambient noise levels for audiometric test rooms. American Journal of Audiology, 9(1), 3–8.

Frank, T., Byrne, D. C., & Richards, L. A. (1988). Bone conduction threshold levels for different bone vibrator types. Journal of Speech and Hearing Disorders, 53, 295–301.

Frank, T., & Crandell, C. C. (1986). Acoustic radiation produced by B-71, B-72, and KH 70 bone vibrators. Ear and Hearing, 7, 344–347.

Frank, T., Durrant, J. D., & Lovrinic, J. H. (1993). Maximum permissible ambient noise levels for audiometric test rooms. American Journal of Audiology, 2, 33–37.

Frank, T., Greer, A. C., & Magistro, D. M. (1997). Hearing thresholds, threshold repeatability, and attenuation values for passive noise-reducing earphone enclosures. American Industrial Hygiene Association Journal, 58, 772–778.

Frank. T., & Holmes, A. (1981). Acoustic radiation from bone vibrators. Ear and Hearing, 2, 59–63.

Frank, T., & Richards, W. D. (1991). Hearing aid coupler output level variability and coupler correction levels for insert earphones. Ear and Hearing, 12, 221–227.

Frank, T., & Richter, U. (1985). Influence of temperature on the output of a mechanical coupler. Ear and Hearing, 6, 206–210.

Frank, T., & Vavrek, M. J. (1992). Reference threshold levels for an ER-3A insert earphone. Journal of the American Academy of Audiology, 3, 51–59.

Frank, T., & Williams, D. L. (1993a). Effects of background noise on earphone thresholds. Journal of the American Academy of Audiology, 4, 201–221.

Frank, T., & Williams, D. L. (1993b). Ambient noise levels in audiometric test rooms used for clinical audiometry. Ear and Hearing, 14(6), 414–422.

Frank, T., & Williams, D. L. (1994). Ambient noise levels in industrial audiometric test rooms. American Industrial Hygiene Association Journal, 55, 433–437.

Frank, T., & Wright, D. C. (1990). Attenuation provided by four different audiometric earphone systems. Ear and Hearing, 11, 70–78.

Franks, J. R., Engle, D. P., & Themann, C. L. (1992). Real-ear attenuation at threshold for three audiometric headphone devices: Implications for maximum permissible ambient noise level standards. Ear and Hearing, 13, 2–10.

Hawkins, D. B., Cooper, W. A., & Thompson, D. J. (1990). Comparisons among SPLs in real-ears, 2 cm^3 and 6 cm^3 couplers. Journal of the American Academy of Audiology, 1, 154–161.

Hood, J. D. (1979). Clinical implications in calibration requirements in bone conduction standardization. Audiology, 18, 36–42.

Jerger, J. (1960). Békésy audiometry in analysis of auditory disorders. Journal of Speech and Hearing Research, 3, 275–287.

Killion, M. C. (1978). Revised estimate of minimal audible pressure: Where is the "missing" 6 dB? Journal of the Acoustical Society of America, 63, 1501–1508.

Killion, M. C. (1984). New insert earphones for audiometry. Hearing Instruments, 35, 38–46.

Lilly, D. J. (1984). Evaluation of the response time of acoustic-immittance instruments. In S. Silman (Ed.), The acoustic reflex (pp. 101–135). New York: Academic Press.

Lilly, D. J., & Prudy, J. K. (1993). On the routine use of Tubephone™ insert earphones. American Journal of Audiology, 2, 17–20.

Margolis, R. (1981). Fundamental of acoustic immittance. In G. Popelka (Ed.), Hearing assessment with the acoustic reflex (pp. 117–143). New York: Grune & Stratton.

Martin, F. N. (1998). Exercises in audiometry: A laboratory manual (pp. 1–5). Boston: Allyn & Bacon.

Morgan, D. E., Dirks, D. D., & Bower, D. R. (1979). Suggested threshold sound pressure levels of modulated (warble) tones in the sound field. Journal of Speech and Hearing Disorders, 44, 37–54.

Occupational Safety and Health Administration. (1983). Occupational noise exposure: Hearing conservation amendment. Federal Register, 48, 9738–9785.

Popelka, G. R. (1984). Acoustic immittance measures: Terminology and instrumentation. Ear and Hearing, 5, 262–267.

Popelka, G. R., & Dubno, J. R. (1978). Comments on the acoustic-reflex response for bone-conducted signals. Acta Otolaryngologica, 86, 64–70.

Richards, W. D., & Frank, T. (1982). Frequency response and output variations of Radioear B-71 and B-72 bone vibrators. Ear and Hearing, 3, 37–38.

Richter, U., & Frank, T. (1985). Calibration of bone vibrators at high frequencies. Audiology Acoustics, 24, 2–12.

Rudmose, W. (1964). Concerning the problem of calibrating TDH-39 earphones at 6 kHz with a 9A coupler. Journal of the Acoustical Society of America, 36, 1049.

Shanks, J. E. (1987). Aural acoustic-immittance standards. Seminars in Hearing: Immittance Audiometry, 8, 307–318.

Shanks, J. E., Wilson, R. H., & Jones, H. C. (1985). Earphone-coupling technique for measuring the temporal characteristics of aural acoustic-immittance devices. Journal of Speech and Hearing Research, 28, 305–308.

Shipton, M. S., John, A. J., & Robinson, D. W. (1980). Air-radiated sound from bone vibration transducers and its implications for bone conduction audiometry. British Journal of Audiology, 14, 86–99.

Walker, G., Dillion, H., & Byrne, D. (1984). Sound field audiometry: Recommended stimuli and procedures. Ear and Hearing, 5, 13–21.

Wilber, L. A., Kruger, B., & Killion, M. C. (1988). Reference thresholds for an ER-3A insert earphone. Journal of the Acoustical Society of America, 83, 669–676.

Wiley, T. L., & Fowler, C. G. (1997). Acoustic immittance measures in clinical audiology. San Diego, CA: Singular Publishing Group.

Wright, D. C., & Frank, T. (1992). Attenuation values for a supra-aural earphone for children and insert earphone for children and adults. Ear and Hearing, 13, 454–459.

Zwicker, E., & Terhardt, E. (1980). Analytical expressions for critical-band rate and critical band-width as a function of frequency. Journal of the Acoustical Society of America, 68, 1523–1525.

Zwislocki, J. J. (1970). An acoustic coupler for earphone calibration (Report LSC-S-7). Syracuse, NY: Laboratory of Sensory Communication, Syracuse University.

Zwislocki, J. J. (1971). An ear-like coupler for earphone calibration. Report LSC-S-9, Laboratory of Sensory Communication. Syracuse, NY: Syracuse University.

Chapter 12

Pure-Tone Tests

Ross J. Roeser and Jackie L. Clark

Pure-tone audiometry is unequivocally the gold standard of every audiological evaluation. Results from pure-tone audiometry are used to make the initial diagnosis of normal or abnormal hearing sensitivity, thereby developing the breadth and depth of audiological diagnostic and (re)habilitation procedures needed for each patient. When results are not within normal limits, pure-tone tests are used to make the diagnosis of the type and degree of hearing loss. Because of the importance of pure-tone data in the diagnostic process, mastering pure-tone audiometry and interpretation of test results is an all-important skill for audiologists.

During pure-tone testing, thresholds are obtained. Test stimuli are referred to as pure tones, because they have one frequency; speech can also be used. The term *threshold* is defined as the lowest intensity at which the patient is able to respond to the stimulus. Because it is impossible to measure the perception of hearing directly, threshold is mathematically defined as the lowest intensity at which the patient responds to the stimulus in a given fraction of trials. The clinical criterion for threshold is typically based on 50%, which means the patient must respond to 2 out of 4 or 3 out of 6 trials. Pure tones are used because they are simple to generate and because they provide valuable diagnostic information on the differential effects of lesions in the peripheral auditory system.

This chapter covers the topic of pure-tone tests. Included are a physical description of pure tones, a description of the equipment used for pure-tone testing, a classification of test results (type and degree of loss), the procedures followed, and an interpretation and description of results. In addition, the use of pure tones for hearing screening is reviewed.

♦ Physical Description of Pure Tones

The two basic physical measures associated with pure tones that should be understood by those performing pure-tone audiometry are frequency and intensity.

Frequency

Sound is normally produced by molecules of air forced to move back and forth by a vibratory source (e.g., a tuning fork), causing waves of compression and rarefaction to form. Frequency specifies the number of back-and-forth oscillations or cycles produced by a vibrator in a given time as molecular movement occurs and the sound is created. The term used to describe frequency, hertz, is named after Heinrich Hertz, abbreviated Hz, and specifies the number of cycles that occur in 1 second. For example, if a vibrator (tuning fork) were set into motion and completed 1000 back-and-forth cycles in 1 second, it would have a frequency of 1000 Hz. Frequency and pitch are related in that as the frequency of a sound increases, the listener perceives a higher and higher pitch. Pitch is the perceptual equivalent of frequency.

Because most sounds contain multiple frequencies, the oscillations that occur are complex. However, when pure tones are generated, only one frequency is present, so the oscillations produced are simple back-and-forth movements. **Figure 12–1** shows the spectrum (intensity × frequency) for a pure tone at 1000 Hz. The only frequency represented in this figure is 1000 Hz, which is clearly shown as a narrow peak at the 1000 Hz nominal value. Pure tones with frequencies lower than 1000 Hz would be shown as a similar narrow peak to the left of the 1000 Hz data,

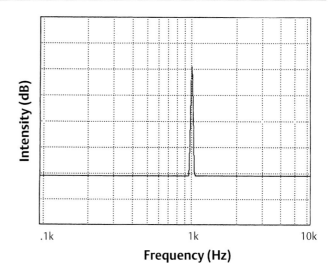

Figure 12–1 Spectrum (frequency × intensity plot) of a 1000 Hz pure tone.

and pure tones higher in frequency than 1000 Hz would be to the right.

> **Pearl**
>
> • The human ear responds to frequencies between 20 and 20,000 Hz. However, it is not equally sensitive to all of these frequencies. The human ear is most sensitive to the mid-frequencies around 1000 Hz.

The human ear responds to frequencies between 20 and 20,000 Hz. Frequencies that are below this range are infrasonic, and those above are ultrasonic. For example, a sound with a frequency of 10 Hz is infrasonic and would not be perceived by the normal ear; a sound with a frequency of 30,000 Hz is ultrasonic and would also not be perceived. Even though the ear responds to frequencies ranging from 20 to 20,000 Hz, only those frequencies between 300 and 3000 Hz are actually critical for the perception of speech. This means that it would be possible for an individual to have essentially no hearing above 3000 Hz and have only marginal difficulty hearing speech in a quiet environment. This observation explains why pure tones are an important component in a thorough assessment of the auditory system.

Pure-tone thresholds are regularly assessed at octave and sometimes at half-octave intervals between the range of 250 and 8000 Hz. The 250 to 8000 Hz frequency range is generally the most audible to the human ear and provides guidelines on how well the individual is able to perceive speech, because the speech frequencies of 300 to 3000 Hz fall within this range. In the typical pure-tone test, thresholds are obtained for the octave frequencies 250, 500, 1000, 2000, 4000, and 8000 Hz. In addition, half octaves

750, 1500, 3000, and 6000 Hz are sometimes tested when hearing loss is present. It is becoming more customary to include 3000 and 6000 Hz in the standard audiometric evaluation, especially when hearing loss is present. Normally, 3000 Hz is tested because of its importance in speech perception and because results from 3000 Hz are used to calculate the percent of hearing impairment as developed by the American Medical Association (AMA) and the American Academy of Otolaryngology–Head and Neck Surgery. Also, 6000 Hz is tested because of its importance in diagnosing noise-induced hearing loss.

Intensity

The physical measurement of what is psychologically perceived as loudness is referred to as intensity, which is determined by the amount of movement or displacement of air particles that occurs as a sound is created. The greater the amount of displacement, the more intense or louder the sound. Intensity is measured in units called decibels, abbreviated dB, a term that means one tenth of a bel (named after Alexander Graham Bell). Technically, the decibel is defined as the logarithmic ratio between two magnitudes of pressure or power.

As indicated by the technical definition, intensity is far more complicated than frequency. To understand the decibel fully requires knowledge of advanced mathematical functions. The decibel is based on a logarithmic function because the ear responds to a very large range of pressure changes. The use of logarithms allows these changes to be expressed by smaller numbers than would be required for a linear function. Excellent references (e.g., Berlin, 1967) are available for the reader to consult for additional information on how to compute decibels using logarithms.

Although the concepts underlying the decibel are somewhat complicated and will not be covered in this chapter, a less difficult concept is that the decibel is a relative unit of measurement. Simply stating, for example, 10 dB or 20 dB has no specific meaning without specifying the reference for the measure. There are three reference levels for the decibel commonly used in audiometric testing: sound pressure level (SPL), hearing level (HL), and sensation level (SL), as follows.

Decibel Sound Pressure Level

Decibel SPL refers to the absolute pressure reference level for the decibel. The pressure reference used to determine dB SPL is 0.000204 dynes/cm². Therefore, 0 dB SPL is equal to a pressure force of 0.000204 dynes/cm², and 10 dB or 20 dB SPL equals 10 or 20 dB above the 0.000204 dynes/cm² force. Because dB SPL is a physical measure, it is not affected by the frequencies present in sound.

Decibel Hearing Level

Decibel HL is the reference to average normal hearing sensitivity. The ear is not sensitive to all frequencies at the same intensity level. That is, hearing sensitivity changes as a function of the frequency of the sound. Therefore, 0 dB

HL represents the dB SPL required to reach threshold sensitivity of the average normal ear at each frequency. Audiometers are calibrated in dB HL, so that any decibel value above 0 dB HL represents a deviation from normal hearing levels. For example, a threshold of 25 dB HL is 25 dB above the normal hearing threshold for that individual for that frequency.

Since the early 1950s, multiple standards have been used to define the absolute SPL levels at which the normal ear responds as a function of frequency (see Chapter 11). At present, all audiometers should conform to the American National Standards Institute (ANSI) 2004 standard.

In some instances, dB hearing threshold level (HTL) will also be used. When dB HTL is used, it implies that the decibel value given was a measured threshold from a patient; that is, the value was an actual level obtained during threshold assessment.

Decibel Sensation Level

Decibel SL is used to specify the intensity of stimuli presented to a given patient relative to the patient's threshold. That is, if a patient has a threshold of 45 dB HL, a signal presented at 20 dB SL would be 20 dB above 45 dB HL (the patient's threshold), or 65 dB HL.

♦ Frequency and Intensity Function of the Human Ear

The ear responds to different absolute intensities, or different SPLs, as a function of frequency. Stated in another way, it takes a different SPL to reach the level at which the normal ear will perceive the sound (threshold level) at different frequencies. **Figure 12–2** illustrates the threshold sensitivity function of the normal ear and gives the ANSI 2004 levels required to reach threshold at each frequency for normal ears (0 dB HL). As shown in this figure, the ear is most sensitive in the midfrequencies, around 1000 to 1500 Hz, indicating that it takes less intensity for sounds to be audible in these frequencies. Because audiometers are calibrated in dB HL, it is not necessary to know the absolute dB SPL/HL difference at each frequency. The audiometer automatically corrects for the dB SPL/HL difference as the frequency is changed.

♦ Pure-Tone Test Equipment: The Audiometer

Pure-tone tests are performed with audiometers. Audiometers are electronic instruments used to quantify hearing sensitivity. Pure-tone audiometers originated from tuning forks, and the frequencies produced by the

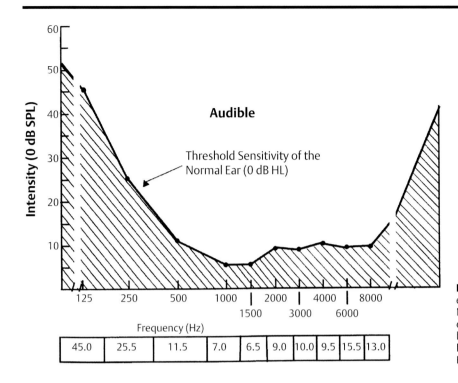

| 45.0 | 25.5 | 11.5 | 7.0 | 6.5 | 9.0 | 10.0 | 9.5 | 15.5 | 13.0 |

Figure 12–2 Threshold sensitivity of the normal ear as a function of frequency. The American National Standards Institute equivalent threshold sound pressure levels (SPLs) shown at the bottom of the figure are required to reach 0 dB hearing level (HL) for a Telephonic Dynamic Headphones (TDH) 39 supra-aural earphone.

first audiometers were similar to those produced by tuning forks. As an example, the frequencies 256, 512, and 1026 Hz were named on the first audiometers. However, today's standard pure-tone audiometers name frequencies with a scale based on the octave and half-octave frequencies of 125, 250, 500, 750, 1000, 1500, 2000, 3000, 4000, 6000, and 8000 Hz.

Like any tool, audiometers vary in degree of sophistication, features offered, and configuration. ANSI (2004) has developed a comprehensive classification system for audiometers that is reviewed in detail in Chapter 11. Based on the institute's facilities, audiometers are classified into standard pure tone, speech, high frequency, or free field equivalent. **Figure 12–3** provides an example of a standard pure-tone audiometer with the major components identified.

Audiometer Types

Standard Pure-Tone and Automatic/Microprocessor Audiometers

Pure-tone and automatic audiometers generate pure-tone stimuli and are used for screening or basic threshold testing. Manual audiometers require the examiner to operate the controls, whereas automatic audiometers are controlled by a microprocessor that responds when the patient signals the system with a handheld switch. Automatic audiometers are commonly used for mass screenings, such as industrial hearing conservation programs. Although these instruments will save time in mass screening programs with cooperative adults, they have limited value in testing children and in diagnostic testing.

Diagnostic Audiometers

Diagnostic audiometers include a variety of features, such as controls for bone-conduction testing, speech testing via monitored live voice or recorded presentation, and stimuli for masking and diagnostic (site-of-lesion) testing.

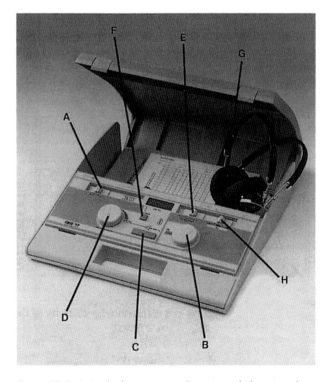

Figure 12–3 A standard pure-tone audiometer with the external components labeled. **Table 12–1** provides a description of each component.

Extended High-Frequency Audiometers

Extended high-frequency audiometers are used for measuring pure-tone hearing thresholds from 8000 to 16,000 Hz. One of the main uses of this type of audiometer is to monitor the onset of possible high-frequency hearing loss from ototoxic medications. The individual susceptibility to ototoxic medication varies greatly (Park, 1996), making the prediction of damage from given dosages of any ototoxic medication virtually impossible to predict; damage also may occur unilaterally (Fausti et al, 1994). Because the damage from many ototoxic medications begins in the very high frequencies and progresses to lower frequencies, monitoring of these very high frequencies can alert the treating physician to impending damage to the speech frequencies. More information regarding ototoxicity and monitoring protocols can be found in Park (1996) and Fausti et al (1994).

In rare cases patients may have hearing loss in the low to mid frequencies but show better hearing around 8000 Hz. In these cases, it is important to test the ultra high frequencies, as the patient may have hearing in these frequencies. If this is the case, the patient may benefit from advanced technology, such as frequency transposition hearing aids.

Due to the acoustic variability encountered with high frequencies, the ANSI (2004) standard describes two circumaural earphone types to be used with high-frequency audiometers. Chapter 10 covers the calibration procedures and instrumentation for high-frequency audiometry.

Special Consideration

- When a severe to profound hearing loss is present, and thresholds at 8000 Hz show improvement greater than 15 to 20 dB, extended high-frequency audiometry (testing above 8000 Hz) should be considered.

Free-field Equivalent Audiometers

Free-field equivalent audiometers are calibrated so that the output of the earphones or bone-conduction oscillator can be expressed in terms of equivalent hearing as if the sound were presented at 0 degree azimuth in the sound field. The output from free-field equivalent audiometers is expressed in SPL, making it more adaptable for comparison of performance for hearing aids.

◆ Audiometer Components

Regardless of the make or model, pure-tone audiometers have certain basic controls and switches in common. These components may vary in appearance and location, but they

Table 12–1   Summary of Components and Functions of Pure-Tone Audiometers

Label	Component	Function
A	Power (on/off) switch	Provides power to the audiometer circuit
B	Frequency selector dial (oscillator)	Selects the frequency of the stimulus
C	Tone interrupter (tone reverse) switch	Activates or inactivates the stimulus
Not shown	Amplifier	Increases the intensity of the signal
D	Attenuator (hearing level dial)	Adjusts the intensity of the stimuli
E	Signal router switch	Selects the device used to present the stimuli
F	Masking level controller	Adjusts the intensity of masking noise
G	Earphones	Present the stimuli via air conduction
Not shown	Bone oscillator	Presents the stimuli via bone conduction
H	Signal selector switch	Selects the type of stimuli to be delivered
Not shown	Loudspeaker	Presents the stimuli in the sound field

perform the same basic functions. **Table 12–1** lists and describes the components shown in **Fig. 12–3**.

Power (On/Off) Switch

Audiometers are equipped with standard three-pronged plugs for 120 V power. After the audiometer has been plugged in, it should be turned on and allowed to "warm up" for ~10 minutes prior to testing. This procedure assures that the proper current has reached all parts of the instrument for optimal functioning. The audiometer should remain in the "on" position for the remainder of the day when additional testing is to be performed, as there is less wear on the electrical components to leave it on all day than to turn it on and off several times during the day.

Pitfall

- Turning audiometers on and off throughout the day causes greater wear on the electronic components than turning them on each day and having them remain on during the entire day they are to be used.

Some portable pure-tone screening audiometers are battery powered. Battery-powered audiometers are useful in situations where conventional power is not available. However, the output from battery-powered audiometers can be unstable, and they should be used only when necessary.

Frequency Selector Dial (Oscillator)

The frequency selector dial changes the frequency of the stimuli in discrete octave and half-octave steps from 125 to 8000 Hz. On many audiometers, the frequency selector dial also shows, by use of smaller numerals on the dial, the maximum output (dB HL or dB HTL) that the audiometer is capable of producing at each test frequency.

Tone Interrupter (Tone Reverse) Switch

The tone interrupter is a button, bar, or lever used either to present or interrupt the test stimuli, depending on the position of the tone reverse switch. The tone reverse switch allows the tone to be "normally on" or "normally off." In the "normally on" position, the tone is turned off by depressing the tone interrupter. In the "normally off" position, the tone is presented by depressing the tone interrupter. In standard pure-tone testing, the tone reverse switch should always be in the "normally off" position. Serious errors can result if the tone reverse switch is in the "normally on" position. The "normally on" position is used only during calibration and for some diagnostic procedures.

Amplifier

The amplifier, an internal component, increases the intensity of the electronic signal. Note that the amplifier delivers maximum intensity to the attenuator; the attenuator controls the output from the transducer (earphone, bone oscillator, or loudspeaker) by reducing the signal from the amplifier.

Attenuator (Hearing Level Dial)

The attenuator or HL dial controls the intensity of test stimuli. The amplifier delivers a constant level signal to the attenuator. The attenuator controls the intensity level of the output signal. Attenuators are resistive devices that control intensity in small steps; most attenuators are designed to operate in 5 dB increments, but some operate in steps of 1 or 2 dB. Because attenuators are resistive devices, the greater the attenuation, the less output is present at the earphone. **Table 12–2** compares the relationship between the HL setting on the attenuator dial, the amount of attenuation, and the output at the audiometer earphone. As shown in this example, at maximum output (110 dB HL), the attenuator dial is at minimum attenuation (0 dB), and the output at the earphone is 116.5 dB SPL. The 6.5 dB difference between the audiometer dial and the output represents the dB HL/dB SPL correction specified by the ANSI 2004 standard for the 1000 Hz tone used in this example. Also shown in **Table 12–2** is that as the output decreases from 110 dB HL to 0 dB HL, the amount of attenuation increases until maximum attenuation is reached at 0 dB HL.

Attenuator (HL) dials have a range from 0 to 110 dB HL or 120 dB HL for air-conduction testing. It should be noted that not all of the test stimuli are capable of being presented at intensities of 110 dB HL. Specifically, 250 and 8000 Hz have limited outputs. Bone-conduction testing is limited to 0 to 40 or 0 to 60 or 70 dB HL, depending on the frequency. For bone-conduction stimuli, the audiometer must deliver more energy to drive the bone-conduction oscillator than to present the stimuli through earphones.

Table 12–2 also shows the linearity of the attenuator dial, that is, the amount of change in output of the audiometer earphone (dB SPL) as the dial is changed in 5 dB steps. In the example shown in **Table 12–2**, the audiometer output is highly linear; the output from the audiometer earphone changes by 5 dB as the attenuator setting is changed in 5 dB steps. Attenuator linearity is not always this exact and must be checked to ensure it is within ANSI standards (see Chapter 11).

Signal Router Switch

Test signals may be delivered to the right or left earphone, bone conduction oscillator, or (in the case of diagnostic audiometers) through loudspeakers. The signal router switch determines which of these devices is activated.

Masking Level Controller (labeled F in **Fig. 12–3**)

When performing air- and bone-conduction threshold audiometry, there is a possibility that test signal will "cross over" to the nontest ear. Whenever the possibility of crossover exists, masking noise must be presented to exclude the nontest ear from participating in the test. The

Table 12–2   Comparison of Attenuator Setting, Decibel Sound Pressure Level, and Output*

Attenuator Setting (dB HL)	Amount of Attenuation	Output from Audiometer Earphone (dB SPL)
110	0	116.5
105	5	111.5
100	10	106.5
95	15	101.5
90	20	96.5
85	25	91.5
80	30	86.5
75	35	81.5
70	40	76.5
65	45	71.5
60	50	66.5
55	55	61.5
50	60	56.5
45	65	51.5
40	70	46.5
35	75	41.5
30	80	36.5
25	85	31.5
20	90	26.5
15	95	21.5
10	100	16.5
5	105	11.5
0	110	6.5

HL, hearing level; SPL, sound pressure level.

*In this example, a 1500 Hz pure tone is used, and the HL/SPL correction is 6.5 dB (see Fig. 11–2).

masking dial controls the intensity of masking signal presented. The topic of clinical masking is covered in detail in Chapter 13.

Earphones

Earphones are designed to transmit test stimuli to each ear individually. Standard earphones are color-coded: red for the right ear and blue for the left ear. Important points regarding earphones are (1) earphones are calibrated to one specific audiometer and should never be interchanged between audiometers unless the equipment is recalibrated, (2) the tension of the headband and resiliency of the earphone cushions are important factors for reliable test results, and (3) placement of the earphones on the patient is one of the most important procedures in audiometric testing.

Figure 12–4 shows schematics and photos of three types of earphones used in pure-tone testing. As shown, in addition to the standard supra-aural cushion, two other types of earphone systems are available: noise excluding (a combination-type system of a supra-aural cushion and a circumaural muff) and insert earphones. The use of noise-excluding earphones provides superior attenuation of ambient background noise, which allows for accurate testing in environments having excessive noise. However, the size and complexity of noise-excluding earphones make them

more difficult to use; thus, they have not been endorsed for widespread use.

Insert-type earphones have the advantage of increased attenuation of background noise (Killion et al, 1985). In addition, they provide increased interaural (between-ear) attenuation, the elimination of ear canal collapse, increased comfort for long test sessions, and better approximate insertion measures when audiometric testing is conducted for hearing aid use. Clinicians should be aware of a small correction factor needed for calibrating insert earphones when used with an audiometer calibrated for standard supra-aural earphones. These values must be added to or subtracted from the threshold obtained at each frequency.

Special Consideration

- Insert earphones eliminate the problem of collapsed ear canals experienced with supra-aural earphones.

Despite the advantages of insert earphones in audiometric testing, recent evidence indicates that only 24% of audiologists report their use in some clinical capacity (Martin et al, 1998). Nevertheless, their benefits certainly make insert

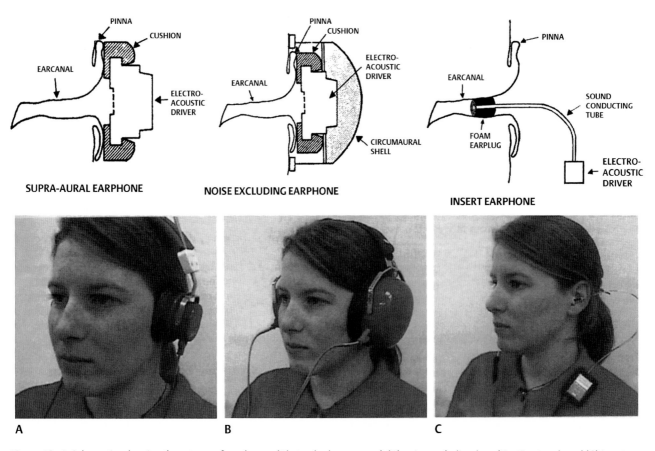

Figure 12–4 Schematics showing three types of earphones: **(A)** standard supra-aural, **(B)** noise-excluding (combination-type), and **(C)** insert.

earphones desirable for routine testing, and there are some situations that require their use, such as when the masking dilemma is encountered (see Chapter 12). If not used routinely, insert earphones are needed for at least part of standard audiometric testing.

Controversial Point

• The use of insert earphones in industrial hearing conservation programs has been questioned because the current standard of the Occupational Safety and Health Administration (OSHA) requires that audiometers used in testing industrial workers have supra-aural earphone cushions.

Bone-Conduction Oscillator

The bone-conduction oscillator is used to obtain threshold measures of bone-conduction sensitivity. There are three types of bone conduction oscillators in use on audiometers: the Pracitronic (Dresden, Germany) KH70 and the Radioear (Radioear Corp., New Eagle, PA) B72 and B71. The most common is the Radioear B71.

Signal Selector Switch

In addition to generating pure tones, diagnostic audiometers are capable of presenting a variety of acoustic signals, including speech, masking noises, and frequency modulated (warbled) tones. The signal selector switch provides a choice of signals to deliver to the patient.

Loudspeakers

Loudspeakers are used to present test stimuli in the sound field. One or more loudspeakers are mounted in a sound-treated room, and test stimuli are presented to the patient at 0, 45, or 90 degrees off center to the right and/or left. As discussed in Chapters 11 and 14, pure-tone stimuli should not be used in sound field testing due to standing waves; special considerations must be taken.

♦ Calibration of Audiometers

Calibration is necessary to ensure that the audiometer is producing a pure tone at the specified frequency and intensity, that the stimulus is present only in the earphone to which it is directed, and that the stimulus is free from unwanted noise, interference, and distortion. This is covered extensively in Chapter 11. Needless to say, the validity of audiometric test data is only as good as the equipment used to obtain them. This emphasizes the need for all audiologists to have a thorough understanding of calibration principles and their application.

Pearl

• If there is access to a sound level meter and coupler, the monthly biological check can be replaced with an electroacoustic measurement of the audiometer output levels. The advantage of physical measurement is that if the outputs are found to be incorrect by more than 3 dB, it may be possible to correct them by changing the audiometer potentiometers.

♦ Pure-Tone Air- and Bone-Conduction Procedures

Pure-tone tests are used to obtain air- and bone-conduction thresholds that will determine the type and degree of the loss.

Pure-Tone Air Conduction

Reliable and valid pure-tone data are critical in diagnostic audiology. Factors that can affect test results and should be considered as part of every pure-tone test include case history/patient information, test environment, listener position, instructions to the patient, ear examination, earphone/bone-conduction oscillator placement, ear selection, frequency sequencing, response strategy, threshold procedure, false-negative and false-positive responses, and infection control procedures.

Case History/Patient Information

Before testing begins, a complete case history should be completed, and the patient's general communication impairment should be assessed. The importance of visual cues to comprehension can be determined by talking to patients outside their visual field or with the examiner's mouth covered. Preliminary information on the degree of hearing loss can be obtained by varying vocal intensity while the examiner's mouth is obscured. Factors that could be helpful during pure-tone threshold testing include whether the patient has tinnitus (a ringing sensation), which is the better ear (e.g., can the patient hear from each ear when using the telephone?), and what types of sounds are the most difficult to hear.

It is important to realize that communicative impairment is complex, idiosyncratic, and does not always correlate with pure-tone findings. For example, some patients with severe or profound losses, because they have learned to compensate with speechreading, may not demonstrate their severe impairment.

Test Environment

Pure-tone threshold audiometry must be performed in a test environment that is free from visual distractions and meets specifications for background noise levels as defined in ANSI

(1991). To meet the standard, it is virtually imperative that a commercially built sound-treated enclosure is used, although some custom-made environments are acceptable. If testing is performed outside soundproof enclosures, sound level measurements are required to determine if the environment meets specifications. An important point is that even if a soundproof enclosure is used, there is a possibility that the environment will not meet minimum background noise specifications. Routinely finding elevated thresholds in the low frequencies (250–500 Hz) is one indication that the test environment is not appropriate for threshold audiometry.

Listener Position

The patient should be seated in such a manner that movements made by the examiner are not observable by the patient, yet gestures made by the patient are observable to the examiner. Some clinicians prefer to have the patient seated so that he or she is facing 90 degrees away from the audiometer. In sound field testing, it is imperative that the listener be positioned correctly in reference to the calibration of the speakers (see Chapter 11).

Instructions to the Patient

Test instructions must be in a language appropriate to the patient and should include the following points:

1. The type of response (i.e., what the patient should do when he or she hears the stimulus)

2. That the objective is to respond even to the faintest stimulus

3. That the patient should respond as soon as the stimulus is perceived and to stop immediately when it is not perceived

4. That each ear will be tested separately and that tones with different "pitches" will be presented

Before proceeding, the patient should be asked if he or she has any questions.

Pearl

- After giving instructions, it is always helpful to ask patients if they have any questions. This will give them the opportunity to ask for repetition or clarification of information that was not heard clearly and/or not understood.

Asking patients if they have questions at the end of instructions is an important clinical protocol for any procedure, because it allows patients to request repetition or clarification of information they may not have understood.

Ear Examination

Before earphone placement, the pinna should be inspected for any active pathology. In addition, the ear canal must be examined with an otoscope for pathology and occlusion, and for the possibility of occlusion resulting from ear canal collapse. When the ear canal is impacted due to excessive cerumen, it must be cleaned, or pure-tone findings will be affected. Even if the canal is partially occluded by 40 to 60% or more, studies have shown that high-frequency thresholds can be reduced by 10 to 14 dB (Roeser et al, 2005). An abnormal otologic finding during inspection of the ear requires that a medical referral be made.

Ear canal collapse during threshold audiometry results from the use of supra-aural earphones. The cartilage of the pinna and ear canal "close off" the opening to the ear canal when the earphones are placed over the ears. Audiometric findings show the presence of conductive pathology when, in fact, none is present. This condition is present in as many as 10% of young children and older adults. Each time earphones are placed on a patient, the possibility of ear canal collapse must be considered.

Depressing the pinna toward the mastoid and observing whether the pinna displacement causes the entrance to the ear canal to narrow or close is one method to check for the possibility of ear canal collapse. Having a supra-aural (doughnut) cushion without the driver mounted in it is helpful to perform this procedure. A simple technique to detect and remedy ear canal collapse during testing with supra-aural earphones is to have the patient hold his or her mouth wide open during testing. The pulling forward and downward of the cartilaginous portion of the external ear canal increases the lumen and will eliminate the closure due to pressure on the pinna. Of course, insert earphones can be used whenever ear canal collapse is suspected.

Earphone/Bone Oscillator Placement

Supra-aural earphones are placed so that the diaphragm of the earphone is directly over the opening to the ear canal. When earphones are placed on the patient, eyeglasses must be removed, and hair should be pushed away from the ear; a lifted earphone can result in a low-frequency transmission loss. With bone-conduction testing, the presence of eyeglasses could increase the likelihood of vibrotactile responses if the oscillator comes in contact with the eyeglass stems.

Earphones are always placed on the patient by the examiner; if the patient readjusts them, the examiner should recheck the earphones before testing proceeds. A small displacement of an earphone away from the ear canal entrance can result in a threshold shift of 25 to 30 dB or more.

Pearl

- Proper earphone placement is important and is required to obtain valid test results. The examiner should place earphones on the patient. If the patient adjusts the earphones after placement, the examiner should verify proper placement before testing begins.

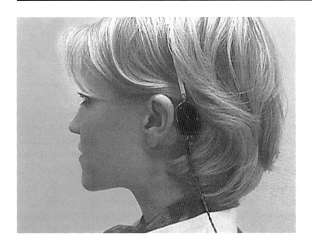

Figure 12–5 Bone-conduction oscillator placed on the mastoid.

The proper use of insert earphones requires them to be placed as comfortably deep into the ear canal as possible. Increased depth increases the real ear and interaural attenuation (Clark and Roeser, 1988) and will help control problems associated with background noise, crossover, and collapsing ear canals.

When placing the bone oscillator on the mastoid, the clinician should make sure that the vibrator does not touch the pinna itself (see **Fig. 12–5**). Before placing the bone vibrator on the mastoid, as much hair as possible should be pulled away, and the oscillator should be placed on the most available part of the mastoid without hair.

Ear Selection

Testing should begin with the better ear as reported by the patient or determined by results from previous tests if they are available. Testing the better ear first allows the patient to respond to stimuli with the least possible distortion and may save time, if masking is needed.

Frequency Sequencing

The American Speech and Hearing Association (ASHA, now the American Speech-Language-Hearing Association) suggested guidelines that stipulate beginning threshold testing at 1000 Hz, because it is one of the midrange frequencies to which the human ear is more sensitive. In addition, a 1000 Hz tone has a pitch that is more familiar to most listeners, it is less affected by background and physiologic noise than low frequencies, and the wavelength in relation to the length of the ear canal makes test–retest reliability better than higher frequencies. After establishing a threshold for the 1000 Hz tone, the next highest octave frequency (2000 Hz) is tested, then 3000, 4000, 6000, and 8000 Hz. Testing at 3000 and 6000 Hz is optional but is most important when hearing thresholds are decreased to any adjacent frequency by 20 dB or more. After 8000 Hz is tested, 1000 Hz is tested for test–retest reliability; threshold is then established for the lower frequencies of 500 and 250 Hz.

Special Consideration

- Because frequencies above 2000 Hz can affect speech intelligibility, clinicians should routinely test 3000 and 6000 Hz when hearing loss is present. Thresholds at 3000 Hz are also needed to calculate AMA/American Academy of Otolaryngology–Head and Neck Surgery (AAO-HNS) percent of hearing impairment.

Response Strategy

Two response strategies to signal the perception of the stimuli that are most commonly used with the cooperative adult patient are a handheld switch/button and hand/finger raising. Using a switch or button provides binary (yes/no) information. Hand or finger raising can provide the same level of information. Instructing patients to raise their hands/fingers on the side corresponding to the ear in which they perceive the test signal helps to identify the location of the signal. In addition, the vigor and latency of the hand/ finger response is often associated with the sensation level at which a patient is perceiving the signal. That is, at high sensation levels, the response is more vigorous and has a shorter latency.

Pearl

- Having patients respond to stimuli using a handheld button provides only binary (yes/no) information. Additional information can be obtained about the subject by observing the amplitude and speed of hand- or finger-raising responses.

Threshold Procedure

Psychoacoustics is the science of establishing the relationship between acoustic stimuli and the sensations that are produced by them. Chapter 10 covers acoustics and psychoacoustic principles in detail. When establishing threshold, the two threshold searching choices are to descend and to ascend. With the descending technique, stimuli are first presented above the patient's threshold, and the intensity is decreased until the patient no longer responds. The ascending technique, in contrast, begins with stimuli that are below the patient's threshold, and the intensity is increased until the patient responds.

It should be noted that the descending and ascending threshold techniques have significant shortcomings. The descending technique is influenced by perseveration, or continuing to respond when the stimuli are no longer perceived (false-positive responses). Conversely, the ascending technique is influenced by inhibition, or failing to respond even when the stimuli are audible (false-negative responses). Because of perseveration and inhibition, the use of an ascending or descending technique alone for hearing threshold assessment can lead to high test–retest variability as well as inaccurate test results.

The modified Hughson-Westlake technique (Carhart et al, 1959) was developed to reduce the influences of perseveration and inhibition. This procedure uses an ascending technique to determine threshold. Each threshold search is preceded by a descending familiarization trial. A familiarization trial is used to reduce the effects of inhibition during the ascending threshold search. An ascending procedure was chosen for determination of threshold because it reduces the possibility that the patient may adapt to the signal or produce inappropriate responses based on the rhythmical patterns of stimulus presentation.

Table 12–3 provides examples of the procedures followed with the modified Hughson-Westlake technique. Familiarization is accomplished by initially presenting a stimulus 1 to 2 seconds in length at a presumed suprathreshold level in the midrange of hearing. This level, normally 40 dB HL, is determined by the audiologist during the pretesting interview with the patient. If a response is obtained, the intensity is decreased in 10 to 20 dB steps, with stimuli presented (for 1–2 seconds) and an off-time varying between 3 and 5 seconds, until no response is obtained. If the patient fails to respond at the initial setting of 40 dB HL, the intensity level is increased in 20 dB steps until a response is obtained (section D of Table 12–3). In Table 12–3, familiarization is shown for each example from the initial presentation at 40 dB HL to the beginning of the threshold search. Broken lines denote the border between the procedures.

Once familiarization has taken place, thresholds are established with an ascending technique in 5 dB steps. When the patient responds to a stimulus presentation, the signal is decreased by 10 dB and then increased in 5 dB steps until the patient responds once again. Threshold is defined as the lowest intensity level at which the patient responds to the stimuli for at least two out of three or three out of six trials.

ASHA's recommended procedure is similar to the modified Hughson-Westlake technique. Familiarization can be accomplished via one of two methods. The first method is to begin with the tone continuously on and increase the intensity until the patient responds. Alternatively, the initial signal presentation is 30 dB HL. If a clear response occurs, threshold measurement should begin. If not, the level is increased to 50 dB HL, then in 10 dB increments until a clear response is elicited, after which the threshold search begins. This method of familiarization eliminates the need for the clinician to make assumptions regarding the patient's hearing ability prior to testing. Search for threshold begins 10 dB below the familiarization response. Each time the patient fails to respond, the level is increased by 5 dB. When a response is present, the level is decreased 10 dB. Threshold is defined as the lowest level at which responses were obtained in 50% of the trials, with a minimum of three responses.

The examples in Table 12–3 show the variety of responses that might be observed during threshold audiometry. Note that for section E the variability in the patient's responses made it impossible to establish a valid threshold. This patient would require reinstruction, retesting, and perhaps special testing.

Throughout testing, stimuli are presented with an on time of 1 to 2 seconds and an off time of at least 3 seconds. This technique takes advantage of the robust neural response to the onset of a stimulus and reduces the potential of auditory adaptation. Stimuli are not presented in regular temporal patterns during testing, and the interval between tones is varied. Otherwise, the patient may simply respond in a rhythmic manner, as opposed to attending to the stimuli.

False-Negative and False-Positive Responses

Two types of false responses can occur during threshold testing: the patient fails to respond when an audible stimulus is

Table 12–3   Examples of Responses during Pure-Tone Threshold Assessment

A Dial dB HL	A Patient Response	B Dial dB HL	B Patient Response	C Dial dB HL	C Patient Response	D Dial dB HL	D Patient Response	E Dial dB HL	E Patient Response
40	+	40	+	40	+	40	−	40	+
35	+	30	+	25	+	60	−	25	+
20	+	15	+	15	+	80	+	10	−
10	−	5	+	5	−	70	−	15	−
15	−	0	+	10	−	75	+	20	+
20	+	0	+	15	−	65	−	10	−
10	−	0	+	20	−	70	−	15	+
15	−	Threshold = 0 dB HL		25	+	75	+	5	−
20	+			15	−	65	−	10	+
10	−			20	+	70	−	0	−
15	−			10	−	75	+	5	−
20	+			15	−	Threshold = 75 dB HL		10	−
Threshold = 20 dB HL				20	+			15	−
				10	−			20	+
				15	−			10	−
				20	+			15	+
				Threshold = 20 dB HL				Threshold = ?	

HL, hearing level.

presented (a false-negative), or the patient responds in the absence of the stimulus (a false-positive). False-negative and false-positive responses are observed as part of the normal threshold procedure, especially when stimuli are presented at or near threshold. Stimuli near threshold are not easily perceived and when patients question the presence or absence of stimuli in the range near threshold, it is normal for them to respond incorrectly. For this reason, it is important that the patient be instructed to respond even when the stimuli are very faint and to be told that it is acceptable to guess when unsure whether or not the tone was presented.

False-negative responses are much less common than false-positive responses during audiometric testing. Some false-negatives reflect a lack of attention to the task due either to neurological deficit or to boredom. In the latter case, the clinician may only need to reinstruct the patient. With neurological deficit, such as traumatic brain injury, the patient may exhibit unusually excessive inhibition to the ascending signal. For these patients, threshold searching might require bracketing in an ascending/descending pattern in 5 dB steps, or defining threshold only using stimuli presented in a descending pattern. If simple reinstruction does not improve performance, and the clinician has little faith in the responses obtained, this impression should be noted on the audiogram or examination report along with a note on the use of any nonstandard techniques.

False-negative responses will occur when individuals are feigning a hearing loss (pseudohypoacusis). These individuals commonly exhibit unreliable responses because they have difficulty maintaining a consistent threshold level (they are unable to monitor their "loudness yardstick"). The special techniques outlined in Chapter 14 should be used for those patients demonstrating pseudohypoacusis.

False-positive responses occur frequently when patients have tinnitus. That is, patients with tinnitus may mistake the pure-tone stimuli for their tinnitus and respond when no stimulus is present. These individuals typically have consistent responses but begin showing false-positives for the frequencies at which tinnitus interference occurs, especially near threshold. Presenting a pulsed pure-tone or warble tone signal for these patients helps them to differentiate the external signal from their constant internal tinnitus.

Special Consideration

- Patients with tinnitus may exhibit a large number of false-positive responses, especially when the test signal is near the tinnitus frequency. For these patients, using a pulsed signal (200 msec on/off) or a warble tone will help them distinguish the test signal from the tinnitus.

Automated Testing

Automated testing has been incorporated into many audiological diagnostic procedures, including middle ear measures, auditory brainstem response (ABR), otoacoustic emissions (OAE), and hearing aid measurement. However, with the exception of industrial hearing screening, pure-tone testing continues to

be performed manually by virtually all audiologists. Because most patients are capable of following the necessary instructions to be tested with automatic equipment, and because there is continued financial pressure to increase the efficiency of audiological testing, there is a clear rationale for developing automated equipment for pure-tone (and speech threshold) testing. In fact, one system has been developed (Otogram, Sonic Innovations, Inc., Salt Lake City, UT), and there is a commercial venture (Hearing Health Network™, Salt Lake City, UT) attempting to reinforce the use of automated audiological testing. Over time, it is likely that equipment will be available for routine pure-tone testing by audiologists.

Infection Control

Physical contact of any instrument used with the patient in the audiological evaluation can result in the spread of infection and/or disease. Supra-aural and especially insert earphones must be cleaned and disinfected between patients. Response switches/buttons should also be given the same attention. Because the clinician will come in physical contact with each patient during audiometric testing, hand washing should occur between each consultation. An excellent source regarding infection control is Bankaitis and Kemp (2003).

Pearl

- Hand washing is the most effective way to prevent the spread of infection and disease.

♦ Pure-Tone Bone Conduction

Comparison of pure-tone air-conduction thresholds with pure-tone bone-conduction thresholds allows for the diagnosis of the type of hearing loss. With bone-conduction testing, the conductive mechanism is bypassed, which provides for a measure of the integrity of the sensorineural mechanism in isolation. When air- and bone-conduction tests are used in combination, the difference between the air- and bone-conduction thresholds can be used to determine the magnitude of the conductive component. It is this difference that indicates whether the hearing loss is conductive, sensorineural, or mixed.

In bone-conduction testing, thresholds are established in much the same manner as air-conduction thresholds. However, instead of using earphones, a single bone-conduction oscillator, secured in a standard headband, is placed on the mastoid or forehead. Prior to the development of audiometers with bone-conduction capabilities, tuning forks were used to diagnose the type of hearing loss.

Modes of Bone-Conduction Transmission

Signals from the bone-conduction oscillator set the bones of the entire skull into motion, stimulating the cochlea in both mastoid bones. As a result, the cochleas of both ears are stimulated, and any responses obtained reflect the auditory sensitivity of the cochlea with the best hearing sensitivity. In bone-conduction testing, it is always important to be aware of the need to mask to prevent the nontest ear from participating in the test (see Chapter 13).

When the skull is set into motion by bone-conduction stimulation, a complex mechanism occurs that involves osseotympanic, inertial, and distortional or compressional stimulation.

Osseotympanic

Inertial properties of the bones composing the skull cause them to vibrate in response to the bone-conduction oscillator. As the mandible moves, it distorts the cartilaginous portion of the external auditory meatus and alternately compresses the air in the meatus. In this manner, skull vibrations radiate into the ear canal. These vibrations are in turn transmitted to the cochlea in the same manner as normal air-conduction stimulation.

Inertial

When the skull is set into motion with a bone-conduction vibrator, the structures of the ossicular chain (including the malleus, incus, and stapes) are not rigidly attached, and there is a lag in their movement relative to skull movement. This lag causes the stapes to move in the oval window in a fashion similar to standard air-conduction stimulation, thus transmitting the signal to the cochlea. This method of stimulation dominates in the low frequencies.

Distortional/Compressional

When the skull is set into motion with a bone-conduction vibrator, the compression of the bones of the skull gives rise to a distortion of the inner ear structures, which in turn produces electromechanical activity in the inner ear, giving rise to the sensation of hearing. The bony structures of the inner ear alternately compress the fluid-filled space of the inner ear. As a consequence of this compression and fluid movement, the basilar membrane movement stimulates the hair cells and results in the sensation of sound. This mode of stimulation is predominant in the high frequencies.

Tuning Fork Tests

Because they provide preliminary diagnostic information, require no special equipment, and are easy to administer, many physicians continue to use tuning forks in their everyday practice. As a result, audiologists must be aware of the tests that are used and their interpretations.

The three tuning fork tests that continue to be used today are the Bing, Rinne, and Weber. Results from these tests are determined by the presence or absence of an occlusion effect. Because the occlusion effect is dependent on low frequencies, with each of these tests a low-frequency tuning fork (256 or 512 Hz) is used.

Table 12–4 provides a summary of three commonly used tuning fork tests. As shown in this table, the Bing test is used for patients who have either a bilateral conductive or sensorineural hearing loss. In this test, the tuning fork is set into vibration, and the handle is placed on the mastoid process. With the tuning fork on the mastoid, the ear canal is alternately occluded and unoccluded by having the patient apply slight pressure on the tragus with his or her finger. The patient is asked if the loudness increases when the ear canal is occluded (Bing positive) or if there is no difference in the loudness of the tone for the occluded or unoccluded ear canal (Bing negative). A Bing positive result means that the occlusion effect was evident and responsible for enhancing the ear's sensitivity for bone-conduction sounds, as seen in patients with normal hearing or sensorineural hearing loss. If the occlusion effect is not evident (Bing negative result), the ear already has a conductive impairment.

Pitfall

- Results from the Bing and Rinne tuning fork tests can be contaminated due to crossover of the bone-conducted test signal to the nontest ear.

Table 12–4 Summary of Commonly Used Tuning Fork Tests

Test	Purpose	Procedure	Results
Bing	Assesses the presence of conductive hearing loss	Tuning fork base is placed on the patient's mastoid while the ear canal is alternately opened and closed by depressing the tragus	If louder when ear closed, the loss is sensorineural; if the same when the ear canal is open and closed, the loss is conductive
Rinne	Compares air conduction to bone conduction sensitivity	Tuning fork is alternately held to the ear, and then the base is placed on the mastoid process	If louder when held to the ear, the loss is sensorineural (Rinne positive); if louder when base is placed on the mastoid process, the loss is conductive (Rinne negative)
Weber	Used for patients reporting unilateral hearing loss	Tuning fork base is placed midline on the patient's forehead	If lateralized to the ear with loss, the loss is conductive; if lateralized to the ear without loss, the loss is sensorineural or mixed

With the Rinne test, the tuning fork is set into vibration and held close to the patient's ear. The patient is then asked to report when he or she can no longer hear the sound produced by the tuning fork. At this point, the handle of the tuning fork is quickly placed against the patient's mastoid process, and the patient is asked if he or she can again hear the tone. If the patient is able to hear the tone produced by the fork for a longer duration by bone conduction than by air conduction, the result is called a Rinne negative, as is observed in patients with a conductive hearing loss. A positive Rinne effect occurs when the patient hears the tone longer by air than by bone conduction, and is indicative of normal hearing or a sensorineural hearing loss.

Care must be taken when interpreting results from the Rinne test, because if the nontest ear has better bone-conduction sensitivity than the test ear, the signal from the mastoid could cross over to the nontest ear and provide an inaccurate diagnosis of conductive pathology.

The Weber is a test of lateralization and is used for patients who report unilateral hearing loss. After the tuning fork is set into vibration, the handle is placed on the forehead, and the patient is asked to report where the signal is heard. Responses are that the signal is heard in the ear with the hearing loss, in the ear with the better hearing, or possibly midline. If the signal lateralizes to the ear with the hearing loss, a conductive hearing loss is indicated, because the improved bone-conduction sensitivity is due to the occlusion effect. If the signal lateralizes to the ear with better hearing, a sensorineural hearing loss is indicated, because the cochlea with the best hearing sensitivity will detect the signal. Patients with normal hearing will report the sound in the midline position.

Once having some utility but no longer in use, the Schwaback test is used to quantify the degree of hearing loss. After the tuning fork is set into vibration and is placed on the mastoid process, the patient is asked to report when he or she no longer hears the tone. At that point, the clinician quickly places the handle of the fork on his or her own mastoid and counts the number of seconds he or she continues to hear the tone. Of course, the success of this test depends on a normal hearing clinician. The results are expressed in terms of the time that the clinician heard the tone beyond that time that the patient's hearing diminished. For example, if the examiner can hear for 10 seconds longer than the patient, the test result is expressed as "diminished 10."

Audiometric tuning fork tests can replace standard tuning fork tests and are done by placing a bone-conduction oscillator set at 35 to 40 dB HL on the patient's forehead. The use of a bone-conduction oscillator for these tests provides greater intensity and frequency control over the stimulus, increasing the reliability and validity of findings.

Pure-tone bone-conduction testing is significantly more sophisticated than tuning fork tests. However, tuning fork tests continue to be used regularly by many physicians to provide a preliminary diagnosis of the type of hearing loss. Though qualitative, tuning fork tests can provide a quick way to validate pure-tone audiometric data. For example, the Weber test should lateralize to the impaired ear with a patient having a unilateral conductive hearing loss. If it does

not, the patient could have ear canal collapse during testing, or masking might have not been used properly. Pure-tone bone-conduction tests provide both quantitative and qualitative information. As a result, tuning forks should not replace but be a complement to bone-conduction audiometry.

Bone-Conduction Tests

The procedure traditionally used for bone-conduction testing is to place the bone oscillator behind the ear on the mastoid bone (see **Fig. 12–5**). However, some clinicians prefer forehead placement. Forehead placement increases test–retest reliability, because frontal bone tissue is relatively homogenous in comparison to mastoid tissue. However, increased test–retest reliability is offset by the fact that 10 to 15 dB additional energy is required to stimulate the cochlea(s) with forehead placement, thereby reducing the dynamic range, or the amount of maximum output, achievable with bone-conduction stimulation. Furthermore, ANSI standards for bone conduction are based on mastoid placement, and no forehead headband arrangements are commercially available that produce the necessary static force recommended by ANSI standards. These latter reasons explain why more than 90% of audiologists continue to use mastoid placement of the bone-conduction vibrator (Martin et al, 1998).

Controversial Point

- Some clinicians advocate forehead bone-conduction oscillator placement because test–retest reliability is increased. However, most audiologists continue to use mastoid placement, because current ANSI standards are calibrated for mastoid placement, and forehead placement reduces the maximum output (dynamic range) for bone-conduction tests.

Pearl

- A routine procedure to improve inter- and intrasubject reliability during bone-conduction testing is to place the bone-conduction oscillator on the mastoid at various locations while asking the patient to identify where the tone appears to be the loudest.

Although bone-conduction testing is invaluable to the diagnostic test battery, there are inherent factors that affect such tests.

1. Variations in the size of the skull and thickness of the skin and bone of the skull are uncontrollable factors. As a result, compared with air-conduction testing, inter- and intrasubject variability is high for bone-conduction testing. With pure-tone air-conduction threshold audiometry, test–retest reliability for a cooperative adult is 5 dB. However with pure-tone bone-conduction threshold

audiometry, test–retest variability can often be 10 or even 15 dB.

2. Because it takes more energy to drive the bone-conduction oscillator, maximum outputs from bone-conduction signals are limited to 40 dB at 250 Hz, 50 dB at 500 Hz, and 60 to 70 dB at 1000 to 4000 Hz. The reduced output means that it is impossible to use bone-conduction results to determine the difference between a sensorineural and mixed loss when air-conduction threshold sensitivity exceeds these maximum output values by more than 10 or 15 dB.

3. Tactile responses will be obtained for bone-conduction stimulation at 250 and 500 Hz at intensities between 35 and 55 dB HL. Whenever low-frequency bone-conduction thresholds are obtained in the 35 to 55 dB range, there is a high probability that the responses were a result of tactile, rather than auditory, stimulation.

4. The interaural attenuation for bone-conduction signals is 0 to 10 dB. As a result, crossover of a bone-conduction signal from one ear to the other occurs even when a slight asymmetrical hearing loss is present, and masking must be used. Without the use of masking, it is possible to make serious errors in diagnosing the type and degree of hearing loss.

5. The effects of environmental noise are greater for bone-conduction threshold testing because thresholds are obtained without occlusion of the external ear canals. With standard pure-tone air-conduction threshold audiometry, the ear canals are occluded with supra-aural earphones. The cushions of the earphones help attenuate the masking effects of ambient background noise in the environment. Bone-conduction testing can be obtained with the ear canals occluded, which is referred to as absolute bone conduction. However, with standard bone-conduction testing, the ear canals are unoccluded, which is referred to as relative bone conduction. Because the ANSI calibration standard for bone-conduction threshold testing is based on relative bone-conduction thresholds (ANSI, 2004), it is not appropriate to occlude the test ear during threshold bone-conduction testing.

Pitfall

• Uncontrollable factors make the variability of bone-conduction threshold testing considerably greater than air-conduction testing. Clinicians must factor this into interpreting audiometric test results.

Although it is recognized that the above factors influence bone-conduction testing, making test–retest reliability significantly greater than air-conduction testing, bone-conduction threshold audiometry is an integral part of the standard diagnostic audiological test battery. Clinicians must be aware that there is greater variability in bone-conduction measures and take this into consideration when interpreting diagnostic test results.

♦ The Audiogram and Audiometric Symbols

The audiogram displays data from the audiological evaluation. As shown in **Fig. 12–6**, frequency is displayed on the abscissa (horizontal axis) and intensity, in dB HL, is displayed on the ordinate (vertical axis). When an audiogram is constructed, one octave on the frequency scale should be equivalent in span to 20 dB on the HL scale. In addition, grid lines of equal darkness and thickness should appear at octave intervals on the frequency scale and at 10 dB intervals on the intensity scale. The ASHA audiogram form records both right and left ear information on one graph with symbols, as shown in **Fig. 12–6A**. Forms with a separate graph depicting each ear, as shown in **Fig. 12–6B**, are common in audiology practice.

Several audiometric symbol systems have been employed by different clinics to record air- and bone-conduction thresholds. This diversity has resulted in confusion and possible misinterpretation when records are exchanged between clinics. For this reason, ASHA has developed a standard system of symbols for audiograms.

As shown, the symbols O and X are used for unmasked air-conduction thresholds; open arrows (carets) with the open end facing to the right and to the left of the frequency indication line are used for unmasked bone-conduction thresholds for the right and left ears, respectively. Triangles and squares are used for right and left masked air-conduction thresholds, respectively. Brackets with the open end facing to the right and to the left are used for masked bone-conduction thresholds for the right and left ears, respectively. Positioning the symbols for bone-conduction tests on the audiogram is easy to remember if the clinician imagines the patient's head on the audiogram facing forward; the open end of the bone-conduction symbols fit over the ears like earphones. The symbol S is used to represent sound field testing.

When no response is obtained at the maximum output of the audiometer, the ASHA guidelines recommend the use of an arrow attached to the lower outside corner of the appropriate symbol, ~45 degrees outward from the frequency axis (pointing down and to the right for left ear symbols and down and to the left for right ear symbols). It is also recommended that the symbol system appear on the audiogram form (see **Fig. 12–6**).

♦ Types of Hearing Loss

Normal Findings

When no hearing loss is present, pure-tone air- and bone-conduction thresholds will be at 0 dB HL at all frequencies. This finding is shown in **Fig. 12–7A**.

Although rare, it is possible to have all thresholds at 0 dB HL. Typically, thresholds for patients with no communication difficulty fall between 0 and 15 or 0 and 25 dB HL. In very few cases, it is possible to find thresholds below 0 dB HL (–5 dB), which would suggest threshold sensitivity that

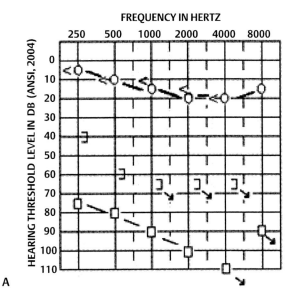

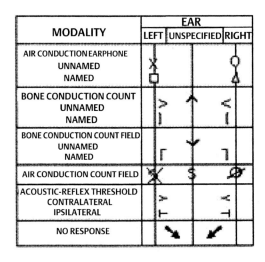

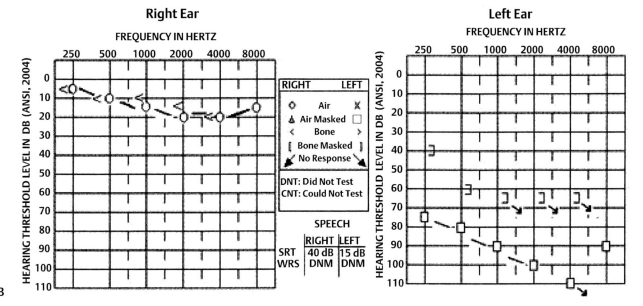

Figure 12–6 Example of an American Speech-Language-Hearing Association audiogram form with **(A)** symbol legend and **(B)** an audiogram form showing data for each ear separately with symbol legend, with the same audiometric data plotted on both. (Data from American National Standards Institute. (2004). American national standard specification for audiometers (S3.6–2004). Washington, DC: Author.)

is significantly better than the normal ear. However, because of the acceptance of the ANSI standard, this is an extremely rare finding, and if it occurs frequently, calibration of the audiometer should be checked.

Although 0 dB HL is the value representing "perfect," normal hearing sensitivity, there is a range of intensities considered to be within normal limits (0–15 dB HL for children, 0–25 dB HL for adults). Those with thresholds in this range should have minimal or little difficulty hearing normal conversational speech, unless other audiological manifestations are present. It should be remembered that any deviation from 0 dB represents a decrease of hearing from the norm; a 10 dB threshold, for example, is a loss of 10 dB compared with the normal reference level.

As pointed out in Chapter 13, pure-tone test findings should be in agreement with results from speech audiometry. The pure-tone average (PTA), or the average threshold of 500, 1000, and 2000 Hz, generally should be within 5 to 10 dB of the speech reception threshold. If this is not the case, the clinician should first make sure the procedures used to perform the test were appropriate, check the equipment used to perform the tests, and then reinstruct the patient. If the PTA and speech threshold results still do not agree, it is possible that the patient is not cooperating (pseudohypoacusis; see discussion below).

By comparing air-conduction to bone-conduction thresholds, three types of organic hearing loss can be defined: conductive, sensorineural, and mixed. **Figure 12–8** shows the difference between these types of hearing loss based on the anatomical site involved. In addition to these three organic types of hearing loss, two other classifications are used: pseudohypoacucis (nonorganic or functional hearing loss) and auditory processing disorder.

Conductive Hearing Loss

The audiometric findings for conductive hearing loss are displayed in **Fig. 12–7B**. As shown, pure-tone bone-conduction thresholds are normal, and pure-tone air-conduction thresholds are abnormal with conductive loss. In addition, measures of middle ear functions will be abnormal with conductive loss. Because the air-conduction signals will actually set the skull into motion at levels of 60 to 70 dB HL, the maximum amount of hearing loss possible due to conductive pathology is 60 to 70 dB. That is, losses greater than 60 to 70 dB cannot be exclusively conductive in nature.

Two behavioral symptoms may separate patients with conductive hearing loss from those with mixed or sensorineural hearing loss. Those with conductive hearing loss will demonstrate no difficulty discriminating speech for a sufficiently loud signal. Moreover, individuals may have softly spoken speech because their own voice is perceived louder than normal due to an "occlusion effect" resulting from the conductive hearing loss. This effect can be easily demonstrated by having normal hearing patients close off their ears by placing their index fingers in their ear canals and then speaking.

Sensorineural Hearing Loss

A pure-tone audiometric pattern for sensorineural loss is shown in **Fig. 12–7C**. With sensorineural hearing loss, air- and bone-conduction thresholds are both elevated and within 10 dB of each other.

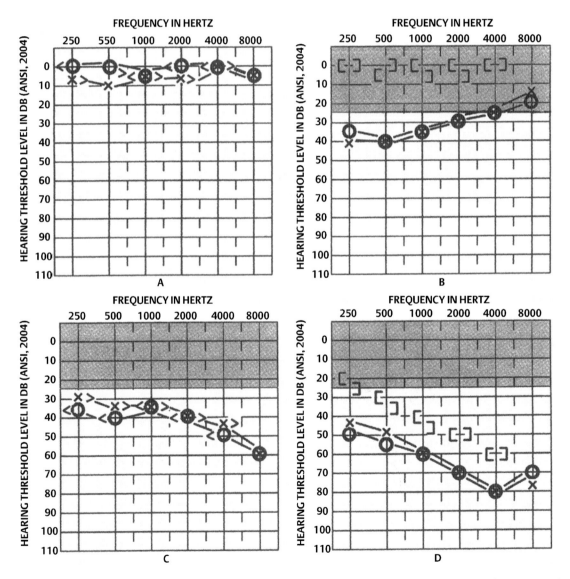

Figure 12–7 Audiometric results showing **(A)** normal hearing, **(B)** conductive hearing loss, **(C)** sensorineural hearing loss, and **(D)** mixed hearing loss. (Data from American National Standards Institute. (2004). American national standard specification for audiometers (S3.6–2004). Washington, DC: Author.)

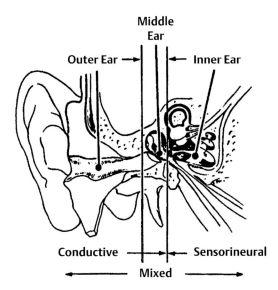

Figure 12–8 The three types of hearing loss classified according to anatomical site of involvement.

Several symptoms characteristic of sensorineural hearing loss are shouting or talking in a loud voice, difficulty discriminating between speech sounds, and recruitment. Shouting or speaking in a loud voice may occur with sensorineural loss because the impaired patient does not have normal hearing by bone conduction. Hence, the patient's own voice or other voices may not be heard, causing these individuals to have difficulty regulating the intensity level of their voice. Not all patients with sensorineural hearing loss speak loudly, and not all patients with a conductive loss speak softly; many learn to regulate their voice levels appropriately. The frequent decrease in word discrimination ability associated with sensorineural hearing loss is due to distortion of the speech signal caused by auditory nerve fiber loss.

The typical sensorineural hearing loss is characterized by better hearing in the low frequencies than in the high frequencies. Consonants contain high-frequency information, whereas vowels are predominantly low in frequency. Therefore, consonant sounds may not be heard or are easily confused. The clinician should keep in mind that, although the speech may be audible, it may not be intelligible.

Another symptom of sensorineural hearing loss, recruitment, refers to a rapid growth in loudness once threshold has been crossed. After the signal is intense enough to be perceived, any further increase in intensity may cause a disproportionate increase in the sensation of loudness. Thus, the individual's dynamic range, or the range of intensities between an individual's threshold and his or her uncomfortable listening level, is limited. Shouting at an individual with sensorineural hearing loss may result only in agitation rather than improved comprehension. Because of the combined effects of recruitment and word discrimination difficulty, individuals with sensorineural hearing loss experience greater difficulty in noisy surroundings than those with normal hearing or a conductive hearing loss.

Mixed Hearing Loss

A pure-tone audiometric pattern for a mixed hearing loss is displayed in **Fig. 12–7D**. With a mixed loss, both air- and bone-conduction thresholds are elevated, but bone-conduction thresholds are better (occur at a lower intensity) than air-conduction thresholds by 10 dB or more. The difference between the two thresholds is referred to as the air–bone gap and represents the amount of conductive loss present.

Pseudohypoacusis

The diagnosis of pseudohypoacusis is made when an individual claims to have a hearing loss, but discrepancies in audiometric test findings and/or behavior suggest that the loss either does not exist at all or does not exist to the degree that is indicated by voluntary test results. Specific information on this classification of impairment and the diagnostic tests available are presented in Chapter 14 of this text.

Auditory Processing Disorder

Auditory processing disorders involve deficits in processing auditory information not attributed to impairment in the peripheral hearing mechanism or intellect. The processing of auditory information involves perceptual, cognitive, and linguistic functions. These functions and the appropriate interactions between these functions result in effective receptive communication. The following are examples of auditory processing abilities (ASHA, 2005):

- Attending, discriminating, and identifying acoustic signals

- Transforming and continuously transmitting information through both the peripheral and central nervous systems

- Filtering, sorting, and combining information at appropriate perceptual conceptual levels

- Storing and retrieving information efficiently; restoring, organizing, and using retrieved information

- Segmenting and decoding acoustic stimuli using phonological, semantic, syntactic, and pragmatic knowledge

- Attaching meaning to a stream of acoustic signals through use of linguistic and nonlinguistic contexts

Pure-tone audiometric tests are severely limited in identifying auditory processing disorders. As a result, specialized tests of central auditory function and auditory processing have been developed. These specialized tests are covered in Chapters 16 and 17.

Auditory Neuropathy

Auditory neuropathy, also referred to as auditory dysynchrony, is a pathologic condition of the auditory system that involves a disruption of synchronous activity in the processing of auditory stimuli, most likely involving the eighth auditory nerve.

With auditory neuropathy, hearing sensitivity can be normal, or hearing loss in the mild to moderate, or even severe, range can be present. Normal cochlear function is present (as evidenced by OAE and/or cochlear microphonic), and the ABR is abnormal or elevated beyond wave I. The primary evidence for auditory neuropathy is that speech recognition is significantly worse than suggested by pure-tone data, sometimes being so impaired that rehabilitation with traditional amplification is unsuccessful. For further information regarding auditory neuropathy, see Starr et al (1996).

♦ Degree of Hearing Loss

The amount of hearing loss shown on the pure-tone audiogram is used to classify the amount of hearing impairment. Hearing impairment is determined by results from audiometric data and is a function of the amount of abnormal or reduced audiological function. Hearing impairment is typically determined by the degree of loss, and results from pure-tone tests are used as the primary means for classifying hearing impairment. No universal schemes are available for classifying the degree of hearing loss from pure-tone tests. For this reason, there is diversity from clinic to clinic in specifying the degree of loss. However, most classification systems are similar.

Because the effects of hearing loss vary according to age, separate systems are used for children and adults. Northern and Downs (1991) provide a common classification system for use with children, as follows:

0 to 15 dB HL: within normal limits

16 to 25 dB HL: slight

26 to 30 dB HL: mild

31 to 50 dB HL: moderate

51 to 70 dB HL: severe

71+: profound

A classification system that is more appropriate with adults is

0 to 25 dB HL: within normal limits

26 to 40 dB HL: mild loss

41 to 55 dB HL: moderate loss

56 to 70 dB HL: moderate to severe loss

71 to 90 dB HL severe loss

91+ dB HL profound loss

These general guidelines for classifying hearing impairment become meaningful with respect to the communication difficulty a patient may experience when they are applied to the PTA of 500, 1000, and 2000 Hz. For example, if thresholds are 45, 50, and 65 dB HL at 500, 1000, and 2000 Hz, respectively, the PTA would be 53 dB, and the loss would fall into the moderate range.

Hearing Disability and Hearing Handicap

Stating that a loss is mild, moderate, or severe based on pure-tone data provides assistance in describing the degree to which an individual will experience difficulty in communicating, but these simple terms do not detail the communicative, social, and emotional effects the loss may cause. In fact, it is impossible to predict the effects hearing loss will have on communicative and social function for an individual patient from pure-tone data. The information presented in **Table 12–5**

Table 12–5   Degree of Communication Difficulty as a Function of Hearing Loss

Communication Difficulty	Level of Hearing Loss (Hz)*	Degree of Loss
Demonstrates difficulty understanding soft-spoken speech; good candidate for hearing aid(s); children will need preferential seating and resource help in school	25–40	Mild
Demonstrates an understanding of speech at 3 to 5 feet; requires the use of hearing aid(s); children will need preferential seating, resource help, and speech therapy	40–55	Moderate
Speech must be loud for auditory reception; difficulty in group settings; requires the use of hearing aid(s); children will require special classes for hearing-impaired, plus all of the above	55–70	Moderate to severe
Loud speech may be understood at 1 foot from ear; may distinguish vowels but not consonants; requires the use of hearing aid(s); children will require classes for hearing impaired, plus all of the above	70–90	Severe
Does not rely on audition as primary modality for communication; may benefit from hearing aid(s); may benefit from cochlear implant; children will require all of the above, plus total communication	90+	Profound

*Pure-tone average: 500 to 2000 Hz.

Source: Goodman, A. (1965). Reference zero levels for pure tone audiometers. ASHA, 7, 262–263.

is a general guide for estimating the communication difficulty presented by hearing losses of varying degrees.

The effect of the hearing loss on communicative function will depend on the type of loss and whether the loss involves one ear, both ears equally, or one ear to a lesser degree. For example, the patient with significant hearing loss in one ear and normal hearing in the other will appear to hear normally, especially in a quiet listening environment. However, when noise is present, patients with unilateral hearing loss will have significant difficulty with speech intelligibility.

The terms *hearing disability* and *hearing handicap* are important in understanding the effects a hearing loss may have on an individual. *Hearing disability* refers to the limitation on function imposed by the hearing loss. *Hearing handicap* is a measure of the effect the hearing loss has on psychosocial function. Seasoned audiologists realize that it is possible for one individual to have a severe hearing impairment with only limited hearing disability or hearing handicap. In contrast, some patients with mild hearing impairment may have severe hearing disability and a hearing handicap.

Because the levels of disability and handicap are so variable between individuals, it is critical that audiologists make an assessment of these variables for each patient. Assessing these variables has the goal of defining the nature and extent of the hearing loss and providing appropriate strategies for rehabilitation.

Disability and handicap are measured with self-assessment scales. Patients are asked to fill out questionnaires addressing how the hearing loss affects them in a variety of listening situations and how it affects their self-perception. These scales are designed to assess the extent of the hearing disability, the social and emotional consequences on the individual, and the extent to which the hearing loss influences quality of life. It is only through this type of analysis that hearing disability and handicap can be determined.

Deaf versus Hard of Hearing

Sometimes the term *deaf* is used to describe individuals having severe or profound hearing loss. However, the term *deaf* is technically reserved for individuals with hearing loss whose auditory sensitivity is so severely impaired that only a few or none of the prosodic and phonetic elements of speech can be recognized. For these individuals, the primary sensory input for communication will be something other than the auditory channel. Few individuals with hearing loss are truly "deaf."

The term *hard of hearing* refers to individuals with hearing loss that can identify enough of the distinguishing features of speech through hearing alone to permit at least partial recognition of spoken language. Individuals classified as hard of hearing rely on the auditory channel as the primary sensory input for communication. With the addition of the visual system (speechreading), individuals who are deaf or hard of hearing may understand even more language, provided the vocabulary and syntax are within the linguistic code.

Describing Pure-Tone Findings

Table 12–6 lists terms that are commonly used to describe pure-tone audiometric findings. It shows the general audiometric configurations they represent.

Clinicians will have their own specific methods of describing audiometric findings, but the general protocol is to describe the degree of loss first, then state the ear(s) in which the loss is present, then use a descriptive term listed

Table 12–6 Common Terms Used to Describe Pure-Tone Audiograms

Term	Description	Audiometric Configuration
Flat	There is little or no change in thresholds (+ or − 20 dB) across frequencies	
Sloping	As frequency increases, the degree of hearing loss increases	
Rising	As frequency increases, the degree of hearing loss decreases	
Precipitous	There is a very sharp increase in the hearing loss between octaves	
Scoop or trough shape	The greatest hearing loss is present in the midfrequencies, and hearing sensitivity is better in the low and high frequencies	
Inverted scoop or trough shape	The greatest hearing loss is in the low and high frequencies, and hearing sensitivity is better in the midfrequencies	
High frequency	The hearing loss is limited to the frequencies above the speech range (2000–3000 Hz)	
Fragmentary	Thresholds are recorded only for low frequencies, and they are in the severe-to-profound range	
4000 to 6000 Hz notch	Hearing is within normal limits through 3000 Hz, and there is a sharp drop in the 4000 to 6000 Hz range, with improved thresholds at 8000 Hz	

Table 12–7   General Format Used to Describe Pure-Tone Threshold Findings

Degree	Ear	Description	Type
Mild	Right ear	Flat	Sensorineural
Moderate	Left ear	Sloping	Conductive
Moderately severe	Bilateral	Rising Precipitous	Mixed
Severe		Scoop or trough shape	
Profound		Inverted scoop or trough shape High frequency Fragmentary 4000–6000 Hz notch	

Example 1: Severe left ear precipitous high-frequency sensorineural hearing loss with normal right ear hearing

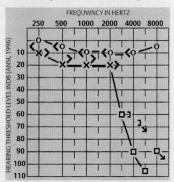

Example 2: Moderate to mild right ear rising mixed and a moderate left ear flat sensorineural hearing loss (Note that the bone-conduction response at 250 Hz is most likely tactile.)

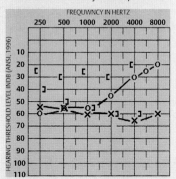

Example 3: Mild right ear rising conductive and profound (fragmentary) left ear (presumed) sensorineural hearing loss (Note that the bone-conduction responses at 250 and 500 Hz are most likely tactile.)

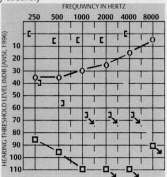

in **Table 12–6** when applicable, and finally state the type of loss. Generally, the ear with the least amount of loss is described first.

Table 12–7 provides examples of pure-tone audiometric findings from three different patients and verbal descriptions for each. Note that in example 1, when the term *high frequency* is used, the implication is that the loss is above the upper limits for speech intelligibility (3000 Hz). In example 2, two different types of losses are shown, and the symbols indicate that masking was used to obtain right ear bone-conduction thresholds and left ear air-conduction thresholds. In example 3, the term *presumed sensorineural hearing loss* was used for the left ear because the patient did not respond to bone-conduction stimuli at the maximum limits of the audiometer, and it is possible that a conductive component is present.

◆ Hearing Screening

Screening programs seek to identify those individuals having a defined disorder as accurately and early as possible and refer them for more comprehensive (diagnostic) testing. The objective is to accurately identify and refer those individuals with the condition (sensitivity) and dismiss individuals without the condition (specificity). This will avoid referring those individuals without the disease for further testing (false-positive results) and missing those with the disease (false-negative results). The goal of hearing screening is to identify those with hearing loss significant enough to interfere with communicative function and refer for medical and/or audiological follow-up, including rehabilitation.

Pitfall

• Factors that will adversely affect results from pure-tone screening tests include patients observing dials, examiner giving visual cues, incorrect adjustment of the headband and earphone placement, vague instructions, noise in the test area, overlong test sessions, and stimulus presentations that are too long or too short.

Pure-tone air-conduction tests have been used for hearing screening of young children and adults for decades. Such tests have proven to be effective in identifying significant hearing loss for populations that are able to make voluntary responses to the pure-tone signal. More recently, advanced audiological procedures have been developed that allow for testing noncooperative populations, such as neonates and infants. **Table 12–8** provides guidelines for hearing screening from birth through 65+ years. Although the procedures for infants and young children do not use pure-tone stimuli, they are included to show the capability that is now available for hearing screening throughout the life span. Chapters 20 and 22 cover the topics of ABR testing and OAE, respectively, and Chapter 23 is a detailed description of neonatal hearing screening.

Table 12–8   Guidelines for Hearing Screening from Birth through 65+ Years

Age	Test Type	Opportunity to Screen	Referral Criteria
Birth to 4	OAE screen[1] ABR screen	• All newborns not screened in hospital • Any child who presents with Parent concern Speech delay Language delay Behavioral problems Social problems School performance problems	Those with high-risk criteria[1] not already screened Those failing OAE or ABR screen Those with 3 continuous months of bilateral otitis media with effusion
4 to 18	Audiometric screen at 20 HL at 1000, 2000, and 4000 Hz[2]	• School hearing screening • Any child who presents with Parental concern Speech delay Language delay Behavioral problems Social problems School performance problems Excessive noise exposure	Rescreen those who fail at any frequency in either ear immediately Rescreen those who fail within 1 to 2 weeks Refer those who fail screen upon second visit
18 to 65	Audiometric screen at 25 dB HL at 500, 1000, 2000, and 4000 Hz	• Periodic health assessment • Parent/family complaint • Poor or declining socialization or work habits • Excessive noise exposure	Rescreen those who fail at any frequency in either ear immediately Rescreen those who fail within 1 to 2 weeks Refer those who fail screen upon second visit
65+	Audiometric screen at 25 dB or 40 dB HL at 500, 1000, 2000, and 4000 Hz (audioscope) Hearing handicap index	• Periodic health assessment • Patient/family complaint • Poor or declining socialization or work habits • Excessive noise exposure • Note that OSHA necessitates threshold testing (not screening)	Counsel those failing 25 dB screen that they have a problem Refer those failing 40 dB screen at any frequency except 4000 Hz Refer those failing hearing handicap index

[1]Joint Committee on Infant Hearing. (1991). 1990 position statement. ASHA Supplementum, 5, 3–6.

[2]American Speech-Language-Hearing Association, Panel on Audiologic Assessment. (1996). Guidelines for audiologic screening. Rockville, MD: Author.

ABR, auditory brainstem response; OAE, otoacoustic emissions; OSHA, Occupational Safety and Health Administration.

Whether the hearing screening program is for infants or the elderly, there are common factors that need consideration. Included are background noise levels in the screening environment, pass-fail criteria, periodicity of testing, criteria for medical follow-up, criteria for audiological follow-up, and record keeping. These topics are covered in Roeser and Clark (2004) and ASHA (1996).

♦ Summary

Accuracy of pure-tone tests is essential in audiometry, as the pure-tone test is the basis of diagnostic audiometry. Test accuracy is dependent on many factors the audiologist should understand, such as the stimulus. The stimulus is composed of a wave of compression and rarefaction alternating at a given rate, or frequency. This pure-tone waveform has an intensity that is described in a logarithmic scale called decibels. It is critical for the clinician to understand the equipment used to present the stimuli, whether they are pure tones, speech, or another acoustic signal. As a specialized piece of equipment, the audiometer allows the clinician to control the intensity, frequency, and duration of the stimulus. The stimulus can be presented via earphones (air conduction) or direct vibrational stimulus (bone conduction). By using both air- and bone-conduction signals, we are able to classify and describe the hearing of our patients. It is equally important for the clinician to have an understanding of the patient and possible patient response modes. Another vital factor in test accuracy is the procedure used to define the patient's thresholds. The presentation must follow standardized procedures to ensure the accuracy and reliability of the results. Results must be properly interpreted and classified. A careful record must be made to describe the hearing loss using standardized methods and recording techniques. Through knowledge of the nature of the test, the test equipment, the test procedures, and careful execution, an accurate assessment of the patient's hearing status can be made.

References

American National Standards Institute. (2004). American national standard specification for audiometers (S3.6–2004). New York: Author.

American Speech-Language-Hearing Association. (2005). Position statement: (Central) auditory processing disorders: The role of the audiologist. Rockville, MD: Author.

American Speech-Language-Hearing Association, Panel on Audiologic Assessment. (1996). Guidelines for audiologic screening. Rockville, MD: Author.

Bankaitis, A. U., & Kemp, R. J. (2003). Infection control in the audiology clinic. St. Louis: Oak Tree Products.

Berlin, C. I. (1967). Programmed instruction in the decibel. In J. L. Northern (Ed.), Hearing disorders (pp. 265–272). Boston: Little, Brown.

Carhart, R., & Jerger, J. F. (1959). Preferred method for clinical determination of pure-tone thresholds. Journal of Speech and Hearing Disorders, 24, 330–345.

Clark, J. L., & Roeser, R. J. (1988). Three studies comparing performance of the ER-3A tubephone with the TDH 50-P earphone. Ear and Hearing, 9(5), 268–273.

Fausti, S. A., Larson, V. D., Noffsinger, D., Wilson, R. H., Phillips, D. S., & Fowler, C. G. (1994). High frequency audiometric monitoring strategies for early detection of ototoxicity. Ear and Hearing, 15(3), 232–239.

Goodman, A. (1965). Reference zero levels for pure tone audiometers. ASHA, 7, 262–263.

Killion, M. C., Wilber, L. A., & Gudmundsen, G. I. (1985). Insert earphones for more interaural attenuation. Hearing Instruments, 36, 34–36.

Martin, F. N., Champlin, C. A., & Chambers, J. A. (1998). Seventh survey of audiometric practices in the United States. Journal of the American Academy of Audiology, 9(2), 95–104.

Northern, J. L., & Downs, M. P. (1991). Hearing and hearing loss in children. In J. Butler (Ed.), Hearing in children (pp. 1–31). Baltimore: Williams & Wilkins.

Park, K. R. (1996). The utility of acoustic reflex thresholds and other conventional audiological test for monitoring cisplatin ototoxicity in the pediatric population. Ear and Hearing, 17(2), 107–115.

Roeser, R. J., & Clark, J. (2004). Screening for auditory disorders. In R. J. Roeser & M. P. Downs (Eds.), Auditory disorders in school children (pp. 96–123). New York: Thieme Medical Publishers.

Roeser, R. J., Lai, L., & Clark, J. L. (2005). Effects of partial ear canal occlusion on pure tone thresholds. Journal of the American Academy of Audiology, 16(9), 740–746.

Starr, A., Picton, T. W., Sininger, Y., Hood, L. J., & Berlin, C. I. (1996). Auditory neuropathy. Brain, 119, 741–753.

Chapter 13

Clinical Masking

Ross J. Roeser and Jackie L. Clark

Diagnostic audiology has the primary goal of identifying etiological factors for hearing loss specific to each patient. To accomplish this goal, the auditory function of each ear must be assessed independent of the contralateral, or opposite, nontest ear (NTE).* That is, when an acoustic signal is presented to the test ear (TE), measures must be taken so that the contralateral, or NTE, ear does not participate in the procedure. Stated differently, audiologists must be aware of prevailing circumstances that may allow the NTE to contribute to the

evaluation of the TE due to "crossover" and be prepared to apply masking when necessary. Crossover occurs when an

---

*The terms nontest ear (NTE), contralateral ear, and opposite ear are used interchangeably throughout this chapter when referring to the ear opposite the test ear (TE). During routine audiometric testing, when needed, masking is introduced into the nontest, or contralateral, ear to prevent crossover.

air-conducted or bone-conducted signal is presented to the test ear at an intensity great enough to stimulate the NTE. Whenever the possibility of crossover exists, the application of appropriate clinical masking procedures is necessary.

Learning to apply masking principles regularly in clinical testing is one of the foremost challenges in audiology; students typically consider the topic of clinical masking a daunting undertaking. However, like all clinical skills, the principles of clinical masking can be mastered easily if they are applied regularly. To become part of routine clinical practice, masking principles must be studied thoroughly and then put into regular practice for several weeks or months.

This chapter provides readers with the principles of clinical masking. Specifically, clinical masking is defined, and considerations for applying masking in clinical testing are covered. Applying masking in diagnostic audiology testing is based on two simple questions: When should masking be used? And, when needed, how much masking is necessary? Specific answers to these questions and examples demonstrating the principles of clinical masking are provided.

Various masking procedures have been put forth, from the "plateau" method described by Hood (1960), to the "absolute" procedures advocated by Studebaker (1967, 1979) and Martin (1997). With the plateau method, clinicians are required to establish masked thresholds with several levels of masking presented to the NTE. The absolute method requires establishing threshold with one level of masking; if the threshold of the test ear does not change establishing a plateau is required only if the threshold of the test ear is affected by the starting level. Thus, the absolute method is time efficient. Until recently, all clinical procedures have based the starting level of the masked signal on the threshold of the NTE (the masked ear). However, Turner (2004a,b) describes a "redux" protocol in which the threshold of the TE is used to calculate the starting level for the NTE. This chapter outlines an absolute masking procedure using the NTE as the basis for determining the starting level, because undermasking can occur if the TE is used as the basis for the starting level.

The masking procedures provided in this chapter are overly conservative, meaning that they will always indicate the need for masking if the potential for crossover occurs. However, there will be situations when these procedures will suggest the need for masking when, in fact, masking is not always necessary. Test results will not be affected by using the guidelines. However, additional testing time will be necessary. New clinicians should follow the masking protocols in this chapter carefully; seasoned clinicians will have the clinical knowledge to modify them when indicated.

♦ What Is Masking?

Simply put, acoustic masking takes place when one sound (the masker) covers up, or makes inaudible, an acoustic signal (the primary auditory signal) a listener is attempting to hear. A more specific definition of masking is "the process by which the threshold of hearing for one sound is raised by the presence of another (masking) sound [and] the amount by which the threshold of hearing for one sound is raised by the

presence of another (masking) sound expressed in decibels" (American National Standards Institute [ANSI], 2004). In our everyday environment, as we listen to meaningful signals around us, we typically encounter masking in the form of unwanted background noise. For example, during class lectures, sounds from air-conditioning/heating systems, audiovisual equipment, conversations outside the classroom, and so forth often interfere with (or mask) the instructor (the primary auditory signal). Masking in our everyday environment is considered interference; in this sense, it is unwanted acoustic energy, an undesirable factor. However, when masking is applied properly during clinical audiometric testing, the masking signal is intentionally delivered to the NTE. Specifically, the appropriate use of masking prevents the inadvertent acoustic stimulation of the NTE resulting from a signal presented to the TE. This phenomenon is called *crossover* and will be discussed in detail later.

Masking versus Effective Masking

The definition of *masking* indicates that, like all other sounds, the intensity of a masking signal is measured in decibels (dB). For example, one could adjust the masking hearing level (HL) dial of an audiometer to 60 dB, and the specified level would then be 60 dB with regard to the audiometer dial for that particular audiometer.

Although the overall intensity of a masking signal can be specified in decibels, the decibel is a relative unit that becomes meaningful only if the reference is specified (see Chapter 10). For masking signals, the meaningful reference is dB effective masking level (dB EM). The term *dB EM* specifies the ability of a masking noise to mask a signal of known frequency and intensity, and is based on the spectrum (intensity and frequency) of the masking noise.

With the example from above, a masking signal delivered to an earphone with the masking dial of an audiometer set at 60 dB will provide 60 dB of masking noise to the specified transducer (earphone or loudspeaker). However, unless the audiometer has been properly calibrated, it is not clear how much acoustic energy can be masked by the masking signal at the 60 dB dial setting for each signal (pure tone or speech) the audiometer generates. That is, the 60 dB dial setting for the masking noise in the example might only mask a 1000 Hz pure tone at 45 dB HL or a speech signal at 50 dB HL. If this were the case, at 1000 Hz, the 60 dB setting on the masking dial would have an EM of 45 dB (i.e., 45 dB EM); for speech, it would be 50 dB EM.

Clinicians should never assume that the masking dial settings on audiometers are calibrated in dB EM. Before masking is used with any audiometer, the effective masking levels of the masking signals must be measured. Measuring EM is also necessary when audiometers are modified as a result of calibration, especially when earphones or loudspeakers are replaced. The procedure for determining the effective masking level of masking signals will be discussed later in this chapter.

Clinical Masking

In routine audiometric testing, as shown in **Fig. 13–1A**, acoustic signals delivered to one ear (the TE) can cross over

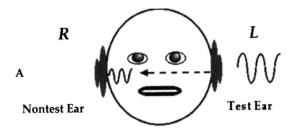

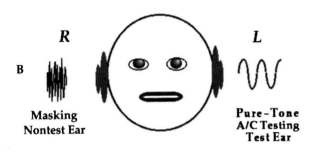

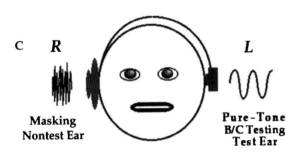

Figure 13–1 In routine audiometric masking, **(A)** a signal delivered to the (left) test ear (TE) will cross over to the nontest ear (NTE) if presented at an intensity greater than the interaural attenuation level plus the bone-conduction (B/C) threshold of the NTE; when needed, the masking signal is delivered to the (right) NTE. **(B)** For air-conduction (A/C) testing, an earphone is placed over the (left) TE, and masking is applied to the (right) NTE through an earphone; **(C)** for bone-conduction testing with mastoid placement, the bone oscillator is placed on the mastoid of the (left) TE, and masking is applied to the (right) NTE through an earphone.

to the NTE. When needed, the masking signal would be introduced into the contralateral ear, or NTE. **Figures 13–1B** and **C** show how masking is applied during air conduction (A/C) and bone conduction (B/C) testing, respectively. **Figure 13–1B** shows an A/C signal being presented to the patient's left (TE) ear and a masking signal delivered to the patient's right (NTE) ear. In **Fig. 13–1C**, a B/C signal is being presented using left mastoid placement of the B/C oscillator, and masking is being delivered to the right ear using a standard supra-aural earphone. When applying masking during B/C testing, the earphone on the nonmasked (TE) ear is placed anterior to the pinna. That is, during B/C testing, the TE is unoccluded, and the masked ear (NTE) is occluded.

B/C thresholds obtained in the unoccluded condition are referred to as relative B/C, whereas B/C thresholds in the occluded condition are absolute B/C. Low-frequency differences between relative and absolute B/C thresholds result from reduction of background noise, changes in physiological noise, and several other factors. As a result, absolute B/C thresholds require less energy than relative B/C thresholds. B/C calibration procedures are based on relative (unoccluded) thresholds. Whenever the ear is occluded with an earphone during masking procedures for B/C testing, it is necessary to account for this difference by taking into account the occlusion effect. The occlusion effect is discussed in more detail later.

Central Masking

It has long been recognized that even with small to moderate amounts of masking noise in the NTE, thresholds of the TE shift by as much as 5 to 7 dB (Wegel and Lane, 1924). The term *central masking* is used to explain this phenomenon and is defined as a threshold shift in the TE resulting from the introduction of a masking signal into the NTE that is not due to crossover (Wegel and Lane, 1924).

Central masking results from an inhibitory response within the central nervous system, behaviorally measured as small threshold shifts in the presence of masking noises (Liden et al, 1959). As a result, the signal intensity level must be increased to compensate for the attenuation effect from the neural activity. Both pure-tone and speech thresholds are affected similarly by the central masking phenomenon (Dirks and Malmquist, 1964; Martin and DiGiovanni, 1979; Studebaker, 1962).

Although the presence of central masking is unequivocal and averages ~5 dB, studies have shown variability in the magnitude of the central masking effect. **Table 13–1** provides data showing the central masking effect for pure-tone A/C and B/C stimuli for the frequencies 500 through 4000 Hz presented between 20 and 80 dB HL. As shown, the range is from 0.2 to 10.6 dB, with an overall average of 3.5 dB and 4.2 dB for A/C and B/C stimuli, respectively. On the basis of data from Dirks and Malmquist (1964), as well as data from other studies (Martin, 1966; Studebaker, 1962), the average

Table 13–1 Central Masking Effect for Pure-Tone Air-Conduction and Bone-Conduction Stimuli between 500 and 4000 Hz Presented at 20 to 80 dB HL

dB	Pure-Tone Air Conduction				Pure-Tone (Mastoid) Bone Conduction			
	500	1000	4000	Mean	500	1000	4000	Mean
20	0.2	1.2	0.6	0.7	0.5	0.9	0.6	0.7
40	1.8	3.0	2.2	2.3	2.9	4.5	1.6	3.0
60	3.6	4.5	3.1	3.7	5.0	5.9	2.1	4.3
80	7.2	8.8	6.2	7.4	7.8	10.6	7.3	8.6
Mean				3.5				4.2

HL, hearing level.

Source: From Dirks, D., & Malmquist, C. (1964). Changes in bone conducted thresholds produced by masking in the non-test ear. Journal of Speech and Hearing Research, 50, 271–278.

threshold shift from central masking has been estimated as 5 dB for pure-tone A/C, B/C, and A/C speech testing.

Some debate the universal recommendation for a central masking correction applied during testing. It is argued, for example, that the general effect is ~5 dB, which would be considered well within test–retest tolerance for threshold measures. In addition, some clinicians find it difficult to recommend an exact correction simply because of the variability found by researchers. For these reasons, some do not correct for central masking during threshold testing. However, Martin (1966) suggests that compensation for central masking is wholly appropriate when testing suprathreshold speech recognition. As such, the presentation level (PL) would be set 5 dB greater than customary to account for the central masking effect. As with threshold measures, some clinicians believe that the 5 dB central masking effect is within test–retest tolerance and therefore do not include a correction factor for suprathreshold speech recognition testing.

♦ The Need for Masking

As stated previously, crossover occurs when the signal presented to one ear travels across the skull and stimulates the NTE. Crossover is encountered in routine testing with patients having unilateral or significant asymmetrical hearing loss, and the test signal must be presented at levels of 45 to 65 dB above the better ear. It is when patients with better hearing sensitivity in one ear are tested that masking is needed most. Crossover results when test signals "leak out" around the earphone cushions and travel around the head to the NTE or through the skull to the NTE (Chaiklin, 1967; Martin and Blosser, 1970).

A shadow curve may result when masking is not used and crossover occurs. Shadow curves are seen when thresholds from the ear with the greater amount of hearing loss mimic thresholds from the normal, or better-hearing, ear. **Figure 13–2** is an example of a shadow curve that would result from a patient with a mild to moderate right ear high-frequency sensorineural hearing loss and no hearing (a profound sensorineural hearing loss) in the left ear. As shown, right ear thresholds are consistent with a mild to moderate high-frequency sensorineural hearing loss, but thresholds from the left ear reveal a moderate to severe mixed hearing loss. For this audiogram, unmasked left ear A/C thresholds are from 50 to 65 dB poorer than those for the right ear. Because of crossover, A/C thresholds for the left ear are "shadowing," or mimicking, the right ear by 50 to 65 dB. Note that the pattern of the left ear unmasked B/C thresholds is nearly identical to that for the right ear.

Figure 13–2 provides clear evidence for the need to mask in audiometric testing. Unmasked A/C and B/C thresholds from the left ear are highly inaccurate. The spurious finding of a conductive component in the left ear suggested medical treatment, when, in fact, a profound loss is present in the left ear. With the application of appropriate masking, the profound sensorineural loss in the left ear would be properly identified.

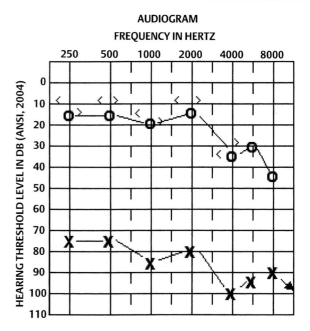

AUDIOGRAM

Figure 13–2 Example of a shadow curve. Note that the thresholds of the left ear are mimicking the bone-conduction thresholds of the right ear at a level equal to 60 to 65 dB, which is the average interaural attenuation level. Data from American National Standards Institute (ANSI). (2004). American national specifications for audiometers (ANSI S3.6). New York: ANSI.

♦ Considerations in Clinical Masking

Two basic considerations in clinical masking are interaural attenuation for A/C and B/C stimuli and the occlusion effect.

Interaural Attenuation

Attenuation of acoustic signals refers to the reduction or weakening of the force or value of energy (intensity) transmitted within some medium. As such, interaural attenuation is the amount of energy lost during the transmission of sound by A/C or B/C across or through the skull to the contralateral ear. Interaural attenuation is measured as a level difference (in decibels) in the signal between ears. For example, if a pure-tone signal is presented through a supra-aural earphone at an intensity of 95 dB HL to the right TE, and 45 dB HL reaches the cochlea of the left NTE, the interaural attenuation would be 50 dB (95 – 45 dB). High interaural attenuation levels are desirable, because the possibility for crossover is reduced. Interaural attenuation values are significantly different for A/C and B/C stimuli.

Air-Conduction Interaural Attenuation

Interaural attenuation during A/C testing varies according to three factors: subject variability, frequency spectrum of the test signal, and earphone transducer type. Subject variability should not be surprising because it is known that interaural attenuation increases as the area of head exposed to the sound waves decreases (Zwislocki, 1953). The amount of

Table 13–2 Mean and Ranges of Interaural Attenuation Values for Pure-Tone Air-Conduction Signals Using Standard Supra-aural Earphones (in dB)

Study	Transducer		250	500	1000	2000	3000	4000	6000	8000	Mean
			Frequency (Hz)								
Chaiklin (1967)	TDH-39	Mean	51	59	69	61	68	70	65	57	62.5
		Range	44–58	54–65	57–66	55–72	56–72	61–85	56–76	51–69	
Coles and Priede (1970)	NA	Mean	61	63	63	63		68			63.6
		Range	50–80	45–80	40–80	45–75		50–85			
Killion et al (1985)	TDH-39	Mean	50	60	60	60	60	65			59.1
		Range	45–65	52–65	52–65	50–68	50–68	52–74			
Liden et al (1959)	NA	Mean	58	60	57	60		61		63	59.2
		Range	45–75	50–70	45–70	45–75		45–75		45–80	
Sklare and Denenberg (1987)	TDH-49	Mean	54	59	62	58	57	65	65		60.0
		Range	45–60	45–75	60–65	45–70	45–70	60–75	50–80		
Zwislocki (1953)	NA	Mean	45	50	55	60		65			55.0
	Overall Mean		55	59	61	60	62	66	65	60	

NA, not reported.

sound vibration ultimately transmitted to the cochlea depends on individual skull properties, including thickness, density, and other such physical features. In addition to physical skull variations, there is also the ever-present test–retest variability naturally occurring in individual subjects.

Table 13–2 lists means and ranges of interaural attenuation values for pure-tone A/C stimuli between 250 and 8000 Hz using standard supra-aural earphones. As shown, the mean values for air-conducted interaural attenuation values are from 45 to 70 dB at octave frequencies from 250 to 8000 Hz, with a range of 40 to 80 dB. To prevent the possibility of crossover contaminating test results and in recognition of the large intersubject variability, the recommended minimal interaural attenuation value for masking during A/C testing is 40 dB (American Speech-Language-Hearing Association [ASHA], 1978; Martin, 1994; Studebaker, 1967). With the conservative interaural attenuation value, the possibility of not masking will be reduced or eliminated when it is called for. However, it should be realized that basing the need for masking during A/C testing on the minimal interaural attenuation value of 40 dB presents the likelihood of applying masking during clinical testing, when, in fact, it may not be needed.

Pearl

- The need for masking for A/C testing is based on the minimum interaural attenuation level for A/C of 40 dB with supra-aural earphones and 50 dB with insert earphones. However, it should be realized that the average interaural attenuation level for A/C is 60 to 65 dB with supra-aural earphones and 50 dB with insert earphones. This conservative approach will result in masking being used when it may not be needed. The application of this rule also implies that clinicians will never fail to use masking when it is needed.

Until recently, virtually all studies on interaural attenuation were performed using supra-aural earphones, because supra-aural earphones have been the standard for audiometric testing. However, the use of insert earphones for routine audiological testing is becoming more commonplace (see Chapter 12). One of the primary advantages of insert earphones related to clinical masking is that they provide increased interaural attenuation. **Table 13–3** displays data showing mean interaural attenuation values for insert earphones for pure tones from 250 to 6000 Hz. As indicated, the range is from 70 to 100 dB, with mean values across frequencies of 80 to 82 dB. The increased interaural attenuation for insert earphones will benefit clinicians during masking procedures. If insert earphones are not used in routine testing, they should be available to clinicians for difficult masking situations, such as the masking dilemma, which is described later.

Bone-Conduction Interaural Attenuation

Interaural attenuation for B/C stimuli is dramatically less than A/C stimuli because both cochleas are encased within each temporal bone of the same skull. Once the skull is set into vibration, both cochleas are stimulated. The B/C oscillator may

Table 13–3 Mean Interaural Attenuation for Insert Earphones for Pure-Tone Stimuli between 250 and 6000 Hz (in dB)

Frequency Study	250	500	1000	2000	3000	4000	6000	Mean
Killion et al. (1985)	95	85	70	75	80			81
Konig (1962)	95	90	83	75	80	82	70	82
Sklare and Denenberg (1987)	100	94+	81	71	69	77	75+	81+

be placed directly on one mastoid process during unmasked B/C testing, but it should not be assumed that the response originates from the TE or even from one ear. As a result, clinicians cannot be certain which cochlea is being tested during unmasked B/C audiometry. In B/C testing, the minimum interaural attenuation is conservatively defined as 0 dB, and crossover should always be considered as likely during unmasked B/C testing.

The Occlusion Effect

Covering (occluding) the ear by any means can lead to a significant enhancement in low-frequency B/C threshold sensitivity. This phenomenon is termed the *occlusion effect*. The occlusion effect is present at 1000 Hz or less and results from occluding the ear canal with an earphone, earplug, earmold, or any other object or substance. Although threshold sensitivity appears to improve during the occlusion effect, the hearing sensitivity of the cochlea does not change. Instead, the signal intensity received at the cochlea is increased. When the skull is set into vibration through osteotympanic bone-conducted sound transmission, sound waves are subsequently generated at the external ear canal and tympanic membrane. These sound waves reach the cochlea through the normal air-conducted route (Martin and Fagelson, 1995). Some radiated energy, especially low frequencies, will escape through the unoccluded external auditory meatus, but when the canal is occluded (as with a supra-aural earphone), low-frequency bone-conducted sound transmission is enhanced.

Individuals with sensorineural hearing loss or normal hearing are most likely to experience an occlusion effect, whereas those individuals with conductive hearing loss will not. This seeming lack of occlusion effect in patients having conductive hearing loss can be attributed to the occlusion effect resulting from middle ear pathology.

Table 13–4 shows the mean occlusion effect (in dB) from several studies for normal-hearing subjects. Occlusion effect

data shown in **Table 13–4** were derived by subtracting B/C thresholds obtained from occluded and unoccluded conditions.

Because the occlusion effect is implicated as influencing thresholds during B/C testing, it is advisable to keep the TE unoccluded, thereby covering the NTE with the earphone only when preparing for masking. However, an occlusion effect can also be found with the earphone placed over the NTE during masked B/C testing. Incremental masking levels, imprecise thresholds, or both could result if inadequate or no consideration is given to the occlusion effect.

♦ Types of Masking Noises

Effectiveness and efficiency of a masking signal depend almost entirely on the critical bandwidth. Critical bandwidth of a masking signal determines the masking efficiency or effectiveness of the signal. The goal is to mask test stimuli with a minimum amount of energy in the masking signal.

Fletcher (1940) was able to calculate a critical bandwidth to determine the necessary range of frequency components in the masker that would surround the test signal. His observations were that some outlying frequency components comprising the masker could be eliminated while still maintaining maximum masking efficiency. It was shortly thereafter that Hawkins and Stevens (1950) investigated dimensions of masking intensity level and the interaction with frequency band. They found that for a test signal to be at a just barely audible level, the overall energy of the masker's critical band had to be equal to the test signal energy. Moreover, they found that those frequencies at or near the test signal had the greatest masking effect. As a result, they concluded that masking effectiveness is decreased when using a broadband masking signal due to the presence of unnecessary masking energy. Masking noise effectiveness thus depends on the signal to be masked and the type of masking noise used.

The early diagnostic audiometers were equipped only with complex masking noise. Considered efficient for its time, the complex noise spectrum was made up of a fundamental signal at 120 Hz and all of the harmonics at multiples of the fundamental. Listeners could hear "beating" or pulsating sounds within the ear because of the discrete frequencies comprised within the signal. Complex noise provided inconsistent frequency and energy levels across frequency. Because of the restricted usefulness of complex noise, today's audiometers are not built with complex noise generators for use in masking.

Three types of masking noises are now available on most audiometers: broadband or white (thermal) noise, narrowband noise, and speech (spectrum) noise. Any of these noise signals can effectively mask a variety of test stimuli when presented at an appropriate intensity. However, to be most effective, a masking signal should be chosen with a

Table 13–4   Mean Occlusion Effect (in dB) for Normal-Hearing Subjects

Study	Frequency (Hz)				
	250	500	1000	2000	4000
Elpern and Naunton (1963)	30.0	20.0	10.0		
Goldstein and Hayes (1965)	12.2	13.1	4.9	0.0	0.0
Hodgson and Tillman (1966)	22.0	19.0	7.0	0.0	0.0
Dirks and Swindeman (1967)	23.7	19.3	7.5	−0.6	0.0
Martin et al (1974)	20.0	15.0	5.0	0.0	0.0
Berger and Kerivian (1983)	20.3	21.6	7.5	−1.3	0.0
Mean	21.3	18.0	6.9	−0.3	0.0
Recommended Occlusion Effect Values		20.0	15.0	5.0	

spectrum as close as possible to the test signal. A basic masking principle is that the most efficient masker produces the greatest threshold shift with the least amount of energy.

Descriptions of each type of masking noise used in audiometric testing follow. Typical spectral plots for these masking noises are illustrated in **Fig. 13–3A–C**.

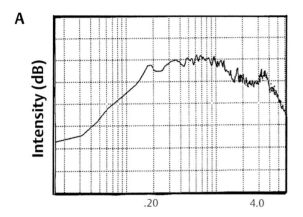

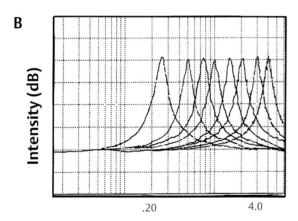

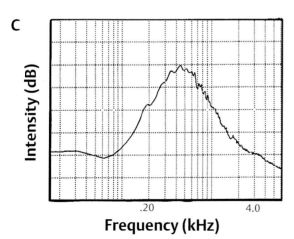

Figure 13–3 Types of masking noise used in audiometric testing. **(A)** Broadband or white (thermal) noise, **(B)** narrowband noise, and **(C)** speech noise.

Broadband or White (Thermal) Noise

Broadband and *white* (or *thermal*) *noise* are terms referring to masking signals having a wide band of frequencies within the range of 100 to 10,000 Hz at approximately equal intensities. However, as shown in **Fig. 13–3A**, the typical acoustic spectrum of white noise maintains a relatively flat frequency response only from 0.2 to 0.6 kHz, at which point the energy is dramatically diminished. For newer supra-aural transducers and insert earphones, the response can extend to 0.8 kHz. The sudden drop in acoustic energy results from the limited frequency response of the transducer; frequency response characteristics vary from transducer to transducer. Despite limited high-frequency response, white noise is still considered a reasonably efficient masker for both pure-tone and speech stimuli.

Narrowband Noise

Narrowband noise is a type of filtered white noise. That is, narrow band noise is a band pass–filtered white noise that allows for discrete shaping of the masking signal into defined bands. Specific noise bands are chosen during testing to contain only the frequencies surrounding the test signal to be masked. ANSI (2004) has provided the standard for the acceptable range of upper and lower cutoff frequencies for narrowband maskers for each test frequency. Filters are adjusted so that the noise band is centered on the same frequency as the pure-tone test signal. As a result, narrowband noises are described by each center frequency; if the narrowband noise is centered at 1000 Hz, it would be defined as a 1000 Hz narrowband noise.

Figure 13–3B shows the acoustic spectrum for narrowband noise signals from 0.025 to 0.8 kHz. This figure clearly illustrates how the center frequency of a narrowband masking signal is changed from low to high frequencies. During pure-tone testing, the center frequency of the masking signal is adjusted to correspond to the pure-tone signal being tested. The use of narrowband noise during pure-tone testing increases the efficiency of the masking signal, thereby requiring less energy to mask the test signal effectively. The increased effectiveness of narrowband noises reduces the necessary energy required to mask the NTE, which increases patient comfort during the masking procedure.

Speech Noise

Speech noise is a type of narrow-band masking signal that has center frequencies within the speech range. Because the primary acoustic energy responsible for speech intelligibility is in the 300 to 3000 Hz range, speech noise is shaped to correspond to this range (**Fig. 13–3C**).

◆ Calibrating Masking Signals

One might incorrectly assume that the calibration reference of the relative average hearing level (i.e., dB HL) used with pure-tone signals is equivalent for masking signals. However, it is not. A more meaningful reference for the effect a masking stimulus will have on a test signal is the EM. ANSI (2004) defines the EM level of a masking signal as the intensity of the masking required to shift the threshold of a test signal during simultaneous presentation with 50% probability of detection. ANSI (2004) also provides the necessary parameters for narrowband noise signals to establish EMs between 125 and 16,000 Hz. As shown in **Table 13–5**, specific critical bandwidths are designated with a lower and upper cutoff frequency for each center frequency specified. In addition, correction factors to add to the reference equivalent threshold sound pressure levels are included to establish EMs for each narrowband noise masking signal. Of course, to establish physical measures of EMs would require sophisticated equipment, including a precision sound level meter, spectral analyzer, and an acoustic coupler, artificial ear, ear simulator, or mechanical coupler.

For most clinicians, it is not feasible to purchase and maintain the necessary calibration equipment to establish EMs for masking signals. Fortunately, most audiometers manufactured within the past few years have masking signals calibrated in EM. However, variability in audiometer masking signals makes it important to verify the EM of masking signals before they are used. The responsibility of verifying and monitoring masking stimuli used during testing lies with the clinician. An alternative to physical calibration of EM is the biological method.

Biological Method of Calibrating Effective Masking Levels

Calibrating EMs with the biological method relies on responses from human ears. Because the biological method is relatively simple to perform, it is commonly used by most clinicians. With the biological method, EMs for normal-hearing subjects are established by calculating the amount (in dB) that a masking signal is able to shift threshold for a test signal, either pure tones or speech, presented at a known hearing level. To determine the EM of a masking signal, the test signal is presented simultaneously with the masking signal through the same (ipsilateral) earphone. The

Table 13–5 Narrowband Masking Noise Calibration Standards with Bandwidths, Center Frequencies, and Corrections to Determine Reference Test Sound Pressure Level (in dB)

Center Frequency (Hz)	Low Cutoff Frequency Correction (Hz)		Upper Cutoff Frequency Correction (Hz)		Critical Bandwidth to RETSP (Hz)	One-Third Octave (dB)*	One-Half Octave (dB)*
	Minimum	Maximum	Minimum	Maximum			
125	105	111	140	149	100	4	4
160	136	143	180	190	100	4	4
200	168	178	224	238	105	4	4
250	210	223	281	297	105	4	4
315	265	281	354	375	105	4	4
400	336	356	449	476	110	4	5
500	420	445	561	595	115	4	6
630	530	561	707	749	125	5	6
750	631	668	842	892	135	5	7
800	673	713	898	951	140	5	7
1000	841	891	1120	1190	160	6	7
1250	1050	1110	1400	1490	190	6	8
1500	1260	1340	1680	1780	225	6	8
1600	1350	1430	1800	1900	240	6	8
2000	1680	1780	2240	2380	300	6	8
2500	2100	2230	2810	2970	385	6	8
3000	2520	2670	3370	3570	480	6	7
3150	2650	2810	3540	3750	510	6	7
4000	3360	3560	4490	4760	685	5	7
5000	4200	4450	5610	5950	915	5	7
6000	5050	5350	6730	7140	1150	5	7
6300	5800	5610	7070	7400	1250	5	6
8000	6730	7130	8980	9510	1700	5	6
9000	7570	8020	10,100	10,700			
10,000	8410	8910	11,220	11,890			
11,200	9420	9980	12,570	13,320			
12,500	10,510	11,140	14,030	14,870			
14,000	11,770	12,470	15,710	16,650			
16,000	13,450	14,250	17,960	19,030			

*Reference effective masking levels are calculated by adding the appropriate values to the reference equivalent threshold sound pressure levels (RETSPLs) at each frequency.

Data from American National Standards Institute. (2004). Specifications for audiometers (ANSI S3.6). New York: Author.

Source: Reprinted with permission from the Acoustical Society of America.

Table 13–6   Demonstration of the Procedure for Calibration of Effective Masking Levels for Pure Tones at 500 and 2000 Hz and for Speech Stimuli

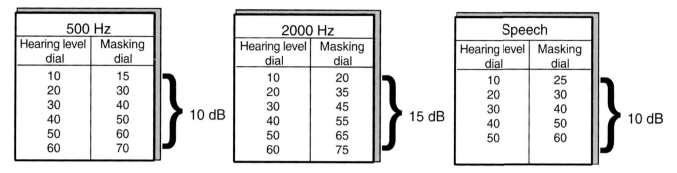

500 Hz	
Hearing level dial	Masking dial
10	15
20	30
30	40
40	50
50	60
60	70

} 10 dB

2000 Hz	
Hearing level dial	Masking dial
10	20
20	35
30	45
40	55
50	65
60	75

} 15 dB

Speech	
Hearing level dial	Masking dial
10	25
20	30
30	40
40	50
50	60

} 10 dB

Correction Factors

Frequency	250	500	1000	2000	3000	4000	6000	Speech
CF		10		15				10

EM of a masking signal is established at the intensity that the test signal is just barely masked by the masking noise. Threshold shifts are recorded for each test signal at several intensities (e.g., 10, 20, and 30 dB HL) until the threshold shifts are linear. The difference between the masker dial setting and the test signal HL level is noted as a correction factor (CF), if needed, to establish the EM. This procedure is completed with three to five subjects. Results are averaged and made available for reference during testing, usually by posting them on the front of the audiometer.

Table 13–6 provides an example of results obtained with the biological method using three types of test stimuli: pure tones at 500 Hz, pure tones at 2000 Hz, and speech. Taking 500 Hz as an example, when the test signal was presented at 10 dB HL, a masking dial level of 15 dB was required to just barely mask the signal in the same earphone. At 20 dB HL, the masking dial level required to mask the 500 Hz signal was 30 dB. Above 20 dB HL, a linear relationship was found between the increases in the amount of test signal and the amount of masking dial increase necessary to mask the test signal. That is, as the test signal was increased in 10 dB steps, the required masking increases were the same. In this case, a correction factor of 10 dB was calculated at 500 Hz. Using this procedure at 2000 Hz and with speech, CFs of 15 dB and 10 dB were calculated for this audiometer, respectively. All additional test signals (250, 500, 750, 2000, 3000, 4000, 6000, and 8000 Hz and speech) would be evaluated in a similar manner, and mean CFs would be posted on the audiometer.

Speech noise is calibrated with reference to the speech recognition thresholds (SRTs). Therefore, EM for speech noise can be calibrated with speech stimuli, as described previously, or it can be estimated by the use of the average EM with speech noise at 500, 1000, and 2000 Hz. Calibration of spondee masking signals would assume that average masked thresholds of three pure tones (500, 1000, and 2000 Hz) are equivalent to the SRT. Research has shown

that when these three pure tones are combined, they best reflect major speech components (Sanders and Rintelmann, 1964). As a result, mean difference values for the average of 500, 1000, and 2000 Hz pure tones can be used for the calibration reference for spondees.

An alternative biological method, the minimum EM level method (MEML), bases mean values on subjects with hearing impairment (Veniar, 1965). The MEML procedure assumes that ears with pathological conditions respond differently to masking than normal ears. Both test and masking signals are presented as in the biological method for pure tones. However, the noise that just barely masks the pure tone in these hearing-impaired subjects is defined as 0 dB MEML.

Certainly, the relative simplicity of obtaining EM with human subjects is an attractive alternative to other methods requiring specialized, and sometimes costly, equipment. However, as demonstrated in **Table 13–6**, the biological method can be time consuming because it requires evaluating several volunteers to implement the calibration procedure. Some degree of inter- and intrasubject variability known to occur is tolerated while establishing threshold, but other threshold variations intrinsically occur as a function of the number of subjects tested. Intersubject threshold variability becomes more pronounced when the subject base is small or unskilled listeners are used. Skilled listeners are preferred because they have less variability in their responses.

◆ The Application of Clinical Masking

Several factors have to be considered when the decision is made to mask during the audiometric evaluation. To this point, underlying theories and principles to conduct audiometric masking have been covered. Because each mode of threshold testing (i.e., A/C, B/C, SRTs, and word recognition testing) has been dealt with individually, the application of masking procedures will be considered for each separate test procedure. During routine audiometric testing the first question to ask is, When is masking needed? Once it has been determined that masking is needed, it becomes necessary to calculate the amount of masking required.

◆ When Is Masking Needed?

> **Pearl**
>
> - Masking principles are based on the minimum interaural attenuation levels of 40 and 50 dB for supra-aural and insert earphones, respectively, for A/C and 0 dB for B/C. Consequently, when these minimum levels are applied, masking will always be used whenever the possibility of crossover is present. Because of the conservative nature of masking rules, strict adherence to them will result in the use of masking, when, in fact, masking may not be necessary.

Through the years clinical practice has established basic rules that guide clinicians in making decisions regarding the application of clinical masking. The following describes masking rules for the essential test battery, including pure-tone A/C, pure-tone B/C, SRT, and word recognition testing.

Pure-Tone Air-Conduction Testing

In pure-tone A/C testing, the determination of when to mask is based on the minimum interaural attenuation for A/C signals. Recall that for supra-aural earphones, the average interaural attenuation level for pure tones is 55 to 65 dB. However, the minimum interaural attenuation level for pure-tone A/C signals with standard supra-aural earphones is 40 dB (see **Table 13–2**). Therefore, to prevent the possibility of crossover during pure-tone A/C testing, masking is needed when the pure-tone A/C threshold of the TE exceeds the pure-tone B/C threshold of the NTE by 40 dB or more. This is a conservative rule in most instances, because crossover will not occur until the difference between the two ears is 55 to 65 dB. However, using 40 dB as the criterion to determine the need for masking will ensure that masking will be employed, especially for those few patients with small interaural attenuation levels. With this conservative rule, it is possible that masking will be used when, in fact, it is not necessary. The use of masking, though, should not affect test results, and it is better to err by masking unnecessarily than by failing to mask when masking is necessary.

Comparing the unmasked pure-tone A/C threshold of the TE to the unmasked pure-tone B/C threshold of the NTE is always the fundamental procedure followed to determine the need for masking in pure-tone A/C testing. The principle underlying the fundamental rule is simply that the pure-tone A/C signal of the TE will cross over to the pure-tone B/C sensitivity of the NTE.

> **Pearl**
>
> - A corollary to the basic rule of when to use masking for pure-tone A/C testing is as follows: masking is needed when the pure-tone A/C threshold of the TE exceeds the pure-tone A/C threshold of the NTE by 40 dB or more.

Although the need for masking in pure-tone A/C testing is based on a comparison of unmasked A/C thresholds of the TE to the B/C sensitivity of the NTE, a corollary to the rule allows for a shortcut in testing. That is, the need for masking can be determined by comparing the pure-tone A/C thresholds for each ear. When there is a difference of 40 dB or more between the two pure-tone A/C thresholds, masking is needed to obtain the threshold of the poorer ear. This corollary applies to A/C testing because B/C thresholds cannot be poorer than A/C thresholds. As a result, when the two A/C thresholds differ by 40 dB or more, the A/C threshold of the poorer ear and the B/C threshold of the better ear likewise will differ by 40 dB or more.

Clinicians must be acutely aware of the fact that it is not possible to assess the need for masking by comparing only the A/C thresholds of the two ears. It is only when thresholds differ by 40 dB or more that the need for masking is inadvertently made known. The ability to determine the need for masking when the two A/C thresholds differ by 40 dB or more is a clinical shortcut that may save time during routine testing. It may be the case during the initial portion of the audiological evaluation that only A/C thresholds are available. In such instances the need for masking can be established when the thresholds from the two ears differ by 40 dB or more.

Figure 13–4A provides an example of when to mask for pure-tone A/C testing; for this example, the masking signal from the audiometer calibrated in **Table 13–6** is used. As shown in **Fig. 13–4A,** the patient's unmasked A/C and B/C thresholds at 1000 Hz are both 10 dB HL for the right ear; for the left ear, pure-tone A/C and B/C thresholds are 60 and 10 dB HL, respectively. It is possible that the left ear A/C threshold (as well as the left ear B/C threshold; see the following discussion) could be a result of crossover because a difference of 50 dB (60–10 dB) exists between the A/C threshold of the left ear and the B/C threshold of the right ear. For this patient, masking would be needed when testing the left ear A/C threshold. That is, masking would be introduced into the right ear while obtaining the threshold at 1000 Hz for the left ear.

The masking corollary for air-conduction testing also applies to this example. Because the pure-tone A/C threshold of the left ear (60 dB HL) differs from the pure-tone A/C of the right ear (10 dB) by 40 dB or more (60–5 dB HL = 55 dB),

A

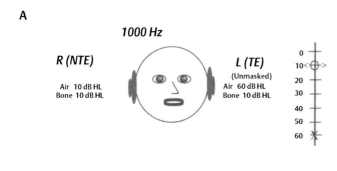

B

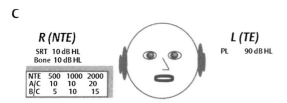

C

Figure 13–4 Audiometric data showing when to mask for **(A)** pure-tone air- (A/C) and bone-conduction (B/C) testing, **(B)** speech recognition threshold (SRT) testing, and **(C)** word recognition testing. HL, hearing level; NTE, nontest ear; PL, presentation level; TE, test ear.

masking would be needed when testing the left ear threshold. This corollary could be applied if only A/C thresholds were available during the test session.

Pure-Tone Bone-Conduction Testing

Pearl

- Masking is needed for pure-tone B/C testing when the B/C threshold differs from the A/C threshold of the same ear by more than 10 dB.

When deciding whether crossover has occurred during pure-tone B/C testing, unmasked A/C thresholds of the TE are compared with unmasked B/C thresholds of the same ear; masking is needed if the difference is greater than 10 dB. That is, masking is needed whenever unmasked results indicate the presence of a conductive component greater than 10 dB.

Recall that the minimum interaural attenuation for B/C stimuli is 0 dB. Assuming that A/C and B/C threshold sensitivity is the same (± 5–10 dB) for each ear, B/C thresholds for each ear will be within 10 dB. However, as the degree of B/C threshold sensitivity of the TE differs from the threshold sensitivity of the NTE, crossover becomes more and more a possibility. When there is a difference in sensorineural sensitivity between the two ears of more than 10 dB, B/C stimuli presented to the poorer-hearing ear will cross over to the better-hearing ear before they are perceived by the ear with poorer hearing. In fact, when the threshold sensitivity of the NTE is better than the TE by 15 dB or more, crossover to the TE is likely.

Special Consideration

- When masking for bone conduction, it is important to make sure that the test ear remains unoccluded by placing the supra-aural earphone off the pinna or by removing the insert earphone from the ear canal. Without this step, thresholds may be influenced by the occlusion effect.

Figure 13–4A provides an example of when masking is needed for pure-tone B/C testing. As shown in this figure, when comparing the unmasked A/C threshold of the left ear (60 dB HL) to the unmasked B/C threshold of the left ear (10 dB HL), the threshold difference (i.e., air–bone gap [ABG]) is 50 dB. The criterion of an ABG of greater than 10 dB is not only met but also exceeded by 40 dB, suggesting that crossover is likely. For this example, it is obvious that crossover affects the test results. With this patient, masking would be introduced into the right ear when testing the left ear B/C threshold at 1000 Hz.

Speech Recognition Threshold Testing

Pearl

- Masking is needed for SRT testing when the PL in the TE exceeds the best B/C threshold in any of the speech frequencies (500, 1000, or 2000 Hz) by 45 dB or more.

Similar to pure-tone A/C and B/C testing, crossover is possible when speech is used as the stimulus. The air-conduction interaural attenuation level for spondees varies between 45 and 55 dB. On the basis of this, the minimum criterion on which to base the need for masking has been established as 45 dB (Konkle and Berry, 1983). As a result, the decision to mask the NTE when obtaining the SRT in the TE is based on a 45 dB difference between the PL in the TE and the best B/C threshold in the speech range (500, 1000, and 2000 Hz) for the NTE. In practice, clinicians must consider the unmasked PL of the SRT in the TE and compare it with the B/C thresholds of the NTE at 500, 1000, and 2000 Hz. If any of the comparisons reveal a difference of 45 dB or greater, masking would be introduced into the NTE, and a masked SRT would be obtained.

Pearl

- A corollary to the basic rule of when to mask for the SRT is that the need for masking exists when the SRT of the TE exceeds the SRT of the NTE by 45 dB or more.

A masking corollary for SRT testing is that masking is needed whenever a 45 dB or more difference exists between the SRT of the TE and the NTE. This corollary is similar to the 40 dB rule used to determine the need for masking in pure-tone A/C threshold testing. As with pure-tone testing, this corollary applies to SRT testing because B/C thresholds cannot be poorer than A/C thresholds. Therefore, when the two SRTs differ by 45 dB or more, the difference between the A/C threshold of the ear with the greater hearing loss (the TE) and the best B/C threshold in the speech frequencies (500, 1000, and 2000 Hz) in the NTE must be 45 dB or more. This corollary has a clear practical application. Some clinicians obtain SRTs for each ear before B/C threshold testing. As a result, if the two SRTs are found to differ by 45 dB or more, the need for masking would be evident without examining B/C threshold test results. An important point is that if the two SRTs do not differ by 45 dB or more, it is not possible to conclude that masking may or may not be needed; the corollary applies only if the SRTs, in fact, differ by 45 dB or more.

Figure 13–4B provides an example of test results requiring masking for SRT testing. In this case, an unmasked SRT of 60 dB is obtained for the left TE, and pure-tone B/C thresholds are 5, 10, and 15 dB for the right NTE at 500, 1000, and 2000 Hz, respectively. Because the 60 dB unmasked SRT in the left ear differs from the best B/C threshold of 5 dB at 500 Hz for the right ear by 55 dB, masking would be required to obtain the SRT in the left ear.

The SRT masking corollary also applies to the data in **Fig. 13–4B**. Note that the unmasked SRT in the left ear differs from the SRT of the right ear by 50 dB. Although the B/C thresholds are also available in **Fig. 13–4B**, it is apparent that masking would be necessary before B/C testing because the two SRTs differ by more than 45 dB.

Word Recognition Testing

Pearl

- Masking is needed for word recognition testing when the PL in the TE exceeds the best B/C threshold in any of the speech frequencies (500, 1000, or 2000 Hz) by 35 dB or more.

Because word recognition testing is undertaken at suprathreshold PLs, there is an increased risk for crossover during word recognition testing. In fact, masking is used during word recognition testing more often than not.

Interaural attenuation levels for monosyllabic words have been reported between 35 and 50 dB. On the basis of these data, the criterion on which masking is based for word recognition testing dB is 35 dB (Konkle and Berry, 1983). To determine the need for masking during testing, clinicians would compare the PL in the TE to the best B/C thresholds in the speech range for the NTE (500, 1000, and 2000 Hz). Masking would be needed if the difference at any one frequency is 35 dB or greater.

Pearl

- A corollary to the basic rule of when to mask for word recognition testing is that the need for masking exists when the PL in the TE exceeds the SRT in the NTE by 35 dB or more.

As with other masking rules, a word recognition corollary exists: masking is needed when the PL in the TE exceeds the SRT in the NTE by 35 dB or more. Once again, this corollary applies because B/C thresholds cannot exceed A/C thresholds, which implies that a 35 dB difference exists between the PL in the TE and the best B/C threshold in the NTE at 500, 1000, and 2000 Hz.

Figure 13–4C provides an example of when masking would be needed for word recognition testing. As shown in this example, a PL of 90 dB HL was chosen. A 90 dB HL presentation level exceeds the best B/C threshold of the NTE by 85 dB, which is a clear indicator for masking. In addition, the PL exceeds the SRT of the NTE by 80 dB HL, also indicating the need for masking. For this patient, the right NTE ear would receive the masking signal when testing word recognition in the left TE.

◆ How Much Masking Is Needed?

General Principles

Over the years, psychoacoustic masking procedures have been developed to address the effects of threshold shifts in the TE resulting from various masking levels in the NTE. The plateau method, described by Hood (1960), provides clear definitions of three important masking levels (**Fig. 13–5**): the minimum amount of masking needed to prevent the possibility of crossover, minimum necessary masking; the range of acceptable effective masking levels in the NTE, plateau; and the point at which any additional masking is too much, or the maximum permissible masking. Any masking that is less than the minimum necessary masking is considered undermasking; masking greater than the maximum permissible is referred to as overmasking. Because of their importance in determining the amount of masking to be used, undermasking, the plateau, and overmasking are discussed in more detail in the following sections.

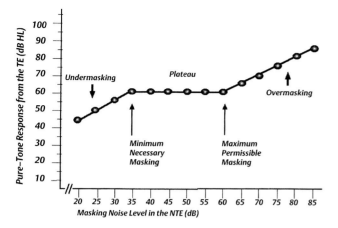

Figure 13–5 Example of the masking plateau showing undermasking, minimum necessary masking, the plateau, maximum permissible masking, and overmasking. HL, hearing level; NTE, nontest ear; TE, test ear.

Undermasking

Considerable variation in terminology for the minimum or sufficient masking levels exists. Examples are *minimum effective masking level* (Liden et al, 1959), *minimum effective masking* (Lloyd and Kaplan, 1978), and *minimum masking level* (Studebaker, 1962). All terms refer to the minimum amount of masking in the NTE that would prevent the possibility of crossover occurring in the TE, or the minimum necessary masking. Any intensity less than the minimum necessary masking level is considered undermasking.

When undermasking occurs, a danger exists that the test signal will still be perceived in the NTE because of an insufficient amount of masking noise presented to the NTE. This situation may inadvertently occur because of equipment calibration errors resulting from an underestimation of the EM or because clinician calculation error resulted in underestimation of the potential interaural attenuation. Obviously, either of these errors can render invalid audiological results.

An undermasking situation will continue to occur during testing as long as it is possible for test stimuli to be perceived in the NTE. For example, **Fig. 13–5** shows a case where masking noise presented below 35 dB in the NTE is at a level that undermasking occurs. For this masking situation, a level of at least 35 dB is required to reach the plateau.

The Plateau

The masking plateau is the intensity range between the minimum necessary masking level and the maximum permissible masking level. The plateau begins at the intensity at which the threshold in the TE remains stable when the masking noise in the NTE is increased. This is the point at which the minimum necessary masking level has been reached. Above this level, the threshold in the TE begins to increase linearly when the intensity of the

masking noise in the NTE is increased and the maximum permissible masking level has been reached. The masking plateau is the range of intensities at which effective masking of the NTE can be achieved while obtaining valid thresholds in the TE.

Figure 13–5 provides data from a hypothetical case where the width of the masking plateau is 25 dB (35–60 dB). As indicated in this figure, introducing less than 35 dB into the NTE would be undermasking, and introducing more than 60 dB would be overmasking. Intensities between 35 and 60 dB would effectively mask the NTE ear without affecting the TE threshold; this range of intensities is the patient's masking plateau. Establishing the plateau during masked threshold assessment provides solid evidence of the TE's true masked response for the test signal.

Masking plateau width will vary from patient to patient. The primary determining factor is the patient's interaural attenuation level. That is, the width of the plateau cannot exceed the magnitude of the interaural attenuation for each patient. From **Table 13–2** it can be seen that the average interaural attenuation level for standard supra-aural earphones ranges from 55 to 65 dB, depending on the test frequency. These data imply that the average masking plateau will be within this range. However, during clinical testing, the interaural attenuation value for a given patient is not known; an assumption is made that it may be as little as 40 dB but will average between 55 and 65 dB.

Factors that can narrow the masking plateau for a given patient include improved interaural attenuation values, reduced A/C thresholds in the NTE (a conductive component), and an increased occlusion effect (Gelfand, 1997). In fact, masking situations exist in which no masking plateau is present. That is, the minimum necessary masking and the maximum permissible masking are the same, and obtaining a masked threshold is not possible. This situation presents a masking dilemma because the level required to just mask the threshold of the masked ear will result in overmasking. The masking dilemma is discussed in more detail later in the chapter.

As pointed out earlier in this chapter, the use of insert earphones has the advantage of increasing the interaural attenuation, from 55 to 65 dB to 69 to 100 dB. By increasing the interaural attenuation, the maximum width of the masking plateau is also increased.

Overmasking

Overmasking occurs when the masking noise in the NTE is at an intensity great enough to influence thresholds in the TE. **Figure 13–5** demonstrates the effects of overmasking. As shown, when the masking noise level in the NTE increases from 60 to 85 dB, the pure-tone threshold in the TE increases linearly. Clearly, beginning at the 65 dB masking noise level, crossover from the masked NTE ear to the TE causes poorer thresholds in the TE. Any time the masking noise level in the NTE is equal to or exceeds the interaural attenuation plus the B/C threshold of the TE, overmasking becomes a certainty (Martin, 1997).

◆ Specific Procedures

Pearl

- To be certain that patients are clear about their expected task, it should be pointed out that they will hear several noises; regardless of their "loudness," the patient's task is to continue to respond only to the very soft pure-tone (i.e., "note" or "beep") signals.

At this point, it should be clear that when the need for masking in the NTE exists, clinicians have a range of intensities at which the masking signal can be presented. The primary question, then, is at what intensity should masking begin, or for each masking situation, what is the starting level for masking?

Establishing the Starting Level

The minimum intensity necessary to mask the NTE has to be at the level that will just affect the threshold of the

NTE. This minimum intensity would be at an effective masking level equal to the threshold of the masked ear, or 0 dB effective level and, as described above, is referred to as the minimum necessary masking. The starting level for masking is set at an intensity slightly above the minimum necessary masking. As a safety factor, 10 to 15 dB is added to the minimum necessary masking to account for the normal threshold sensitivity variability. By adding the 10 to 15 dB safety factor, one ensures that the masking signal is at an effective level just above the threshold of the masked ear. During testing, the factors needed to calculate the starting level for pure-tone A/C testing are the threshold of the NTE (the masked ear) and the safety factor of 10 to 15 dB. In addition, unless the audiometer masking signals are calibrated in EM, a CF is included in the calculation. When masking is needed, the examiner begins by introducing the masked signal into the NTE at an effective level 10 or 15 dB above the threshold of the NTE. As described below, the patient's response to the masked signal presented at the starting level determines the procedures to be followed.

The same basic principle is followed for pure-tone B/C testing. However, because B/C threshold calibration is based

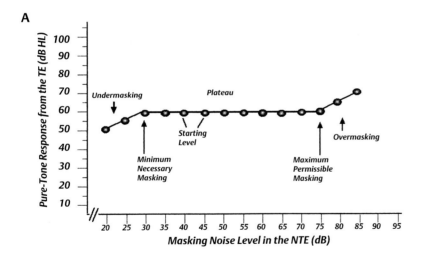

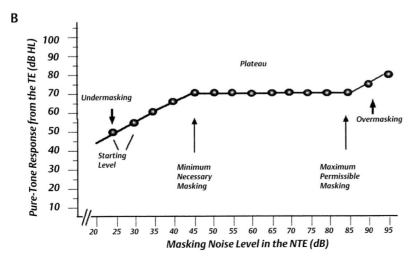

Figure 13–6 Examples of two possible outcomes when masking: **(A)** when the starting level exceeds the minimum necessary masking and is within the masking plateau, and **(B)** when the starting level is below the minimum necessary masking.

on unoccluded ears, and one ear is occluded with an ear-phone during B/C testing with masking, the occlusion effect is factored into the formula to determine the starting level for B/C testing.

Two possible outcomes exist once the starting level of masking is introduced into the NTE. The two are illustrated in **Fig. 13–6A** and **B**. First, it is possible that the unmasked threshold does not change significantly when the masking starting level is introduced into the NTE. This finding would indicate that the unmasked threshold was, in fact, not a re-sult of crossover (a "crossover threshold") or that the un-masked threshold was valid. In **Fig. 13–6A**, the starting level of masking was determined to be 40 to 45 dB. The 40 to 45 dB level was found to be greater than the intensity required for the minimum necessary masking and within the mask-ing plateau. In this case, the threshold of the TE did not in-crease when the starting level of masking was introduced into the NTE.

Another possibility is that the starting level chosen is in-adequate to prevent crossover. Stated differently, the possi-bility exists that the starting level is not within the masking plateau. **Figure 13–6B** shows that when a starting level of 25 to 30 dB was introduced into the NTE, it was necessary to continue increasing the masking intensity above the starting level to find the masking plateau. In this case, re-sponses from the TE shifted to 70 dB HL before the mini-mum necessary masking of 45 dB HL was achieved and the masking plateau was found.

Specific procedures to establish the starting levels and necessary follow-up protocols for each of the basic audio-logical tests are discussed in more detail later in the chapter.

Determining Masking Levels for Pure-Tone Air-Conduction Testing

Pearl

- To calculate the starting level for pure-tone A/C threshold testing, add the threshold of the NTE, plus the CF (if needed), plus a safety factor of 10 to 15 dB.

Starting level (PT A/C) = threshold of the NTE + CF + safety factor (10–15 dB)

Figure 13–7A–C provides an example of when masking would be needed for pure-tone A/C testing and the three possible outcomes for masked findings. As shown, for each of the three examples, the unmasked right ear A/C thresh-old at 2000 Hz is 55 dB HL; left ear A/C and B/C thresholds are 10 dB HL and 5 dB HL, respectively. The 50 dB differ-ence between the A/C threshold of the right ear and the B/C threshold of the left ear is greater than the 40 dB min-imum criterion to establish the need for masking when the right ear A/C threshold is obtained. For this patient, when testing the right ear A/C threshold, the starting level

for the left ear (NTE) would be at an effective level equal to 10 to 15 dB above the threshold of the left ear. Because the NTE A/C threshold is 10 dB HL for this patient, the starting level for masking would be at an effective level of 20 to 25 dB (10 dB HL threshold plus the 10 to 15 dB safety factor).

Assuming the same audiometer used to calculate the cor-rection factors in **Table 13–6** was used to test this patient, the factors required to calculate the starting level are

A/C NTE	+	Safety factor (SF)	+	Correction factor (CF)
			=	Starting level
(10 dB)	+	(10–15 dB)	+	(15 dB)
			=	35–40 dB dial setting

The correction factor was calculated by use of the proce-dures described earlier in this chapter.

Once the starting level of masking is introduced into the NTE, the procedure then is to determine whether the un-masked threshold of the TE was affected by introducing masking noise into the NTE. That is, while masking is intro-duced into the NTE, threshold sensitivity is assessed in the TE. Recall that central masking will affect thresholds in the TE by an average of 5 dB. The implication of this factor is that when masking is used in the NTE, it is likely that thresholds in the TE will change by 5 dB as a result of cen-tral masking.

Pearl

- During masking, patients may occasionally need rein-struction. Some indicators are frequent positive re-sponses (both false and true), pure-tone thresholds con-tinue to increase and never reach plateau, and the patient ceases to respond to the audible pure-tone stimulus be-cause the masking noise is "annoyingly" loud.

Three outcomes are possible when masking is used: (1) masking does not affect thresholds in the TE by more than 5 dB; (2) masking does affect thresholds in the TE by more than 5 dB, and a plateau is found; and (3) masking does af-fect thresholds in the TE by more than 5 dB, but it is not possible to find a plateau.

Outcome 1: Masking Does Not Affect the A/C Threshold in the TE by More than 5 dB

If the unmasked pure-tone A/C threshold does not vary from the masked threshold by more than 5 dB, the unmasked threshold is assumed to be valid and is recorded as a masked threshold. In this case, if the masked threshold is either 55 or 60 dB, this level would be accepted and recorded as a valid threshold and recorded as a masked threshold (**Fig. 13–7A**).

Outcome 2: Masking Does Affect the A/C Threshold in the TE by More than 5 dB, and a Plateau Is Established

If the masked threshold shifts by 10 dB or more when the masking starting level is introduced into the NTE, it

2000 Hz

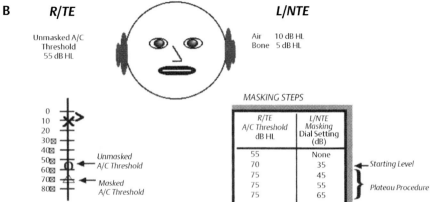

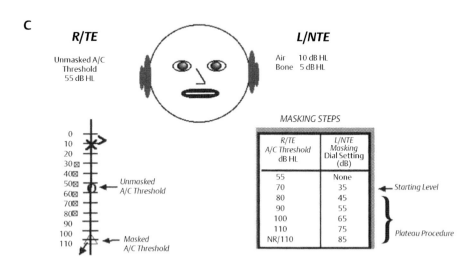

Figure 13–7 Example of when masking would be needed for pure-tone air-conduction testing and the three possible outcomes: **(A)** masking does not affect thresholds in the test ear (TE) by more than 5 dB; **(B)** masking does affect thresholds in the TE by more than 5 dB or more, and a plateau is found; **(C)** masking does affect threshold in the TE by more than 5 dB, but a plateau is not found. A/C, air conduction; HL, hearing level; NR, no response; NTE, nontest ear.

becomes necessary to find the masked plateau. When masking is used and the threshold in the TE shifts by 10 dB or more, the masked plateau is established as follows:

1. The threshold in the TE is reestablished by increasing the test signal in 10 dB increments.

2. Once a response to the pure-tone signal is obtained, the masking noise in the NTE is increased in 10 dB steps, and the threshold of the TE is reestablished.

3. This procedure is followed until the threshold in the TE does not change while the masking noise is increased in three consecutive 10 dB steps (the plateau is reached).

4. Once the plateau is reached, the masked threshold has been found. To account for the central masking effect, 5 dB is subtracted from the masked threshold, and this value is recorded on the audiogram form as a masked threshold.

Controversial Point

- Some clinicians use 10 dB steps to reach the plateau, whereas others prefer 15 dB steps.

As seen in **Fig. 13–7B**, the initial unmasked threshold of 55 dB HL shifted to 70 dB HL by introducing a starting level of 35 dB masking (35 dB dial/20 dB EM). With successive increases of masking in the left ear (NTE), the right ear (TE) threshold increased to 75 dB HL and was unchanged when the masking signal in the NTE was increased from 40 to 55 dB. At this point, the plateau has been reached, and the masked threshold is 75 dB HL. The correction of –5 dB for central masking is accounted for, and the masked threshold is recorded at 70 dB HL.

Outcome 3: Masking Does Affect A/C Thresholds in the TE by More than 5 dB, but a Plateau Is Not Established

A possible masking outcome is that successive increases in the masking signal in turn increase the threshold in the TE to the limits of the audiometer without establishing a plateau. The implication is that stimuli in the TE were consistently crossing over to the NTE, and the increases in masking made them imperceptible in the NTE. When this finding occurs, it is assumed that the TE threshold is beyond the limits of the audiometer, and a "no response" symbol is recorded at the audiometer's limits (**Fig. 13–7C**).

Determining Masking Levels for Pure-Tone Bone-Conduction Threshold Testing

Factors that are used to calculate the starting levels for pure-tone B/C testing are the same as for pure-tone A/C,

---

Pearl

- To calculate the starting level for pure-tone B/C threshold testing, add the threshold of the NTE, plus the CF (if needed), plus a safety factor of 10 to 15 dB, plus the occlusion effect (when applicable).

  Starting level (PT B/C)   = Threshold of the NTE + CF
  + Safety factor (10–15 dB)
  + Occlusion effect

---

with the exception that the occlusion effect must be added when applicable. Recall that the occlusion effect is the enhancement of B/C thresholds when the external ear canal is occluded. Because a masking earphone is placed over the NTE during the masking procedure, and because the minimum interaural attenuation level for B/C is 0 dB, thresholds obtained with masking can be influenced by the occlusion effect. **Table 13–4** shows the mean occlusion effect within the midintensity range of 60 dB to be 20, 15, and 5 dB at 250, 500, and 1000 Hz, respectively. These values are added to the masking levels whenever pure-tone B/C testing is performed at these frequencies.

Figure 13–8A–C provides examples of when masking would be needed for pure-tone B/C testing and the three possible outcomes for masked findings. For each of the three examples, the right ear masked A/C threshold at 500 Hz is 70 dB HL with an unmasked B/C threshold of 5 dB HL; left ear A/C and B/C thresholds are 10 and 5 dB HL, respectively. The 65 dB difference between the A/C threshold of the right ear and the B/C threshold of the right ear is greater than the 10 dB minimum criterion required to establish the need for masking when the right ear B/C threshold is obtained. (An unmasked conductive component greater than 10 dB is present.)

Assuming the same audiometer used to calculate the correction factors in **Table 13–6** was used to test this patient, factors required to calculate the starting level when testing the right ear B/C thresholds at 500 Hz are

A/C NTE + Safety + Correction + Occlusion = Starting level
            factor (SF)   factor (CF)   effect (OE)

(10 dB)   + (10–15 dB) + (10 dB)   + (15 dB)   = 45–50 dB
                                                      dial setting

As shown in **Table 13–6**, 15 dB was added to the calculation for the occlusion effect because the test frequency is 500 Hz.

As with A/C testing, when the starting level is introduced into the NTE, the procedure is to determine whether the unmasked threshold in the TE is influenced by the introduction of masking in the NTE. Three possible outcomes may occur.

500 Hz

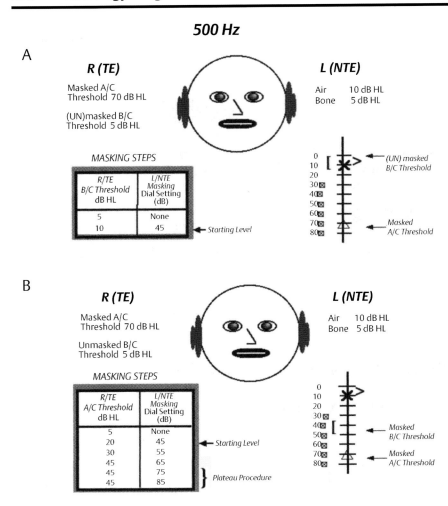

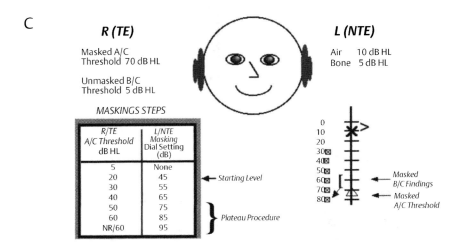

Figure 13–8 Example of when masking would be needed for pure-tone bone-conduction (B/C) testing and the three possible outcomes: **(A)** masking does not affect B/C thresholds in the test ear (TE) by more than 5 dB; **(B)** masking does affect B/C thresholds in the TE by more than 5 dB, and a plateau is found; **(C)** masking does affect B/C thresholds in the TE by more than 5 dB, but a plateau is not found. A/C, air conduction; HL, hearing level; NR, no response; NTE, nontest ear.

Outcome 1: Masking Does Not Affect the B/C Threshold in the TE by More than 5 dB

If the unmasked threshold does not shift by more than 5 dB, the unmasked threshold is assumed to be valid and is recorded as a masked threshold. In this case, a masked B/C threshold of either 5 or 10 dB HL would be accepted as valid and recorded as a masked threshold. This result is shown in **Fig. 13–8A**.

Outcome 2: Masking Does Affect the B/C Threshold in the TE by More than 5 dB, and a Plateau Is Established

When masking is introduced at the starting level into the NTE, and B/C thresholds shift by at least 10 dB, the plateau is found in the same manner described previously. In the example in **Fig. 13–8B**, the 5 dB HL unmasked B/C threshold shifts to 20 dB HL when the starting level is used. Subsequent 10 dB increases in the masking level result in threshold shifts in the TE to a level of 45 dB HL. With two 10 dB incremental increases of the masking noise, the TE threshold remains constant at 45 dB HL, indicating that the plateau has been established. To account for central masking, the masked threshold is recorded as 40 dB HL.

Outcome 3: Masking Does Affect the B/C Threshold in the TE by More than 5 dB, but a Plateau Is Not Established

One additional outcome is that the B/C thresholds in the TE do not plateau at the maximum levels of the audiometer. **Figure 13–8C** provides an example of this finding. The unmasked B/C threshold of 5 dB shifts as the masking levels increase from the initial starting level of 40 or 45 dB to 90 dB. At the masking level of 90 dB, the patient does not respond to the test signal at the maximum limits of the audiometer for B/C at 60 dB HL. In this case, a "no response" B/C symbol is recorded at 60 dB HL.

Determining Masking Levels for Speech Recognition Threshold Testing

> **Pearl**
>
> • To calculate the starting level for SRT testing, subtract 35 dB from the PL of the unmasked SRT in the TE, and add the average ABG in the speech frequencies of the NTE (if any).
>
> Starting level (SRT) = PL (TE) – 35 dB* + average ABG (NTE)
>
> *(45 dB minimum interaural attenuation level – 10 dB safety factor)

Principles for calculating masking levels for speech stimuli are the same as for pure tones, with a slight variation in the procedure. An acoustic method using a subtraction procedure is recommended for speech stimuli (Studebaker, 1979). To use the subtraction procedure, the minimum interaural attenuation levels for the speech stimuli must be taken into account. The subtraction procedure is based on the assumption that speech in the TE can be prevented from crossing to the NTE effectively if the level of noise in the NTE is above the minimum interaural attenuation level. A safety factor of 10 dB is added to the noise to account for patient variability. For SRT testing, the starting level is determined by subtracting 35 dB from the PL of the unmasked SRT (45 dB minimum interaural attenuation level – 10 dB safety factor).

The acoustic method is quite adequate as long as no conductive component is present in the NTE. If a conductive component exists, the masking signal must be increased by the average level of the conductive component (the ABG). Otherwise the intensity of the masking signal will be inadequate, and undermasking will result.

Figure 13–9A and **B** provides examples of masking for SRT testing without and with ABGs present in the NTE, respectively. For each example, the audiometer used to calculate the correction factors in **Table 13–6** was used to test this patient. For **Fig. 13–9A**, no significant ABGs are present in the NTE. The factors required to calculate the starting level are

(PL (TE) − IA SRT)	+ CF	+ NTE Avg. ABG	= Starting level (SRT)
(75 dB HL − 35 = 40)	+ 10 +	0	= 50 dB dial setting

where IA is interaural attenuation. This starting level would be introduced into the NTE, and the masked threshold would be established in the same manner as for pure-tone thresholds. That is, with masking, either the unmasked threshold would change by 5 dB or less, a plateau would be found, or the SRT would shift to the maximum limits of the audiometer. When the masked SRT is found, the result would be recorded on the audiogram form.

When an ABG is present in speech frequencies of the NTE, calculating the starting level for SRT testing must factor in the conductive component. **Figure 13–9B** provides an example when an ABG is present. The factors required to calculate the starting levels for SRT testing when an ABG is present are

(PL (TE) − IA SRT)	+ CF	+ NTE Avg. ABG	= Starting level (SRT)
(75 dB HL − 35 = 40)	+ 10 +	15	= 65 dB dial setting

Once again, this starting level would be introduced into the NTE. With masking, either the unmasked threshold would change by 5 dB or less, a plateau would be found, or the SRT would shift to the maximum limits of the audiometer. Results would be entered on the audiogram form.

Determining Masking Levels for Word Recognition Testing

As with SRT testing, masking levels during word recognition testing use the acoustic method. However, unlike

Speech Recognition Threshold Testing

A WITHOUT Air–Bone Gap

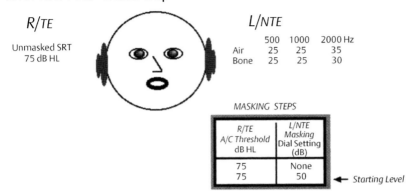

B WITH Air–Bone Gap

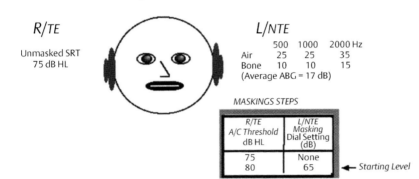

Figure 13–9 Example of when to mask for speech recognition threshold testing when **(A)** an air–bone gap (ABG) in the speech frequencies is absent in the nontest ear (NTE) and **(B)** an ABG in the speech frequencies is present in the NTE. A/C, air conduction; HL, hearing level; SRT, speech recognition threshold; TE, test ear.

Pearl

- To calculate the starting level for word recognition testing, subtract 25 dB from the PL in the TE, and add the average ABG in the speech frequencies of the NTE (if any).

    Starting level (word recognition tests) = PL (TE) − 25 dB* + average ABG (NTE)

    * (45 dB minimum interaural attenuation level − 20 dB safety factor)

threshold procedures, the PL of test stimuli during word recognition testing remains constant. Consequently, the intensity of the masking stimulus is the same throughout the procedure. Another difference between masking for SRT and word recognition testing is that the recommended

safety factor is increased to 20 dB (Studebaker, 1979). The intensity level of the masking in the NTE is based on subtracting 25 dB from the PL of the monosyllabic words in the TE. The 25 dB level is derived from the minimum interaural attenuation level for speech (45 dB) minus the safety factor of 20 dB.

Similar to SRT testing, when a conductive component is present in the speech range of the masked (NTE) ear, the average difference (ABG) between the A/C and B/C thresholds at 500, 1000, and 2000 Hz is added to the masking level.

Figure 13–10A and **B** illustrates examples of masking for word recognition testing without and with ABGs present in the NTE, respectively. For each example, the audiometer used to calculate the correction factors in **Table 13–6** was used to test this patient.

No ABGs are present in the speech frequencies for the NTE for the patient in **Fig. 13–10A**. The factors required to calculate the starting level are

Word Recognition Testing

A WITHOUT Air–Bone Gap

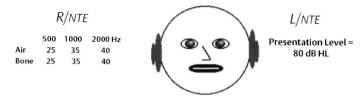

R/NTE

	500	1000	2000 Hz
Air	25	35	40
Bone	25	35	40

L/NTE

Presentation Level = 80 dB HL

Masking Level in NTE = 65 dB

B WITH Air–Bone Gap

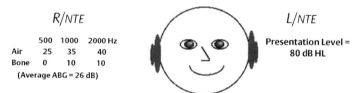

R/NTE

	500	1000	2000 Hz
Air	25	35	40
Bone	0	10	10

(Average ABG = 26 dB)

L/NTE

Presentation Level = 80 dB HL

Masking Level in NTE = 90 dB

Figure 13–10 Example of when to mask for word recognition testing when **(A)** an air–bone gap (ABG) in the speech frequencies is absent in the nontest ear (NTE) and **(B)** an ABG in the speech frequencies is present in the NTE. ABG, air–bone gap; TE, test ear.

(PL (TE) − IA SRT) + CF + NTE Avg. ABG = Starting level
                                              (word recognition)
(80 dB HL − 25 = 55 dB HL) + 10 + 0 = 65 dB dial setting

This 65 dB masking level would be presented to the right (NTE) ear throughout the test procedure. When the masked word recognition score is established, the result would be recorded on the audiogram form as a masked score.

Figure 13–10B provides an example of masking for word recognition testing when an ABG is present. Those factors required to calculate the starting level for word recognition testing when an ABG is present are

(PL (TE) − IA SRT) + CF + NTE Avg. ABG = Starting level
                                           (word recognition)
(80 dB HL − 25 = 55 dB HL) + 10 + 25 = 90 dB dial setting

The 90 dB masking level would be introduced into the NTE. Once completed, the masked word recognition score is entered on the audiogram form.

The Masking Dilemma

A masking dilemma occurs when it is impossible to mask the NTE effectively without exceeding the maximum permissible masking level. Whenever a bilateral conductive hearing loss of 35 dB or more is present, a masking dilemma is

possible. As the extent of conductive hearing loss increases in the NTE, the likelihood of the masking dilemma becomes greater until the point at which the patient's interaural attenuation level is reached. Because the average interaural attenuation ranges between 55 and 65 dB, the masking dilemma is a certainty for most patients when a conductive component is present in the masked (NTE) ear in the 55 to 65 dB range. Recall that some patients will have interaural attenuation levels lower than the average 55 to 65 dB range, possibly as low as 40 dB. This implies that the masking dilemma will be present for a few patients when the masked (NTE) ear has a conductive component as low as 40 dB.

Figure 13–11 displays audiometric results from a patient having a moderate to severe bilateral conductive hearing loss. Because the bilateral conductive components exceed 50 to 55 dB, a masking dilemma is posed in this case. As an example, the starting level when testing the right ear pure-tone A/C threshold at 1000 Hz (masking the left [NTE] ear) would be

A/C NTE	+	SF	+	CF	=	Starting level
(55 dB)	+	(10–15 dB)	+	(15 dB)	=	80–85 dB dial setting

Masking presented to the NTE at the 80 to 85 dB dial setting is at an effective level of 65 to 70 dB (80–85 dB dial setting minus the 15 dB CF). If this patient had an average interaural attenuation level between 55 and 65 dB, a masking

AUDIOGRAM

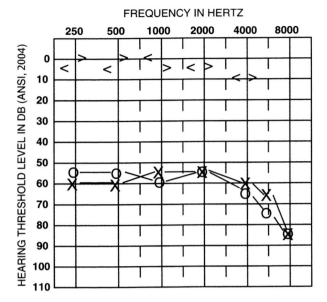

Figure 13–11 Example of a masking dilemma with a patient having a moderate to severe bilateral conductive hearing loss.

noise in the NTE would cross to the TE, and overmasking would result. For this patient, the result of introducing masking into either ear will shift thresholds in the TE when attempting to find the plateau. In fact, thresholds will be shifted to the maximum limits of the audiometer, a finding that is impossible because the unmasked results on the audiogram must reflect the threshold sensitivity of at least one ear. Thresholds for both ears cannot shift when masking is used.

When confronted with a masking dilemma, clinicians should use insert earphones to obtain thresholds. Insert earphones increase the interaural attenuation levels from an average of 55 to 65 dB to an average of 80 dB (see **Table 13–3**). Increased interaural attenuation will allow for the use of greater masking levels in the NTE without crossover to the TE.

Masking with Special Populations

Masking can be confusing for children and adults with cognitive impairment, because it is difficult for them to differentiate between and/or respond to the two simultaneously presented acoustic signals. A modified plateau method can be used as a time-saving approach for these patients. The patient should be instructed that two sounds will be presented; the signal in the TE will be the same "whistles" or "beeps" that the patient has already been listening to, and the other will be a "windy noise" that he or she should ignore. Introduce the masking signal into the NTE at the calculated starting level. If the patient responds to the masking signal, instruct him or her once again to wait until only the "whistle/beeps" are heard in the TE. A pure tone is then presented in the TE

at a suprathreshold level of 30 dB above the unmasked threshold. The patient should respond at this intensity and should then be reinstructed if no response is made. If reliable responses are obtained at the 30 dB SL level, the masking signal is increased by 20 dB, and the pure tone is presented again at 30 dB SL. Depending on whether the patient responds or not, one of two steps should be followed:

1. If the patient responds, the likelihood is that the unmasked threshold is valid, and the masking signal is increased 20 dB above the starting level. If the patient responds to the pure tone, the pure-tone stimulus is incrementally decreased by 10 dB until no response occurs. The last response is considered the masked threshold.

2. If the patient does not respond, either the unmasked threshold resulted from crossover, or the patient has difficulty responding to two signals presented simultaneously. The pure tone is increased to 50 dB SL. The patient should respond at this intensity and then be reinstructed if no response is made. If the patient responds to the pure tone, the pure-tone stimulus is incrementally decreased by 10 dB until no response occurs. The last response is considered the masked threshold. If, however, the patient does not respond, seeking a masked threshold may not be possible for this individual.

Although the above procedure is helpful with some children as well as adults with cognitive impairment, obtaining masked thresholds for others may be impossible. For these cases, the use of insert earphones is especially important due to their increased interaural attenuation (see Chapter 12), and using additional diagnostic tests, including immittance measures, otoacoustic emissions, and auditory brainstem response, becomes critical. When masked thresholds cannot be obtained, clinicians should always indicate that masking was attempted without success on the audiogram and in the report.

◆ Case Studies

Case Study No. 1

Results from three patients are presented in **Figs. 13–12** through **13–14** to illustrate the masking principles presented in this chapter. Unmasked results for the data in **Fig. 13–12** show a moderate to severe right ear mixed hearing loss and a moderate to severe left ear high-frequency sensorineural hearing loss. Although many of today's audiometers do not require CFs, to become familiar with factoring them into the calculation, the two examples will use the following CFs (in dB):

Hz	250	500	1000	2000	3000	4000	6000	8000	Speech
dB	10	5	15	5	10	15	20	5	0

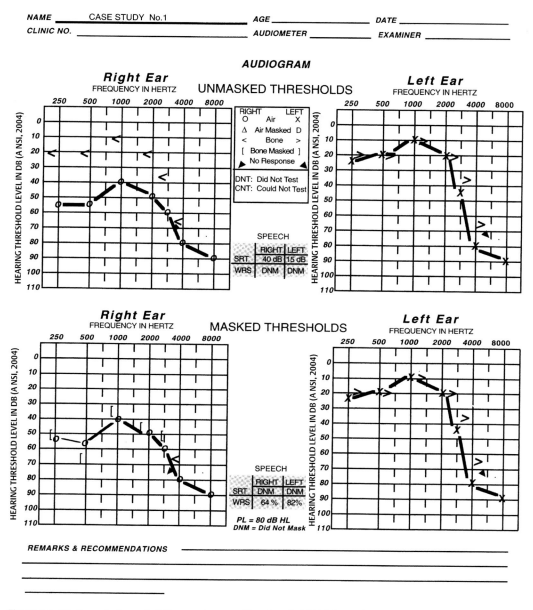

Figure 13–12 Case study no. 1. SRT, speech recognition threshold; WRS, word recognition score.

The starting levels (in dB) for masking required for the data in **Fig. 13–12** are as follows:

♦ When obtaining right ear pure-tone A/C thresholds, no masking is needed.

♦ When obtaining left ear pure-tone A/C thresholds, no masking is needed.

♦ When obtaining right ear pure-tone B/C thresholds:

Hz	A/C NTE	+	SF	+ CF	+ OE	=	Starting level
250 =	25	+	10–15	+ 10	+ 20	=	65–70
500 =	20	+	10–15	+ 5	+ 15	=	50–55
1000 =	10	+	10–15	+ 15	+ 5	=	40–45
2000 =	20	+	10–15	+ 5	+ 0	=	35–40
3000 =	45	+	10–15	+ 10	+ 0	=	65–70
4000 =	No masking is needed						

♦ When obtaining left ear pure-tone B/C thresholds, no masking is needed.

♦ When obtaining the right ear SRT, no masking is needed.

♦ When obtaining the left ear SRT, no masking is needed.

♦ When obtaining the right ear word recognition score:

Avg. ABG NTE*
PL (TE)	− 25 dB	+ (500, 1000, 2000 Hz)	+ CF	= Masking level
80 dB HL	− 25 dB +	0	+ 0	= 55 dB

♦ When obtaining the left ear word recognition score:

Avg. ABG NTE*
PL (TE)	− 25 dB	+ (500, 1000, 2000 Hz)	+ CF	= Masking level
80 dB HL	− 25 dB +	30	+ 0	= 85 dB

Once masking is introduced into the NTE for threshold measures, and the patient's responses do not change by more than 5 dB, the threshold is accepted as valid and recorded on the audiogram form as masked results. For word recognition tests, the level is held constant throughout the procedure.

Case Study No. 2

In **Fig. 13–13**, unmasked findings suggest a mild bilateral conductive hearing loss. For this patient, the starting levels (in dB) would be

♦ When obtaining right ear pure-tone A/C thresholds, no masking is needed.

♦ When obtaining left ear pure-tone A/C thresholds, no masking is needed.

♦ When obtaining right ear pure-tone B/C thresholds:

Hz	A/C NTE	+	SF	+	CF	+	OE	=	Starting level
250	= 35	+	10–15	+	10	+	20	=	75–80
500	= 35	+	10–15	+	5	+	15	=	65–70
1000	= 40	+	10–15	+	15	+	5	=	70–75
2000	= 35	+	10–15	+	5	+	0	=	50–55
4000	= 35	+	10–15	+	15	+	0	=	60–65

♦ When obtaining left ear pure-tone B/C thresholds:

Hz	A/C NTE	+	SF	+	CF	+	OE	=	Starting level
250	= 30	+	10–15	+	10	+	20	=	70–75
500	= 30	+	10–15	+	5	+	15	=	60–65
1000	= 35	+	10–15	+	15	+	5	=	65–70
2000	= 30	+	10–15	+	5	+	0	=	45–50
4000	= 25	+	10–15	+	15	+	0	=	50–55

---

* The average ABG at 500, 1000, and 2000 Hz is based on unmasked findings. If masked findings were available, there would be no ABG at 500, 1000, and 2000 Hz, and the masking level would be 55 dB.

♦ When obtaining the right ear SRT, no masking is needed.

♦ When obtaining the left ear SRT, no masking is needed.

♦ When obtaining the right ear word recognition score:

Avg. ABG NTE*
PL (TE)	− 25 dB	+ (500, 1000, 2000 Hz)	+ CF	= Masking level
80 dB HL	− 25 dB +	35	+ 0	= 90 dB

♦ When obtaining the left ear word recognition score:

Avg. ABG NTE*
PL (TE)	− 25 dB	+ (500, 1000, 2000 Hz)	+ CF	= Masking level
80 dB HL	− 25 dB +	30	+ 0	= 85 dB

Case Study No. 3

Pearl

• When masked results from one ear shift significantly, there may be no need to mask findings from the contralateral ear.

Unmasked audiometric results in **Fig. 13–14** show a moderate to severe right ear and severe to profound left ear mixed hearing loss. This case is presented to illustrate that if masked results from one ear shift significantly, there is no need to mask findings from the other ear. For this patient, masking would be used when testing left ear thresholds first because the severity of the loss in the left ear makes the likelihood of crossover greater for the left ear than the right ear.

The starting levels (in dB) used when testing the left ear are as follows:

♦ When obtaining left ear pure-tone A/C thresholds:

Hz	A/C NTE	+	SF	+	CF	=	Starting level
250	= 50	+	10–15	+	10	=	70–75
500	= 60	+	10–15	+	5	=	75–80
1000	= 65	+	10–15	+	15	=	90–95
2000	= 60	+	10–15	+	5	=	75–80
3000	= 60	+	10–15	+	10	=	80–85
4000	= 40	+	10–15	+	15	=	65–70
6000	=	No masking is needed					
8000	=	No masking is needed					

♦ When obtaining left ear pure-tone B/C thresholds:

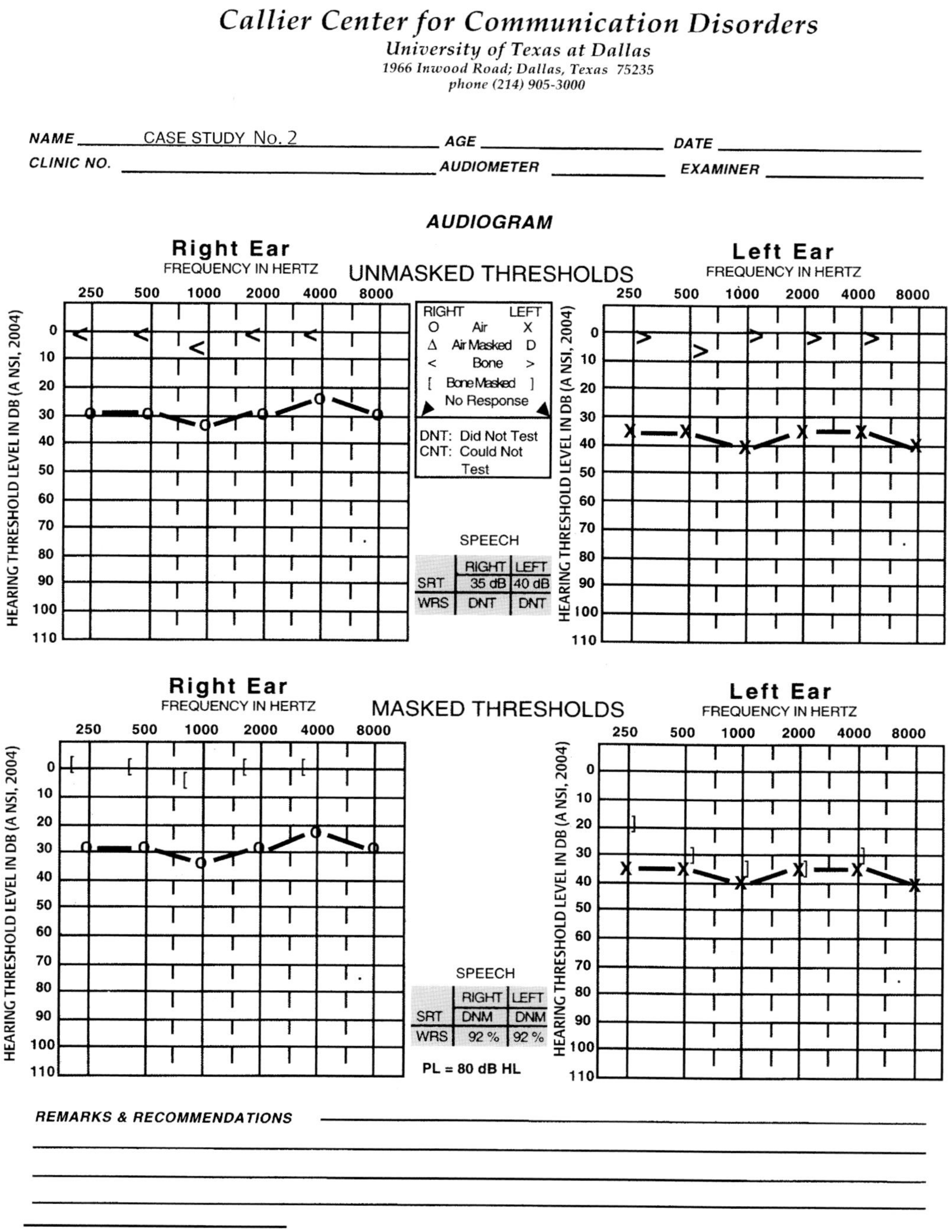

Callier Center for Communication Disorders
University of Texas at Dallas
1966 Inwood Road; Dallas, Texas 75235
phone (214) 905-3000

NAME ___CASE STUDY No. 2___ AGE _____ DATE _____

CLINIC NO. _____ AUDIOMETER _____ EXAMINER _____

AUDIOGRAM

UNMASKED THRESHOLDS

Right Ear — FREQUENCY IN HERTZ

Left Ear — FREQUENCY IN HERTZ

	RIGHT		LEFT
O	Air		X
Δ	Air Masked		D
<	Bone		>
[	Bone Masked		]
▶	No Response		◀

DNT: Did Not Test
CNT: Could Not Test

SPEECH

	RIGHT	LEFT
SRT	35 dB	40 dB
WRS	DNT	DNT

MASKED THRESHOLDS

Right Ear — FREQUENCY IN HERTZ

Left Ear — FREQUENCY IN HERTZ

SPEECH

	RIGHT	LEFT
SRT	DNM	DNM
WRS	92 %	92 %

PL = 80 dB HL

REMARKS & RECOMMENDATIONS _____

Figure 13–13 Case study no. 2. SRT, speech recognition threshold; WRS, word recognition score.

Hz	A/C NTE	+	SF	+	CF	+	OE	=	Starting level
250 =	50	+	10–15	+	10	+	20	=	90–95
500 =	60	+	10–15	+	5	+	15	=	90–95
1000 =	65	+	10–15	+	15	+	5	=	95–100
2000 =	60	+	10–15	+	5	+	0	=	75–80
3000 =	60	+	10–15	+	10	+	0	=	80–85
4000 =	40	+	10–15	+	15	+	0	=	65–70

♦ When obtaining the left ear SRT:

Avg. ABG NTE

$$PL\,(TE) - 35\,dB + (500, 1000, 2000\,Hz) + CF = Masking\ level$$
$$80\,dB\ HL - 35\,dB + 45 + 0 = 85\,dB$$

♦ When obtaining the left ear word recognition score, this test cannot be performed due to the severity of the loss.

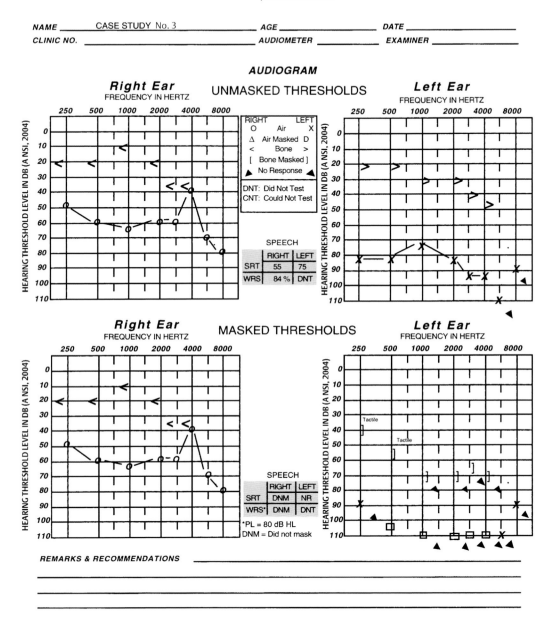

Figure 13–14 Case study no. 3. SRT, speech recognition threshold; WRS, word recognition score.

As illustrated in **Fig. 13–14,** the use of masking when testing the left ear caused pure-tone and speech thresholds to shift to the profound level. Consequently, even though the masking rules would suggest the need for masking when testing the right ear, data from the right ear are known to be valid. That is, unmasked findings always reflect the performance of the better ear. When one ear is eliminated through the use of masking, the resulting unmasked data must reflect findings from the remaining ear.

Data in case study no. 3 represent an advanced masking concept. This and others will become secondhand once the masking principles outlined in this chapter become familiar to the clinician.

◆ Summary

The proper use of masking during clinical audiometry ensures the examiner that test results reflect the performance of the test ear only. This chapter describes the principles used in clinical masking. The questions of when to mask and how much masking to use are addressed. By following the masking principles in this chapter, one is assured that diagnostic test results from the test ear are valid.

References

American National Standards Institute (ANSI). (2004). American national specifications for audiometers (ANSI S3.6). New York: ANSI.

American Speech-Language-Hearing Association. (1978). Guidelines for manual pure-tone audiometry. ASHA, 20, 297–301.

Berger, E. H., & Kerivan, J. E. (1983). Influence of physiological noise and the occlusion effect on the measurement of real-ear attenuation at threshold. Journal of the Acoustical Society of America, 74, 81–94.

Chaiklin, J. B. (1967). Interaural attenuation and cross-hearing in air conduction audiometry. Journal of Auditory Research, 7, 413–424.

Coles, R. R. A., & Priede, V. M. (1970). On the misdiagnosis resulting from incorrect use of masking. Journal of Laryngology and Otology, 84, 41–63.

Dirks, D., & Malmquist, C. (1964). Changes in bone conducted thresholds produced by masking in the non-test ear. Journal of Speech and Hearing Research, 50, 271–278.

Dirks, D., & Swindeman, J. G. (1967). The variability of occluded and unoccluded bone-conduction thresholds. Journal of Speech and Hearing Research, 10, 232–249.

Elpern, B. , & Naunton, R. F. (1963). The stability of the occlusion effect. Archives of Otolaryngology, 77, 376–384.

Fletcher, H. (1940). Auditory patterns. Reviews of Modern Physics, 12, 47–65.

Gelfand, S. A. (1997). Essentials of audiology. New York: Thieme Medical Publishers.

Goldstein, D. P., & Hayes, C. S. (1965). The occlusion effect in bone-conduction hearing. Journal of Speech and Hearing Research, 25, 137–148.

Hawkins, J. E., & Stevens, S. S. (1950). Masking of pure tones and of speech by white noise. Journal of the Acoustical Society of America, 22, 6–13.

Hodgson, W. R., & Tillman, T. (1966). Reliability of bone conduction occlusion effects in normals. Journal of Auditory Research, 6, 141–153.

Hood, J. D. (1960). The principle and practice of bone-conduction audiometry: A review of the present position. Laryngoscope, 70, 1211–1228.

Killion, M. C., Wilber, L. A., & Gundmundson, G. I. (1985). Insert earphones for more interaural attenuation. Hearing Instruments, 36(2), 34–38.

Konig, E. (1962). On the use of hearing aid type earphones in clinical audiometry. Acta Otolaryngologica, 55, 331–341.

Konkle, D. F., & Berry, G. A. (1983). Masking in speech audiometry. In D. F. Konkle & W. F. Rintleman (Eds.), Principles of speech audiometry (pp. 285–319). Baltimore, MD: University Park Press.

Liden, G., Nilsson, G., & Anderson, H. (1959). Masking in clinical audiometry. Acta Otolaryngologica, 50, 125–136.

Lloyd, L. L., & Kaplan, H. (1978). Audiometric interpretation: A manual of basic audiometry. Baltimore, MD: University Park Press.

Martin, F. N. (1966). Speech audiometry and clinical masking. Journal of Auditory Research, 6, 199–203.

Martin, F. N. (1994). Introduction to audiology (5th ed.). Needham Heights, MA: Allyn & Bacon.

Martin, F. N. (1997). Introduction to audiology (6th ed). Boston: Allyn & Bacon.

Martin, F. N., & Blosser, D. (1970). Cross hearing air conduction or bone conduction. Psychonomic Science, 20, 231–239.

Martin, F. N., Butler, E. C., & Burns, P. (1974). Audiometric Bing test for determination of minimum masking levels for bone conduction tests. Journal of Speech and Hearing Disorders, 39, 148–152.

Martin, F. N., & Di Giovanni, D. (1979). Central masking effects on spondee thresholds as a function of masker sensation level and masker sound pressure level. Journal of the American Audiology Society, 4, 141–146.

Martin, F. N., & Fagelson, M. (1995). Bone conduction reconsidered. Tejas, 20, 26–27.

Sanders, J. W., & Rintelmann, W. F. (1964). Masking in audiometry. Archives of Otolaryngology, 80, 541–556.

Sklare, D. A., & Denenberg, L. J. (1987). Interaural attenuation for Tubephone insert earphones. Ear and Hearing, 8, 298–300.

Studebaker, G. A. (1962). On masking in bone conduction testing. Journal of Speech and Hearing Research, 5, 215–227.

Studebaker, G. A. (1967). Clinical masking of the nontest ear. Journal of Speech and Hearing Disorders, 32, 360–371.

Studebaker, G. A. (1979). Clinical masking. In W. F. Rintelmann (Ed.), Hearing assessment (pp. 51–100). Baltimore, MD: University Park Press.

Turner, R. G. (2004a). Masking redux: 1. An optimized masking method. Journal of the American Academy of Audiology, 15, 17–28.

Turner, R. G. (2004b). Masking redux: 2. A recommended masking protocol. Journal of the American Academy of Audiology, 15, 29–46.

Veniar, F. A. (1965). Individual masking levels in pure-tone audiometry. Archives of Otolaryngology, 82, 518–521.

Wegel, R. L., & Lane, G. I. (1924). The auditory masking of one pure tone by another and its probable relation to the dynamics of the inner ear. Physiological Reviews, 23, 266–285.

Zwislocki, J. (1953). Acoustic attenuation between ears. Journal of the Acoustical Society of America, 25, 752–759.

Chapter 14

Speech Audiometry

Linda M. Thibodeau

Evaluation of speech processing is an important component of the diagnostic audiological evaluation for variety of reasons. First, speech thresholds provide validating data for pure-tone thresholds. Second, at suprathreshold levels, speech recognition scores contribute to decisions regarding site-of-lesion and development of rehabilitation strategies.

Over time, the terminology used for speech audiometry has changed as speech perception research with patients has expanded from a clinical to a psychoacoustic framework. Consequently, a discussion of speech audiometry must begin with a clear taxonomy of terminology, followed by a review of those critical aspects of speech in relation to diagnostic information using various evaluative techniques. Although this chapter will focus on the diagnostic application of speech audiometry, it must be realized that just as speech processing is an important step in the diagnostic process, it is equally important in the rehabilitative process. Therein lies the ultimate challenge for audiologists: to provide technology and behavioral strategies that will allow patients with impaired hearing to maximize their communicative functioning.

To assess speech processing adequately, several decisions regarding the signal, presentation format, and response task must be made. These decisions affect the analysis and interpretation of the results. Factors influencing such decisions include age of the patient, purpose of the evaluation, and available time for testing. Clinicians must evaluate the relative importance of these variables for each patient and determine the most efficient means of obtaining the desired information.

Information presented in this chapter will provide the framework for decisions regarding the signal, presentation format, and response task with evidence supporting the most efficient and sensitive procedures that can be used both diagnostically and rehabilitatively. In addition, common problems in the evaluation of speech processing will be addressed, with suggestions given for avoiding those pitfalls. Typically, these problems arise from a mismatch between the selected materials, procedure, or response task and the patient's capabilities. Therefore, it is imperative to begin with a clear rationale for why evaluation of speech processing is necessary, followed by a review of how the various evaluation procedures can influence results. Finally, a review of the possible tests and procedures available for different age groups is provided.

◆ Terminology

Typically, evaluation of speech processing at threshold levels has resulted in obtaining a speech awareness or detection threshold (SAT/SDT) or speech recognition (or reception) threshold (SRT), and evaluation at suprathreshold levels has resulted in obtaining a speech discrimination score (SDS) or word discrimination score (WDS). However, as the many facets of speech processing are considered, it becomes apparent that more precise terminology is needed. Ideally, the same taxonomy would apply to both diagnostic and rehabilitative services.

Controversial Point

- In speech audiometry, the preferred term to specify the threshold for speech is the *speech detection threshold* (American Speech-Language-Hearing Association [ASHA], 1988), although some audiologists still use *speech awareness threshold*. The preferred term to specify the threshold for speech understanding is the *speech recognition threshold*, although some audiologists still use *speech reception threshold*.

A clearly established hierarchy of four levels of auditory processing used by Erber (1982) in auditory training can be applied to the diagnostic battery. The four levels of processing are awareness, discrimination, identification/recognition, and comprehension. Currently available tests in speech audiometry fall into either awareness or identification/ recognition. A brief review of how the clinical measures fall into this hierarchy is provided below, and greater discussion is given in the section entitled "Level of Auditory Ability Assessed."

Awareness Those tests that require the patient to indicate simply that a sound was detected, such as the SDT and SAT.

Discrimination Those tests that require the patient to detect a change in the acoustic stimulus. Currently, there are no tests of speech discrimination used in traditional speech audiometry.

Identification/recognition Those tests that require the patient to attach a label to the stimulus either by pointing to a corresponding picture/object or by repeating the stimulus orally or in writing. Routine clinical assessments in speech audiometry include measures at threshold levels, or an SRT, and measures at suprathreshold levels, using words (word recognition score [WRS]) or sentences (sentence recognition score [SRS]).

Comprehension Those tests that require the patient to attach meaning to the stimulus by answering questions verbally or in writing, or by pointing to a picture that conveys the associated meaning. Auditory comprehension is not assessed in traditional speech audiometry.

Controversial Point

- The general term used to specify identification/recognition of speech at suprathreshold levels in this chapter is *speech recognition score*. When known stimuli are discussed, the term *word recognition score* is applied for word stimuli, and *sentence recognition score* is applied for sentence stimuli. Some audiologists continue to use the less accurate term *speech discrimination score* for all measures of identification/recognition of speech at suprathreshold levels.

◆ Rationale for Evaluating Speech Processing

Typically, speech-processing evaluations are included in the routine audiological exam to determine the extent to which altered thresholds disrupt perception of complex signals. Evaluation of responses to pure-tone information does not allow for complete understanding of a patient's deficit. Consequently, evaluation of speech processing should be included not only in the diagnostic battery but also in the hearing aid fitting process. In some pathologies, abnormal speech processing may be the most significant diagnostic factor. Furthermore, two patients with the same degree of hearing loss may demonstrate very different speech-processing abilities. In other words, two patients may have the same reduction in absolute sensitivity (i.e., thresholds) but vary in their differential sensitivity, or processing of suprathreshold information. This may lead to different hearing aid fittings for these two patients because one may benefit more from advanced noise reduction processing to help compensate for suprathreshold processing deficits. Furthermore, rehabilitation for these two patients may differ in that the one with the greater speech-processing deficit would require more emphasis on repair strategies and possible environmental modifications. Thus, the rationale for the evaluation of speech processing includes three areas: relative effects of reduced absolute and differential sensitivity, contributions to differential diagnosis, and application to hearing aid fittings and auditory rehabilitation.

Relative Effects of Reduced Absolute and Differential Sensitivity

When audibility of the signal is reduced, the effects on recognition of specific speech features can be well predicted by the absolute thresholds for pure tones (Dubno and Levitt, 1981). The reduction in absolute sensitivity is routinely represented on the audiogram and may be interpreted relative to the long-term speech spectrum commonly referred to as the "speech banana." The relationship of thresholds to the speech banana shown in **Fig. 14–1** is often used in counseling the patient with hearing loss regarding the speech sounds that will be difficult to perceive. In general, a reduction in audibility of low-frequency information interferes with perception of cues for nasality, whereas a reduction in audibility of high-frequency information interferes with perception of cues for sibilants and fricatives. However, speech processing involves more than just audibility of the signal, as illustrated in two case studies presented by Skinner et al (1982). They identified two patients with similar thresholds but very different speech recognition scores and attributed the difference in scores to differences in suprathreshold processing.

Pearl

- *Differential sensitivity* refers to the ability to detect changes in intensity, frequency, and temporal aspects of the signal, all of which are potential cues for speech recognition.

AUDIOGRAM

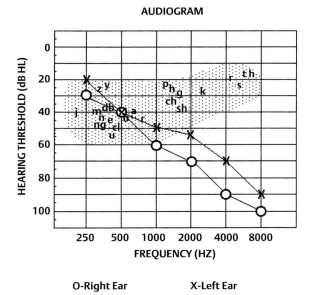

O-Right Ear   X-Left Ear

Figure 14–1 Relationship of a patient's threshold to the "speech banana."

The relationship between differential sensitivity and threshold sensitivity varies widely. Evaluation of differential sensitivity is not routinely included in the clinical audiological battery. Psychoacoustic studies have shown moderate to strong correlations between speech recognition and frequency resolution (Thibodeau and Van Tasell, 1987; Tyler, Wood, and Fernandes, 1982) and temporal resolution (Festen and Plomp, 1983; Tyler, Summerfield, Wood, and Fernandes, 1982). Therefore, when speech-processing performance is lower than expected based on threshold information, the reduced performance may be related to a reduction in differential sensitivity.

In the typical clinical assessment of speech processing, the effects of reduced absolute and differential sensitivity cannot be separated. Unless the signal is spectrally shaped to ensure complete audibility, the combined effects of these deficits will be represented in a single score. The degree to which amplification can compensate for reduced speech recognition is based in part on improvements in speech recognition with increased audibility. For example, if a patient's speech recognition score improves 25% when the presentation level is increased from 60 to 90 dB HL (hearing level), the potential benefits of amplification are strongly supported.

One way to quantify changes in absolute sensitivity is through a procedure known as the articulation index (AI; French and Steinberg, 1947). The AI is calculated based on a person's hearing sensitivity relative to the long-term average speech spectrum. More credit is given for audibility of high frequencies because of their significant contribution to speech intelligibility. Someone with an AI of 0.90 would have access to 90% of the speech information and excellent speech recognition, whereas someone with an AI of 0.50 will have considerably more difficulty. By comparing one's performance to that predicted by the AI, described in more detail below, one can gain an estimate of the speech-processing problems that may remain even after audibility is restored and thereby provide more appropriate counseling.

Contributions to Differential Diagnosis

In addition to determining the effects of reduced absolute and differential sensitivity, evaluation of speech processing is a critical part of the differential diagnostic battery. Although there is a wide range of speech-processing abilities across auditory pathologies, the assessment is particularly informative in the diagnostic process when performed at more than one intensity level (Jerger and Jerger, 1971). When evaluating speech processing, the type and degree of the hearing loss, age of the patient, and linguistic sophistication must be considered. Because of the variety of speech materials and assessment procedures, there are limited normative data across these variables of age, type, and degree of loss for interpretation of a single score. Some experts argue that speech audiometry is of limited diagnostic value because of the wide dispersion of performance scores (Bess, 1983). There are general trends reported in the literature that contribute to the differential diagnostic process of general site of lesion rather than specific etiology. For example, it has been shown that patients with conductive losses have excellent recognition of single words (> 90%) when presented at comfortable listening levels. However, patients with losses of the same degree but sensorineural in nature generally will have reduced speech recognition (Hood and Poole, 1971).

To evaluate the significance of reduced speech recognition scores, audiologists should compare speech recognition performance to that expected for patients with similar degrees of the hearing loss. One useful set of data is provided by Dubno and colleagues (1995), who determined the 95% confidence limit for maximum recognition of specific speech materials for patients with sensorineural hearing loss of varying degrees, as discussed below. When speech recognition is outside the 95% confidence limit for that degree of loss, it may be indicative of retrocochlear pathology and the need for further evaluation.

Perhaps the greatest diagnostic significance of speech audiometry is the reduction in speech recognition with increasing intensity, or the "rollover" effect that occurs with retrocochlear pathologies (Dirks et al, 1977; Jerger and Jerger, 1971). A discrepancy in performance between scores from a patient's two ears or between word and sentence recognition is also suggestive of retrocochlear pathology. To increase the diagnostic significance of speech audiometry, the test battery must be expanded to include testing across different intensity levels, types of materials, and/or competing backgrounds.

Pearl

- Rollover occurs when the speech recognition score decreases more than 20% from the maximum performance obtained at a lower intensity level. This is consistent with retrocochlear pathology (Jerger and Jerger, 1971).

Application to Hearing Aid Fittings and Auditory Rehabilitation

Speech audiometry plays a significant role in the recommendation for amplification. Pure-tone thresholds unquestionably may indicate the need for amplification, and it can quickly be determined that average conversational speech is not completely audible using techniques such as the AI (Mueller and Killion, 1990), described below. However, the evaluation of speech processing as part of the hearing aid fitting also involves examining the relationship of average conversational speech to a patient's dynamic range, as shown in **Fig. 14–2**. For this patient exhibiting a flat hearing loss of 70 dB HL and uncomfortable listening levels of 90 dB HL, the gain required to amplify average conversational speech so that it is suprathreshold yet below the patient's uncomfortable listening levels is only 25 dB at 2 kHz. This results in the speech information at 2 kHz being ~9 dB SL (sensation level) and below the 90 dB HL discomfort level. If, instead, a half-gain rule were applied at 2 kHz, this

patient would receive 35 dB of gain that would result in the speech information being amplified beyond the discomfort level or being unfavorably limited by the hearing aid.

Unless patients and their significant others indicate through informal discussion or formal handicap measures that the loss of hearing interferes with their daily communication, a hearing aid evaluation may not be warranted. When daily communication is affected, the results of speech audiometry help to determine potential hearing aid benefit. For example, if speech recognition improves when stimuli are presented at a more intense level than typical conversational speech, the patient is likely to benefit from amplification. Conversely, if the speech recognition deteriorates at increased intensity levels, perhaps resulting from a reduced dynamic range, the prognosis for successful use of amplification is more guarded, and the need for alternate communication strategies is emphasized.

Once it has been determined that amplification will be of potential benefit, the perception of speech through the hearing aid(s) must be assessed. The audibility of speech may be determined through a procedure called "live speech mapping." This is a measure of the aided output in the ear canal through a real-ear system while someone is speaking to the patient. The speaker may be the audiologist or a family member. The real-ear equipment will average the output, and it can be displayed relative to prescribed targets. Also, by looking at the plot of the speech output relative to the patient's thresholds, the audibility of normal conversational speech can be verified. Furthermore, the speaker may present soft and loud speech for verification (Ross and Smith, 2005).

In addition to audibility of speech, patients must be assured that speech is as intelligible as it was without amplification. It is possible to provide amplification that restores audibility of the signal but results in reduced recognition (Van Tasell and Crain, 1992). It is important that perceptible and significant gains in recognition in quiet and/or in noise are achieved. Such gains may not be realized at the initial fitting (Gatehouse, 1993) but should be assessed during a trial period.

Audiologists must document gains in speech recognition performance for patients to justify the fitting of amplification. Improved performance relative to the unaided condition can easily be documented except perhaps in cases of mild, high-frequency hearing loss. Showing the benefits of new technology, compared with the patient's present hearing aid(s), may be more difficult. Research with new hearing aid circuits, including digital signal processing, has often failed to show clinically significant differences in speech recognition over traditional amplification, despite patients' subjective preference for the newer technology (Prinz et al, 2002; Wood and Lutman, 2004). As hearing aid technology has moved beyond the basic premise of restoring audibility, the demands for more sensitive speech assessment procedures have increased. For example, the benefits of circuits designed to address poor frequency resolution may not be evident by measuring the percent of correct recognition of word lists but require a more sensitive measure, such as the discrimination of high-frequency second-formant transitions (Thibodeau and Van Tasell, 1987). Likewise, the benefit

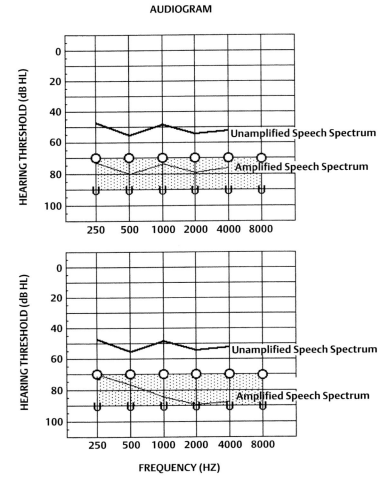

Figure 14–2 Relationship of unamplified (heavy line) and amplified (thin line) average speech spectrum to a patient's dynamic range (shaded region). Speech spectrum is from Pascoe (1975). The upper audiogram illustrates 25 dB gain, and the lower one represents application of a half-gain rule.

of advanced noise reduction strategies will require more sensitive, yet time efficient, speech evaluation procedures. Perhaps the greatest challenge and impetus for change in speech audiometry practices will be the development of more sophisticated speech materials to allow assessment of hearing aid benefit.

◆ Variables in Speech Evaluation Paradigms

Speech Acoustics

To select appropriate speech materials and evaluate the results obtained, the importance of the acoustics of the signal being presented must be considered. A brief review of the

long- and short-term characteristics of the speech signal will be provided; an in-depth review of speech acoustics relative to hearing loss may be found in Van Tasell (1986). When assessing speech processing, one must know the typical level of conversational speech that a patient will encounter in everyday life. By averaging conversational speech levels over time, the long-term speech spectrum can be determined (Olsen et al, 1987), as shown in **Fig. 14–2**. It is important to note, for reasons given below, that the most intense portion of the spectrum is in the 0.5 kHz region. The average overall level of speech is ~74 dB SPL (sound pressure level; Benson and Hirsh, 1953), which corresponds to 61 dB HL on the audiometer for insert phones and 54 dB HL for Telephonics Dynamic Headphones (TDH) 39 earphones (Telephonics Corporation, Huntington, NY; American National Standards Institute [ANSI], 2004). When a measure of speech processing at conversational levels is desired, 50 dB HL is the typical level used.

Special Consideration

- It is important to note that when speech stimuli are administered at 30 dB above a patient's threshold, all of the speech sounds may not, in fact, be audible.

Regarding the short-term characteristics of speech, the intensity range from the weakest to the most intense phoneme is ~30 dB (Fletcher, 1970). Vowels are more intense and longer in duration than consonants and, consequently, more intelligible. During the typical speech assessment, the weak consonants are often inaudible for persons with hearing loss of a moderate or greater degree. Particularly, patients with high-frequency hearing loss may find low-intensity fricatives and sibilants inaudible even at an overall presentation level of 80 dB HL, as shown in **Fig. 14–3**. For a patient with a severe sensorineural loss above 1 kHz, the high-frequency consonants in the shaded region will not be audible even when speech is delivered at 80 dB HL from the audiometer. Therefore, true maximum speech recognition may not be observed in the typical clinical evaluation because the speech signal is not spectrally shaped to compensate for the hearing loss when presented through the audiometer.

Knowing the types of speech cues most likely to be misperceived is useful when analyzing error types. Through analysis of consonant confusion matrices obtained from normal-hearing persons who listened to speech through a variety of filtering conditions, it was determined that voicing and manner cues are carried across the frequency spectrum. However, place of articulation is cued primarily in high-frequency information (Dubno and Levitt, 1985). Therefore, one would expect a patient with a high-frequency hearing loss to have the most difficulty with place information. These error patterns were confirmed by Olsen and Matkin (1979), who also reported that consonant errors were likely to be substitutions rather than omissions. When omissions did occur, they were most likely for final consonant sounds.

Recent advances in hearing aid technology may have effects on the temporal characteristics of the speech signal (e.g., adaptive compression), making it important to know the temporal characteristics of sounds, syllables, and pauses between words in sentences. To evaluate the effects of technology that alter the signal in the temporal domain, the duration of the stimuli must be considered in relationship to temporal processing. For example, to evaluate the effects of a compression system that is designed to vary the release time relative to the duration of the signal that set it into compression, speech stimuli must be used that will allow observation of this effect. It is unlikely that presenting lists of monosyllabic words of relatively equal duration would reveal the effects of such a circuit, whereas, presenting connected speech in the presence of background noise with an average duration between words of 200 msec might reveal differences between an adaptive release time circuit and one with a fixed release time less than 150 msec.

Temporal characteristics of importance to these decisions include not only the duration of speech sounds but also the duration of pauses between words and syllables. Pickett (1999) provides an overview of how the duration of individual sounds depends on their position relative to pauses, syllables, stress, linguistic content, and acoustic features. For example, vowels can range from 52 to 212 msec but average 130 msec when in a stressed syllable and 70 msec in an unstressed syllable (Klatt, 1976). In addition, vowels are ~20 msec shorter when followed by a voiceless stop consonant (Umeda, 1975). Consonants vary from 25 msec for a stop consonant such as /t/ preceding a stressed vowel, to 86 msec for a nasal consonant such as /m/ in the initial stressed syllable of a word. As with vowels, consonant duration is

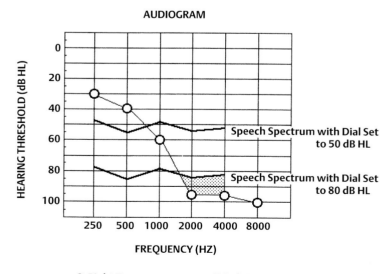

Figure 14–3 Audibility of speech for a patient with a severe high-frequency hearing loss. Speech spectrum is from Pascoe (1975). The shaded region represents the portion of the speech spectrum that is not audible even at a higher presentation level on the audiometer.

~20 to 40 msec longer in words having higher content meaning (Umeda, 1977). Consonants such as /s/ can range from a duration of more than 200 msec at the end of a phrase to 50 msec in a consonant cluster.

Syllable duration is also influenced by stress and proximity to pauses. Initial syllables range from 130 to 483 msec, whereas final syllables preceding a pause range from 243 to 516 msec (Crystal and House, 1990). Pauses that occur between syllables, words, and sentences are related to speaking rate. For conversational speech, the rate is typically 200 words per minute. When speakers are instructed to speak "clearly," the rate is typically 100 words per minute (Picheny et al, 1989). Pauses account for ~20% of the time during reading and up to 50% of the time in conversation (Klatt, 1976).

Given a speaking rate of 200 words per minute and a pause rate of 50%, the average word and pause duration would be 150 msec each. It is argued that hearing aids with fast-acting compression circuits (i.e., release times of 40 to 50 msec) would potentially allow background noise to be amplified during pauses (Teder, 1993). Therefore, evaluation of such circuits or adaptive release time circuits must include speech stimuli of appropriate durations for the electroacoustic effect, or lack thereof, to be experienced.

Level of Auditory Ability Assessed

Unfortunately, speech processing is often assessed without regard for the cognitive demands required by the auditory processing task. This is particularly important when testing children, so that low scores are not interpreted as impaired performance when a child is not capable of performing at that level of auditory processing. As mentioned earlier, evaluation of speech processing can be considered in terms of a hierarchy of auditory processing that is often used as a guide for establishing auditory training activities (Erber, 1982). It is necessary to relate traditional audiological tests to the hierarchy to illustrate the misconceptions associated with the typical speech test erroneously called "word discrimination."

Pearl

- Speech assessments can be performed at various levels of processing, including awareness, discrimination, identification/recognition, and comprehension.

Audiological tests at the simplest level of processing (awareness) are known as speech awareness or detection thresholds. In an infant, this may be a change in some observable behavior, such as eye widening, sucking, or general body movement. For the toddler, the awareness response may be a turn to the sound source, which is then reinforced by a visual stimulus. Preschoolers may respond to speech via play audiometry, where a block is dropped in a bucket upon hearing speech.

Although auditory discrimination, the next level of auditory processing proposed by Erber (1982), can be evaluated

in many ways, there are no tests of discrimination routinely used in the audiological battery. The evaluation of discrimination, that is, one's ability to detect a change in the acoustic stimulus, is accomplished in young infants by using a dishabituation response recorded as a change in sucking or heart rate (Eimas et al, 1971). In toddlers, the dis-habituation response may be a head turn. When paired with appropriate visual training, children's speech discrimination may be tested with the oddity paradigm as young as 4 years of age. By age 5 or 6, a same/different paradigm is often used to evaluate discrimination. For adults, discrimination of speech features has most often been measured using an ABX procedure, in which the listener determines if the first (A) or second (B) stimulus is the same as the last one (X). In all of these procedures, the patient is required to respond only when a change has been perceived in some acoustic dimension of the stimulus, such as the intensity, frequency, or timing. Patients may respond by changing an ongoing response when an auditory change is noted, by indicating which item in a stimulus sequence is different, or by comparing two stimuli and indicating if they were identical or not. Therefore, when assessing auditory discrimination, the patient is merely comparing stimuli. Using the term *word discrimination* to refer to the evaluation of speech processing during the audiological exam is not accurate because the typical clinical procedure requires the patient to repeat what is heard, which is the next level of auditory processing, identification or recognition.

The next level, auditory identification/recognition, may be accomplished by selecting an object, pointing to a picture, or producing the stimulus in written or verbal form. Patients must recognize the sequence of sounds and then associate it with some previous experience. Recognition tasks differ from the next level of processing in that no semantic processing is required. That is, the patient may be able to imitate the word *laud* but not be able to define it or use it in a sentence. Typical audiological speech assessments at the recognition level of processing include the SRT and the WRS and SRS. It is important to note that audiologists typically perform recognition tests as a function of intensity level. A recognition test is usually administered at the threshold level and at one or more suprathreshold levels. It is becoming increasingly common to also include another recognition test at a suprathreshold level in the presence of background noise.

Auditory comprehension, the final level of auditory processing in Erber's (1982) hierarchy, is not routinely assessed during the clinical audiological battery. However, in some cases, assessment of auditory comprehension may be accomplished most efficiently in a sound-treated room with the precise presentation level known to be audible for the patient. For example, following simple commands or answering the "5W" questions ("who," "what," "when," "where," and "why") at a fixed intensity level in a sound booth removes the possibility of errors resulting from distractions or intensity variations with live-voice presentation. Because evaluation of auditory comprehension is not within the scope of this chapter, the reader is referred to Johnson and colleagues (1997), who discuss this level of auditory processing and associated materials in detail.

Response Format

There are two general types of response formats: open and closed set. For closed-set tasks, the patient will have objects, pictures, or printed stimuli from which to choose. For open-set tasks, there are three response options: repeat the stimuli orally, write the stimuli on paper, or type the stimuli on a keyboard. Response formats largely depend on the age of the patient. Younger children are more likely to respond in closed-set formats because of limited vocabulary and oral/graphic skills, whereas older patients with normal speech production are likely to repeat the stimuli, which is the most time-efficient format.

A closed-set task results in the greatest scoring accuracy because the response is clearly indicated. If time permits, obtaining a written response can be more accurate than receiving a verbal one. Interpretation of the verbal response may be influenced by the articulation of the patient and by the bandwidth and signal-to-noise ratio (SNR) of the monitoring system. Furthermore, there is a tendency for the examiner to err in favor of accepting an incorrect verbal response (Merrell and Atkinson, 1965). When testing young children whose articulation skills are still developing, two examiners may be needed: one to deliver the stimuli and monitor responses through the talkback system, and the other to manipulate response choices and monitor responses from within the test room (see Chapter 15).

Speech Stimuli

Possible types of speech stimuli range from nonsense syllables to connected speech. **Table 14–1** contains a summary of the relative advantages and disadvantages of the types of speech materials as presented by Tyler (1994). Two major factors influencing selection of the material are patient age and the purpose of the evaluation.

Once the vocabulary level is determined, the purpose of the assessment will dictate the materials to be used. If the goal is to determine which acoustic features can be identified, a representative sample of speech sounds that is not influenced by phonemic or syntactic constraints is necessary. For example, a patient may hear *boke* and respond that the word is *broke* or *boat* because these phonemic combinations are possible in English as opposed to *bsoke* or *bopke*. Because familiarity with the language and one's ability to guess influence responses when whole words are used, a true assessment of "hearing" speech features must be done using nonsense syllables, such as the Nonsense Syllable Test (Levitt and Resnick, 1978).

When evaluating a patient's ability to use context, speech stimuli that differ in semantic relationships will be needed. One such test is Speech Perception in Noise (SPIN; Bilger et al, 1984), which is composed of sentences with the final word either semantically related (high probability) or not related (low probability) to the remainder of the sentence. Differences in the scores on the high- and low-probability lists reflect the degree to which the patient benefits from semantic context.

Another purpose of speech assessment may be to determine the minimum intensity level required for 50% speech recognition, that is, the speech recognition threshold. This preferred term is synonymous with the traditional term *speech reception threshold* (ASHA, 1988). For this test, it is necessary for the stimuli to be as homogeneous as possible with respect to time and intensity so that intelligibility is equivalent across the words in the list. Young and colleagues (1982) recommended the following list of 15 spondaic words that were determined to be homogeneous in SPL:

inkwell	baseball	toothbrush
playground	workshop	northwest
sidewalk	doormat	mousetrap
railroad	grandson	drawbridge
woodwork	eardrum	padlock

Pearl

- First and foremost in selecting speech evaluation materials, the vocabulary level must be appropriate; otherwise the test will reflect the effects of language as well as hearing abilities.

Pearl

- A common purpose for assessing speech recognition performance is to predict how much difficulty that person may have in the real world as a result of the hearing loss.

Table 14–1 Relative Merits of Different Types of Speech Materials

Speech Stimulus	Advantages	Disadvantages
Nonsense syllables	Examine phonetic errors; use of closed set; linguistic knowledge not an influence	Perceived poor face validity; no evaluation of context or coarticulation effects
Words	High face validity; relatively easy to adapt to closed set, requiring picture-pointing response, short administration time	Some words may be overused and not truly open set; familiarity with language may be an influence
Sentences/phrases	High face validity; includes coarticulation effects; allows for evaluation of temporal effects	Influenced by linguistic knowledge; requires more time to administer and possibly score
Paragraph	Highest face validity; can be used for judgments of intelligibility and quality	More time to administer; possible confound if familiar with the topic

Source: Adapted from Tyler, R. (1994). The use of speech-perception tests in audiological rehabilitation: Current and future research needs. Journal of the Academy of Rehabilitative Audiology, 27, 47–66, with permission.

To predict real-world performance, ideally the stimuli must have great face validity and be a subset of what the patient will encounter in the real world. Much effort has been spent on developing lists that are phonetically balanced, representative words encountered in English. For historical reviews of these studies, the reader is referred to Bess (1983) and Penrod (1994). The question of whether a sample of single words will be predictive of performance with sentences has been raised. Boothroyd and Nittrouer (1988) and Olsen et al (1997) have shown that the scores on tests of single-word recognition are predictive of performance on sentence recognition. Their results support the notion that speech recognition is a generalized skill and that scores on all speech recognition tests are related. Therefore, audiologists may choose from a variety of available speech stimuli to assess speech recognition, but such decisions will be influenced by a trade-off between time and reliability.

A survey of 218 audiologists across the United States by Martin et al (1998) revealed that word lists, rather than sentence lists, were used by 92% of the respondents. Common speech recognition lists were the Central Institute for the Deaf W-22 (CID W-22) (48%) and the Northwestern University 6 (NU-6) (44%), the origins of which are described by Penrod (1994). Interestingly, comparison with similar surveys conducted since 1985 showed that the use of CID W-22 lists was declining, whereas the NU-6 lists were increasing in popularity. Most audiologists (56%) administer half lists (25 words) to each ear. Bess (1983) reviews the controversy in the literature in the 1960s and 1970s regarding the issues surrounding using half lists, including disruption of the phonetic balance of the list and reduced reliability with fewer stimulus presentations. However, the size of the list to present must be determined based on the purpose of testing. If a half list is presented to determine a general estimate of speech recognition ability, one must interpret the score according to the critical difference range for 25-word lists, as described below. When pathology results in slight changes in speech recognition, the percent correct measures at a fixed intensity level are probably not as sensitive as an adaptive procedure.

Thornton and Raffin (1978) showed that the sensitivity of a speech measure is proportional to the number of trials administered. They developed a probabilistic model based on speech recognition as a binomial distribution; that is, the variability in performance is highest in the middle range of scores and lowest at the extreme ranges of scores (0 and 100%). If a recognition test stimulus is scored as correct or incorrect and the total score reflects the percentage of the items perceived correctly, then test scores may be compared with the critical differences determined by Thornton and Raffin for a given number of test items, as shown in **Table 14–2**. For example, if an initial test score was 80% on a 50-item list, a subsequent score would have to fall outside the range of 64 to 92% to be considered significantly different at the 95% confidence level. In other words, there is a 95% probability that on repeated tests, a patient having a score of 80% will receive a score between 64 and 92%. However, if a 25-item list were presented, the subsequent score would have to be lower than 56% or higher than 96% to be significantly different. If a 10-item

Table 14–2   Critical Differences for Speech Recognition Scores[*]

Initial Speech Recognition Score (%)	100 Items	50 Items	25 Items	10 Items
90	81–96	76–98	72–100	50–100
80	68–89	64–92	56–96	40–100
70	57–81	52–86	48–92	30–90
60	47–73	42–78	36–84	20–90
50	37–63	32–68	28–76	10–90
40	27–53	22–58	16–64	10–80
30	19–43	14–48	12–56	10–70
20	11–32	8–36	4–44	0–60
10	4–19	2–24	4–32	0–50

[*] For a given number of test items, values within each range are not significantly different from the initial speech recognition score ($p > .05$).

Source: Adapted from Thornton, A. R., & Raffin, M. J. M. (1978). Speech discrimination scores modified as a binomial variable. Journal of Speech and Hearing Research, 21, 507–518, with permission.

list were presented, the critical difference range increases to 40 to 100%.

One solution to the trade-off dilemma has been proposed by Olsen et al (1997), who suggest using isophonemic word lists comprised of 10 consonant-vowel-consonants (CVCs) that are scored by phonemes rather than whole word correct. Two lists of 10 words each can be presented monaurally in approximately 2 minutes, less time than required for 25 monosyllables. If the two scores are not significantly different according to the Thornton and Raffin (1978) critical differences, the two can be averaged to represent the speech recognition performance for that ear. If variability is high and the two scores are different, additional lists will be required.

Presentation Mode

Speech audiometry stimuli can be presented by monitored live voice or recorded voice. Use of live voice is convenient and allows for flexibility and reduced administration time. Live-voice presentation is often used for determination of the SRT, despite the ASHA (1988) recommendation to use recorded materials. Fewer audiologists use live-voice presentation for suprathreshold speech recognition testing (82% vs 94% of surveyed audiologists; Martin et al, 1998). Live voice may be more acceptable for threshold testing because the patient is responding primarily to the intense vowel sounds that are generally equated by monitoring the peaks on the volume unit (VU) meter. However, for suprathreshold recognition testing, performance depends more on receiving less intense consonant information that cannot be monitored by the fast action of the VU meter. Furthermore, the SRT contributes less to the differential diagnosis and is primarily used to confirm the pure-tone testing results. However, the speech recognition score contributes to the site-of-lesion determination, and, therefore, greater precision is required.

Pearl

- For determining the speech recognition score, it is imperative that prerecorded stimuli are presented that have been equated for intensity, so that scores reflect true performance of the patient and not variations in the speaker.

Increased reliability of performance with taped rather than live-voice presentation has been consistently demonstrated (Brandy, 1966; Hood and Poole, 1980), yet it warrants reiteration according to the results of the most recent practice survey. Martin et al (1998) reported that 82% of audiologists responding to the survey are still using monitored live-voice presentation. Reasons for this most likely include the greater flexibility for the examiner and perhaps lack of equipment. It is hoped that the move toward recorded presentation will increase as manufacturers are more likely to include compact disc players with audiometers that facilitate access to particular lists.

A study that clearly illustrates the problems associated with live-voice testing for speech recognition was performed by Brandy in 1966. Speech recognition scores for 25-word lists were obtained from 24 patients with normal hearing. Half of the patients listened to three different recordings from the same talker, and the other half listened to three randomizations of one recording of the same talker. Variation in scores across the three different recordings by the same talker was significant (9.76%), whereas variation in scores for the same recording was nonsignificant (3.3%). Given the inherent variability in speech recognition testing even when recorded materials are used, as illustrated by Thornton and Raffin (1978), monitored live-voice testing must be done in situations deemed last resort. Such situations include (1) equipment limitations so great that even a cassette player or compact disc player is not available and

(2) testing patients that demand frequent interaction to maintain attention and complete the test.

Often live-voice testing is considered more expedient. However, stretching this logic, the time argument could also be used to rationalize the use of tuning forks for pure-tone audiometry. Audiologists agree that this would not be a very sensitive or reliable measure of hearing. In addition, it would be difficult to determine the degree of hearing loss without reference to some calibrated standard for normal hearing. The same criterion for precision is also required for reliable speech-processing measures.

Pearl

- It has been argued that if limited time precludes the use of taped speech materials, then time should be preserved by not administering speech tests at all (Stach, 1998).

Presentation Level

Depending on the purpose of the speech recognition assessment, the stimuli may be presented at the level of average conversation, the most comfortable listening level for the patient, or the level necessary to achieve maximum performance. To contribute to the differential diagnostic process, several presentation levels may be necessary to determine which one affords the patient the maximum opportunity for clear recognition and to determine if performance declines with increased intensity (i.e., rollover).

Pearl

- Evaluation of speech recognition at several intensity levels is referred to as a performance intensity (PI) function.

The shape of the PI function is unique not only for a given patient but also for the type of material used. PI functions for nonsense syllables, words, and sentences are shown in **Fig. 14–4.** The function for sentences is the steepest where

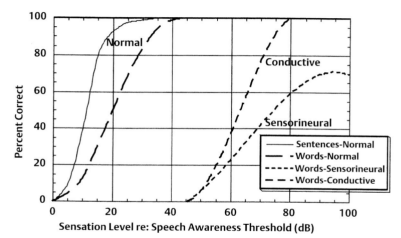

Figure 14–4 Performance intensity functions for sentences and words for patients with normal hearing and for words for patients with conductive and sensorineural hearing loss. Adapted from Hood, J. D., & Poole, J. P. (1971). Speech audiometry in conductive and sensorineural hearing loss. Sound, 5, 30–38, with permission.

each dB of intensity results in ~10% increase in recognition. However, for words, each dB increase results in about a 4% increase.

By obtaining a PI function, audiologists can determine the maximum performance for each patient, referred to as PBmax, when phonetically balanced monosyllabic word lists are used. To evaluate the significance of the PBmax score, it may be compared with data obtained from patients with similar degrees of sensorineural hearing (Dubno et al, 1995), as described in "Interpretation of Results." If the PBmax is disproportionately low relative to others with similar hearing loss, it is suggestive of retrocochlear pathology.

It is often not clinically feasible to evaluate speech processing at several intensity levels. Therefore, in an attempt to achieve PBmax and determine if rollover is present, testing may begin at a high level, such as 80 dB HL, unless this level is less than the SRT + 30 dB (80 dB HL < SRT + 30). If the 80 dB HL level is adequate, and the measured score is 84% or higher when a half list is used, further testing to determine PBmax is not necessary. The reason is that even if the maximum possible score of 100% was obtained at a lower intensity, the difference score of 16% is less than the 20% criterion difference to be considered rollover (Jerger and Jerger, 1971). However, if a score below 84% is achieved, it could mean one of two things: a higher presentation level is needed to achieve PBmax because of reduced audibility of the signal, or a lower presentation level is needed because the score reflects rollover.

The decision to present a second list at an intensity level above or below 80 dB HL will be determined by the pure-tone average (PTA). If the PTA is above 40 dB HL, it is likely that a higher presentation level is necessary to achieve PBmax because the AI predicts that the entire spectrum may not have been audible at 80 dB HL presentation level. However, if the PTA is less than 40 dB HL, the AI predicts that the speech information should have been audible, and a lower presentation level would determine if the low score was suggestive of rollover.

Pitfall

- When using a high-intensity presentation level during speech audiometry, the probability for crossover is high, and masking may be needed (see Chapter 13).

Evaluation of speech recognition for rehabilitation purposes should include presenting stimuli at an average conversational level (50 dB HL) to demonstrate to the patient the effects of reduced audibility and potential for improvement with amplification. It may also be helpful to determine the recognition performance at the patient's most comfortable loudness (MCL). These results may facilitate patient counseling regarding the gradual adjustment to amplification of speech to levels above the MCL that may be required to receive maximum benefit.

Calibration for Speech Stimuli

Presentation of complex signals requires different calibration procedures than those used for pure-tone testing.

Table 14–3   Sound Pressure Levels for Normal Hearing of Speech for Various Transducers

Transducer*	dB SPL for Normal Hearing of Speech**	dB HL Equivalent
Earphone: TDH 39	19.5	0
Earphone: TDH 49	19.5	0
Earphone: TDH 50	20.0	0
Insert phone: EAR 3A	12.5	0
Sound field speaker: 0 degree azimuth	16.5	0
Sound field speaker: 45 degrees azimuth	12.5	0

*All TDH earphones are mounted in MX-41/AR cushions.

**All earphone values are determined in an NBS 9A 6 cc coupler with the exception of EAR 3A insert phone values, which were measured in a dB-0138 2 cc coupler.

HL, hearing level; SPL, sound pressure level.

Source: Data from American National Standards Institute. (2004). American National Standards specifications for audiometers (ANSI S3.6–2004). New York: Author.

Because speech is a dynamic signal that results in difficulty determining a precise level, a steady 1 kHz tone is used for calibration of speech levels. The audiometer level is set so that the output from the earphone is 20 dB above the HL dial value for a TDH-50 earphone. That is, 0 dB HL, or normal hearing for speech, is equivalent to 20 dB SPL (ANSI, 2004). SPLs for normal hearing for speech are provided in **Table 14–3**. When recorded materials are produced, a calibration tone precedes the stimuli. This tone is generally recorded at a level that is equivalent to the frequent peaks of the speech signal unless otherwise specified. The calibration tone should be set to peak at 0 V on the VU meter.

When calibrating for sound field testing, factors that must be accounted for include distance from the speaker, azimuth, ear canal resonance, head shadow, and standing waves. Reference levels for speech recognition at 0 and 45 degrees azimuth are 16.5 dB SPL and 12.5 dB SPL, respectively (ASHA, 1991). Because pure-tone signals can combine and cancel when presented in rooms with reflective surfaces resulting in standing waves, the calibration stimulus for speech in the sound field is speech-weighted noise. Even though the threshold for speech will be lower in the sound field than under phones because of the advantages of ear canal acoustics, the calibration values are such that the sound field and earphone testing are equated. In other words, when the audiometer is calibrated properly for sound field and earphone testing, the average SRTs obtained monaurally under phones and in the sound field essentially should be equal given normal test–retest variability.

Procedures

There are several different measures used in speech audiometry. If assessing awareness of speech, the procedure will be an adaptive one to determine the level at which speech is just barely audible. For assessment of speech recognition, there are at least three choices: (1) present speech stimuli at a fixed presentation level and measure the percent correctly identified; (2) present running speech at a fixed presentation level and measure intelligibility by percentage; and (3) present words or sentences in an adaptive paradigm and determine the intensity level necessary to achieve 50% correct recognition. The first method to assess speech recognition has been used by a majority of audiologists since at least 1972 (Martin et al, 1998). With regard to connected speech, equivalent passages have been developed for patients to rate intelligibility and are known as the Connected Speech Test (Cox and McDaniel, 1989). However, these have been used primarily for hearing aid comparisons. Adaptive procedures have been shown to be sensitive measures of the effects of hearing loss configuration or selective amplification (Van Tasell and Yanz, 1987). One advantage of adaptive tests over a fixed presentation level is reducing ceiling and floor effects. There is currently only one commercially available clinical test of speech recognition with normative data employing an adaptive procedure, the Hearing in Noise Test (HINT), in which the patient repeats sentences presented with a fixed-level background noise (Nilsson et al, 1994). Originally designed for the assessment of binaural hearing in noise in the sound field, this test has not been used as a routine clinical assessment of monaural speech recognition.

Other procedures are required for the determination of the loudness of speech, which include MCL and uncomfortable loudness level (UCL, ULL). These levels are typically determined with an adaptive procedure where the patient is asked to judge the loudness of running speech as the level is adjusted. Hawkins (1984) recommends using an ascending method of limits to determine the UCL. He defines it as that level between the patient's judgments of "loud, but OK" and "uncomfortably loud."

Analysis of Results

For suprathreshold measures of speech recognition, percent correct scores are generally reported. However, if a closed set is used, the probability of guessing must be considered. For example, chance performance on a test with a response set of 4 items is 25%. Rather than whole-word scoring for open-set testing, Olsen et al (1997) suggest scoring by phonemes. Perhaps a more useful summary of performance would be to analyze error patterns by means of a confusion matrix. Error patterns associated with various configurations of hearing loss as reported in the literature (Bilger and Wang, 1976) could be used for comparison purposes to determine if a patient's error patterns were typical for his or her hearing loss. If not, additional counseling may be needed. Unfortunately, such an analysis is not available as a convenient clinical tool at this time.

If an adaptive procedure is used, then some average value will be determined based on a given number of reversals. For example, HINT (Nilsson et al, 1994) involves varying the level of the sentences and averaging the levels at which the

response changed from correct to incorrect or vice versa. If a simple up-down procedure is used, the threshold represents the level at which 50% correct performance would be achieved.

Interpretation of Results

Regardless of presentation, stimuli, response format, and analysis, the results are most valuable if they can be compared with normative values for interpretation. To compare results, one must use procedures identical to those used with the standardization sample. It is evident from PI functions (**Fig. 14–4**) that considerable variation in performance occurs across presentation level and speech stimuli. Therefore, standardized procedures are needed against which to compare speech recognition scores. Despite the variety of clinical materials available for assessing speech recognition, there are few with normative databases on standardized procedures. It is often assumed that the norm for comparison is the level achieved by persons with normal hearing. If testing were performed in quiet using common English vocabulary, the predicted norm would be 100%. This may be acceptable if test conditions allow the entire speech spectrum to be audible, but generally this is not the case. Therefore, it is important to assess how missing high-frequency information would affect a score on a speech recognition test. Two simplified clinical procedures are described below to facilitate interpretation of speech recognition by accounting for audibility: a Count-the-Dot audiogram and a Speech Recognition Interpretation (SPRINT) chart.

Special Consideration

- Some speech recognition materials are available in Spanish and French (**Table 14–4**); however, normative data to aid interpretation of results are limited. Further information regarding issues in cultural diversity is given in Chapter 15.

One way to compare speech performance based on audibility of the signal is to use the Count-the-Dot audiogram, which is based on the AI developed by French and Steinberg (1947), with modifications by several researchers for clinical applications (Humes, 1991; Mueller and Killion, 1990; Pavlovic, 1989). The AI ranges from 0 to 1 and represents the proportion of the speech spectrum that is available to convey information to the patient. It is computed from acoustical measurements of the speech spectrum, the effective masking spectrum of any noises, the relative importance of frequency regions, and the auditory dynamic range of the patient. These measurements can be made in each of 15 one-third-octave bands throughout the speech range.

Pearl

- The articulation index reflects the audibility of the speech spectrum and represents the proportion that is available to the patient.

Table 14–4 Hierarchy of Speech Perception Measures

Code	Test	Author	Recommended Age	Stimuli	Presentation Format	Response	Norms
Awareness							
SDT	Speech detection threshold	ASHA (1988)	Birth to 3 years	Monosyllabic words	Live voice	Behavioral change	Northern and Downs (1991)
Discrimination							
ADT	Auditory Discrimination Test	Wepman (1973)	5–8 years	Monosyllabic word pairs	Live voice	Respond verbally, same/different	Yes
Identification							
SRT	Speech recognition threshold	ASHA (1988)	3–adult	Spondees	Tape or CD[1,6]	Repeat the word or point to pictures	ANSI (2004)
GFW	GFW Diagnostic Auditory Discrimination Test	Goldman et al (1974)	3–adult	Monosyllabic words presented in quiet	Tape[4]	Point to one of two pictures	Included in manual, based on age
WIPI	Word Intelligibility by Picture Identification	Ross and Lerman (1970; rev. 2004)	4–6 years	Four equivalent lists of 25 monosyllabic words each	Tape or CD[1]	Point to one of six pictures	Papso and Blood (1989), Sanderson-Leepa and Rintelmann (1976)
NU-CHIPS	Northwestern University Children's Perception of Speech	Elliott and Katz (1980)	3–5 years	50 monosyllabic words	Tape or CD[1]	Point to one of four pictures	Included in manual
PSI	Pediatric Speech Intelligibility Test	Jerger and Jerger (1982)	3–6 years	20 monosyllabic words and two sentence formats in two lists of 10 sentences each	Tape or CD[1]	Point to one of five pictures	Jerger and Jerger (1982)
TAC	Test of Auditory Comprehension	Trammel (1981)	4–17 years	Environmental sounds, words, stereotypic messages arranged in 10 subtests	Tape[2]	Point to one of three pictures	Included in manual, based on PTA and age
PBK	Phonetically balanced kindergarten word lists	Haskins (1949)	6–12 years	50 monosyllabic words	Tape or CD[1]	Repeat the words	Sanderson-Leepa and Rintelmann (1976)
BKB SIN	Bamford-Kowal-Bench Speech in Noise	Etymotic Research (2005)	5–14 years	Sentences	CD[7]	Repeat the sentence	Included in manual
HINT-C	Hearing in Noise Test for Children	Nilsson et al (1996)	6–12 years	Sentences	CD[5]	Repeat the sentence	Included in manual
HINT	Hearing in Noise Test	Nilsson et al (1994)	13 years and up	Sentences	CD[5]	Repeat the sentence	Included in manual
Quick SIN	Quick Speech in Noise	Etymotic Research (2001)	12 years and up	Sentences	CD[7]	Repeat the sentence	Included in manual
PAL PB 50	Psychoacoustics Laboratory phonetically balanced 50-word lists	Eagan (1948)	12 years and up	Monosyllabic words	Tape or CD[1]	Repeat the words	Yellin et al (1989)
CID W-22	Central Institute for the Deaf W-22	Hirsh et al (1952)	12 years and up	Monosyllabic words	Tape or CD[1]	Repeat the words	See text re using, Yellin et al (1989)

(Continued)

Table 14–4   *(Continued)*

NU-6	Northwestern University 6	Tillman and Carhart (1966)	12 years and up	Monosyllabic words	Tape or CD[1]	Repeat the words	Dubno et al (1995)
SPIN	Revised Speech Perception in Noise	Bilger et al (1984)	12 years and up	High and low predictability sentences	Tape[3]	Repeat the final word of the sentence	Included in manual
SSI	Synthetic Sentence Identification	Speaks and Jerger (1965)	12 years and up	Sentences that do not convey meaning	Tape or CD[1,6]	Identify the sentence from a list of ten	Jerger (1973)

[1]Available from Auditec of St. Louis, 2515 South Big Bend Boulevard, St. Louis, MO 63143; 314–781–8890, http://www/auditec.com.

[2]Portions are available from Foreworks Publications, Box 33493, Portland, OR 97292; 503–653–2614; http://www.foreworks.com/fore.html.

[3]Available from University of Illinois, Department of Speech and Hearing Science, 901 South Sixth Street, Champaign, IL, 61820; 217–333–2230.

[4]Available from American Guidance Service, 4201 Woodland Road, Circle Pines, MN 55014–1796; 800–328–2560.

[5]Available from Bio-logic Systems Corp, One Bio-logic Plaza, Mundelein, IL 60060; 800–272–8075; www.blsc.com/hearing/hint.html.

[6]Comparable materials in Spanish and French are available from Auditec of St. Louis, 2515 South Big Bend Boulevard, St. Louis, MO 63143; 314–781–8890; http://www/auditec.com.

[7]Available from: Etymotic Research, Inc., 61 Martin Lane, Elk Grove Village, IL 60007; www.etymotic.com.

ANSI, American National Standards Institute; ASHA, American Speech-Language-Hearing Association; CD, compact disc; PTA, pure-tone average.

Formally, the AI is defined as

$$AI = P_{I=1,15} BI(i) \ BE(i),$$

where *P* is a proficiency factor, considered to represent practice effects of the patient and precision with which test materials are enunciated; *BI* (band importance) is a weight chosen to represent the relative contribution of a given frequency band (*i*) to speech transmission under ideal conditions; and *BE* (band efficiency) is a measure of the proportion of the speech signal in a given band (*i*) that is above the patient's masked threshold and below the loudness discomfort level. Initial validation studies showed that the effects on speech recognition performance of varying frequency/gain characteristics by filtering or adding noise to the signal were well predicted by the AI for normal-hearing persons (French and Steinberg, 1947; Kryter, 1962). Standard normal curves (ANSI, 2002) relating speech recognition to AI are shown in **Fig. 14–5**.

Clinical adaptations of this procedure were developed so that the AI could be easily determined by plotting one's hearing thresholds on an audiogram, which had the relative weights of the speech information across the frequency range represented by dots. An example of the Count-the-Dot audiogram is shown in **Fig. 14–6**. This may be used as a reference against which to compare one's performance and determine if there are effects of the hearing loss on speech recognition beyond those accounted for by loss of audibility. Because the AI accounts for reduced absolute sensitivity, one may predict a speech recognition score after calculating the AI and by using the function in **Fig. 14–5**. The degree to which one's score deviates from that predicted by the AI reflects difficulties resulting from reduced differential sensitivity. For example, an AI of 0.2 predicts that the normal-hearing persons would achieve only ~50% correct speech recognition for single words. If the person with hearing impairment achieves less than this, then it may be concluded that the person was not able to use suprathreshold speech information as efficiently as normals. This may be the result of reduced differential sensitivity, such as poor frequency or temporal resolution (Pavlovic, 1984).

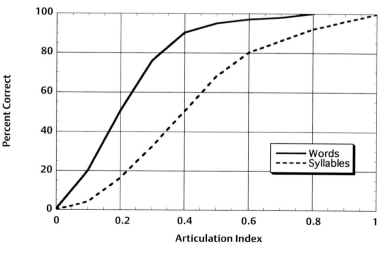

Figure 14–5 Articulation index function for words and syllables. Adapted from American National Standards Institute. (2002). Methods for the calculation of the speech intelligibility index (ANSI S3.5–1997, R2002). New York: Author with permission; and French, N. R., & Steinberg, J. C. (1947). Factors governing the intelligibility of speech sounds. Journal of the Acoustical Society of America, 19, 90–119, with permission.

COUNT-THE-DOT
AUDIOGRAM

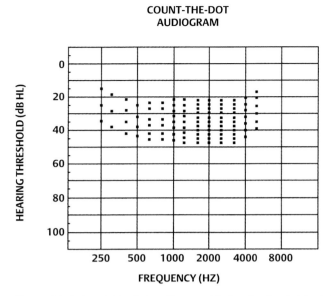

Figure 14–6 Count-the-Dot audiogram. HL, hearing level. Adapted from Mueller, H. G., & Killion, M. C. (1990). An easy method for calculating the articulation index. Hearing Journal, 43, 14–17, with permission.

Another way to evaluate performance is to use the SPRINT charts shown in **Figs. 14–7** and **14–8**. As mentioned earlier, performance can be compared within a patient through the use of the binomial distribution for speech developed by Thornton and Raffin (1978). They determined the degree to which a second speech recognition score must vary from an initial score to be significantly different at various confidence levels; the data in **Figs. 14–7** and **14–8** are based on a 95% level of confidence. To facilitate interpretation in the audiological setting, the SPRINT charts may serve as a reference sheet. The two charts were developed to quickly interpret the significance of the difference between two scores for 25- and 50-word lists. Vertical arrows represent the 95% confidence differences for percentage scores (Thornton and Raffin, 1978). If the intersection of the plot of the two scores, using the abscissa for the first score and the right ordinate for the second score, falls within the bounds of the arrow, then the two scores are not significantly different. It can easily be seen in both figures that the critical difference ranges are largest in the midrange of scores (40–60%) and decline at the upper and lower ranges of performance. For example, in **Fig. 14–7**, by looking at the arrow above the 40% score, it can be seen

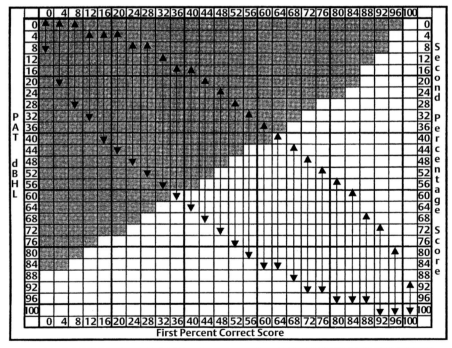

95% Confidence Limit for PBmax on NU6 25-word list. Plot score according to PTA on left ordinate and percent correct score on the abscissa. If it falls in the shaded area, it is considered disproportionately low. (Adapted from Dubno et al., 1995)

95% Critical differences for 25-word list. Plot first and second score according to the abscissa and right ordinate. If it falls within the arrow, the two scores are not significantly different (Adapted from Thornton & Raffin, 1978)

Copyright by Linda M. Thibodeau, 1999

Figure 14–7 Speech Recognition Interpretation (SPRINT) chart for 25-word NU-6 lists. HL, hearing level; PTA, pure-tone average.

Speech Recognition Interpretation Chart
(SPRINT)

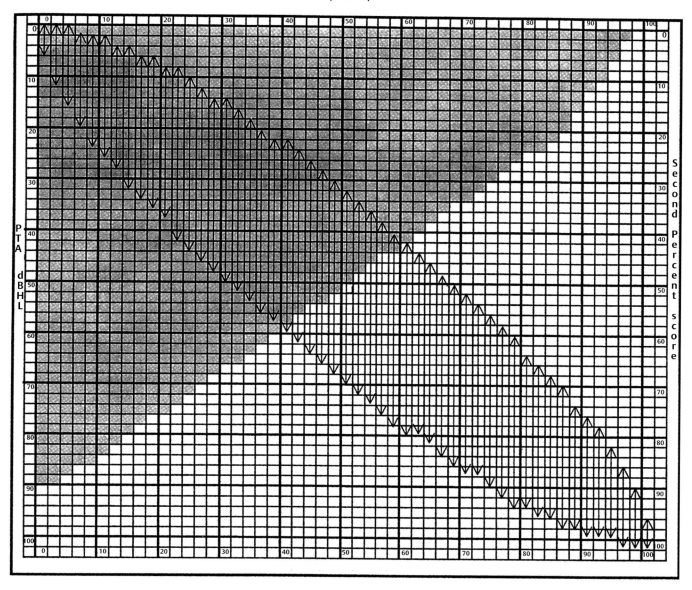

95% Confidence Limit for PBmax on NU6 50-word list. Plot score according
to PTA on left ordinate and percent correct score on the abscissa.
If it falls in the shaded area, it is considered disproportionately low.
(Adapted from Dubno et al.,1995)

95% Critical differences for 50-word list. Plot first and second score
according to the abscissa and right ordinate. If it falls within the arrow, the two
scores are not significantly different. (Adapted from Thornton & Raffin, 1978)

Copyright by Linda M. Thibodeau, 1999

Figure 14–8 Speech Recognition Interpretation (SPRINT) chart for 50-word NU-6 lists. HL, hearing level; PTA, pure-tone average.

that a second score on a 25-word list would have to be below 16% or above 64% to be significantly different (a range of 48%). However, for a score of 88%, the critical difference range is only 68 to 96% (a range of 28%). In addition, it is clear that the range of differences is greater for 25 words than 50 words. For example, if the score is 40%, and 25 stimuli are used (**Fig. 14–7**), the range within the 95% level of confidence is 48% (16–64%), but if 50 stimuli are used (**Fig. 14–8**), the range is 36% (22–58%).

Pearl

- Scores obtained using a 50-word list that differ by 20% or more will always be significantly different relative to 95% confidence limits established by Thornton and Raffin (1978). For a 25-word list, use 25%.

Figs. 14–7 and **14–8** can also be used to estimate whether a single speech recognition score agrees with expected values according to pure-tone sensitivity for 25- and 50-word lists, respectively. Data for these comparisons were based on the 95% confidence limits of the PBmax for NU-6 word lists from a sample of 407 ears with a wide range of pure-tone averages (PTAs; 0.5, 1.0, and 2.0 kHz) (Dubno et al, 1995). When a patient's PBmax is below that predicted based on the PTA, it may be concluded that word recognition is significantly impaired relative to most patients with equivalent hearing loss. To determine this on the SPRINT chart, the score represented on the abscissa is plotted as a function of the PTA represented on the left ordinate. If it falls within the shaded region, the percent correct score is considered disproportionately low for that degree of hearing loss. For example, if the patient's PTA is 52 dB HL, and a 25-word list was used (**Fig. 14–7**), the 95% confidence limit is 48%. Any score below 48% would fall in the shaded region and be considered abnormally low for that PTA. For PTA values not listed in the SPRINT chart (e.g., 62 dB HL), round up to the next higher PTA (e.g., 64 dB HL) for a conservative interpretation. When speech recognition scores fall below expected values, further diagnostic testing is warranted, and specific counseling during the rehabilitation process regarding coping strategies is needed.

One may also want to compare group speech recognition scores. If the dependent variable is a percent correct score, an arc–sine transform is necessary prior to any statistical analysis of the results (Studebaker, 1985). This transform adjusts for the disparate variances that exist in perception scores in which less variability is observed at the extremes than in the midrange of performance. Based on the number of words in the list, the scores ranging from 0 to 100% may be transformed from 0 to 120%.

Interpretation of results also involves comparison across measures for accuracy checks and predictive purposes. Examining the interrelationships among speech measures can be helpful in determining if performance falls within expected ranges. For example, the SDT is generally 10 to 12 dB below the SRT (Eagan, 1948).

Pearl

- SDT is within ± 10 dB of the 0.5 kHz threshold unless the patient's audiogram rises in the higher frequencies, in which case the SDT will be ± 5 dB of the best threshold (Frisina, 1962).

Appropriate tests for each age level are presented in the following section with consideration of the factors mentioned above. Only those tests for which normative data are available are included so that interpretation of performance is possible.

◆ Speech Audiometry Measures

Audiological assessments involving speech will be discussed according to the hierarchy of auditory processing beginning with awareness, followed by discrimination and identification. Following this general discussion, typical patterns of results by pathology and assessment options by age group will be presented. **Table 14–4** contains the hierarchy of speech perception measures of interest. For the suprathreshold tests, only those that have recorded versions available and have published data to which results can be compared are discussed. For a comprehensive review of speech recognition tests, the reader is referred to Roeser (1996) and Mendel and Danhauer (1997). Measures used to assess auditory comprehension level are not included in this review because this assessment at this level of performance does not exclusively lead to a differential diagnosis of a certain auditory pathology. Although a central auditory processing problem may contribute to difficulties in auditory comprehension, such problems may be identified through more commonly used testing at the identification level of processing. Speech measures used to assess loudness perception of speech are also reviewed as they relate to hearing aid fitting.

Awareness

The intensity level at which one becomes aware of the presence of speech is determined in much the same way as for pure-tone thresholds. An SDT is usually obtained for patients who are not able to repeat words, a skill that is necessary for SRT. Although referring to the same threshold, the preferred term is SDT because it is a more accurate description of the task (ASHA, 1988). Assessment of SDT can be useful to confirm the validity of pure-tone thresholds based on the relationships that have been observed. SDTs reflect hearing abilities primarily in the 250 to 0.5 kHz region because that is the most intense region in the speech signal to which a patient first responds. Frisina (1962) reported that the SDT was highly correlated with the threshold at 0.5 kHz in students with significant hearing loss (r = .84 to .98 across age groups). Average SDT was 2 to 6 dB better than the average threshold at 0.5 kHz. Frisina advised that if the difference exceeded 10 dB, the validity of either measure should be questioned. However, if the audiogram rises in the higher frequencies, one would expect the SDT to be within ± 10 dB of the best threshold.

SDT may be determined by presenting speech in an ascending or descending manner. A descending approach is preferable, but if response validity is questionable, an ascending approach may be used as an exploratory search for the first response to speech. Generally, the level is changed by 20 dB per presentation until a reversal is observed (i.e., no response if descending and a positive response if ascending). Familiar words, nonsense syllables, or connected speech may be presented at each level. When a reversal is noted, the intensity level is also changed in the reverse direction, and a bracketing procedure is initiated using 10 dB down, 5 dB up (descending approach) and 10 dB up, 5 dB down (ascending approach). Bracketing around threshold continues until the lowest level is determined at which a response is obtained on half of the trials presented.

Discrimination

Despite numerous procedures to evaluate discrimination in the research setting, there is only one test of true discrimination in which the patient is asked to detect a change in auditory information. First developed for children in 1958, then revised in 1973 by Wepman, the Auditory Discrimination Test (ADT) includes 40 pairs of monosyllabic words. The pairs are presented orally to children ages 5 to 8 years, who are instructed to respond verbally whether the pairs are the same or different. Ten of the 40 pairs are the same, and the remaining word pairs contain phonemes within the same phonetic category. For example, monosyllables with stop consonants were paired with others with stops (e.g., *cat* and *pat*) to assess discrimination of primarily spectral cues rather than spectral and temporal cues. Performance may be compared with a chart where a rating scale value is determined ranging from +2, which indicates "very good development," to −2, which means below the "level of the threshold of adequacy."

Identification

Most of the speech tests routinely used in the audiological test battery assess performance at the identification level. Typically, the patient is asked to repeat nonsense syllables, words, or sentences or to point to pictures in response to standardized stimuli. Speech recognition performance at three intensity levels is of interest: at threshold, at 30 to 40 dB SL, and at 80 to 90 dB HL.

Speech Recognition at Threshold Level

ASHA (1988) recommended a procedure for assessment of SRT that includes presenting spondee words without a carrier phrase. Martin and Weller (1975) found no effect of using a carrier phrase on the SRT. Patients should be familiarized with the test list so that the effects of audibility of the signal are being measured, not familiarity of the vocabulary (Tillman and Jerger, 1959). Testing is begun at a

level 30 to 40 dB above the estimated speech recognition threshold. Words are presented at decrements of 10 dB or increments of 20 dB for correct and incorrect responses, respectively, until a level is reached at which two consecutive words are missed. Intensity level is then increased by 10 dB to begin the threshold determination. Two spondees are presented at each 2 dB decrement until five of six words are repeated incorrectly. Testing may also be done using 5 dB decrements until both words at a given intensity level are missed. Threshold is determined by subtracting the number of correct responses from the starting level and adding a correction factor of 1 dB (2 dB if 5 dB decrements were used) necessary when estimating threshold at the 50% point on the psychometric function with 2 dB steps. Martin and colleagues (1998) reported that ~90% of audiologists are using 5 dB decrements, and 60% do not use the ASHA recommended criterion of missing five of six words. Instead, they follow an abbreviated procedure shown by Martin and Dowdy (1986) to yield results similar to the ASHA procedure. The researchers recommend presenting one spondee starting at 30 dB HL and at 10 dB decrements thereafter until an incorrect response is obtained. If the response is incorrect or absent at 30 dB HL, increase to 50 dB HL, and use 10 dB increments thereafter until a correct response is obtained. Bracketing techniques require presenting one word at each level by incrementing in 5 dB steps for incorrect responses and decrementing in 10 dB steps for correct responses until three correct responses have been obtained at a given level. Threshold is the lowest level at which a minimum of three correct responses were obtained. The SRT is generally 10 to 12 dB greater than the SDT (Eagan, 1948).

Speech Recognition at Suprathreshold Levels

Tests that have been developed and can be interpreted relative to normative data include the NU-6 and Pschoacoustics Laboratory phonetically balanced 50-word lists (PAL PB 50), the Goldman-Fristoe-Woodcock (GFW) Test of Auditory Discrimination, and the revised SPIN, HINT, Hearing in Noise Test for Children (HINT-C), Synthetic Sentence Identification (SSI) sentence lists, Quick Speech in Noise (Quick SIN), and Bamford-Kowal-Bench Speech in Noise (BKB SIN; see **Table 14–4** for references). For comparison to normative data, recorded materials for specific presentation levels must be used as described below for each test. When prescribed procedures cannot be used, the modification must be noted, and cautions regarding interpretation should be stated.

PAL PB 50 monosyllabic word lists were created by Eagan (1948) in an attempt to have all the phonetic elements represented in proportions as they exist in English. Although not commonly used clinically (Martin et al, 1998), the 20 lists of 50 words each were used by Yellin et al (1989) with 324 patients. By presenting lists at increasing intensity levels, the maximum percent correct score (PBmax) was determined. Interpretation of the PBmax scores for 25-word, PAL PB 50 lists according to high-frequency pure-tone average (HF-PTA: 1, 2, and 4 kHz) can be made by using tables provided by Yellin et al (1989). For HF-PTAs between 20 and 80 dB HL, the following formula based on the Yellin et al data can be used to determine the lower limit of performance for PAL PB 50 word lists:

$$\text{Lower limit score} = 89.15 + (\text{HF-PTA})(-1.03)$$

If a word recognition score falls below this limit, it is considered disproportionately low for that degree of hearing loss, and further testing to rule out retrocochlear pathology, as well as an otologic referral, is warranted.

Although normative data are not available for the most often used speech recognition test, CID W-22s (Martin et al, 1998), data provided by Yellin et al (1989) with PAL PB 50 lists may be used for interpretation of CID W-22 scores with limitations. Because the more difficult words were eliminated (resulting in 4 lists of 50 words each), the scores on the CID W-22 lists will generally be higher than those obtained with PAL PB

50 lists (Hirsh et al, 1952). Therefore, if the speech recognition score obtained with W-22 words falls below the 95% lower boundary determined for the PAL-50 word lists, it is surely disproportionately low for that degree of hearing loss based on HF-PTA. If the score falls at the 95% confidence limit or above, interpretation is compromised.

In an attempt to improve upon the phonetic balance of the lists, Tillman and Carhart (1966) developed the NU-6 word lists, which also consist of 200 monosyllabic words divided into four phonemically balanced lists. These lists are the second most frequently used material for assessing speech recognition (Martin et al, 1998). Interpretation of PBmax scores obtained using 25-word, NU-6 lists, as a function of three-frequency PTA (0.5, 1.0, and 2.0 kHz), can be done by using **Table 14–5** from Dubno et al (1995). For PTAs between 20 and 72 dB HL, the following formula based on

Table 14–5   Diagnostic Significance of Speech Audiometry*

Hearing Status	SRT	WRS (NU-6 Lists)	SRS (SSI)	PBmax vs SSImax	PI function	UCL for Speech
Normal hearing	SRT ± 10 dB = PTA	88% or higher on 25-word list presented at 30 dB above SRT	100% at MCR of 0 dB	PBmax = SSImax	No decline > 20% in performance as intensity is increased	UCL – SRT > 100 dB
Conductive hearing loss	SRT ± 10 dB = PTA	88% or higher on 25-word list presented at 30 dB above SRT	100% at MCR of 0 dB	PBmax = SSImax	No decline > 20% in performance as intensity is increased	UCL – SRT > 100 dB
Cochlear hearing loss	SRT ± 10 dB = PTA	Reduced re that expected for PTA (Figs. 14–7 and 14–8)	Flat: Reduced by same degree as WRS Sloping: Reduced by same degree as WRS	Flat: PBmax = SSImax Rising: PBmax – SSImax = 2% Sloping 2 kHz: PBmax = SSImax Sloping 1 kHz: PBmax – SSImax = –12% Sloping 0.5 kHz: PBmax – SSImax = –20%	No decline > 20% in performance as intensity is increased	UCL – SRT < 100 dB Recruitment
Retrocochlear hearing loss	SRT ± 10 dB = PTA	Disproportionately low re that expected for PTA (Figs. 14–7 and 14–8)	Eighth nerve: Rollover—decline in PI function > 20% on affected side Central: Rollover can be present on side opposite lesion	Eighth nerve: PBmax = SSImax Central: PBmax – SSImax > 2% in the side opposite the lesion	Eighth nerve: Rollover—decline in PI function > 20% on affected side Central: Rollover can be present on side opposite lesion	UCL – SRT < 100 dB Derecruitment
Presbycusis	SRT ± 10 dB = PTA	Disproportionately low re that expected for PTA (Figs. 14–7 and 14–8)	Reduced usually more than PBmax	PBmax – SSImax > 10%	Rollover: decline in PI function > 20%	UCL – SRT < 100 dB

*Classifications based on Thornton and Raffin (1978), Dubno et al (1995), Jerger and Jerger (1971), Jerger and Hayes (1977), and Jerger et al (1978).

MCR, message-to-competition ratio; NU-6, Northwestern University 6; PBmax, highest score on phonetically balanced word list; PI, performance intensity; PTA, pure-tone average; SRS, sentence recognition score; SRT, speech recognition threshold; SSImax, highest score on Synthetic Sentence Identification in the ipsilateral competing condition at 0 dB message-to-competition ratio; UCL, uncomfortable loudness level; WRS, word recognition score.

the Dubno et al data can be used to determine the lower limit of performance for NU-6 25-word lists:

$$\text{Lower limit score} = 110.05 + (\text{PTA})(-1.24)$$

If a word recognition score falls below this limit, it is considered disproportionately low for that degree of hearing loss. As described earlier, SPRINT charts in **Figs. 14–7** and **14–8** may be used to interpret NU-6 scores obtained with 25 and 50 words, respectively. The PBmax scores that are below the 95% confidence limit are represented by the shaded bar for each PTA value.

Although not traditionally used in the audiological evaluation, the GFW Diagnostic Auditory Discrimination Test is another exam of auditory recognition that is designed for ages 3 to adult and can be very useful because of the extensive normative data. This test consists of three parts that are administered via audiocassette tape and earphones (Goldman et al, 1974). Part 1 consists of a closed-response task of 100 monosyllabic stimuli, each pictured with a perceptually similar foil (i.e., two pictures per page). If performance is poor on part 1, the next two parts are given, which allows for more specific description of sound confusions. Although normative data for the GFW Diagnostic Auditory Discrimination Test were not obtained in a sound suite at a specified presentation level, the performance levels for normal-hearing patients would allow the clinician to assess the relative effects of reduced absolute and differential sensitivity. If the taped stimuli are presented at a comfortable level for the patient, and the score is within 2 standard deviations (SDs) of the mean value for that age group, it can be concluded that the patient does not have significant deficits in differential sensitivity. However, if the score is significantly below that of the normative sample, then it may be concluded that the performance was the result of the combined effects of reduced absolute and differential sensitivity. One way to attempt to partial out these effects would be to conduct the test with amplification that has been adjusted to maximize the AI (Rankovic, 1995).

Tests of speech recognition employing sentence stimuli that have normative data include SPIN, HINT, SSI, and Quick SIN. Bilger et al (1984) developed the revised SPIN test to assess the patient's use of semantic context by comparing final-word recognition scores from high- and low-predictability sentence lists presented with a 12-talker babble competing signal. Stimuli consist of eight lists of 50, five- to eight-word sentences in which the final word is a monosyllabic noun. Sentences are presented at a fixed signal-to-babble ratio of +8 dB, with the sentences 50 to 55 dB above a patient's threshold for the babble. Norms were developed on 128 persons, ages 19 to 69, with sensorineural hearing loss ranging from mild to severe. A table is provided in the manual with the range of acceptable number correct scores for the high-context sentences as a function of the low-context sentences. One's ability to use the context information was found to be independent of the degree of hearing loss. The 95% confidence limits for the low- and high-predictability sentences are ± 0.95 and ± 0.68, respectively, which suggests that this test is very sensitive to changes in performance.

HINT consists of 25 equivalent lists of 10 sentences composed of 4 to 6 words each that are presented in an adaptive procedure to determine reception thresholds for sentences (RTSs; Nilsson et al, 1996). Norms were developed for sound field testing with speech always at 0 degree azimuth and the speech-spectrum noise at 0, 90, or −90 degrees azimuth. Norms are also available for testing under headphones or insert phones. Speech noise is presented at 65 dBA, with the level of the sentences decreased or increased if the sentence was repeated correctly or incorrectly, respectively. To use the HINT normative data, the results of the test administered with a particular sound room, audiometer, and loudspeakers must be compared with the norms collected in a laboratory setting. Results may vary because of differences in room acoustics resulting from size and the reflective surfaces. For adult normal-hearing patients, the RTS in quiet is 16.62 dBA, and the SNRs are −2.82, −9.07, and −10.42 dB for RTS in noise at 0, 90, and −90 degrees, respectively. To compare two scores, the 95% confidence limit values are ± 1.48, ± 1.2, and ± 1.42 dB in quiet, noise at 0 degree, and noise at each side, respectively.

The SSI test was developed to overcome some of the problems with single-word tests, such as the lack of a dynamic signal resembling connected speech, and with sentence tests, such as the influence of nonauditory factors (e.g., memory and context). Speaks and Jerger (1965) developed a set of 7-word sentences in which every successive 3 words are related syntactically but not semantically to be presented in a closed-set format in the presence of a competing single talker. The competing message can be presented ipsilateral to the sentences (SSI-ICM) or contralateral to the sentences (SSI-CCM). Sentences are presented at 50 dB above the PTA or SRT. For SSI-ICM, sentences are presented at a series of message-to-competition (MCR) ratios beginning at +10 and decreasing until the percent correct identification drops to 20%. Jerger (1973) reported that adults with normal hearing will achieve 100, 80, 55, and 20% identification on the SSI-ICM with MCRs of 0, −10, −20, and −30 dB, respectively. However, on the SSI-CCM, persons with normal hearing perform very well with MCRs as high as 40 dB. SSI-CCM has been most useful in differential diagnosis of retrocochlear pathology.

The Quick SIN is a sentence recognition test in which the SNR necessary for 50% recognition is measured in a background of babble (Killion et al, 2004). There are 12 equivalent lists of 6 sentences each presented in prerecorded SNRs on CD-ROM ranging from 0 to 25 dB in 5 dB steps. A list takes about 1 minute to administer. Scoring of the five key words yields an estimate of SNR loss that is accurate to ± 2.7 dB when results from two lists are averaged (95% confidence). Some lists are recorded with high-frequency emphasis to estimate the benefit of using amplification to restore high-frequency information. Alternatively, some lists are low-pass filtered to simulate high-frequency hearing loss. The manual provides interpretation of the SNR loss and suggests rehabilitative approaches. For example, an SNR loss of 10 dB is considered "moderate," and directional microphones may be of help (Etymotic Research, 2001).

Loudness Perception

There are two common tests of loudness judgments that contribute useful information to the differential diagnostic as well as rehabilitative process. Unusual sensitivity to loud sounds is consistent with recruitment observed with cochlear pathology. Judgments of loudness are also important in hearing aid fitting strategies. For example, one strategy is to amplify speech to the patient's MCL level. A patient's UCL level or loudness discomfort level (LDL) must always be considered when fitting amplification so that the output limiting of the hearing aid can be set to a level that allows maximum receipt of the dynamic range of speech without sacrificing maximum comfort.

Pitfall

- Measuring UCL with running speech will reflect loudness perception primarily in the 0.5 kHz region where the most intense energy in the speech signal is contained. Frequency-specific UCL measures, particularly in the region of the hearing loss, may provide more useful diagnostic information.

MCL and UCL are typically determined with running speech so that the patient judges the loudness of the fluctuating intensities in the speech signal. Presentation usually begins ~20 dB above the SRT, and the patient is asked to judge the loudness of the stimuli. Hawkins (1984) suggested a 9-point rating scale to help patients define the ranges of responses they may use. Choices range from "very soft" to "comfortable, but slightly loud" to "painfully loud." At each presentation level, one of the descriptions is selected that best describes the loudness. Hawkins recommended a bracketing procedure using 10 dB steps to increase intensity and 5 dB steps to decrease intensity until the desired loudness level (MCL or UCL) is determined on two out of four trials. Cox (1981) has shown that UCLs are typically 3 dB lower on the first trial than compared with subsequent measures of UCL. Therefore, if a single estimate is obtained, one may consider it a conservative estimate of the patient's true UCL.

◆ Speech Audiometry in Differential Diagnosis

An overview of characteristic patterns of speech recognition for words and sentences and expectations for uncomfortable listening levels for patients with conductive, sensorineural, and retrocochlear pathology is presented. These patterns are summarized in **Table 14–5** by pathology and typical speech test. The reader is referred to **Figs. 14–7** and **14–8** for more specific interpretations of word recognition scores and to Chapter 1 for more discussion of differential diagnosis of retrocochlear pathology.

Normal Hearing

For persons with normal hearing, there are predictable relationships among various measures of speech processing, as shown in **Table 14–5**. SDT should agree with pure-tone thresholds at 0.5 kHz, and SRT should agree with PTA within ± 10 dB. For all suprathreshold speech recognition measures, persons with normal hearing are expected to perform near 100% correct when age-appropriate materials are used. Speech recognition with words and sentences should be relatively equal. UCLs should be ~100 dB above the SRT.

Conductive Hearing Loss

Patients with conductive hearing losses perform similar to normal-hearing persons once the intensity of the signal is increased to overcome the reduction in audibility. Recognition of words and sentences should be near 100%. The UCL will also be ~100 dB above the SRT.

Sensorineural Hearing Loss

Patients with sensorineural hearing loss generally have reduced speech recognition consistent with the degree of loss. Expected performance on NU-6 lists is illustrated in **Figs. 14–7** and **14–8**. There is no significant decline (> 20%) in speech recognition as intensity level is increased. However, there are characteristic patterns of PBmax and SSImax depending on the configuration of the hearing loss, as outlined in **Table 14–5**.

Retrocochlear Hearing Loss

Patients with retrocochlear hearing loss have three significant characteristics in their speech performance. Their speech recognition for single words is poorer than that expected based on their PTA (**Figs. 14–7** and **14–8**). Recognition performance declines with increased intensity, and there is a discrepancy between recognition of words and sentences. Typical patterns for eighth nerve and central lesions are provided in **Table 14–5**.

◆ Speech Audiometry for Special Age Groups

Toddlers (2–4 Years)

Speech Awareness

Speech audiometry is often administered first in the young pediatric assessment because the toddler is more likely to respond to speech than pure tones (Eagles and Wishik, 1961). Discussion will be divided into two sections depending on whether the child has imitation skills. Test format will be more informal for the child who is not yet able to repeat words because the vocabulary will be more restricted and individually tailored. Because of the customization of these tests, presentation must be live voice; if possible, ear specific responses should be obtained. Insert earphones may be preferable for ear-specific information because of their small size. If earphones are not tolerated, the child should be seated at the calibrated location from the loud-speaker (ASHA, 1991) at 0 degree azimuth.

Often, the first measure for the toddler who cannot yet repeat words is the SDT. Some audiologists prefer to start below threshold, calling the child's or caregiver's name with 10 dB increases in intensity until an observable response is obtained. A carrier phrase should be used, such as "Where is..." or "Show me the...." Starting below threshold, presentations should continue until the minimum level is determined at which an observable response was obtained twice.

If conditioned orientation reflex (COR) audiometry procedures can be used (see Chapter 15), the clinician would start with names at a suprathreshold level. Although this would normally be 40 dB HL, if hearing loss is present or suspected, initial stimuli should be presented at 70 dB HL or higher until a response is obtained. When it is determined that the child is conditioned to the task, the level is lowered in 20 dB steps until there is no response, at which time it is raised in 5 dB steps until a response is obtained again. Bracketing then begins where the level is reduced in 10 dB steps and increased in 5 dB steps until the lowest level is determined at which a response is obtained twice. Minimum response levels for speech may be interpreted relative to those reported by Northern and Downs (1978) in **Table 14–6**.

Speech Recognition at Threshold Levels

A measure of speech recognition would be completed with vocabulary familiar to the child as reported by the caregiver. Most likely this will involve asking the child to point to body parts or get familiar objects/toys using live-voice presentation at 30 to 40 dB SL (sensation level). If possible, it is desirable to use spondees, two-syllable words presented with equal stress. Griffing and colleagues (1967) developed the Verbal Auditory Screening for Preschool Children (VASPC), a screening procedure that involves determining the SRT based on 12 spondaic words that were pictured on a board. Although the identification of 12 common words, easily recognizable in pictures, was a useful contribution to the pediatric test battery, the VASPC was not found to be a sensitive screening tool (Mencher and McCulloch, 1970; Ritchie and Merklein, 1972).

Table 14–6 Minimum Response Levels for Speech and Warbled Pure Tones Reported by Northern and Downs (1978)

Age (months)	Speech (dB HL) (SD)	Warbled Pure Tones (dB HL) (SD)
0–1	40–60	78 (6)
1–4	47 (2)	70 (10)
4–7	21 (8)	51 (9)
7–9	15 (7)	45 (15)
9–13	8 (7)	38 (8)
13–16	5 (5)	32 (10)
16–21	5 (1)	25 (10)
21–24	3 (2)	26 (10)

HL, hearing level; SD, standard deviation.

In some instances when a child cannot be tested with headphones, speech awareness/recognition may be evaluated through the use of the bone-conduction vibrator. Calibration of speech through the bone vibrator should be verified from the audiometer manufacturer's documentation. When calibrated properly, there are high correlations between the bone-conducted PTA threshold (0.5, 1.0, and 2.0 kHz) and the bone-conducted SRT (Merrell et al, 1973). Comparison of speech processing through the bone vibrator and through the earphones may be necessary to approximate the air–bone gap when pure-tone thresholds cannot be obtained.

Speech Recognition at Suprathreshold Levels

As with the SRT procedure, speech recognition at suprathreshold levels must be performed with words within the child's receptive vocabulary. Besides using a closed set of familiar words, such as body parts, toys, objects, or pictures, there are at least two formal measures designed for children below age 4.

Elliott and Katz (1980) designed the Northwestern University Children's Perception of Speech (NU-Chips) test for preschoolers ages 3 to 5. Four randomizations of a 50-word list are used with two picture books of 50 monochrome plates of four pictures each. Book A is used for forms A and B and Book B for C and D. Some of the foils on each page are phonemically similar to the test stimulus. Commercially available monosyllabic word lists are presented via tape or CD-ROM at 30 to 40 dB SL with either a male or female talker.

Another test for young children is the Pediatric Speech Intelligibility (PSI) test by Jerger and colleagues (Jerger et al, 1980, 1981; Jerger and Jerger, 1982). This closed-response test for children ages 3 to 6 includes one list of 20 monosyllabic words and two lists of 10 sentences in two syntactic formats ("Show me the rabbit putting on his shoes" and "The rabbit is putting on his shoes"). The child is instructed to choose one of five pictures of animals that corresponds to the stimulus. Unlike the word test, performance on the sentence test varies with receptive language age, with format 2 being reserved for children with higher language functioning. The test may be presented with competition using a +4 dB MCR for the word test and 0 dB MCR for the sentence tests. Jerger and Jerger (1982) reported that the PI functions for the words and sentences in quiet was 8 to 10 dB and for words and sentences in competition was 10 to 12 dB. At a presentation level of 50 dB SPL (30 dB HL), normal-hearing children achieve 100% performance on the words and the sentences in both quiet and in noise.

Children (4–12 Years)

Speech Recognition at Threshold Levels

By age 4, children should be able to imitate words and complete a traditional SRT procedure by pointing to familiar pictures. Testing may be done live voice to tailor the spondees to the child's vocabulary. Testing should follow the ASHA (1988) recommended procedures or Martin and Dowdy (1986) modification as described earlier.

Pearl

- A procedure to use for the occasional child who presents a nonorganic hearing loss is to begin presenting spondees at the intensity level that elicits imitation from the child. For each spondee that is repeated correctly, lower the intensity 1 dB. Usually the child is unable to discern that the intensity level is changing, and shortly after, he or she is responding at a level expected for children with normal hearing. At that point, the child should be congratulated on having excellent hearing and encouraged to maintain the excellent attention to the task.

Speech Recognition at Suprathreshold Levels

As mentioned earlier, the NU-Chips test is appropriate for children through age 5. A widely used test with children ages 4 to 6 is the Word Intelligibility by Picture Identification (WIPI) (Ross and Lerman, 1970); however, there are limited normative data available to assist in interpretation of these scores. The revised version includes updated pictures for 25% of the words (Ross et al, 2005). Research with the original version was conducted by Sanderson-Leepa and Rintelmann (1976), who presented the WIPI in the sound field to 12 normal-hearing children in each age group 3.5, 5.5, 7.5, and 9.5 years old. At a 32 dB sensation level re SRT, the mean percent correct was 91.7, 97.3, 98.7, and 99.0, respectively. Standard deviations ranged from 6.26% for the youngest to 1.8% for the oldest. Papso and Blood (1989) also evaluated the original WIPI in the sound field with 30 normal-hearing children from 4 to 5 years. In quiet, the average percent correct was 94.3 (SD = 4.5), compared with an adult control group who achieved 100%. However, in multitalker noise at a +6 signal-to-noise ratio, the children scored 67.6% (SD = 12.0), and the adults scored 94.9% (SD = 3.5). These data document that children as young as 3.5 years old should be able to perform near 90% (+/− 6%) correct on the WIPI. Furthermore, if the WIPI is administered in the presence of babble (+6 dB signal-to-noise ratio), one would expect approximately a 30% decline in performance.

For children older than 6 years, the phonetically balanced kindergarten (PBK) lists are most often used. Similar to the open-set format used with adults, these lists have vocabulary from the spoken vocabulary of kindergartners (Haskins, 1949). Sanderson-Leepa and Rintelmann (1976) found that normal-hearing preschoolers performed significantly lower than 5- to 6-year-olds, verifying the appropriateness of the PBKs for use with kindergartners.

The only auditory processing test with normative data on children with hearing loss is the Test of Auditory Comprehension (TAC; Trammel, 1981). Although the test is no longer published, it is the most comprehensive assessment tool for children with hearing loss, and it is still being used. Designed to complement an auditory training curriculum, the TAC includes 10 subjects ranging from awareness to comprehension in background noise. A profile of performance is provided in the areas of discrimination, memory sequencing, and figure–ground perception. Tape-recorded

stimuli are presented at a comfortable listening level, and the child responds by selecting the corresponding monochrome picture from a set of three choices. Performance can be interpreted against normative data provided in the manual according to degree of hearing loss from moderate to severe-profound and age from 4 to 17 years.

Clinicians are often seeking a measure of speech recognition in noise for the school-aged child because referrals for suspected auditory processing problems are frequently made at this age. As mentioned earlier, there are normative data for the PSI and WIPI for children up to age 6 listening to speech in noise. Rupp (1980) provided data for recognition of PBK lists presented in white noise at a 0 dB signal-to-noise ratio at the most comfortable listening levels for children in kindergarten through fifth grade. Performance in the sound field ranged from 34% to 49% correct for kindergartners and fifth graders, respectively.

The HINT-C is an adaptation of the HINT for use with children ages 6 to 12 (Nilsson et al, 1996). Results from testing 84 children revealed that a more favorable signal-to-noise ratio was needed for children to achieve the same performance level as adults. Although there are no norms for testing children under headphones, average differences between scores for children and adults are provided in the manual for testing in quiet and with noise at 0 and 90 degrees azimuth. For example, at 0 degree azimuth, an average adult achieves an RTS at −2.82 dB. The average difference for a 7-year-old child is 2.18 dB, so one would expect an RTS at 0.64 dB (−2.82 + 2.18 = 0.64). In other words, the average adult can repeat sentences correctly 50% of the time when the speech is 2.82 dB below the noise, but the average 7-year-old needs the speech to be just above the noise to perform at the same level.

Another adult test of speech recognition in noise that has been adapted for use with children ages 5 to 14 years is the Quick SIN. This version for children is called the BKB SIN because the Bamford et al sentences are recorded at signal-to-noise ratios from 25 to 0 in 5 dB steps. There are 18 list pairs of 8 to 10 sentences, each with 5 key words for scoring in each sentence. For a valid score, a pair of lists must be presented that takes ~3 minutes. The scores from the pair are averaged to yield the SNR loss. The manual provides data that show how SNR values, reliability, and critical differences improve as a function of age (Etymotic Research, 2005).

Pitfall

- There are limited materials with normative data available to assess speech recognition in children. Audiologists must carefully select the most sensitive materials with normative data that are appropriate for the child.

Geriatrics (65 + Years)

Evaluation of speech recognition in the elderly involves the same procedures as for adults with two considerations: shorter stimuli may be necessary because of memory difficulties, and comparison to normative values will be different to account for the normal reductions in audibility with aging. Clinical experience has shown that the elderly are more successful with monosyllabic stimuli than sentence materials. NU-6 lists are appropriate to use with the elderly and can be interpreted according to the Dubno et al (1995) values for disproportionate speech recognition. Of their subject pool, 86% were older than 60 years of age, with the oldest being 82 years of age. If a closed-set response task is needed, the GFW Test of Auditory Discrimination includes normative data up to age 70 years (Goldman et al, 1970; Goldman et al, 1974), and the GFW Diagnostic Auditory Discrimination Test includes normative data up to age 87 years. These two tests require the patient to choose one of two pictures that corresponds to the stimulus. One advantage of these latter two tests is the sound confusion analysis that may be particularly helpful to assess benefits of an auditory training program or monitor hearing aid adjustment.

♦ Summary

There are at least three objectives of speech audiometry: (1) to determine the effects of hearing loss on absolute and differential sensitivity, (2) to contribute to the differential diagnostic process, and (3) to facilitate the hearing aid fitting process. To accomplish these objectives, several decisions regarding the evaluation process must be made, including the level of processing to be assessed, response format, stimuli, presentation mode and level, calibration, procedures, and analysis and interpretation of results. Because these choices may dramatically influence the results, audiologists must have a clear understanding of the options and the resulting information that may be obtained.

When choosing the appropriate procedures for speech audiometry, it is imperative to consider sensitive and valid measures of performance. In addition, there is limited benefit to the patient to evaluate speech recognition if performance is not evaluated relative to a normative database. It is no longer acceptable to report that "word recognition was poorer than expected based on pure-tone thresholds" without indicating how such a conclusion was reached. Tools such as the Count-the-Dot audiogram and the SPRINT charts should be readily available for the audiologist's use in the interpretation of test scores. There is certainly a need for further development of more sensitive assessment procedures with normative data across a wide range of hearing impairments.

Pearl

- Audiologists can interpret speech recognition scores through the use of tools such as the Count-the-Dot audiogram and the SPRINT charts.

References

American National Standards Institute. (2002). Methods for the calculation of the speech intelligibility index (ANSI S3.5–1997, R2002). New York: Author.

American National Standards Institute. (2004). American National Standards specifications for audiometers (ANSI S3.6–2004). New York: Author.

American Speech-Language-Hearing Association. (1988). Guidelines for determining threshold level for speech. ASHA, 30, 85–89.

American Speech-Language-Hearing Association. (1991). Sound field measurement tutorial. ASHA, 33, 25–37.

Benson, R. C., & Hirsh, I. J. (1953). Some variables in audio spectrometry. Journal of the Acoustical Society of America, 2, 449–453.

Bess, F. (1983). Clinical assessment of speech recognition. In D. Konkle & W. Rintelmann (Eds.), Principles of speech audiometry (pp. 127–201). Baltimore, MD: Academic Press.

Bilger, R. C., Nuetzel, J. M., Rabinowitz, W. M., & Rzeczkowski, C. (1984). Standardization of a test of speech perception in noise. Journal of Speech and Hearing Research, 27, 32–48.

Bilger, R. C., & Wang, M. D. (1976). Consonant confusions in patients with sensori-neural hearing loss. Journal of Speech and Hearing Research, 19, 718–740.

Boothroyd, A. , & Nittrouer, S. (1988). Mathematical treatment of context effects in phoneme and word recognition. Journal of the Acoustical Society of America, 84, 101–114.

Brandy, W. T. (1966). Reliability of voice tests of speech discrimination. Journal of Speech and Hearing Research, 9, 461–465.

Cox, R. (1981). Using LDL to establish hearing aid limited levels. Hearing Instruments, 32, 16–20.

Cox, R. M., & McDaniel, D. M. (1989). Development of the speech intelligibility rating (SIR) test for hearing aid comparisons. Journal of Speech and Hearing Research, 32, 347–352.

Crystal, T. H., & House, A. S. (1990). Articulation rate and the duration of syllables and stress groups in connected speech. Journal of the Acoustical Society of America, 88, 101–112.

Dirks, D., Kamm, D., Bower, D., & Betsworth, A. (1977). Use of performance intensity functions for diagnosis. Journal of Speech and Hearing Disorders, 42, 311–322.

Dubno, J. R., Lee, F. S., Klein, A. J., Matthews, L. J., & Lam, C. F. (1995). Confidence limits for maximum word-recognition scores. Journal of Speech and Hearing Research, 38, 490–502.

Dubno, J. R. & Levitt, H. (1981). Predicting consonant confusions from acoustic analysis. Journal of the Acoustical Society of America, 69, 249–261.

Eagan, J. (1948). Articulation testing methods. Laryngoscope, 58, 955–991.

Eagles, E. L., & Wishik, S. M. (1961). A study of hearing in children. Transactions—American Academy of Ophthalmology and Otolaryngology, 65, 261–282.

Eimas, P. D., Siqueland, E. R., Juscyzk, P., & Vigorito, J. (1971). Speech perception in infants. Science, 171, 303–306.

Elliott, L., & Katz, D. (1980). Development of a new children's test of speech discrimination. St. Louis: Auditec.

Erber, N. (1982). Auditory training. Washington, DC: Alexander Graham Bell Association for the Deaf.

Etymotic Research. (2001). QuickSIN speech-in-noise test. St. Louis: Auditec.

Etymotic Research. (2005). BKB SIN speech-in-noise test. St. Louis: Auditec.

Festen, J. M., & Plomp, R. (1983). Relations between the auditory functions in impaired hearing. Journal of the Acoustical Society of America, 73, 652–662.

Fletcher, S. G. (1970). Acoustic phonetics. In F. S. Borg & S. G. Fletcher (Eds.), The hard of hearing child (pp. 57–84). New York: Grune & Stratton.

French, N. R., & Steinberg, J. C. (1947). Factors governing the intelligibility of speech sounds. Journal of the Acoustical Society of America, 19, 90–119.

Frisina, R. D. (1962). Audiometric evaluation and its relation to habilitation and rehabilitation of the deaf. American Annals of the Deaf, 107, 478–481.

Gatehouse, S. (1993). Role of perceptual acclimatization in the selection of frequency responses for hearing aids. Journal of the American Academy of Audiology, 4, 296–306.

Goldman, R., Fristoe, M., & Woodcock, R. (1970). G-F-W test of auditory discrimination. Circle Pines, MN: American Guidance Service.

Goldman, R. , Fristoe, M., & Woodcock, R. (1974). G-F-W diagnostic auditory discrimination test. Circle Pines, MN: American Guidance Service.

Griffing, T. S., Simonton, K. M., & Hedgecock, L. D. (1967). Verbal auditory screening for preschool children. Transactions—American Academy of Ophthalmology and Otolaryngology, 71, 105–111.

Haskins, H. (1949). A phonetically balanced test of speech discrimination for children. Unpublished master's thesis, Northwestern University, Evanston, IL.

Hawkins, D. (1984). Selection of a critical electroacoustic characteristic: SSPL90. Hearing Instruments, 35, 28–32.

Hood, J. D., & Poole, J. P. (1971). Speech audiometry in conductive and sensorineural hearing loss. Sound, 5, 30–38.

Hood, J. D., & Poole, J. P. (1980). Influence of the speaker and other factors affecting speech intelligibility. Audiology, 19, 434–455.

Humes, L. E. (1991). Understanding the speech-understanding problems of the hearing impaired. Journal of the American Academy of Audiology, 2, 59–69.

Jerger, J. (1973). Audiological findings in aging. Advance in Oto-rhino-laryngology, 20, 115–124.

Jerger, J., & Jerger, S. (1971). Diagnostic significance of PB word functions. Archives of Otolaryngology, 93, 573–580.

Jerger, J., Speaks, C., & Trammel, J. L. (1968). A new approach to speech audiometry. Journal of Speech and Hearing Disorders, 33, 318–328.

Jerger, S., & Jerger, J. (1982). Pediatric speech intelligibility test: Performance-intensity characteristics. Ear and Hearing, 3, 325–334.

Jerger, S., Jerger, J., & Lewis, S. (1981). Pediatric speech intelligibility test: 2. Effect of receptive language age and chronological age. International Journal of Pediatric Otorhinolaryngology, 3, 101–118.

Jerger, S., Lewis, S., Hawkins, J., & Jerger, J. (1980). Pediatric speech intelligibility test: 1. Generation of test materials. International Journal of Pediatric Otorhinolaryngology, 2, 217–230.

Johnson, C., Benson, P., & Seaton, J. (1997). Educational audiology handbook. San Diego, CA: Singular Publishing Group.

Killion, M. C., Niquette, P. A., & Gudmundsen, G. I. (2004). Development of a quick speech-in-noise test for measuring signal-to-noise ratio loss in normal-hearing and hearing-impaired listeners. Journal of the Acoustical Society of America, 116(4), 2395–2405.

Klatt, D. H. (1976). Linguistic uses of segmental duration in English: Acoustic and perceptual evidence. Journal of the Acoustical Society of America, 59, 1208–1221.

Klatt, D. H. (1980). Software for a cascade/parallel formant synthesizer. Journal of the Acoustical Society of America, 67, 971–995.

Kryter, K. (1962). Methods for the calculation and use of the articulation index. Journal of the Acoustical Society of America, 43, 1689–1697.

Levitt, H., & Resnick, S. B. (1978). Speech reception by the hearing impaired: Methods of testing and the development of new tests. Scandinavian Audiology Supplementum, 6, 107–130.

Martin, F. N., Champlin, C. A., & Chambers, J. A. (1998). Seventh survey of audiometric practices in the United States. Journal of the American Academy of Audiology, 9, 95–104.

Martin, F.N., & Dowdy, L. K. (1986). A modified spondee threshold procedure. Journal of Audiology Research, 26, 115–119.

Martin, F. N., & Weller, S. M. (1975). The influence of the carrier phrase on the speech reception threshold. Journal of Communication Pathology, 7, 39–44.

Mencher, G. T., & McCulloch, B. F. (1970). Auditory screening of kindergarten children using the VASC. Journal of Speech and Hearing Disorders, 35, 241–247.

Mendel, L., & Danhauer, J. (1997). Audiologic evaluation and management and speech perception assessment. San Diego, CA: Singular Publishing Group.

Merrell, H. B., & Atkinson, C. J. (1965). The effect of selected variables on discrimination scores. Journal of Audiology Research, 5, 285–292.

Merrell, H. B., Wolfe, D. L., & McLemore, D. C. (1973). Air and bone conducted speech reception thresholds. Laryngoscope, 83, 1929–1939.

Mueller, H. G., & Killion, M. C. (1990). An easy method for calculating the articulation index. Hearing Journal, 43, 14–17.

Nilsson, M., Soli, S. D., & Gelnett, D. (1996). Development and norming of a hearing in noise test for children. House Ear Institute Internal Report, 5, 115–128

Nilsson, M., Soli, S., Sullivan, J. (1994). Development of the Hearing in Noise Test for the measurement of speech reception threshold in quiet and in noise. Journal of the Acoustical Society of America 95, 1085–1099.

Northern, J., & Downs, M. (1978). Hearing in children. Baltimore, MD: Williams & Wilkins.

Olsen, W. O., Hawkins, D., & Van Tasell, D. J. (1987). Representations of the long-term spectra of speech. Ear and Hearing, 8, 100S–108S.

Olsen, W. O., & Matkin, N. (1979). Speech audiometry. In W. Rintelmann (Ed.), Hearing assessment. Baltimore, MD: University Park Press.

Olsen, W. O., Van Tasell, D. J., & Speaks, C. E. (1997). The Carhart Memorial Lecture, American Auditory Society, Salt Lake City, Utah 1996: Phoneme and word recognition for words in isolation and in sentences. Ear and Hearing, 18, 175–188.

Papso, C. F., & Blood, I. M. (1989). Word recognition skills of children and adults in background noise. Ear and Hearing, 10, 235–236.

Pascoe, D. P. (1975). Frequency response of hearing aids and their effects on the speech perception of hearing-impaired subjects. Annals of Otology, Rhinology, and Laryngology, 84(5, pt. 2, suppl. 23), 5–40.

Pavlovic, C. V. (1984). Use of the articulation index for assessing residual auditory function in listeners with sensorineural hearing impairment. Journal of the Acoustical Society of America, 75, 1253–1258.

Pavlovic, C. V. (1989). Speech spectrum considerations and speech intelligibility predictions in hearing aid evaluations. Journal of Speech and Hearing Disorders, 54(1), 3–8.

Penrod, J. (1994). Speech threshold and word recognition/discrimination testing. In J. Katz (Ed.), Handbook of clinical audiology (pp. 147–164). Baltimore, MD: Williams & Wilkins.

Picheny, M. A., Durlach, N. I., & Braida, L. D. (1989). Speaking clearly for the hard of hearing: 3. An attempt to determine the contribution of speaking rate to differences in intelligibility between clear and conversational speech. Journal of Speech and Hearing Research, 32, 600–603.

Pickett, J. M. (1999). The acoustics of speech communication: Fundamentals, speech perception theory, and technology (pp. 86–89). Boston: Allyn & Bacon.

Prinz, I., Nubel, K., & Gross, M. (2002). Digital vs. analog hearing aids for children: Is there a method for making an objective comparison possible? HNO, 50(9), 844–849.

Rankovic, C. M. (1995). Derivation of frequency-gain for maximizing speech reception. Journal of Speech and Hearing Research, 38, 913–929.

Ritchie, B. C., & Merklein, R. A. (1972). An evaluation of the efficiency of the Verbal Auditory Screening Test for Children (VASC). Journal of Speech and Hearing Research, 15, 280–286.

Roeser, R. (1996). Audiology desk reference. New York: Thieme Medical Publishers.

Ross, M., & Lerman, J. (1970). A picture identification test for hearing impaired children. Journal of Speech and Hearing Research, 13, 44–53.

Ross, M., Lerman, J., & Cienkowski, K. (2005). Word intelligibility by picture identification. St. Louis: Auditec.

Ross, T., & Smith, K. (2005). How to use live speech as part of a hearing instrument fitting and verification process. Hearing Review, 12, 40–46.

Rupp, R. (1980). Discrimination of PB-K's in noise (PBKN). St. Louis: Auditec.

Sanderson-Leepa, M. E., & Rintelmann, W. F. (1976). Articulation functions and test–retest performance of normal hearing children on three speech discrimination tests: WIPI, PBK-50, and NU Auditory Test No. 6. Journal of Speech and Hearing Disorders, 41, 503–519.

Skinner, M. W., Karstaedt, M. M., & Miller, J. D. (1982). Amplification bandwidth and speech intelligibility for two listeners with sensori-neural hearing loss. Audiology, 21, 251–268.

Speaks, C., & Jerger, J. (1965). Method for measurement of speech identification. Journal of Speech and Hearing Research, 8, 185–194.

Stach, B. (1998). Word-recognition testing: Why not do it well? Hearing Journal, 51, 10–16.

Studebaker, G. (1985). A "rationalized" arc sine transform. Journal of Speech and Hearing Research, 28, 455–462.

Teder, H. (1993). Compression in the time domain. American Journal of Audiology, 2, 41–46.

Thibodeau, L. M., & Van Tasell, D. J. (1987). Tone detection and synthetic speech discrimination in band-reject noise by hearing-impaired listeners. Journal of the Acoustical Society of America, 82, 864–873.

Thornton, A. R., & Raffin, M. J. M. (1978). Speech discrimination scores modified as a binomial variable. Journal of Speech and Hearing Research, 21, 507–518.

Tillman, T. W., & Carhart, R. (1966). An expanded test for speech discrimination utilizing CNC monosyllabic words: Northwestern University Auditory Test No. 6 (Tech. Rep. No. SAM-TR-66–55). Brooks Air Force Base, TX: U.S. Air Force School of Aerospace Medicine.

Tillman, T. W., & Jerger, J. (1959). Some factors affecting the spondee threshold in normal-hearing subjects. Journal of Speech and Hearing Research, 2, 141–146.

Trammel, J. (1981). Test of auditory comprehension. Portland, OR: Foreworks Publications.

Tyler, R. (1994). The use of speech-perception tests in audiological rehabilitation: Current and future research needs. Journal of the Academy of Rehabilitative Audiology, 27, 47–66.

Tyler, R., Summerfield, A., Wood, E., & Fernandes, M. (1982). Psychoacoustic and phonetic temporal processing in normal and hearing impaired listeners. In G. van den Brink & F. Bilsen (Eds.), Psychophysical, physiological, and behavioural studies in hearing (pp. 458–465). Delft, Netherlands: Delft University Press.

Tyler, R. S., Wood, E. J., & Fernandes, M. (1982). Frequency resolution and hearing loss. British Journal of Audiology, 16, 45–63.

Umeda, N. (1975). Vowel duration in American English. Journal of the Acoustical Society of America, 58, 434–445.

Umeda, N. (1977). Consonant duration in American English. Journal of the Acoustical Society of America, 61, 846–858.

Van Tasell, D. J. (1986). Auditory perception of speech. In J. Davis & E. Hardick (Eds.), Rehabilitative audiology for children and adults (pp.13–58). New York: Macmillan.

Van Tasell, D. J., & Crain, T. R. (1992). Noise reduction hearing aids: Release from masking and release from distortion. Ear and Hearing, 13, 114–121.

Van Tasell, D. J., & Yanz, J. L. (1987). Speech recognition threshold in noise: Effects of hearing loss, frequency response, and speech materials. Journal of Speech and Hearing Research, 30, 377–386.

Wepman, J., & Reynolds, W. (1973). Wepman's auditory discrimination test (ADT), second edition. Los Angeles, CA: Western Psychological Services.

Wood, S. A., & Lutman, M. E. (2004). Relative benefits of linear analogue and advanced digital hearing aids. International Journal of Audiology, 43(3), 144–155.

Yellin, M. W., Jerger, J., & Fifer, R. C. (1989). Norms for disproportionate loss in speech intelligibility. Ear and Hearing, 10, 231–234.

Young, L. L., Jr., Dudley, B., & Gunter, M. B. (1982). Thresholds and psychometric functions of the individual spondaic words. Journal of Speech and Hearing Research, 25, 586–593.

Chapter 15

Audiologic Evaluation of Special Populations

Angela G. Shoup and Ross J. Roeser

Audiologists provide diagnostic assessments for a variety of patient populations. In addition to evaluating normally developing children and normal adults, an audiologist may provide diagnostic assessment for newborns only hours of age, infants who are days or weeks old, children or adults who are mentally challenged, elderly patients with dementia or even Alzheimer's disease, patients who have had strokes, and patients with pseudohypoacusis or hyperacusis. This chapter covers the topic of diagnostic tests for patients with special needs, including infants and young children (0–5 years), the elderly, those with developmental disabilities, those with dementia, those with visual impairment, adults with cognitive deficits (aphasia and Alzheimer's disease), those with pseudohypoacusis, and those with hyperacusis.

♦ Considerations in Evaluating Special Populations

It is incumbent on clinicians to view each patient as an individual, making careful behavioral observations, asking questions when necessary, and truly listening to responses. For some patients, the standard audiologic test environment and procedures may be unachievable. Skilled clinicians will recognize when changes are needed and modify diagnostic test protocols appropriately within acceptable clinical guidelines. Clinician flexibility in the testing session may translate into redesigning the environment for optimum results, changing the order in which tests are completed, and obtaining nontraditional responses during the diagnostic procedures. This approach to the evaluation process is even more important when the patient has multisensory deficits or handicaps in addition to hearing loss. Consideration is given in this chapter to evaluating normally developing patients across the life span and patients who present challenges because of existing medical/cognitive/developmental/psychological conditions. It is often difficult for clinicians to develop proficiency in testing patients with special needs because of the heterogeneity of patient populations and infrequency in encountering these patients in the traditional audiology clinic. For these reasons, it is important for clinicians to have a thorough understanding of the deviations in test protocols that are acceptable and how these acceptable deviations may affect test results and their interpretation.

Cognitive Status

Although chronological age is a factor when selecting appropriate testing techniques for patients with special needs, mental age and neurological status are more important. When assessing infants, gestational age is calculated to determine the "corrected" age. Knowing the corrected age allows for more accurate interpretation of physiological responses, such as the auditory brainstem response (ABR). Review of case history information and observation of the individual will assist the clinician in estimating the capabilities of the patient, and thus selecting test procedures that will be more successful. Clinicians who have a "feel," through subjective observations, for the mental/developmental age of the patient can interpret behavioral responses more accurately.

Cross-Check Principle

A test battery approach is especially useful with special populations. When limited information is obtained from traditional tests, converging evidence acquired from a carefully selected test battery helps in developing a "picture" of the patient's auditory capabilities so that appropriate recommendations can be made. Obtaining valid information through this approach was first proposed by Jerger and Hayes (1976) and was labeled the "cross-check principle." This principle takes into consideration that many patients may be able to provide only limited behavioral audiometric information, and the validity may be questioned. When this occurs, clinicians may use another test procedure such as an objective measure (i.e., immittance, otoacoustic emissions, ABR) to verify the behavioral results or to provide additional information about auditory status.

Patients from Diverse Cultural Backgrounds: A Growing Need

Language barriers and differences in rules of interaction may influence testing protocols for patients from diverse cultural backgrounds. When faced with evaluating or treating culturally diverse patients, most clinicians readily consider concerns about difficulty caused by language differences. Appropriate

communication with patients from diverse cultural backgrounds requires understanding not only of spoken language but also accepted mannerisms and behaviors (cultural pragmatics). For example, many cultures consider direct eye contact to be rude. Other cultures consider the head to have special religious significance, so the clinician should seek approval before touching the head in any way (Nellum-Davis, 1993). Language and basic rules for interaction are not the only barriers to successful service delivery; more important barriers may include a lack of recognition and understanding of varying values and beliefs. Ethnocentrism has been defined as "an attitude or outlook in which values derived from one's own cultural background are applied to other cultural contexts where different values are operative" (LeVine and Campbell, 1972, p. 1). In many cases, this is taken a step further when an individual considers all cultural values or beliefs that are different to be wrong or unacceptable. Clinicians can become impatient and develop negative impressions about parents who hesitate to follow through with recommendations for amplification or specific intervention strategies. Before judging too harshly, clinicians should try to learn about and understand the patients' cultural beliefs about health care and disease. For example, some Asian-American patients may believe that the hearing loss or other disease or disorder is due to a curse or a gift from God (Cheng, 1993). Many cultures, including Native Americans and Hispanics, may believe in folk remedies or religious ceremonies for treatment and be hesitant to pursue "Western medicine."

Pitfall

- Although in many cases the patient will have a friend or family member with him or her who speaks English as well as the patient's language, the use of informal interpreters such as family or friends is generally discouraged for many reasons. First, when an acquaintance of the patient serves as the interpreter, the patient's privacy may be violated. Second, the clinician cannot verify the competence of an informal interpreter. Third, when a child is used, the resulting "role reversal" may jeopardize traditional family values by undermining parental respect and authority (Smart and Smart, 1995).

When a non-English-speaking patient enters the clinic for diagnostic assessment, procuring the services of a language interpreter should be considered. The rules for communicating through a language interpreter are the same as for when a sign-language interpreter is needed for hearing-impaired patients. Clinicians should remember to speak to the patient, not the interpreter, pause after statements to allow the interpreter to present the information to the patient, and allow the patient time to ask questions.

The Audiology Home

A cornerstone for providing audiologic care to those with special needs is the Audiology Home (Jerger et al, 2001).

The Audiology Home provides those with hearing loss and special needs with multidisciplinary assessment and intervention services under the supervision of a case manager, preferably through one facility but often through several facilities and/or providers. The advantage of centralized management, or "one-stop shopping," is that it allows for coordination of services and integration of information, which is often needed due to the multifaceted needs of those with hearing loss and special needs. It is not unusual for special needs patients with hearing loss and their families to require the services of audiologists, speech-language pathologists, psychologists, physicians, counselors, and educators. It is through the Audiology Home that the information provided by these professionals is coordinated and integrated into treatment strategies to provide maximum benefit.

◆ Infants and Young Children (0–5 Years)

Appropriate audiologic evaluation of the very young infant has become increasingly important with the advent of universal newborn hearing screening programs (Chapter 23). Physiologic test procedures provide much information in the evaluation of pediatric patients (Chapters 18, 20, 21, and 22). In behaviorally evaluating pediatric patients, knowledge and understanding of development, including auditory, gross motor, fine motor, self-help, and social skills, are important. Not only can this information facilitate interaction with the child and selection of appropriate tests, but the clinician can also be alerted to possible concerns that may require referral to another professional. A clear understanding of appropriate age-specific behaviors can be obtained from subjective observation and parent or caregiver reports. Questions should be asked about auditory behavior and general development through either a case history or a simple questionnaire or checklist. Test protocols are selected on the basis of the neurodevelopmental age of the child, with the procedures falling roughly within the following categories: 0 to 6 months, 6 to 24 months, and 2 to 5 years. **Table 15–1** summarizes test procedures for evaluating infants and children. Many of these procedures also assess auditory sensitivity in developmentally delayed older patients.

When reporting test results in pediatric patients, a distinction exists between threshold and minimal response level. Because of developmental improvement in responses

Table 15–1   Summary of Audiologic Evaluation Procedures for Infants and Young Children

Test	Technique	Developmental Age Range	Advantages	Disadvantages
Behavioral observation audiometry	Conditioning: none Reinforcement: none	0–6 months	No specialized equipment needed; can be used with children who cannot be conditioned	Rapid habituation; only sensitive to patients with severe to profound hearing losses; not sensitive to unilateral hearing loss; large intersubject and intrasubject variability
Conditioned orientation reflex/ visual reinforcement audiometry	Conditioning: head turn Reinforcement: lighted/ animated toy and social	6–30 months	Can present stimuli through speakers, earphones, or bone oscillator; less inter- and intrasubject variability; can obtain minimal response levels close to threshold; sensitive to even mild hearing losses	Some infants cannot be conditioned until about 12 months of age; many infants will not tolerate earphones or will not turn their heads when wearing earphones; specialized equipment is required
Tangible reinforcement operant conditioning audiometry (TROCA)	Conditioning: press button/lever Reinforcement: candy, cereal, small toys, etc.	30 months–4 year	Accurate thresholds can be obtained reliably; stimuli can be presented through speakers, earphones, or bone oscillators	May require numerous sessions; patient habituates when satiated by reinforcer; reinforcers may not be appropriate/safe
Conditioned play audiometry	Conditioning: play activity Reinforcement: play activity and social; may also use visual reinforcement	30 months–4 year	Accurate thresholds can be reliably obtained; can be accomplished with traditional equipment; stimuli can be presented through speakers, earphones, or the bone oscillator	May have to change activities many times to keep child's interest; child may need to be reconditioned when activities change

Table 15–2 Auditory Behavior Index for Infants: Stimulus and Level of Response

Age	Noisemakers (approximate dB SPL)	Warbled Pure Tones (dB HL)	Speech (dB HL)	Expected Response
0–6 weeks	50–70	78	40–60	Eye widening, eye blink, stirring or arousal from sleep, startle
6 weeks–4 months	50–60	70	47	Eye widening, eye shift, eye blink, quieting, rudimentary head turn by 4 months
4–7 months	40–50	51	21	Head turn on lateral plane toward sound; listening attitude
7–9 months	30–40	45	15	Direct localization of sounds to side, indirectly below
9–13 months	25–35	38	8	Direct localization of sounds on side, directly below, indirectly above
13–16 months	25–30	32	5	Direct localization of sound on side, above and below
16–21 months	25	25	5	Direct localization of sound on side, above and below
21–24 months	25	26	3	Direct localization of sound on side, above and below

HL, hearing level; SPL, sound pressure level.

Source: Adapted from Northern, J. L., & Downs, M. P. (1984). Hearing in children (3rd ed.). Baltimore, MD: Williams & Wilkins.

to sound, the term *minimal response level* was recommended by Matkin (1977) for describing audiologic test results in young children. At an early age, the softest level to which an infant responds may not, in fact, be the infant's threshold. Attention, motivation, and other factors influence when an infant chooses to respond. The auditory behavior index (ABI) in **Table 15–2** can be used as a simple guideline that summarizes development of auditory behavior to a variety of stimuli from birth to 24 months.

Test Environment

Audiologic test environments for infants and young children must meet the same criteria as for adults. These include adequate lighting, ventilation, and ambient noise levels that meet current standards of the American National Standards Institute (ANSI). In addition, when designing an audiologic test environment for infants and young children, special attention must be paid to safety. Appropriately sized furniture with rounded edges rather than sharp corners should be used. Speakers mounted securely will prevent accidental displacement by a playful child. A nonthreatening environment is also a concern when selecting furniture and decorations.

Test rooms will need to be larger for testing children than those used for testing adults only. The sound room should be large enough to accommodate not only a chair for the child or for the caregiver to hold the child, if needed, but also a pediatric table and chairs for conducting play audiometry. Flexibility is important; thus, it is necessary to be able to arrange the testing booth for procedures with the clinician in or out of the room.

Test Stimuli

Each test procedure has a choice of stimuli, which may include pure tones or warbled pure tones; speech; filtered speech; white, narrowband, or speech noise; or environmental sounds. Obviously, for frequency specificity, pure tones or warbled pure tones are preferable. However, for some patients, obtaining valid responses to pure tones is not achievable, and the clinician must use other types of stimuli that will be successful in evoking a response from the infant.

Pearl

- The ABI may also be useful in identifying infants at risk for developmental delay (Northern and Downs, 1984). Because the ABI provides developmentally appropriate responses to sound, the type of response observed may be used as an indication of the child's physiological or cognitive status.

Although some general information can be inferred when using stimuli other than pure tones, caution must be used in interpretation. For example, when narrowband noise is used, the spectral characteristics must be known. Some audiometers produce narrowband noises that have very wide filter skirts, which may provide spurious data when precipitous hearing losses are found, usually in the high frequencies. The type of stimulus used should be clearly noted on the audiogram, and the limitations on interpretation of stimuli that are not frequency specific should be stressed. Because other professionals may not be aware of the importance of frequency-specific information, it is the responsibility of the audiologist to ensure that clinical data are presented properly for interpretation.

Special Consideration

- When testing infants and young children, speech stimuli should be presented initially because the likelihood of a response is greater. When using pure tones, 500 and 2000 Hz are presented first so that if the child habituates, information is available about threshold sensitivity in the low- and high-frequency speech range.

Order of stimulus presentation is determined by the child's responsiveness. Children usually respond more readily to speech stimuli. Consequently, when evaluating infants and young children, speech is used as the initial stimulus in testing to obtain a general idea of auditory sensitivity. Speech is usually used first when conditioning a child for a specific type of response. Quite often a child may not participate for a complete audiometric examination. For this reason, once speech testing is finished, high-frequency (2000 Hz) and low-frequency (500 Hz) stimuli are presented so that responses in the speech range are confirmed. If the child is willing to continue with testing, other frequencies can then be evaluated. Similarly, if the child will wear earphones, ear-specific responses can be obtained. With this hierarchical approach, if the child becomes uncooperative, sensitivity for speech and some ear-specific data are available.

Pearl

- For difficult-to-test patients, it is helpful to have immittance and otoacoustic emission equipment available in the sound room so that the test order can be modified quickly. Once the child is comfortable in a specific test environment, time can be saved and the possibility of acquiring more complete information can be enhanced if the child is not moved to a different location.

0 to 6 Months

Behavioral assessment of auditory sensitivity traditionally has been difficult to accomplish in newborns. For this reason, observation of responses to sound may be used to corroborate parent reports or findings from physiologic tests (see Chapters 18, 20, and 22), but behavioral measures are not generally used to estimate thresholds. Minimal response levels obtained in young infants may be elevated. Special procedures have been reported that may improve the sensitivity of behavioral testing for young infants less than 6 months of age (Delaroche et al, 2004; Werner et al,

1993). The difficulty lies in being able to obtain responses in infants that are reacting to sound more reflexively than intentionally. To elicit and interpret responses from very young infants successfully, the environment must be carefully controlled to eliminate extraneous distractions. In addition, the clinician must understand the capabilities of the patient and the developmentally appropriate responses to sound. Furthermore, the effects of attention on these responses must be considered to promote the appropriate state for testing.

Behavioral Observation Audiometry

The sensitivity of behavioral observation audiometry (BOA) is low and will usually only identify infants with a severe to profound hearing loss. BOA uses various types of sounds to elicit generalized responses. Although the stimuli for BOA are often noisemakers of various frequencies and intensities, an audiometer can be used for improved frequency specificity and control of intensity. For this type of evaluation, the infant is positioned in the sound field with at least one speaker for stimulus presentation. Although it is preferable for the infant to sit alone, the infant may be held in the caregiver's lap with a second audiologist positioned closely to observe changes in behavior. The caregiver must be cautioned not to move or cue the infant during testing. Test stimuli are presented through loudspeakers beginning at 0 dB HL (hearing level) and ascending in 10 dB steps until a response is observed. Stimuli may include speech, warbled tones, and narrowband noise. Behavior changes may include an increase or decrease in sucking on a pacifier, change in respiration, searching, eye movement, and body movement. This response must be repeated. Time intervals between stimulus presentation should be varied to avoid patterning. It is important to observe the child between stimuli to determine how often the behavior occurs without stimulus presentation. If it is uncertain that the child is responding, the intensity should be increased, and the behavior should be more pronounced if the child is responding. If no responses are observed at low intensities, an intense stimulus should be presented to elicit a startle response. Because no reinforcement is used, the response rapidly habituates.

Unfortunately, with BOA, the audiometric information obtained is limited. Because the stimuli are often presented through speakers, responses provide insight into the status of the better ear only. In addition, several types of behaviors are accepted as "responses" and likely are obtained using a range of intensities, even in normal-hearing infants. Consequently, inter- and intrasubject variability of BOA is high (Thompson and Wilson, 1984). Such variation may be due to differences in the rate of development among infants. Bias can introduce error because of the subjective nature of judging the presence or absence of a response. As stated earlier, the major limitation of BOA is that the minimal response levels are usually suprathreshold, and typically only infants with severe to profound hearing loss are identified with BOA.

6 to 24 Months

Visual Reinforcement Audiometry and Conditioned Orientation Reflex

Infants between 4 and 7 months will begin to turn their heads (localize) on a lateral plane in response to sound (see **Table 15–2**). When developed, this skill can become part of a protocol to obtain more reliable behavioral responses. Two audiometric tests that rely on the localization response are visual reinforcement audiometry (VRA) and conditioned orientation reflex (COR) audiometry. VRA requires the infant to respond with a head turn toward a sound source. These head turns are then reinforced by presenting an attractive three-dimensional animated toy so that the child can see it. Only one sound source is required for VRA, but two are needed for COR.

To respond successfully for COR, the infant must hear the stimulus, localize the source, and make a head turn in the correct direction. Learning to respond to the appropriate speaker may be especially difficult for infants with middle ear disease and unilateral hearing loss. Infants who are developmentally delayed or are premature may be unable to complete such an assessment until much later (Moore et al, 1992).

Some special equipment is needed for VRA and COR testing. For VRA, the sound room must have at least one speaker for sound field presentation of test stimuli. For COR, the sound room has to be designed with two speakers, usually placed at 90 and 270 degrees (Hayes and Northern, 1996). To provide visual reinforcement, animated toys are mounted on top of the speakers (**Fig. 15–1A**). Ideally, boxes with dark Plexiglas covers are placed over the toys so that the toys are invisible until lighted. A control switch is available to light the box and provide reinforcement when the child localizes the sound to the speaker.

A step-by-step procedure for COR is as follows (**Fig. 15–1**):

1. The child is seated alone in a chair or high chair, or on a parent's lap, between the two speakers. The child is distracted by looking at pictures or playing with a quiet toy (**Fig. 15–1A**).

2. An auditory stimulus is presented at ~70 dB above the child's expected threshold, and the box containing the toy is illuminated (**Fig. 15–1B**). If the child localizes the toy visually, he or she is reinforced by the audiologist in the sound room by praise. This conditioning continues, and the auditory stimuli are alternated between speakers, with the auditory and visual stimuli presented simultaneously for a period of 3 to 4 seconds.

3. Once the child is conditioned, the auditory stimuli are presented without visual reinforcement (**Fig. 15–1C**). The illuminated toy in the box is activated only as a reward to the child when a response is observed. This procedure is

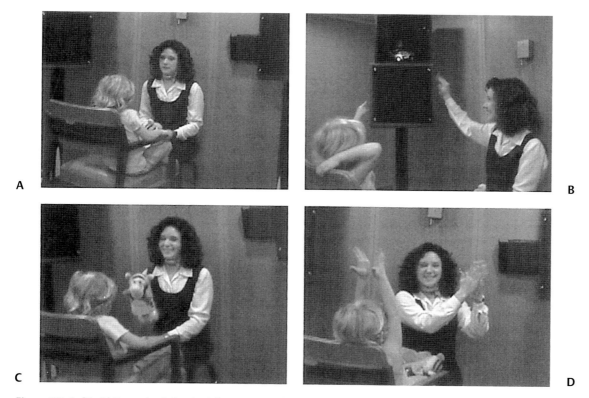

A

B

C

D

Figure 15–1 (A–D) Example of visual reinforcement audiometry/conditioned orientation reflex being performed in a sound field (see text for explanation).

continued, decreasing the intensity of the auditory stimuli until the child does not respond, and the minimal response level is obtained (**Fig. 15–1D**).

Appropriate positioning of the infant in the sound room is critical for VRA/COR to be conducted properly. Calibration of the sound presented from the speakers is affected by position in the room. The infant must be seated between the two speakers as close to the point of calibration as possible. Providing earplugs for the parent or caregiver helps eliminate unwanted test participation at low intensities and protects hearing at high intensities when eliciting startle responses. An option to prevent cueing is to place earphones on the caregiver and present a low-level masking noise during the test session.

Two clinicians may be used for VRA/COR testing: one audiologist remains in the sound room with the child and one in the control room at the audiometer. Communication between examiners during testing is imperative and can be accomplished through a microphone/earphone talk-forward system between the two rooms. The bone oscillator can also be placed on the clinician inside the test room, and communication between the two audiologists can take place by presenting speech through the bone oscillator.

The audiologist working with the child in the test room has the responsibility for conditioning the infant to respond to the signal; controlling the child's attention by creating a distraction to keep the child looking at midline between trials, indicating when a response has occurred, and offering social reinforcement as needed. The audiologist in the booth can indicate infant responses with a handheld signaling switch.

When two audiologists are not available, it is possible to carry out VRA/COR by using the child's caregiver or a volunteer in the sound room to control attention and observe the child. This modification requires a short training session before testing is performed, reminding the observer to be careful not to inadvertently give the child any cues. There are also commercially available systems that allow a single clinician to conduct VRA/COR assessments in a more efficient manner with control of both the stimulus and the reinforcement from within the sound booth.

Many infants will not tolerate earphones, and some develop "neck freeze" when earphones are placed. These children will not turn their heads to the sound until the earphones are removed. Other infants, however, are able to be assessed with VRA/COR through earphones. When such cooperative patients are identified, the audiologist should preferably utilize insert earphones, and the same type of procedure detailed above can be followed. The audiologist should remember that even infants who will not tolerate earphones may tolerate a bone oscillator for a limited amount of time. In such cases, general information about the contribution of sound transmission through the middle ear to any identified auditory impairment may be estimated.

Results obtained with VRA and COR are more reliable than with BOA due to less inter- and intrasubject variability. As a result, comparison of individual test results can be made to normative clinical data.

2 to 5 Years

Conditioned Play Audiometry

Conditioned play audiometry (CPA) is the method of choice for children from ~30 months to 5 years of age. From ~25 months to 30 months, infants are often more difficult to test. They habituate rapidly to VRA and typically are not yet ready to participate in CPA. Clinicians must be especially flexible and patient when attempting to obtain valid information about auditory sensitivity in this age group.

CPA involves conditioning children to engage in some activity whenever they perceive a sound. Often, the tasks are organized in a hierarchical fashion from simple to complex. This enables the child to be conditioned with a fairly simple task; the task difficulty is then increased as the child becomes restless or bored. For example, the audiologist may first condition the child to place blocks in a bucket until interest is lost. Then, the task can be changed to a more difficult one, such as stacking rings on a stick. When selecting these games, the composition of the game pieces is an important consideration. The pieces need to be of an appropriate size for a child to manipulate easily and also not too visually interesting.

Initially when conditioning for CPA, the audiologist may need to guide the child's hand to assist. Assistance stops once the child begins responding independently. A step-by-step procedure is as follows (**Fig. 15–2**):

1. With the help of the audiologist, the child holds an object, such as a block, close to but not touching his or her ear (**Fig. 15–2A**).

2. An auditory stimulus that is expected to be above the child's threshold is presented, and the audiologist directs the child's hand to make a response, such as dropping an object (a block) in a container (**Fig. 15–2B**). Initially, the stimulus can be a high-intensity pure tone delivered from the headset of a portable audiometer placed on a table near the child. Reinforcement through praise is given once the child performs the response.

3. The conditioning continues until the child performs the behavior independently. In a normally developing child, three to five consecutive trials should be sufficient.

4. Earphones are placed on the child, and testing proceeds with 2000 Hz and 500 Hz first, then 4000 and 1000 Hz for each ear (**Fig. 15–2C**). Other frequencies may be assessed if the child remains cooperative.

It may be difficult to condition some children to sound. If this is the case, the child may first be conditioned to a stimulus in another sensory modality. Thorne (1967) suggested presenting a somatosensory stimulus, such as having the child hold the bone vibrator in one hand and a block in the other with the two objects touching. When a 500 Hz stimulus is presented through a bone oscillator at the limits of the equipment, the child will feel the vibration with his or

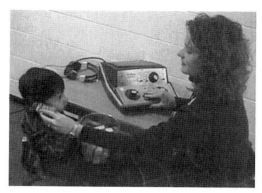

A

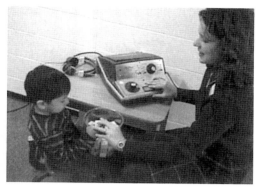

B

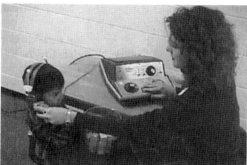

C

Figure 15–2 (A–C) Conditioned play audiometry is performed by conditioning the child to perform a motor task, such as dropping a block in a bucket, when the auditory stimuli are perceived. Note that the audiometer is located outside the child's peripheral vision (see text for explanation).

her hand. The child is then taught to drop the block in the bucket each time this sensation occurs (**Fig. 15–3A**). After the child begins responding consistently, the bone vibrator is transferred to the mastoid, and the child is conditioned to drop the block in response to the auditory stimulus (**Fig. 15–3B**). Finally, earphones are placed on the child, and responses are obtained to pure-tone air-conducted stimuli (**Fig. 15–3C**).

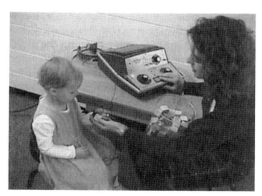

A

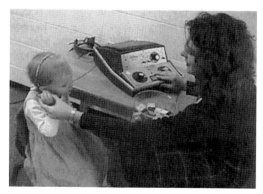

B

C

Figure 15–3 (A–C) Tactile stimulation using a low-frequency (250 or 500 Hz) bone-conducted stimulus at high intensities can assist in conditioning a child during conditioned play audiometry (see text for explanation).

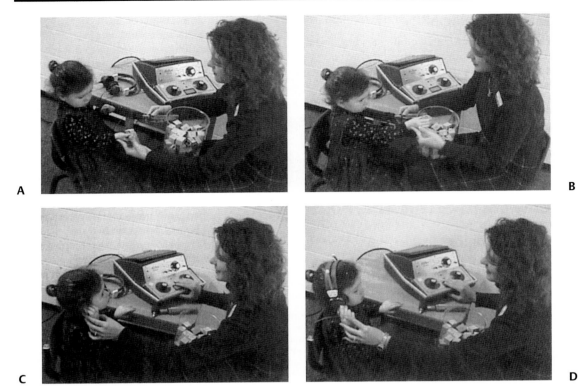

Figure 15–4 Play audiometry reinforcement using a flashlight is performed **(A,B)** by having the child initially respond to a visual stimulus (flashlight or otoscope light). **(C,D)** After the child is conditioned to the visual stimulus, conditioning to an auditory stimulus is attempted.

A similar procedure called play audiometry reinforcement using a flashlight (PARF) is easily accomplished in the traditional setting with a flashlight or otoscope (Roeser and Northern, 1981). For PARF, the child is given an object, and a flashlight or otoscope is held next to it (**Fig. 15–4A**). Each time the light is turned on, the child is conditioned to drop the block in the bucket (**Fig. 15–4B**). Once the child is able to carry out the task with the light, earphones are placed on a table, and a 1000 Hz stimulus is presented at a high intensity (**Fig. 15–4C**). The child is then reconditioned to provide the appropriate response to the sound. Finally, earphones are placed on the child, and testing with pure tones is performed (**Fig. 15–4D**).

Use of visual and tactile stim uli for CPA is beneficial because they are more concrete than auditory stimuli, and children will condition more readily when they are used. This allows the examiner to determine whether the child can be conditioned to the tasks involved in CPA. If a child can be conditioned to respond to light or tactile stimuli but cannot be conditioned to an auditory stimulus, hearing loss is probable.

Tangible Reinforcement Operant Conditioning Audiometry

Tangible reinforcement operant conditioning audiometry (TROCA) has also been recommended for use with children from 3 to 5 years of age and for use with patients having developmental disabilities. TROCA has some similarities to CPA, but the primary reinforcement is automatically dispensed when the child makes a correct response. The reinforcer is one desired by the child, often in the form of food, such as cereal or candy.

TROCA is rarely used in the traditional audiology clinic for a variety of reasons. A primary disadvantage is that numerous short test sessions are required, during which time the child is conditioned. Most clinical situations do not afford the luxury of this type of conditioning, and test results are delayed, often for weeks or even months, while the child is conditioned. Edible reinforcers can contain sugar that will increase hyperactive behavior. To avoid these difficulties, some audiologists have used small toys or coins as reinforcers. However, small toys or coins may inadvertently be swallowed by the child.

Speech Thresholds and Word Intelligibility

Whereas a speech awareness threshold is often the only response to speech in very young infants, speech recognition thresholds can be evaluated for older infants and children. A child can be conditioned to point to objects (baseball, cow, etc.) or pictures if the child is too shy to speak or if articulation is unclear. If children are unfamiliar with the objects or pictures that are available, they can be instructed to point to body parts.

Tests that have been developed specifically for use in evaluating word intelligibility in young children include the Northwestern University Children's Perception of Speech (NU-Chips; Elliott and Katz, 1980) and the Word Intelligibility by Picture Identification (WIPI) test (Ross and Lerman, 1970). Recommended for testing children as young as 3 years, the NU-Chips consists of four alternative forced-choice black-and-white pictures in a book. The WIPI is appropriate for use with children from 4 to 5 years of age and has six multicolor foils from which to choose. Word intelligibility in older children with good articulation may be evaluated with the phonetically balanced kindergarten 50-word list (PBK 50) (Haskins, 1949).

Physiological Tests

Because responses obtained from behavioral tests with infants and children are often not reliable, objective physiological evaluations have gained popularity. Click-evoked ABRs are not frequency specific, and as a result, tone burst protocols and auditory steady-state responses (ASSRs) are becoming more widely used. Although differences exist between adult and infant ABRs, thresholds can be obtained at similar intensity levels. Differences in ABR and behavioral thresholds in infants are believed to be due to a combination of sensory and nonsensory factors (Werner et al, 1993).

Otoacoustic emissions offer a quick means of verifying the integrity of the inner ear when middle ear function is normal, thereby adding power to the infant and child test battery. The importance of otoacoustic emissions in assessment of peripheral auditory status has increased the need for effective middle ear measures in infants. Traditionally, immittance measurements in infants have been equivocal. Tympanometry suggesting middle ear fluid (type B) may be of value in infants, but the presence of normal tympanometric results in young infants may be erroneous. Tympanometry with higher frequency probe tones rather than the traditional 226 Hz probe tone may increase the usefulness of tympanometry. Furthermore, evaluation of acoustic reflexes may be included. If the infant has present acoustic reflexes, normal middle ear function can be inferred. See Chapters 18, 20, and 22 for more information about these physiological test procedures.

Auditory Neuropathy/Auditory Dys-synchrony

Although physiological tests are valuable in assessing difficult to test patients, the audiologist must remember that these measures provide indicators of function at various levels of the auditory system but are not tests of "hearing." For example, some patients may exhibit auditory neuropathy/dys-synchrony. Physiological test results for these patients are consistent with normal cochlear outer hair cell function, as evidenced by present otoacoustic emissions, in the presence of abnormal nervous system function. Abnormal nervous system function is identified by a characteristically abnormal ABR (Berlin et al, 1998) or the absence of the acoustic reflex when otoacoustic emissions are present.

Complicated prognoses exist for these patients who can have varied auditory perceptual capabilities in spite of the physiological test results. Some of these patients will function essentially normally. Others may have difficulty understanding speech in difficult listening environments. Still others may have varying degrees of loss of sensitivity to pure tones and/or an inability to comprehend speech. If auditory neuropathy/dys-synchrony is identified soon after birth, the physiological findings may improve over time, with some of these patients demonstrating maturation to a normal ABR after several months. For other early identified patients, there may be no significant change over time with the ABR remaining abnormal and otoacoustic emissions continuing to be present. Other patients may continue to have an abnormal ABR, and the otoacoustic emissions may also disappear over time. Because the presence of otoacoustic emissions in light of abnormal ABR and/or middle ear reflexes in these patients can be diagnostically useful, middle ear disease can complicate testing and monitoring.

Treatment options differ because of the variability in functional capabilities of patients with diagnostic indicators consistent with auditory neuropathy/auditory dys-synchrony. For those who do evince auditory perceptual dysfunction, traditional amplification is often not beneficial. Cochlear implantation is a viable treatment option for some of these patients (Rapin and Gravel, 2003). Because the physiological indices of auditory neuropathy/auditory dys-synchrony may change over time, monitoring is especially important in very young patients with such indicators.

◆ The Elderly

Many elderly patients do not pursue evaluation for hearing impairment. In some cases, this is due to denial or the lack of perception of disability, which may be related to the insidious nature of the hearing loss. It is not uncommon for the elderly person to be unaware of how to obtain appropriate audiologic testing and habilitation. This often occurs with the infirm or institutionalized elderly. In cases of impaired cognition, senility, or dementia, caregivers may incorrectly interpret the symptoms of hearing loss as manifestations of the cognitive dysfunction.

Appropriate evaluation of and intervention for possible hearing impairment are important for improving the quality of life in elderly patients. Although hearing loss has been found to have no effect on measures of activities of daily living (Rudberg et al, 1993), hearing loss does have a negative impact on the elderly. These include social isolation and depression (Weinstein and Ventry, 1982), paranoia (Rosch, 1982), and an increased decline in cognitive function when combined with senility and Alzheimer's disease (Weinstein and Amsell, 1986).

Considerations in Diagnostic Testing

When assessing elderly patients, concomitant sensory and physical problems may affect diagnostic testing. For example, many elderly patients may experience visual impairment, have mobility limitations, or have cognitive impairment, all of which may affect the reliability of test results (Phillips et al, 1993). As individuals age, the rate of information processing decreases. This factor must be considered when structuring the test environment and carrying out test procedures. Audiologists should allow for slower information processing during instruction and explanation of test results and recommendations. Because the capacity of working memory also decreases with age, information presented in short packages will be more readily understood by the elderly patient. Speech comprehension by elderly people improves with exaggeration of stress. In fact, modification of speech in this manner to improve comprehension by elderly patients has been termed *Elderspeak* (Kemper, 1991).

Elderly patients are more conservative in responding to auditory stimuli; thus, they may wait for a sound to be clearly audible before indicating its presence, rather than respond to the softest sound heard (Rees and Botwinick, 1971). For this reason, many elderly patients may need to be (re)instructed to be more aggressive during threshold assessment to ensure that the degree of hearing loss is not overestimated.

For Medicare enrollees as of January 1, 2005, the Centers for Medicare and Medicaid services added an initial preventive physical examination (IPPE). This initial evaluation, conducted by a physician or qualified nonphysician provider, is to be completed within the first 6 months of enrollment in Medicare Part B and includes, among other systems to be evaluated, a screening for hearing and balance impairment. The screening is to be in the form of a questionnaire. Individuals identified as "at risk" by the questionnaire can then be referred for more thorough evaluation.

The Welch Allyn (Skaneateles Falls, NY) Audioscope 3 is used in some nursing homes and physicians' offices for identifying elderly patients who should be referred for additional testing. A handheld device that resembles an otoscope, the Audioscope 3 emits pure tones at three possible screening levels (20, 25, or 40 dB) at 500, 1000, 2000, and 4000 Hz. Nurses or physicians instruct patients to respond when they hear the tones; when the screening is not passed, the patient is referred for diagnostic testing. Studies have found the Audioscope to have a sensitivity of 94% and a specificity of 72 to 90%. Use of the Audioscope in conjunction with a hearing handicap scale, such as the Hearing Handicap Inventory for the Elderly—Screening Version (HHIE-S), has been demonstrated to yield a test accuracy of 83% for noninstitutionalized elderly patients (Lichtenstein et al, 1988).

◆ The Mentally/Physically Challenged

Developmental Disabilities

Developmental disorders include disabilities evident in childhood, such as mental retardation, cerebral palsy, learning difficulties, problems with motor skills, visual impairment, and other physical deficits. Because approximately one third of hearing-impaired children in special education classes have multiple disabilities, the demand for audiologists to have a working knowledge of the various developmental disabilities and their impact on diagnostic audiologic tests has increased (Young, 1994). Unfortunately, the various challenges and difficulties experienced when testing patients with multiple handicaps may result in many of the patients having hearing loss being inadequately or improperly diagnosed. This section will focus on patients with developmental disabilities that may have an impact on the audiologic evaluation.

Mental Retardation

Mental retardation is defined by diagnostic criteria from the fourth edition, text revision, of the American Psychiatric Association (APA)'s *Diagnostic and Statistical Manual of Mental Disorders* (*DSM-IV-TR;* American Psychiatric Association, 2000) as "significantly subaverage intellectual functioning" with "significant limitations in adaptive functioning" (**Table 15–3**). To fit the *DSM-IV-TR* definition, the onset of mental retardation must occur before 18 years of age.

Mental retardation can occur in isolation, but in many cases it is associated with other anomalies in one of many syndromes (Green, 2003). Hearing loss is an associated factor in some of these syndromes. Although in many cases the syndrome a patient has may not be identified, in cases where the syndrome is known, the audiologist can review information to determine expected hearing loss and the likelihood of progression for deciding on an appropriate monitoring schedule (Green, 2003).

In evaluating patients with mental retardation, the developmental age of the patient is considered when selecting

Table 15–3   Indicators of Impairments in Present Adaptive Functioning

Communication
Self-care
Home living
Social/interpersonal skills
Use of community resources
Self-direction
Functional academic skills
Work
Leisure
Health
Safety

Note: For diagnosis of mental retardation, deficits must be evident in at least two of the areas.

Source: American Psychiatric Association. (2000). DSM-IV-TR: Diagnostic and statistical manual of mental disorders (4ᵗʰ ed), text revision. Washington, DC: Author.

appropriate test procedures (**Table 15–1**). The incidence of cerumen impaction is high in the mentally retarded population, so careful otoscopic evaluation should be performed routinely in any audiometric evaluation or hearing screening (Crandell and Roeser, 1993).

Cerebral Palsy

Vining et al (1976, p. 644) defined cerebral palsy as "a nonprogressive disorder of motion and posture due to brain insult or injury occurring in the period of early brain growth (generally under 3 years of age)." Some risk factors for cerebral palsy are low birth weight, multiple births, hyperbilirubinemia, neonatal difficulties, and a maternal history of complications in pregnancy.

In 1897, Sigmund Freud first proposed a classification system for cerebral palsy, including hemiplegia, general cerebral spasticity, paraplegic spasticity, centralized chorea and bilateral athetosis, and bilateral spastic hemiplegia (Vining et al, 1976). Some types of cerebral palsy are more likely than others to have associated sensorineural hearing loss. Prevalence of hearing loss will depend on the causative factor for the cerebral palsy. For example, patients with choreoathetoid cerebral palsy may have hearing loss as a result of kernicterus, which occurs in some infants with hyperbilirubinemia when unconjugated bilirubin deposits in the brain. This condition leads to various neurological impairments and is a risk factor for both cerebral palsy and sensorineural hearing loss.

Considerations in Diagnostic Testing   Although audiologists do not need to be able to classify the specific type of cerebral palsy, they should be aware that the patient may exhibit some degree of hypertonicity, hyperreflexia, contractures, and extensor plantar reflex (Babinski's sign; Vining et al, 1976). In general, patients with spastic cerebral palsy will move very stiffly and may even exhibit difficulty in moving at all. Involuntary, uncontrolled bodily movements are more characteristic of those with athetoid cerebral palsy. These involuntary body movements often make it difficult to determine whether the patient has responded solely to the presence of the test signal. In addition, these movements may introduce some degree of masking noise, which can affect threshold measurements. Movement artifacts may also make physiological assessments of auditory status, such as otoacoustic emissions, acoustic reflexes, and ABRs, difficult.

Special Consideration

- Many patients with cerebral palsy may have associated visual defects. Before attempting VRA, audiologists should obtain information about the patient's visual status. If uncorrected visual deficits exist, VRA may not be the assessment tool of choice.

Response modes should vary depending on patient capabilities. One may find that eye movements or eye blinks are the only means for the patient to signal a response. Modified play procedures may be useful with adult patients who understand the process but are physically incapable of responding with traditional response modes. For example, some adult patients may find it easier to release an object that has been placed in their hand when hearing a tone than to raise their hand or push a button.

Down Syndrome

Down syndrome is also termed trisomy 21, in reference to its chromosomal abnormality etiology. Patients with Down syndrome have recognizable physical characteristics, including upward slanting eyes, epicanthic folds, small noses, low nasal bridges, protruding tongues, broad hands and fingers, and short stature (Gath, 1978). In addition, Down syndrome patients exhibit varying degrees of mental handicap that can affect their ability to participate in age-appropriate audiometric testing.

Because anatomical malformations of the auditory system have been reported from the pinna through the central auditory system, it is estimated that hearing loss occurs in 40 to 70% of Down syndrome patients (Bilgin et al, 1996). Hearing loss may be conductive, mixed, or sensorineural. Down syndrome patients have pinnas that are smaller and lower set than in the normal population (Aase et al, 1973). Ear canals are often stenotic, and malformations of middle ear structures have been noted (Bilgin et al, 1996). As a result, Down syndrome patients have more problems with excessive cerumen and concomitant conductive hearing loss (Maroudias et al, 1994). In addition, ossicular malformations and structural differences in the middle ear, eustachian tube, and nasopharynx have been reported (Sando and Takahashi, 1990), which may be partially responsible for the increased incidence of otitis media with effusion in this population (Selikowitz, 1993).

Although reported inner ear malformations include both the cochlear and the vestibular systems, these structural differences are minor (Bilgin et al, 1996). A greater concern exists with the incidence of early onset sensorineural hearing loss (Keiser et al, 1981) similar to presbycusis. Walford (1980), in fact, suggested that patients with Down syndrome exhibit "accelerated aging," which not only includes the auditory system but also the visual system and cognitive function.

One important consideration in evaluating patients with Down syndrome is the selection of test procedures that are developmentally appropriate. A young Down syndrome child may be best evaluated with VRA, whereas an older Down syndrome patient may be successfully evaluated with CPA even into adulthood. However, caution is called for when interpreting test results because patients with Down syndrome have questionable response validity as a result of excessive false-positive responses (Diefendorf et al, 1995). Furthermore, slightly elevated thresholds may be due, in part, to increased inattentiveness and other nonsensory factors in Down syndrome children (Werner et al, 1996).

Pearl

- Greenberg et al (1978) suggested the use of the Bayley Scales of Infant Development (BSID) before audiometric assessment of Down syndrome children to determine the mental age equivalent. Their research revealed that Down syndrome patients do not successfully complete VRA until the BSID mental age of 10 to 12 months.

Although excessive cerumen and stenotic ear canals may make immittance measurements more difficult in patients with Down syndrome, it is still recommended. Acoustic reflex testing may not be useful with Down syndrome patients because reports have found them to be absent or elevated in many with normal middle ear function and adequate hearing (Schwartz and Schwartz, 1978).

Special Consideration

- Because of concern about possible conductive hearing loss in children with Down syndrome, it has been recommended that, minimally, a sound field and bone conduction speech recognition threshold/speech awareness threshold (SRT/SAT) be obtained when complete air- and bone-conduction results are not available (Diefendorf et al, 1995).

Management of patients with Down syndrome should include careful monitoring of auditory status even after treatment of middle ear pathological conditions. Residual conductive hearing loss requiring additional medical intervention has been reported in many patients even after placement of tympanostomy tubes (Selikowitz, 1993). For children with Down syndrome and chronic hearing loss, appropriate habilitation procedures are needed while the child continues to experience hearing difficulties. Amplification should be considered until the medical condition can be resolved. In some cases the medical intervention may not be successful in alleviating the hearing loss, and in other cases a concomitant sensorineural hearing loss may be present. In adult patients, monitoring of hearing is recommended due to possible early onset of presbycusis.

Attention Deficit/Hyperactivity Disorder

In delineating the criteria for diagnosis of attention deficit/hyperactivity disorder (ADHD), the *DSM-IV-TR* separates the symptoms on the basis of whether they are primarily due to inattention or hyperactivity-impulsivity. There are also three subtypes described. To be diagnosed with ADHD, combined type, a child must have exhibited a minimum of six of the symptoms of inattention and six

Table 15–4   Symptoms for Attention Deficit/Hyperactivity Disorder

Inattention
Fails to give close attention to details or makes careless mistakes
Difficulty sustaining attention/persisting with tasks to completion
Appear as though mind is elsewhere/does not listen
Frequent shifts in attention/failure to follow tasks through to completion
Difficulty organizing tasks and activities
Avoidance of activities that demand sustained self-application and mental effort
Work habits disorganized with scattered and poorly maintained papers/materials
Easily distracted by irrelevant stimuli
Often forgetful

Hyperactivity
Fidgetiness/squirming
Failure to remain seated when expected to do so
Excessive inappropriate running/climbing
Difficulty playing/engaging quietly in leisure activities
Appearing to be often "on the go"
Talking excessively

Impulsivity
Impatience
Difficulty awaiting turn
Frequently interrupting others

Source: American Psychiatric Association. (2000). DSM-IV-TR: Diagnostic and statistical manual mental disorders (4th ed), text revision. Washington, DC: Author.

of the symptoms of hyperactivity-impulsivity for at least 6 months (**Table 15–4**). For ADHD, predominantly inattentive type, there should be at least six of the symptoms of inattention but fewer than six symptoms of of hyperactivity-impulsivity, and for ADHD, predominantly hyperactive-impulsive type, there should be at least six symptoms of hyperactivity-impulsivity but fewer than six symptoms of inattention present. The combined type is believed to be most common in children and adolescents. For all types, the symptoms must also be evident in more than one setting (e.g., home and school) and to a degree that is considered maladaptive. Furthermore, some of the symptoms must be evident before the age of 7 and cannot be accounted for by another type of mental disorder.

Sometimes the audiologist or otolaryngologist may be the initial referral for a child with attention deficit disorder (ADD)/ADHD. Often, the parents are concerned that a hearing problem may be causing their child to do poorly in school or misbehave. Because patients with ADD/ADHD are easily distracted and have difficulty remembering, brief instructions should be given so that it is clear about what is expected in the test situation. Distractions in the test environment should be kept to a minimum. If the test session will be long (as in an evaluation for central auditory processing deficits), frequent breaks are called for, and careful monitoring of the attentional state throughout testing is needed. Tones and speech should be presented during periods when movement is minimal and the child praised when sitting still to listen.

Table 15–5 Criteria for Diagnosis of Autistic Disorder*

Impairment in Social Interaction
Marked impairment in the use of multiple nonverbal behaviors to regulate social interaction
Failure to develop peer relationships appropriate to developmental level
Lack of spontaneous seeking to share enjoyment, interests, or achievements with others
Lack of social or emotional reciprocity

Impairment in Communication
Delay in, or total lack of, the development of spoken language
For those who do speak, marked impairment in the ability to sustain a conversation
Stereotyped and repetitive use of language or idiosyncratic language
Lack of varied, spontaneous make-believe play or social imitative play appropriate to developmental level

Restricted, Repetitive, and Stereotyped Patterns of Behavior, Interests, and Activities
Encompassing preoccupation with one or more stereotyped and restricted patterns of interest that is abnormal either in intensity or focus
Inflexible adherence to specific, nonfunctional routines or rituals
Stereotyped and repetitive motor mannerisms
Persistent preoccupation with parts of objects

*A total of at least 6 must be evident for a diagnosis of autism to be made.
Source: American Psychiatric Association. (2000). DSM-IV-TR: Diagnostic and statistical manual of mental disorders (4th ed), text revision. Washington, DC: Author.

Autism

Patients with autism are characterized by the symptoms listed in **Table 15–5**. In addition to these indicators, autism is suspected if a child has delayed social interaction, limited language use in social communication, or symbolic/imaginative play before the age of 3 (American Psychiatric Association, 2000). Because of unresponsiveness to sound, it is not unusual for an audiologist to be the first professional to evaluate a young autistic child. Parents may be confused about their child's inconsistent responses to various sound stimuli. For example, a child with autism may not seem to hear a loud sound such as a train nearby but become distressed at softer, less noticeable sounds. An audiologist may want to use the Checklist for Autism in Toddlers (CHAT; Egelhoff et al, 2005) or have the parent and/or teachers complete the Gilliam Autism Rating Scale (GARS; Gilliam, 1995) if autism is suspected (Lindsay, 2005).

Considerations in Diagnostic Testing   Although these children may seem to be less reactive than normal, they can actually "shut down" with stimulation overload. If an autistic child is not responding in a test environment, the environment/test stimuli may need to be simplified. Sensory integration therapy has been successfully used by speech-language pathologists and occupational therapists in working with autistic patients. Clinicians can use some of the principles found in sensory integration therapy to improve testing autistic children. Touching the child unexpectedly during testing should be avoided; when touching is necessary, firm pressure should be used because light, unexpected

touches are known to be overstimulating to autistic children (Quill, 1995). Because autistic patients may be tactilely hypersensitive, having the parents introduce the child to earphones at home prior to testing may be useful (Cloppert and Williams, 2005). Slow, rhythmic vestibular stimulation has been found to be calming for autistic children, so one may want to place the child in a rocking chair during testing (Quill, 1995).

Some authors have suggested that autistic children do not have a simple sensory deficit but rather an attentional problem (Lovaas et al, 1971). Such children may have difficulties selectively attending to specific stimuli. Unlike many children who perform better with multisensory cues for play audiometry or VRA conditioning, children with autism may exhibit stimulus overselectivity (Lovaas et al, 1971). As a result, when testing a child with autism, it is best to limit the number of cues.

In fact, concern about overstimulation or problems with selective attention in autistic children led to the suggestion that the use of ear protectors to reduce auditory stimulation in classroom settings may improve the behavior of some autistic children and their performance on tasks requiring concentration (Fassler and Bryant, 1971). Hypersensitivity to sound has also been indicated in individuals with autism (Downs et el, 2005; Rosenhall et al, 1999).

Downs et al (2005) recommend that in addition to traditional audiometric testing, auditory behaviors should be assessed with a tool such as the Children's Auditory Performance Scale. With this tool, parents may rate their child with autism as having more difficulty with auditory memory, auditory attention, listening in noise, and listening while involved in another activity (Downs et al, 2005).

Patients with Dementia

According to the diagnostic criteria from *DSM-IV-TR* (APA, 2000), dementia can occur as a result of vascular problems, human immunodeficiency virus, head trauma, Parkinson's disease, Huntington's disease, Creutzfeldt-Jakob disease, normal-pressure hydrocephalus, hypothyroidism, brain tumor, vitamin B_{12} deficiency, intracranial radiation, substance use (alcohol, drug abuse, or medications), or a combination of these factors. All patients with dementia will exhibit some type of memory impairment that results in difficulty learning new information or recalling information. These patients may also have aphasia, apraxia, agnosias, and problems with various higher-level tasks. Two patient populations with dementia commonly seen in audiology practices are those with brain injury and Alzheimer's disease.

Brain injuries can occur in a variety of ways, such as head trauma or stroke. The type of deficits observed depends on the area of the brain affected. **Table 15–6** lists aphasia syndromes produced by strokes within the various areas of the brain. As shown, depending on the area of the lesion, spontaneous speech, comprehension, repetition, naming, reading comprehension, and writing are affected differently. To evaluate patients with brain injury appropriately, it is helpful to know which brain functions are impaired and intact, so as to capitalize on the intact capabilities of the patient. For example, if it is known that the patient has a lesion to

Table 15–6   Aphasia Syndromes Produced by Strokes

Syndrome	Area of Lesion	Spontaneous Speech	Comprehension	Repetition	Naming	Reading Comprehension	Writing
Wernicke's aphasia	Posterior portion of superior temporal gyrus (Wernicke's area)	Fluent	Poor	Poor	Poor	Poor	Poor
Pure word deafness	Both primary auditory cortices, or connection between them and Wernicke's area	Fluent	Poor	Poor	Good	Good	Good
Broca's aphasia	Frontal cortex rostral to base of primary motor cortex (Broca's area)	Nonfluent	Good	Poor*	Poor	Good	Poor
Global aphasia	Broca's area and Wernicke's area	Nonfluent	Poor	Poor	Poor	Poor	Poor
Conduction aphasia	Area of parietal lobe superior to lateral fissure	Fluent	Good	Poor	Good	Good to poor	Good
Anomic aphasia	Various parts of parietal or temporal lobes	Fluent	Good	Good	Poor	Good to poor	Good to poor
Transcortical sensory aphasia	Connections between speech areas and posterior association cortex	Nonfluent or even absent	Poor	Good	Poor	Poor†	Poor
Transcortical motor aphasia	Supplementary motor area	Nonfluent	Good	Good	Poor	Good	Poor

*May be better than spontaneous speech.

†Patient may be able to read words without comprehending them.

Source: Adapted from Carlson, N. R. (1986). Physiology of behavior (3rd ed). Boston: Allyn & Bacon.

both primary auditory cortices with pure word deafness, written instructions for pure-tone testing can be provided. Patients with Broca's aphasia will not be able to repeat words for word intelligibility testing, but comprehension is usually good; therefore, a picture-pointing task may be a more valid indicator of auditory comprehension.

Patients with Alzheimer's disease have progressive memory loss and cognitive dysfunction. In addition, central changes in sensory systems, including those subserving vision, olfaction, and audition, have been documented. Lesions have been documented in patients with Alzheimer's disease in the auditory system at the inferior olivary nucleus (Iseki et al, 1989), the lateral lemniscus (Ishii, 1966), the inferior colliculus, the medial geniculate body, and auditory primary and association cortices (Sinha et al, 1993). Other than those changes that can be attributed to normal aging, the peripheral auditory system does not seem to be similarly affected in these patients (Sinha et al, 1996). The other deficits experienced by patients with Alzheimer's disease contribute to difficulty in obtaining reliable audiologic test results.

Considerations in Diagnostic Testing

In general, when evaluating patients with dementia, short, simple instructions should be used. Modeling appropriate

behaviors or responses in the test session is especially helpful. For example, for patients with Wernicke's aphasia, demonstrating otoscopy and tympanometry rather than describing the procedure is more appropriate. Obviously, a complete case history is the best means to provide information about the patient's lesion and expected deficits. Obtaining information from caregivers about the patient's general behavior and capabilities will aid in making appropriate modifications to test procedures and facilitate obtaining valid test results.

Visual Impairment

The prevalence of visual impairment in patients with hearing loss has been estimated at ~38 to 58% (Campbell et al, 1981), with a higher incidence in patients with conditions known to cause hearing and visual impairment, such as congenital rubella, neonatal sepsis, and Rh incompatibility (Woodruff, 1986). Within this group are patients with visual and auditory impairment severe enough to be referred to as "deaf-blind." Patients labeled as deaf-blind are usually not deaf or blind but exhibit varying degrees of each sensory impairment.

When working with patients who may have visual and hearing impairment, the audiologist should allow them to become familiar with the test situation through their preferred modality. Although this will usually be tactile, the audiologist should also be aware that many of these patients may be defensive (Mascia and Mascia, 2003).

Testing of infants, as previously discussed, often involves the use of visual reinforcement. When evaluating infants with visual impairment, one recommended modification is to use vibrotactile rather than visual reinforcement (Spradlin, 1985). If CPA is considered, selecting items that are tactually interesting and easily discriminated is an important consideration. In addition, equipping the sound room with adjustable lighting and removing the dark Plexiglas covers from the visual reinforcers to increase visibility are important considerations for visually impaired patients (Gustin, 1997). Gustin (1997) also suggests that the visual reinforcers be portable to allow them to be moved closer to the child for testing.

◆ Pseudohypoacusis

Pseudohypoacusis was a term originally coined by Carhart (1961) to denote a situation in which a patient exhibits hearing loss inconsistent with audiologic test results or medical findings. Patients with pseudohypoacusis can be divided into two categories (Sohmer et al, 1977). The first category consists of those patients who deliberately, or consciously, feign hearing loss. This category would include patients who expect to receive financial or psychological gain for their hearing loss. Patients who have decreased auditory function caused by an "unconscious, psychogenic process" make up the second category (Spraggs et al, 1994). The term *conversion deafness*, although its existence is controversial (Goldstein, 1966), has been applied to the second group. Conversion disorders can take many forms, including hearing loss, visual impairment, and motor impairments.

Pseudohypoacusis in children seems to reach a peak between the ages of 10 and 12 (Andaz et al, 1995) and often is connected to social or academic problems (Bowdler and Rogers, 1989). Children who exhibit nonorganic disabilities are often introverted (Aplin and Rowson, 1986) and may actually be reporting other functional impairments, such as visual problems. Broad (1980) even suggested that children with functional hearing loss may be using malingering as a psychological self-defense mechanism. In fact, children who are suffering from abuse have been reported to exhibit functional hearing loss (Drake et al, 1995).

Although some adult patients have been identified with cases of conversion deafness (Wolf et al, 1993), most reported cases of pseudohypoacusis in adults are believed to be volitional. Cases of functional hearing loss have been noted in industrial (Harris, 1979) and military (Gold et al, 1991) populations. Feigning hearing loss may be attempted for financial gain, as in many workmen's compensation cases, or to avoid work responsibilities.

When evaluating patients with suspected pseudohypoacusis, one must remember that organic causes of hearing loss are more prevalent than nonorganic causes, and thus

must first be considered and ruled out. Furthermore, a nonorganic overlay can coexist with some degree of organic hearing impairment, in which case the degree of the true hearing impairment must be determined.

Identification of pseudohypoacusis is extremely important not only to ensure that the patient receives appropriate intervention but also to avoid potentially harmful intervention. Placement of high-power hearing aids on a child who has a functional hearing loss can cause organic damage. More importantly, candidates for invasive management procedures, such as cochlear implants, have been found to exhibit functional hearing loss or nonorganic overlays (Spraggs et al, 1994).

Diagnostic Testing

Informal Observations and the Basic Audiologic Evaluation

In the initial encounter with a new patient, careful attention should be paid to general behavior and communicative competence. Patients with pseudohypoacusis may exhibit a variety of almost stereotypical behaviors. For example, a patient may make exaggerated attempts to understand the clinician, such as straining to hear, leaning forward, and making exaggerated motions to lip read. Other patients may have little or no difficulty understanding the clinician in nontest conversation but provide audiometric test results that are inconsistent with the ease observed during informal communication.

In most cases, success in obtaining valid test results in patients who exhibit pseudohypoacusis is determined in the first few moments of testing. The initial, informal observation of communicative behavior provides a starting point. As testing progresses further without determining valid threshold levels, the more difficult it becomes to encourage an uncooperative patient to provide truthful responses. Once a patient has convinced the clinician, family members, physician, and so forth that the functional hearing loss is organic, the patient often becomes more determined to continue to demonstrate the hearing loss.

Pearl

- An informal technique to use with young or naive patients with pseudohypoacusis is to set the audiometer at an intensity significantly below the voluntary SRT, and with monitored live voice ask general questions, such as How old are you? What grade are you in? and Where do you go to school?

In conventional audiometric testing, the patient with pseudohypoacusis will often provide extremely inconsistent responses. Therefore, when it is difficult to obtain a threshold because of inconsistent responding, pseudohypoacusis should be suspected. This inconsistency is also evident in comparing tests obtained at different times.

Expected test–retest reliability for audiometric pure-tone and speech tests is 5 to 10 dB. Patients who exhibit pseudohypoacusis are often unable to repeat threshold measures within this degree of reliability. Thus, whenever thresholds differ more than 10 dB from one test session to the next, the possibility of pseudohypoacusis should be considered. However, some organic conditions of the auditory system can result in threshold variability, and clinicians must take this into account before assuming that pseudohypoacusis is present.

In a standard audiometric evaluation, the SRT to spondaic words is compared with the pure-tone average (PTA) at 500, 1000, and 2000 Hz. If the difference between the SRT and PTA exceeds 8 dB, pseudohypoacusis should be suspected. When patients attempt to feign hearing loss, a universal finding is that the SRT will be better than the PTA because speech is perceived as being louder than pure tones. As a result, the patient will respond at lower intensities to speech than pure tones. Lack of agreement between the SRT and PTA is typically the first indication of pseudohypoacusis during the diagnostic audiologic evaluation.

Pearl

- Patients with pseudohypoacusis will often provide atypical responses on speech threshold test measures. For example, a patient may provide only one syllable of a spondee word or get all of the words right at one time and then miss all of them later.

When pseudohypoacusis is considered a possibility for any patient, an ascending approach is advised to establish threshold. The reason is that if a descending approach is used, the patient will be given the opportunity to develop a loudness "yardstick" to be used as a reference.

Use of an ascending approach in conjunction with a descending approach can be an easy method for evaluating patients suspected of having pseudohypoacusis. In cooperative listeners, thresholds derived from ascending tones should be comparable to those derived from descending tones. However, patients with pseudohypoacusis can have thresholds that are 20 to 30 dB better for ascending tones than for descending tones (Harris, 1958). A difference in responses obtained with these two types of presentation is one clinical indicator of pseudohypoacusis.

Many patients with pseudohypoacusis feign a unilateral hearing loss. Within the basic audiometric evaluation, clues are available to suggest that the unilateral impairment is not organic. Because of crossover, when a patient has a unilateral loss with significant threshold differences between ears, sounds presented to the impaired ear at 50 to 65 dB above the threshold of the better ear will be heard by the better ear. The patient will respond until masking is presented to the normal ear (see Chapter 12). This unmasked audiometric configuration is called a shadow curve. When a patient is feigning unilateral hearing loss and no responses are obtained with sound to the "impaired" ear, it is clear that a discrepancy is present. The absence of a shadow curve with unilateral hearing loss is indicative of pseudohypoacusis.

Tests for Pseudohypoacusis

Special tests have been developed for evaluating patients with pseudohypoacusis. Although many are still in use, some are primarily of historical interest. Many of the tests that are no longer used require specialized equipment or proved to be too difficult. **Table 15–7** lists selected tests for pseudohypoacusis. Note that the asterisks identify those tests that are presented for historical purposes.

Special Consideration

- When establishing pure-tone or speech recognition thresholds, an ascending approach is first used whenever pseudohypoacusis is suspected.

Pure-Tone and Speech Stenger Tests   When auditory stimuli are presented to both ears simultaneously, with the stimulus to one ear being louder than the other, only the louder sound will be perceived by the patient (Newby, 1979). For example, with normal-hearing listeners, a sound presented to one ear at 50 dB and to the other at 15 dB will be perceived as a

Table 15–7   Tests for Pseudohypoacusis

Procedure	Hearing Loss for Test Is Applicable	Type of Test
Basic audiometry	Unilateral/bilateral	Qualitative
Test–retest threshold reliability	Unilateral/bilateral	Qualitative
SRT/PTA agreement	Unilateral/bilateral	Qualitative
Speech threshold/ PTA agreement	Unilateral	Qualitative
Failure to demonstrate shadow curve		
Tests for Pseudohypoacusis		
Stenger (minimum contralateral interference level) test	Unilateral	Quantitative
Doerfler-Stewart test*	Unilateral/bilateral	Qualitative
Lombard reflex*	Unilateral/bilateral	Qualitative
Delayed auditory feedback*	Unilateral/bilateral	Qualitative
Swinging story/varying intensity story test (VIST)	Unilateral/bilateral	Qualitative
Immittance measures	Unilateral/bilateral	Quantitative
Otoacoustic emissions	Unilateral/bilateral	Quantitative
Auditory evoked potentials		
Electrocochleography	Unilateral/bilateral	Quantitative
ABR	Unilateral/bilateral	Quantitative
Middle latency response	Unilateral/bilateral	Quantitative
Late components	Unilateral/bilateral	Quantitative

*Historical tests not routinely used in daily audiological practice.

ABR, auditory brainstem response; PTA, pure-tone average; SRT, speech recognition threshold.

Source: Adapted from Roeser, R. J. (1986). Diagnostic audiology (p. 43). Austin, TX: Pro-Ed.

monaural sound in one ear only. Responses can be elicited with pure-tone or speech stimuli; this is known as the Stenger phenomenon.

The Stenger phenomenon is useful for evaluating patients who exhibit unilateral hearing loss. This task is very difficult for a patient to manipulate. Speech or pure tones are presented 10 dB above threshold in the better ear and 10 dB below the reported threshold in the ear exhibiting hearing loss. Normally, the patient will perceive the stimulus in the better ear because it is 10 dB above threshold. If patients are providing valid responses, they will respond. However, for patients with pseudohypoacusis, the sound in the "unilaterally impaired ear" will be louder, and they will only hear sound in the "impaired" ear. Therefore, they will refuse to respond, and pseudohypoacusis may be inferred.

In this application, the Stenger phenomenon is a simple and powerful diagnostic tool for determining pseudohypoacusis in patients exhibiting unilateral hearing loss. However, an additional procedure can be used to glean information about the probable true thresholds in the "impaired" ear. For this additional information, the audiologist must calculate the minimum contralateral interference level (MCIL). After obtaining a positive Stenger test, the intensity of the stimulus to the "impaired" ear is then reduced in 5 dB steps. Eventually, the patient will perceive the stimulus in the better ear and will respond. The level at which the patient responds is the MCIL. True threshold for the "impaired" ear is calculated by subtracting 10 to 15 dB from the level presented to the ear with the nonorganic hearing loss when the patient first responded. This allows quantitative information for the "impaired" ear.

Doerfler-Stewart Test   When feigning hearing loss, patients attempt to use a loudness yardstick to decide to which stimuli they will respond. The Doerfler-Stewart test (Doerfler and Stewart, 1946) capitalizes on this behavior by attempting to confuse the patient with removal of this yardstick. This is accomplished by presenting background noise while obtaining an SRT; the presentation of the background noise disrupts the loudness yardstick (Doerfler and Stewart, 1946).

The first step in performing the Doerfler-Stewart test is to obtain a binaural SRT in quiet. Presentation level of the spondaic words is then increased 5 dB SL (sensation level) in each ear, and noise is delivered binaurally at 0 dB SL and then increased in intensity until the patient can no longer repeat the spondaic words. This intensity is the noise interference level (NIL). Next, the clinician increases the level of the noise to 20 dB above the NIL. At this level, the SRT is reestablished by gradually decreasing the level of the noise until an additional SRT is obtained in quiet. Finally, the patient's threshold for the noise is obtained, which is termed the noise detection threshold (NDT).

With normative data provided by Martin (1975), the relationships between the three SRTs, the NIL, and the NDT are used to determine whether pseudohypoacusis is present. In general, pseudohypoacusis may be suspected if the SRTs in quiet and noise differ by more than 5 dB, if the noise interferes with speech at a level lower than established norms, if the NDT is better than the SRT, or if the NDT is at a lower level than masking should occur for speech. Because the

Doerfler-Stewart test is performed binaurally, it cannot be used for patients with unilateral hearing loss.

Lombard Reflex   The Lombard reflex is based on the observation that in the presence of background noise, patients will increase the intensity of their speech to be heard (Newby, 1979). If a patient is reading a prepared text, and noise is presented at a level too soft for the patient to hear, either because of the very soft level of the noise or the presence of hearing loss, the intensity of the patient's speech should not be affected. If noise is presented at low to moderate levels to a patient who is feigning a severe hearing loss, however, the intensity of speech will be modified, and the clinician may suspect pseudohypoacusis.

Pearl

- The "yes-no" method is helpful in testing young patients thought to demonstrate pseudohypoacusis (Frank, 1976). The patient is instructed to say "yes" whenever the pure tone is heard and "no" when it is not. Patients demonstrating pseudohypoacusis will often respond "no" to stimuli below voluntary threshold.

The test is performed by asking the patient to read from a prepared text while wearing earphones. Background noise is presented at a low sensation level and then gradually increased. Pseudohypoacusis may be present if the intensity of speech increases in the presence of noise at lower levels than expected for the reported hearing loss.

Physiological Tests   As with all patients with special needs, many of the physiological assessment tools discussed in other chapters in this book are useful for evaluating patients with suspected pseudohypoacusis. With immittance measures (acoustic reflex) and otoacoustic emissions testing (Chapters 17 and 21), information indicating the expected degree of hearing loss can be obtained. For example, if otoacoustic emissions are present, the patient should not exhibit more than a mild hearing loss (except in some special cases of patients with auditory neuropathy/auditory dys-synchrony). Acoustic reflex thresholds alone can provide some indices of auditory function in that reported auditory threshold cannot be poorer than threshold for the acoustic reflex. Finally, in cases in which true thresholds cannot be obtained, electrophysiological evaluations may be needed. Material on auditory evoked potentials is covered in Chapters 18 to 20.

◆ Hyperacusis

Hyperacusis means "oversensitive hearing." Patients with hyperacusis manifest severe loudness discomfort to everyday environmental sounds presented at normal intensities.

Hyperacusis dolorosa has been suggested as a general term for patients having discomfort to moderately loud sound levels regardless of their hearing sensitivity (Mathisen, 1969). However, Brandy and Lynn (1995) differentiate between two types of hyperacusic patients: threshold hyperacusis was suggested for patients with better hearing than age-related hearing sensitivity norms and suprathreshold hyperacusis for patients having discomfort to sounds less than 65 dB sound pressure level (SPL) when hearing sensitivity was normal. Whether hearing sensitivity is within normal levels or not, it is clear that audiologists will, on rare occasions, encounter patients who report extreme hypersensitivity to everyday environmental sounds.

No clear etiological factors have been identified for hyperacusis. Various disorders, such as Bell's palsy, temporomandibular joint problems, central nervous system damage, Meniere's disease, hypothyroidism, autism, and noise exposure, have been associated with this rare disorder. However, a universal relationship does not appear to exist between any one abnormality and hypersensitivity to sound.

Patients with extreme hyperacusis may become incapacitated, with the disorder affecting virtually all aspects of the patient's social and occupational life. Although only limited data support a physiological basis for hyperacusis (Brandy and Lynn, 1995), audiologists should not dismiss the disorder as being purely psychological and do nothing. As part of the treatment program, referral to The Hyperacusis Network (444 Edgewood Drive, Green Bay, WI 54302) should be considered. Treatments for hyperacusis have included vitamin therapy, antidepressants, tranquilizers, β-blockers, biofeedback, and counseling. Desensitization therapy has been successful in treating hyperacusic patients (Jastreboff et al, 1996).

♦ Summary

Providing diagnostic audiologic tests for patients with special needs is one of the foremost challenges for the clinical audiologist. This chapter reviews test procedures that have been developed over the years for patients with special needs. Through proper application of available audiologic procedures, comprehensive diagnostic audiologic data can be successfully obtained from all patients, even those with special needs.

References

Aase, J. M., Wilson, A. C., & Smith, D. W. (1973). Small ears in Down syndrome: A helpful diagnostic aid. Journal of Pediatrics, 82, 845–847.

American Psychiatric Association. (2000). DSM-IV-TR: Diagnostic and statistical manual of mental disorders (4th ed), text revision. Washington, DC: Author.

Andaz, C., Heyworth, T., & Rowe, S. (1995). Nonorganic hearing loss in children: a 2-year study. ORL Journal of Otorhinolaryngology and Related Specialties, 57(1), 33–35.

Aplin, D.Y., & Rowson, V. J. (1986). Personality and functional hearing loss in children. British Journal of Clinical Psychology, 25(Pt. 4). 313–314.

Berlin, C. I., Bordelon, J., St. John, P., Wilensky, D., Hurley, A., Kluka, E., & Hood, L. J. (1998). Reversing click polarity may uncover auditory neuropathy in infants. Ear and Hearing, 19, 37–47.

Bilgin, H., Kasemsuwan, L., Schachern, P. A., Paparella, M., & Le, C.T. (1996). Temporal bone study of Down syndrome. Archives of Otolaryngology—Head and Neck Surgery, 122, 271–275.

Bowdler, D. A., & Rogers, J. (1989). The management of pseudohypoacusis in school-age children. Clinical Otolaryngology, 14(3), 211–215.

Brandy, W. T., & Lynn, J. M. (1995). Audiologic findings in hyperacusic and nonhyperacusic subjects. American Journal of Audiology, 4(1), 46–51.

Broad, R. D. (1980). Developmental and psychodynamic issues related to cases of childhood functional hearing loss. Child Psychiatry and Human Development, 11(1), 49–58.

Campbell, C. W., Polomeno, R. C., Elder, J. M., Murray, J., & Altosaar A. (1981). Importance of an eye examination in identifying the cause of congenital hearing impairment. Journal of Speech and Hearing Disorders, 46, 258–261.

Carhart, R. (1961). Tests for malingering. Transactions of the American Academy of Ophthalmology and Otolaryngology, 65, 32–39.

Carlson, N. R. (1986). Physiology of behavior (3rd ed). Boston: Allyn & Bacon.

Cheng, L. L. (1993). Asian-American cultures. In D.E. Battle (Ed.), Communication disorders in multicultural populations (pp. 38–77). Boston: Andover Medical Publishers.

Cloppert, P., & Williams, S. (2005). Evaluating an enigma: What people with autism spectrum disorders and their parents would like audiologists to know. Seminars in Hearing, 26(4), 253–258.

Crandell, C., & Roeser, R J. (1993). Incidence of excessive/impacted cerumen in individuals with mental retardation: A longitudinal investigation. American Journal of Mental Retardation, 97, 568–574.

Delaroche, M., Thiebaut, R., & Dauman, R. (2004). Behavioral audiometry: Protocols for measuring hearing thresholds in babies aged 4–18 months. International Journal of Pediatric Otorhinolaryngology, 68, 1233–1243.

Diefendorf, A. O., Bull, M. J., Casey-Harvey, D., Miyamoto, R., Pope, M.L., Renshaw, J.J., Schreiner, R.L., & Wagner-Escobar, M. (1995). Down syndrome: A multidisciplinary perspective. Journal of the American Academy of Audiology, 6(1), 39–46.

Doerfler, L. G., & Stewart, K. (1946). Malingering and psychogenic deafness. Journal of Speech and Hearing Disorders, 11, 181–186.

Downs, D., Schmidt, B., & Stephens, T. J. (2005). Auditory behaviors in children and adolescents with pervasive developmental disorders. Seminars in Hearing, 26(4), 226–240.

Drake, A. F., Makielski, K., McDonald-Bell, C., & Atcheson, B. (1995). Two new otolaryngologic findings in child abuse. Archives of Otolaryngology—Head and Neck Surgery, 121(12), 1417–1420.

Egelhoff, K., Whitelaw, G., & Rabidoux, P. (2005). What audiologists need to know about autism spectrum disorders. Seminars in Hearing, 26(4), 202–209.

Elliott, L., & Katz, D. (1980). Development of a new children's test of speech discrimination. St. Louis, MO: Auditec.

Fassler, J., & Bryant, N. D. (1971). Disturbed children under reduced auditory input: A pilot study. Exceptional Children, 38(3), 197–204.

Frank, T. (1976). Yes-no test for nonorganic hearing loss. Archives of Otolaryngology, 102, 162–165.

Gath, A. (1978). Down syndrome and the family. New York: Academic Press.

Gilliam, J. E. (1995). Gilliam Autism Rating Scale (GARS). Austin, TX: Pro-Ed.

Gold, S. R., Hunsaker, D. H., & Haseman, E. M. (1991). Pseudohypoacusis in a military population. Ear, Nose and Throat Journal, 70(10), 710–712.

Goldstein, R. (1966). Pseudohypacusis. Journal of Speech and Hearing Disorders, 31(4), 341–352.

Green, G. E. (2003). Evaluation of neurologic syndromes with mental retardation and auditory sequelae. Seminars in Hearing, 24(3), 179–188.

Greenberg, D. B., Wilson, W. R., Moore, J. M., & Thompson, G. (1978). Visual reinforcement audiometry (VRA) with young Down syndrome children. Journal of Speech and Hearing Disorders, 43, 448–458.

Gustin, C. (1997). Audiologic testing of children with a visual impairment. Hearing Journal, 50(4), 70–75.

Harris, D. A. (1958). A rapid and simple technique for the detection of nonorganic hearing loss. Archives in Otolaryngology, 68, 758–760.

Harris, D. A. (1979). Detecting non-valid hearing tests in industry. Journal of Occupational Medicine, 21(12), 814–820.

Haskins, H. (1949). A phonetically balanced test of speech discrimination for children. Unpublished master's thesis.

Hayes, D., & Northern, J. L. (1996). Infants and hearing. San Diego, CA: Singular Publishing Group.

Iseki, E., Matsushita, M., Kosaka, K., Kondo, H., Ishii, T., & Amano. N. (1989). Distribution and morphology of brain stem plaques in Alzheimer's disease. Acta Neuropathologica (Berlin), 78(2), 131–136.

Ishii, T. (1966). Distribution of Alzheimer's neurofibrillary changes in the brainstem and hypothalamus of senile dementia. Acta Neuropathologica (Berlin), 6(2), 181–187.

Jastreboff, P. J., Gray, W. C., & Gold, S. L. (1996). Neurophysiological approach to tinnitus patients. American Journal of Otology, 17, 236–240.

Jerger, J., & Hayes, D. (1976). The cross-check principle in pediatric audiometry. Archives of Otolaryngology, 102, 614–620.

Jerger, S., Roeser, R. J., & Tobey E. (2001). Management of hearing loss in infants: The UTD/Callier Center position statement. Journal of the American Academy of Audiology, 12, 329–336.

Keiser, H., Montague, J., Wold, D., Maune, S., & Pattison, D. (1981). Hearing loss of Down syndrome adults. American Journal of Mental Deficiency, 85(5), 467–472.

Kemper, S. (1991). Language and aging: Enhancing caregiver's effectiveness with "Elderspeak." Experimental Aging Research, 17(2), 80.

LeVine, R. A., & Campbell, D. T. (1972). Ethnocentrism: Theories of conflict, ethnic attitudes, and group behavior. New York: John Wiley & Sons.

Lichtenstein, M. J., Bess, F. H., & Logan, S. A. (1988). Validation of screening tools for identifying hearing-impaired elderly in primary care. Journal of the American Medical Association, 259(19), 2875–2878.

Lindsay, R. L. (2005). Medical perspectives on autism spectrum disorders. Seminars in Hearing, 26(4), 191–201.

Lovaas, O. I., Schreibman, L., Koegel, R., & Rehm, R. (1971). Selective responding by autistic children to multiple sensory input. Journal of Abnormal Psychology, 77(3), 211–222.

Maroudias, N., Economides, J., Christodoulou, P., & Helidonis, E. (1994). A study on the otoscopical and audiological findings in patients with Down syndrome in Greece. International Journal of Pediatric Otorhinolaryngology, 29, 43–49.

Martin, F. N. (1975). Introduction to audiology. Englewood Cliffs, NJ: Prentice-Hall.

Mascia, J., & Mascia, N. (2003). Methods and strategies for audiological assessment of individuals who are deaf-blind with developmental disabilities. Seminars in Hearing, 24(3), 211–222.

Mathisen, H. (1969). Phonophobia after stapedectomy. Acta Otolaryngologica, 68, 73–77.

Matkin, N. (1977). Assessment of hearing sensitivity during the preschool years. In F. Bess (Ed.), Childhood deafness (pp. 145–167). New York: Grune & Stratton.

Moore, J. M., Thompson, G., & Folsom, R. C. (1992). Auditory responsiveness of premature infants utilizing visual reinforcement audiometry (VRA). Ear and Hearing, 13(3), 187–194.

Nellum-Davis, P. (1993). Clinical practice issues. In D. E. Battle (Ed.), Communication disorders in multicultural populations (pp. 306–316). Boston: Andover Medical Publishers.

Newby, H. (1979). Audiology (4th ed). Englewood Cliffs, NJ: Prentice-Hall.

Northern, J. L., & Downs, M. P. (1984). Hearing in children (3rd ed.). Baltimore, MD: Williams & Wilkins.

Phillips, C. D., Chu, C. W., Morris, J. N., & Hawes, C. (1993). Effects of cognitive impairment on the reliability of geriatric assessments in nursing homes. Journal of the American Geriatrics Society, 41, 136–142.

Quill, K. A. (1995). Teaching children with autism: Strategies to enhance communication and socialization. New York: Delmar Publishers.

Rapin, I., & Gravel, J. (2003). Auditory neuropathy: Physiologic and pathologic evidence calls for more diagnostic specificity. International Journal of Pediatric Otorhinolaryngology, 67, 707–728.

Rees, J. N., & Botwinick, J. (1971). Detection and decision factors in auditory behavior of the elderly. Journal of Gerontology, 26(2), 133–136.

Roeser, R. J., & Northern, J. L. (1981). Screening for hearing loss and middle ear disorders (pp. 98–121). In F. N. Martin (Ed.), Hearing disorders in children. Austin, TX: Pro-Ed.

Roeser, R. J. (1986). Diagnostic audiology (p. 43). Austin, TX: Pro-Ed.

Rosch, P. J. (1982). Prepare your practice to keep pace with the aging patient population. Physical Management, 22, 28–45.

Rosenhall, U., Nordin, V., Sandstrom, M., Ahlsen, G., & Gillberg, C. (1999). Autism and hearing loss. Journal of Autism and Developmental Disorders, 29(4), 349–357.

Ross, M., & Lerman, J. (1970). A picture identification test for hearing-impaired children. Journal of Speech and Hearing Research, 13, 44–53.

Rudberg, M. A., Furner, S. E., Dunn, J. E., & Cassel, C. K. (1993). The relationship of visual and hearing impairments to disability: An analysis using the longitudinal study of aging. Journal of Gerontology, 48(6), M261–M265.

Sando, I., & Takahashi, H. (1990). Otitis media in association with various congenital diseases. Annals of Otology, Rhinology and Laryngology, S148, 13–16.

Schwartz, D. M., & Schwartz, R. H. (1978). Acoustic impedance and otoscopic findings in young children with Down syndrome. Archives of Otolaryngology, 104, 652–656.

Selikowitz, M. (1993). Short-term efficacy of tympanostomy tubes for secretory otitis media in children with Down syndrome. Developmental Medicine and Child Neurology, 35, 511–515.

Sinha, U. K., Hollen, K. M., Rodriguez, R., & Miller, C. A. (1993). Auditory system degeneration in Alzheimer's disease. Neurology, 43(4), 779–785.

Sinha, U. K., Saadat, D., Linthicum, F. H., Hollen, K. M., & Miller, C. A. (1996). Temporal bone findings in Alzheimer's disease. Laryngoscope, 106, 1–5.

Smart, J. F., & Smart, D. W. (1995). The use of translators/interpreters in rehabilitation. Journal of Rehabilitation, 61(2), 14–20.

Sohmer, H., Feinmesser, M., Bauberger-Tell, L., & Edelstein, E. (1977). Cochlear, brain stem, and cortical evoked responses in nonorganic hearing loss. Annals of Otology, Rhinology and Laryngology, 86(2, Pt. 1). 227–234.

Spradlin, J. (1985). Auditory evaluation. In M. Bullis (Ed.), Communication development in young children with deaf-blindness: Literature review I (pp. 49–61). Monmouth, OR: Teaching Research Publications.

Spraggs, P. D., Burton, M. J., & Graham, J. M. (1994). Nonorganic hearing loss in cochlear implant candidates. American Journal of Otology, 15(5), 652–657.

Thompson, G., & Wilson, W. (1984). Clinical application of visual reinforcement. Seminars in Hearing, 5, 85–99.

Thorne, B. (1967). Conditioning children for pure tone testing. Journal of Speech and Hearing Disorders, 27, 84–85.

Vining, E. P., Accardo, P. J., Rubenstein, J. E., Farrell, S. E., & Roizen, N. J. (1976). Cerebral palsy: A pediatric developmentalist's overview. American Journal of Diseases in Children, 130(6), 643–649.

Walford, R. L. (1980). Immunology and aging. American Journal of Clinical Pathology, 74, 247–253.

Weinstein, B. E., & Amsel, L. (1986). Hearing loss and senile dementia in the institutionalized elderly. Clinical Gerontology, 4, 3–15.

Weinstein, B. E., & Ventry, I. M. (1982). Hearing impairment and social isolation in the elderly. Journal of Speech and Hearing Research, 25, 593–599.

Werner, L. A., Folsom, R. C., & Mancl, L. R. (1993). The relationship between auditory brain stem response and behavioral thresholds in normal-hearing infants and adults. Hearing Research, 68, 131–141.

Werner, L. A., Mancl, L. R., & Folsom, R. C. (1996). Preliminary observations on the development of auditory sensitivity in infants with Down syndrome. Ear and Hearing, 17, 455–468.

Wolf, M., Birger, M., Ben Shoshan, J., & Kronenberg, J. (1993). Conversion deafness. Annals of Otology, Rhinology and Laryngology, 102(5), 349–352.

Woodruff, M. E. (1986). Differential effects of various causes of deafness on the eyes, refractive errors, and vision of children. American Journal of Optometry and Physiological Optics, 63(8), 668–675.

Work Groups for the DSM-IV Text Revision. (2000). Diagnostic and Statistical Manual of Mental Disorders (4th ed), text revision. (DSM-IV-TR). Washington, DC: American Psychiatric Association.

Young, C. V. (1994). Developmental disabilities. In J. Katz (Ed.), Handbook of clinical audiology (4th ed., pp. 521–533). Philadelphia: Williams & Wilkins.

Chapter 16

Diagnosing (Central) Auditory Processing Disorders in Children

Robert W. Keith

The diagnosis and remediation of (central) auditory processing disorders [(C)APD] in children and adults is one of the more fascinating areas in the audiologist's scope of practice. No other clinical entity presents a more complex set of symptoms to challenge the audiologist. The wide range of intellectual, behavioral, educational, psychological, medical, and social issues associated with (C)APD require that the audiologist be widely read in a variety of subjects.

The purposes of this chapter are to introduce students and audiologists to the broad construct of (C)APDs,[1] to define various issues related to it, and to discuss the diagnostic approach to children who are thought to be at risk for

(C)APD. Assessment techniques evolve, sometimes quickly, and some of the tests described here may fall into disuse as others take their place. It is hoped that the information provided here will be useful in the future as a foundation, despite these changes. In addition, Chapter 3 of this text presents a clinical perspective on the anatomy and physiology of the central auditory system and should be reviewed in concert with the material in this chapter.

◆ Some Important Definitions

One of the challenges of testing for auditory processing disorders in children is to determine whether an individual is experiencing a primary auditory processing disorder, attention deficit disorder, language disorder, or learning disorder. In many cases these problems coexist, and it may not be possible to determine which problem is primary and which is secondary. Nevertheless, it is in the child's best interest to understand the relationships that exist. For clarification, the following definitions of these entities are taken from the

fourth edition of the *Diagnostic and Statistical Manual of Mental Disorders (DSM-IV*; American Psychiatric Association, 1994).

Attention Deficit/Hyperactivity Disorder

The essential feature of attention deficit/hyperactivity disorder (ADHD) is a persistent pattern of inattention and/or hyperactivity that is more frequent and severe than is typically observed in individuals at a normal level of development. There are three subtypes of ADHD based on the predominant symptom pattern: ADHD combined type, predominantly inattention type, and predominantly hyperactive-impulsive type. The prevalence of ADHD is estimated at 3 to 5% in school-age children. Diagnosis of ADHD is based on six or more of nine symptoms of inattention or six or more of nine symptoms of hyperactivity, as listed in **Table 16–1**.

Learning Disorders

In the *DSM-IV*, learning disorders cover reading, mathematics, and written expression. A diagnosis is made when achievement on individually administered standardized

Table 16–1   Diagnostic Criteria for Attention Deficit/Hyperactivity Disorder

A. Either (1) or (2):

(1) Six or more of the following symptoms of inattention have persisted for at least 6 months to a degree that is maladaptive and inconsistent with developmental level:

Inattention

(a) Often fails to give close attention to details or makes careless mistakes in schoolwork or other activities
(b) Often has difficulty sustaining attention in tasks or daily activities
(c) Often does not seem to listen when spoken to directly
(d) Often does not follow through on instructions and fails to finish schoolwork, chores, or duties in the workplace (not due to oppositional behavior or failure to understand instructions)
(e) Often has difficulty organizing tasks and activities
(f) Often avoids, dislikes, or is reluctant to engage in tasks that require sustained mental effort, such as schoolwork or homework
(g) Often loses things necessary for tasks or activities (e.g., toys, school assignments, pencils, books, or tools)
(h) Is often easily distracted by extraneous stimuli
(i) Is often forgetful in daily activities

(2) Six or more of the following symptoms of hyperactivity-impulsivity have persisted for at least 6 months to a degree that is maladaptive and inconsistent with developmental level:

Hyperactivity

(a) Often fidgets with hands or feet or squirms in seat
(b) Often leaves seat in classroom or in other situations in which remaining seated is expected
(c) Often runs about or climbs excessively in situations in which it is inappropriate (in adolescents or adults, may be limited to subjective feelings of restlessness)
(d) Often has difficulty playing or engaging in leisure activities quietly
(e) Is often "on the go" or often acts as if "driven by a motor"
(f) Often talks excessively

Impulsivity

(g) Often blurts out answers before questions have been completed
(h) Often has difficulty awaiting turn
(i) Often interrupts or intrudes on others (e.g., butts into conversation or games)

B. Some hyperactive-impulsive or inattentive symptoms that caused impairment were present before age 7 years.

C. Some impairment from the symptoms is present in two or more settings (e.g., at school and at home).

D. There must be clear evidence of clinically significant impairment in social, academic, or occupational functioning.

E. The symptoms do not occur exclusively during the course of a pervasive developmental disorder, schizophrenia, or other psychotic disorder and are not better accounted for by another mental disorder (e.g., mood, anxiety, dissociative, or personality disorder).

Source: American Psychiatric Association. (1994). DSM-IV: Diagnostic and statistical manual of mental disorders (4th ed). Washington, DC: Author.

tests in one or more of the areas given here is substantially below that expected for age, schooling level, and intelligence. "Substantially below" is usually defined as a discrepancy of more than 2 standard deviations (SDs) between achievement and intelligence quotient (IQ). If a sensory deficit is present (e.g., hearing loss), the learning difficulties must be in excess of those usually associated with the deficit.

Associated features of learning disorders include demoralization, low self-esteem, and deficits in social skills. The prevalence of learning disorders range from 2 to 10%, with ~5% of students in public schools in the United States identified as having a learning disorder.

Communication Disorder

Communication disorders listed in the *DSM-IV* include expressive language disorder, mixed receptive-expressive language disorder, phonological disorder, stuttering, and communication disorder. Prevalence estimates average around 3% of school-age children for each category. Phonological disorders decrease in prevalence to 0.5% by the age of 17 years. Linguistic features of an expressive language disorder are many, including limited vocabulary, difficulty in acquiring new words, shortened sentences, simplified grammatical structure, and slow rate of language development. Expressive language disorder may be either acquired or developmental. Both are described as neurologically based, although the acquired type (usually) has a known neurological insult, whereas the neurological insult for the developmental type is not known.

The essential feature of a mixed receptive-expressive language disorder is impairment in both receptive and expressive language scores. The comprehension deficit is the primary feature that differentiates this from expressive language disorder. The child may intermittently appear not to hear or to be confused or not paying attention when addressed. Deficits in various areas of sensory information processing are common, especially in temporal auditory processing (e.g., processing rate, association of sounds and symbols, sequence of sounds and memory, and attention to and discrimination of sounds). Other associated disorders are ADHD and developmental coordination disorder, among others.

The essential features of a phonological disorder include failure to use developmentally expected sounds that are appropriate for age and dialect. Audiologists may be more familiar with the earlier diagnostic term *developmental articulation disorder*.

(Central) Auditory Processing Disorder

It is instructive to note that the *DSM-IV* does not include a diagnostic category of auditory processing disorder. In recent years, there has been increased awareness of this disorder among professionals, accompanied by an increase in demand for diagnostic services by parents, as well as a need for the development of appropriate remediation procedures. Nevertheless, in many situations it is difficult to obtain services for children diagnosed with (C)APD because a specific diagnostic code does not exist.

One of the difficulties in diagnosing (C)APD is the lack of consensus on the definition of the disorder. Other difficulties are caused by the inability to clearly separate (C)APD from other the disorders described above. For example, Cacace and McFarland (1998) argued that there is not sufficient empirical evidence to validate the proposition that (C)APD is a modality-specific perceptual dysfunction. Their argument was based on whether the definition of (C)APD is to be inclusive (e.g., see the definition in American Speech-Language-Hearing Association [ASHA], 2005) or exclusive of all language and attentional processes that service acoustic signal processing (see, e.g., Jerger and Musiek, 2000).

In the ninth revision of the *International Classification of Diseases* (*ICD-9*; American Medical Association [AMA], 1996), diagnosis code was established for auditory processing disorders (389.14, Central Hearing Loss). However, until (C)APD is formally recognized by the *DSM-IV* guidelines in the same way as ADHD, learning disorders, and communication disorders, it will be difficult for audiologists to obtain reimbursement for testing. Using the *DSM-IV* guidelines as a model (First et al, 1995), this author proposes a method for differential diagnosis of (C)APD, as shown in **Table 16–2**.

Table 16–2   A Proposal for a Differential Diagnosis of (Central) Auditory Processing Disorders

Auditory processing disorder must be differentiated from . . .	In contrast to the disorder, the other condition . . .
Normal variations in auditory processing abilities	Is not substantially below what is expected for a child's age level
Peripheral hearing impairment	Is characterized by a unilateral or bilateral conductive or sensorineural hearing loss of any degree, from mild to severe
Language impairment	Is characterized by a phonological impairment, limited vocabulary, difficulty in acquiring new words, shortened sentences, simplified grammatical structure, and slow rate of language development
Learning disorder	Is characterized by an impairment confined to a specific area of academic achievement (i.e., reading, arithmetic, writing skills)
Borderline intellectual functioning	Is characterized by a degree of intellectual impairment
Attention deficit/hyperactivity disorder	Is a persistent pattern of inattention and/or hyperactivity that is more frequent and severe than is typically observed in individuals at a normal level of development

If the *DSM-IV* (First et al, 1995) had diagnostic criteria of auditory processing disorder, it would read something like the following:

1. Behaves as if a peripheral hearing loss were present, despite normal hearing (Bellis, 1996, p.107)

2. Difficulty with auditory discrimination, expressed as diminished ability to discriminate among speech sounds (phonemes)

3. Deficiencies in remembering phonemes and manipulating them (e.g., on tasks such as reading, spelling, and phonics, as well as phonemic synthesis and analysis) (Katz et al, 1992, p. 84)

4. Difficulty understanding speech in the presence of background noise

5. Difficulty with auditory memory, either span or sequence; unable to remember auditory information or follow multiple instructions

6. Demonstrates scatter across subtests, with domains assessed by speech-language and psychoeducational tests and with weaknesses in auditory-dependent areas (Bellis, 1996, p. 107)

7. Poor listening skills, characterized by decreased attention to auditory information and distractible or restless in listening situations

8. Inconsistent responses to auditory information (sometimes responds appropriately, sometimes not) or inconsistent auditory awareness (one-to-one conversation is better than in a group) (Hall and Mueller, 1997, p. 555)

9. Receptive and/or expressive language disorder; may have a discrepancy between expressive and receptive language skills

10. Difficulty understanding rapid speech or persons with an unfamiliar dialect

11. Poor musical abilities, does not recognize sound patterns or rhythms; poor vocal prosody in speech production

The model proposes that a child must exhibit at least 4 of these symptoms to receive a diagnosis of (C)APD. Additionally, the symptoms must be present for at least 6 months. The symptoms must deviate from mental age; that is, the behavior is considerably more frequent and intense than that associated with most children of the same age. If these criteria are met, it would be reasonable to conclude that the child has an auditory processing disorder.

Pearl

• The reader should remember that the proposed models for differential diagnoses of (C)APD and diagnostic criteria for (C)APD exist in the mind of this author only. The models are proposed in an attempt to demonstrate how things might be if (C)APD existed in the DSM-IV guidelines.

◆ Further Definition of (Central) Auditory Processing Disorder

In 1995, the ASHA Task Force on Central Auditory Processing Consensus Development met to define *central auditory processing* (a term that was changed to *(central) auditory processing*; see discussion below) and its disorders (ASHA, 1996). A second purpose was to define how the disorders can be identified and ameliorated through intervention.

According to the task force, central auditory processes are the auditory system mechanisms and processes responsible for the following behavioral phenomena:

◆ Sound localization and lateralization

◆ Auditory discrimination

◆ Auditory pattern recognition

◆ Temporal aspects of audition, including

  ◆ Temporal resolution

  ◆ Temporal masking

  ◆ Temporal integration

  ◆ Temporal ordering

◆ Auditory performance decrements with competing acoustic signals

◆ Auditory performance decrements with degraded acoustic signals

According to the ASHA statement, these mechanisms and processes are presumed to apply to nonverbal as well as verbal signals and to affect many areas of function, including speech and language. They have neurophysiological as well as behavioral correlates. Furthermore, many neurocognitive mechanisms and processes are engaged in recognition and discrimination tasks. Some are specifically dedicated to acoustic signals, whereas others (e.g., attentional processes, long-term language representations) are not. With respect to these nondedicated mechanisms and processes, the term *central auditory processes* refers particularly to their deployment in the service of acoustic signal processing.

The ASHA consensus statement defines a (C)APD as an observed deficiency in one or more of the behaviors listed above. For some persons, (C)APD is presumed to result from the dysfunction of processes and mechanisms dedicated to audition; for others, (C)APD may stem from some more general dysfunction, such as an attention deficit or neural timing deficit, that affects performance across modalities. It is also possible for (C)APD to reflect coexisting dysfunctions of both sorts. Subsequently, a conference held at the Callier Center in Dallas, Texas, focused on several aspects of (C)APD, including definition, screening, diagnosis, and future research (Jerger and Musiek, 2000). Among other considerations, the working group agreed to promote the use of the term *auditory processing disorder* rather than the previously used *central auditory processing disorder*. The purpose of the change was to "avoid the imputation of anatomic loci" and to emphasize the interactions of disorders at peripheral and central sites. During those discussions, a panel of experts broadly defined APD as "a deficit in the processing of information that is specific to the auditory modality." The statement continues: "The problem may be exacerbated in unfavorable acoustic environments, and may be associated with difficulties in listening, speech understanding, language development and learning." In its pure form, however, APD was conceptualized as a deficit in the processing of auditory input. The construct of an "auditory-specific" disorder helped focus examiners to consider that other types of childhood disorders exhibit behaviors that are similar to those with APD. They include, for example, reading and learning disabilities, language impairment, and cognitive disorders. Therefore, to effectively differentiate between APD and other disorders, the audiologist must consider several listener variables when conducting auditory tests. The variables include, among others, attention, fatigue, hearing sensitivity, intellectual and developmental age, motivation, motor skills, native language, and language experience. When these factors are not recognized, the examiner may make an erroneous diagnosis of an auditory processing problem. In the end, the participants felt that a test approach that focused on behavioral tests and supplemented by electrophysiologic and electroacoustic testing held the greatest promise as a test battery for APDs.

In 2005, the ASHA Working Group on Auditory Processing Disorders (ASHA, 2005) issued a technical report that focused on the audiologist's role in the diagnosis and intervention of persons with (C)APD. When considering the terminology recommended by the previous conferences, the working group embraced the original concept of the need for a multidisciplinary team approach to assessment and intervention. However, the group stated that the term *APD* was confusing to some, and agreed to use *(C)APD* with the understanding that the terms are to be considered synonymous. Finally, the working group confirmed the opinion that (C)APD is a deficit in neural processing of auditory stimuli that is not due to higher order language or cognitive or related factors. Although (C)APD may coexist with other disorders, including attention deficit disorder (ADD), language impairment, and learning disability, it is not the result of these other disorders.

♦ A Note on the Development of Specific Subgroups of Central Auditory Disorders

Jerger and Allen (1998) point out that the lack of specificity of central auditory test batteries "can complicate the remediation and management of children diagnosed as having (C)APD on the basis of such measures." Their philosophical position is that "our goals should be reoriented toward determining the normalcy/abnormalcy of the component processes involved in spoken word recognition." In practical terms, that philosophy translates into determining subtypes of auditory processing disorders in children. Some effort is being made in that regard at the time of this writing, although more is required. For example, based on the Staggered Spondee Word (SSW) test results, Katz and Wilde (1994) developed a model that can be used for understanding the (C)APD and devising a remediation program. Their model includes four categories: phonemic decoding, tolerance-fading memory, integration, and organization. Bellis (1996, p. 193) describes four categories of disorders: auditory decoding deficit, integration deficit, association deficit, and output-organization deficit. Both Katz and Wilde and Bellis recommend management suggestions based on the (C)APD category to which the child is assigned.

Experience has shown that models for categorizing subgroups of auditory processing disorders should be viewed with some caution. Subgroup categories are simplistic, often without clear definition or agreement of what tests or test findings place a child in a certain category. Whether those categories are valid and whether subjects can be reliably placed into one of the category choices are questionable. Gustafson and Keith (2005) reviewed 159 patient files to examine the relationship among tests of speech-language pathology and auditory processing. The lack of significant correlations among measures indicated a lack of construct validity for the Buffalo model. The results suggested that a "cookbook" approach to management using the Buffalo model should be conducted with caution in managing children with APD. In spite of questions raised by Gustafson and Keith, the work done by Katz and others represents an early effort to systematize the assessment and remediation of (C)APD that will have long-term benefits for clinicians. Keith and Cunningham-Fallis (1998) proposed that decisions for remediation should be based on results of central auditory tests. **Table 16–3** provides examples of this model.

Table 16–3 Remediation Algorithm Based on Results of Central Auditory Test Findings

Disorder	Remediation
Disorder of temporal processing	Perceptual training (modify speaker rate, auditory discrimination, phonemic/phonologic training, computer-assisted remediation (e.g., FastForWord and Earobics)
Disorder of auditory figure ground or other monaural degraded speech test	Reduce noise in environment Classroom management, including preferential seating Use of FM system or other assistive listening device
Disorders of binaural separation/maturation	Receptive and expressive language remediation usually provided by a speech-language pathologist

FM, frequency modulation.

◆ Use of Standard Scores in Determining Subject Profiles

As stated in the previous section, Bellis (1996) proposed that one diagnostic criterion for determining whether APD exists is demonstrated by scatter across subtests with domains assessed by speech-language and psychoeducational tests, as well as weaknesses in auditory-dependent areas. The scatter alluded to can be demonstrated by comparing standard score findings among tests of auditory processing, language, and cognition. For example, when subtest scores vary substantially, a scatter exists. When significant subtest scatter exists, it suggests that the child has areas of strength and weakness that need to be explored. In situations where one modality is substantially below others, the finding can help lead the examiner to a diagnosis of auditory processing versus language or cognitive deficit. Examination of standard scores allows direct comparison of performance between tests (e.g., between tests of cognition, language, and auditory processing) or change in performance as measured on tests performed longitudinally on a single individual. In most tests using standard scores, the average score or mean is 100, with an SD of 15. For subtests within a battery, the average score is 10, with a standard deviation of 3 (Keith, 2000b). Therefore, standard scores of 100 (or 10) are always at the 50th percentile, and a standard score that is 1 SD above the mean (i.e., 115 or 13) is always at the 84% percentile level. Similarly, a standard score that is 1 SD below the mean (i.e., standard score of 85 or 7) is always at the 16th percentile level. Finally, a standard score of 130/16 (+2 SD) is always at the 98th percentile level, and a standard score of 70/4 (−2 SD) is always at the 2nd percentile level (see **Table 16–4**). Further expansion of the relationships that exist among composite and subtest standard score and percentile ranks is shown in **Table 16–5**.

For example, to determine subject profiles using standard scores, compare the test results obtained across modality (IQ, language, auditory). When there is a composite discrepancy of >15 standard scores, then the discrepancy indicates areas of specific weakness leading to a differential diagnosis. Comparison of standard scores can lead to two basic patterns: (1) no standard score discrepancy with high or low performance across all modalities, or (2) standard score discrepancy with low standard scores in one modality that

Table 16–4 Composite Standard Scores: Corresponding Distances from the Mean and Percentile Ranks*

Composite Standard Score	Distance from the Mean	Percentile Rank
145	+3 SD	100
130	+2 SD	98
115	+1 SD	84
100	Mean	50
85	−1 SD	16
70	−2 SD	2
55	−3 SD	0

* For subtest standard scores, the mean is 10, and the standard deviation (SD) is 3.

identifies a specific deficit. Common diagnoses include intellectual deficit, specific language impairment, specific auditory processing deficit, and intellectual deficit with co-existing specific language impairment. Within auditory test battery subtests, comparison of standard scores can lead to three basic patterns: (1) no standard score discrepancy, (2) standard score discrepancy with poor scores identifying specific auditory processing deficit, or (3) no standard score discrepancy with substantial abnormality of ear advantage. Examples of using standard score discrepancies to identify specific modality deficits are shown in **Fig. 16–1A** and **B**.

When considering the model of standard score analysis to determine subject profile, it is important to consider a dissenting voice indicating that methodological problems in research and practice cause subtest analysis results to be more "illusory" than real and to represent more of "a shared professional myth than clinically astute detective work" (Watkins, 2003). Watkins' analysis was limited to subtests of IQ tests. Whether the caveat applies to other analyses remains to be seen.

◆ Auditory Neuropathy (Auditory Dys-synchrony)

An auditory problem apparently related to, but different from, a typical auditory processing disorder is auditory neuropathy. There was growing awareness among audiologists

Table 16–5 Conversion of Composite Standard Score and Subtest Standard Score to Percentile Rank

Standard Score	Subtest Score	% Rank	Standard Score	Subtest Score	% Rank	Standard Score	Subtest Score	% Rank	Standard Score	Subtest Score	% Rank
145	19	> 99	107	—	68	97	—	42	87	—	19
140	18	> 99	106	—	66	96	—	39	86	—	18
135	17	99	105	11	63	95	9	37	85	7	16
130	16	98	104	—	61	94	—	34	80	6	9
125	15	95	103	—	58	93	—	32	75	5	5
120	14	91	102	—	55	92	—	30	70	4	2
115	13	84	101	—	53	91	—	27	65	3	1
110	12	75	100	—	50	90	8	25	60	2	< 1
109	—	73	99	—	47	89	—	23	55	1	> 1
108	—	70	98	—	45	88	—	21			

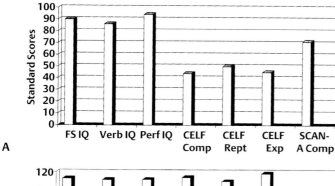

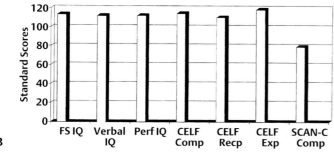

Figure 16–1 Determining subject standard score profile using standard scores. **(A)** A subject with specific language impairment indicated by Clinical Evaluation of Language Function (CELF) standard scores is more than 15 standard scores below the cognitive and SCAN-A scores. **(B)** A subject with specific auditory processing disorder indicated by SCAN-C composite standard score is more than 20 points below the intelligence quotient (IQ) and CELF scores. FS, full scale.

in the 1980s and 1990s of a group of children who fell under a variety of labels, including central auditory dysfunction, brainstem auditory processing syndrome, auditory neural synchrony disorder, and auditory neuropathy. The basis of this disorder appears to be some combination of problems between the axon terminal of the inner hair cell and the dendrite of the spiral ganglion neurons or the axons of the spiral ganglion neuron with the auditory nerve in their course to the brainstem (Stein et al, 1996). Starr et al (1996) provided further information to suggest that auditory neuropathy is an auditory nerve disorder. According to Sininger et al (1995) and Hood (1998), the symptoms seen in auditory neuropathy include the following:

♦ Mild to moderate elevation of auditory thresholds to pure tones by air and bone conduction

♦ Present otoacoustic emissions (OAE)

♦ Reversal of cochlear microphonics on change of signal phase

♦ Absent acoustic reflexes to ipsilateral and contralateral tones

♦ Absent to severely abnormal auditory brainstem response (ABRs) in response to high-level stimuli and inability to suppress OAE

♦ Word recognition ability poorer than expected for pure-tone hearing loss configuration

♦ Absent masking level differences (MLDs)

Sininger et al (1995) state further that one of the characteristics of auditory neuropathy is that intervention appropriate for sensory hearing loss, such as conventional amplification, is not beneficial in many cases, although it is in some. Stein

et al (1996) point out the dilemma raised by a failed screening ABR and passed OAE when OAE are used in infant hearing screening programs, as recommended by the U.S. National Institutes of Health. Those children may be considered to have "normal hearing" when auditory neuropathy is present. The problems of auditory neuropathy are beyond the scope of this chapter, but the reader should be aware of its existence. Furthermore, Sininger et al (1995) state that auditory neuropathy and (C)APD are different entities because "(C)APD is characterized by normal hearing, while auditory neuropathy involves the peripheral auditory system and hearing loss." According to Starr et al (1996), auditory neuropathy "could be one etiology for some cases with the disorder known as central auditory processing disorder," especially those in whom pure-tone thresholds were elevated. Subsequently, the term *auditory dys-synchrony* was proposed to describe individuals with symptoms previously described as having auditory neuropathy.

Rapin and Gravel (2006) suggest that proliferation of the term *auditory neuropathy* resulted in the diagnosis being made without neurologic corroboration, purely on the basis of audiological criteria that included atypical or absent ABRs, preserved OAE and/or cochlear microphonic, and worse speech discrimination than predicted by the behavioral audiogram. In that case, Rapin and Gravel state, the diagnosis is inappropriate because the diagnosis should be made only when pathology demonstrates involvement of the spiral ganglion neurons or their axons. Their model proposing anatomically based nomenclature of nonconductive hearing losses is shown in **Table 16–6.**

In addition, Rapin and Gravel (2006) maintain that the differential diagnosis of electrophysiologic testing and imaging of the cochlea, eighth cranial nerve (CN VIII), and the brain

Table 16–6 Proposed Anatomically Based Nomenclature of Nonconductive Hearing Losses

Anatomical Site of Pathology	Proposed Nomenclature
Hair cell	Sensory hearing loss
Spiral ganglion cells/CN VIII	Auditory neuropathy
Central auditory pathway (cochlear nucleus–inferior colliculus–medial geniculate body–auditory cortex)	Central hearing loss
Spiral ganglion cells/CN VIII and/or central auditory pathway (when the locus of pathology is undetermined)	Neural hearing loss
Hair cells and/or spiral ganglion cells/CN VIII and/or central auditory pathway (when the locus of pathology is undetermined)	Sensorineural hearing loss

CN VIII, eighth cranial nerve.

Source: Rapin, I., & Gravel, J. S. (2006) Auditory neuropathy: A biologically inappropriate label unless acoustic nerve involvement is documented. Journal of the American Academy of Audiology, 17, 147–150.

are now possible to make the distinctions among the types of pathologies described in **Table 16–6**. Both electrophysiology and cochlear imaging will reduce the "erroneous and confusing" use of the term *auditory neuropathy* for cases where there is tenuous or nonexistent evidence that the pathology involves the spiral ganglion cells and CN VIII selectively. When that link cannot be established, Rapin and Gravel suggest that the term *neural hearing loss* is preferable to *auditory neuropathy* as it is currently applied. For those reasons, the use of OAE and ABR alone are inadequate to diagnose auditory neuropathy, according to these authors.

♦ Referral Guidelines

In addition to the diagnostic criteria for (C)APD listed earlier, some of the following behaviors appear to be characteristic of children with auditory processing disorders:

1. They are often male. According to Arcia and Conners (1998), there are two theories proposed to explain this phenomenon. According to one theory, girls have a relatively higher threshold to insult than boys. Another is that boys have a relatively more genetic variability. They might be affected more frequently than girls because their relatively slower development results in a longer period than girls have of immaturity and susceptibility to insult.

2. They have normal pure-tone hearing thresholds. Some have a significant history of chronic otitis media that has been treated or resolved.

3. They generally respond inconsistently to auditory stimuli. They often respond appropriately, but at other times they seem unable to follow auditory instructions.

4. They may have difficulty with auditory localization skills. This may include an inability to tell how close or far away the source of the sound is, and an inability to differentiate soft and loud sounds. There have been frequent reports that these children become frightened and upset when they are exposed to loud noise, and often hold their hands over their ears to stop the sound.

5. They may listen attentively but have difficulty following long or complicated verbal commands or instructions.

6. They frequently request that information be repeated.

7. They have poor listening skills. They require a substantial amount of time to answer questions. They have difficulty relating what is heard to the words seen on paper. They may be unable to appreciate jokes, puns, or other humorous twists of language.

In addition to specific auditory behaviors, many of these children have significant reading problems, are poor spellers, and have poor handwriting. They may have articulation or language disorders. In the classroom, they may act out frustrations that result from their perceptual deficits, or they may be shy and withdrawn because of the poor self-concept that results from multiple failures.

These examples are only a few of the behaviors that are associated with (C)APD. Not every child with an auditory processing problem will exhibit all of the behaviors mentioned. The number of problems experienced by a given child will be an expression of the severity of the (C)APD, with symptoms ranging from mild to severe.

The reader will recognize that the behaviors listed here are not unique to children with (C)APD. They are common to children with peripheral hearing loss, attention deficit disorders, allergies, and other problems. It should not bother clinicians to find similar behaviors among children with various auditory and language-learning disorders. Children (and adults) are capable of a limited repertoire of responses to the problems of life. However, children with similar behaviors may have very different underlying causes and do not represent a homogenous group. It is the clinician's task to determine the true underlying deficit or deficits among children with similar behaviors and to recommend the appropriate remediation approach for each child.

♦ Questionnaires

Checklists of Central Auditory Processing

Several checklists exist to assist school personnel in identifying children who may benefit from central auditory testing. Unfortunately, some have never been validated, including the Fisher (1976) checklist and a checklist developed by Willeford and Burleigh (1985, 1994). Sanger et al (1985) developed the Checklist of Classroom Observations for Children with Possible Auditory Processing Problems. This 23-item questionnaire was devised for educators to record and rate their observations of children's behavior throughout a typical day. Teachers rate the behaviors according to the frequency observed. Behaviors addressed include inattentiveness, reading or spelling problems, and recurring ear infections.

One tool useful in reviewing children's behavior is the Children's Auditory Performance Scale (CHAPS) developed by Smoski and colleagues (1992) to systematically collect and quantify the observed listening behaviors of children. CHAPS is a scaled questionnaire for children 7 years and older. Questions include 36 items concerning listening behavior in noise, quiet, ideal conditions, and multiple speakers, as well as questions about memory and attention. The responder ranks the child with seven responses that range from "less difficulty" to "cannot function at all." The results are calculated to provide a total and average condition score for each of the six categories and a total condition score. The questionnaire is normed to include an "at-risk range" and a "passing range." Fifty-five percent of children in the standardization sample who fell in the at-risk range required some sort of special support of accommodations to succeed in school. According to the authors, the clinical applications of this scale are to identify children who should be referred for an auditory processing evaluation, and to prescribe and measure the effects of therapeutic intervention. At this writing, CHAPS is available through the Educational Audiology Association (www.edaud.org).

A Checklist of Attention and Hyperactivity

The text *Conners' Rating Scales—Revised* (Conners, 1997) has been widely used for diagnosis of ADD with or without hyperactivity based on the *DSM-IV* construct of those disorders. According to Collett et al (2003), these scales can "reliably, validly, and efficiently measure *DSM-IV*–based ADHD symptoms and have great utility in research and clinical work." This screening tool asks caregivers to rank the child's behaviors on questions of restlessness, distractibility, impulsivity, and so on. The items are designed to differentiate children with ADD from those who do not have the disorder. When concern is high, the audiologist will want to determine whether reported behaviors are due to ADD or problems with central auditory processing. When an APD is ruled out and ADD or ADHD is suspect, referral to the appropriate professional for diagnosis is appropriate, because the diagnosis of ADD/ADHD is outside the scope of practice of audiologists.

◆ Case History

The assessment should begin with careful observation of the child, with particular attention to the auditory behavior patterns described previously in this chapter. Care should be taken to identify strengths as well as weaknesses and to note performance in other modalities, including vision, motor coordination, tactile response, speech, and language.

When possible, an in-depth history from the child's caregiver should be taken. Many years ago Rosenberg (1978) called the case history "the first test" because of the value of the information obtained. He pointed out that a carefully

taken history can be extremely useful in differentiating among various problems, can supplement results from auditory tests, and can help in making decisions about the child's educational management.

The case history should be taken systematically to avoid missing important information. The person taking the history should provide an opportunity for the caregiver to state his or her concerns about the child, to describe the child's behaviors, and to express any other related concerns. Specific facts that should be requested include information about (1) the family; (2) the mother's pregnancy; (3) conditions at birth; (4) the child's growth and development, health, and illnesses; (5) general behavior and social-emotional development; (6) speech and language development; (7) hearing and auditory behavior; and (8) educational progress. The specific questions asked of parents will depend on the setting in which the testing is being done and the purpose of the examination. Areas to be investigated in the history when a (C)APD is suspected are given in **Table 16–7**.

◆ Assessment: Prior to Central Auditory Testing

Testing for Peripheral Hearing Loss, Including Conductive and Sensorineural Impairment

Before any attempt is made to diagnose a child as having (C)APD, it is necessary to rule out the presence of a peripheral hearing loss of the conductive or sensorineural type. Neijenhuis and colleagues (2004) found that scores of subjects with mild sensorineural hearing loss were significantly poorer than those of subjects with normal hearing on five of six tests in an auditory processing test battery. In contrast to previous studies in the literature, these authors found that dichotic digit and pattern-recognition tests were greatly affected by mild hearing loss. Therefore, comprehensive audiometry, including pure-tone air- and bone-conduction threshold tests, speech audiometry, and tests of middle ear function (see Chapters 12, 14, and 18), should be administered prior to the central auditory tests. Recent evidence indicates the additional value of obtaining OAE (see Chapter 24) prior to testing.

In general, central auditory testing is done when hearing is within normal limits, defined as thresholds between 0 and 15 dB HL (hearing level) for the frequencies 500 through 4000 Hz and within 5 dB for adjacent octave frequencies. When a unilateral hearing loss is present, only monaural sensitized speech tests can be administered.

Pitfall

- Care must be taken to identify any conductive or sensorineural hearing loss prior to central auditory testing. Unrecognized peripheral hearing loss will contaminate central auditory test results and invalidate findings.

Table 16–7 Information Model for Taking a Case History

Area	Information Needed
Family history	History of any family member's difficulty in school achievement; the language spoken in the home
Pregnancy and birth	Unusual problems during pregnancy or delivery; abnormalities present in the child at birth
Health and illness	Childhood illnesses, neurological problems, history of seizure, psychological trauma, head trauma or injury, middle ear disease, allergies; drugs or medications prescribed by the physician
General behavior and social-emotional development	Age-appropriate play behavior, social isolation, impulsiveness, withdrawal, aggression, tact, sensitivity to others, self-discipline
Speech and language development	Evidence of articulation or receptive/expressive language disorder; ability to communicate ideas verbally; ability to formulate sentences correctly; appropriateness of verbal expression to subject or situation
Hearing and auditory behavior	Ability to localize sounds auditorialy; ability to identify the sound with its source; reaction to sudden, unexpected sound; ability to ignore environmental sounds; tolerance to loud sounds; consistency of response to sound; need to have spoken information repeated; ability to follow verbal instructions, listen for appropriate length of time, remember things heard, pay attention to what is said, comprehend words and their meaning, understand multiple meanings of words and abstract ideas; discrepancies between auditory and visual behavior
Nonauditory behavior	Motor coordination: gross, fine, and eye–hand; hand dominance; visual perception; spatial orientation; any unusual reaction to touch
Educational history and progress	History of progress in school; reading, math, musical and art ability

Source: Keith, R. W. (1995) Development and standardization of SCAN-A: Test of auditory processing disorders in adolescents and adults. Journal of the American Academy of Audiology, 6, 286–292.

When children have a recent history of otitis media, a single hearing test may not be adequate. Fluctuating hearing loss associated with allergies or colds makes it unwise to administer central auditory tests based on a previous hearing test. As an additional comment about conductive hearing loss, until recently little information was available on the long-term effects of early and prolonged otitis media with static or fluctuating hearing loss on central auditory abilities. There is evidence that otitis media can cause auditory learning problems and is not the innocuous disease that it was once considered to be (Menyuk 1992). The residual effects can be central auditory processing problems that may cause language and learning delays that persist long after the middle ear disease has been resolved (Gravel and Ellis, 1995). Therefore, children with histories of frequent colds or chronic middle ear disease should be carefully watched for signs of an APD.

Other Factors to Consider When Diagnosing (Central) Auditory Processing Abilities

- The consensus panel members who attended the Callier Center conference (Jerger and Musiek, 2000) recognized that when assessing children suspected of having an APD, one is likely to encounter other processes and functions that may confound the interpretation of test results. To differentiate APD from other disorders with similar symptomatology, the examiner must consider the following relevant listener variables:

- Attention
- Auditory neuropathy/auditory dys-synchrony

- Subject fatigue
- Intellectual and developmental age
- Medications
- Motivation
- Motor skills
- Native language, language experience, language age
- Response strategies and decision-making style

Failure to account for these factors when administering and interpreting an APD test battery can lead to an erroneous diagnosis and remediation plan.

Behavioral Tests of (Central) Auditory Processing Abilities

Some Background Information on Sensitized Speech Test Central auditory testing has a rich history going back to the early 1950s. Many of the principles developed at that time are relevant to today's practicing audiologist. Some examples of early work in central auditory testing include Calearo and Antonelli's investigations into sensitized speech testing in the 1950s (summarized by Calearo and Antonelli, 1973), Matzker's (1959) early work on binaural fusion, Berlin et al's (1973) research on dichotic consonant vowel performance, Katz's SSW test (Katz, 1962), and Jerger's Distorted Speech test (1960) and the Speech with Alternating Masking index (1964). Calearo and Antonelli (1973) summarized several principles that explain how auditory messages are handled by the normal central nervous system (CNS). They include

♦ Channel separation. A signal delivered to one ear is kept distinct from a different signal in the other ear. The reader should note that some authors maintain that all dichotic tests involve binaural separation of information presented to the two ears (e.g., Calearo and Antonelli, 1973), whereas others separate dichotic tests into those that involve separation of information presented at the two ears and those that involve integration of information across the corpus callosum (e.g., Medwetsky, 2002; Musiek and Pinheiro, 1985). It is important to note this evolution of terminology to understand that authors may have a different meaning for the same terms.

♦ Binaural fusion. When a single auditory message is divided into segments, and they are delivered binaurally and simultaneously, fusion (or integration of the message) will take place at the brainstem level, and the subject will experience only one message.

♦ Contralateral pathways. Auditory messages from one ear cross at the brainstem level and reach the temporal lobe of the opposite side.

♦ Hemispheric dominance for language. Although one cerebral hemisphere (usually the left) is verbally dominant, the other hemisphere appears to possess limited verbal abilities. We now understand that linguistic information reaching the nondominant hemisphere (the right hemisphere from information presented to the left ear) crosses to the dominant language hemisphere through the densely myelinated fibers in the splenium of the corpus callosum.

Related to the above, some additional principles apply to central auditory assessment:

♦ Most diseases affecting central hearing pathways produce no loss in threshold sensitivity. Therefore, pure-tone tests generally do not identify (C)APD.

♦ Undistorted speech audiometry is not sufficiently challenging to the central auditory nervous system to identify the presence of a central auditory lesion/disorder.

♦ Only tests of reduced acoustic redundancy (distorted speech materials called sensitized speech tests by Teatini, 1970) are sufficiently challenging to the auditory nervous system to identify a central auditory lesion/disorder.

Controversial Point

• Some authors maintain that all dichotic tests involve binaural separation of information presented to the two ears. They consider tests of auditory integration as brainstem phenomenon conducted using incomplete message sets presented to the two ears. Other authors distinguish between dichotic tests that involve separation of information presented at the two ears and those that involve integration of information across the corpus callosum. Readers should be aware of the different meaning of integration used in the literature.

The rationale for sensitized speech testing was further described by Jerger (1960) as the "subtlety principle," where the subtlety of the auditory manifestation increases as the site of lesion progresses from peripheral to central. More recently, Phillips (1995) described these processes in a somewhat different way as "patterns of convergence and divergence in the ascending auditory pathway."

Sensitized speech tests use various means of distortion of the speech stimuli to reduce the intelligibility of the message. Distortion can be accomplished by reducing the range of frequencies in the speech signal, by filtering (filtered speech testing), by reducing the intensity level of speech above a simultaneously presented background noise (auditory figure ground testing), by interrupting the speech at different rates, and by increasing the rate of presentation (time-compressed speech). The basic principle of sensitized speech testing is that a distorted message can be understood by persons with normal hearing and a normal central auditory system. However, when a central auditory disorder is present, speech intelligibility is poor. The construct of sensitized speech testing is extremely powerful and forms the basis of all behavioral speech tests of central auditory function.

Transition from Site of Lesion to Auditory Learning Disabilities   The reader will recognize that most of the distortions of speech used in the diagnosis of site of lesion in adult subjects are also used to identify (C)APD in children. An excellent example is the SSW test (Katz, 1962) that was originally designed to identify cortical lesions in adults. Later, the test was successfully applied to identifying (C)APD in children. Bornstein and Musiek (1984) stated that

> [m]any of the tasks that were developed to identify site of central auditory nervous system pathology in adults have been used to assess performance of children with various communication problems. Although medically significant pathology affecting the auditory system may be present in children, the primary use of these tasks is to describe a child's performance and how it relates to behavior and communication development. Performance difficulties on these tasks may reflect a dysfunction or a maturational delay of the central auditory nervous system that precludes adequate perception and therefore optimum speech and language development.

One of the difficulties that occurred in the transition to (C)APD testing was the continued use of terms inferring the existence of an auditory "lesion" to describe test findings, when no specific lesion existed. The language of central auditory lesion frightened and confused parents. More recently, descriptions of auditory performance are based on neuromaturation, hemispheric function, developmental delays, relationships with language impairment and learning disorders, and so on. Also, terminology that describes auditory abilities and disorders is more useful in the design of remediation strategies for affected children.

Special Consideration

• Terminology that describes auditory abilities and disorders is more useful in the design of remediation strategies for affected children than terms inferring the existence of an auditory "lesion."

♦ The Test Battery Approach to Central Auditory Testing

There have been some attempts to develop algorithms for approaching central auditory assessment (e.g., Bellis, 1996; Hall and Mueller, 1997, ch. 11; Matkin and Hook, 1983; Willeford and Burleigh, 1985, ch. 14). Because there was no standard approach to testing, audiologists chose from a variety of tests based on their best understanding of the disorder. The disparity of approaches left the professional and the consumer confused about auditory processing disorders and remediation.

The report "Central Auditory Processing: Current Status of Research and Implications for Clinical Practice" (ASHA, 1996) recommended a central auditory test battery based on those mechanisms and processes that are responsible for central auditory processing. The assessment recommended by the panel includes

- Case history
- Observation of auditory behaviors
- Audiologic test procedures
- Pure tones, speech recognition, and immittance
- Temporal processes
- Localization and lateralization
- Low-redundancy monaural speech
- Dichotic stimuli
- Binaural interaction procedures
- Speech-language pathology measures

The panel recommendations provide a framework for a systematic approach to the diagnosis of central processing disorders. That framework standardizes test battery approaches and reduces confusion for consumers and professionals alike. The panel also points out that some measures of auditory function have questionable validity and reliability and have inadequate normative data. The need for understanding the statistical properties of tests that are chosen for central auditory testing cannot be overemphasized. Readers are urged to learn about these concepts and apply them to their clinical practice. There are many reasons for using standardized tests. They include the ability to properly interpret test results and determine with confidence the child's auditory processing abilities. Results from standardized tests can be compared directly to results obtained by other professionals, including speech language pathologists and psychologists. Additionally, parents of affected children can be very sophisticated (through information available on Web sites and other sources) in asking questions about properties of tests being administered to their children. As professionals, it is imperative that we be able to answer those questions. The consensus conference held at the Callier Center for Communication Disorders in Dallas (Jerger and Musiek, 2000) proposed a minimal test battery for the audiological diagnosis of

APD. The participants recommended that an approach focusing on behavioral tests and supplemented by electrophysiologic and electroacoustic testing held the greatest promise as a test battery for APDs. Although audiologists may choose to use additional tests, the set of procedures suggested as the minimum necessary test battery included

- Pure-tone audiometry
- Performance-intensity functions for word recognition
- A dichotic task (e.g., dichotic digits, words, or sentences)
- Duration pattern sequence test
- Temporal gap detection
- Immittance audiometry
- OAE
- ABR and middle latency response

Subsequently, several authors (Katz et al, 2002) expressed concerns about the specifics of the recommendations made by the consensus committee. These authors cited lack of appropriate norms, insufficient literature support for the test battery, inadequate documentation of the sensitivity and specificity of the tests, and the fact that they were not in common use by audiologists. A primary concern was the emphasis on physiological measures recommended by the consensus committee and the lack of comment on treatment and management recommendations. A basic philosophical concern expressed by Katz et al was the concentration on "factors associated with children's learning and listening difficulties" instead of identifying whether "pathological/ physiological auditory variations are present." In a reply to those concerns, Jerger and Musiek (2002) maintain that it is important to consider diagnosis and treatment as separate issues. In addition, they state, "electrophysiological and electroacoustic measures are indispensable components of a diagnostic test battery for APD." The ASHA technical paper on the role of audiologists was not specific in the recommendation of a diagnostic test battery (ASHA, 2005). Instead, the paper lists the types of tests that can be used by audiologists for central auditory assessment. The list parallels the recommendations of the first ASHA consensus conference and is included in the summary below. At the time of this writing, however, there is no universal agreement on a specific test battery including the role of electrophysiology in the assessment of persons with APD. There is agreement that the test battery should be individually designed, based on the presenting complaints and circumstances of the individual who is to be tested.

♦ Suggested Central Auditory Tests

Temporal Processes

According to the ASHA consensus statement, central auditory processes include temporal aspects of audition. The diagnosis of a (C)APD is accomplished using a variety of indices, including behavioral auditory measures, such as tests of temporal processes—ordering, discrimination, resolution (e.g., gap detection), and integration.

There are many reasons for assessing temporal processing during a central auditory test battery. According to Thompson and Abel (1992), the ability to process basic acoustic parameters such as frequency and duration may predict speech intelligibility. Discrimination of a change in frequency is essential for distinguishing place of articulation in stop consonants and manner in stops and glides. The acoustic cue for place in stops is formant transition (i.e., a rapid change in frequency over a limited time interval). Discrimination of a change in duration likely underlies the recognition of voice contrasts in stops, timing of silent bursts in fricatives, and differentiation of vowel length. Thus, deficits in ability to "hear" small differences in timing aspects of ongoing speech create speech discrimination errors, even though hearing thresholds may be normal. According to Bornstein and Musiek (1984), temporal perceptual impairment has negative linguistic implications for children. For example, duration cues play a role in phoneme identification and in providing linguistic cues.

In research conducted over many years, Tallal and associates (Tallal, 1996; see also Merzenich et al, 1996) contend that dysfunction of higher level speech processing, necessary for normal language and reading development, may result from difficulties in the processing of basic sensory information. One component of basic sensory information is the role that temporal processing plays in relation to identification of brief phonetic elements presented in speech contexts. Tallal et al (1996) state that, "rather than deriving from a primarily linguistic or cognitive impairment, the phonological and language difficulties of language-learning impaired children may result from a basic deficit in processing rapidly changing sensory inputs" (p. 81). They propose that temporal deficits disrupt normal development of an efficient phonological system and that these phonological processing deficits result in subsequent failure to speak and read normally. Briefly, the researchers found that processing of rapidly occurring acoustic information is critically involved in the development and maintenance of language. In fact, language-impaired children differ considerably from normally developing children in the rate at which they access sensory information. Tallal et al's findings led to the development of the computerized remediation program called Fast ForWord (Scientific Learning Corp., Dover, DE).

Rosen (2003) examined the empirical evidence relevant to theories that relate APD to a core deficit in specific language impairment and dyslexia. He notes that, although auditory deficits are more common in specific language impairment/specific reading disability (SLI/SRD) groups, they are far from universal. Many people with dyslexia have normal auditory processing, and there are auditory processing deficits in persons with normal language and literacy skills. Thus, Rosen concludes that auditory deficits, including temporal processing disorders, appear to be associated with these problems but are not the cause. In spite of these controversies, it is important to identify those individuals who have an APD in the temporal domain. The following are measures available to make that diagnosis.

The Auditory Fusion Test—Revised (AFT-R) (McCroskey and Keith, 1996) is designed to measure temporal resolution, which is one aspect of audition discussed by the ASHA (1995) consensus panel. The method of evaluating temporal resolution in the AFT-R is through determination of the auditory fusion threshold. The auditory fusion threshold is measured in milliseconds and is obtained by having a listener attend to a series of pure tones presented in pairs. The silent time interval (the interpulse interval) between each pair of tones increases and decreases in duration. As the silent interval changes, the listener reports whether the stimulus pairs are heard as one or two tones. The auditory fusion threshold is the average of the points at which the two tones, for the ascending and descending interpulse interval (IPI) series, are perceptually fused and heard as one. This stimulus protocol is sometimes called "gap detection."

Among the underlying assumptions for this test procedure is the understanding that (1) the acoustic signals that comprise a spoken language have a basis in time, (2) the learning of these temporally bound acoustic signals requires a listening system that can detect the smallest time segment that is part of the spoken language code, and (3) individuals whose auditory systems have varying degrees of temporal processing disorders will exhibit varying kinds of verbal disabilities.

The Random Gap Detection Test (RGDT; Keith, 2000c) was designed as a modification of the AFT-R. Following a practice trial, the six subtests include the frequencies 500, 1000, 2000, and 4000 Hz, a click stimulus of 230 μs, and a randomized gap-in-noise test. The stimulus intervals range from 0 to 40 msec, with interstimulus intervals recorded with gaps randomly assigned. Stimulus pairs are recorded with a 4.5 second interval to allow subjects time to respond. Normative data found no difference between data obtained on the AFT-R and the RGDT.

The gaps-in-noise (GIN) test (Musiek et al, 2005) was also developed as a measure of temporal resolution. Four equivalent lists present a series of 4 second noise segments in which are embedded gaps. The gap durations included in the test are 2, 3, 4, 5, 6, 8, 10, 12, 15, and 20 msec. As with other tests, subjects are instructed to indicate when they hear the gaps embedded in noise. Musiek et al (2005) found that the GIN test is sensitive to the presence of lesions of the central auditory pathways. The tests described here help to identify a temporal processing disorder that may be related to language learning and/or reading problems. They are viewed as tests of temporal integrity at the level of the cortex. Even though they are cortical measures, they have a low linguistic and cognitive load; for example, the listener must simply respond by indicating whether one or two tone pulses were heard.

Pattern Recognition Testing

The duration patterns test (Musiek et al, 1990) is a sequence of three consecutive 1000 Hz tones with one differing by being either longer (L), 500 msec, or shorter (S), 200 msec, in duration than the other two tones in the sequence. The tones have a rise/fall time of 10 msec and an interstimulus interval of 300 msec. Six different sequences—LLS, LSL, LSS,

SLS, SLL, and SSL—are used in the test. A total of 30 to 50 three-tone sequences are presented monaurally or binaurally at 50 dB re: spondee threshold (ST). Prior to testing, 5 to 10 practice items are provided to each subject to ensure his or her understanding of the task (Hurley and Musiek, 1997). The subject responds to each stimulus presentation with a verbal description of the sequence heard, pointing response, and/or humming. A percent correct score is computed, with performance below 70% considered abnormal by some investigators; however, normative data are limited, especially for children (Hall and Mueller, 1997, p. 535). According to Musiek et al (1990), the duration patterns test is sensitive to cerebral lesions while remaining unaffected by peripheral hearing loss.

Localization and Lateralization

The ASHA consensus conference recommended inclusion of tests of localization and lateralization in a central auditory test battery on the basis of the relationship between brainstem function and neural coding of sound time structure (Phillips, 1995). For example, according to Phillips, determining the location of a sound source requires "temporal processing" in that an acoustic cue underlying the spatial perception is the relative timing of signals arriving at the two ears. Localization refers to the perception of the direction a sound comes from in space, for the case of free-field stimulation. Lateralization refers to the perceived place a sound seems to occupy within the head, for the case of stimulation using earphones (Watson, 1994). Although these phenomena have been extensively studied by psychoacousticians, little clinical research on abnormalities of localization and lateralization has occurred. Jerger and Harford (1960) described abnormalities of simultaneous median plane localization in patients with brainstem lesions.

Devers and colleagues (1978) studied "dynamic auditory localization" in children who were from regular classrooms and children from self-contained learning disability classrooms. By having the children track a moving sound in a geometric (triangular) pattern, they found significant differences between the two groups of children. Devers et al proposed that results suggested a difference in binaural integration abilities of the children with learning disabilities. They cautioned against concluding that a causal relationship exists between the poor tracking ability and the learning disability. Nevertheless, this research provided early insights into perceptual problems that may be experienced by children with (C)APD.

Although there is growing interest in children with "hyperacusis," a frequent complaint among children with learning disabilities, little is known about this disorder. Marriage (1996) defines hyperacusis as abnormal loudness discomfort caused by sounds that would be acceptable to most listeners. The symptoms are typically an aversion to loud sound of any kind, with apparent lowering of the loudness discomfort threshold in persons with normal hearing. The author of this chapter uses the term *dysfunctional three-dimensional auditory space* to describe the apparent inability of some children to recognize how near or far away a sound source, and their constant fear of loud sounds.

Clearly, more research is needed to understand these problems of localization, lateralization, and hyperacusis among children with (C)APD.

Low-Redundancy Monaural Speech

The purposes of assessing low-redundancy monaural speech during a central auditory test battery are as follows. Speech in noise testing, commonly called auditory figure–ground (AFG) testing, has been administered for many years on patients with all types of lesions. Results have found that AFG testing can identify abnormalities in auditory function but cannot precisely determine the site of lesion in the auditory system (Olsen et al, 1975). Similarly, it is generally known that results of low-pass filtered word testing are poorer for the ear contralateral to a temporal lobe lesion compared with the ipsilateral side. However, brainstem lesions may result in decreased performance on the ipsilateral or contralateral ear. Thus, as Rintlemann (1995) correctly stated, "It is difficult to establish good correlation between test results and the locus of the brain stem pathology. Hence, the primary purpose of these tests is in identifying lesions of the central auditory system rather than localizing them." The same general comment can be made for other degraded speech tests, including interrupted and time-compressed speech. A current view of low-redundancy monaural speech testing is to determine *functional disorders of auditory communication*, a term coined by Bergman et al (1987).

One of the most common complaints among children with auditory processing disorders is their inability to communicate when background noise is present. Therefore, speech-in-noise testing may be indicated to identify when the child's ability to communicate in the presence of noise is substantially below what is expected for a child's age level. For that reason, it may be beneficial to use different competing signals (e.g., a single speaker vs multitalker speech babble background) at different signal-to-noise (S/N) ratios (e.g., +8, +4, and 0 dB S/N). Research finds that linguistic materials (e.g., multitalker speech babble background noise) are more effective maskers than speech-spectrum noise (SSN), even though the SSN has the same long-term spectrum and amplitude as the meaningful multitalker competing message (Sperry et al, 1997). Other research finds that white noise and narrowband noise are also less effective than speech babble for masking speech. There is a great deal of variability among normal subjects in their ability to discriminate speech in a noise background. Therefore, when speech-in-noise testing is done to identify auditory processing disorders, it is important to know the normal performance cut-off for the S/N ratio and type of noise used in the test.

Two methods of assessing AFG abilities are to use normed tests that utilize a fixed signal-to-noise ratio represented in SCAN-C and SCAN-A (Keith, 1995, 2000a) and a variable S/N ratio represented by Quick Speech in Noise (Quick SIN) and Bamford-Kowal-Bench Speech in Noise test (BKB SIN; Nyquette, 2005; Nyquette et al, 2001). Other differences in the test approach are stimuli that are single words (e.g., the SCAN batteries) versus sentences (e.g., the Quick SIN and the BKB SIN). When sentence material is used, subjects have the additional benefit of linguistic content to identify the signal. The two approaches allow the audiologist to determine whether the individual's speech perception in noise is normal or not and to determine the S/N ratios at which the individual can function. Additionally, the two approaches allow the audiologist to determine whether a subject benefits from context when listening to speech in noise.

Using a different approach to AFG testing, the Listening in Spatialized Noise test (LISN) produces a three-dimensional auditory environment under headphones (Cameron et al, 2006b). The signal is a story presented at 0 or ± 90 degree azimuth. Various measures assess the extent to which either spatial, vocal, or spatial and vocal cues combined increase a listener's ability to comprehend the story. Following the establishment of normative data, Cameron and colleagues (2006a) found that children with documented APD performed significantly poorer on all LISN measures than age-matched controls. The test is not auditory specific because it requires subjects to report what parts of the story they heard, taxing memory, sequencing, and other linguistic skills. Those issues are addressed in the LISN-S that is under investigation by Cameron and her colleagues. In the LISN-S, the subject is required to simply repeat the sentence without understanding or remembering it.

Few tests of central auditory function are designed to be administered to very young children. One test that includes competing messages that is available for children younger than 6 years is the Pediatric Speech Intelligibility (PSI) test (Jerger, 1987). The PSI consists of monosyllabic word and sentence material with both ipsilateral and contralateral competing messages. Testing is performed by presenting a sentence or word target and requiring the child to point to the picture corresponding to the sentence or word that was heard. The test is said to be insensitive to developmental differences in cognitive skills and receptive language abilities while sensitive to the presence of lesions of the central auditory pathways, as well as auditory processing disorders.

Pearl

Some tests of low-redundancy monaural speech include:

- Pediatric Speech Intelligibility (PSI) test (Jerger, 1987)

- Auditory figure–ground and filtered words subtests of SCAN-C (Keith, 2000) and SCAN-A (Keith, 1995)

- Quick SIN (Nyquette et al, 2001) and BKB SIN (Nyquette, 2005)

- High- and low-pass filtered speech (Veterans Affairs, 1992)

- Time-compressed speech (Keith, 2002; Veterans Affairs, 1992)

- Another resource for prerecorded central auditory tests is Auditec (St. Louis, MO)

In addition to the use of careful subject histories (Chermak and Tucker, 2002), one proposal for differentiating children with auditory figure–ground problems and those with ADHD is to administer tests of AFG and auditory vigilance. The rationale for this test approach is that children with (C)APD will have difficulty on the AFG but not on tests of auditory vigilance. Children with ADHD will have problems with vigilance but not AFG. When both (C)APD and ADHD exist, it may not be possible to separate these comorbid conditions (Riccio et al, 1996). The Auditory Continuous Performance Test (ACPT; Keith, 1994) was designed to measure a child's selective attention (indicated by correct responses to specific linguistic cues) and sustained attention (indicated by a child's ability to maintain attention and concentration on a task for an extended period of time). The child listens to a series of familiar monosyllabic words presented at one per second over 11 continuous minutes. Instructions are to respond each time the child hears the target word *dog* that is presented randomly throughout the test. Errors of omission (misses) and commission (false alarms) are scored. Early validation studies found that the ACPT (Keith, 1994) correctly identified ADHD 70% of the time. Subsequently, Briggs (1998) found that the ACPT correctly identified 86% of children with ADHD.

Another degraded speech task commonly used to identify functional disorders of communication during central auditory testing is the filtered word test. Originally designed to identify temporal lobe tumors in adult patients (Calearo and Antonelli, 1973), low-pass filtered word testing is currently used to identify auditory processing disorders in children and adults with (C)APD. Obviously, except for telephones and sound systems with poor frequency ranges, filtered speech is seldom encountered in the real world. The rationale for testing is that individuals with normal hearing who find it difficult to understand filtered words probably have difficulty understanding degraded speech of many kinds. The inability to understand speech in spite of acoustic distortions in everyday situations provides obstacles to communication for persons so affected.

Low-pass filtered word tests are a category of tests in which speech is degraded by removing part of the frequency spectrum. Some authors consider this a test of auditory closure that is defined as the ability to understand the whole word or message when part is missing. Early research (Willeford, 1977) showed reduced performance on filtered word testing in children who are poor listeners who have central auditory dysfunction. Many authors verified Willeford's early studies. Presumably the child with (C)APD is unable to understand when there are acoustic distortions of speech, resulting in poor listening abilities in acoustic environments that are less than optimal.

Filtered word tests are available with different cut-off frequencies and filter slopes (Bornstein et al, 1994; Keith 1995a, 2000). Because filtered word test results are particularly vulnerable to high-frequency hearing loss, it is important to rule out peripheral hearing loss prior to testing. In addition, as with all central auditory testing, it is important to know the mean and range of scores obtained on normal subjects for the filter conditions used.

Dichotic Stimuli

Dichotic speech testing is typically administered to determine hemispheric dominance for language, shown by asymmetrical ear responses, and to assess neuromaturational development of the auditory system. Dichotic listening tests involve the simultaneous presentation of different acoustic stimuli to the two ears. Commonly used stimuli include consonant-vowel (CV) nonsense syllables incorporating the six stop consonants paired with the vowel /a/, digits from 1 through 10 except for 7, words, spondees, and sentences. With the exception of the SSW test, the dichotic signals are recorded with simultaneous alignment of onset and off times. Tests are administered at comfortable listening levels under earphones. The listener is required to repeat or write what is heard. There are two types of listening instructions given to subjects, free recall and directed ear testing. Free recall allows the subject to respond to whatever was heard in either ear. Directed ear testing requires the subject to report what was heard in the right or the left ear first. Tests vary on whether they require reporting of what was heard in one or both ears. When instructions require the subject to respond to both stimuli, the first ear reported will show better scores and higher reliability than the second ear. Because the right ear performance is typically better in young subjects, reflecting the ear-to-dominant hemisphere relationship, children will usually report what is heard in the right ear first under free recall conditions. Therefore, directed ear listening provides better estimates of the true ear score difference and reliability of test scores in the left ear. Directed ear listening provides additional diagnostic information. For example, Obrzut et al (1981) found that children with learning disabilities exhibited a marked switch in ear advantage on directed right and directed left ear first responses. That is, they yielded a right ear advantage when directed to respond from the right ear first, and a left ear advantage when directed to respond from the left ear first.

In general, for normal subjects, all dichotic test results show a right ear advantage under free recall and directed ear testing. A right ear advantage is typically present whether the child is right or left handed. For one thing, handedness does not necessarily indicate hemispheric dominance for language (Knox and Roeser, 1980). Furthermore, years ago Satz (1976) reported that a strong REA is an extremely probable predictor of left hemispheric specialization for speech and language function. However, Satz found that a left ear advantage rarely predicts right hemispheric function for language only. The greater the linguistic content of the signal (going from consonant vowels to words, spondees, and sentences), the larger the right ear advantage (the larger the difference between the right and left ear scores). As the central auditory nervous system matures, the left ear scores improve, and the right ear advantage gets progressively smaller. At age 11 or 12 years, the auditory system is adultlike in terms of performance on dichotic testing. These principles are shown in **Fig. 16–2**, where typical results of a normal 6-year-old child are shown for dichotic CV syllables, words from SCAN-C (Keith, 2000a), spondees from the SSW (Katz, 1977), and competing sentences (Willeford, 1962). Typical findings for a normal 11-year-old are shown in **Fig. 16–3**. The figure shows improvement in both left and right ear scores, with narrowing of the ear

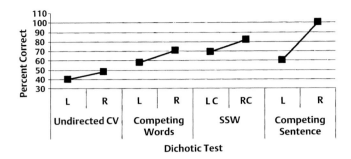

Figure 16–2 Typical results of dichotic listening tests expected from a normal 6-year-old. Responses are reported for dichotic consonant-vowel (CV) tests for undirected ear listening conditions. The SCAN-C competing words test, competing conditions of the Staggered Spondee Word (SSW) test, and the Competing Sentence Test of the Willeford battery are obtained under directed ear listening conditions. There are no published data available for directed ear CV testing in 6-year-olds. L, left; LC, left competing; R, right; RC, right competing.

difference for all but dichotic CV test results that remain essentially unchanged from childhood through adulthood.

The interpretation of abnormal dichotic speech tests follows (Keith and Anderson, 2006):

1. Poor overall performance

2. Enhanced right ear advantage in the directed-right condition and enhanced left ear advantage in the directed-left condition

3. A marked left ear advantage for both directed-right and directed-left ear conditions

Abnormal performance on dichotic tests indicates delays in auditory maturation, underlying neurological disorganization, or damage to auditory pathways. Left ear advantages for all test conditions indicate the possibility of damage to the auditory reception areas of the left hemisphere, or failure to develop left hemisphere dominance for language. These abnormalities are related to a wide range of specific learning disabilities, including (central) auditory processing, language, learning, and reading disorders. Longitudinal testing will help the audiologist

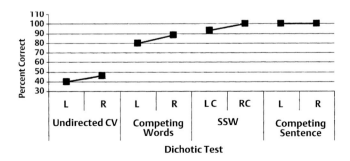

Figure 16–3 Typical results of dichotic listening tests expected from a normal 11-year-old. The tests reported are the same as those shown in Fig. 16–2. L, left; LC, left competing; R, right; RC, right competing; SSW, Staggered Spondee Word test.

discern whether maturation is occurring. If repeat testing after an appropriate interval (e.g., a year) shows little or no change in dichotic test scores, it is likely that the central auditory system is damaged or disordered. The greater the disorder, the more likely that residual deficits will remain in later years.

Pearl

Some tests of dichotic listening include:

- Dichotic words (SCAN-C and SCAN-A; Keith, 1994, 1995)
- Dichotic spondees (SSW; Katz, 1962)
- Dichotic sentences (SCAN-C and SCAN-A; Keith, 1994, 1995)
- Dichotic syllables, digits, sentences (Veterans Affairs, 1992)

Binaural Interaction Procedures

Masking Level Differences

The MLD refers to the difference between thresholds obtained under two binaural masking paradigms termed *homophasic* and *antiphasic*. According to Wilson and colleagues (1994), a homophasic condition is one in which the signals in two channels are in phase with one another, and the noises in two channels are in phase with one another (S_oN_o). An antiphasic condition is one in which either the signals or the noises in the two channels are 180 degrees out of phase ($S_oN\pi$ or $S\pi N_o$). Masking level differences have been used for many years in psychoacoustic research and in the clinical evaluation of brainstem function. MLDs are determined by obtaining binaural masked thresholds for either pure tones or speech under homophasic and antiphasic conditions. The thresholds for the homophasic (e.g., noise in phase at the two ears and signal in phase at the two ears) minus the antiphasic conditions (e.g., noise in phase at the two ears and signal out of phase at the two ears) is the MLD. This effect is sometimes called the binaural release from masking. The MLD can be 10 to 15 dB for pure tones and is frequency dependent, with the largest effects in the lower frequencies (300–600 Hz). The MLD for speech is smaller than for pure tones (Wilson et al, 1994). Subjects must have normal hearing to maximize the MLD, because peripheral hearing loss has a substantial effect on reducing the size of the MLD. Brainstem lesions can reduce or eliminate the MLD (Olsen and Noffsinger, 1976). Early research by Sweetow and Reddell (1978) found reduced MLDs in children with suspected auditory perceptual problems. The tonal MLDs were effective in discriminating children with auditory perceptual dysfunction from normal children, but speech MLDs were not. Current interest in the MLD is directed at the fact that it is a nonlinguistic task that may identify dysfunction in the processing of auditory information at brainstem levels. These dysfunctions, when better understood, may underlie certain auditory processing disorders that are related to auditory, language, and learning disorders.

Pearl

- The test of MLDs for spondaic words is available through Veterans Affairs (Veterans Affairs, 1992). Several commercial diagnostic audiometers provide capability of MLD testing.

Electrophysiologic Assessment of Central Auditory Function

Some mention should be made of electrophysiologic procedures in central auditory testing. The ASHA task force on central auditory processing (ASHA, 1996) determined that electrophysiologic procedures "may also be useful" in the diagnosis of (C)APD. To quote further from that document, "The auditory brainstem response is well known and applied routinely to detect brainstem lesions. The middle, late, and event-related potentials are still in the development stage but can be of considerable value in certain clinical situations." Taking a more assertive stand, the Dallas Consensus Conference (Jerger and Musiek, 2000) chose to include ABR and middle latency response (MLR) as part of the routine test battery (see Chapter 21). That position was challenged by Katz et al (2002), and there is continuing controversy on the routine use of these tests in routine testing for auditory processing disorders.

◆ Language Testing: What the Audiologist Needs To Know

Audiologists who work in the area of (C)APD need to know about language and its disorders. There are a range of basic principles with which the audiologist should become familiar. For example, the audiologist must have an understanding of language skill development to formulate meaningful recommendations. They should familiarize themselves with typical language milestones and have a working understanding of approximate age and sequence of emergence. It is essential that the audiologist also have an appreciation for the functional aspects of language that are at the core of communicative competence. The following information comprises a brief outline on aspects of language that will be a helpful reminder for audiologists.

The operative concepts addressed in this chapter are

- ◆ Discrimination
- ◆ Phonology
- ◆ Receptive language
- ◆ Expressive language
- ◆ Prosody
- ◆ Pragmatics

Discrimination

Children must have the ability to discriminate fine differences between speech sounds (phonemes) to form the basis for phonemic decoding, and ultimately comprehension. Discrimination allows the listener to recognize meaningful segments of language that comprise words and sentences and also allows the listener to tune out distractions and background noise, bringing the relevant information into the foreground. Through this process, information can be selected for comprehension and stored in short- and long-term memory. Studies have found that infants as young as 3 months demonstrate behaviors that suggest the ability to discriminate between minimally contrasted sound pairs such as /p/ and /b/. The ability to discriminate between speech sounds is essential to the development of receptive comprehension and expression of such sounds within the phonological system.

Phonology

The phonological system is comprised of the sound patterns of language, which combine to form meaningful segments of language. Within the age range of 18 to 28 months, children should demonstrate competence in the production of most vowel sounds and the consonant sounds /n/, /m/, /p/, and /h/. Following the emergence of these speech sounds, children will usually begin to produce /f/, /ng/, /w/, /t/, /k/, /b/, /g/, and /d/. These sounds generally develop over a longer period of time and require refinement through the ages of 3 to $3^1/_2$. Other sounds, such as /s/, /r/, /sh/, /ch/, /zh/, /v/, /z/, and /th/, may take several years to develop, with mastery occurring as late as 6 to 7 years old.

Receptive Language

Receptive language is the input system of language that takes in information through the senses. Children typically follow a developmental progression marked by the following milestones: by 1 month, infants should respond to voice, and by 2 months they should visually track movement. By 3 months, infants begin to coo in response to a pleasant or familiar voice, and by 4 months they should localize a sound source by head movements. By 5 months, most infants respond to their own name, and by 6 months they should recognize some commonly used words, such as *daddy, bye-bye,* and *mama.* At 7 months, infants generally show interest in the sounds of objects and by 8 months can recognize the names of some common objects. At 9 months, infants should follow simple directions, and by 10 months they should understand *no* and *stop.* By 11 to 12 months, infants begin to understand simple questions and recognize action words, names of objects, people, and pets. Between 13 and 18 months, children should understand some new words each week and should be able to identify pictures in a book. They should be able to point to a few body parts and should be able to identify some common objects when they are named. From 19 to 24 months, children should recognize many common objects and pictures when they are named, should begin to understand possessive forms, and should follow many simple directions. By 25 to 30 months, children generally can understand prepositions, questions, personal pronouns, and the use of common objects. By 31 to 36 months, they should be able to listen to simple stories, follow a two-part direction, and understand turn taking. It is the progression through these developmental stages that should be emphasized, not a strict or arbitrary adherence to age levels. Ages should serve only as a guide, especially when working with children who have disabilities.

Expressive Language

Although there is variability in individual rate of acquisition, most children follow a developmental sequence that encompasses the following skills. During the first month, infants cry and produce vowel-like sounds. By 2 months, primary caretakers can generally recognize different kinds of cries that signal different needs. By 3 months, infants begin to make "cooing" sounds primarily in the back of the oral cavity and may occasionally use consonant sounds such as /m/, /p/, and /b/. By 4 to 6 months, most infants develop greater control over their oral structures and begin to combine consonants and vowels in "babbling" patterns. Between 6 and 11 months, infants continue to babble, repeating sequences of sounds in reduplicated patterns. First words should emerge between 12 and 18 months, and most children begin combining words into two-word groups between the ages of 2 and $2^1/_2$. Beyond this stage, language skills should expand rapidly toward sentence usage by the age of 3 to $3^1/_2$.

Prosody

Speech is shaped by the prosodic features of stress, duration, and loudness. These features are important for early discrimination of speech and nonspeech sounds. Prosodic features complement the linguistic signal and aid the listener in his or her interpretation of grammatical and semantic functions, as well as emotional intent and social cues. Early prosodic development can be seen in infants' differentiated cries, with later evidence appearing in intonated babbling patterns. As children approach first word usage, it is often possible to detect inflection patterns of "jargon," which approximate the prosodic features of adult speech.

Pragmatics

Interaction is the key in language development and usage. The area of pragmatics addresses the functional, communicative parameters that govern language usage within an interactive context. The development of social or pragmatic skills begins long before the emergence of first words. Eye contact should begin within the first month, closely followed by early turn taking during face-to-face interaction. This provides a foundation for later turn taking during conversation. Young children should be able to focus jointly with a communicative partner on a topic or object of interest. Communicative or pragmatic function of language is also illustrated by the child's use of language to signal a variety of functions. These social/semantic functions include requesting an object, requesting an action, protesting, requesting a social routine, requesting comfort, greeting, requesting permission, commenting, requesting information, and providing information. It is the child's ability to develop language as a social and interactive tool (taking precedence over phonological and syntactic development) that forms the basis of communicative competence.

◆ Language Testing

Language tests are designed to assess areas of strength and weakness for aspects of language described above. Nonstandardized language sampling and standardized language measures are both used by speech-language pathologists for assessment. That information is used in the development of remediation programs for children with central auditory processing and language disorders. The ASHA (1996) consensus statement on (C)APD points out that clinicians should be cautious in attributing language/learning difficulties to (C)APD in any simple fashion. Clinicians should not infer the existence of (C)APD solely from evidence of learning disability or language impairment or vice versa.

◆ Interpreting Test Results

In the preceding sections, definitions of central auditory processing and related attention, language, and learning disorders have been provided. The purpose of providing this information is to assist the audiologist in understanding what an auditory processing disorder is and what it is not. A brief review of the ASHA consensus statement finds that careful examination of the child's history, observation of auditory behaviors, and review of the results of audiologic procedures are used to identify deficits in auditory processing. Audiologic test results should be reviewed to develop an auditory profile. Does the child have difficulty listening under conditions of degraded speech as shown by tests of time compressed speech or filtered words? Is there difficulty understanding speech in the presence of background noise? If so, what kind of noise, and what signal-to-noise ratio is necessary for adequate understanding? Are there apparent problems in the neurologic pathways, as indicated by difficulty in localization or lateralization, or tests of masking level differences? Is there indication of delays in maturation or damage to the auditory nervous system shown by poor performance or abnormal ear advantages on dichotic tests? Does the child have problems of auditory discrimination because of a temporal processing disorder? Does the temporal processing disorder compromise understanding speech presented at rapid rates?

Audiologic findings are viewed in conjunction with results of speech-language pathology, psychology, learning disabilities, and other specialties. Only when findings are integrated can meaningful remediation programs be designed. The combination of test results will be used to determine whether the child will benefit from direct perceptual training, compensation for auditory deficits, or cognitive training.

Acknowledgments   Appreciation is expressed to my speech-language pathologist colleague Melinda Chalfonte-Evans, who helped in writing comments on what audiologists should know about language.

References

American Medical Association. (1996). International classification of diseases (9th rev. clinical modification). Washington, DC: Author.

American Psychiatric Association. (1994). DSM-IV: Diagnostic and statistical manual of mental disorders (4th ed.) Washington, DC: Author.

American Speech-Language-Hearing Association. (1996). Central auditory processing: Current status of research and implications for clinical practice. American Journal of Audiology, 5, 51–55.

American Speech-Language-Hearing Association. (2005). (Central) auditory processing disorders: The role of the audiologist [position statement]. Washington, DC: Author.

Arcia, E., & Conners, C. K. (1998). Gender differences in ADHD? Developmental and Behavioral Pediatrics, 19, 77–83.

Bellis, T. J. (1996) Assessment and management of central auditory processing disorders in the educational setting. San Diego, CA: Singular Publishing Group.

Bergman, M., Hirsch, S., Solzi, P., & Mankowitz, Z. (1987). The threshold-of-interference test: A new test of interhemispheric suppression in brain injury. Ear and Hearing, 8, 147–150.

Berlin, C., Lowe-Bell, S., Cullen, J., Thompson, C., & Loovis, C. (1973). Dichotic speech perception: An interpretation of right ear advantage and temporal offset effects. Journal of the Acoustical Society of America, 53, 699–709.

Bornstein, S. P., & Musiek, F. E. (Eds.). (1984), Implications of temporal processing for children with learning and language problems. San Diego, CA: College Hill Press.

Bornstein, S. P., Wilson, R. H., & Cambron, N. K. (1994). Low- and high-pass filtered Northwestern University auditory test no. 6 for monaural and binaural evaluation. Journal of the American Academy of Audiology, 5, 259–264.

Briggs, S. (1998). The auditory continuous performance test as part of an attention deficit-hyperactivity disorder test battery. Communication sciences and disorders. Unpublished masters thesis. University of Cincinnati, Cincinnati, OH.

Cacace, A. T., & McFarland, D. J. (1998). Central auditory processing disorder in school-aged children: A critical review. Journal of Speech and Hearing Research, 41, 355–373.

Calearo, M. D., & Antonelli, A. R. (1973). Disorders of the central auditory nervous system. In M. Paparella & D. Shumrick (Eds.), Otolaryngology (pp. 407–425). Philadelphia: Saunders.

Cameron, S., Dillon, H., & Newall, P. (2006a). The Listening in Spatialized Noise test: An auditory processing disorders study. Journal of the American Academy of Audiology, 17, 306–320.

Cameron, S., Dillon, H., & Newall, P. (2006b). The Listening in Spatialized Noise test: Normative data for children. International Journal of Audiology, 45, 99–108.

Chermak, G., & Tucker, E. (2002). Behavioral characteristics of auditory processing disorder and attention-deficit hyperactivity disorder: Predominantly inattentive type. Journal of the American Academy of Audiology, 13, 332–338.

Collett, B. R. Ohan, J. L., & Myers, K. M. (2003). Ten-year review of rating scales: 5. Scales assessing attention-deficit/hyperactivity disorder. 42(9), 1015–1037.

Conners, C. K. (1997). Conners' rating scales (rev.). North Tonawanda, NY: Multi-Health Systems.

Devers, J. S., Hoyer, E. A., & McCroskey, R. L. (1978). Dynamic auditory localization by normal and learning disability children. Journal of the American Audiology Society, 3, 172–178.

First, M. B., Frances, A. & Pincus, H. A. (1995). DSM-IV handbook of differential diagnosis. Washington, DC: American Psychiatric Association.

Fisher, L. (1976). Auditory problems checklist. Tampa, FL: Educational Audiology Association.

Gravel, J., & Ellis, M. A. (1995). The auditory consequences of otitis media with effusion: The audiogram and beyond. Seminars in Hearing, 16, 44–58.

Gustafson, T. J., & Keith, R. W. (2005). Relationship of auditory processing categories as determined by the Staggered Spondee Word Test (SSW) to speech-language and other auditory processing test results. Journal of Educational Audiology, 12, 1–20.

Hall, J. W., & Mueller, H. G. (1997). Audiologists' desk reference. San Diego, CA: Singular Publishing Group.

Hood, L. J. (1998). Auditory neuropathy: What is it and what can we do about it? Hearing Journal, 51, 10–18.

Hurley, R. M., & Musiek, F. M. (1997). Effectiveness of three central auditory processing (CAP) tests in identifying cerebral lesions. Journal of the American Academy of Audiology, 8, 257–262.

Jerger, J. (1960). Observations on auditory behavior in lesions of the central auditory pathways. Archives of Otolaryngology, 71, 797.

Jerger, J. (1964). Auditory tests for disorders of the central auditory mechanisms. Springfield, IL: Charles C Thomas.

Jerger, J., & Harford, E. (1960). Alternate and simultaneous binaural balancing of pure tones. Journal of Speech and Hearing Research, 3, 15–30.

Jerger, J., & Musiek, F. (2000). Report of Consensus Conference on the Diagnosis of Auditory Processing Disorders in School-Aged Children. Journal of the American Academy of Audiology, 11, 467–474.

Jerger, S. (1987). Validation of the Pediatric Speech Intelligibility test in children with central nervous system lesions. Audiology, 26.

Jerger, S., & Allen, J. S. (1998). How behavioral tests of central auditory processing may complicate management. Nashville, TN: Bill Wilkerson Center Press.

Katz, J. (1962). The use of staggered spondaic words for assessing the integrity of the central auditory nervous system. Journal of Auditory Research, 2, 327–337.

Katz, J., Johnson, C., Brandner, C., et al. (2002). Clinical and research concerns regarding the 2000 APD consensus report and recommendations. Audiology Today, 2, 13–19.

Katz, J., Stecker, S., & Henderson, D. (1992) Central auditory processes: A transdisciplinary view. St. Louis, MO: Mosby Year Book Publishers.

Katz, J., & Wilde, L. (1994). Auditory processing disorders. In J. Katz (Ed.), Handbook of clinical audiology (4th ed., pp. 490–502). Baltimore, MD: Williams & Wilkins.

Keith, R. W. (1994). The Auditory Continuous Performance Test. San Antonio, TX: The Psychological Corp.

Keith, R. W. (1995). Development and standardization of SCAN-A: Test of auditory processing disorders in adolescents and adults. Journal of the American Academy of Audiology, 6, 286–292.

Keith, R. W., & Anderson, J. (Eds.). (2006). Dichotic listening tests. San Diego, CA: Plural Publishing.

Keith, R. W., & Cunningham-Fallis, R. L. (1998). How behavioral tests of central auditory processing influence management. In F. Bess (Ed.), Children with hearing impairment: Contemporary trends (pp. 137–145). Nashville, TN: Bill Wilkerson Center Press.

Keith, R. W. (2000a). Development and standardization of SCAN-C: Test for auditory processing disorders in children—revised. Journal of the American Academy of Audiology, 11, 438–445.

Keith, R. W. (2000b). SCAN-C: Test for auditory processing disorders in children—revised. San Antonio, TX: The Psychological Corp.

Keith, R. W. (2000c). Random Gap Detection Test (RGDT). St. Louis: Auditec.

Keith, R. W. (2002). Time Compressed Sentence Test. Examiner's manual. St. Louis: Auditec.

Knox, C., & Roeser, R. J. (1980). Cerebral dominance in normal and dyslexic children. Seminars in Speech, Language, and Hearing, 1, 181–194.

Marriage, J. (1996). Hyperacusis in Williams syndrome. Manchester, England: University of Manchester Press.

Matkin, N. D., & Hook, P. E. (1983). A multidisciplinary approach to central auditory evaluations. Baltimore, MD: University Park Press.

McCroskey, R. L., & Keith, R. W. (1996) Auditory fusion threshold test (rev.). St. Louis: Auditec.

Medwetsky, L. (2002). Central auditory processing. In J. Katz (Ed.), Handbook of clinical audiology (5th ed., pp. 495–531). Philadelphia, PA: Lippincott Williams & Wilkins.

Menyuk, P. (Ed.). (1992). Relationship of otitis media to speech processing and language development. St. Louis: Mosby Year Book.

Merzenich, M. M., Jenkins, W. M., Johnston, P., Schreiner, C., Miller, S. L., & Tallal, P. (1996). Temporal processing deficits of language learning impaired children ameliorated by training. Science, 271, 77–81.

Musiek, F. E., Baran, J. A., & Pinheiro, M. L. (1990). Duration pattern recognition in normal subjects and patients with cerebral and cochlear lesions. Audiology, 29, 304–313.

Musiek, F., & Pinheiro, M. (1985). Dichotic speech tests in the detection of central auditory function. Baltimore: Williams & Wilkins.

Musiek, F. E., Shinn, J., Jirsa, R., et al. (2005). The GIN (Gaps in Noise) test performance in subjects with confirmed central auditory nervous system involvement. Ear and Hearing, 26, 608–617.

Neijenhuis, K., Tschur, H., & Snik, A. (2004). The effect of mild hearing impairment on auditory processing tests. Journal of the American Academy of Audiology, 15, 6–16.

Nyquette, P. A. (2005). BKB-SIN Speech-in-Noise test. Elk Grove Village, IL Etymotic Research.

Nyquette, P., Gudmunsen, G., & Killion, M. (2001). QuickSIN Speech-in-Noise Test. Elk Grove Village, IL: Etymotic Research.

Obrzut, J., Hynd, G., Obrzut, A., & Pirozzolo, F. (1981). Effect of directed attention on cerebral asymmetries in normal and learning disabled children. Developmental Psychology, 17, 118–125.

Olsen, W. O., & Noffsinger, D. (1976). Masking level differences for cochlear and brain stem lesions. Annals of Otology, Rhinology and Laryngology, 86, 820–825.

Olsen, W. O., Noffsinger, D., & Kurdziel, S. (1975). Speech discrimination testing in quiet and in white noise by patients with peripheral and central lesions. Acta Otolaryngologica, 80, 375–382.

Phillips, D. P. (1995). Central auditory processing: A view from auditory neuroscience. American Journal of Otology, 16, 338–352.

Rapin, I., & Gravel, J. S. (2006). Auditory neuropathy: A biologically inappropriate label unless acoustic nerve involvement is documented. Journal of the American Academy of Audiology, 17, 147–150.

Riccio, C. A., Cohen, M. J., Hynd, G. W., & Keith, R. W. (1996). Validity of the Auditory Continuous Performance Test in differentiating central processing auditory disorders with and without ADHD. Journal of Learning Disabilities, 29, 561–566.

Rintelmann, W. F. (1995). Monaural speech tests in the detection of central auditory disorders. Baltimore, MD: Williams & Wilkins.

Rosen, S. (2003). Auditory processing in dyslexia and specific language impairment: Is there a deficit? What is its nature? Does it explain anything? Journal of Phonetics, 31, 509–527.

Rosenberg, P. D. (1978). Case history: The first test. In J. Katz (Ed.), Handbook of clinical audiology (2nd ed.). Baltimore, MD: Williams & Wilkins.

Sanger, D. D., Freed, J. M., & Decker, TN. (1985). Behavioral profile of preschool children suspected of auditory language processing problems. Hearing Journal, 38, 17–20.

Satz, P. (1976). Cerebral dominance and reading disability: An old problem revisited. Baltimore, MD: University Park Press.

Sininger, Y. S. H., Hood, L., Starr, A., Berlin, C., & Picton, T. W. (1995). Hearing loss due to auditory neuropathy. Audiology, 7, 11–13.

Smoski, W. J., Brunt, M. A., & Tannahill, J. D. (1992). Listening characteristics of children with central auditory processing disorders. Language, Speech, and Hearing Services in Schools, 23, 145–152.

Sperry, J. L., Wiley, T. L., & Chial, M. R. (1997). Word recognition performance in various background competitors. Journal of the American Academy of Audiology, 8, 71–80.

Starr, A., Picton, T. W., Sininger, Y., Hook, L. J., & Berlin, C. I. (1996). Auditory neuropathy. Brain, 119, 741–753.

Stein, L., Tremblay, K., Pasterak, J., Banerjee, S., Lindermann, K., & Kraus, N. (1996). Brainstem abnormalities in neonates with normal otoacoustic emissions. Seminars in Hearing, 17, 197–213.

Sweetow, R. W., & Reddell, R. D. (1978). The use of masking level differences in the identification of children with perceptual problems. Journal of the American Audiology Society, 4, 52–56.

Tallal, P., Miller. S. L., Bedi, G., et al. (1996). Language comprehension in language-learning impaired children improved with acoustically modified speech. Science, 271(5245), 81–84.

Teatini, G. P. (Ed.). (1970). Sensitized speech tests: Results in normal subjects. Odense, Denmark: Danavox Foundation.

Thompson, M. E., & Abel, S. M. (1992). Indices of hearing in patients with central auditory pathology: 2. Choice response time. Scandinavian Audiology Supplementum, 35, 17–22.

Veterans Affairs (1992). Tonal and speech materials for auditory perceptual assessment.

Watkins, M. W. (2003). IQ subtest analysis: Clinical acumen or clinical illusion? Scientific Review of Mental Health Practice, 2.

Watson, C. S. (1994, October). How does basic science show that central auditory processing is critical to audition? The view from psychoacoustics. Paper presented at the American Speech-Language-Hearing Association Consensus Development Conference, Albuquerque, NM.

Willeford, J. (1977). Assessing central auditory behavior in children: A test battery approach. New York: Grune & Stratton.

Willeford, J., & Burleigh, J. (1985). Handbook of auditory processing disorders in children. Orlando, FL: Grune & Stratton.

Willeford, J., & Burleigh, J. (Eds.). (1994). Sentence procedures in central testing. Baltimore, MD: Williams & Wilkins.

Wilson, R. H., Zizz, C. A., & Sperry, J. L. (1994). Masking level difference for spondaic words in 2000-msec bursts of broadband noise. Journal of the American Academy of Audiology, 5, 236–242.

Chapter 17

Diagnosing Auditory Processing Disorders in Adults

Brad A. Stach

The central auditory nervous system is a highly complex network that analyzes and processes neural information from both ears and transmits the processed information to the auditory cortex and other areas within the nervous system. Auditory processing ability is usually defined as the capacity with which the central auditory nervous system transfers information from the eighth cranial nerve (CN VIII) to the auditory cortex. An auditory processing disorder (APD) is an impairment in this function of the peripheral and central auditory nervous systems.

As discussed in chapter 16, the term *(central) auditory processing disorder* [(C)APD] historically was used to describe the hearing disorder associated with dysfunction of the auditory nervous system. Here, *central* referred to the nervous system, as opposed to peripheral, which was used to describe disorders of the cochlea and conductive mechanisms. Clinically, (C)APD was most often described by measures of suprathreshold hearing ability. Despite efforts to distinguish peripheral from central disorder, it is not always clear whether reduced suprathreshold performance is attributable to changes in cochlear function or in peripheral or central

nervous system function. Complicating matters further, some disorders occur at the peripheral-central junction, and the identification of the contributing component is not readily distinguishable. As a result, general agreement has been reached to refer to these suprathreshold hearing disorders as auditory processing disorders (APDs) rather than attributing to them a locus of dysfunction. Nevertheless, APD is a term that refers to disorders reflecting changes in auditory nervous system function.

The ability of the central auditory nervous system to process sound was evaluated historically for diagnostic purposes to identify specific lesions or disease processes of the nervous system. Numerous measures of auditory nervous system function were scrutinized for what they could reveal about the presence of such neurologic disorders. These diagnostic site-of-lesion efforts formed a basis for the assessment of central auditory disorders today, which is much more focused on describing communication disorder than on diagnosing specific neurologic disease.

If the role of audiologic evaluation is defined as the assessment of hearing in a broad sense, it is easy to understand why many clinicians and researchers embrace the importance of evaluating more than just the sensitivity of the ears to faint sounds and the ability of the ear to recognize single-syllable words presented in quiet. Although both measures provide important information to the audiologic assessment, they fail to offer a complete picture of an individual's auditory ability. Certainly, the complexity of auditory perception, as evidenced in the ability to follow a conversation in a noisy room or the effortless ability to localize sound, requires more than the rudimentary assessment of hearing sensitivity and speech recognition to adequately characterize what it takes to hear. Neither do these measures adequately describe the possible disorders that a person might have. As a result, it is becoming increasingly common for assessment of central auditory ability to be included as a routine component of the basic audiologic evaluation.

In recent decades, techniques that were once used to assist in the diagnosis of neurologic disease have been adapted for use in the assessment of communication impairment that occurs as a result of APDs. Speech audiometric measures that are sensitized in certain ways, along with other psychophysical measures designed to challenge the auditory nervous system, are now commonly used to evaluate auditory processing ability. A typical battery of tests might include the assessment of speech recognition across a range of signal intensities, the assessment of speech recognition in the presence of competing speech signals, the measurement of dichotic listening, and an assessment of temporal processing capacity. Results of such an assessment provide an estimate of auditory processing ability and a more complete profile of a patient's auditory function and handicap (Chmiel and Jerger, 1996; Golding et al, 2006; Jerger, Oliver, and Pirozzolo, 1990). Such information is often useful in providing guidance regarding appropriate amplification strategies or other rehabilitation approaches (Chmiel et al, 1997; Stach et al, 1985, 1991). The use of frequency modulated (FM) systems and other devices designed to enhance the signal-to-noise ratio (SNR) has proven effective in some patients with APD. The value of this information has led many clinicians to evaluate suprathreshold auditory ability as a routine component of any thorough assessment of hearing.

Auditory evoked potentials and other electrophysiologic measures may also be useful in the diagnosis of APD. These techniques are described in Chapter 21. This chapter will describe behavioral tests that have been developed over the years for the assessment of central auditory processing.

◆ Purposes of Assessing Auditory Processing

The aim of auditory processing assessment is to evaluate the ability of the auditory nervous system to process acoustic signals. Advanced speech audiometric and other behavioral measures are used to assess auditory nervous system function, often referred to as auditory processing ability. At least two important reasons exist for doing so:

(1) to assist the medical profession in identifying specific lesions of the auditory system and (2) to describe a communication disorder.

Identification of a Specific Lesion

It was in the 1950s that speech audiometric measures were first used successfully to identify lesions of the central auditory nervous system (Bocca et al, 1954). Speech recognition measures, including monotically presented words sensitized by low-pass filtering and dichotic testing, were found to be effective in identifying patients with temporal lobe lesions and other neurologic disorders. From those beginnings, speech audiometric measures, along with other behavioral techniques, were designed and evaluated for their effectiveness in identifying lesions of the auditory nervous system.

Refinement of these behavioral measures ensued throughout the 1960s and '70s, bringing with it an enhanced understanding of the function of the auditory nervous system and the impact of neurologic disorder on that function. Much of the design of our approach today is a direct result of concepts that were formulated during these early efforts.

During the 1980s, the importance of the diagnostic, site-of-lesion role of central auditory testing diminished with the advent of radiologic imaging techniques and the refinement of auditory evoked potential assessment. As ever smaller lesions were being detected by the progressively increasing accuracy of these imaging and evoked potential measures, the sensitivity of auditory processing tests diminished accordingly. As a result, the role of central auditory assessment in the identification of specific lesions changed from one of diagnosis to one of screening.

Although measures of auditory processing ability remain useful diagnostically in helping to identify the presence of neurologic disorders, particularly in a screening role, they are now used more often to assess the functional impact of such a disorder and to monitor the course of the disease process.

> **Pearl**
>
> • The real value of APD measures lies not in screening for medical problems but in quantifying the impact of a neurologic disorder on communication ability.

Description of a Communication Disorder

As measures of auditory processing ability were being refined for diagnostic, site-of-lesion purposes, their value in providing insight into a patient's auditory abilities beyond the level of cochlear processing became increasingly clear. These same behavioral measures designed to identify lesions could be used to assess and quantify a hearing disorder resulting from an impaired central auditory nervous system. That is, their value in quantifying functional deficits became apparent as they were being applied in an effort to identify structural deficits. These functional deficits, referred to collectively as APDs, were found to be readily quantifiable with the same strategies used for diagnosis.

Today, assessment of auditory processing ability is used for several purposes. It serves as a screener for retrocochlear neurologic disorder, and it is useful in quantifying the consequences of such neurologic disorder. In addition, the measurement of auditory processing serves as a metric of suprathreshold hearing ability, which permits a more complete understanding of communication function. As a result, it is valuable in quantifying hearing impairment resulting from functional deficits in the auditory nervous system. Finally, assessment of auditory processing ability assists in defining how a patient will hear after a peripheral hearing sensitivity loss has been corrected with hearing aids.

Pearl

Testing auditory processing ability:

- Screens for retrocochlear disorders.
- Measure suprathreshold hearing.
- Helps define communication ability after the peripheral loss has been corrected with hearing aids.

◆ The Nature of Auditory Processing Disorders

Although a tendency exists to think of hearing impairment as the sensitivity loss that can be measured on an audiogram, there are other types of hearing impairment that may or may not be accompanied by sensitivity loss. These other impairments result from disease, damage, or degradation of the central auditory nervous system in adults or delayed or disordered auditory nervous system development in children.

A disordered auditory nervous system, regardless of cause, will have functional consequences that can vary from a subclinical to a substantial, easily measurable auditory deficit. Auditory nervous system impairments tend to be divided into two groups, depending on the nature of the underlying disorder, even though the functional consequences may be similar. When an impairment is caused by an active, measurable disease process, such as a tumor or other space-occupying lesion, or from damage due to trauma or stroke, it is often referred to as a retrocochlear disorder. That is, retrocochlear disorders result from structural lesions of the nervous system. When an impairment is due to developmental disorder or delay or from diffuse changes such as the aging process, it is often referred to as an APD. That is, APDs result from "functional lesions" of the nervous system. The term *APD* is also used to describe the functional consequence of a retrocochlear disorder.

The consequences of both types of disorders are similar from a hearing perspective, but the disorders tend to be treated differently because of the consequences of diagnosis and the likelihood of a significant residual communication disorder. Retrocochlear disorders are those that are often addressed first by medical management. Any residual communication disorder is often a secondary consideration because of the immediate health threat of most retrocochlear disease, which must be treated first. APDs often are seen as communication disorders and are either the residual consequence of a retrocochlear disorder or the consequence of diffuse changes or disorders that are not amenable to medical management. Both types of disorders are likely to present similar audiologic findings, and their treatment as a communication disorder is not likely to differ. The functional deficit to the patient will be similar regardless of the underlying cause.

Symptoms

Some adults with APDs will have normal hearing sensitivity. Others, especially those who are elderly, will have some degree of peripheral hearing sensitivity loss upon which the central auditory disorder is imposed. In the former group, the most common symptom is that of a hearing disorder in the presence of normal hearing sensitivity. Such patients will describe difficulty hearing in certain listening situations despite their ability to detect faint sounds. In the latter group, the most common symptom will be a hearing disorder that seems to be disproportionate to the degree of hearing sensitivity loss. Regardless of category, adults with APDs share common difficulties along a continuum of severity.

The most common symptom of APD is difficulty extracting a signal of interest from a background of noise. Although the basis for the disorder is not always clear, it most often results in an inability to structure auditory space appropriately. This spatial hearing deficit usually translates into difficulty hearing in noise. Typical environments in which difficulties occur include parties, restaurants, and in the car. Another common symptom is difficulty localizing a sound source, especially in the presence of background noise. Perhaps as a consequence of these symptoms, patients and their families are also likely to describe behaviors such as inattentiveness and distractibility.

These symptoms, of course, are not unlike those of patients with peripheral hearing sensitivity loss. It should be no surprise that an auditory disorder, regardless of its locus, would result in similar perceived difficulties.

Pearl

- A distinguishing feature of APD is the inability to extract sounds of interest from noisy environments despite an ability to perceive the sounds with adequate loudness.

Signs

Clinical findings in patients with APDs reflect impairments in those functions attributable to the central auditory nervous system. That is, tests of central auditory processing have been designed to try to assess those functions uniquely attributable

Table 17–1 Clinical Signs of Auditory Processing Disorder

Categories of Reduced Function

Absolute speech recognition
Recognition of frequency-altered speech
Recognition of speech in competition
Recognition of speech at high-intensity levels
Temporal processing
Localization
Lateralization
Dichotic listening
Binaural processing
Acquired suprathreshold asymmetry

to the auditory nervous system rather than to the cochlea. Indeed, one important clinical challenge is to rule out or control the influences of the cochlea or cochlear hearing loss. A list of common clinical signs is shown in **Table 17–1.**

Following is a description of many of the diverse clinical signs of APD. Although the clinical signs attributable to a central disorder may provide insight into the basis and locus of the underlying disorder, the symptoms related to the various signs seem to be reasonably similar across patients. That is, whether a disorder is identified as a problem in temporal processing, dichotic listening, or localization, the functional consequence to the patient tends to be difficulty with spatial hearing in adverse listening environments. Indeed, development of these various measures did not evolve from a systematic plan to assess the central auditory mechanism; rather, it evolved from efforts to challenge the integrity of the central nervous system by measuring functions that are attributable to it.

Subtlety and Bottleneck Principles

As a general rule, the more peripheral a lesion, the greater its impact will be on auditory function (the bottleneck principle). Conversely, the more central the lesion, the more subtle its impact will be (the subtlety principle). One might conceptualize this by thinking of the nervous system as a large oak tree. If one of its many branches were damaged, overall growth of the tree would be affected only subtly. Damage to its trunk, however, could have a significant impact on the entire tree. A well-placed lesion on the auditory nerve can substantially impact hearing, whereas a lesion in the midbrain is likely to have more subtle effects.

Pearl

- The bottleneck principle holds that the more peripheral a lesion, the greater its impact on auditory function. The subtlety principle holds that the more central the lesion, the more subtle its impact on auditory function.

Perhaps the best illustration of the bottleneck principle comes from reports of cases with lesions that effectively disconnect the cochlea from the brainstem. These cases demonstrate the presence of severe or profound hearing loss and very poor speech recognition despite normal cochlear function, as indicated by normal otoacoustic emissions (OAE) or CN VIII action potentials. In cases involving lesions of the cerebellopontine angle secondary to tumor (Cacace et al, 1994; Kileny et al, 1998), multiple sclerosis (Stach and Delgado-Vilches, 1993), and miliary tuberculosis (Stach et al, 1998), results have shown how a strategically placed lesion at the bottleneck can substantially affect hearing ability. The bottleneck in the case of the auditory system is, of course, CN VIII as it enters the auditory brainstem.

One specific type of auditory nervous system disorder is *auditory neuropathy* (Starr et al, 1996), a term used to describe a condition in which cochlear function is normal, and CN VIII function is abnormal. The underlying nature of auditory neuropathy is a dys-synchrony of neural discharge, resulting in significant hearing disorder. It is distinguishable from disorders caused by space-occupying lesions in that imaging results of the nerve and brainstem are normal. Although hearing sensitivity loss varies in degree in cases of auditory neuropathy, speech perception is often significantly worse than expected based on audiometric thresholds (Hood et al, 2003; Madden et al, 2002), exemplifying the consequences of a disorder at the level of the bottleneck.

If the bottleneck is unaffected, then lesions at higher levels will have effects on auditory processing ability that are more subtle (e.g., Baran et al, 2004; Musiek et al, 2004). These effects tend to become increasingly subtle as the lesions are located more centrally in the system. For example, whereas a lesion at the bottleneck can cause a substantial hearing sensitivity loss, a brainstem lesion often results in only a mild low-frequency sensitivity loss (Jerger and Jerger, 1980), and a temporal lobe lesion is unlikely to affect hearing sensitivity at all. Similarly, speech recognition of words presented in quiet can be very poor in the case of a lesion at the periphery but will be unaffected by a lesion at the level of the temporal lobe (e.g., Allen et al, 1996).

Reduced Absolute Speech Recognition

Speech recognition, even in quiet, can be affected by auditory nervous system disorder, particularly if the disorder occurs at or near the bottleneck. Although more subtle in nature, absolute speech recognition can also be affected by more diffuse disorders. A disproportionate decline in word recognition with age, beyond that which might be predicted from degree of cochlear hearing loss, is known as phonemic regression. Although largely refuted over the years as explainable by the peripheral hearing loss, more recent evidence (Gates et al, 2003) tends to support the notion that at least some of the decline in speech recognition in quiet can be attributable to age-related changes in the auditory nervous system.

Controversial Point

- The extent to which decline in the absolute word recognition score (WRS) is attributable to aging per se, rather than to an associated cochlear hearing loss, is an ongoing argument.

Reduced Recognition of Frequency-Altered Speech

Another hallmark sign of APD is a reduction in recognition of speech materials that have been altered in the frequency domain. It has been known for over 50 years that reducing the informational content, or redundancy, of speech targets by low-pass filtering creates a challenge to an impaired auditory nervous system that is not present in an intact system (Boca et al, 1954). As a result, patients with auditory processing disorder are likely to perform more poorly on a low-pass filtered speech test than those with normal hearing ability.

Reduced Recognition of Speech in Competition

One of the most important consequences of APD is an inability to extract signals of interest from a background of noise. This can be measured directly with several different speech audiometric techniques. Results show that patients with APDs have significant difficulty identifying speech in the presence of competition. In general, the more meaningful or speechlike the competition, the more it will interfere with the perception of speech (Larsby et al, 2005; Sperry et al, 1997; Stuart and Phillips, 1996).

Much of the early work in this area focused on monaural perception of speech targets in a background of competition presented to the same ear. Other results have shown deficits in patients with APDs when competition is presented to the opposite ear or when both targets and competition are presented to both ears in a sound field.

Reduced Speech Recognition at High-Intensity Levels

In cases of normal auditory processing ability, speech recognition performance increases systematically as speech intensity is increased to an asymptotic level, representing the best speech understanding that can be achieved in that ear. In some cases, however, a paradoxical rollover effect exists, in which performance declines substantially as speech intensity increases beyond the level producing the maximal performance score. In other words, as speech intensity increases, performance rises to a maximum level, then declines, or "rolls over," sharply as intensity continues to increase. This rollover effect is commonly observed when the site of the hearing loss is retrocochlear, in the auditory nerve or the auditory pathways in the brainstem (Jerger and Jerger, 1971; Miranda and Pichora-Fuller, 2002).

Reduced Temporal Processing

Impairment in processing in the time domain is also a common sign in central auditory disorders. Temporal processing deficits have been identified based on several measures, including time compression of speech, duration pattern discrimination, duration difference limens, and gap detection. Some researchers believe that deficits in temporal processing are the underlying cause of, and the primary contributors to, many of the other measurable deficits associated with APDs.

Disordered Localization and Lateralization

The ability to localize acoustic stimuli spatially generally requires auditory system integration of sound from both ears. Some patients with central auditory disorders have difficulty locating the directional source of a sound. Disorders of the central auditory nervous system have been associated with deficits in ability to localize the source of a sound in a sound field or to lateralize the perception of a sound within the head.

Deficits in Dichotic Listening

Most people with intact auditory nervous systems are able to identify different signals presented simultaneously to both ears. If the signals are linguistic in nature, most individuals will experience a slight right ear advantage in dichotic listening ability. APDs, particularly those caused by impairment of the corpus callosum and auditory cortex, often results in dichotic deficits characterized by substantial reduction in left ear performance.

Other Deficits in Binaural Processing

The binaural auditory system is an exquisite detector of differences in timing of sound reaching the two ears. This helps in localizing low-frequency sounds, which reach the ears at different points in time. Abnormality in the processing of phase cues is a common sign of APD that occurs as a result of impairment in the lower auditory brainstem.

A different kind of deficit in binaural processing is referred to as binaural interference. Under normal circumstances, binaural hearing provides an advantage over monaural hearing. This so-called binaural advantage has been noted in loudness judgments, speech recognition, and evoked potential amplitudes. In contrast, in cases of binaural interference, binaural performance is actually poorer than the best monaural performance. In such cases, performance on a perceptual task with both ears can actually be poorer than performance on the better ear in cases of asymmetric perceptual ability. It appears that the poorer ear actually reduces binaural performance below the better monaural performance. Binaural interference has been reported in elderly individuals (Jerger et al, 1993) and in patients with multiple sclerosis (Silman, 1995). The functional consequence of binaural interference may be to reduce the potential benefit of binaural hearing aids when hearing with both ears is poorer than hearing with one ear.

Acquired Suprathreshold Asymmetry

Asymmetry in peripheral hearing sensitivity can have a disproportionate effect on processing by the poorer hearing, or deprived ear, caused presumably by changes in central auditory function as a consequence of the asymmetry. Some asymmetry occurs naturally as a result of greater cochlear disorder in one ear than the other. In such cases, evidence is mounting that processing by the poorer ear is adversely affected beyond that which might be expected if the loss were symmetric (Silverman and Emmer, 1993).

Pitfall

- The detrimental effects of asymmetry on the central auditory nervous system can be created by fitting a hearing aid to one ear of a person with symmetrical hearing loss.

Asymmetry can also occur by fitting a hearing aid on one ear only, so-called late-onset auditory deprivation (Silman et al, 1984, 1992; Silverman and Silman, 1990). Late-onset auditory deprivation refers to an apparent asymmetric decline in speech recognition ability in the unaided ear of a person who was fitted with only one hearing aid. That is, in a patient fitted with one hearing aid, speech recognition ability in that ear remains constant over time, while the same ability in the unaided ear begins to show signs of deterioration. As long as hearing is symmetric in both ears, this decline is not apparent. However, once a hearing aid is fitted in one ear, resulting in asymmetric hearing, ability appears to decline in the disadvantaged ear. Although this reduction may be reversible if the unaided ear is aided within a reasonable time frame, in some patients the decline in speech understanding may not recover (Gelfand, 1995). As a result, a binaural interference phenomenon may occur, wherein binaural ability is actually poorer than the better monaural ability.

◆ Causes of Central Auditory Disorders

There are two primary causes of APDs in adults. One is neuropathology of the peripheral and central auditory nervous system, resulting from tumors or other space-occupying lesions or from damage due to trauma or stroke. The other is from diffuse changes in brain function, usually related to the aging process. A list of potential causes of APD is given in **Table 17–2**.

Disorders Caused by Neuropathology

A retrocochlear disorder is caused by a change in neural structure of some component of the peripheral or central auditory nervous system. The effect that this structural change will have on function depends primarily on lesion size, location, and impact. For example, a retrocochlear lesion may or may not affect auditory sensitivity. A tumor on CN VIII can cause a substantial sensorineural hearing loss, depending on how much pressure it places on the nerve, the damage that it causes to the nerve, and the extent to which it damages the cochlea. A tumor in the temporal lobe, however, is quite unlikely to result in any change in hearing sensitivity; although, it may result in a more subtle suprathreshold hearing disorder.

Retrocochlear neuropathological conditions can occur at any level in the peripheral and central auditory nervous system pathway. The likely causes and consequence of retrocochlear disorders are delineated below.

Table 17–2 Causes of Auditory Processing Disorder

Locus of Disorder	Pathology
CN VIII	Cochleovestibular schwannoma
	Neurofibromatosis 2 (NF2)
	Lipoma
	Meningioma
	Neuritis
	Diabetic neuropathy
	Auditory neuropathy/dys-synchrony
Brainstem	Infarct
	Glioma
	Multiple sclerosis
Cortex	Cerebrovascular accident
	Tumor
	Trauma
Diffuse	Meningitis
	Toxicity
	Deprivational effects of peripheral pathology
	Degenerative effects of biologic aging

CN VIII, eighth cranial nerve.

CN VIII Nerve Disorders

The most common neoplastic growth affecting the auditory nerve is a cochleovestibular schwannoma. The more generic terms *acoustic tumor* and *acoustic neuroma* typically refer to a cochleovestibular schwannoma. Other terms used to describe this type of tumor are *acoustic neurinoma* and *acoustic neurilemoma*.

A cochleovestibular schwannoma is a benign, encapsulated tumor composed of Schwann's cells arising from CN VIII. Schwann's cells serve to produce and maintain the myelin that ensheathes the axons of CN VIII. This tumor arising from the proliferation of Schwann's cells is benign in that it is slow growing; is encapsulated, often avoiding local invasion of tissue; and does not disseminate to other parts of the nervous system. Acoustic tumors are unilateral and most often arise from the vestibular branch of CN VIII. Thus, they are sometimes referred to as vestibular schwannomas.

The effects of a cochleovestibular schwannoma depend on its size, location, and extent of the pressure it places on CN VIII and the brainstem. Auditory symptoms may include tinnitus, hearing loss, and unsteadiness. Depending on the extent of the tumor's impact, it may cause headache, motor incoordination from cerebellar involvement, and involvement of adjacent cranial nerves. For example, involvement of CN VIII can cause facial numbness, involvement of CN VII can cause facial weakness, and involvement of CN IV can cause diplopia.

Among the most common symptoms of cochleovestibular schwannoma are unilateral tinnitus and unilateral hearing loss. The hearing disorder varies in degree depending on the location and size of the tumor. Hearing sensitivity can range from normal to a profound hearing loss. Speech recognition ability typically is disproportionately poor for the degree of hearing loss. If the tumor is affecting CN VIII function, its effects are unlikely to be subtle because of the bottleneck principle.

A cochleovestibular schwannoma on CN VIII can also cause retrograde cochlear dysfunction (Mahmud et al, 2003). That is, the presence of a tumor on CN VIII can result in changes in the structure of the cochlea, caused by the formation of proteinaceous material in the cochlear space. Thus, although the primary site of the lesion may be CN VIII, its influence may be more peripheral. Clinical signs will vary from those consistent with retrocochlear disorder, when the influence of the tumor is primarily on nerve function, to those consistent with cochlear disorder, when the influence is primarily on the labyrinth. It may be that the clinical picture progresses from the former to the latter as the tumor persists.

One other important form of schwannoma is neurofibromatosis. This tumor disorder has two distinct types. Neurofibromatosis 1 (NF1), also known as von Recklinghausen's disease, is an autosomal dominant disease characterized by café au lait spots and multiple cutaneous tumors, with associated optic gliomas, peripheral and spinal neurofibromas, and, rarely, acoustic neuromas. In contrast, neurofibromatosis 2 (NF2) is characterized by bilateral cochleovestibular schwannomas. The schwannomas are faster growing and more virulent than the unilateral type. This is also an autosomal dominant disease and is associated with other intracranial tumors. Hearing loss in NF2 is not particularly different from a unilateral type of schwannoma, except that it is bilateral and often progresses more rapidly.

In addition to cochleovestibular schwannomas, several other types of tumors, cysts, and aneurysms can affect CN VIII and the cerebellopontine angle, where CN VIII enters the brainstem. These other neoplastic growths, such as lipoma and meningioma, occur more rarely than cochleovestibular schwannomas. The effect of these various forms of tumor on hearing is often indistinguishable.

In addition to acoustic tumors, other disease processes can affect CN VIII function, including cochlear neuritis, diabetic cranial neuropathy, and auditory neuropathy/dys-synchrony.

Not unlike any other cranial nerve, CN VIII can develop neuritis, or inflammation of the nerve. Although rare, acute cochlear neuritis can occur as a result of a direct viral attack on the cochlear portion of the nerve. This results in degeneration of the cochlear neurons in the ear. Hearing loss is sensorineural and often sudden and severe. It is accompanied by poorer speech understanding than would be expected from the degree of hearing loss. One specific form of this disease occurs as a result of syphilis. Meningoneurolabyrinthitis is an inflammation of the membranous labyrinth and CN VIII that occurs as a predominant lesion in early congenital syphilis or in acute attacks of secondary and tertiary syphilis.

Diabetes mellitus is a metabolic disorder caused by a deficiency of insulin, with chronic complications including neuropathy and generalized degenerative changes in blood vessels. Neuropathies can involve the central, peripheral, and autonomic nervous systems. When neuropathy from diabetes affects the auditory system, it usually results in vestibular disorder and hearing loss consistent with retrocochlear disorder.

Auditory neuropathy is a specific disorder of the auditory nerve that results in a loss of synchrony of neural firing.

Because of the nature of the disorder, it is also referred to as auditory dys-synchrony (Berlin et al, 2001). The cause of auditory neuropathy is often unknown, although it may be observed in cases of syndromic peripheral pathologies. Auditory neuropathy is diagnosed on the basis of a constellation of clinical findings. Although in its purest form it is considered to be of neural origin, the clinical constellation has also been reported in patients with peripheral inner hair cell loss in the cochlea. When the cause does appear to be neural, suprathreshold hearing can be affected significantly.

Brainstem Disorders

Brainstem disorders that affect the auditory system include infarcts, gliomas, and multiple sclerosis. Brainstem infarcts are localized areas of ischemia produced by interruption of the blood supply. Auditory disorder varies depending on the site and extent of the disorder (Musiek and Baran, 2004).

Gliomas are tumors composed of neuroglia, or supporting cells of the brain. They develop in various forms, depending on the types of cells involved, including astrocytomas, ependymomas, glioblastomas, and medulloblastomas. Any of these can affect the auditory pathways of the brainstem, resulting in various forms of retrocochlear hearing disorder, including hearing sensitivity loss and speech perception deficits.

Multiple sclerosis is a demyelinating disease. It is caused by an autoimmune reaction of the nervous system that results in small scattered areas of demyelination and the development of demyelinated plaques. During the disease process, there is local swelling of tissue that exacerbates symptoms, followed by periods of remission. If the demyelination process affects structures of the auditory nervous system, hearing disorder can result. There is no characteristic hearing sensitivity loss that emerges as a consequence of the disorder, although all possible configurations have been described. Speech perception deficits are not uncommon in patients with multiple sclerosis (Stach, Delgado-Vileches, and Smith-Farach, 1990).

APDs associated with brainstem lesions will vary, depending on the level at which they occur in the brainstem, as well as the extent of the lesion's influence. Generally, the higher in the brainstem, the more subtle are the effects of the lesion. In lower brainstem lesions, performance on difficult monotic tasks is typically poor in the ear ipsilateral to the disorder. In addition, abnormalities are often found in measures of binaural release from masking. In higher brainstem lesions, performance on difficult monotic tasks can be abnormal in both the ipsilateral and contralateral ears. Brainstem lesions have also been associated with reduction in localization, lateralization, and temporal processing abilities.

Cortical Disorders

One of the more common cortical pathologies is caused by cerebrovascular accident, or stroke, which results from an interruption of blood supply to the brain due to aneurysm, embolism, or clot. This, in turn, causes a sudden loss of function related to the affected portion of the brain. Any other disease processes, lesions, or traumas that affect the central nervous system can affect the auditory nervous system as well. When the temporal lobe is involved, audition may be affected, although more typically, receptive language processing is affected, whereas hearing perception is relatively spared.

Auditory processing disorders associated with temporal lobe lesions include poor dichotic performance, some reduction in performance on difficult monotic tasks, typically in the ear opposite to the lesion, impaired localization ability, and reduced temporal processing ability.

Bilateral temporal lobe lesions are an exception to the subtlety principle. In such cases, "cortical deafness" can occur, resulting in symptoms that resemble auditory agnosia or profound hearing sensitivity loss (Hood et al, 1994; Jerger et al, 1969, 1972).

Functional Disorders of Aging

Changes in structure and function occur throughout the peripheral and central auditory nervous systems as a result of the aging process (Chisolm et al, 2003). Structural degeneration occurs in the cochlea and in the central auditory nervous system pathways. Evidence of neural degeneration has been found in the auditory nerve, brainstem, and cortex.

Anatomical and physiologic aging of the auditory system results from at least two processes (Willott, 1996). One is the central effects of peripheral pathology, or those that are secondary to the deprivational effects of cochlear hearing loss. The other is the central effects of biologic aging of the nervous system structures themselves. As with all other structures of the body, the brain undergoes changes related to the aging process. These central effects of biologic aging include a loss of neuronal tissue; loss of dendritic branches, reducing the number of synaptic contacts; changes in excitatory and inhibitory neurotransmitter systems; and other degenerative changes.

Whereas the effect of structural change in the auditory periphery is to attenuate and distort incoming sounds, the major effect of structural change in the central auditory nervous system is the degradation of auditory processing. Hearing impairment in the elderly, then, can be quite complex, consisting of attenuation of acoustic information, distortion of that information, and/or disordered processing of neural information (Pichora-Fuller and Souza, 2003). In its simplest form, this complex disorder can be thought of as a combination of peripheral cochlear effects (attenuation and distortion) and central nervous system effects (APD). The consequences of peripheral sensitivity loss in the elderly are similar to those of younger hearing-impaired individuals. The functional consequence of structural changes in the central auditory nervous system is APD.

Pearl

- The functional consequences of cochlear hearing loss in patients who are elderly appear to be similar to those of younger individuals. The functional consequence of structural changes in the central auditory nervous system with aging is APD.

Auditory processing ability is usually defined operationally on the basis of behavioral measures of speech understanding. Degradation in auditory processing has been demonstrated most convincingly by the use of "sensitized" speech audiometric measures. Age-related changes have been found on degraded speech tests that use both frequency (Bocca, 1958) and temporal alteration (Price and Simon, 1984; Sticht and Gray, 1969). Tests of dichotic performance have also been found to be adversely affected by aging (Gelfand et al, 1980; Jerger et al, 1995; Jerger, Stach, Johnson, et al, 1990). In addition, aging listeners do not perform as well as younger listeners on tasks that involve the understanding of speech in the presence of background noise (Helfer and Wilber, 1990; Jerger and Hayes, 1977; Pestalozza and Shore, 1955; Wiley et al, 1998). Some aging patients also experience binaural interference (Jerger et al, 1993).

In addition to reduced performance on speech audiometric measures, temporal processing deficits (Fitzgibbons and Gordon-Salant, 1996) have been described on measures of precedence (Cranford and Romereim, 1992; Roberts et al, 2003), duration difference limens (Fitzgibbons and Gordon-Salant, 1996), duration discrimination (Phillips et al, 1994), and gap detection (Moore et al, 1992; Roberts and Lister, 2004; Schneider et al, 1994).

◆ Factors Influencing Diagnostic Assessment

The measurement of auditory processing ability in adults is typically performed with a test battery approach that assesses absolute speech recognition ability, speech recognition in competition, dichotic listening, and temporal processing ability. Within each of these categories, there is substantial variation in test usage across clinical sites. In addition, there are new developments in testing strategies that hold promise to enhance the ability to quantify central auditory function.

Regardless of the test or test battery used in the assessment of auditory processing ability, there are some factors that influence both the selection of testing tools and the approaches used, as well as the success with which they are likely to be implemented. One of the most important factors in speech audiometric testing is the way in which information content of the test materials is manipulated. Other factors that are critical are those related to hearing sensitivity loss and cognitive ability of the patients being tested.

Informational Content

As neural impulses travel from the cochlea through CN VIII to the auditory brainstem and cortex, the number and complexity of neural pathways expand progressively. The system, in its vastness of pathways, includes a certain level of redundancy or excess capacity of processing ability. Such redundancy serves many useful purposes, but it also makes the function of the central auditory nervous system somewhat impervious to our efforts to examine it. For example, a patient can have a rather substantial lesion of the auditory brainstem or cortex and still have normal hearing and normal word recognition ability. To be able to assess the impact of such a lesion, the speech audiometric measures must be sensitized in some way before we can adequately examine the brain and understand its function and disorder.

Pearl

- Intrinsic and extrinsic redundancies combine to make the function of the central auditory nervous system somewhat impervious to our efforts to examine it. Nevertheless, if a neurologic system with reduced intrinsic redundancy is presented with speech materials with reduced extrinsic redundancy, then the abnormal processing caused by the neurologic disorder will be revealed.

Redundancy in Hearing

There is a great deal of redundancy associated with our ability to hear and process speech communication. Intrinsically, the central auditory nervous system has a rich system of anatomical, physiologic, and biochemical overlap. Among other functions, such intrinsic redundancy permits multisensory processing and simultaneous processing of different auditory signals. Another aspect of intrinsic redundancy is that the nervous system can be altered substantially by neurologic disorder and still maintain its ability to process information.

Extrinsically, speech signals contain a wealth of information due to phonologic, syntactic, and semantic content and rules. Such extrinsic redundancy allows a listener to hear only part of a speech segment and still understand what is being said. For example, consonants can be perceived from the coarticulatory effects of vowels even when the acoustic segments of the consonants are not heard. An entire sentence can be perceived from hearing only a few words that are embedded into a semantic context.

Extrinsic redundancy increases as the content of the speech signal increases. Thus, nonsense syllables are least redundant; continuous discourse is most redundant. The immunity of speech perception to the effects of hearing sensitivity loss varies directly with the amount of redundancy of the signal. The more redundancy inherent in the signal, the more immune that signal is to the effects of hearing loss. Stated another way, perception of speech that has lower redundancy is more likely to be affected by the presence of hearing loss than is perception of speech with greater redundancy.

Extrinsic and Intrinsic Redundancy Relationship

The issue of redundancy plays a role in the selection of speech materials. In assessing the effects of a cochlear hearing impairment on speech perception, signals that

Table 17–3   Relationship of Intrinsic and Extrinsic Redundancy to Speech Recognition Ability

Intrinsic		Extrinsic		Speech Recognition
Normal	+	Normal	=	Normal
Normal	+	Reduced	=	Normal
Reduced	+	Normal	=	Normal
Reduced	+	Reduced	=	Abnormal

have reduced redundancy can be used. Nonsense syllables or monosyllable words are sensitive to peripheral hearing impairment and are useful in quantifying its effect. Sentential approximations and sentences, in contrast, are not. Redundancy in these materials is simply too great to be affected by most degrees of hearing impairment.

In assessing the effects of a disorder of the central auditory nervous system on speech perception, however, the situation becomes more difficult. Speech signals of all levels of redundancy provide too much information to a central auditory nervous system that itself has a great deal of redundancy. Even if the intrinsic redundancy is reduced by neurologic disorder, the extrinsic redundancy of speech may be sufficient to permit normal processing. The solution to assessing central auditory nervous system disorders is to reduce the extrinsic redundancy of the speech information enough to reveal the reduced intrinsic redundancy caused by neurologic disorder. This concept is shown in **Table 17–3**. Normal intrinsic and extrinsic redundancies result in normal processing. Reducing the extrinsic redundancy, within limits, will have little effect on a system with normal intrinsic redundancy. Similarly, a neurologic disorder that reduces intrinsic redundancy will have little impact on perception of speech with normal extrinsic redundancy. However, if a system with reduced intrinsic redundancy is presented with speech materials that have reduced extrinsic redundancy, then the abnormal processing caused by the neurologic disorder will be revealed.

Methods of Reducing Extrinsic Redundancy

To reduce extrinsic redundancy, speech signals must be sensitized in some way. **Table 17–4** shows some methods for sensitizing test signals. In the frequency domain, speech can be sensitized by removing high frequencies, or low-pass filtering, thus limiting the phonetic content of the speech targets. Speech can be sensitized in the time domain by time compression, a technique that removes

Table 17–4   Methods for Sensitizing Speech Audiometric Measures

Domain	Technique
Frequency	Low-pass filtering
Time	Time compression
Intensity	High-level testing
Competition	Speech in noise
Binaural	Dichotic measures

segments of speech and compresses the remaining segments to increase speech rate. In the intensity domain, speech can be presented at sufficiently high levels at which disordered systems cannot seem to process effectively. Another very effective way to reduce redundancy of a signal is to present it in a background of competition. Yet another way to challenge the central auditory system is to present different, but similar, signals to both ears simultaneously in a dichotic paradigm.

Patient Factors

One of the most limiting factors in the selection of test measures of APD is the influence of hearing sensitivity loss on the ability to interpret test outcome. Another is the influence of cognitive competence on the complexity of the task that can be administered.

Hearing Sensitivity Loss

A significant confounding variable in the measurement of auditory processing ability is the presence of cochlear hearing impairment. In cases where hearing loss is present, signals that have enhanced redundancy need to be used so that hearing sensitivity loss does not interfere with interpretation of the measures. That is, materials should be used that are not affected by peripheral hearing impairment so that assessment can be made of processing at higher levels of the system. The issue is usually one of interpretation of test scores. For example, nonsense-syllable perception is usually altered by peripheral hearing impairment, and any effects of central nervous system disorder might not be revealed because they are difficult or impossible to separate from the effects of the hearing sensitivity loss. Use of sentences would likely overcome the peripheral hearing impairment, but their redundancy would be too great to challenge nervous system processing, even if it is disordered.

Pitfall

- A significant confounding variable in the assessment of auditory processing ability is the presence of hearing sensitivity loss. If the effects of the loss on a measure are unknown or uncontrollable, then interpretation of results will often be equivocal.

In some cases, the presence of hearing sensitivity loss simply precludes test interpretation, and testing cannot be performed effectively. For example, the consonant-vowel (CV) nonsense syllables used in the dichotic CV test are notoriously influenced by even a slight amount of cochlear hearing loss. The same has been reported for dichotic digits (Neijenhuis et al, 2004). If the test is used in a patient with hearing sensitivity loss, then poor performance cannot be interpreted as a dichotic deficit because the performance level could also be attributed to the cochlear hearing loss. As another example, the masking level difference (MLD)

test of binaural release from masking is an excellent test of lower brainstem function. However, the same performance abnormality attributable to a brainstem disorder can be obtained in a patient with a mild degree of low-frequency hearing loss. Thus, interpretation of the test is equivocal in the presence of hearing sensitivity loss.

In other cases, however, the influence of cochlear hearing loss on the speech measure is known, which may allow adequate interpretation. For example, absolute performance on one speech-in-competition measure, the Synthetic Sentence Identification (SSI) test, can be compared with normative databases on degree of hearing loss (Yellin et al, 1989). In this way, a patient's performance can be compared with expectations for someone with a cochlear hearing loss of the same degree. If performance is within the expected range, then auditory processing ability is classified as normal. If performance falls below the expected range, then performance on the test is considered abnormal, consistent with an APD. As another example, expectations of performance on a dichotic measure, the dichotic digits test, can be adjusted to more accurately assess central auditory ability in the presence of hearing loss (Musiek, 1983a,b). Without knowing the expected influence of hearing sensitivity loss, performance on these tests could not be interpreted accurately.

Special Consideration

- When the influences of hearing sensitivity loss and audiometric configuration on speech recognition scores are known, tests of auditory processing ability can be interpreted in the presence of hearing impairment.

The easiest solution to the issue of cochlear hearing loss is to use highly redundant speech signals to overcome the hearing sensitivity loss and then to sensitize those materials enough to challenge central auditory processing ability. The targets can be sensitized by adding background competition, testing at high intensity levels, and so on.

The issue of hearing sensitivity loss and its influence on measuring auditory processing ability is particularly challenging in the aging population. Much of the reduction in speech recognition ability, particularly in quiet, that is attributable to the aging process can actually be explained by degree of hearing sensitivity loss. That being said, reduction in auditory processing ability, as measured with speech recognition in competition, can be attributed to central auditory aging when hearing sensitivity loss is adequately controlled during test interpretation.

For example, several studies have addressed the role of peripheral sensitivity loss in declining speech understanding with age. One study attempted to estimate the prevalence of APD in a clinical population (Stach et al, 1990) and to assess the possibility that increased peripheral sensitivity loss was, in fact, the cause of increased speech audiometric abnormalities. Seven hundred patient files, 100 patients from each of seven half-decades, were evaluated. In the study, APD was operationally defined on the basis of speech audiometric test results. Absolute test scores were compared against empirically established norms (Yellin et al, 1989) for hearing loss. This permitted accurate interpretation of scores despite the presence of peripheral hearing loss that occurs with age. Hearing loss was then matched across age groups. Despite equivalent peripheral sensitivity loss across groups, the prevalence of APD increased systematically with age. These results serve to emphasize that APD cannot be explained simply as an artifact of peripheral sensitivity loss.

In another study (Jerger, Jerger, and Pirozzolo, 1991), a battery of speech audiometric tests and a battery of neuropsychologic measures were administered to 200 elderly individuals with varying degrees of sensitivity loss. Although results showed a predictable influence of hearing sensitivity loss on most measures, a significant amount of the total variance in SSI performance was attributable to knowledge of subject age.

As a final example, another study (Jerger, 1992) analyzed speech audiometric scores from 137 older subjects across four age groups that were matched for degree of pure-tone sensitivity loss. Results showed a statistically significant decline in SSI score as a function of age that could not be explained on the basis of hearing sensitivity loss.

These examples serve to illustrate that APD can be assessed in patients with hearing sensitivity loss but that great care must be taken in doing so if the influences of peripheral and central effects are to be isolated.

Absolute Speech Recognition

The need to control for, or at least understand, absolute speech recognition is much the same concept as the influence of hearing sensitivity loss. Absolute speech recognition in quiet will have some influence on speech recognition in noise, and interpretation of the latter cannot be made without adequate knowledge of the former. This concept is perhaps easiest to illustrate in cases of asymmetry. Suppose, for example, that absolute speech recognition scores for sentence materials were 100 and 70% for the right and left ears, respectively. A competing sentence dichotic measure is then performed and shows an asymmetry in dichotic performance, with the left ear score being poorer than the right. Is this a dichotic deficit or simply a reflection of the monotic asymmetry? Similarly, speech-in-noise scores should not be compared with normative data if speech-in-quiet scores are not known or somehow anchored to expected levels.

Special Consideration

- Absolute speech recognition in quiet will have some influence on speech recognition in noise, and interpretation of the latter cannot be made without adequate knowledge of the former.

Cognitive Competence

Can the patient perform the perceptual task? It seems like such an easy question. Not unlike the issue of hearing sensitivity loss, this question often arises when assessing the aging population. Are these changes in speech recognition ability attributable to true APD, or are they simply a reflection of reduced capacity to perform the task brought on by senescent changes in cognition? The answer seems to be that for most of the perceptual tasks in the auditory processing test battery, task-related demands are low enough to not be influenced by reductions in memory or cognition. In others, however, there is evidence that reduced scores can be related to the task rather than to an auditory problem.

What, then, is the role of cognitive ability in declining speech understanding with age? Jerger and colleagues (Jerger, Stach, Pruitt, et al, 1989) suggested that speech audiometric tests of central function were not necessarily related to cognitive disability. Audiological data were analyzed from 23 patients with a neuropsychological diagnosis of dementia. Among the cognitive deficits found in these patients were those of memory, tolerance of distraction, mental tracking and sequencing, and cognitive flexibility. Despite such deficits, 12 of the 23 subjects (52%) yielded speech audiometric results consistent with normal auditory processing ability. Although the APD found in the remaining 11 subjects could be related to cognitive deficits, it might also be the case that results on the neuropsychological evaluation were confounded by the effects of APD. That is, in these 11 subjects, the relative contribution of auditory and cognitive deficits could not be separated. In any event, the fact that some patients with dementia could perform well on behavioral speech audiometric tests argues against the explanation that APDs can be explained as easily by subtle cognitive decline as by an auditory deficit.

In another study, Jerger and colleagues (Jerger, Oliver, and Pirozzolo, 1989) measured both auditory and cognitive status in 130 older subjects. They found that auditory processing ability and cognitive function were congruent in only 64% of subjects, indicating that the two measures are relatively independent. That is, APDs can occur in those individuals with normal cognitive status, and cognitive decline can occur in those with normal auditory processing ability.

Pearl

- Disorders of cognitive ability and disorders of central auditory processing can be independent entities, yet each may influence interpretation of measures of the other.

These results suggest that, in general, speech audiometric measures are independent of significant cognitive decline. However, the story is not quite that simple. In other studies of the aging process that used dichotic measures, some performance deficits were found to be task related (Hallgren et al, 2001; Jerger, Stach, Johnson, et al, 1990). This suggests that dichotic results could be overinterpreted as deficits if care is not taken to limit these nonauditory influences. Patients were asked to perform a dichotic measure in two ways. One was a free-recall mode, in which the patient's task was to identify both sentences in either order. The other was a focused-recall task, in which the patient was asked to identify only those sentences perceived in the right ear. The task was then repeated for the left ear. Results showed that several elderly patients had difficulty on the free-recall task but improved when the task was simplified. It appears that short-term memory problems were influencing the results on this dichotic measure. When the task was simplified, some patients still showed deficits, but they appeared to be truly auditory in nature. Care must be taken when selecting tests for clinical populations that include older individuals to ensure that task-related performance issues are well understood and controlled.

The processes involved in auditory processing and other, more supramodal cognitive functions overlap to an extent that they cannot always be measured independently. As an example, one study (Gates et al, 2002) suggests the intriguing notion that APD precedes the onset of Alzheimer's disease. Nevertheless, the quantification of a specific auditory processing deficit as an independent entity can be very useful in designing strategies for treatment of hearing disorder.

Pitfall

- Memory and other supramodal cognitive factors can cause task-related deficits that are not reflective of auditory ability, especially on measures of dichotic listening.

Influence of Medication and Other Drugs

Performance on any behavioral measure, particularly on those that are designed to stress the auditory system, can be adversely influenced by some medications and intoxicants. Performance can be reduced temporarily from acute drug use or intoxication, or it can be reduced permanently from chronic exposure to toxins. As an example of the former, patients who have ingested alcohol prior to the evaluation can perform poorly on measures of central auditory processing ability. As an example of the latter, workers who are exposed to industrial toxins for several years will show permanent changes in auditory processing ability.

Procedural Factors

Procedural factors can certainly influence the successful implementation of a central auditory processing test battery. Most commercially available tests have been designed to control many of these factors. Nevertheless, applicability of certain tests and test materials can be limited, especially in older patients.

Speech versus Nonspeech Stimuli

There are merits and controversies related to the use of speech and nonspeech targets and competition. Regarding targets, the more speechlike the signal, the more redundant the informational content. This helps in overcoming hearing loss but requires sensitizing to challenge the central auditory system. The less speechlike the targets, the easier they are to control, but the more distant they are from being readily generalized to communication ability.

Regarding competition, the issue is related to how interfering the competitor can be. White noise or multitalker babble tends to act like a masker without much interference other than that which is achieved acoustically. The more speechlike and meaningful the competition, the more interfering it is likely to be, and the more effective it will be in challenging the auditory processing system (Larsby et al, 2005; Sperry et al, 1997; Stuart and Phillips, 1996). For this reason, competition consisting of single talkers, double talkers, or even noise that has been temporally altered to resemble speech has been used effectively to provide interference with the perceptual task.

Special Consideration

- The more speechlike the competition, the more interfering it will be in assessing speech in noise, and the more valuable it will be as a competitor in APD assessment.

Response Modes

Another procedural factor that can influence outcomes is whether speech audiometric measures are open or closed set in nature. There are at least two advantages to closed-set measures. First, the use of closed-set responses generally allows the "anchoring" of performance at a known level. For example, if performance on a measure in quiet is 100% on a closed-set measure, then it is readily assured that the patient has the language, cognition, memory, and attention to perform the particular task. Once competition is added or some other sensitizing is done to the targets, the tester is assured that the patient has the capacity to perform the task. A second advantage can be achieved when testing is being performed on adults with limited language ability, such as those with aphasia. In such cases, picture-pointing tasks can be used, wherein the patient has a limited number of foils from which to choose the correct answer, and the language level may be low enough to overcome the effects of aphasia (S. Jerger et al, 1990).

Monaural versus Binaural versus Dichotic

Assessing all three conditions—monaural speech recognition, binaural ability, and dichotic listening—is often of value. Each has the potential to provide insight about the presence and nature of an APD. In isolation, each reveals only a portion of the system's ability to process information.

Task Complexity

Complexity of the perceptual or response tasks tends to add a variable that can be difficult to control (Shinn et al, 2005).

As learned in the example of elderly listeners' difficulty with free recall of dichotically presented sentences, if a task is to be applicable to all ages of adults, then it must take into consideration task-related limitations of aging patients. Tasks that require perceptual judgments, adaptive psychophysical procedures, and measures that tax memory can all add confounding variables to the assessment of APD in older adults.

♦ Some Diagnostic Measures of Auditory Processing Disorders

Following are descriptions of some available measures of central auditory processing ability. Although not exhaustive, those that are described are among the measures that have stood the test of time or that hold promise as effective measures for clinical testing.

Monaural Measures

Monaural measures of auditory processing ability are typically speech audiometric measures that are in some way sensitized in an effort to challenge the central auditory mechanisms. Monaural speech audiometric measures include high-level word recognition testing, time-compressed speech, low-pass filtered speech, and speech in competition. Other monaural measures include nonspeech assessment of temporal processing ability.

Word Recognition in Quiet

Interpretation of word recognition measures is based on the predictable relation of maximum word recognition scores to degree of hearing loss (Dubno et al, 1995; Gates et al, 2003; Yellin et al, 1989). If the maximum score falls within a predetermined range for a given degree of hearing loss, then the results are considered to be within expectation for a cochlear hearing loss. If the score is poorer than expected, then word recognition ability is considered to be abnormal for the degree of hearing loss and consistent with retrocochlear disorder.

One modification of this original word recognition paradigm has been the exploration of speech perception across the patient's entire dynamic range of hearing rather than at just a single suprathreshold level. The goal here is to determine a maximum score regardless of test level. To obtain a maximum score, lists of words or sentences are presented at three to five intensity levels, extending from just above the speech threshold to the upper level of comfortable listening. In this way, a performance intensity (PI) function is generated for each ear. In most cases, the PI function rises systematically as speech intensity is increased to an asymptotic level representing the best speech understanding that can be achieved in the test ear. In some cases, however, there is a paradoxical rollover effect, in which the function declines substantially as speech intensity increases beyond the level producing the maximal performance score. In

other words, as speech intensity increases, performance rises to a maximum level, then declines or "rolls over" sharply as intensity continues to increase. This rollover effect is commonly observed when the site of the hearing loss is retrocochlear in the auditory nerve or the auditory pathways in the brainstem (Jerger and Jerger, 1971).

Pearl

- The use of high-level speech recognition testing is a way of sensitizing speech audiometric measures by challenging the auditory system at high-intensity levels. Reduced performance at high-intensity levels is not uncommon in disordered central auditory nervous systems.

The use of PI functions is a way of sensitizing speech by challenging the auditory system at high-intensity levels. Because of its ease of administration, many audiologists use it routinely as a screening measure for retrocochlear disorders.

Sensitized Speech

One of the first measures of auditory processing ability was the low-pass filtered speech test. In this test, single-syllable words are low-pass filtered below 500 Hz to eliminate higher frequency information and the redundancy that it provides. Most listeners with normal hearing sensitivity and normal auditory nervous systems can perceive these targets accurately, despite the severity of filtering. However, patients with APDs require more redundancy and tend to perform poorly on these measures. Results in patients with temporal lobe lesions showed poorer scores in the ear contralateral to the lesion (Boca et al, 1954), and patients with brainstem lesions showed ipsilateral, contralateral, and bilateral ear effects (Calearo and Antonelli, 1968).

Time compression of speech targets is another way to reduce the redundancy. Time compression effectively speeds up speech by eliminating segments of the speech signal and compressing the remaining speech into a smaller time window. This results in rapid speech that is unaltered in the frequency and amplitude domains. Processing of time-compressed speech has been shown to be abnormal in patients with brainstem lesions (Calearo and Antonelli, 1968), cortical disorder (Kurdziel et al, 1976), and in aging populations (Sticht and Gray, 1969).

Although redundancy can be reduced by low-pass filtering or time compression, these methods have clinical limitations because of their susceptibility to the effects of cochlear hearing loss. That is, hearing sensitivity loss of cochlear origin may affect scores on these measures in a manner that does not permit the interpretation of central auditory system integrity. As a result, test results are generally only interpretable on individuals who have normal hearing sensitivity, which does not give these measures widespread clinical applicability in adult populations.

Perhaps the most successfully used sensitized speech measures are those in which competition is presented as a means of stressing the auditory system. There are any number of measures of speech-in-noise that have been developed over the years, among them the Speech Perception in Noise (SPIN) test and Hearing in Noise Test (HINT). SPIN (Kalikow et al, 1977) has as its target a single word that is the last in a sentence. In half of the sentences, the word is predictable from the context of the sentence; in the other half, the word is not predictable. These signals are presented in a background of multitalker competition. HINT (Nilsson et al, 1994) uses sentence targets and an adaptive paradigm to determine the threshold for speech recognition in the presence of background competition. Although these and numerous other measures are useful in assessing speech recognition in competition, their use for assessment of APD has been limited by both a lack of validation in the target population and, importantly, the challenge of interpretation in the presence of cochlear hearing loss.

One measure of suprathreshold ability that has stood the test of time is the SSI test (Jerger et al, 1968). The SSI uses sentential approximations that are presented in a closed-set format. The patient is asked to identify the sentence from a list of 10. Sentences are presented in the presence of single-talker competition. Testing typically is performed with the signal and the competition at the same intensity level, a message-to-competition ratio of 0 dB. The SSI has some advantages inherent in its design. First, because it uses sentence materials, it is relatively immune to hearing loss. Said another way, the influence of mild degrees of hearing loss on identification of these sentences is minimal, and the effect of more severe hearing loss on absolute scores is known. Second, it uses a closed-set response, thereby permitting practice that reduces learning effects and ensures that a patient's performance deficits are not task related. Third, the single-talker competition, which has no influence on recognition scores of those with normal auditory ability, can be quite interfering to sentence perception in those with central auditory processing ability. Reduced performance on the SSI has been reported in patients with brainstem disorders (Jerger and Jerger, 1975; S. Jerger and Jerger, 1983) and in the aging population.

Temporal Processing

Various measures of temporal processing have been used to assess central auditory ability. One measure is known as the Auditory Duration Patterns Test (ADPT; Musiek et al, 1990). The ADPT is a sequence of three 1000 Hz tones, one of which varies from the others in duration. The duration of a tone is either longer (500 msec) or shorter (200 msec). The patient's task is to identify the pattern of tones as long-long-short, long-short-long, short-short-long, and so on. Practice items can be given prior to testing to eliminate learning effects. Abnormal performance has been reported in patients with temporal lobe disorder (Hurley and Musiek, 1997; Musiek et al, 1990).

Another promising measure is the Gaps-in-Noise (GIN) test. Broadband noise segments in which silent intervals, or gaps, are randomly placed are presented to patients. The patients' task is to identify the gaps, which range in duration from 2 to 20 msec, and a gap detection threshold is

determined. Abnormal performance has been reported in patients with confirmed central auditory nervous system disorders (Musiek et al, 2005).

Other measures of temporal processing have shown changes related to the aging process (Fitzgibbons and Gordon-Salant, 1996). These measures include assessment of temporal resolution by gap detection or modulation detection and assessment of duration discrimination by duration difference limen determination. Results on these psychophysical measures from the aging population show the potential for their usefulness in assessing central auditory processing ability in the time domain (Roberts and Lister, 2004).

Binaural Measures

One important aspect of auditory processing ability is the manner in which both ears work together to integrate and separate information. Measures of binaural ability include assessment of the manner in which the ears process phase cues, integrate information, lateralize and localize the source of sound, and extract signals of interest from background competition.

Masking Level Difference

One behavioral diagnostic measure that has stood the test of time is a measure of lower brainstem function known as the masking level difference. The MLD measures binaural release from masking due to interaural phase relationships. The binaural auditory system is an exquisite detector of differences in timing of sound reaching the two ears. This helps in localizing low-frequency sounds, which reach the ears at different points in time. The concept of binaural release from masking reveals how sensitive the ears are to these timing, or phase, cues.

The MLD test is the clinical strategy designed to measure binaural release from masking. To carry out the MLD, a 500 Hz interrupted tone is split and presented in phase to both ears. Narrowband noise is also presented, at a fixed level of 60 dB HL (hearing level). Using the Békésy tracking procedure, threshold for the in-phase tones is determined in the presence of the noise. Then the phase of one of the tones is reversed, and threshold is tracked again. The MLD is the difference in threshold between the in-phase and the out-of-phase conditions. For a 500 Hz tone, the MLD should be greater than 7 dB and is usually around 12 dB.

Abnormal performance on the MLD is consistent with brainstem disorder (Hannley et al, 1983; Olsen and Noffsinger, 1976). Care must be taken in interpreting MLD results in the presence of hearing loss, because the MLD shift is reduced with reduced hearing thresholds (Jerger et al, 1984).

Special Consideration

- Care must be taken in interpreting MLD results in the presence of hearing loss, especially when losses occur at 500 Hz or thresholds at 500 Hz are asymmetric.

Binaural Integration

Efforts have been made to assess how the two ears can work together to integrate partial information from each into a binaural perception of the whole. Two such efforts include the measures of binaural fusion and binaural resynthesis.

Binaural fusion is a measure in which words, usually monosyllables, are pass-band filtered into a low-pass band and a high-pass band. In the original description of the binaural fusion test, the low-pass band was from 500 to 800 Hz and the high-pass band from 1815 to 2500 Hz (Matzker, 1959). The low-pass band is presented to one ear and the high-pass band to the other. Recognition of either band in isolation is generally poor. However, normal listeners are capable of fusing the two pass bands when they are presented binaurally and can recognize the words with a high level of accuracy. Abnormally poor binaural fusion scores have been reported in some patients with brainstem disorder (Smith and Resnick, 1972) and in some patients with temporal lobe disorder.

Another test of binaural integration, often referred to as binaural resynthesis, is the Rapidly Alternating Speech Perception (RASP) test (Bocca and Calearo, 1963), wherein a sentence stimulus is alternated between the ears every 300 msec. The segments presented to one ear are minimally intelligible under normal conditions. The segments from both ears fuse together into an easily recognizable message under normal circumstances. Abnormal performance on the RASP test has been associated with disorders at the level of the lower brainstem (Musiek and Geurkink, 1982).

Precedence

The precedence effect in sound localization is measured by presenting identical clicks from two speakers on opposite sides of the subject's head. The onset of clicks from one speaker is presented earlier than that from the other speaker. With proper delays, normal subjects perceive a fused image originating from the leading speaker. The precedence effect has been shown to be abnormal in elderly individuals (Cranford and Romereim, 1992) and in patients with multiple sclerosis (Cranford et al, 1990). Emerging strategies for precedent effect assessment, including the measurement of lag burst thresholds (Roberts et al, 2003), hold intriguing promise for routine clinical implementation.

Localization

Localization ability is usually measured in a sound field and expressed as the accuracy of identifying a signal source. Numerous strategies for measuring localization ability have been implemented over the years, but few have proven to be practical clinically. Nevertheless, poor localization ability has been associated with auditory nervous system disorders at the level of the brainstem (Hausler et al, 1983; Stephens, 1976) and cortex (Sanchez-Longo and Forster, 1958; Stephens, 1976).

One of the more promising strategies for assessment of localization ability is the three-dimensional (3-D) auditory test of localization (Koehnke and Besing, 1997). Using virtual reality techniques and digital signal processing technology,

3-D assessment of sound-source localization can be made under earphones, with the source being externalized to various spatial locations outside the head. This and other virtual reality techniques promise to bring the measurement of localization ability under control to an extent that it can be implemented clinically for assessment of this important aspect of auditory processing ability.

Other Measure of Spatial Hearing

Measurement of the precedent effect and virtual sound localization can be used to assess spatial hearing. These and a growing number of other virtual strategies are emerging to address this very important notion of the ability to accurately hear in auditory space (Koehnke and Besing, 2001). We may yet learn that deficits in spatial hearing ability are the underlying cause of most problems hearing in background noise experienced by those with APD.

Another promising strategy for the assessment of spatial hearing is the cued discourse technique (Jerger, Johnson, et al, 1991). Identical ongoing speech signals are presented from speakers opposite the right and left ear. The speech signal is a single talker reading a story written in the first person. The same story is presented from both speakers with a delay of 1 minute in one of the speakers. The patient's task is to count the number of times that the personal pronoun *I* is perceived from the speaker that is being cued. The number of errors is counted, and the opposite speaker is cued. Following completion, multitalker babble is introduced from an overhead speaker, and the process is repeated over a range of SNRs. Results of the cued discourse measure have shown significant asymmetries in patients with APDs (Jerger, Johnson, et al, 1991) and in the aging population (Jerger and Jordan, 1992). The listening situation is a challenging one, and the technique seems likely to assist in quantifying disorders in those patients with obscure and difficult-to-measure auditory complaints.

Dichotic Measures

Another effective approach to assessing central auditory processing ability is the use of dichotic tests. In the dichotic paradigm, two different speech targets are presented simultaneously to the two ears. The patient's task is usually either to repeat back both targets in either order or to report only the target heard in the precued ear. In this latter case, the right ear is precued on half the trials and the left on the other half. Two scores are determined, one for targets correctly identified from the right ear, the other for targets correctly identified from the left ear. The patterns of results can reveal auditory processing deficits, especially those due to disorders of the temporal lobe and corpus callosum. Dichotic tests have been constructed using nonsense syllables, monosyllabic words, spondaic words, sentences, and synthetic sentences.

Dichotic CVs

Consonant-vowel nonsense syllables have been used as dichotic stimuli (Berlin et al, 1972), presented either simultaneously or in a manner that staggers the presentation from

30 to 90 msec. Simultaneous presentation yields normal scores of ~60 to 70% correct identification. In the staggered condition, scores are better for the lagging ear than for the leading ear. Regardless of method, abnormal results on the dichotic CV test have been reported in patients with temporal lobe lesions (Olsen, 1983), temporal lobectomy (Berlin et al, 1972), and hemispherectomy.

Dichotic Digits

Dichotic listening has been assessed for many years with a paradigm that uses digits as stimuli (Kimura, 1961). More recent efforts (Musiek, 1983a) have rekindled interest in use of the digits test to assess dichotic performance. In its current version, the dichotic digits test consists of 40 pairs of digits, delivered simultaneously to both ears. The patient's task is to identify the digits in a free-recall mode (i.e., in any order). One advantage of the dichotic digits test is its relative resistance to the effects of peripheral hearing loss. Abnormal performance on the dichotic digits test has been reported in patients with brainstem lesions (Musiek 1983b), temporal lobe lesions (Hurley and Musiek, 1997; Kimura, 1961; Musiek, 1983b), and as a result of the aging process (Wilson and Jaffe, 1996). Although the predominant findings have shown contralateral ear effects, many patients with brainstem and temporal lobe lesions will also show abnormal ipsilateral performance.

Staggered Spondaic Word Test

The Staggered Spondaic Word (SSW) test (Katz, 1962) is one in which a different spondaic word is presented to each ear, with the second syllable of the word presented to the leading ear overlapping in time with the first syllable of the word presented to the lagging ear. Thus, the leading ear is presented with one syllable in isolation (noncompeting), followed by one syllable in a dichotic mode (competing). The lagging ear begins with the first syllable presented in the dichotic mode and finishes with the second syllable presented in isolation. The right ear serves as the leading ear for half of the test presentations. Error scores are calculated for each ear in both the competing and noncompeting modes. A correction can be applied to account for hearing sensitivity loss. Abnormal SSW performance has been reported in patients with brainstem (Musiek, 1983b), corpus callosum (Baran et al, 1986), and temporal lobe lesions (Olsen, 1983).

Competing Sentence Test

The competing sentence test uses short natural sentences that average six to seven words in length. The sentence presented to the target ear is generally set at an intensity level 15 dB below the level of the sentence presented to the nontarget ear. Sentences are generally scored as correct if the meaning and content of the sentence were identified appropriately. Abnormal competing sentence test performance has been reported in patients with temporal lobe lesions (Musiek, 1983b), predominantly on the ear contralateral to the lesion.

Dichotic Sentence Identification Test

The Dichotic Sentence Identification (DSI) test (Fifer et al, 1983) uses synthetic sentences from the SSI test, aligned for presentation in the dichotic mode. The response is a closed set, and the subject's task is to identify the sentences from among a list on a response card. The DSI was designed in an effort to overcome the influence of hearing sensitivity loss on test interpretation and was found to be applicable for use in ears with a pure-tone average (PTA) of up to 50 dB HL and asymmetry of up to 40 dB. Abnormal DSI results have been reported in aging patients (Jerger et al, 1994; Jerger, Stach, Johnson, et al, 1990).

◆ Toward a Cogent Clinical Strategy

With such a wide array of diagnostic options, the challenge of deciding which to use for clinical assessment can be a daunting one. Several test batteries have been applied over the years (e.g., Medwetsky, 2002; Musiek et al, 1994) with varying degrees of success.

A test battery will be described briefly here in an effort to illustrate one approach to the diagnosis of APD that has proven successful clinically (Jerger and Hayes, 1977; Stach, Spretnjak, and Jerger, 1990). The approach that is used to diagnose APD is based on the assumptions that (1) APD is an auditory perceptual problem, not a cognitive or linguistic problem; (2) it can be operationally defined on the basis of speech audiometric measures; and (3) tests can be administered in a manner that limits the influences of cochlear hearing loss, language, and cognition on interpretation of results. Though it is by no means the only strategy that exists, it is successful for several reasons. First, the measures have been validated in populations of patients with confirmed neurologic disease processes, making them useful for diagnostic screening purposes and applicable for describing APD as a communication disorder (Jerger and Jerger, 1975; S. Jerger and Jerger, 1983). Second, the measures can be used with the majority of patients in a manner that is clinically efficient. Third, the approach has a reasonable degree of specificity in that factors unrelated to central auditory disorders seldom result in poor performance on the measures used. Fourth, the approach is effective, to the extent possible, in controlling the influences of cochlear hearing loss on test interpretation. In addition, the measures can be applied in a manner that controls the cognitive influences of factors such as memory, thereby isolating auditory disorder from supramodal influences on test interpretation.

Pearl

- The key factors in any successful test battery approach are the efficient and effective controls over cochlear sensitivity loss, absolute speech recognition ability, and supramodal influences.

Applying such a clinical strategy to any number of existing tests of APD would likely enhance their usefulness in a test battery as well. The key factors are the efficient and effective controls over cochlear sensitivity loss, absolute speech recognition ability, and supramodal influences.

A Test Battery Approach

The test battery described here includes word recognition testing in quiet, the SSI test (Jerger et al, 1968) with ipsilateral competing message, and the DSI test (Fifer et al, 1983). APD is operationally defined on the basis of patterns of speech audiometric scores.

Word recognition testing is performed in quiet across a range of intensity levels, providing a PI function. The maximum WRS is compared with empirically derived normative scores based on degree of hearing sensitivity loss. These normative scores are based on the performance of a large number of patients with cochlear hearing loss and no evidence of retrocochlear disorder. If performance equals or exceeds the lower limits of normal, then the score is considered to be appropriate for that degree of hearing loss and consistent with normal hearing, conductive hearing loss, or sensorineural hearing loss of cochlear origin. If performance is below the lower limits of normal, then the score is considered to be abnormal for that degree of hearing loss, consistent with retrocochlear disorder. A PI function is obtained to look for rollover. A small amount of rollover (< 20%) can be attributable to cochlear hearing loss. A more significant rollover is consistent with retrocochlear disorder.

The SSI test is administered monaurally, with ipsilateral competition at a message-to-competition ratio of 0 dB. This test is also administered across a range of intensity levels to determine a PI function. Interpretation is based on maximum score comparison to established norms based on degree of hearing loss, the amount of rollover, and the discrepancy between speech recognition of words in quiet and the sentences in competition. Excessive reduction in sentence recognition in competition in comparison to word recognition scores obtained in quiet is a finding that is often consistent with retrocochlear disorder.

The DSI test is generally presented at a single intensity level. If hearing sensitivity is normal, sentences are delivered at 50 dB HL to both ears. If a hearing loss exists, the level is increased in both ears. Testing is always performed at equal HL in both ears. Often, dichotic performance is evaluated under two task conditions: free recall and focused recall. In the free-recall condition, the patient is asked to identify both sentences regardless of the ear in which they are heard. In the focused-recall condition, the patient is asked to identify only those sentences identified in a specified ear, and then the other ear is tested. Results are consistent with a dichotic deficit when scores on the focused-recall condition show significant asymmetry or reduced scores in both ears.

In terms of screening for retrocochlear disorder, general patterns have emerged as being consistent with lesions at a certain level within the auditory system. These patterns are summarized in **Table 17–5**. When a hearing loss is

Table 17–5 Expected Patterns of Abnormality Related to Auditory Processing Disorder on a Battery of Tests*

Site	WRSmax	WRS PI	SSImax	SSI PI	DSI
Cochlea	–	–	–	–	–
CN VIII	+	+	+	+	–
Brainstem	–	±	+	+	–
Temporal lobe	–	–	±	±	+

* These include maximum word recognition (WRSmax) scores presented in quiet, performance intensity function of word recognition scores in quiet (WRS PI), maximum Synthetic Sentence Identification scores (SSImax), performance intensity function of SSI scores (SSI PI), and scores on the Dichotic Sentence Identification (DSI) test. Predicted performance on these measures would be –, normal or predictable from the degree of hearing sensitivity loss; ±, sometimes abnormal, depending on the site, size, and extent of influence of the lesion; or +, abnormal.

CN VIII, eighth cranial nerve.

cochlear, word recognition and SSI scores will be consistent with the degree of loss, and little if any rollover will occur on the PI function. DSI scores will be normal.

When a hearing loss is sensorineural due to a CN VIII lesion, suprathreshold word recognition ability is likely to be substantially affected. Maximum scores are likely to be poorer than predicted from the degree of hearing loss, and rollover of the PI function is likely to occur. SSI scores are also likely to be depressed. Abnormal results will occur in the ear ipsilateral to the lesion. Dichotic measures will be normal.

When a hearing disorder occurs as a result of a brainstem lesion, suprathreshold word recognition ability is likely to be affected. WRSs in quiet may be normal, or they may be depressed or show rollover. SSI scores are likely to be depressed or show rollover in the ear ipsilateral to the lesion. Dichotic measures will likely be normal.

When a hearing disorder occurs as the result of a temporal lobe lesion, hearing sensitivity is unlikely to be affected, and WRSs are likely to be normal. SSI scores may or may not be abnormal in the ear contralateral to the lesion. DSI scores are most likely to show a deficit due to the temporal lobe lesion, usually characterized by a substantial left ear deficit.

In patients with APD and no identifiable neuropathology, patterns of results are similar to those of patients with brainstem and/or temporal lobe lesions. In an elderly patient, for example, it is not uncommon to observe reduced maximum SSI scores with rollover and reduced dichotic performance.

Controlling for Hearing Sensitivity Loss

One of the benefits of this type of test battery approach is that it can be used in patients with a wide range of hearing sensitivity loss. That is, scores can be interpreted in the presence of a hearing loss, because the influence of the loss on speech recognition scores is known or controllable.

The influence of hearing sensitivity loss is controlled in several ways. First, as stated previously, maximum scores

Table 17–6 Lower Limits of Maximum Synthetic Sentence Identification Scores for Different Degrees of Cochlear Hearing Sensitivity Loss as Quantified by the Pure-Tone Average of Thresholds at 500, 1000, and 2000 Hz

PTA (dB)	SSImax (%)
0	86
5	81
10	76
15	71
20	66
25	61
30	56
35	51
40	46
45	41
50	36
55	31
60	26
65	21
70	16
75	11
80	6
≥85	0

PTA, pure-tone average; SSImax, maximum Synthetic Sentence Identification.

Source: Adapted from Yellin, M. W., Jerger, J., & Fifer, R. C. (1989). Norms for disproportionate loss of speech intelligibility. Ear and Hearing, 10, 231–234, with permission.

can be compared with normative databases on degree of hearing loss. This can be done for both word recognition and SSI scores. An example of the normative data for the SSI test is shown in **Table 17–6**. Thus, if a patient with a PTA of 35 dB HL has a maximum SSI score of 70%, the result is consistent with what could be expected from a hearing loss of that magnitude. However, if the maximum score was 30%, then performance would be interpreted as poorer than that which would be attributable to the hearing loss alone, implicating a retrocochlear disorder as a contributor to the performance deficit.

A second way of controlling the influence of hearing sensitivity loss is by establishing a PI function. If maximum scores approach 100%, then the hearing loss is not influencing absolute word recognition ability. Should rollover occur at higher intensity, the reduced performance could not be attributable to any influence of sensitivity loss on absolute performance.

Another way of managing hearing loss influence is by testing at more than one message-to-competition ratio. For example, one strategy used with the SSI test is to begin testing at a favorable ratio of +10 dB. If a patient scores 100%, then the hearing sensitivity loss is not interfering with perception of the sentence. A reduced score at a reduced message-to-competition ratio, then, is more appropriately attributable to a problem in auditory processing ability. A similar strategy can be used in dichotic testing. Each ear can be assessed in isolation to determine absolute sentence recognition ability. Any reduction in scores with dichotic presentation can then be attributed to a dichotic deficit rather than any peripheral influences.

Controlling Supramodal Influences on Test Interpretation

Nonauditory, or supramodal, influences are controlled in much the same way as the influence of cochlear sensitivity loss. Good performance at one intensity level and poorer performance at a higher intensity level are difficult to explain on the basis of a cognitive or language deficit. Similarly, good performance at one message-to-competition ratio and poorer performance at another are difficult to attribute to these nonauditory influences. Often performance will be asymmetric as well, forcing the unlikely argument necessary to explain ear asymmetry on the basis of a cognitive or language deficit. That is, can there be a left ear cognitive deficit? Can there be a left ear language deficit? Obviously, the likelihood of asymmetry resulting from a cognitive or language deficit is small. An argument would also have to be made to explain the rollover of the PI function. It seems unlikely that a patient might somehow be cognitively more impaired at higher intensity levels than at lower intensity levels.

Using this type of test battery approach, with words and sentences presented at various intensity levels and message-to-competition ratios, it is possible to ensure that the patient is cognitively capable of carrying out the task, linguistically capable of carrying out the task, and has the attentional ability to carry out the task. Any deficit, then, could be attributable to an APD.

Thus, use of PI functions, various message-to-competition ratios, and word-versus-sentence comparisons permits the assessment of auditory processing ability in a manner that reduces the likelihood of nonauditory factors influencing the interpretation of test results. Clinical experience with this diagnostic strategy has been encouraging. In conjunction with thorough immittance, OAE, and auditory evoked potential measurements, the use of well-controlled speech audiometric measures has proven to be quite powerful in defining the presence or absence of an APD.

◆ Illustrative Cases

The following cases illustrate results from two patients, one with retrocochlear disorder secondary to brainstem lesions and the other with APD secondary to auditory nervous system aging.

Auditory Processing Disorder in Neuropathology

Patient 1 has auditory complaints secondary to multiple sclerosis. The patient is a 34-year-old woman. Two years prior to her evaluation, she experienced an episode of diplopia, accompanied by a tingling sensation and weakness in her left leg. These symptoms gradually subsided and reappeared in slightly more severe form a year later. Ultimately, she was diagnosed with multiple sclerosis. Among various other symptoms, she had vague hearing complaints, particularly in the presence of background noise.

Immittance audiometry is consistent with normal middle ear function, characterized by a type A tympanogram, normal static immittance, and normal right and left uncrossed reflex thresholds. However, crossed reflexes are absent bilaterally. This unusual pattern of results is consistent with a central pathway disorder of the lower brainstem.

Pure-tone audiometric results are shown in **Fig. 17–1A**. The patient has a mild low-frequency sensorineural hearing loss bilaterally, a finding that is not uncommon in brainstem disorder (Jerger and Jerger, 1980; Stach, Delgado-Vilches, and Smith-Farach, 1990).

Suprathreshold speech recognition performance is abnormal in both ears. Although word recognition scores are normal when presented in quiet, scores on sentence recognition in the presence of competition are abnormal, as shown in **Fig. 17–1B**. Dichotic scores were normal.

Auditory evoked potentials are also consistent with abnormality of brainstem function. On the left, no waves were

identifiable beyond component wave II, and on the right, none were identifiable beyond wave III.

Multiple sclerosis is a disease that involves the formation of demyelinating plaques within the white matter of the brainstem. When the plaques occur in or near the auditory pathways, function can be disrupted. In this case, the speech audiometric results showed a classic pattern of brainstem disorder. Recognition of words in quiet was normal. The measure was not sensitized, and the signals contained too much redundancy to challenge the impaired nervous system. Had the lesions been more peripheral at the juncture of CN VIII and the brainstem, these scores may well have been significantly reduced. Because neural information coursed through the bottleneck without disruption, perception of undistorted speech remained normal. In contrast, sentence recognition in competition was reduced bilaterally. This is likely due to bilateral lesions, with the ipsilateral ear affected on both sides. Dichotic performance remains normal because the temporal lobes and

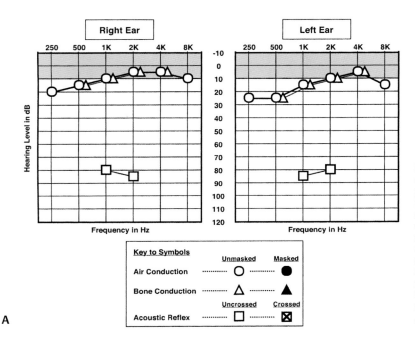

Figure 17–1 Hearing consultation results in a 34-year-old woman with multiple sclerosis. **(A)** Pure-tone audiometric results show mild low-frequency sensorineural hearing loss bilaterally. **(B)** Speech audiometric results during exacerbation of the disease process show that word recognition in quiet is normal, but sentence recognition in competition is abnormal. **(C)** Speech audiometric results during remission show relatively normal processing ability. DSI, Dichotic Sentence Identification test; SAT, speech awareness threshold; S/N, signal-to-noise ratio; SSI, Synthetic Sentence Identification test; SSI$_M$, maximum SSI score; ST, spondee threshold; WRS, word recognition score; WRS$_M$, maximum WRS. (Data from ANSI, 1996.)

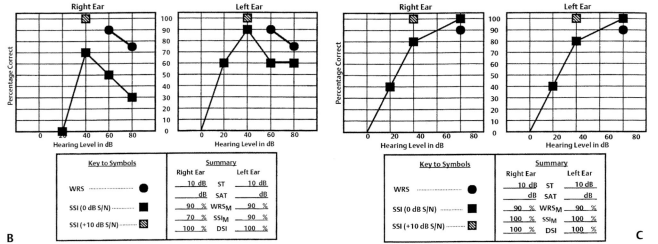

corpus callosum remain intact. Once again, these undistorted signals are perceived clearly at the level of the temporal lobe because of the redundancy of the signal.

One other characteristic of multiple sclerosis is that it goes through periods of exacerbation and remission. Results in **Fig. 17–1B** were obtained during a period of exacerbation of the disease process. Results in **Fig. 17–1C** were obtained 3 months later during a period of remission. SSI scores returned to near-normal levels as function of the brainstem improved.

Auditory Processing Disorder in Aging

Patient 2 has a long-standing sensorineural hearing loss. The patient is a 78-year-old woman with bilateral sen-

sorineural hearing loss that has progressed slowly over the past 15 years. She has worn hearing aids for the past 10 years and has an annual audiologic reevaluation each year. Her major complaints are in communicating with her grandchildren and trying to hear in noisy restaurants. Although her hearing aids worked well for her at the beginning, she is not receiving the benefit from them that she did 10 years ago.

Immittance audiometry is consistent with normal middle ear function, characterized by a type A tympanogram, normal static immittance, and normal crossed and uncrossed reflex thresholds bilaterally.

Pure-tone audiometric results are shown in **Fig. 17–2A**. The patient has a moderate, bilateral, symmetric, sensorineural

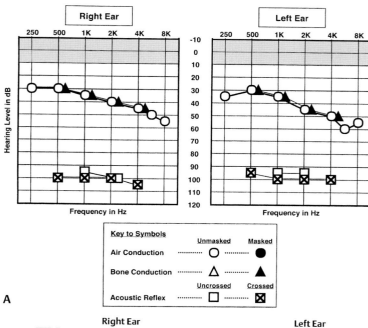

Figure 17–2 Hearing consultation results in a 78-year-old woman with long-standing, progressive hearing loss. **(A)** Pure-tone audiometric results show bilateral, symmetric, moderate, sensorineural hearing loss. **(B)** Speech audiometric results show reduced word recognition in quiet, consistent with the degree and configuration of cochlear hearing loss. Sentence recognition in competition is substantially reduced. **(C)** Dichotic performance is reduced in the left ear, regardless of task complexity. DSI, Dichotic Sentence Identification test; SAT, speech awareness threshold; SSI, Synthetic Sentence Identification test; SSI$_M$, maximum SSI score; ST, spondee threshold; WRS, word recognition score; WRS$_M$, maximum WRS. (Data from ANSI, 1996.)

	Right Ear	Left Ear
Free Recall	100	60
Focused Recall	100	40

hearing loss. Hearing sensitivity is slightly better in the low frequencies than in the high frequencies.

Speech audiometric results are consistent with those found in older patients. Word recognition scores are reduced, but not below a level predictable from the degree of hearing sensitivity loss. However, speech recognition in the presence of competition is substantially reduced, as shown in **Fig. 17–2B**, consistent with the patient's age. Performance on the SSI at +10 dB message-to-competition ratio was 100% bilaterally. However, at a 0 dB ratio, performance was substantially reduced. In addition to these monotic deficits, the patient shows evidence of a dichotic deficit, with reduced performance in the left ear. Results are shown in **Fig. 17–2C**. Performance on a free-recall task was reduced, with performance reduced even further on the focused-recall task.

Results of a hearing handicap assessment show that the patient has communication problems a significant proportion of the time in most listening environments, especially those involving background noise.

These results are not uncommon in many aging patients with hearing disorders. Word recognition in quiet is consistent with the degree of hearing loss. Speech perception in the presence of competition is reduced beyond what might be expected from the hearing sensitivity loss. In addition, dichotic performance is abnormal on the left ear.

◆ Summary

Auditory processing ability is usually defined as the capacity with which the central auditory nervous system transfers information from the eighth nerve to the auditory cortex. APD is an impairment in this function of the central auditory nervous system.

A disordered auditory nervous system, regardless of cause, will have functional consequences that can vary from subclinical to a substantial, easily measurable auditory deficit. A distinguishing feature of APD is the inability to extract sounds of interest in noisy environments despite an ability to perceive the sounds with adequate loudness. There are two primary causes of APD in adults. One is neuropathology of the peripheral and central auditory nervous systems, resulting from tumors or other space-occupying lesions or from damage due to trauma or stroke. The other is from diffuse changes in brain function, usually related to the aging process.

The aim of auditory processing assessment is to evaluate the ability of the central auditory nervous system to process acoustic signals. Advanced speech audiometric and other behavioral measures can be used to assess central auditory nervous system function to assist in the screening of specific lesions of the auditory system and to describe a communication disorder. The measurement of auditory processing ability in adults is typically carried out with a test battery approach that assesses absolute speech recognition ability, speech recognition in competition, dichotic listening, and temporal processing ability. Monaural speech audiometric measures include high-level word-recognition testing, time-compressed speech, low-pass filtered speech, and speech in competition. Other monaural measures include nonspeech assessment of temporal processing ability. Measures of binaural ability include assessment of the manner in which the ears process phase cues, integrate information, lateralize and localize the source of sound, and extract signals of interest from background competition. Another effective approach to assessing auditory processing ability is the use of dichotic tests. With such a wide array of diagnostic options, the challenge of deciding which to use for clinical assessment can be a daunting one.

There are several factors that influence the selection of testing tools and approaches as well as the success with which they are likely to be implemented. One of the most important factors in speech audiometric testing is the way in which information content of the test materials is manipulated. Other factors that are critical are those related to hearing sensitivity loss and cognitive ability of the patients being tested. Indeed, the key factors in any successful test battery approach are the efficient and effective controls over cochlear sensitivity loss, absolute speech recognition ability, and supramodal influences. The use of performance-intensity functions, various message-to-competition ratios, and word-versus-sentence comparisons permits the assessment of auditory processing ability in a manner that reduces the likelihood of cochlear hearing loss and nonauditory factors influencing the interpretation of test results. In conjunction with thorough immittance, otoacoustic emission, and auditory evoked potential measurements, the use of well-controlled speech audiometric measures has proven to be quite powerful in defining the presence or absence of an APD.

References

Allen, R. L., Cranford, J. L., & Pay, N. (1996). Central auditory processing in an adult with congenital absence of left temporal lobe. Journal of the American Academy of Audiology, 7, 282–288.

Baran, J. A., Bothfeld, R. W., & Musiek, F. E. (2004). Central auditory deficits associated with compromise of the primary auditory cortex. Journal of the American Academy of Audiology, 15, 106–116.

Baran, J. A., Musiek, F. E., & Reeves, A. G. (1986). Central auditory function following anterior sectioning of the corpus callosum. Ear and Hearing, 7, 359–362.

Berlin, C., Hood, L., & Rose, K. (2001). On renaming auditory neuropathy as auditory dys-synchrony. Audiology Today, 13(6), 15–17.

Berlin, C. I., Lowe-Bell, S. S., Jannetta, P. J., & Kline, D. G. (1972). Central auditory deficits of temporal lobectomy. Archives of Otolaryngology, 96, 4–10.

Bocca, E. (1958). Clinical aspects of cortical deafness. Laryngoscope, 68, 301–309.

Bocca, E., & Calearo, C. (1963). Central hearing processes. In J. Jerger (Ed.), Modern developments in audiology (pp. 337–370). New York: Academic Press.

Bocca, E., Calearo, C., & Cassinari, V. (1954). A new method for testing hearing in temporal lobe tumours. Acta Otolaryngologica, 44, 219–221.

Cacace, A. T., Parnes, S. M., Lovely, T. J., & Kalathia, A. (1994). The disconnected ear: phenomenological effects of a large acoustic tumor. Ear and Hearing, 15, 287–298.

Calearo, C., & Antonelli, A. R. (1968). Audiometric findings in brain stem lesions. Acta Otolaryngologica, 66, 305–319.

Chisolm, T. H., Willott, J. F., & Lister, J. J. (2003). The aging auditory system: Anatomic and physiologic changes and implications for rehabilitation. International Journal of Audiology, 42(Supplement 2), 3–10.

Chmiel, R., & Jerger, J. (1996). Hearing aid use, central auditory disorder, and hearing handicap in elderly persons. Journal of the American Academy of Audiology, 7, 190–202.

Chmiel, R., Jerger, J., Murphy, E., Pirozzolo, F., & Tooley-Young, C. (1997). Unsuccessful use of binaural amplification by an elderly person. Journal of the American Academy of Audiology, 8, 1–10.

Cranford, J. L., Boose, M., & Moore, C. A. (1990). Tests of precedence effect in sound localization reveal abnormalities in multiple sclerosis. Ear and Hearing, 11, 282–288.

Cranford, J. L., & Romereim, B. (1992). Precedence effect and speech understanding in elderly listeners. Journal of the American Academy of Audiology, 3, 405–409.

Dubno, J. R., Lee, F. S., Matthews, L. J., & Lam, C. F. (1995). Confidence limits for maximum word-recognition scores. Journal of Speech and Hearing Research, 38, 490–502.

Fifer, R. C., Jerger, J. F., Berlin, C. I., Tobey, E. A., & Campbell, J. C. (1983). Development of a dichotic sentence identification test for hearing-impaired adults. Ear and Hearing, 4, 300–305.

Fitzgibbons, P. J., & Gordon-Salant, S. (1996). Auditory temporal processing in elderly listeners. Journal of the American Academy of Audiology, 7, 183–189.

Gates, G. A., Beiser, A., Rees, T. S., D'Agostino, R. B., & Wolf, P. A. (2002). Central auditory dysfunction may precede the onset of clinical dementia in people with probable Alzheimer's disease. Journal of the American Geriatrics Society, 50, 482–488.

Gates, G. A., Feeney, M. P., & Higdon, R. J. (2003). Word recognition and the articulation index in older listeners with probable age-related auditory neuropathy. Journal of the American Academy of Audiology, 14, 574–581.

Gelfand, S. A. (1995). Long-term recovery and no recovery from the auditory deprivation effect with binaural amplification: Six cases. Journal of the American Academy of Audiology, 6, 141–149.

Gelfand, S. A., Hoffman, S., Waltzman, S. B., & Piper, N. (1980). Dichotic CV recognition at various interaural temporal onset asynchronies: Effect of age. Journal of the Acoustical Society of America, 68, 1258–1261.

Golding, M., Taylor, A., Cupples, L., & Mitchell, P. (2006). Odds of demonstrating auditory processing abnormality in the average older adult: The Blue Mountain Hearing Study. Ear and Hearing, 27, 129–138.

Hallgren, M., Larsby, B., Lyxell, B., & Arlinger, S. (2001). Cognitive effects in dichotic speech testing in elderly persons. Ear and Hearing, 22, 120–129.

Hannley, M., Jerger, J. F., & Rivera, V. M. (1983). Relationships among auditory brain stem responses, masking level differences and the acoustic reflex in multiple sclerosis. Audiology, 22, 20–33.

Hausler, R., Colburn, S., & Marr, E. (1983). Sound localization in subjects with impaired hearing: Spatial-discrimination and interaural-discrimination tests. Acta Otolaryngologica Supplementum, 400, 1–62.

Helfer, K. S., & Wilber, L. A. (1990). Hearing loss, aging, and speech perception in reverberation and noise. Journal of Speech and Hearing Research, 33, 149–155.

Hood, L. J., Berlin, C. I., & Allen, P. (1994). Cortical deafness: A longitudinal study. Journal of the American Academy of Audiology, 5, 330–342.

Hood, L. J., Berlin, C. I., Bordelon, J., & Rose, K. (2003). Patients with auditory neuropathy/dys-synchrony lack efferent suppression of transient evoked otoacoustic emissions. Journal of the American Academy of Audiology, 14, 302–313.

Hurley, R. M., & Musiek, F. E. (1997). Effectiveness of three central auditory processing (CAP) tests in identifying cerebral lesions. Journal of the American Academy of Audiology, 8, 257–262.

Jerger, J. (1992). Can age-related decline in speech understanding be explained by peripheral hearing loss? Journal of the American Academy of Audiology, 3, 33–38.

Jerger, J., Alford, B., Lew, H., Rivera, V., & Chmiel, R. (1995). Dichotic listening, event-related potentials, and interhemispheric transfer in the elderly. Ear and Hearing, 16, 482–498.

Jerger, J., Brown, D., & Smith, S. (1984). Effect of peripheral hearing loss on masking level difference. Archives of Otolaryngologica, 110, 290–296.

Jerger, J., Chmiel, R., Allen, J., & Wilson, A. (1994). Effects of age and gender on dichotic sentence identification. Ear and Hearing, 15, 274–286.

Jerger, J., & Hayes, D. (1977). Diagnostic speech audiometry. Archives of Otolaryngologica, 103, 216–222.

Jerger, J., & Jerger, S. (1971). Diagnostic significance of PB word functions. Archives of Otolaryngologica, 93, 573–580.

Jerger, J., & Jerger, S. (1975). Clinical validity of central auditory tests. Scandinavian Audiology, 4, 147–163.

Jerger, J., Jerger, S., Oliver, T., & Pirozzolo, F. (1989). Speech understanding in the elderly. Ear and Hearing, 10, 79–89.

Jerger, J., Jerger, S., & Pirozzolo, F. (1991). Correlational analysis of speech audiometric scores, hearing loss, age, and cognitive abilities in the elderly. Ear and Hearing, 12, 103–109.

Jerger, J., Johnson, K., Jerger, S., Coker, N., Pirozzolo, F., & Gray, L. (1991). Central auditory processing disorder: A case study. Journal of the American Academy of Audiology, 2, 36–54.

Jerger, J., & Jordan, C. (1992). Age-related asymmetry on a cued-listening task. Ear and Hearing, 13, 272–277.

Jerger, J., Lovering, L., & Wertz, M. (1972). Auditory disorder following bilateral temporal lobe insult: Report of a case. Journal of Speech and Hearing Disorders, 37, 523–535.

Jerger, J., Oliver, T. A., & Pirozzolo, F. (1990). Impact of central auditory processing disorder and cognitive deficit on the self-assessment of hearing handicap in the elderly. Journal of the American Academy of Audiology, 1, 75–80.

Jerger, J., Silman, S., Lew, H. L., & Chmiel, R. (1993). Case studies in binaural interference: Converging evidence from behavioral and electrophysiologic measures. Journal of the American Academy of Audiology, 4, 122–131.

Jerger, J., Speaks, C., & Trammel, J. L. (1968). A new approach to speech audiometry. Journal of Speech and Hearing Disorders, 33, 319–328.

Jerger, J., Stach, B. A., Johnson, K., Loiselle, L. H., & Jerger, S. (1990). Patterns of abnormality in dichotic listening in the elderly. In J. H. Jensen (Ed.), Proceedings of the 14th Danavox Symposium on Presbyacusis and Other Age-Related Aspects (pp. 143–150). Odense, Denmark: Danavox.

Jerger, J., Stach, B., Pruitt, J., Harper, R., & Kirby, H. (1989). Comments on speech understanding and aging. Journal of the Acoustical Society of America, 85, 1352–1354.

Jerger, J., Weikers, N., Sharbrough, F., & Jerger, S. (1969). Bilateral lesions of the temporal lobe: A case study. Acta Otolaryngologica Supplementum, 258, 1–51.

Jerger, S., & Jerger, J. (1980). Low frequency hearing loss in central auditory disorders. American Journal of Otology, 2, 1–4.

Jerger, S., & Jerger, J. (1983). Neuroaudiologic findings in patients with central auditory disorder. Seminars in Hearing, 4, 133–159.

Jerger, S., Oliver, T. A., & Martin, R. C. (1990). Evaluation of adult aphasics with the pediatric speech intelligibility test. Journal of the American Academy of Audiology, 1, 89–100.

Kalikow, D. N., Stevens, K. N., & Elliott, L. L. (1977). Development of a test of speech intelligibility in noise using sentence materials with controlled word predictability. Journal of the Acoustical Society of America, 61, 1337–1351.

Katz, J. (1962). The use of staggered spondaic words for assessing the integrity of the central auditory system. Journal of Auditory Research, 2, 327–337.

Kileny, P. R., Edwards, B. M., Disher, M. J., & Telian, S. A. (1998). Hearing improvement after resection of cerebellopontine angle meningioma: Case study of the preoperative role of transient evoked otoacoustic emissions. Journal of the American Academy of Audiology, 9, 251–256.

Kimura, D. (1961). Some effects of temporal lobe damage on auditory perception. Canadian Journal of Psychology, 15, 157–165.

Koehnke, J., & Besing, J. (1997). Clinical application of 3-D auditory tests. Seminars in Hearing, 18, 345–354.

Koehnke, J., & Besing, J. M. (2001). The effects of aging on binaural and spatial hearing. Seminars in Hearing, 22(3), 241–254.

Kurdziel, S., Noffsinger, D., & Olsen, W. (1976). Performance by cortical lesion patients on 40 and 60% time-compressed materials. Journal of the American Audiology Society, 2, 3–7.

Larsby, B., Hällgren, M., Lyxell, B., & Arlinger, S. (2005). Cognitive performance and perceived effort in speech processing tasks: Effects of different noise backgrounds in normal-hearing and hearing impaired subjects. International Journal of Audiology, 44, 131–143.

Madden, C., Rutter, M., Hilbert, L., Greinwald, J. H., & Choo, D. I. (2002). Clinical and audiological features in auditory neuropathy. Archives of Otolaryngology–Head and Neck Surgery, 128, 1026–1030.

Mahmud, M. R., Khan, A. M., & Nadol, J. B. (2003). Histopathology of the inner ear in unoperated acoustic neuroma. Annals of Otology, Rhinology and Laryngology, 112, 979–986.

Matzker, J. (1959). Two methods for the assessment of central auditory function in cases of brain disease. Annals of Otology, Rhinology and Otolaryngology, 68, 115–119.

Medwetsky, L. (2002). Central auditory processing testing: A battery approach. In J. Katz (Ed.), Handbook of clinical audiology (5th ed, pp. 510–524). Baltimore, MD: Lippincott Williams & Wilkins.

Miranda, T. T., & Pichora-Fuller, M. K. (2002). Temporally jittered speech produces performance intensity, phonetically balanced rollover in young normal-hearing listeners. Journal of the American Academy of Audiology, 13, 50–58.

Moore, B. C. J., Peters, R. W., & Glasberg, B. R. (1992). Detection of temporal gaps in sinusoids by elderly subjects with and without hearing loss. Journal of the Acoustical Society of America, 92, 1923–1932.

Musiek, F. E. (1983a). Assessment of central auditory dysfunction: The dichotic digit test revisited. Ear and Hearing, 4, 79–83.

Musiek, F. E. (1983b). Results of three dichotic speech tests on subjects with intracranial lesions. Ear and Hearing, 4, 318–323.

Musiek, F. E., & Baran, J. A. (2004). Audiological correlates to a rupture of a pontine arteriovenous malformation. Journal of the American Academy of Audiology, 15, 161–171.

Musiek, F. E., Baran, J. A., & Pinheiro, M. L. (1990). Duration pattern recognition in normal subjects and patients with cerebral and cochlear lesions. Audiology, 29, 304–313.

Musiek, F. E., Baran, J. A., & Pinheiro, M. L. (1994). Neuroaudiology case studies. San Diego, CA: Singular Publishing Group.

Musiek, F. E., Charette, L., Morse, D., & Baran, J. A. (2004). Central deafness associated with a midbrain lesion. Journal of the American Academy of Audiology, 15, 133–151.

Musiek, F. E., & Geurkink, N. A. (1982). Auditory brain stem response and central auditory test findings for patients with brain stem lesions: A preliminary report. Laryngoscope, 92, 891–900.

Musiek, F. E., Shinn, J. B., Jirsa, R., Bamiou, D., Baran, J. A., & Zaidan, E. (2005). GIN (Gaps in Noise) test performance in subjects with confirmed central auditory nervous system involvement. Ear and Hearing, 26, 608–618.

Neijenhuis, K., Tschur, H., & Snik, A. (2004). The effect of mild hearing impairment on auditory processing tests. Journal of the American Academy of Audiology, 15, 6–16.

Nilsson, M., Soli, S. D., & Sullivan, J. A. (1994). Development of the Hearing in Noise test for the measurement of speech reception thresholds in quiet and in noise. Journal of the Acoustical Society of America, 95, 1085–1099.

Olsen, W. O. (1983). Dichotic test results for normal subjects and for temporal lobectomy patients. Ear and Hearing, 4, 324–330.

Olsen, W. O., & Noffsinger, D. (1976). Masking level differences for cochlear and brain stem lesions. Annals of Otology, 85, 820–825.

Pestalozza, G., & Shore, I. (1955). Clinical evaluation of presbycusis on the basis of different tests of auditory function. Laryngoscope, 65, 1136–1163.

Phillips, S. L., Gordon-Salant, S., Fitzgibbons, P. J., & Yeni-Komshian, G. H. (1994). Auditory duration discrimination in young and elderly listeners with normal hearing. Journal of the American Academy of Audiology, 5, 210–215.

Pichora-Fuller, M. K., & Souza, P. E. (2003). Effects of aging on auditory processing of speech. International Journal of Audiology, 42(2), S11–S16.

Price, P. J., & Simon, H. J. (1984). Perception of temporal differences in speech by "normal-hearing" adults: Effect of age and intensity. Journal of the Acoustical Society of America, 76, 405–410.

Roberts, R. A., Koehnke, J., & Besing, J. (2003). Effects of noise and reverberation on the precedence effect in listeners with normal hearing and impaired hearing. American Journal of Audiology, 12, 96–105.

Roberts, R. A., & Lister, J. J. (2004). Effects of age and hearing loss on gap detection and the precedence effect: Broadband stimuli. Journal of Speech, Language, and Hearing Research, 47, 965–978.

Sanchez-Longo, L. P., & Forster, F. M. (1958). Clinical significance of impairment of sound localization. Neurology, 8, 119–125.

Schneider, B. A., Pichora-Fuller, M. K., Kowalchuk, D., & Lamb, M. (1994). Gap detection and the precedence effect in young and old adults. Journal of the Acoustical Society of America, 95, 980–991.

Shinn, J. B., Baran, J. A., Moncrieff, D. W., & Musiek, F. E. (2005). Differential attention effects on dichotic listening. Journal of the American Academy of Audiology, 16, 205–218.

Silman, S. (1995). Binaural interference in multiple sclerosis: Case study. Journal of the American Academy of Audiology, 6, 193–196.

Silman, S., Gelfand, S. A., & Silverman, C. A. (1984). Effects of monaural versus binaural hearing aids. Journal of the Acoustical Society of America, 76, 1357–1362.

Silman, S., Silverman, C. A., Emmer, M. B., & Gelfand, S. A. (1992). Adult-onset auditory deprivation. Journal of the American Academy of Audiology, 3, 390–396.

Silverman, C. A., & Emmer, M. B. (1993). Auditory deprivation from and recovery in adults with asymmetric sensorineural hearing impairments. Journal of the American Academy of Audiology, 4, 338–346.

Silverman, C. A., & Silman, S. (1990). Apparent auditory deprivation from monaural amplification and recovery with binaural amplification: Two case studies. Journal of the American Academy of Audiology, 1, 175–180.

Smith, B. B., & Resnick, D. M. (1972). An auditory test for assessing brain stem integrity: Preliminary report. Laryngoscope, 82, 414–424.

Sperry, J. L., Wiley, T. L., & Chial, M. R. (1997). Word recognition performance in various background competitors. Journal of the American Academy of Audiology, 8, 71–80.

Stach, B. A., & Delgado-Vilches, G. (1993). Sudden hearing loss in multiple sclerosis: Case report. Journal of the American Academy of Audiology, 4, 370–375.

Stach, B. A., Delgado-Vilches, G., & Smith-Farach, S. (1990). Hearing loss in multiple sclerosis. Seminars in Hearing, 11, 221–230.

Stach, B. A., Jerger, J. F., & Fleming, K. A. (1985). Central presbyacusis: A longitudinal case study. Ear and Hearing, 6, 304–306.

Stach, B. A., Loiselle, L. H., & Jerger, J. F. (1991). Special hearing aid considerations in elderly patients with auditory processing disorders. Ear and Hearing, 12(Suppl.), 131S–138S.

Stach, B. A., Spretnjak, M. L., & Jerger, J. (1990). The prevalence of central presbyacusis in a clinical population. Journal of the American Academy of Audiology, 1, 109–115.

Stach, B. A., Westerberg, B. D., & Roberson, J. B. (1998). Auditory disorder in central nervous system miliary tuberculosis: A case report. Journal of the American Academy of Audiology, 9, 305–310.

Starr, A., Picton, T. W., Sininger, Y., Hood, L. J., & Berlin, C. I. (1996). Auditory neuropathy. Brain, 119, 741–753.

Stephens, S. D. G. (1976). Auditory temporal summation in patients with central nervous system lesions. In S. D. G. Stephens (Ed.), Disorders of auditory function (pp. 243–252). London: Academic Press.

Sticht, T. G., & Gray, B. B. (1969). The intelligibility of time-compressed words as a function of age and hearing loss. Journal of Speech and Hearing Research, 12, 443–448.

Stuart, A., & Phillips, D. P. (1996). Word recognition in continuous and interrupted broadband noise by young normal-hearing, older normal-hearing, and presbyacusic listeners. Ear and Hearing, 17, 478–489.

Wiley, T. L., Cruickshanks, K. J., Nondahl, D. M., Tweed, T. S., Klein, R., & Klein, B. E. K. (1998). Aging and word recognition in competing message. Journal of the American Academy of Audiology, 9, 191–198.

Willott, J. F. (1996). Anatomic and physiologic aging: A behavioral neuroscience perspective. Journal of the American Academy of Audiology, 7, 141–151.

Wilson, R. H., & Jaffe, M. S. (1996). Interactions of age, ear, and stimulus complexity on dichotic digit recognition. Journal of the American Academy of Audiology, 7, 358–364.

Yellin, M. W., Jerger, J., & Fifer, R. C. (1989). Norms for disproportionate loss of speech intelligibility. Ear and Hearing, 10, 231–234.

Chapter 18

Middle Ear Measures

Jackie L. Clark, Ross J. Roeser, and Marissa Mendrygal

Objective measurements of the outer and middle ear were reportedly performed as early as 1867 for the purpose of quantifying impedance characteristics of the ear (Wiley and Block, 1985). For the next century, there were sporadic reports dealing with objective measures of middle ear function, but little clinical utility was developed by these early studies. By the mid 1900s, "impedance audiometry" was incorporated into the standard audiological test battery.

Although there was a flurry of developmental studies on the clinical application of middle ear measures in the 1960s through the early '80s, few noteworthy clinical middle ear measures have been developed in the past 20 years. That is not to say that more sophisticated and more technologically advanced measures of middle ear function are not being explored; however, many of these advanced procedures have yet to find their way into routine clinical practice.

This chapter reviews the basic principles and clinical application of procedures used in middle ear measures and provides readers with a review of the current status in several advanced areas of middle ear measurement.

Immittance Measures

The terminology used for measures of middle ear function has changed over the past several years and can be confusing. The following definitions should help clarify this confusion.

Impedance

Impedance generally refers to the opposition to the flow of energy in a system (the outer and middle ear). Impedance is expressed in ohms and is made up of several components that are influenced by the mass, stiffness, and frictional resistance present in the system. As described below, immittance measures are the product of the complex impedance of the ear. The term *impedance measures* was first used to describe the clinical procedures involved in testing middle ear function.

Admittance

Admittance refers to the ease with which acoustic energy is transmitted (in the outer and middle ear), expressed in mhos (*mho* is *ohm* spelled backward). *Admittance* and *compliance* are terms that are used synonymously.

Immittance

Immittance middle ear measures are electronically or electroacoustically based on the measurement of impedance or admittance. Thus, the term *immittance* was created to encompass both techniques (American Speech-Language-Hearing Association [ASHA], 1979, 1990).

Compliance

Compliance is the inverse of stiffness as it relates to the ease of acoustic energy transmission and is used synonymously with the term *admittance* or *static admittance*. However, *static admittance* is the suggested terminology (ASHA, 1990; Margolis and Heller, 1987). Compliance and static admittance are measured in equivalent volumes of air using cubic centimeters or milliliters (1 cubic centimeter is the same volume as 1 milliliter: $1 \, cc^3 = 1 \, mL$).

Immittance measures are based on the principle that when a known quantity of acoustic energy (sound) is delivered to the ear canal, some of the energy is transferred through the middle ear and delivered to the cochlea, where it is perceived as sound, while some of the energy is reflected by the tympanic membrane and external ear structures. The amount of reflected energy will vary depending on the impedance of the system. Immittance measures are influenced by the complex impedance of the ear, which comprises the interaction between magnitude and phase, or resistance and reactance. These multiple variables can be measured and described through a system referred to as vector analysis, which provides two-dimensional graphic representations of impedance and admittance functions, with rectangular and polar notations. A mathematical summary of vector analysis is presented by Margolis and Hunter (2000), as they show how acoustic stimulation affects the complex impedance components of the outer and middle ear system.

Although complex impedance components are involved in quantifying the immittance characteristics of middle ear function, stiffness is by far the dominant factor affecting middle ear measures. That is, when an acoustic signal is delivered to the ear canal, stiffness is the dominant factor determining how much energy is absorbed and delivered to the inner ear and how much is reflected. More energy is reflected when a system is stiffer or less compliant (or less flaccid/mobile). Another way to consider the same information is that when the structures in the outer and middle ear stiffen, less energy will be transferred through the middle ear and admitted into the inner ear, resulting in more energy being reflected. Conversely, when a system is less stiff (or more compliant), the system will reflect less energy, and more energy will be admitted. Once again, recall that stiffness and compliance (or static admittance) are reciprocally related; as one increases, the other decreases.

The primary application of middle ear measures is to identify and classify architectural and functional defects within the auditory system, including the external auditory canal, tympanic membrane, middle ear space, and brainstem neural pathways. Findings provide valuable diagnostic information regarding the patient's auditory system from the external ear canal through the brainstem. When used in conjunction with other diagnostic audiological procedures, immittance measures will help identify and monitor tympanic membrane immobility associated with otitis media, confirm the diagnosis of auditory neuropathy, provide diagnostic information regarding facial nerve lesions, diagnose perforations of the tympanic membrane, and detect the presence of otosclerosis.

Because little cooperation is required from the patient, tests of middle ear function can be performed on those who may not be testable with behavioral procedures. Although a highly useful clinical procedure, immittance measures do not eliminate the need for behavioral and/or electrophysiologic diagnostic testing. A patient can have findings well within normal limits on immittance measures and still manifest severe bilateral sensorineural hearing loss.

Although procedures used to administer immittance tests are relatively simple and can be learned in a matter of hours, the difficulty with admittance testing lies in interpretation. To properly interpret the diagnostic value of the results from the admittance test battery, a thorough understanding of the auditory system and the principles of admittance is required. Such understanding includes a comprehensive knowledge of the acoustic and physiologic principles underlying the admittance technique and auditory system, as well as the various pathologic conditions that may affect the auditory system.

◆ The Immittance Instrument

Sometimes inappropriately called an "immittance audiometer" or an "immittance bridge," the immittance instrument is used to measure middle ear function and is made up of sophisticated components that carry out complex operations. Because immittance measures do not assess hearing, it is misleading to refer to the equipment as an "audiometer." The term *immittance bridge* was adopted because the instrument circuit used to contain an electronic component called a Wheatstone bridge, but the terminology is inaccurate with the development of microprocessing technology, which has automated this once manually operated equipment.

Figure 18–1 shows a microprocessor-based diagnostic immittance instrument. This instrument allows the user to perform simple screening testing as well as advanced diagnostic procedures and can be used in automatic or manual modes. **Figure 18–2A** and **B** shows the probe placed in the right ear canal ear and a contralateral probe placed in the left ear for acoustic reflex testing. Immittance data are obtained from the ear with the probe (the probe ear); the contralateral ear is stimulated with an acoustic signal to determine if acoustic reflexes can be recorded from the probe ear. As discussed later in this chapter, during the acoustic reflex test, an ipsilateral acoustic reflex stimulus is delivered to the probe ear (ipsilateral reflex-eliciting ear),

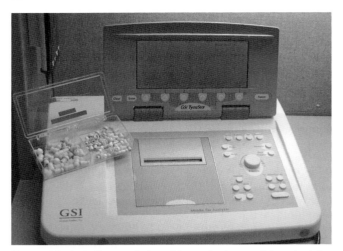

Figure 18–1 A diagnostic immittance instrument (see text for description).

and a contralateral acoustic stimulus is delivered to the ear opposite the probe ear (contralateral reflex-eliciting ear). The probe ear choice can then be changed and the procedure repeated. In **Fig. 18–2**, the ipsilateral acoustic reflex signal is being delivered while immittance measures are being recorded from the probe right ear (ipsilateral reflex-eliciting ear). Next, the contralateral acoustic reflex signal is delivered to the left ear (contralateral reflex-eliciting ear) while the acoustic reflex elicited from the stimulus presented to the left ear is being recorded in the (contralateral) probe right ear. To prevent confusion when describing immittance results, it is helpful to reference results according to the probe ear chosen. For example, a patient having a contralateral acoustic reflex from the probe right condition implies that the acoustic signal was delivered to the left ear while immittance of the right ear was being measured.

Figure 18–3 is a schematic showing the role for each component in the immittance instrument. As illustrated in the diagram, the cavity between the probe tip of the immittance instrument and the external ear canal and tympanic membrane is closed. The physical dimensions of the area under the probe tip will vary depending on the physical size of the ear canal, as well as the insertion depth of the probe tip. As shown in **Fig. 18–3**, the probe is placed into the ear canal using a probe tip (3) to obtain a hermetic seal. The probe tip is connected to the immittance instrument, which has four components: an oscillator (1) and loudspeaker (2a), which are used to introduce a probe tone into the ear canal; an air pump and manometer (4a), which are used to change the air pressure in the ear canal for dynamic measures of the eardrum and middle ear structures; a microphone (5a) and system analyzer (6), which are used to compute immittance measures; and an ipsilateral reflex eliciting system (7a and 7b), which are used to introduce a signal into the ear canal to elicit the ipsilateral acoustic reflex.

The immittance probe apparatus measures the stiffness or static admittance of the middle ear system in the following way: a probe tone set at 220/226 Hz (this can vary in frequency; see discussion of multifrequency tympanometry later in this chapter) is generated from the oscillator (1), emitted from the loudspeaker (2a), and introduced into the external ear canal through the port in the probe tip (2b). Depending on the state of the ear canal and middle ear, some energy is absorbed and transmitted (admitted) to the inner ear, and some energy is reflected. The reflected energy is sent through a second port in the probe tip (5b) and delivered to the microphone (5a), and the system analyzer (6) identifies various aspects of the response (energy voltage, intensity, etc.) resulting from the signal. These measures can be made with the tympanic membrane in a resting (static) state or in a dynamic state by increasing and decreasing the air pressure in the ear canal with the air pump (4a) while measuring it with the manometer (to obtain a tympanogram). Changes also occur in the system due to middle ear (stapedial) muscle contraction in response to an intense signal delivered to either the probe ear (7) or the ear contralateral to the probe ear (not shown), which can be recorded by the system analyzer (6).

Acting like a small sound pressure measuring device, the immittance instrument is capable of determining the state of

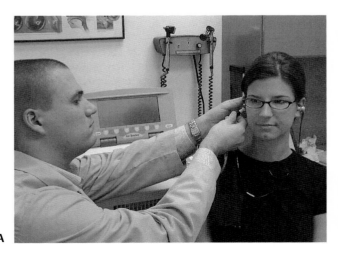

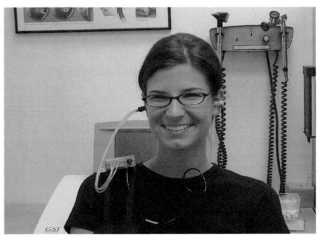

A   B

Figure 18–2 (A) Placement of the probe into the external auditory canal. **(B)** Placement of the instrument for obtaining the immittance values in the probe right ear; the left ear canal has an insert earphone placed into it for stimulation of the contralateral acoustic reflex.

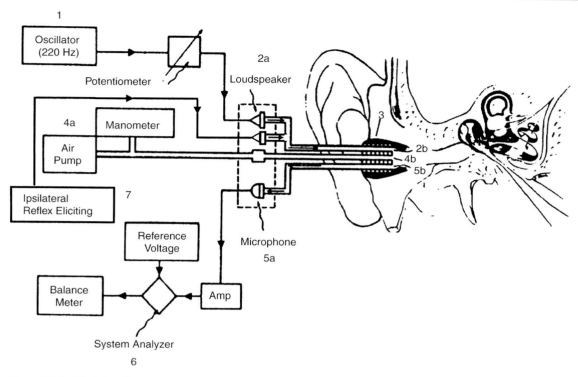

Figure 18–3 Principles of immittance measurement in the probe ear (see text for description).

the middle ear. Reflected energy measured from the probe tone is recorded by the microphone, and the system analyzer is able to determine the functional state of the ear. A higher amount of reflected energy means that the system is stiffer or less compliant than normal, whereas a low amount indicates the system is less stiff or more compliant. Conditions such as otitis media and ossicular chain fixation result in high stiffness or low static admittance; in such cases, the reflected energy would be higher than normal. Conversely, low stiffness or high static admittance would be caused by conditions such as a disarticulation of the ossicular chain or a scarred, flaccid tympanic membrane. Under these conditions, more energy would pass through the middle ear than normal, so the amount reflected would be less than in a normal ear.

Most immittance instruments use microprocessors, which allow for rapid assessment of middle ear function (typically, less than 1 minute per ear). Following data collection, the information is displayed on a screen, and a hard copy can be printed. An example of data from immittance measures from a microprocessor-based immittance system is provided in **Fig. 18–4**, which will be described in more detail below.

◆ Routine Immittance Measures

Two basic immittance procedures are used to assess middle ear function: the tympanogram and the acoustic reflex. Although each test provides significant information by itself,

both procedures are considered when interpreting the results and developing a diagnosis. Moreover, diagnostic information from immittance measures is strengthened when results from all audiologic test procedures are interpreted together.

Tympanogram

Tympanograms are graphic displays of eardrum mobility as a function of mechanically varying the air pressure (see **Fig. 18–5**) in a hermetically sealed external ear canal. Tympanometry originally measured eardrum mobility in cubic centimeters of compliance, but systems now measure eardrum mobility in milliliters of admittance. Tympanometric morphology provides diagnostic information, but additional measures of tympanometric width or gradient, static admittance or tympanogram height, and ear canal volume (described below) provide absolute tympanometric values for objective classification.

A tympanogram is plotted by introducing a positive air pressure (+200 daPa) into the probe ear and reducing it to a negative pressure, typically in the −200 daPa to −300 daPa range. Admittance (compliance) of the ear is obtained based on the amount of reflected energy. The shape of a tympanogram is affected by various disorders in the outer and middle ear, which is affected primarily by the stiffness of the system; this in turn affects mobility or static admittance. When the reflected energy varies from a known normal range, many disorders affecting the outer and middle ear can be detected.

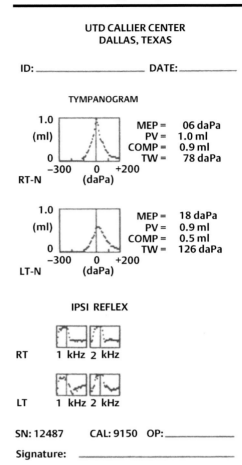

UTD CALLIER CENTER
DALLAS, TEXAS

ID: _____ DATE: _____

TYMPANOGRAM

MEP =   06 daPa
PV =   1.0 ml
COMP =   0.9 ml
TW =   78 daPa

MEP =   18 daPa
PV =   0.9 ml
COMP =   0.5 ml
TW =   126 daPa

IPSI REFLEX

RT   1 kHz   2 kHz

LT   1 kHz   2 kHz

SN: 12487   CAL: 9150   OP: _____

Signature: _____

REMARKS:

Figure 18–4 Example of printed findings obtained from a microprocessor-based immittance instrument. Results shown would indicate normal middle ear function bilaterally (see text for description).

To understand how varying air pressure in the external auditory canal affects the amount of reflected energy from the tympanic membrane, one must understand the pressure/admittance (compliance) principle. **Fig. 18–5** illustrates

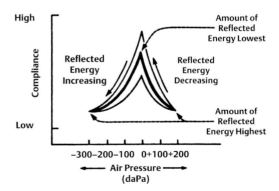

Figure 18–5 Schematic representation of how varying air pressure in the external ear canal affects the stiffness of the eardrum and the reflected energy of the probe tone (see text for description).

this principle in a normal ear. Recall that stiffness and admittance (compliance) are reciprocally related and that by measuring one of these characteristics, the other can be derived. In **Fig. 18–5**, the amount of reflected energy is at its lowest point when the pressure in the external auditory canal is at atmospheric pressure (0 daPa). Under this condition, in the normal ear (1) there is equal pressure between the external and middle ear cavities; (2) the amount of energy absorbed by the tympanic membrane and middle ear structures from the probe tone is at the highest level; and (3) the amount of reflected energy from the probe tone is at its lowest level, which means that the static admittance is at its highest point. However, when either a positive or negative pressure is introduced into the external ear canal, the force exerted on the normal tympanic membrane stretches and stiffens it. As the system stiffens, a concomitant decrease in admittance (compliance) increases the amount of reflected energy. In **Fig. 18–5**, the amount of reflected energy is greatest at +200 daPa and −300 daPa, which indicates that static admittance is at its lowest point at these two distinct air pressure values for this ear.

Figure 18–6 provides an example of how a tympanogram is manually recorded using an absolute scale. Air pressure is introduced into the ear canal at +200 daPa. The positive pressure establishes a stiff system with low static admittance, and the amount of reflected energy is greater than at atmospheric pressure. At this point (1 in **Fig. 18–6**), the first reading is measured at 1.4 mL. This reading also represents the equivalent physical volume of the system. In the normal ear, the static admittance obtained at +200 daPa will be low. Air pressure is then gradually reduced from +200 daPa until it reaches the point where the amount of reflected energy is the lowest and the static admittance is the highest. This reading is the point of maximum static admittance and indicates that the air pressure between the external ear canal and middle ear cavity are equal (2 in **Fig. 18–6**). This point is also referred to as the tympanometric peak pressure (TPP). In the normal ear, the point of maximum static admittance is at or near atmospheric pressure, 0 to −50 daPa. Finally, a third reading (3 in **Fig. 18–6**) is obtained at a more negative pressure, ~200 daPa less pressure than the point of maximum static admittance, or −200 daPa, to complete the tympanometric configuration. When the three points are connected, the resulting tympanometric pattern can be classified according to normal or various abnormal middle ear conditions.

Classifying Tympanograms

Several systems have been proposed to classify tympanograms. The classic (descriptive) method was given by Jerger (1970) and is, by far, the most widely used because of its simplicity. The absolute system is a method for quantifying tympanometric shapes based on norms for objective interpretation. **Table 18–1** provides a comparison between the classic (descriptive) immittance method and the absolute (microprocessor-based) method.

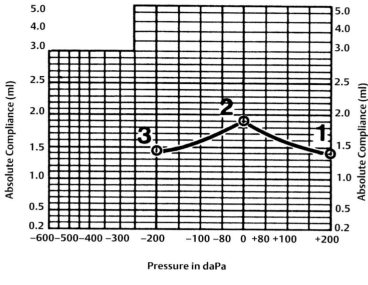

O = Right Ear   X = Left Ear

Pressure in daPa

Figure 18–6 Example of a manually plotted tympanogram (see text for description).

Pearl

• The morphology and absolute values must be taken into consideration when classifying tympanograms properly.

Classic (Descriptive) Method   The classic system comprises three types—A, B, and C—which in turn are subcategorized (see **Fig. 18–7**). The three type A classifications have peak pressures within the range of normal (i.e., +50 to −200 daPa), but different amounts of compliance and static admittance. Type A suggests normal tympanic membrane mobility based on normal pressure and normal compliance of the system. The subclassifications of Types A_d and A_s represent abnormally high and low static admittance, respectively. Type B classifications

represent little or no static admittance in the conductive system, regardless of the air pressure in the external ear. This is the most abnormal tympanogram that can be found. Type C classification is characterized by compliance and static admittance values within the range of normal limits, but abnormal negative pressure in the middle ear exists. **Table 18–2** provides diagnostic implications for each of the descriptions represented by the Jerger system.

Absolute Method   Although the classic method for describing tympanograms is simple, it is subjective, and not all tympanograms fall into the three main classifications. The absolute method quantifies tympanogram classifications using TPP, tympanometric width (TW) or tympanometric gradient (GR), static admittance (peak Y) or tympanogram height, and ear canal volume (V_{ea}).

Table 18–1   Summary of Immittance Tests and Comparison of Classic and Absolute (Microprocessor-Based) Methods of Classifying Tympanograms

Procedure	Purpose	Classic Units of Descriptive Measurement	Absolute Units of Descriptive Measurement
Tympanogram	Assess the pressure/compliance function of the TM	Types A, A_s, cc^3/mL* A_d, B, and C	Tympanometric peak pressure (TPP) daPa Tympanic width (TW) daPA Gradient (GR)
Tympanogram height	Classification of the tympanogram	Static cc^3/mL* compliance	Static mmho or admittance cc^3/mL* (peak Y)
Physical volume	Measure the equivalent volume of the space between probe tip and TM	Physical cc^3/mL* volume test	Equivalent cc^3/mL* ear canal volume (V_{ea})

*Cubic centimeters and milliliters are identical volumes (1 cc^3 = 1 mL).

TM, tympanic membrane.

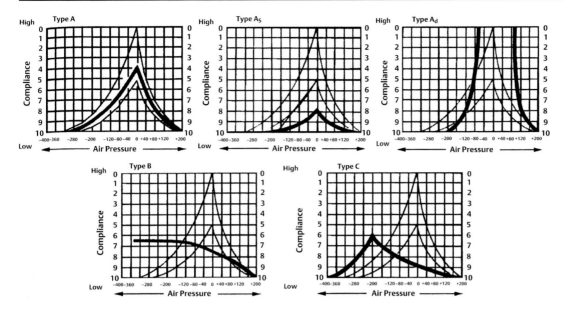

Figure 18–7 The classic classification of tympanograms. (After Jerger, 1970.)

Controversial Point

• Differences of opinion exist as to the point at which negative TPP is considered abnormal. Some researchers have suggested −150 daPa, especially in patients who are monitored for chronic middle ear pathology, whereas others continue to adhere to the theoretical models of −200 daPa.

TPP is a direct measure of the air pressure in the middle ear at which the peak of the tympanogram occurs. Negative pressure occurs when the gas (air) is absorbed by mucosa in the middle ear due to eustachian tube closure. Negative TPP is indicative of the early stages of otitis media; positive TPP is found in the early stages of acute otitis media. **Table 18–3** provides mean norms for TPP, as well as the three other absolute immittance measures. Normal

Table 18–2   Tympanogram Types and Their Description Using the Classic and Absolute Systems

Tympanogram Type	Compliance (mL)	Static Admittance	Peak Pressure (daPa)	Clinical Audiologic Findings
Type A	0.4 to 1.5	0.27 to 2.8	+50 to −150	Represents normal middle ear function; the peak (point of maximum compliance) occurs within normal static admittance limits and at pressures between +50 to −150 mm H$_2$0
Type A$_s$	0.4 to 1.5	< 0.27	+50 to −150	Represents abnormal stiffness in the middle ear system, resulting in a fixation of the ossicular chain as in otosclerosis; static admittance measures are abnormally low
Type A$_d$	0.4 to 1.5	> 2.8	+50 to −150	Represents a flaccid tympanic membrane resulting from scar tissue or a possible disarticulation of the middle ear ossicles; compliance measures are abnormally high
Type B (perf)	> 1.5	< 0.27	No peak	Represents some pathological condition exists in the middle ear; static compliance (admittance) measures are abnormally low, but initial compliance values are high
Type B (o.m.)	< 0.4	< 0.27	No peak	Represents restricted tympanic membrane mobility and would indicate that some pathological condition exists in the middle ear; static compliance measures are abnormally low
Type C	0.4 to 1.5	0.27 to 2.8	−200 or worse	Represents significant negative pressure in the middle ear cavity (considered significant for treatment when more negative than −200 mm H$_2$O); this may indicate a precursor or resolution of otitis media; compliance measures are usually within normal limits

perf, tympanic membrane perforation; o.m., otitis media.

Table 18–3 Mean Norms and 90% Ranges for Immittance Measures

Tympanometric Peak Pressure	Tympanometric Width/Gradient	Static Admittance/ Compliance (Peak Y)	Ear Canal Volume
Borderline: 100 to 200 daPa Abnormally negative: more than −200 daPa	Children mean = 100 daPa 90% range = +60 to −150 daPa Adult mean = 80 daPa 90% range = 50 to 110 daPa	Children mean = 0.5 mmho/cc³/mL* 90% range = 0.2 to 0.9 mmho/cc³/mL* Adult mean = 0.8 mmho/cc³/mL* 90% range = 0.3 to 1.4 mmho/cc³/mL*	Children mean = 0.7 cc³/mL* 90% range = 0.4 to 1.0 cc³/mL* Adult mean = 1.1 cc³/mL* 90% range = 0.6 to 1.5 cc³/mL*

*Cubic centimeters and milliliters are identical volumes (1 cm³ = 1 mL).

Source: Adapted from American Speech-Language-Hearing Association Committee on Audiometric Evaluation. (1990). Guidelines for screening for hearing impairment and middle-ear disorders. ASHA; 32(Supplement 2), 17–24; with permission.

middle ear pressure ranges between +50 and −200 daPa. As shown in **Table 18–3**, between −100 and −200 daPa, middle ear function is borderline abnormal; beyond −200 daPa, middle ear function is abnormal. Research has shown that large fluctuations can be found in TPP; abnormal TPP in the absence of other middle ear anomalies does not reflect significant changes in middle ear function, and abnormal TPP cannot be observed reliably with an otoscope. Because some studies have shown that TPP is not a good predictor of middle ear effusion (Fiellau-Nikolajsen, 1983; Nozza et al, 1994), this measure is not used as a sole criterion for a medical referral.

Pitfall

- Abnormal negative middle ear pressure in children observed on tympanograms is not always an indication of an obstructed eustachian tube. Rather, this finding may be a result of middle ear evacuation as a result of sniffing.

TW (or GR) describes the width (and slope) of the sides of the tympanogram surrounding the peak. TW is calculated by measuring the pressure range from the tympanogram corresponding to a percentage of reduction in static admittance from the maximum peak admittance. The procedure is as follows: (1) the peak (maximum) static admittance is obtained (e.g., 1.0 cc³/mL); (2) peak admittance values are reduced by a percentage (e.g., 50%) and noted on the positive and negative tails on the tympanogram; (3) a line is drawn connecting the points noted on the positive and negative tails of the tympanogram (at 0.5 cc³/mL); and (4) the distance between the positive and negative tympanogram points is measured in daPa. The current norms provided in **Table 18–3** are based on a 50% criterion (ASHA, 1979, 1990).

TW/GR measures appear to be sensitive to middle ear diseases that are not detected by other immittance measures or otoscopy (Fiellau-Nikolajsen, 1983; Nozza et al, 1994). Normative data have been established with several studies involving 3- to 10-year-olds (Hunter et al, 1992; Shanks et al, 1992). It should be noted that when

tympanograms are flat (type B), the TW/GR cannot be measured properly.

Static admittance (peak Y) or tympanogram height can also be referred to as static compliance (see **Table 18–1**). Static admittance provides objective information on the height of the tympanogram by quantifying its peak relative to the tail value (obtained at +200 daPa); the process of obtaining static admittance measures also provides data on the equivalent volume measure of the external and, possibly, middle ear.

Static admittance measurement can be explained using the volume principle, which states that the absolute size of a cavity of known physical characteristics (e.g., a hard wall cavity) can be determined by knowing the amount of reflected energy from an input signal of known intensity. **Figure 18–8** illustrates this concept, showing a fixed volume cavity A with a reflected sound pressure level (SPL) value that is high compared with cavities B and C. In cavity B (**Fig. 18–8**), the same input acoustic signal is used, but the output SPL is reduced due to the increased volume in the larger cavity. With a larger cavity, there is more absorption, which causes less resistance, and, as a result, less energy reflection occurs. In cavity C (**Fig. 18–8**), the same input acoustic signal is also used, but output SPL is reduced due to an even larger cavity. Based on this simple principle, the absolute volume of a cavity can be determined as long as the physical characteristics of the cavity are specified. When the physical characteristics of the cavity cannot be specified, such as when measures are being taken from different ears, the term *equivalent volume* is used. Equivalent volume readings refer to measures that are obtained from cavities of unknown physical characteristics, but the readings appear to be consistent with those expected from known hard wall cavities. For example, if a reading of 1.4 mL was obtained from a patient's ear canal, it would indicate that the ear canal had a volume equivalent to a hard wall cavity 1.4 mL in size. Thus, an equivalent volume of 1.4 mL was obtained.

Static admittance is measured by introducing a positive pressure into the external auditory canal. In a normal ear, the increased stiffness of the tympanic membrane sets up an artificial acoustic "wall." Under this condition, the volume of the cavity from the probe tip of the immittance instrument to the eardrum is measured in volume units

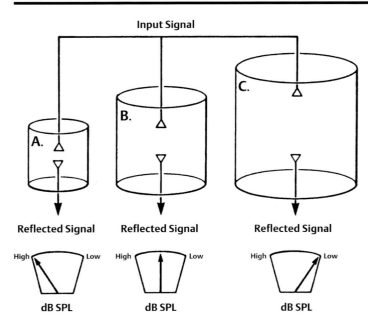

Input Signal

Reflected Signal   Reflected Signal   Reflected Signal

High ⌐   ⌐ Low   High ⌐   ⌐ Low   High ⌐   ⌐ Low

dB SPL   dB SPL   dB SPL

Figure 18–8 The effects of volume change on the input/output function of an acoustic signal for **(A)** a small cavity, **(B)** a medium cavity, and **(C)** a large cavity. SPL, sound pressure level.

(cubic centimeters or milliliters) equivalent to a cavity of known physical characteristics. Once pressure is removed, the tympanic membrane returns to its natural resting place, and the artificial acoustic wall will no longer be present. Under this condition, the cavity from the probe tip, including the external canal and middle ear space, is again measured in equivalent units.

To obtain static admittance, the probe tip is placed into the external ear canal, which directs the probe tone into the ear canal, and a pressure of +200 daPa is introduced. The positive air pressure serves to stretch and stiffen the tympanic membrane, resulting in a large amount of reflected energy. An admittance (compliance) reading is obtained, which gives an equivalent volume (cubic centimeters or milliliters) at this positive air pressure setting. When the eardrum is intact, this reading is the equivalent volume of the external ear canal (sometimes referred to as the C_1 reading). Air pressure is then adjusted from +200 daPa to the point of maximum static admittance (at or near 0 daPa in the normal ear), and a second reading is made (sometimes referred to as the C_2 reading). This reading is the equivalent volume of the combined outer and middle ear system. Static admittance is calculated by subtracting the first reading (C_1) from the second reading (C_2). This derived value represents the equivalent volume of the middle ear system. That is, by subtracting the equivalent volume of the ear canal only (C_1) from the equivalent volume of the ear canal and middle ear, represented by the value obtained at maximum compliance (C_2), the equivalent volume of only the middle ear remains. In **Fig. 18–6**, the static admittance is 0.5 mL (C_2 = 1.9 mL; C_1 =1.4 mL; $C_2 - C_1$ = 1.9 − 1.4). With microprocessing immittance units, the calculations are performed automatically, and the resulting admittance values are displayed digitally.

Table 18–3 provides the mean normal values and 90% ranges for static admittance for children and adults separately. As shown, for children the mean value is +0.5

mmho/cc³/mL, with a range of 0.2 to 0.9 mmho/cc³/mL. For adults, the mean value is 0.8 mmho/cc³/mL, with a range of 0.3 to 1.4 mmho/cc³/mL.

Ear canal volume measures are diagnostically significant when equivalent volumes exceed expected norms in the presence of a flat tympanogram. In such cases, the static admittance measure helps to detect eardrum perforation or determine whether a pressure equalization (PE) tube (surgically placed in an eardrum) is patent (open). In addition, when equivalent volumes are significantly less than the expected norms in the presence of a flat tympanogram, the admittance measure helps detect an occlusion in the external ear canal. The measure is sometimes called the physical volume test (PVT), but the American National Standards Institute (ANSI; 2002) and International Electrotechnical Commission (IEC; 2004) standards refer to this measure as ear canal volume.

Special Consideration

- Large physical ear canal volume measures in the presence of a flat tympanogram are consistent with tympanic membrane perforations and/or open tympanostomy tubes. However, physical ear canal volumes (C1) and static admittance may be well within normal limits in the presence of active draining or significant middle ear disease.

The PVT is accomplished by introducing positive air pressure into the external auditory canal. If a pressure seal is obtained, the equivalent volume is measured at +200 daPa (the C_1 reading; see **Fig. 18–5**). Mean ear canal volume norms and 90% ranges are provided in **Table 18–3** for children and adults separately. For children, the mean is 0.7 cc³/mL with a 90% range of 0.4 to 1.0 cc³/mL. For adults, the mean is 1.1 cc³/mL with a 90% range of 0.6 to 1.5 cc³/mL.

The diagnosis of a perforated tympanic membrane or, if a PE tube had been placed, the decision that it is patent (open) is made if the reading is unusually high, often exceeding 4.0 to 5.0 cc³/mL in adults with a flat (type B) tympanogram. In **Fig. 18–6**, V_{ea} = 1.4 mL. The size and shape of the probe tip and its placement in the ear canal will influence the ear canal volume reading. This may result in some test–retest variability but should not change the interpretation of the test significantly.

When testing an ear with a perforation or open PE tube, a hermetic seal may not be possible, or the pressure may suddenly release when introducing a positive pressure into the external ear canal. This finding would indicate that the eustachian tube is functioning. When a PE tube is present, and ear canal volume is normal or below normal, the diagnosis is that the PE tube is blocked.

Changing Probe Tone Frequency

The probe tone frequency of 226 Hz is used for standard clinical practice because this frequency is most effective for general identification of abnormalities of the tympanic membrane (e.g., perforation or retraction), middle ear conditions (e.g., effusion and abnormal pressure), and eustachian tube dysfunction in many patient populations. However, decades of research and a plethora of literature reports have shown that this single-frequency tympanogram is sometimes inadequate for diagnosing high-impedance pathologic conditions affecting the ossicular chain, such as neoplasms, otosclerosis, and ossicular fixation. As a result, multifrequency tympanometry using probe tones that sweep through frequencies 200 to 2000 Hz has been suggested as a way to improve diagnosis of abnormal conditions.

Controversial Point

- Despite a plethora of information on the added sensitivity of multifrequency tympanometry in identifying middle ear disease, clinicians have not embraced its routine use.

Early works by Liden (1969) and Colletti (1976, 1977) provided the basis for diagnostic interpretation of multifrequency tympanometry. In a series of studies, the researchers describe tympanograms with multiple peaks as V, W, and inverted *V* as a function of probe tone frequency changes (see **Fig. 18–9**). The clinical application of multifrequency tympanometry is based on the ability to distinguish between low- and high-resonant frequencies with the contributions of mass, stiffness, and resistance of the disorder. Hunter and Margolis (1992) provide a broad review of the clinical applications for multifrequency tympanometry.

Some diagnostic immittance instruments currently provide the option of using more than one probe tone frequency. However, despite the evidence supporting improved sensitivity in audiologic diagnoses, especially with those middle ear pathologies presenting severely restricted tympanic membrane mobility, clinicians have failed to embrace the use of multifrequency tympanometry for routine use. Apparently, the added diagnostic effectiveness of multifrequency tympanometry has not provided adequate justification for the additional expense in equipment and time for routine clinical use. An exception is pediatric populations, which is described later.

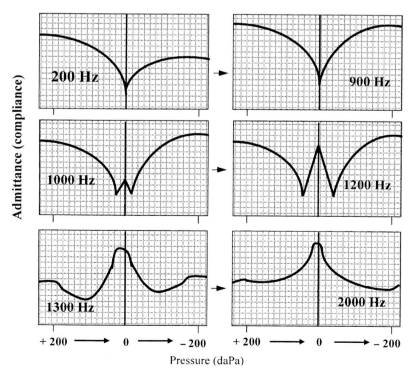

Figure 18–9 Multifrequency tympanometry recordings.

Acoustic Reflex Arc

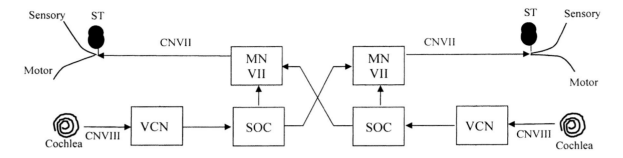

Figure 18–10 Schematic of the acoustic reflex neural pathways. CN VII, seventh cranial nerve; CN VIII, eighth cranial nerve; MNVII, motor nucleus of the seventh cranial nerve; SOC, superior olivary complex; ST, stapedius muscle; VCN, ventral cochlear nucleus.

The Acoustic Reflex

In a normal ear, when an acoustic stimulus is delivered to the ear canal at an intensity between 70 and 90 or 100 dB HL (hearing level), one small muscle in the middle ear, the stapedius, contracts and creates the phenomenon referred to as the acoustic reflex. Because the stapedius muscle is attached to the stapes, upon contraction, movement occurs in the ossicular chain, which, in turn, results in a stiffening of the tympanic membrane. The immittance instrument detects an acoustic reflex by measuring changes in the reflected energy occurring from the tympanic membrane stiffening during stapedial contraction. A repeatable change in the amount of reflected energy is an indication of an acoustic reflex. The acoustic reflex provides clinicians with one of the single most powerful differential diagnostic audiological procedures because of the ease of administration and amount of information obtained.

Figure 18–10 illustrates the neural mechanisms mediating the acoustic reflex. As shown, neural impulses from the eighth cranial nerve (CN VIII) from each cochlea are directed to the ipsilateral ventral cochlear nucleus (VCN in **Fig. 18–10**) and to the superior olivary complex (SOC in **Fig. 18–10**). They then cross the brainstem (decussate) and are sent to the motor nucleus (MN) of CN VII (facial), where the descending path provides innervation of the stapedius muscle and then facial sensory and motor functions (CN VII in **Fig. 18–10**). Of significant clinical importance is the bilateral aspect of the acoustic reflex; stimulating one ear (the ipsilateral ear) will elicit an acoustic reflex in both the ipsilateral and contralateral ears. As described later in the chapter, comparing reflexes from both ears while stimulating one ear has considerable diagnostic value.

When interpreting acoustic reflex data, the fact that the immittance procedure does not directly measure middle ear muscle contraction must be taken into account because three conditions affect the ability to record stapedius muscle contraction: a middle ear disorder, hearing loss in the stimulated ear, and interruption of neural innervation of the stapedius muscle.

Middle Ear Disorder

Mechanical conditions in the middle ear can obliterate the recording of an acoustic reflex. For example:

1. Otosclerosis will cause the footplate of the stapes to adhere to the bone surrounding the oval window, increasing the stiffness of the ossicular chain.

2. Middle ear fluid will cause the tympanic membrane and middle ear structures to lose all compliance, and stapedius muscle contraction cannot influence the immobility of the middle ear system.

3. Disarticulation will result in loss of energy transfer across the ossicular chain to the tympanic membrane.

4. Perforation will cause the probe tone to be presented directly to the middle ear space, giving a large equivalent volume reading. Any changes in the system caused by contraction of the stapedius muscle cannot be recorded by the immittance system.

When abnormal middle ear pressure is present, acoustic reflex measures are taken with the ear canal pressure adjusted to match the middle ear pressure as determined by the tympanogram. Equalizing pressure puts the tympanic membrane at or near the point of maximum compliance, increasing the likelihood that the reflex will be detected if it occurs.

The fact that middle ear disorders can obliterate the recording of an acoustic reflex means that the reflex may occur but not be recorded due to mechanical abnormalities of the middle ear. This makes it all the more important to have clinicians view all components of the immittance test battery for accurate diagnosis. As an example, contradictory findings would exist if the tympanogram indicated there was little or no compliance (type B) and an acoustic reflex was recorded.

Hearing Loss in the Stimulated Ear

Acoustic reflex thresholds are assessed by varying the intensity of the pure-tone reflex-eliciting stimuli in the 70 to 100 dB HL range and noting the lowest intensity at which the reflex occurs. Once a threshold is established at one frequency, the intensity is recorded, and other frequencies can then be assessed. However, in immittance screening, only one frequency is typically tested at a fixed intensity of ~100 dB HL.

The presence of reflexes within normal intensity limits is consistent with normal middle ear and brainstem function and suggests that auditory sensitivity is not significantly impaired. However, acoustic reflexes may occur within the expected normal intensity range at all frequencies when mild or moderate-to-severe sensorineural hearing loss is present. Partial or elevated reflexes may also be recorded. *Partial* means that a reflex is present at some frequencies tested and absent at others, and *elevated* refers to reflex thresholds exceeding 100 dB HL. Partial or elevated reflex thresholds may indicate the presence of a hearing loss at those frequencies at which they are absent.

A diagnosis of recruitment is made when sensorineural hearing loss is known to exist and acoustic reflexes are elicited at or less than 50 dB sensation level (SL), indicating a cochlear lesion. Because acoustic reflexes can be recorded at reduced sensation levels, when pure tones are used, they cannot predict hearing threshold sensitivity with absolute assurance. Hearing threshold sensitivity must be assessed behaviorally or electrophysiologically if there are questions regarding hearing loss.

If middle ear function is normal, and a mild to moderate sensorineural hearing loss less than 40 to 60 dB HL is present, absent acoustic reflexes will suggest a sensorineural hearing loss without recruitment. Such a finding implies a diagnosis of retrocochlear pathology. Absent reflexes have also been observed in individuals with normal or near-normal hearing, which may indicate middle ear disease or neurological involvement of CN VIII, such as in auditory neuropathy (see below), or CN VII. If the facial nerve is involved, the absence of acoustic reflexes when middle ear function is normal suggests a lesion in the neural pathway prior to stapedius muscle innervation; the presence of an acoustic reflex in such patients suggests a lesion following stapedius muscle innervation.

Interruption of Neural Innervation of the Stapedius Muscle

Brainstem lesions affecting the acoustic reflex pathway can interrupt neural impulses that elicit acoustic reflexes from ipsilateral and/or contralateral stimulation.

Feeney and colleagues (2004) evaluated a newer measurement technique, wideband reflectance, for measuring acoustic stapedius reflex thresholds. With wideband reflectance, complex stimuli in the 125 to 10,000 Hz range, resembling "chirplike" sounds, are introduced into the ear canal with a specially calibrated probe tip. Rather than measuring differences for a single probe tone frequency, the wideband procedure measures energy reflectance and admittance for the complex signal. Feeney et al (2004) found that the wideband reflectance technique was more successful than the single probe tone technique in recording the acoustic reflex, and thresholds were on average 3 dB more sensitive. They concluded that the wideband reflectance technique holds promise as a clinical procedure for measuring acoustic reflexes for normal-hearing subjects who fail to show reflexes with the standard clinical procedure.

Ipsilateral/Contralateral Comparison

Comparison of ipsilateral and contralateral acoustic reflexes provides a powerful diagnostic audiologic tool. Jerger and Jerger (1977) developed a classification system that categorizes findings into six distinct patterns (see **Table 18–4**). As

Table 18–4   Ipsilateral-Contralateral, Acoustic Reflex Pattern Interpretation with Left Side Involvement

Reflex Pattern Name	Hz	Visual (Probe Ear) R	Visual (Probe Ear) L	Verbal	Clinical Interpretation
Normal	Crossed	☐	☐	Normal for both ears	1. Normal
	Uncrossed	☐	☐		
Vertical	Crossed	☐	■	Abnormal whenever probe is in the affected ear	1. Mild middle ear disorder (in the left ear)
	Uncrossed	☐	■		2. CN VII (facial nerve) disorder (on the left side)
Diagonal	Crossed	■	☐	Abnormal with sound to the affected ear	1. Right nerve disorder (on the left side)
	Uncrossed	☐	■		2. Severe cochlear loss (in the left ear)
Inverted L-shape	Crossed	■	■	Abnormal on both ears to crossed stimulation, abnormal on affected ear to uncrossed stimulation	1. Unilateral middle ear disorder (in the left ear)
	Uncrossed	☐	■		2. Intra-axial brainstem disorder eccentric to one side (left side)
					3. Combined CN VII and CN VIII disorder
Horizontal	Crossed	■	■	Abnormal to crossed stimulation on both ears	1. Extra-axial and/or intra-axial brainstem disorder
	Uncrossed	☐	☐		
Unibox	Crossed	■	☐	Abnormal with sound to affected ear on crossed stimulation only	1. Extra-axial and/or intra-axial brainstem disorder
	Uncrossed	☐	☐		

☐ = Reflex present

■ = Reflex absent

CN VII, seventh cranial nerve; CN VIII, eighth cranial nerve.

Source: Adapted from Jerger, S., & Jerger, J. (1977). Diagnostic value of cross vs uncrossed acoustic reflexes: eighth nerve and brain stem disorders. Archives of Otolaryngology, 103, 445–453, with permission.

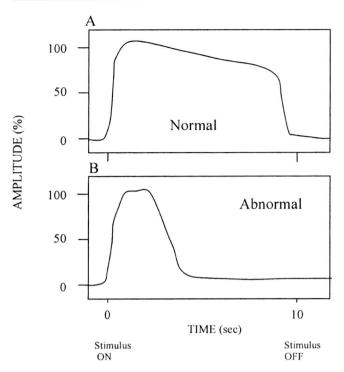

Figure 18–11   **(A)** Normal and **(B)** abnormal findings on the acoustic reflex decay test.

shown, these patterns are based on open or filled box patterns. Normal results are represented by open boxes for all four conditions. Cochlear, CN VII, CN VIII, or brainstem sites of lesion are represented by vertical, diagonal, inverted L-shape, horizontal, and unibox patterns. It should be noted that the findings in **Table 18–4** are from left side involvement; the patterns would be reversed if the right side were involved.

Acoustic Reflex Decay

If the acoustic reflex stimulus is presented continuously over an extended period (10 seconds or longer) in the normal ear, the muscle contraction in the acoustic reflex will be sustained at maximum or near-maximum amplitude throughout stimulation. This function is evaluated during the acoustic reflex decay test. Acoustic reflex decay is assessed with low-frequency stimuli (500 and 1000 Hz) because, for unclear reasons, at higher frequencies acoustic reflex amplitudes may decrease in less than 10 seconds even in normal ears. The standard procedure is to present the stimulus contralaterally at 10 dB SL (re: the threshold of the acoustic reflex of test ear), or between 90 and 105 dB HL for 10 seconds. **Figure 18–11A** illustrates acoustic reflex functions when a signal is maintained constant over the 10 second period. In patients with normal reflex function, there will be a clearly maintained amplitude response over the 10 second period. However, abnormal reflex decay will be marked by an inability to maintain full amplitude for the duration of the stimulation. As shown in **Fig. 18–11B**, the amplitude of the reflex decreases to less than half the maximum amplitude within 5 seconds.

Abnormal reflex decay can be observed in patients with either cochlear or CN VIII pathological conditions, such as space-invading tumors and Bell's palsy. When the decay occurs within 5 seconds or at frequencies less than 1000 Hz, results are suggestive of CN VIII dysfunction. This test has a high degree of sensitivity to retrocochlear pathologies, and because of its ease of administration, the acoustic reflex decay is considered a valuable diagnostic test. However, some concern exists about presenting acoustic stimuli for extended periods at high intensities. For this reason, the acoustic reflex decay test should be administered judiciously while never exceeding 105 dB HL presentation levels for any frequency. When deemed necessary, it is best to administer the test at the end of the test session, especially after threshold testing. This way, behavioral thresholds will not be affected by the intense stimulation required for reflex decay. If concerns should arise regarding temporary or permanent threshold shifts caused by the intense stimulation, reliable behavioral test results will be recorded.

◆ Case Studies

The following four case studies (**Figs. 18–12** through **18–15**) provide examples of audiologic and immittance findings for frequently observed types of middle ear pathologies. For each patient, otoscopic examination revealed an ear canal free from occluding debris.

Case 1

Figure 18–12 provides expected findings for a patient having either a tympanic membrane perforation or a tympanostomy tube that is open (patent). Masked, pure-tone thresholds show a mild conductive hearing loss in the right ear and normal threshold sensitivity in the left ear. Immittance measures show normal tympanic membrane static admittance for the left ear (type A) but little or no static admittance for the right ear (type B). The excessively large physical volume (V_{ea}) measure for the right ear (C_1 at +200 mm H_2O = 3.5 mL) is commensurate with a tympanic membrane perforation/open tympanostomy tube. Acoustic reflexes are absent for the contralateral and ipsilateral probe right conditions due to the abnormal mechanical condition of the right ear resulting from the perforation/tympanostomy tube. They are also absent for the contralateral probe left condition due to the hearing loss in the right ear. Acoustic reflexes are present for this patient only in the ipsilateral probe left condition. If this patient had a tympanostomy tube, and the physical volume measure (V_{ea}) was not large, the clinical indication would be that the tube is blocked.

Case 2

The data in **Fig. 18–13** are expected findings for a patient with bilateral ossicular chain ossification, most commonly associated with otosclerosis. This patient presents with a moderate bilateral conductive hearing loss. Both tympanograms show peak pressure (TPP) at atmospheric pressure, with severely reduced tympanic membrane static admittance bilaterally (type A_s). Acoustic reflexes are absent contralaterally and present ipsilaterally in the left ear.

Case Study #1

PURE TONE AUDIOMETRY

Type of Test: (Reg) Play VRA BOA
Transducer: TDH 50 (ER 3A) SF

Reliability: (Good) Fair Poor

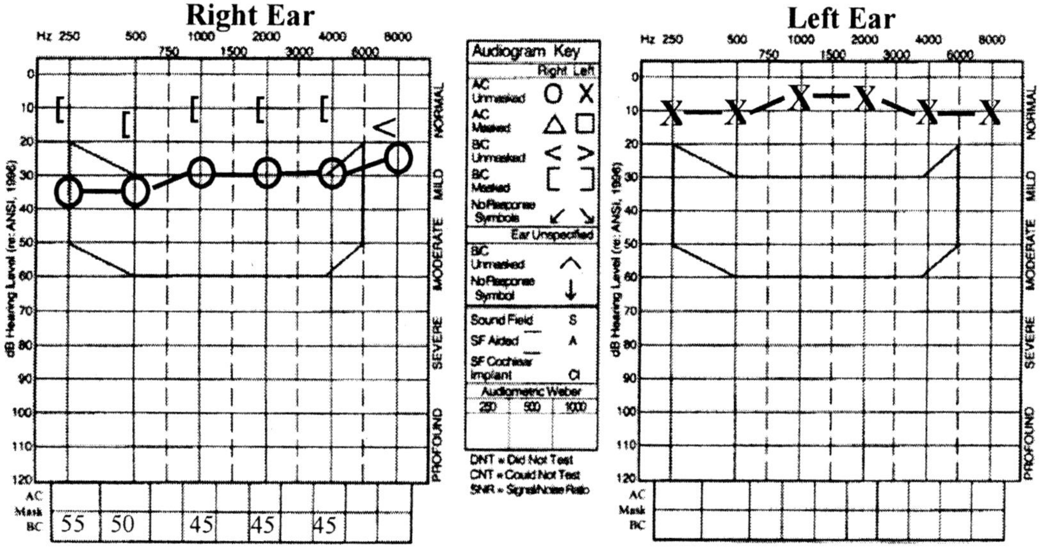

Right Ear

Left Ear

Audiogram Key

	Right	Left
AC Unmasked	O	X
AC Masked	△	□
BC Unmasked	<	>
BC Masked	[	]
No Response Symbols	↙	↘

BC Unmasked	<
No Response Symbol	→
Sound Field	S
SF Aided	A
Implant	CI

DNT = Did Not Test
CNT = Could Not Test
SNR = Signal-to-noise Ratio

Audiometric Weber
250 500 1000 2000

Speech Audiometry

	SAT	SRT	PTA	MCL	ULL	SRS%	
		30	31			96	40SL	Right Ear
		10	6			100	40 SL	Left Ear

IMMITTANCE

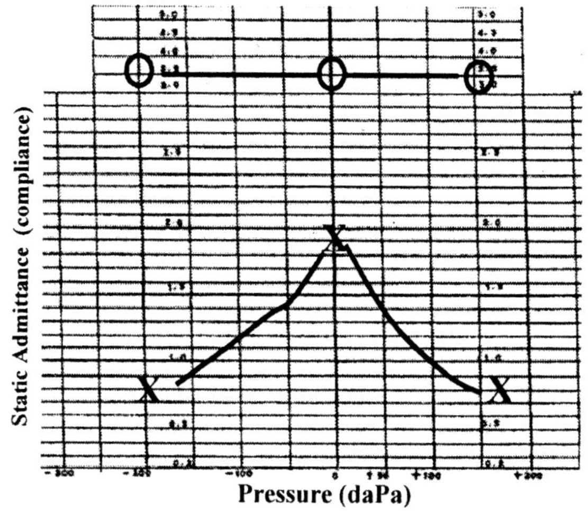

Static Admittance (compliance)

Pressure (daPa)

Ac. Reflex Data		500	1000	2000	4000	Hz
Probe Right	Con	NR	NR	NR	NR	
	Ipsi		NR	NR		
Probe Left	Con	NR	NR	NR	95	
	Ipsi		85	85		

NR = No Response

Figure 18–12 Audiological and immittance findings from a patient with a tympanic membrane perforation in the right ear. AC, air conduction; BC, bone conduction; BOA, behavioral observation audiometry; MCL, most comfortable level; PTA, pure-tone average; SAT, speech awareness threshold; SF, sound field; SL, sensation level; SRS, speech recognition score; SRT, speech recognition threshold; ULL, uncomfortable loudness level; VRA, visual reinforcement audiometry.

Case Study #2

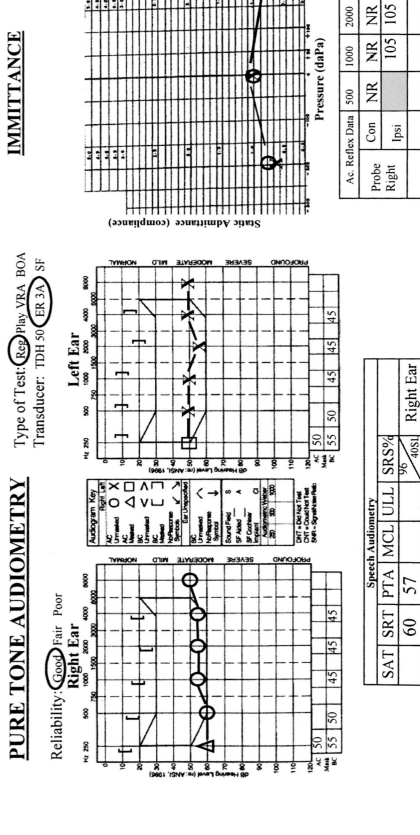

PURE TONE AUDIOMETRY

Type of Test: (Reg) Play VRA BOA

Transducer: TDH 50 (ER 3A) SF

Reliability: (Good) Fair Poor

IMMITTANCE

Static Admittance (compliance)

Pressure (daPa)

Ac. Reflex Data		500	1000	2000	4000	Hz
Probe Right	Con	NR	NR	NR	NR	
	Ipsi		105	105		
Probe Left	Con	NR	NR	NR	NR	
	Ipsi		105	105		

NR = No Response

Speech Audiometry

	SAT	SRT	PTA	MCL	ULL	SRS%	
		60	57			96 / 40SL	Right Ear
		50	52			100 / 40 SL	Left Ear

Figure 18–13 Audiological and immittance findings from a patient with bilateral ossicular chain fixation, most likely due to otosclerosis. AC, air conduction; BC, bone conduction; BOA, behavioral observation audiometry; MCL, most comfortable level; PTA, pure-tone average; SAT, speech awareness threshold; SF, sound field; SL, sensation level; SRS, speech recognition score; SRT, speech recognition threshold; ULL, uncomfortable loudness level; VRA, visual reinforcement audiometry.

Case 3

The audiometric findings in **Fig. 18–14** are similar to those for case 1, showing a mild right ear conductive hearing loss and normal hearing in the left ear, but the immittance data are different. Tympanograms show normal tympanic membrane static admittance for the left ear (type A) but little or no static admittance for the right ear (type B), with a C_1 value in the range of normal limits. As with the patient in case 1, acoustic reflexes are present only in the ipsilateral probe left condition. These findings are typical for a patient with otitis media in the right ear.

Case 4

The data in **Fig. 18–15** show normal right ear threshold sensitivity and a moderate rising to mild conductive hearing loss in the left ear. The tympanogram for the right ear shows normal tympanic membrane static admittance (type A) but excessively high static admittance for the left ear (type A_d). Acoustic reflexes are present only for the probe right ipsilateral condition. These findings would suggest ossicular chain disarticulation for the left ear.

◆ Special Considerations and Disorders

Tympanometry in Infants

An abundance of clinical and research data clearly documents that tympanometric recordings from newborns differ widely from those of older infants, toddlers, and children. In fact, when low-frequency probe tones (220 Hz) are used for tympanometry with normal newborns, acoustic conductance and susceptance will show three different patterns, rather than the normal type A pattern (Himelfarb et al, 1979). Low-frequency probe tone findings from infants are thought to be a result of incomplete ossification of the external auditory canals and ossicular chain mechanisms, as well as tympanic membrane orientation (Keefe et al, 1993).

Pearl

- Tympanograms obtained on infants less than 6 months of age using the standard 226 Hz probe tone frequency are not sensitive to middle ear disorders; higher frequency probe tones are needed with this population.

As a consequence, tympanograms on newborns obtained with the standard 226 Hz probe tone cannot accurately reflect the condition of the middle ear (Paradise et al, 1976). In some instances, a newborn's underossified and overly compliant canal will render tympanometric values that would suggest normal tympanic membrane mobility in the presence of medically diagnosed otitis media with effusion.

Fortunately, tympanograms with higher frequency probe tones, in the 660 to 1000 Hz range, are accurate in evaluating outer and middle ear status of infants from birth to 6 months of age (Marchant et al, 1986).

Screening for Middle Ear Disorders

Historic and current literature is replete with studies showing the advantages and disadvantages of immittance screening for middle ear disorders in schoolchildren. Support for immittance screening is provided by the known fact that pure-tone screening alone is not sensitive to middle ear disorders. The advantages of including immittance measures in screening programs are seen with an increased sensitivity in identifying children with middle ear disease and a possible reduction in the number of children requiring pure-tone retesting prior to referral. Because there is compelling evidence that significant delays in speech and language development and educational retardation may be related to chronic middle ear disease in children, especially during the early years, there is added interest in identifying children with middle ear disorders as early as possible.

Pitfall

- Despite the high prevalence of middle ear disorders in children, immittance screening is not recommended by national organizations because of the high false-positive rates.

Many programs testing toddlers and young children have incorporated middle ear screening into their protocol, using pure-tone tests along with tympanometry and acoustic reflexes. Margolis and Hunter (1999) present a detailed description of a screening program that incorporates case history, visual inspection of the ear canal, pure-tone screening, and immittance measures. It should be emphasized that regular audiometric screening with immittance measures included is encouraged for special populations, including Native Americans; those with sensorineural hearing loss, developmental delay, and mental impairment; and children with craniofacial anomalies, including cleft palate and Down syndrome (Bluestone et al, 1986). Concomitant effects of middle ear disease places many young children, who would have a higher preponderance of middle ear disease, at significantly greater risk for speech and language delay.

Despite the compelling data supporting screening for middle ear disorders in young populations, various agencies and guidelines have recommended against mass screening for middle ear disorders (Bess, 1980). Unfortunately, the increased sensitivity of immittance measures alone can result in excessively high numbers of false-positive identifications.

Large Vestibular Aqueduct Syndrome

Singly, the most prevalent etiology associated with sudden onset or progressive childhood hearing loss is large (enlarged)

Case Study #3

IMMITTANCE

Static Admittance (compliance)

Pressure (daPa)

Ac. Reflex Data		500	1000	2000	4000	Hz
Probe Right	Con	NR	NR	NR	NR	
	Ipsi		NR	NR		
Probe Left	Con	NR	NR	NR	NR	
	Ipsi		85	85		

NR = No Response

PURE TONE AUDIOMETRY

Reliability: (Good) Fair Poor

Type of Test: (Reg) Play VRA BOA

Transducer: TDH 50 (ER 3A) SF

Right Ear

Left Ear

Speech Audiometry

	SAT	SRT	PTA	MCL	ULL	SRS%	
Right Ear		30	31			96 40SL	
Left Ear		10	7			100 40 SL	

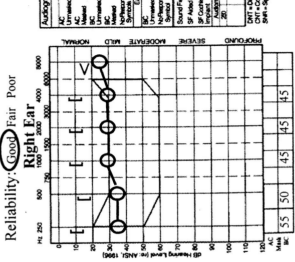

Figure 18–14 Example of audiologic and immittance findings from a patient with otitis media in the right ear. AC, air conduction; BC, bone conduction; BOA, behavioral observation audiometry; MCL, most comfortable level; PTA, pure-tone average; SAT, speech awareness threshold; SF, sound field; SL, sensation level; SRS, speech recognition score; SRT, speech recognition threshold; ULL, uncomfortable loudness level; VRA, visual reinforcement audiometry.

Case Study #4

PURE TONE AUDIOMETRY

Type of Test: (Reg) Play VRA BOA

Transducer: TDH 50 (ER 3A) SF

Reliability: (Good) Fair Poor

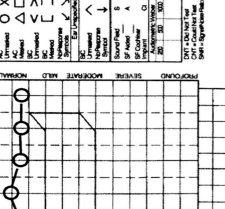

IMMITTANCE

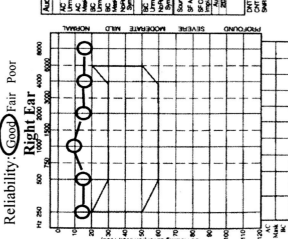

Ac. Reflex Data

		500	1000	2000	4000	
Probe Right	Con	NR	NR	NR	NR	
	Ipsi		85	85		Hz
Probe Left	Con	NR	NR	NR	NR	
	Ipsi		NR	NR		

NR = No Response

Speech Audiometry

	SAT	SRT	PTA	MCL	ULL	SRS%	
		15	13			96 / 40SL	Right Ear
		45	43			100 / 40 SL	Left Ear

Figure 18–15 Audiologic and immittance findings from a patient with ossicular chain disarticulation in the left ear. AC, air conduction; BC, bone conduction; BOA, behavioral observation audiometry; MCL, most comfortable level; PTA, pure-tone average; SAT, speech awareness threshold; SF, sound field; SL, sensation level; SRS, speech recognition score; SRT, speech recognition threshold; ULL, uncomfortable loudness level; VRA, visual reinforcement audiometry.

vestibular aqueduct syndrome (LVAS or EVS), accounting for 15 to 20% of these children (Arcand et al, 1991; Emmett, 1985). Typically, diagnosis is made in the early years of childhood with either an associated inner ear anomaly (e.g., hypoplastic cochlea, Mondini-Alexander dysplasia or variant), or congenital disorders (e.g., Pendred's syndrome, CHARGE, Alagille syndrome, branchio-oto-renal syndrome) or in complete isolation (Arcand et al, 1991; Temple et al, 1999). Although progressive hearing loss is common with children manifesting LVAS, minor trauma, infection, or activities involving a Valsalva's maneuver can precipitate decreased hearing sensitivity (Can et al, 2004; Govaerts et al, 1999).

Sensorineural hearing loss is most prevalent in LVAS. However, air–bone gaps with fluctuating daily tympanometric findings (e.g., types A, B, and C) and unremarkable otoscopic observations have been documented (Clark and Roeser, 2005). It is believed that these inconsistent findings can be the result of decreased mobility of the stapes resulting from increased perilymphatic pressure, stapes fixation, or an incomplete transmission of the ossicles/ossicular discontinuity because of incomplete bone formation around the inner ear (Nakashima et al, 2000; Shirazi et al, 1994; Valvassori, 1983).

Because of the apparent conductive component at the cochlea, a medical misdiagnosis of otitis media with effusion can easily delay the eventual finding of LVAS for many months or years. Fortunately, LVAS is the most common radiographically detectable malformation found in children that typically coexists with other anatomical structural abnormalities in patients with early onset of hearing loss (Okumura et al, 1995). As a result, all children with newly identified hearing loss should have both radiographic imaging and genetic testing to confirm the diagnosis and provide input into treatment. Hearing aid use and cochlear implants have been shown to be effective for children with LVAS (Clark and Roeser, 2005).

Auditory Neuropathy/Dys-synchrony

Auditory neuropathy, which is sometimes referred to as auditory dys-synchrony, involves a disruption of auditory function due to axonal or demyelinating conditions at the inner hair cells of the cochlea, auditory neurons in the spinal ganglion, CN VIII fibers, or any combination of these sites (Berlin et al, 1998; Starr et al, 1996). The diagnostic findings with auditory neuropathy are consistent with normal outer hair cell function in the presence of abnormal neural function at the level of CN VIII (vestibulocochlear), likely not a single underlying cause. Behaviorally, patients identified with auditory neuropathy will have difficulty understanding simple sentences in quiet and in noise, and in extreme cases, they will have markedly delayed speech and language development than would be predicted from hearing thresholds. Some of the underlying etiologies include hyperbilirubinemia, premature birth, genetics, hereditary motor sensory neuropathy, Charcot-Marie-Tooth neuropathy syndrome, mitochondrial disorder, and ischemic hypoxic neuropathy.

Although auditory neuropathy is unequivocally diagnosed when otoacoustic emissions are present and auditory brainstem response (ABR) waveforms are poorly formed and/or reverse polarity, absent or elevated acoustic reflexes are becoming recognized as another hallmark in identification. Despite normal tympanic membrane mobility (i.e., type A), individuals with auditory neuropathy will typically have absent acoustic reflexes in the presence of normal cochlear function.

Recent research of a large group of patients identified with auditory neuropathy showed universally absent ipsilateral and contralateral acoustic reflexes (Berlin et al, 2005). With a suggested 40% incidence of auditory neuropathy in the neonatal intensive care unit (Rea and Gibson, 2003), there is more of a rationale to include ipsilateral acoustic reflex assessment of at least 1000 and 2000 Hz in any perinatal hearing screening program that depends solely upon otoacoustic emissions (OAE) assessments. A higher probe frequency to measure middle ear reflexes may be considered for newborn screening programs that use OAE only. In such programs, ABR testing should be considered when acoustic reflexes are not recorded.

◆ Summary

Technological advances have made the measurement of middle ear function through immittance measures a routine part of the diagnostic audiological test battery. Immittance measures provide an effective and efficient method for quantifying the state of the middle ear, as well as auditory and brainstem function. Through the use of microprocessing systems, the procedure can be administered in a matter of minutes for each ear. However, immittance measures should be considered a part of the audiological test battery, not replacing behavioral or electrophysiologic measures. Immittance measures are of considerable value when testing infants and special populations, but modifications of the standard protocol should be considered for these populations.

References

American National Standards Institute. (2002). Specifications for instruments to measure aural acoustic impedance and admittance [ANSI S3.39–1987 (R2002)]. New York: Author.

American Speech-Language-Hearing Association Committee on Audiometric Evaluation. (1979). Guidelines for acoustic immittance screening of middle ear function. ASHA, 21, 283–288.

American Speech-Language-Hearing Association. (1990). Guidelines for screening for hearing impairment and middle-ear disorders. ASHA, 32(Suppl. 2), 17–24

Arcand, P., Desrosiers, M., Dube, J., & Abela, A. (1991). The large vestibular aqueduct syndrome and sensorineural hearing loss in the pediatric population. Journal of Otolaryngology, 20, 247–250.

Berlin, C. I., Bordelon, J., St. John, P., Wilensky, D., Hurley, A. Kluka, E., & Hord, L. (1998). Reversing click polarity may uncover auditory neuropathy in infants. Ear and Hearing, 19, 37–47.

Berlin, C. I., Hood, L. J., Morlet, T., Wilensky, D., St. John, P., Montgomery, E., & Thibodaux, M. (2005). Absent or elevated middle ear muscle reflexes in the presence of normal otoacoustic emissions: A universal finding in 136 cases of auditory neuropathy/dys-synchrony. Journal of the American Academy of Audiology, 16, 546–553.

Bess, F. H. (1980). Impedance screening for children: A need for more research. Annals of Otology, Rhinology and Laryngology Supplement, 89 (3, Pt. 2), 228–232.

Bluestone, C. D., Fria, T. J., Arjona, S. K., Casselbrant, M. L., Schwartz, D. M., Ruben, R. J., Gates, G. A., et al. (1986). Controversies in screening for middle ear disease and hearing loss in children. Pediatrics, 77, 57–70.

Can, I. H., Gocmen, H., Kurt, A., & Samim, E. (2004). Sudden hearing loss due to large vestibular aqueduct syndrome in a child: Should exploratory tympanotomy be performed? International Journal of Pediatric Otorhinolaryngology, 68, 841–844.

Clark, J. L., & Roeser, R. J. (2005). Large vestibular aqueduct syndrome: A case study. Journal of the American Academy of Audiology, 16, 822–828.

Colletti, V. (1976). Tympanometry from 200 to 2000 Hz probe tone. Audiology, 15, 106–119.

Colletti, V. (1977). Multifrequency tympanometry. Audiology, 16, 278–287.

Emmett, J. R. (1985). The large vestibular aqueduct syndrome. American Journal of Otology, 6, 387–415.

Feeney, M. P., Keefe, D. H., & Sanford, C. A. (2004). Wideband reflectance measures of the ipsilateral acoustic stapedius reflex threshold. Ear and Hearing, 25, 421–430.

Fiellau-Nikolajsen, M. (1983). Tympanometry and secretory otitis media: Observations on diagnosis, epidemiology, treatment, and prevention in prospective cohort studies of three-year-old children. Acta Otolaryngologica Supplementum, 394, 1–73.

Govaerts, P. J., Casselman, J., Daemers, K., De Ceulaer, G., Somers, T., & Offeciers, F. E. (1999). Audiological findings in large vestibular aqueduct syndrome. International Journal of Pediatric Otorhinolaryngology, 51, 157–164.

Himelfarb, M. Z., Popelka, G. R., & Shanon, E. (1979). Tympanometry in normal neonates. Journal of Speech and Hearing Research, 22, 179–191.

Hunter, L. L., & Margolis, R. H. (1992). Multifrequency tympanometry: Current clinical application. American Journal of Audiology, 1, 33–43.

Hunter, L. L., Margolis, R. H., Daly, K., & Giebink, G. (February 1992). Relationship of tympanometric estimates of middle ear volume to middle ear status at surgery. Paper presented at the midwinter research meeting of the Association for Research in Otolaryngology, St. Petersburg Beach, FL.

International Electrotechnical Commission. (2004). Electroacoustics—audiological equipment: 5. Instruments for the measurement of aural acoustic impedance/admittance [IEC 60645-5 (2004-11)]. Geneva: Author.

Jerger, J. (1970). Clinical experience with impedance audiometry. Archives of Otolaryngology, 92, 311–324.

Jerger, S., & Jerger, J. (1977). Diagnostic value of cross vs uncrossed acoustic reflexes: Eighth nerve and brain stem disorders. Archives of Otolaryngology, 103, 445–453.

Keefe, D. H., Bulen, J. C., Arehart, K. H., & Burns, E. M. (1993). Ear-canal impedance and reflection coefficient in human infants and adults. Journal of the Acoustical Society of America, 94, 2617–2638.

Liden, G. (1969). The scope and application of current audiometric tests. Journal of Laryngology and Otology, 83, 507–520.

Marchant, C. D., McMillan, P. M., Shurin, P. A., Johnson, C. E., Turczyk, V. A., Feinstein, J. C. & Panek, D. M. (1986). Objective diagnosis of otitis media in early infancy by tympanometry and ipsilateral acoustic reflex thresholds. Journal of Pediatrics 109: 590-595.

Margolis, R. H., and Hunter, L. L. (1999). Tympanometry—Basic principles and clinical applications. In F. E. Musiek & W. F. Rintelmann (Eds.), Contemporary Perspectives on Hearing Assessment (pp. 89–130). Boston: Allyn and Bacon.

Margolis, R. H., & Hunter, L. L. (2000). Acoustic immittance measurements. In R. Roeser, M. Valente, & H. Hosford-Dunn (Eds.), Audiology: Diagnosis (pp. 381–423). New York: Thieme Medical Publishers.

Nakashima, T., Ueda, H., Furuhashi, A., Sato, E., Asahi, K., Naganawa, S., Beppu, R. (2000). Air-bone gap and resonant frequency in large vestibular aqueduct syndrome. American Journal of Otology, 21, 671–674.

Nozza, R. J., Bluestone, C. D., Kardatzke, D., & Bachman, R. (1994). Identification of middle ear effusion by aural acoustic admittance and otoscopy. Ear and Hearing, 15, 310–323.

Okumura, T., Takahashi, H., Honjo, I., Takagi, A., & Mitamura, K. (1995). Sensorineural hearing loss in patients with large vestibular aqueduct. Laryngoscope, 105, 289–293.

Paradise, J. L., Smith, G. C., & Bluestone, C. D. (1976). Tympanometric detection of middle ear effusion in infants and young children. Pediatrics, 58, 198–210.

Rea, P. A., & Gibson, W. P. (2003). Evidence for surviving outer hair cell function in congenitally deaf ears. Laryngoscope, 113, 2030–2034.

Shanks, J. E., Stelmachowicz, P. G., Beauchaine, K. L., & Schulte, L. (1992). Equivalent ear canal volumes in children pre- and post-tympanostomy tube insertion. Journal of Speech and Hearing Research, 35, 936–941.

Shirazi, A., Fenton, J. E., & Fagan, P. A. (1994). Large vestibular aqueduct syndrome and stapes fixation. Journal of Laryngology and Otology, 108, 989–990.

Starr, A., Picton, T. W., Sininger, Y., Hood, L. J., & Berlin, C. I. (1996). Auditory neuropathy. Brain, 119, 741–753.

Temple, R. H., Ramsden, R. T., Axon, P. R., & Saeed S. R. (1999). The large vestibular aqueduct syndrome: The role of cochlear implantation in its management. Clinical Otolaryngology and Allied Sciences, 24, 301–306.

Valvassori, G. E. (1983). The large vestibular aqueduct and associated anomalies of the inner ear. Otolaryngological Clinics of North America, 16, 95–101.

Wiley, T. L., & Block, M. G. (1985). Overview of basic principles of acoustic immittance measurements (pp. 423–437). In J. Katz (Ed.), Handbook of clinical audiology (3rd ed.) New York: Williams & Wilkins.

Chapter 19

Electrocochleography

John A. Ferraro

The transduction of acoustic energy in the auditory periphery involves the generation of stimulus-related, bioelectrical potentials in the cochlea. As the term implies, electrocochleography (ECochG) is a method for recording these potentials. The product of ECochG is referred to as an electrocochleogram (ECochGm). As shown in **Fig. 19–1**, the ECochGm in response to broadband click stimuli may include the cochlear microphonic (CM), cochlear summating potential (SP), and the whole nerve or compound action potential (AP) of the auditory nerve. These three components may be recorded independently or in various combinations.

Historically, attempts to record the CM from humans date back almost to the time of its discovery in the cat by Wever and Bray in 1930 (see Perlman and Case, 1941). Although the SP was described in animals in 1950 (Davis et al, 1950; von Bekesy, 1950), its recording in humans received little to no attention until the mid to late 1970s (e.g., Eggermont, 1976; Gibson et al, 1977). The first recordings of human auditory nerve APs are credited to Ruben et al (1960).

Although available to the hearing scientist for over a half century, ECochG's emergence as a clinical tool did not begin until the 1970s. Renewed and increased attention to all auditory evoked potentials (AEPs) during this period was due in part to the discovery and application of the auditory brainstem response (ABR). Another important factor, which has facilitated the recent clinical popularity of ECochG in particular, is the development and refinement of noninvasive recording techniques. Ruben and his coworkers (1960), for example, performed their AP measurements on patients undergoing middle ear surgery. Within a few years, nonsurgical techniques that involved passing a needle electrode through the tympanic membrane (TM) to rest on the cochlear promontory were introduced (e.g., Aran and LeBert, 1968; Yoshie et al, 1967). This transtympanic (TT) approach to ECochG is still used in Europe and other countries outside the United States. However, invasive recording methods have not been well accepted in the United States for a variety of reasons to be discussed later. Fortunately, the components that constitute an ECochGm can also be measured noninvasively from extratympanic (ET) sites such as the ear canal or the lateral surface of the TM. Pioneering work in this area was performed by Sohmer and Feinmesser (1967), Coats and Dickey (1970), and Cullen et al (1972), among others. A more thorough discussion

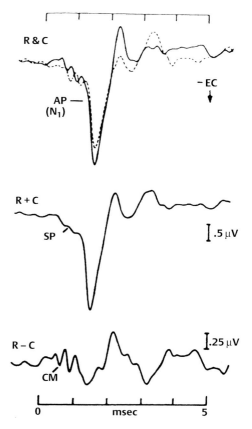

Figure 19–1 Components of the human electrocochleogram evoked by click stimuli. Top tracings show responses to rarefaction (R) and condensation (C) polarity clicks. Adding separate R and C responses (middle tracing) enhances the cochlear summating potential (SP) and auditory nerve action potential (AP), which are not phase-locked to the stimulus. Subtracting R and C responses (bottom tracing) enhances the cochlear microphonic (CM). (From American Speech-Language-Hearing Association. (1988). The short latency auditory evoked potentials: A tutorial paper by the Working Group on Auditory Evoked Potential Measurements of the Committee on Audiologic Evaluation. Washington, DC: ASHA, p. 9, with permission. Based on data from Coats, A. C. (1981). The summating potential and Meniere's disease. Archives of Otolaryngology, 104, 199–208 .)

and description of ECochG recording approaches is presented in the Recording Techniques section of this chapter.

The technical capability to record cochlear and auditory nerve potentials in humans has led to a variety of clinical applications for ECochG, including the following:

♦ Diagnosis/assessment/monitoring of Meniere's disease/ endolymphatic hydrops (MD/ELH) and the assessment/ monitoring of treatment strategies for these disorders

♦ Enhancement of wave I of the ABR

♦ Measurement and monitoring of cochlear and auditory nerve function during surgery involving the auditory periphery

♦ Diagnosis of auditory neuropathy/dys-synchrony

Although other uses for ECochG have been described, the above four applications appear to be the most clinically popular ones at the time of this writing and will therefore receive the majority of attention in this chapter. The intention here is to provide background information and reference material for the practitioner who currently uses ECochG in the laboratory, clinic, and/or operating room, or is interested in doing so.

♦ Salient Features of the Cochlear Microphonic, Cochlear Summating Potential, and Action Potential

Detailed descriptions of the CM, SP, and AP are abundant in the hearing science literature and beyond the scope of this chapter. The reader is encouraged to review this literature to gain a better understanding and appreciation of the specific features of these potentials and their relevance to hearing function. Indeed, this knowledge is essential to the clinical application of ECochG. The following section summarizes the salient features of the CM, SP, and AP, especially with reference to their recording in humans.

Cochlear Microphonic

At least in animals, the CM is perhaps the most thoroughly investigated inner ear potential. However, as a clinical tool in humans, the SP and AP have received more attention than the CM. The historical popularity of the CM in the laboratory has been facilitated by the relative ease with which it can be recorded and its considerable magnitude compared with other electrical phenomena associated with hearing. These features are not necessarily helpful for human recordings, however, in part because of the CM's characteristics. That is, the CM is an alternating current (AC) voltage that tends to mirror the waveform of the acoustic stimulus. This feature makes it difficult to separate true CM from stimulus artifact in clinical, noninvasive recordings. In addition, the effectiveness of the CM in the differential diagnosis of inner ear/auditory nerve disorders has yet to be established because changes in this component tend to reflect general, as opposed to specific, cochlear pathology.

The current inadequacy of the CM as a clinical tool may be more attributable to our incomplete understanding of its specific features than to the features themselves. For a time, the CM was considered to be primarily a by-product of cochlear processing. It is now thought that the CM may provide the input to the motor activity of the organ of Corti's outer hair cells (Evans and Dallos, 1993) and represent the generator potential for the inner hair cells (Dallos, 1997).

Newer knowledge about the CM may expand its usefulness in the clinic. For example, Bian and Chertoff (1998) derived indices of mechanical to electrical transduction from the CM. Some of the indices were able to distinguish between cochlear pathologies even though auditory thresholds were similar. These findings suggest that new analytic approaches to quantifying the CM may prove useful in the differential diagnosis of inner ear pathology. In addition, it has long been known that measurement of cochlear potentials at the round window (the most dominant component of which is the CM) in animals is sensitive to changes in middle ear transmission characteristics (Gerhardt et al, 1979; Guinan and Peake, 1967). This feature may prove useful for intraoperative monitoring and predicting outcome for patients undergoing middle ear surgery.

The mysteries of cochlear transduction processes are being unraveled at a rapid pace. In addition, the noninvasive techniques for recording the bioelectrical events associated with these processes are becoming more sensitive. As new knowledge and technology in this area are applied to humans, the CM will most assuredly assume a more prominent role in clinical ECochG. A vivid example of this prediction is the very recent use of the CM in the diagnosis of auditory neuropathy/auditory dys-synchrony, which has evolved since the first edition of this textbook. The current chapter has been amended to include a discussion of this application (see Clinical Applications section).

Cochlear Summating Potential

The SP is a complex response that comprises several components. Like the CM, the SP is stimulus-related and generated by the hair cells of the organ of Corti. Also like the CM, the SP is a reflection of the displacement-time pattern of the cochlear partition. Whereas the CM reflects the stimulus waveform, however, the SP displays a rectified, direct current (DC) version of this pattern more representative of the stimulus envelope (Dallos, 1973). The SP manifests itself as a shift in the CM baseline, the direction (or polarity) of which is dictated by an interactive effect between stimulus parameters (i.e., frequency and intensity) and the location of the recording electrode. The relationship between the CM and SP waveforms is illustrated in **Fig. 19–2**. When recorded extratympanically (i.e., from the TM or ear canal), the SP is often seen as a downward (negative) deflection that persists for the duration of the acoustic stimulus.

Because of its complexity, the SP is probably the least understood cochlear potential, and its role in hearing function remains unclear. However, as a DC response to an AC stimulus, the SP is thought to represent the sum of various nonlinearities associated with transduction processes in the cochlea (Dallos et al, 1972). Thus, the magnitude of the SP may be a reflection of the amount of distortion that accompanies or is produced by these processes. This characteristic has made the SP useful for certain clinical conditions. In particular, it is now well documented that the ECochGms of patients with MD/ELH often display SPs that are enlarged in comparison to the SPs of normal-hearing subjects, or patients with cochlear disorders other than MD/ELH (Coats, 1981; Dauman et al, 1986; Ferraro and Krishnan, 1997;

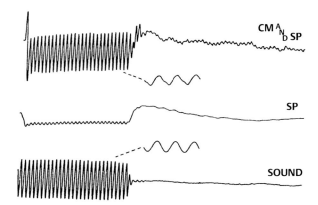

Figure 19–2 Relationship among the waveforms of the acoustic stimulus (sound) and resultant cochlear microphonic (CM) and summating potential (SP). Insets show details of the CM and sound tracings via an expanded time base. (From Durrant, J. D. (1981). Auditory physiology and an auditory physiologist's view of tinnitus. Journal of Laryngology and Otology, 4(Suppl.), 21–28, with permission.)

Ferraro et al, 1983; Gibson et al, 1977). Conventional rationale for this finding is that an increase in endolymph volume creates additional distortion within the system, which is reflected in the SP. Whether the nature of this increased distortion is mechanical (Gibson et al, 1977) and/or electrical (Durrant and Dallos, 1974) has not been resolved, and other factors such as biochemical and/or vascular changes may also be responsible for an enlarged SP. Regardless of the specific pathophysiology, measurement of the SP to help diagnose, assess, and monitor MD/ELH has emerged as a primary application for modern-day ECochG.

Action Potential

The AP recorded via ECochG represents the summed response of several thousand auditory nerve fibers that have fired in synchrony. When evoked by click stimuli, the term *whole nerve AP* is sometimes applied because, theoretically, the "square" waveform of the click has a flat spectrum that contains all frequencies and therefore stimulates the entire basilar membrane. A stimulus with a narrower bandwidth, such as a tone burst, excites a more limited segment of the membrane to produce a "compound AP." In reality, although both of the above describers for the AP can be misleading, "whole nerve," in particular, is a true misnomer because the spectrum of the acoustic click that reaches the cochlea is far from flat and substantially narrower in bandwidth than the spectrum of the electrical pulse driving the transducer. Furthermore, synchronicity of neural firings is essential to producing a well-defined AP. Maximum synchrony, in turn, occurs at the onset of the stimulus, even for tone bursts. If this onset is abrupt, the response will be dominated by neural contributions from the basal, high-frequency end of the normal cochlea (Kiang, 1965). Thus, the entire nerve is not excited in response to click stimuli, nor is the segment of the basilar membrane excited by tonal stimuli necessarily limited to that which codes for the signal's frequency.

The AP, like the CM (or unlike the SP), is an AC voltage. However, unlike either of the cochlear potentials whose waveforms reflect the displacement-time pattern of the cochlear partition, the AP waveform is characterized by a series of brief, predominantly negative peaks representative of the pattern of resultant neural firings. At suprathreshold stimulus levels, the first and largest of these peaks is referred to as N_1. N_1 is virtually the same component as wave I of the ABR and, as such, arises from the distal portion of the auditory nerve (Moller and Janetta, 1983). AP peaks beyond N_1 (e.g., N_2 and N_3) are analogous to corresponding ABR components (i.e., waves II and III) but have received little if any clinical attention in ECochG.

For clinical purposes, the most useful features of the AP relate to its amplitude and latency. The former is a reflection of the number of nerve fibers firing. However, because the afferent fibers of the auditory nerve primarily innervate the inner hair cells (Spoendlin, 1966), AP amplitude also can be viewed as a reflection of inner hair cell output. AP latency represents the time between stimulus onset and the peak of N_1. This measure is analogous to the "absolute latency" for ABR components and incorporates stimulus travel time from the output of the transducer to the inner ear, traveling wave propagation time along the basilar membrane, and the time associated with the synchronization of neural impulses that produce the AP peaks. As with all waves of the ABR, reductions in signal intensity at suprathreshold levels for the AP are accompanied by changes in the N_1, including amplitude reduction leading to eventual disappearance into the electrical noise floor and latency prolongation.

Since its initial recording in humans in 1960, the AP has been the most widely studied component of the ECochGm. Early interest in the AP, however, was directed toward the development of an electrophysiological index of hearing status in children (Cullen et al, 1972). This effort was overshadowed by the advent of the ABR for such purposes, primarily because wave V of the ABR appeared to be more sensitive and easier to measure than the AP-N_1. As AEP applications and technology have evolved over the years, the use of the AP to assess and monitor cochlear and auditory nerve function has received renewed attention, especially in surgical settings. In addition, the use of a combined AP-ABR approach for assessing

retrocochlear status in hard-of-hearing subjects is gaining popularity. Currently, perhaps the most popular application of the AP involves the measurement of its amplitude in comparison to that of the SP in patients suspected of having MD/ELH. As described earlier, an enlarged SP often characterizes the ECochGms of patients with MD/ELH. The clinical consistency of this finding, however, improves considerably when the SP amplitude is compared with the amplitude of N_1 to form the SP/AP amplitude ratio (Coats, 1981; Eggermont, 1976). It is widely reported that an enlarged SP/AP amplitude ratio to click stimuli is a positive ECochG finding for ELH.

◆ Administering Electrocochleography

Recording Techniques: Transtympanic versus Extratympanic

As mentioned in the opening of this chapter, there are two general approaches for recording ECochG: transtympanic and extratympanic. TT ECochG is an invasive procedure that involves passing a needle electrode through the TM to rest on the cochlear promontory. During surgeries that expose the middle ear space, TT recordings can also be made with a ball electrode on the round window via the surgical field. Needle and ball electrodes used for TT ECochG are shown in **Figure 19–3**. ET recordings are performed with an electrode resting against the skin of the ear canal or surface of the TM. For the latter recording site, the procedure is also referred to as tympanic (or TM) ECochG (Ferraro and Ferguson, 1989), even though this approach is still considered to be ET. Although ET ECochG can be performed using a needle electrode in the skin of the ear canal, this option is rarely, if ever, chosen. Therefore, virtually all ET recordings tend to be noninvasive. Four examples of ET electrodes are shown in **Fig. 19–4**.

Both TT and ET approaches to ECochG have advantages and disadvantages. The primary advantage of the TT approach is the close proximity of the recording electrode to the response generators. This "near field" situation produces large components with relatively little signal averaging.

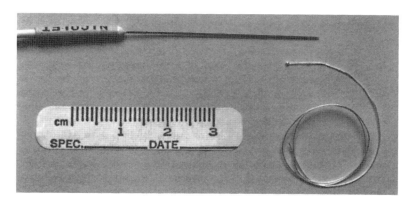

Figure 19–3 Needle (promontory placement) and ball-tipped (round window placement) electrodes used for transtympanic electrocochleography.

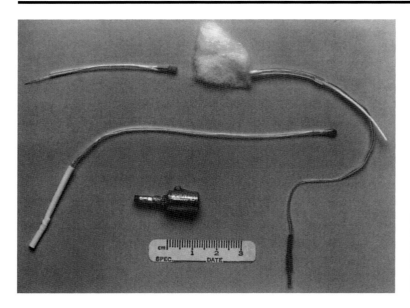

Figure 19–4 Electrodes used for extratympanic electrocochleography: Modified (and home-made) version of Stypulkowski-Staller tymptrode (top left), Lilly wick electrode (top right), and Bio-logic Systems Corp. (Mundelein, IL) ECochGtrode (middle) are placed at the surface of the tympanic membrane. Etymotic Research Inc. (Elk Grove, IL). Gold-foil TIP-trode (bottom) rests in the outer portion of the ear canal.

Pitfall

- The major limitations of TT ECochG relate to its invasiveness. Such procedures require the assistance of a physician and are therefore limited to a medical setting. In addition, penetrating the TM with a needle is not accomplished without some degree of pain/discomfort to the patient, even when local anesthetics are used. These disadvantages certainly have limited the use of TT ECochG in the United States.

By comparison, ECochG responses recorded from ET sites require more signal averaging and tend to be smaller in amplitude than their counterparts measured from the promontory or round window.

The biggest advantage associated with ET approaches is that they can be performed in nonmedical settings with minimal to no discomfort for the patient. This latter condition also obviates the need for sedation/local anesthesia. By virtue of these advantages, ET ECochG is becoming increasingly popular among audiologists and even physicians who perform this test. Another factor that has contributed to the growing popularity of ET ECochG relates to advances in electrode design (discussed in the following section) and the practice of using the TM as a recording site. The TM offers a practical compromise between ear canal and TT placements with respect to component amplitudes and signal averaging time (Ferraro, Blackwell, et al, 1994; Ferraro, Thedinger, et al, 1994; Ruth et al, 1988; Schoonhoven et al, 1995). In addition, the waveform features essential to interpreting the TT ECochGm tend to be preserved in TM recordings (Ferraro, Thedinger, et al, 1994).

Pitfall

- Unfortunately, placement of an electrode on the highly sensitive TM can sometimes result in more patient discomfort than is customary for other, noninvasive ET approaches (but certainly not as much as is usually associated with TT ECochG).

Controversial Point

- Given the advantages and disadvantages of both approaches, the decision to perform ET or TT ECochG often depends on the traditional practices, personnel, and attitudes of the clinic. Obviously, TT recordings are dependent on the availability of a physician who has the time and interest to perform the examination. Although a physician is not needed for ET ECochG, placing an electrode on the TM is certainly a more delicate maneuver than attaching surface electrodes to the scalp or resting them in the ear canal. With proper instruction and materials, however, this procedure is easily learned and well within the scope of professional practice for audiologists.

Recording Parameters

Selection of recording parameters for ECochG will vary according to the components of interest. Because these components generally occur within a latency epoch of 5 msec following stimulus onset, they can be considered to be in the family of early- or short-latency AEPs (Picton et al, 1974). They are, in fact, the earliest (shortest) members of this family. As relatives, ECochG components and the ABR can be recorded using similar parameters. A notable

Table 19–1 Electrocochleography Recording Parameters

Electrode Array

Primary (+)	Ear canal/tympanic membrane/ promontory/round window
Secondary (−)	Contralateral earlobe/mastoid process/ear canal
Common	Nasion/ipsilateral earlobe

Signal Averaging Settings

Time base	5–10 msec
Amplification factor	50,000–100,000 times (ET) 5000–25,000 times (TT)
Bandpass filter	5–3000 Hz
Repetitions	1000–1500 (ET) 100–200 (TT)

Stimuli

Type	BBC, TB
Duration (BBC)	100 μs electrical pulse
Envelope (TB)	2 msec linear rise/fall, 5–10 msec plateau
Polarity	Rarefaction and condensation (BBC), alternating (TB)
Repetition rate	11.3/second
Level	85 dB HL (115 dB pe SPL)

BBC, broadband click; ET, extratympanic; HL, hearing level; pe SPL, peak equivalent sound pressure level; TB, tone burst; TT, transtympanic.

exception occurs in the selection of the bandpass of the preamplifier for ECochG when the SP is of interest. That is, the high-pass filter setting must be close to zero to accommodate a DC component. Other differences between ECochG and ABR recording parameters involve the electrode array and the number of samples to be averaged. For ECochG, the latter is dependent on the choice of recording approaches, with TT requiring considerably fewer repetitions than ET. **Table 19–1** illustrates suitable parameters for recording the SP and AP together, which are the components of interest when ECochG is used in the diagnosis of MD/ELH. A description of these parameters with rationale is provided later in the chapter.

Electrode Array

Many clinicians/researchers use an electrode array that displays the AP as a downward (negative) deflection. To accomplish this task, the primary electrode, that is, the electrode connected to the (+) noninverted input of the differential preamplifier, should rest in the ear canal, or on the TM, promontory, or round window (depending on the choice of ET or TT recording approaches). Sites for the secondary (−) electrode include the vertex of the scalp, high forehead, or contralateral earlobe or mastoid process.

Pearl

- We prefer the earlobe or mastoid as the secondary (−) electrode site for ECochG simply because electrodes tend to be easier to attach and secure to these sites.

Choices for "ground" or "common" sites include the nasion and ipsilateral earlobe or mastoid. Reversing the + and − inputs to the preamplifier shifts the polarity of the ECochGm by 180 degrees. This array would display the AP-N_1 as a positive peak, which might be preferable for comparisons to conventional ABR recordings.

It often is the case that the test battery for a given patient includes both ECochG and measurement of the ABR. These recordings can be accomplished using five electrodes: a TM electrode (because our choice is TM ECochG) and surface electrodes attached to both earlobes (or mastoid processes), the high forehead (or vertex), and nasion. A common electrode configuration for this approach is TM (+)-to-contralateral earlobe (−) for ECochG, and high forehead or vertex (+)-to-ipsilateral earlobe (−) for ABR, with the common electrode at the nasion for both arrays.

Time Base

As indicated earlier in the chapter, ECochG components represent the earliest voltage changes to occur in the ear in response to acoustic stimulation. For brief transient stimuli such as clicks, the time base (or signal averaging window) must therefore be set to capture the electrophysiological activity occurring within the first few milliseconds following stimulus onset. For click stimuli, a time base of 10 msec allows for visualization of the ABR components that follow N_1. For longer duration stimuli such as tone bursts, the time base should extend beyond the duration of the stimulus envelope so that the entire response is observable within the averaging window (remember that both the SP and CM persist for the duration of the stimulus). For example, a 20 msec window could be used if the stimulus were a 1000 Hz tone burst with a 2-cycle rise/fall time and a 10-cycle plateau (i.e., a 14 msec envelope).

Amplification Factor

Preamplification is applied to help maximize the signal-to-noise ratio for a given recording condition. The amount of amplification needed for suitable recordings of the SP and/or AP for ET measurements generally ranges between 50,000 and 100,000 times, whereas the factor for TT recordings can be 5 to 10 times smaller. In part, selection of this parameter is based on the level of the electrical noise floor, which incorporates several elements (e.g., myogenic and electroencephalographic activity, electrical artifact from the equipment, and/or testing environment). The sensitivity setting of the signal averager's analog-to-digital converter also must be taken into account. Thus, amplification/sensitivity settings may vary from laboratory to laboratory and also among evoked potential units from different manufacturers. However, the manipulation of these variables to provide settings appropriate to recording conditions is easily accomplished in most commercial instruments.

Bandpass Filter

As mentioned earlier, when the SP is of interest, the bandpass of the preamplifier filter must be wide enough to allow for the amplification of a DC component. To record the SP-AP complex, the bandpass must also include the fundamental frequency of the AP, which is ~1000 Hz.

Pitfall

- Recording the SP and AP together presents a dilemma in that the amplification systems generally employed for ECochG are not designed for DC signals. Thus, the selection of a bandpass to accommodate both the SP and AP represents a compromise that introduces some degree of distortion to both components.

When using such a wide bandpass, the DC (SP) component is frequency filtered, and recording of the AC (AP) component may be distorted by the presence of low-frequency noise.

Pearl

- Practically speaking, the click-evoked SP tolerates a certain degree of filtering because it is a brief duration transient and therefore not a true DC component (Durrant and Ferraro, 1991).

Repetitions

In general, the number of stimulus repetitions needed to evoke a well-defined ECochGm will vary with recording conditions and also the subject's degree of hearing loss. The former depends on the recording approach, with TT ECochG requiring considerably fewer averages than ET ECochG does. For subjects with hearing loss in the 1000 to 4000 Hz range, more repetitions may be necessary than usually needed for normal-hearing subjects or those with low-frequency losses.

Special Consideration

- When sensorineural hearing loss in the mid- to high frequencies exceeds 50 to 60 dB HL, the use of ECochG recorded from the TM or other ET sites to help diagnose or assess MD/ELH is questionable.

The basis for the preceding special consideration is that hearing losses of this magnitude generally involve (i.e., reduce the output of) the population of hair cells that produce the ECochGm. On the other hand, when hearing loss of similar or greater magnitude precludes the identification of wave I in the presence of wave V in the conventionally recorded ABR, ECochG can be very useful. Ferraro and Ferguson (1989), for example, have shown that the AP-N_1 is usually recordable under such conditions and can be substituted for ABR wave I to determine the I–V interwave interval.

Stimuli

As mentioned earlier, the broadband click tends to be the most popular stimulus for short-latency AEPs because it excites synchronous discharges from a large population of neurons to produce well-defined peaks. In addition, 100 μs is a popular choice for the duration of the driving rectangular pulse because the first spectral null for a click of this duration occurs at 10,000 Hz (i.e., 0.01 μs). Thus, the signal theoretically contains equal energy at all frequencies below this value. In reality, the frequency range of the transducer is usually lower than 10,000 Hz, and the outer and middle ears filter the acoustic signal further. As described earlier in this chapter, the spectrum of the acoustic signal reaching the cochlea is not flat, nor as wide as 10,000 Hz.

Pitfall

Unfortunately, the brevity of the click makes it a less than ideal stimulus for studying cochlear potentials.

Because the duration of both the CM and SP are stimulus dependent, both components appear only as brief deflections when evoked by clicks (**Fig. 19–1**). Despite this limitation, the use of clicks has proven to be very effective in evoking the SP-AP complex for certain ECochG applications, even though the duration of the SP is abbreviated under these conditions (Durrant and Ferraro, 1991).

Although the click continues to remain popular, several studies have also advocated the use of tonal stimuli for ECochG (Ferraro, Blackwell, et al, 1994; Ferraro, Thedinger, et al, 1994; Levine et al, 1992; Margolis et al, 1995). Tonal stimuli generally provide for a higher degree of frequency specificity than clicks. This feature can be useful for monitoring cochlear status in progressive disorders (such as MD/ELH) where hearing is usually not affected at all frequencies during the initial stages. In addition, the use of extended-duration stimuli, such as tone bursts, improves the visualization of the SP and CM (Durrant and Ferraro, 1991).

Pitfall

A problem related to the use of tonal stimuli for ECochG (and other AEPs) is the lack of standardization regarding stimulus parameters.

Most studies employ tone bursts of only one or two frequencies; stimulus envelopes are different, and there is no standardized approach to defining stimulus intensity. These inconsistencies make it difficult to compare data across laboratories/clinics. For tone bursts, we prefer an envelope with a linear rise–fall time of 2 msec and a 10 msec plateau. Shorter plateaus (e.g., 5 msec) can sometimes be used to avoid interference by ABR components (Levine et al, 1992).

Stimulus polarity relates to the initial deflection of the transducer diaphragm and is an important factor for ECochG. Presenting clicks or tone bursts in alternating polarity inhibits the presence of recorded signals that are phase-locked to the stimulus, such as stimulus artifact and CM. The former can sometimes be large enough to obscure early ECochG components, and the latter generally overshadows both the SP and AP. Thus, the use of alternating polarity stimuli is preferable if the SP amplitude and SP/AP amplitude ratio are measurements of interest, such as when ECochG is used in the diagnosis of MD/ELH. On the other hand, several studies have now shown that recording separate responses to condensation and rarefaction clicks may provide useful clinical information. In particular, certain subjects with MD/ELH display abnormal latency differences between AP-N_1 latencies to condensation versus rarefaction clicks (Levine et al, 1992; Margolis et al, 1995; Orchik et al, 1997).

Controversial Point

- What is the appropriate polarity for delivering click stimuli? In deference to the studies described above, measurement of separate responses to condensation and rarefaction clicks should be used to assess the AP-N1 latency difference. These responses can be added together off-line to derive the SP amplitude and SP/AP amplitude ratio.

For ECochG, as with most signal-averaged AEPs, it is important that the cochlear/neural response to one stimulus be complete before the next stimulus is presented. For click-evoked, short-latency AEPs, this requirement allows for considerable latitude in the selection of the stimulus repetition rate. However, increasing this rate beyond 10 to 30 per second may cause some adaptation of the AP. Rates on the order of 100 per second cause maximal suppression of the AP while leaving the SP relatively unaffected. Gibson et al (1977) and Coats (1981) applied this approach to maximize visualization of the SP. Unfortunately, the use of very fast stimulus repetition rates has not proven to be very successful in the clinic, in part because the AP contribution is not completely eliminated, and the SP may also be reduced. In addition, rapid clicks presented at loud levels tend to be annoying to patients.

When ECochG is performed to help diagnose MD/ELH, the signal should be intense enough to evoke a well-defined SP-AP complex. For this application, stimulus presentation should begin at a level near the maximum output of the stimulus generator. Unfortunately, as mentioned earlier, there is a lack of standardization for AEP stimuli regarding signal calibration and dB reference. Common references include dB hearing level (HL, or hearing threshold level [HTL], or normalized hearing level [nHL]), dB sensation level (SL), and dB peak equivalent sound pressure level (pe SPL). As in conventional audiometry, dB HL is based on the mean behavioral threshold of a group of hearing subjects with normal hearing, whereas dB SL is the number of decibels above an individual threshold. Decibel pe SPL is determined by matching the SPL of a transient signal to that of a continuous sinusoid and therefore represents the only physical measure of intensity of the three common references. It may be necessary to calibrate ECochG signals in both HL and pe SPL. The average behavioral threshold of a group of normal-hearing subjects to the various stimuli used for ECochG (e.g., clicks and tone bursts) is represented in dB HL. For dB pe SPL, an oscilloscope is used to match the level of the click to that of a 1000 Hz continuous sinusoid. Consistent with the findings of Stapells et al (1982), 0 dB HL for clicks corresponds to ~30 dB pe SPL.

Pearl

- Masking of the contralateral ear is usually not a concern for conventional ECochG since the magnitude of any electrophysiological response from the non-test ear is very small. In addition, ECochG components are generated prior to crossover of the auditory pathway.

A final note regarding stimuli relates to stimulus artifact, which can be quite large for ECochG because of the nature of ET (especially TM) electrodes. These wire devices also serve as antennae that are very receptive to electromagnetic radiation from the transducer and other electrical sources in the environment. The following suggestions are offered to help reduce stimulus artifact:

- Use a tubal insert transducer.
- Separate the transducer from the electrode cables as much as possible.
- Braid the electrode cables.
- Test subjects in a shielded sound booth with the examiner and AEP unit located outside the booth.
- Plug the AEP unit into an isolated socket equipped with a true-earth ground.
- Use a grounded cable for the primary electrode (such cables are commercially available).
- Turn off the lights in the testing room, and unplug unnecessary electronic equipment (it also may be necessary to turn off the lights in the examiner's room).
- Consider encasing the transducer in grounded mu metal shielding.

We have found the above guidelines to be particularly important when attempting to record the CM for the purpose of diagnosing auditory neuropathy/auditory dyssynchrony (to be discussed in more detail later).

Preparing for Electrocochleography

Selection of Recording Approach

As described in the previous section, the selection of recording approaches to ECochG generally depends on reasons related to the traditional practices and attitudes of the clinic as well as the availability of qualified personnel to perform the examination.

Pitfall

- Unfortunately, a factor that usually is not considered in the selection of ET versus TT approaches is the attitude of the patient.

Given an informed choice (i.e., an explanation of options with advantages and disadvantages of each), most patients will select ET ECochG for obvious reasons. Taking all of the above factors into account, the approach to ECochG in many clinics is limited exclusively to ET methods even though personnel and resources may be available to perform TT recordings.

Pearl

- Virtually all ET recordings in the author's clinic/laboratory are made from the TM because of the advantages this site offers over other ET locations (i.e., along the ear canal).

The benefits TM ECochG offers over other ET approaches include increased component amplitudes, more stable/repeatable responses, and reduced testing time because less signal averaging is needed (Ferraro and Ferguson, 1989; Ruth et al, 1988; Stypulkowski and Staller, 1987). Given our preference for TM ECochG, the following information emphasizes this particular approach.

Instructions to the Patient

Most patients are unfamiliar with ECochG and confused as to what it is, why they need it, and how it will be performed. The term *electrocochleography* sometimes adds to this confusion. Instructions to the patient can begin on the way to the testing room with an assurance that the procedure is noninvasive and painless, and will take ~1 hour. They can even sleep through it if they wish. Engaging patients in conversation at this point and watching them walk also provides some insight regarding their hearing and balance status. Once in the sound booth, the patient rests in a supine position on a reclining chair (reclined to the maximum) that provides good support for the whole body, especially the head, neck, and upper back. Eyeglasses and/or earrings are removed (usually by the patient), and food, chewing gum, candy, and so on must be swallowed or discarded. When the patient is comfortable and attentive, ECochG is described as a method for recording the electrical responses of the inner ear to click-type sounds. It also helps to explain that his or her doctor has requested this examination to assess whether or not too much fluid in the inner ear is the cause for the symptoms. The patient is then informed that surface electrodes will be attached to the scalp,

a small, cotton-tipped electrode will be inserted along the ear canal to rest on the TM, and an earplug will be used to hold the electrode in place and deliver the clicks.

Special Consideration

- Patients should be cautioned that the TM electrode might feel strange and may even be a little uncomfortable, but that it should not be particularly painful.

The procedures for preparing the skin and placing the surface electrodes are described while performing these tasks (for more detailed instructions on how to prepare the skin for surface electrodes, see Ferraro, 1997). Otoscopy is performed before inserting the TM electrode to assess the patency of the ear canal and appearance of the TM. Cerumen removal may be necessary to visualize the TM and clear a pathway along the ear canal large enough for the electrode. Once the surface electrodes have been placed and otoscopy performed, the TM electrode can be constructed and placed.

Special Consideration

If either the ear canal or TM appears abnormal or damaged, ECochG should not be performed, and the referring physician should be notified of such conditions.

Construction of the Tympanic Membrane Electrode (Tymptrode)

The photograph of ET electrodes in **Fig. 19–4** includes the tymptrode (originally described by Stypulkowski and Staller, 1987, and modified by Ferraro and Ferguson, 1989), the Lilly wick electrode (Lilly and Black, 1989), and the TM-ECochGtrode manufactured by Bio-logic Systems Corp. (Mundelein, IL). The latter two electrodes are commercially available. The tymptrode can be fabricated using "store bought" materials, such as those listed here (see Ferraro, 1992, 1997):

- Medical-grade silicon (Silastic) tubing (0.058 inch inner diameter, 0.077 inch outer diameter)
- Teflon-insulated silver wire (0.008 inch bare diameter, 0.011 inch insulated diameter)
- Soft cotton (until recently, the author used foam rubber for the electrode tip, as pictured in **Fig. 19–4**, but now uses cotton, which is more comfortable for the patient)
- Electrode gel (not paste or cream)
- Fine, needle-nosed forceps
- A 1 cc disposable tuberculin syringe with needle
- Copper microalligator clip soldered to the end of an electrode cable

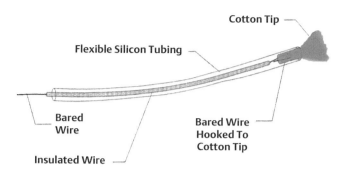

Figure 19–5 Construction of the tymptrode.

Briefly, the procedure for constructing the tymptrode involves cutting the wire and tubing into segments a few centimeters longer than the ear canal, with the wire ~2 cm longer than the tubing. The fine forceps are used to scrape the insulation off both ends of the wire (a crucial step), which is then threaded through the tubing. One end of the wire protruding from the tubing remains bare; the other end is hooked to the end of a small plug (~2 × 3 mm) of soft cotton. Once again using the fine forceps, the end of the cotton plug hooked to the wire is tucked into the tubing, leaving a small portion of the cotton protruding from the tip. **Figure 19–5** is a labeled drawing of a tymptrode constructed as described here. Tymptrodes, at this stage, can be fabricated and stockpiled for indefinite periods of time. Immediately prior to use, the cotton tip of the tymptrode must be impregnated with electrode gel. This step is accomplished by filling the tuberculin syringe with gel and injecting the entire piece of cotton until it is thoroughly saturated (including that portion of the cotton within the tubing attached to the wire). Attach the microalligator clip of the electrode cable to the other (bare) end of the wire, and the tymptrode is ready for insertion.

Pearl

- Both ears should be tested, even if unilateral disease is suspected. Comparison between affected and unaffected sides can provide important diagnostic information. The affected side should be tested first in case the patient becomes restless as the examination progresses.

Placing the Tymptrode

To gain the assistance of gravity when placing the tymptrode, the patient is instructed to gently roll over onto his or her side so that the test ear is facing up. The tymptrode is then inserted into the entrance of the ear canal and gently advanced (by hand or using the fine forceps) until the gelled, cotton tip makes contact with the TM. The latter is confirmed via otoscopy and electrophysiological monitoring. It also helps to ask the patient when he or she feels the electrode touching the TM.

Pitfall

- Even with an otoscope, it is sometimes difficult to actually see the point of contact between the tymptrode tip and the TM.

Pearl

Monitoring the electrophysiological noise floor during electrode placement helps to achieve proper contact with the TM.

As the electrode is being advanced into the ear canal, the raw electroencephalogram (EEG)/noise floor is displayed on-screen. Large, spurious, and cyclic or peak-clipped voltages (i.e., an open-line situation) characterize this electrical activity. When proper contact of the tymptrode tip with the TM is achieved, the noise floor drops dramatically and becomes more stable. Using both visual and electrophysiological monitoring provides the best opportunity for achieving proper contact with the TM on the first try.

Once the tymptrode is in contact with the TM, the foam tip of the sound delivery tube is compressed and inserted into the ear canal alongside the tymptrode tubing.

Special Consideration

- Care must be taken during this stage to not push the electrode farther against the TM when inserting the earplug, as this can cause some discomfort to the patient. However, the tymptrode is relatively soft and flexible, which allows the tip to compress or bend at the TM rather than penetrate the membrane.

Only a portion of the transducer earplug needs to be inserted into the canal to achieve proper stimulation for evoking the ECochGm. To minimize discomfort, we usually cut off a portion of the earplug (about one third), which makes it easier to insert without disturbing the tymptrode. **Figure 19–6** is a schematic representation of the tymptrode and sound delivery tube in the ear canal.

Interpreting an Electrocochleogram

As with most AEPs, measures of component amplitude and latency form the bases for interpreting the ECochGm. **Figure 19–7** depicts a normal ECochGm to click stimuli recorded from the TM. Stimulus level was 80 dB HL, and click polarity was alternated to favor the SP and AP at the expense of inhibiting the CM. Component amplitudes can be measured from peak to peak (left panel) or by using a baseline reference (right panel).

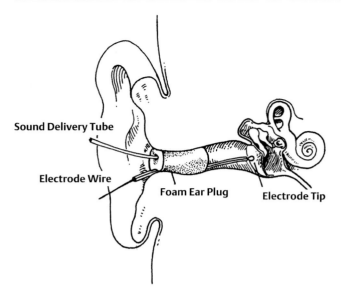

Figure 19–6 Illustration of the tymptrode in position and held in place by the foam ear tip of the sound delivery tube. (Adapted from Ferraro, J. A. (1992). Electrocochleography: How, Part I. Audiology Today, 4, 26–28, with permission.)

Controversial Point

- Should SP and AP amplitudes be measured from peak to peak or by using a baseline reference? The method of choice in our laboratory for TM and other ET approaches is peak to peak because of the considerable lability of the baseline amplitude for ET recordings. However, the choice of methods really does not matter as long as you are consistent within and between subjects, and normative values have been established for the method you have chosen.

Using peak-to-peak values from our laboratory, normal SP amplitudes measured at the TM using 80 dB HL clicks generally range from 0.1 to 1.0 μV s, with a mean of 0.4 μV. AP amplitudes can be as large as 5.0 μV, although our mean value is ~2.0 μV. AP-N_1 latency is measured from stimulus onset to the peak of N_1 and, as mentioned earlier in this chapter, should be identical to the latency of ABR wave I. At 80 dB HL, normal N_1 latencies generally range from 1.3 to 1.7 msec, with a mean of ~1.5 msec. These values have been corrected for the 0.9 msec delay attributable to stimulus travel time through the sound tube of the tubal insert transducer. Although labeled in **Fig. 19–7**, N_2 has received little interest for ECochG applications.

Also as shown in **Fig. 19–7**, SP and AP amplitudes are made from the leading edge of both components. The resultant values are used to derive the SP/AP amplitude ratio, which is a key measure when ECochG is used to help diagnose and monitor MD/ELH. (Normal SP/AP amplitude ratios in our laboratory range from ~10 to 40%, with a mean value of 25%.)

Figure 19–8 depicts a normal electrocochleogram evoked by an 80 dB HL, 2000 Hz tone burst (2 msec rise/fall, 10 msec plateau, alternating polarity). As opposed to click-evoked responses where the SP appears as a small shoulder preceding the AP, the SP to tone bursts persists as long as the stimulus. The AP and its N_1, in turn, are seen at the onset of the response. SP amplitude is measured with reference to baseline amplitude at the midpoint of the waveform to minimize the influence of the AP. Thus, the polarity of the SP depends on whether the voltage at midpoint is above (positive SP) or below (negative SP) the baseline voltage. **Figure 19–9** illustrates tone burst SPs at several frequencies recorded from both the TM and promontory (TT) of the same normal-hearing subject. Note that for both recording approaches, the polarities of the SPs at 500 and 8000 Hz are slightly positive, whereas negative SPs are seen at 1, 2, and 4 kHz. This feature tends to vary across frequencies, recording approaches, and within and across subjects.

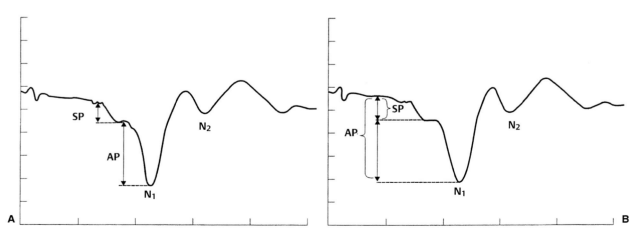

Figure 19–7 Normal electrocochleogram from the tympanic membrane to clicks presented in alternating polarity at 80 dB HL (hearing level). The amplitudes of the summating potential (SP) and action potential (AP) can be measured from peak-to-trough **(A)**, or with reference to a baseline value **(B)**. Amplitude/time scale is 1.25 μV/1 msec per gradation. Insert phone delay is 0.90 msec.

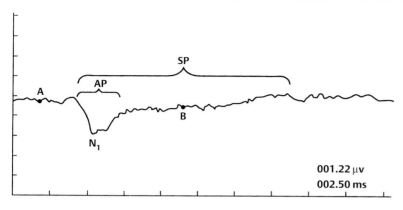

Figure 19–8 Normal electrocochleogram from the tympanic membrane to a 2000 Hz tone burst presented in alternating polarity at 80 dB HL (hearing level). Action potential (AP) and its first negative peak (N₁) is seen at the onset of the response. Summating potential (SP) persists as long as the stimulus. SP amplitude is measured at midpoint of response (point B), with reference to a baseline value (point A). Amplitude (microvolts)/time (milliseconds) scale at lower right. (From Ferraro, J. A., Blackwell, W., Mediavilla, S. J., & Thedinger, B. (1994). Normal summating potential to tone bursts recorded from the tympanic membrane in humans. Journal of the American Academy of Audiology, 5, 17–23, fig. p. 19, with permission.)

Pearl

- An important aspect illustrated in Fig. 19–9 is that the amplitudes of tone burst SPs are very small, which renders the actual polarity of the SP in normal listeners somewhat inconsequential.

Another noteworthy aspect of **Fig. 19–9** is that, although the magnitudes of the TM responses are approxi-

mately one quarter the size of the promontory responses (note amplitude scales), the corresponding patterns of the TM and TT recordings at each frequency are virtually identical.

In **Fig. 19–10**, mean SP amplitudes recorded from the TMs of 20 normal-hearing subjects are plotted as a function of tone burst frequency. All mean values are slightly positive and range between 0.10 and 0.22 μV. Standard deviations (SDs, indicated by the bars) are comparatively large and range from 0.18 to 0.22 across frequencies.

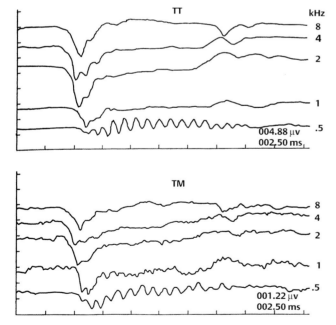

Figure 19–9 Electrocochleograms evoked by tone bursts of different frequencies presented at 80 dB HL (hearing level). Stimulus frequency in kilohertz indicated at the right of each waveform. Amplitude (microvolts)/time (milliseconds) scale at lower right. TM, tympanic membrane; TT, transtympanic. (From Ferraro, J. A., Blackwell, W., Mediavilla, S. J., & Thedinger, B. (1994). Normal summating potential to tone bursts recorded from the tympanic membrane in humans. Journal of the American Academy of Audiology, 5, 17–23, fig. p. 20, with permission.)

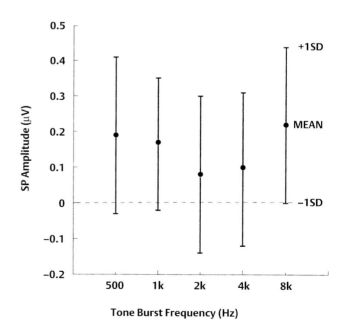

Figure 19–10 Mean summating potential (SP) amplitudes measured from the tympanic membrane of 20 normal ears as a function of tone burst frequency. Bars represent ± 1 standard deviation (SD). Stimulus level was 80 dB HL (hearing level). (From Ferraro, J. A., Blackwell, W., Mediavilla, S. J., & Thedinger, B. (1994). Normal summating potential to tone bursts recorded from the tympanic membrane in humans. Journal of the American Academy of Audiology, 5, 17–23, fig. p. 21, with permission.)

Pitfall

• Comparison of tone burst–ECochG data among studies is difficult at best due to a lack of consistency and standardization regarding such aspects as recording approach and parameters, measurement techniques, stimulus calibration, and selection of stimulus parameters. Unfortunately, this situation necessitates the establishment of laboratory/clinic-specific norms for tone burst data.

◆ Clinical Applications of the Electrocochleogram

Meniere's Disease/Endolymphatic Hydrops

Although much has been learned about MD (or idiopathic ELH) since its initial description in the literature over 135 years ago, the true pathophysiology of this disorder continues to elude us. As a result, neither a cure nor an effective treatment strategy that works for all patients has been developed. The symptoms upon which diagnosis of MD/ELH is based include recurrent, spontaneous vertigo, hearing loss, aural fullness, and tinnitus (Committee on Hearing and Equilibrium, American Academy of Otolaryngology–Head and Neck Surgery, 1995). However, the presence and severity of these symptoms tend to vary over time both among and within patients. The capricious nature of this disorder makes it difficult to diagnose and evaluate with a high degree of specificity and/or sensitivity.

As mentioned earlier in this chapter, ECochG has emerged as one of the more powerful tools in the diagnosis, assessment, and monitoring of MD/ELH, primarily through the measurement of the SP and AP. Examples of this application are shown in **Figs. 19–11** through **19–13**. The upper tracings in both **Figs. 19–11** (click-evoked ECochGms) and **19–12** (tone burst–evoked ECochGms) were measured from the promontory (TT), whereas the lower waveforms represent TM recordings. **Figure 19–13** displays TM tracings to tone bursts from the right (affected) and left (unaffected) sides of an MD/ELH patient. For the click-evoked ECochGms in **Fig. 19–11**, the SP/AP amplitude ratios (based on absolute SP and AP amplitudes) were ~1.0 and 2.0 for the TT and TM recordings, respectively. Both values are enlarged beyond the normal limits. Thus, despite different recording approaches that led to different values for the SP/AP amplitude ratio, both TT and TM ECochGms were positive for MD/ELH. Also notable in **Fig. 19–11** is the instability of the TM waveforms' baseline voltages compared with those of the TT recordings. As mentioned previously, this instability is the reason some clinicians prefer to measure absolute as opposed to baseline-referenced component amplitudes. Had the SP and AP amplitudes been measured with respect to a baseline voltage, SP/AP amplitude ratios would have been ~0.50 (TT) and 0.75 (TM).

As mentioned earlier in this chapter, the SP/AP amplitude ratio is a more consistent feature across and within subjects than the individual amplitudes of either component (Eggermont, 1976). Coats (1986), however, noted that this ratio does not represent a simple linear relationship. In normal patients, for example, fourfold increases in AP amplitude may be accompanied by twofold decreases in SP amplitude. This relationship is illustrated in **Fig. 19–14**, wherein SP amplitudes have been normalized to AP amplitudes to derive the 95% confidence interval of normal values (dashed line). Any SP/AP amplitude ratio above the confidence interval is considered to be abnormal.

SP amplitudes for the tone burst ECochGms in **Fig. 19–12** vary slightly across frequencies. However, a pronounced SP

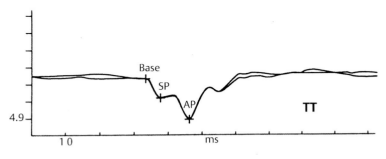

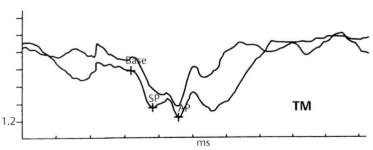

Figure 19–11 Abnormal responses to clicks recorded from the promontory (transtympanic) and tympanic membrane (TM) of the affected ear of the same patient. Both TT and TM responses display an enlarged summating potential (SP)/action potential (AP) amplitude ratio, which is a positive finding for endolymphatic hydrops. "Base" indicates reference for SP and AP amplitude measurements. Stimulus onset delayed by ~2 msec. (From Ferraro, J. A., Thedinger, B., Mediavilla, S. J., & Blackwell, W. (1994). Human summating potential to tone bursts: Observations on TM versus promontory recordings in the same patient. Journal of the American Academy of Audiology, 6, 217–224, fig. p. 27, with permission.)

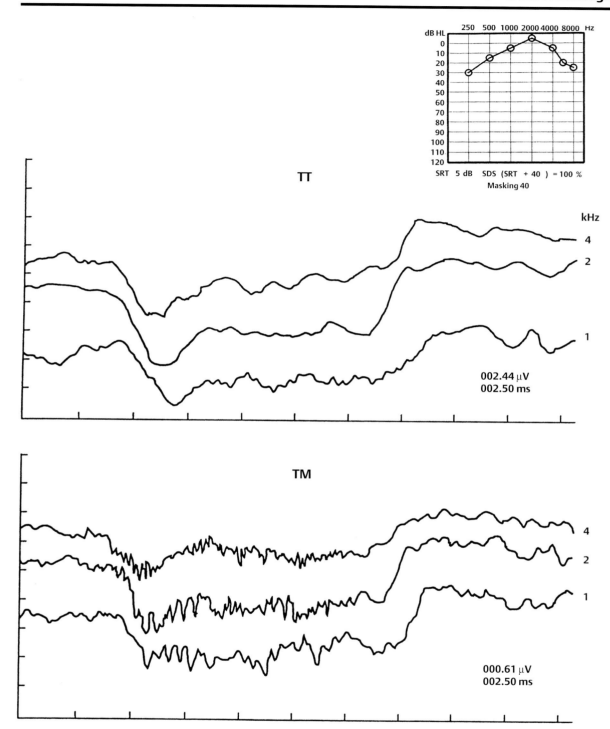

Figure 19–12 Abnormal responses to tone bursts recorded from the promontory (TT) and tympanic membrane (TM) of the affected ear of the same patient. All tracings show an enlarged summating potential trough, which is a positive finding for endolymphatic hydrops. Tone burst frequency in kilohertz indicated at the right of each tracing. Amplitude (microvolts)/time (milliseconds) scale at lower right. Pure-tone au-diogram at upper right. (From Ferraro, J. A., Thedinger, B., Mediavilla, S. J., & Blackwell, W. (1994). Human summating potential to tone bursts: Observations on TM versus promontory recordings in the same patient. Journal of the American Academy of Audiology, 6, 217–224, fig. p. 26, with permission.)

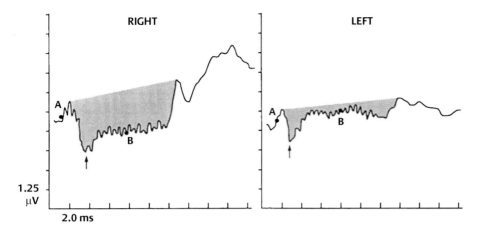

Figure 19–13 Comparison of TM electro-cochleograms between the affected (right) and unaffected (left) sides of a patient with endolymphatic hydrops. Stimulus was a 1000 Hz tone burst (2 msec rise/fall, 10 msec plateau) presented at 90 dB HL (hearing level). Shaded areas include the action potential and summating potential (SP) components. SP amplitude measured at point B with reference to point A. Arrows indicate AP-N_1. (From Ferraro, J. A. (1993). Electrocochleography: Clinical applications. Audiology Today, 5, 36–38, fig. p. 37, with permission.)

trough is seen at all frequencies and in all tracings, once again, regardless of recording approach. It also should be noted for tone burst responses that the measurement of interest is the magnitude of the SP trough rather than the SP/AP amplitude ratio. Indeed, the AP component to tone bursts may not even be visible in the face of an abnormally enlarged SP. As shown in **Fig. 19–13**, enlargement of the SP trough can be even more dramatic when the affected and unaffected sides are displayed together.

The reported incidence of an enlarged SP and SP/AP amplitude ratio in the general Meniere's population is only ~60 to 65% (Coats, 1981; Gibson et al, 1977) This situation makes the diagnostic utility of ECochG somewhat questionable, particularly for patients whose symptoms are not "classic" and for whom the clinical profile is unclear (Campbell et al, 1992). Thus, researchers continue to seek ways to improve the sensitivity of ECochG (i.e., the percentage of MD/ELH patients who display ECochGms that are positive for this disorder).

Pearl

- One way to make ECochG more sensitive is to test patients when they are experiencing symptoms of MD/ELH.

Ferraro et al (1985), for example, found positive ECochGms in over 90% of patients who were symptomatic at the time of testing and whose symptoms included aural fullness and hearing loss.

Pitfall

- Unfortunately, the practicality of testing patients when they are symptomatic is questionable, given the fluctuating nature of the disorder, especially in its early stages. In addition, many patients are unwilling or unable to complete an examination during a vertiginous attack.

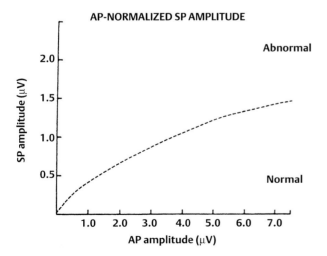

AP-NORMALIZED SP AMPLITUDE

Figure 19–14 Relationship between individual summating potential (SP) and action potential (AP) amplitudes to click stimuli. Dashed line represents 95% confidence limit for normal SP/AP amplitude ratio. (From Ferraro, J. A., & Ruth, R. A. (1994). Electrocochleography. In: J. Jacobson (Ed.), Auditory evoked potentials: Overview and basic principles (pp. 101–122). Boston: Allyn & Bacon, fig. p. 112, with permission.)

Other approaches to increasing the sensitivity of ECochG have been directed toward the parameters associated with recording and interpreting the ECochGm. An example of such a method involves measuring the AP-N_1 latency difference between responses to condensation versus rarefaction clicks (as described earlier in this chapter). **Figure 19–15** exemplifies this procedure. The AP-N_1 latency difference (LD) between clicks of opposite polarity for this MD/ELH patient was 0.75 msec. The upper limit of the LD in normal subjects from this study was 0.38 msec. The basis for comparing AP-N_1 latencies to clicks of opposite polarity relates to changes in the velocity of the traveling wave in an endolymph-loaded cochlea. That is, the up-and-down movement of the cochlear partition under such conditions may be abnormally restricted (or enhanced) in one direction over the other. If this condition occurs, the velocity of the traveling wave (on which the AP-N_1 latency is dependent) will differ if the initial movement of the cochlear partition is upwards (as with rarefaction clicks) versus downwards (as with condensation clicks).

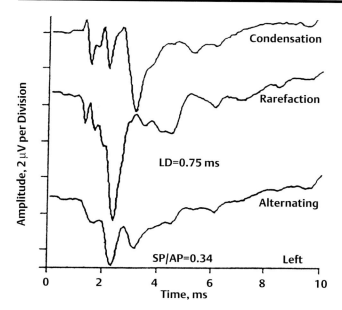

Figure 19–15 Electrocochleogram from a Meniere's patient evoked with condensation (top tracing) and rarefaction (middle tracing) polarity clicks. The latency difference of 0.75 msec between AP-N₁ components is a positive finding for endolymphatic hydrops because it is greater than 0.38 msec. This feature is obscured if the condensation and rarefaction tracings are combined to derive the response to alternating clicks (bottom tracing). AP, action potential; LD, latency difference; SP, summating potential. (From Margolis, R. H., Rieks, D., Fournier, M., Levine, S. M. (1995). Tympanic electrocochleography for diagnosis of Meniere's disease. Archives of Otolaryngology—Head and Neck Surgery, 121, 44–55, fig. p. 52, with permission.)

Another interesting feature in **Fig. 19–15** is that when responses to rarefaction and condensation clicks are combined (lowest tracing), the AP-N₁ latency difference is obscured. What appears instead is an SP-AP complex that looks to be abnormally wide or prolonged. Morrison et al (1980) reported a widening of the SP-AP duration in Meniere's patients over 25 years ago. Prolongation of the complex was attributed to an "after-ringing" of the CM caused by ELH. In light of more recent studies, however, it may be more likely that differences in AP-N₁ latency to condensation versus rarefaction clicks produced what appeared to be a widened SP-AP complex to the alternating clicks used by Morrison et al.

Even though the underlying mechanisms may be unclear, the preceding studies suggest that the duration of the SP-AP complex may be important to consider in the interpretation of the ECochGm. Ferraro and Tibbils (1997) explored this notion by combining both amplitude and duration features of the response to measure the "area ratio" between the SP and AP. **Figure 19–16** displays representative tracings from this study. The waveforms in the left panel are from a normal-hearing subject, whereas the right tracings are from a patient suspected of having MD/ELH. The shaded portions of the top tracings in both panels represent the SP area, which was defined by the onset of the SP (baseline) and that point in the tracing

where the waveform returned to the baseline amplitude. It should be noted that despite the label, this measurement included the areas of components other than the SP, such as the AP-N₁, and often -N₂. The shaded portions of the lower tracings represent the area of the AP-N₁. The results from this study revealed that MD/ELH patients with enlarged SP/AP amplitude ratios also have enlarged SP/AP area ratios. However, enlarged area ratios also were seen in several patients suspected of having MD/ELH, but whose SP/AP amplitude ratios were within normal limits. These findings suggest that use of the SP/AP area ratio may improve the sensitivity of ECochG. Subsequent research using data from 138 patients with MD/ELH has shown that measurement of the SP/AP area ratio significantly improves the diagnostic sensitivity of ECochG in comparison to the SP/AP amplitude ratio (Devaiah et al, 2003).

An important aspect regarding the use of ECochG in the evaluation of MD/ELH is the association between the results of an examination and the subsequent diagnosis and treatment of the patient. An outcome study to examine this aspect was conducted in 1997 (Murphy et al, 1997). Chi-square analysis was applied to a database established from 103 patients referred for ECochG to help diagnose or rule out MD/ELH. Fifty patients from this study had negative ECochGms. Despite these results, 24 of these patients were still diagnosed as having MD/ELH. This finding translates to a sensitivity factor (or true-positive rate) for ECochG of 68%. On the other hand, 51 of the 53 patients who had positive ECochGms received a diagnosis of MD/ELH. The specificity factor (true-negative rate) derived from this finding is ~93%. The results from this outcome study simply help to confirm empirical observations from several other studies. Namely, ECochG is a fairly sensitive, yet highly specific tool in the evaluation of MD/ELH. Additional outcome studies comparing the various features of the ECochGm used to help diagnose MD/ELH with the eventual diagnosis are under way using a much larger clinical population. These features include the SP and AP amplitudes and durations to clicks and tone bursts, N₁-latency, and the SP/AP amplitude and area ratios.

Finally, another AEP approach to diagnosing MD/ELH has recently surfaced that deserves attention in this chapter. Although this method utilizes the ABR and not ECochG per se, it is based on changes that occur in the cochlea during hydropic conditions that affect the timing of neural potentials. Described by Don et al (2005), this method measures the difference between wave V absolute latency in response to clicks presented alone versus clicks delivered in the presence of a 500 Hz pink noise masker. The difference between wave V latencies under these two conditions was found to be significantly shorter for Meniere's patients versus normal-hearing subjects, indicating that the presence of endolymphatic hydrops lessens the effectiveness of the pink noise masker. The commercially available software for applying this approach will allow for a comparison to other techniques currently used to diagnose Meniere's disease (e.g., ECochG).

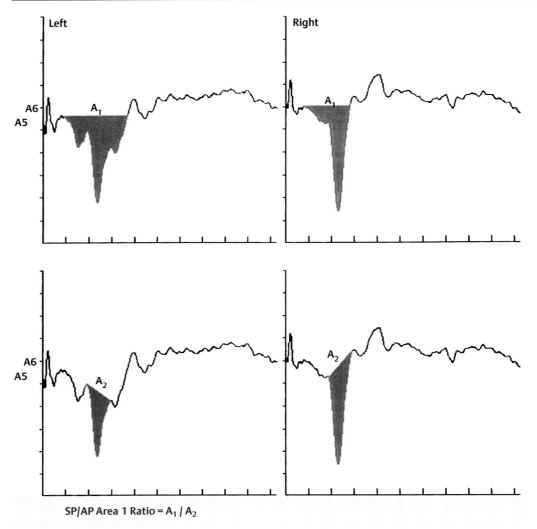

SP/AP Area 1 Ratio = A₁ / A₂

Figure 19–16 Method for measuring the areas of the summating potential (SP) and action potential (AP) to click stimuli to derive the SP/AP area ratio. Shaded portions represent the area of each component. Electrocochleogram in the left panel is from a normal subject. Electrocochleogram in the right panel is from a patient suspected of having Meniere's disease and displays an enlarged SP area (and SP/AP area ratio).

Pearl

- As a final note regarding the specificity of ECochG, enlarged SP/AP amplitude ratios also have been reported for perilymphatic fistulas (Ackley et al, 1994; Kobayashi et al, 1993). Thus, the fluid pressure of the scala media may be the underlying feature to which ECochG is specific. That is, increased pressure in the scala media leading to a positive ECochGm may be caused by ELH or by reduced pressure in the scalae vestibuli and/or tympani (as in a fistula).

Enhancement of Wave I

Identification of waves I, III, and V and the subsequent measurement of the I–III, I–V, and III–V interwave intervals (IWIs) are crucial to the interpretation of the ABR, especially

in the diagnosis of retrocochlear disorders. However, when the ABR is recorded conventionally with surface electrodes on the scalp and earlobes (or mastoid processes), wave I is among the first components to disappear as stimulus intensity is lowered from suprathreshold levels (Fria, 1980; Schwartz and Berry, 1985). Wave I may be reduced, distorted, or absent, despite the presence of an identifiable wave V in subjects with hearing loss, including those with acoustic tumors (Cashman and Rossman, 1983; Hyde and Blair, 1981). This situation significantly reduces the diagnostic utility of the ABR because the I–V and III–V IWIs are immeasurable. Under all of the above and other "less than optimal" recording conditions (e.g., noisy electrical and/or acoustical environment, restless subject), simultaneous recording of the AP-N₁ via ECochG and the ABR has been shown to be beneficial (Ferraro and Ferguson, 1989; Ferraro and Ruth, 1994). Specifically, the amplitude of the AP-N₁ (or

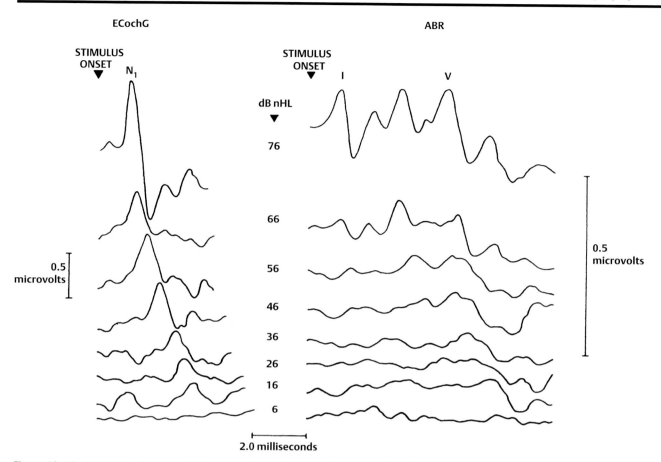

Figure 19–17 Comparison between AP-N$_1$ recorded from the tympanic membrane (TM; left tracings) and conventional auditory brainstem response (ABR; right tracings) in a normal-hearing subject. Note the disparity between electrocochleography (ECochG) and ABR amplitude scales, which illustrates how much larger the TM recordings are. Threshold of N$_1$ and wave V are the same (6–16 dB nHL [normalized hearing level]). Wave I in the conventional ABR disappears between 26 and 36 dB nHL. (From Ferraro, J. A., & Ferguson, R. (1989). Tympanic ECochG and conventional ABR: A combined approach for the identification of wave I and the I–V interwave interval. Ear and Hearing, 3, 161–166, fig. p. 163, with permission.)

wave I) recorded from the TM is larger than corresponding amplitudes measured from the mastoid process or ear canal regardless of stimulus level. **Figure 19–17** displays TM-ECochG (left panel) and ABR (right panel) recordings from a normal-hearing individual. The electrode array for ECochG is vertex (+)-to-TM (−), which displays the AP-N$_1$ as a positive peak in accordance with the conventional display of the ABR. The filter bandpass for ECochG also is conventional to the ABR (i.e., 100–3000 Hz) because the SP is not of interest. Corresponding amplitude scales highlight the disparity in magnitudes between ECochG and ABR components. Of particular importance, however, is that the visual detection thresholds of N$_1$ and wave V are the same (16 dB nHL), whereas wave I in the conventional ABR becomes poorly defined at 46 dB nHL, and is absent at 26 dB nHL. **Figure 19–18** from the same study illustrates how the combined ECochG-ABR is applied in a subject with considerable hearing loss. Wave I is absent in the presence of wave V in the conventionally recorded ABR for this patient (top tracings). However, when the ABR is recorded using a vertex (+)-to-TM (−) electrode array (bottom tracings), N$_1$ is identifiable, permitting the measurement of the N$_1$-V IWI. A mean value widely reported

for the conventionally recorded I–V IWI is 4.0 msec (± 0.5 msec). In the face of high-frequency hearing loss however, slightly shorter I–V IWIs are often observed because the absolute latency of wave I may be more delayed than the corresponding latency of wave V. In addition, the second component of N$_1$ (which is analogous to N$_2$ or wave II) becomes dominant at low stimulus levels. These observations indicate that the upper limit of the I–V IWI established from normal listeners may not apply to patients with significant hearing loss, including those with retrocochlear lesions. These individuals are the very ones for whom the combined ECochG-ABR approach would be applicable. Additional research using the combined approach in hard-of-hearing patients with and without retrocochlear lesions is needed to address this issue.

Recording the ABR using an "electrocochleographic" approach (i.e., from the ear canal) also can be helpful in the assessment of newborn/infant hearing status (Ferraro and Gaddam, 2004). **Figure 19–19** illustrates an intensity series of ABR tracings from a newborn. The upper waveforms in each set of two were recorded using a high-forehead (+)-to-ipsilateral ear canal (−) electrode configuration. The

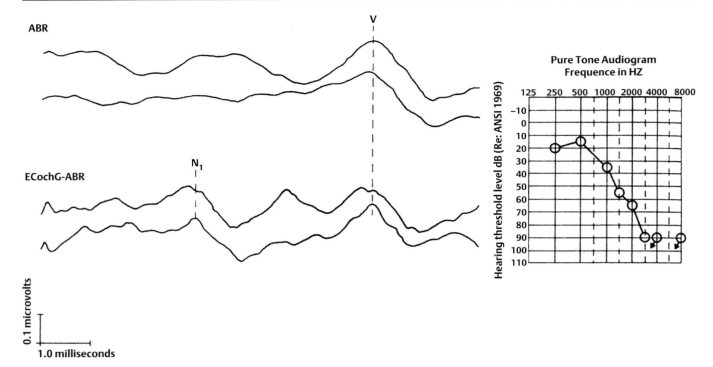

Figure 19–18 ABR recorded with a vertex (+)-to-ipsilateral earlobe(−) electrode array, and electrocochleography (ECochG)–auditory brainstem response (ABR) recorded with a vertex (+)-to-ipsilateral tympanic membrane (−) electrode array from a patient with hearing loss (audiogram at right). Wave I is absent in the conventional ABR tracings, whereas N_1 is recordable with the ECochG-ABR approach. (From Ferraro, J. A., & Ferguson, R. (1989). Tympanic ECochG and conventional ABR: A combined approach for the identification of wave I and the I–V interwave interval. Ear and Hearing, 3, 161–166, fig. p. 165, with permission.)

lower tracings in each set were recorded conventionally (i.e., using the mastoid as the secondary electrode site). The ear canal electrode was a commercially available TIP-trode (Etymotic Research Inc., Elk Grove, IL) cut down to approximately one third of its normal length. Reducing the

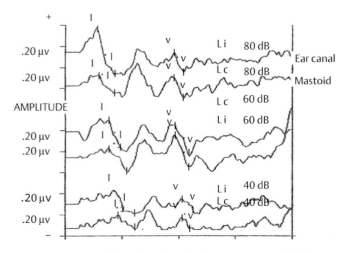

Figure 19–19 Two-channel auditory brainstem response (ABR) tracings from a newborn at three stimulus levels (80, 60, 40 dB HL) recorded using high forehead (+)-to-ear canal (−) (top tracing of each pair) and high forehead (+)-to-mastoid (−) electrode configurations. The amplitudes of wave I in the ear canal recordings are larger than the mastoid recordings at all levels.

size of the TIPtrode made it suitable for insertion into the neonatal ear canal. As can be seen from the tracings, recording the ABR from the ear canal enhanced the amplitude of wave I at all three stimulus levels.

Intraoperative Monitoring

Intraoperative monitoring of inner ear and auditory nerve status during surgeries that involve the peripheral auditory system has become an important application for ECochG. Such monitoring usually is done to help the surgeon avoid potential trauma to the ear/auditory nerve in an effort to preserve hearing (Ferraro and Ruth, 1994). In addition, intraoperative ECochG recordings may be helpful in identification of anatomical landmarks such as the endolymphatic sac (Gibson and Arenberg, 1991). Finally, ECochG monitoring has been examined as a method to help predict postoperative outcome, especially for patients undergoing endolymphatic decompression/shunt surgery for the treatment of MD/ELH (Arenberg et al, 1993; Gibson et al, 1988; Gibson and Arenberg, 1991; Mishler et al, 1994; Wazen, 1994). Examples of the above applications for intraoperative ECochG monitoring are presented in the following sections.

Hearing Preservation

Figure 19–20 illustrates a series of intraoperative ECochGms recorded from a patient undergoing vestibular neurectomy for treatment of intractable vertigo. These responses were

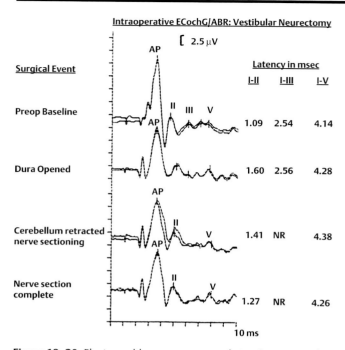

Figure 19–20 Electrocochleograms measured at various events during vestibular neurectomy surgery. Auditory brainstem response (ABR) components also are visible. Preservation of all components throughout surgery indicates preservation of the cochlear nerve. ECochG, electrocochleography. (From Musiek, F. E., Borenstein, S. P., Hall, J. W. III, & Schwaber, M. K. (1994). Auditory brainstem response: Neurodiagnostic and intraoperative applications. In J. Katz (Ed.), Handbook of clinical audiology (4th ed., pp. 351–374). Baltimore, MD: Williams & Wilkins, fig. p. 369, with permission.)

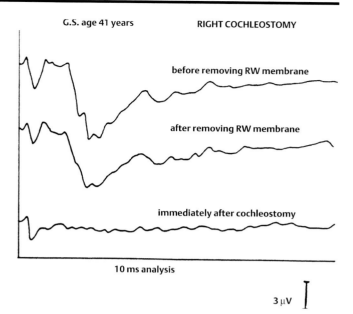

Figure 19–21 Electrocochleograms measured during cochleostomy surgery involving removal of the round window (RW) membrane. All components disappeared immediately after puncturing the cochlear duct. (From Gibson, W. P. R., & Arenberg, I. K. (1991). The scope of intraoperative electrocochleography. In I. K. Arenberg (Ed.), Proceedings of the Third International Symposium and Workshops on the Surgery of the Inner Ear (pp. 295–303). Amsterdam: Kugler Publications, p. 299, with permission.)

measured from the promontory and also include ABR components. The presence of the AP throughout the surgery indicates that hearing was preserved during the procedure, which was verified postoperatively. Combining both ECochG and ABR measures also allows for monitoring of auditory brainstem status in addition to cochlear/auditory nerve function.

Figure 19–21 displays serial tracings from an ear in which a cochleostomy was performed for treatment of intractable vertigo. In this example, the AP disappeared when the cochlear duct was opened, which was predictive of the patient's total loss of hearing above 2 to 3 kHz following surgery.

Based on a review of recent literature, three important questions should be considered regarding the use of ECochG (and other AEP) intraoperative monitoring for the purpose of preserving hearing. First, will trauma to the ear be reflected in the ECochGm? There is ample evidence from several studies (including the example in **Fig. 19–20**) that the answer to this question is yes. Second, are changes in the ECochGm that reflect trauma to the ear reversible? That is, if the ear is damaged as indicated by the ECochGm, can the surgical approach be altered in time to correct or at least mitigate the problem? The answer to this question is not always, because the auditory nerve is very unforgiving. It is not unusual to lose the AP (and hearing) very rapidly, especially when the surgical field includes the cochlear blood supply, such as during the removal of an acoustic neuroma. Animal studies have shown that cessation of cochlear blood flow will result

in complete abolishment of the AP within 30 to 45 seconds (Perlman et al, 1959). When this situation occurs, ECochG monitoring to preserve hearing is akin to locking the gate after the horse has left the corral. Because time is of the essence in such situations, direct nerve as opposed to farfield, signal-averaged monitoring should be applied.

The third question to consider regarding intraoperative monitoring to preserve hearing is whether or not the surgical approach can be altered at all if the ECochGm indicates trauma to the ear. The answer to this question is once again not always. During acoustic tumor removal, for example, it may be the case that complete resection of the tumor is not possible without compromising the nerve. Thus, hearing may be lost regardless of monitoring.

The above questions are not posed to discourage the use of intraoperative ECochG monitoring to preserve/protect hearing. Rather, they are presented merely as issues to consider when applying the procedure.

Identification of Anatomical Landmarks

Although controversial in its own right, decompression or shunting of the endolymphatic sac is an option for patients who fail nonsurgical approaches for treatment of MD/ELH. During such surgeries, instantaneous measurements of the mechanoelectrical processes of the inner ear can be achieved via ECochG. As described earlier, these measurements can alert the surgeon to imminent damage to the cochlea. However, identifying the endolymphatic sac with certainty is not an easy task, especially in MD when congenital abnormalities and unusual anatomical variations may be present (Arenberg,

A.T.   Approx   80 dB HL Click

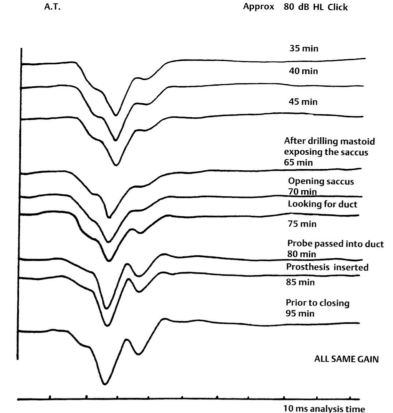

35 min

40 min

45 min

After drilling mastoid
exposing the saccus
65 min

Opening saccus
70 min
Looking for duct

75 min

Probe passed into duct
80 min

Prosthesis inserted

85 min

Prior to closing
95 min

ALL SAME GAIN

10 ms analysis time

Figure 19–22 Electrocochleograms measured at various events during endolymphatic sac surgery. "Probe passed into duct" tracing shows a reduction in the summating potential. This alteration helped to differentiate the location of the endolymphatic duct from surrounding tissue. (From Gibson, W. P. R., & Arenberg, I. K. (1991). The scope of intraoperative electrocochleography. In I. K. Arenberg (Ed.), Proceedings of the Third International Symposium and Workshops on the Surgery of the Inner Ear (pp. 295–303). Amsterdam: Kugler Publications, p. 300, with permission.)

1980). As indicated in **Fig. 19–22**, ECochG may be helpful in these situations. The uppermost tracings display an enlarged SP and SP/AP amplitude ratio. However, the SP becomes smaller and remains that way after a metal probe is passed into the endolymphatic duct (bottom three tracings). Probing of surrounding tissue did not alter the ECochGm.

Prediction of Postoperative Outcome

Several recent studies have indicated that intraoperative monitoring of ECochG may be helpful in predicting the postoperative status of patients. **Figures 19–19** and **19–20** represent examples of this application. That is, maintenance of the AP during surgery is predictive of postoperative preservation of hearing, whereas disappearance of the AP indicates that some, if not all, hearing may be lost. This latter occurrence should be interpreted very cautiously.

Special Consideration

- Both reduction and abolition of ECochG and ABR components can occur during surgical retraction of the nerve/brainstem/cerebellum that recovers when the retractor is repositioned or removed. Thus, disappearance of the AP may not always be indicative of hearing loss.

Another feature of the ECochGm that has been used to predict postoperative outcome is changes in the SP/AP amplitude ratio during endolymphatic sac surgery. Reductions in the ratio when the sac is open or shunted are interpreted as prognostic indicators of successful outcome (i.e., improvement in symptoms, including hearing status). However, the long-term predictive value of intraoperative ECochG (or ECochG in general) remains questionable. **Figure 19–23** displays selected tracings measured from a patient undergoing endolymphatic shunt decompression surgery. A noticeable reduction in the SP/AP amplitude ratio to click stimuli, as well as the SP amplitude to tone bursts, was observed when the sac was decompressed. Likewise, this patient reported an improvement in symptoms following surgery. **Figure 19–24** displays the intraoperative ECochGm from another patient. In this example, the SP amplitude and SP/AP amplitude ratio remained enlarged throughout surgery. Yet this patient, too, reported considerable improvement in symptoms following surgery.

Many of the statements found in the literature regarding the predictive value of intraoperative ECochG monitoring are based on anecdotal observations. Long-term studies that include a comparison of pre-, peri-, and postoperative data (ECochG and other tests) are needed to fully assess this application.

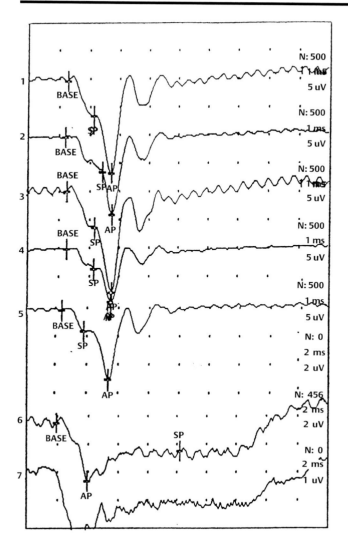

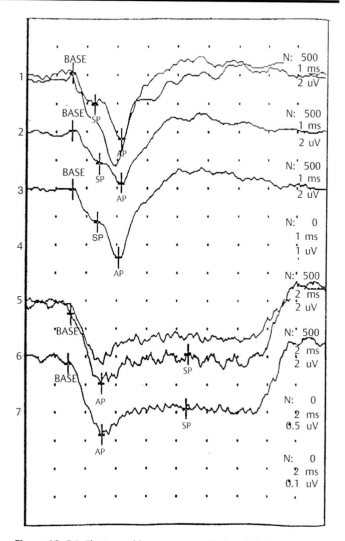

Figure 19–23 Electrocochleograms recorded during endolymphatic shunt surgery: baseline tracing (1), drilling on mastoid (2), probing for endolymphatic duct (3), inserting prosthesis (4), closing (5). Tracing 5 shows a reduction in the summating potential (SP)/action potential (AP) amplitude ratio compared with tracing 1. Tracings 1 through 5 are in response to clicks, whereas tracings 6 and 7 were recorded to tone bursts at the onset of surgery. This patient reported improvement in symptoms following surgery.

Figure 19–24 Electrocochleograms recorded to clicks (tracings 1–4), and 2000 Hz tone bursts (5–7) during endolymphatic shunt surgery. Summating potential (SP)/action potential (AP) amplitude ratio remained enlarged throughout surgery, yet this patient also reported improvement in symptoms following surgery.

Controversial Point

- Can intraoperative ECochG monitoring be used to predict patient outcome following surgery? In the author's experience, ECochG is more analogous to a "thermometer" rather than a "barometer" of inner ear function. That is, ECochG is a useful tool for measuring the acute status of the ear at the time of testing, but not necessarily for predicting long-term cochlear/auditory nerve function.

Auditory Neuropathy/Dys-synchrony

As indicated earlier in this chapter, the use of the ECochG (actually, an ECochG approach to recording the ABR) has

attracted recent interest for the diagnosis of auditory neuropathy/dys-synchrony. In particular, the presence of CM in the absence of ABR components may be an indicator of auditory neuropathy/dys-synchrony (Starr et al, 2001). **Figure 19–25** illustrates this approach. In these tracings, the ABR was recorded in response to condensation (C) and rarefaction (R) clicks from a normal-hearing child and from a 4-year-old with auditory neuropathy. The normal tracings display ABR components along with CM and SP, which can be enhanced or reduced by adding or subtracting responses to C and R clicks. The top tracings in the auditory neuropathy recordings (C and R) illustrate early activity (whose phase is dependent on stimulus polarity) but no discernible ABR components. When these tracings are added together (C + R), the CM is canceled, leaving only the SP component, which is independent of stimulus phase. When the tracings are subtracted (C – R), the CM is enhanced. The implication

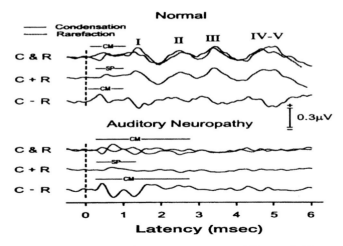

Figure 19–25 Auditory brainstem response (ABR) recorded in response to condensation (C) and rarefaction (R) clicks from a normal child and a 4-year-old with auditory neuropathy. The normal tracings illustrate ABR components along with cochlear microphonic (CM) and cochlear summating potential (SP), which can be enhanced or reduced by adding or subtracting responses to C and R clicks. In the auditory neuropathy tracings, CM and SP are seen in the absence of ABR components. (From Starr, A., Sininger, Y., Nguyen, T., Michalewski, H. G., Oba, S., & Abdala, C. (2001). Cochlear receptor (microphonic and summating potentials, otoacoustic emissions) and auditory pathway (auditory brainstem potentials) activity in auditory. Ear and Hearing, 22, 91–99, fig. p. 93, with permission.)

here is that the presence of CM and/or SP (i.e., cochlear potentials) in the absence of subsequent ABR (neural) components is a positive finding for auditory neuropathy.

Although the above approach holds promise as a diagnostic indicator for auditory neuropathy/dys-synchrony, caution must be exercised in the interpretation of the CM. That is, electromagnetic artifact from the stimulus transducer also introduces cyclic activity that mirrors the acoustic waveform

and reverses its phase with stimulus polarity. **Figure 19–26** illustrates this condition. These tracings were sent to us by a local practitioner along with other test results for a second opinion. The subject in question was a 3-year-old child who displayed no measurable hearing via behavioral testing and absent otoacoustic emissions. The presence of cyclic activity in the ABR waveforms that reversed polarity with the stimulus was initially interpreted as CM, and the child's diagnosis included suspicion of auditory neuropathy. We viewed the tracings as being contaminated by stimulus artifact and could not support this diagnosis.

Pitfall

- The utility of the CM in the diagnosis of auditory neuropathy/dys-synchrony is limited because of the difficulty in separating CM from stimulus artifact in conventional AEP recordings.

Pearl

- One key to distinguishing CM from stimulus, electromagnetic artifact is the time of onset of the cyclic activity. That is, stimulus artifact is seen at the very onset of the waveform (as seen in **Fig. 19–26**). The CM, on the other hand, appears after a brief (1–1.5 msec) latency period due to stimulus travel time through the sound tube and outer and middle ears. Another important safeguard for recording CM involves repeating measurements with the sound tube in place but clamped. Stimulus artifact will persist under this condition, but true CM disappears. We also have found that shielding the stimulus transducer with mu metal and using a grounded electrode cable help to minimize electromagnetic artifact when attempting to record the CM.

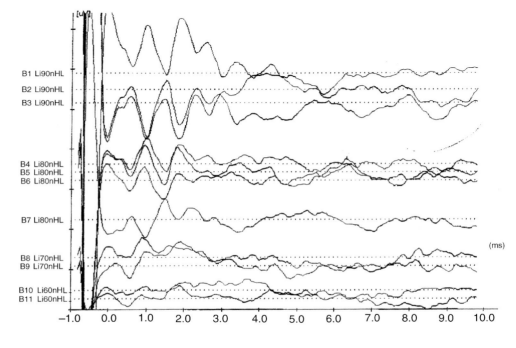

Figure 19–26 Auditory brainstem response (ABR) tracings of a 4-year-old child referred to our clinic for a second opinion regarding the diagnosis of auditory neuropathy. The basis for diagnosing auditory neuropathy was the perceived presence in these tracings of cochlear microphonic (CM) in the absence of ABR components. We could not support the diagnosis of auditory neuropathy, as stimulus artifact, which also reverses polarity with the stimulus, appears throughout the response.

Other Applications

As indicated in the introductory section of this chapter, currently the four most popular applications for ECochG are those described above (i.e., diagnosis/evaluation of MD/- ELH, identification/enhancement of wave I, intraoperative monitoring, and diagnosis of auditory neuropathy/dys-synchrony). However, other uses, such as estimation of hearing thresholds, have been reported. Laureano et al (1995), for example, found significant correlation between AP and behavioral thresholds to mid- to high-frequency tone bursts. As described earlier, Ferraro and Ferguson (1989) found no differences between TM-recorded AP and conventionally recorded wave V thresholds in normal-hearing individuals. Wave V threshold, of course, often is used to estimate hearing sensitivity in infants and other difficult-to-test populations.

Despite the above studies, it is unlikely that ECochG will emerge as a tool of choice for estimating hearing sensitivity. In most cases, other electrophysiological and behavioral approaches that tend to be more accurate, less time-consuming, and easier to administer are available. This is not to say, however, that the relationship between ECochG and hearing status should not continue to be studied. Lilly (1997), for example, has reported on the utility of ECochG for estimating hearing reserve in cochlear implant candidates. Schoonhoven et al (1995) found a relationship between the slopes of AP input–output functions measured from the TM and cochlear recruitment. Keith et al (1992) used ECochG to assess the integrity of the inner ear prior to stapedectomy surgery in a patient who was unable to be tested behaviorally.

◆ Summary

The evaluation of inner ear and auditory nerve function via ECochG continues to be useful for a variety of clinical applications. This basic premise persists in the face of continued controversy regarding how ECochG is recorded, interpreted, and applied. Increased attention to resolving these controversies and to expanding current applications is apparent in the recent literature, and these efforts bode well for the future of ECochG. It truly is the case that ECochG provides a window through which the physiology and pathophysiology of the human auditory periphery can be studied in the laboratory, clinic, and operating room. We may not yet fully understand what we are seeing through this window or even how or where to look. However, the key to unlocking these mysteries most certainly involves our ability to make the window larger, as well as our resolve to continue looking through it.

References

Ackley, R. S., Ferraro, J. A., & Arenberg, I. K. (1994). Diagnosis of patients with perilymphatic fistula. Seminars in Hearing, 15, 37–41.

American Speech-Language-Hearing Association. (1988). The short latency auditory evoked potentials: A tutorial paper by the Working Group on Auditory Evoked Potential Measurements of the Committee on Audiologic Evaluation. Washington, DC: ASHA.

Aran, J. M., & LeBert, G. (1968). Les responses nerveuse cochleaires chez l'homme, image du fonctionnement de l'oreille et nouveau test d'audiometrie objectif. Revue de Laryngologie, Otologie, 89, 361–365.

Arenberg, I. K. (1980). Abnormalities, congenital abnormalities and unusual anatomic variations of the endolymphatic sac and vestibular aqueduct: Clinical, surgical and radiographic correlations. American Journal of Otology, 2, 118–149.

Arenberg, I. K., Gibson, W. P. R., & Bohlen, H. K. H. (1993). Improvements in audiometric and electrophysiologic parameters following nondestructive inner ear surgery utilizing a valved shunt for hydrops and Meniere's disease. Proceedings of the Sixth Annual Workshops on Electrocochleography and Otoacoustic Emission, International Meniere's Disease Research Institute, pp. 545–561.

Bian, L., & Chertoff, M. (1998). Similar hearing loss, different physiology: Characterizing cochlear transduction in pure tone or salicylate damaged ears. Abstracts of the Twenty-First Midwinter Research Meeting of the Association for Research in Otolaryngology. p. 84.

Campbell, K. C. M., Harker, L. A., & Abbas, P. J. (1992). Interpretation of electrocochleography in Meniere's disease and normal subjects. Annals of Otology, Rhinology and Laryngology, 101, 496–500.

Cashman, M., & Rossman, R. (1983). Diagnostic features of the auditory brainstem response in identifying cerebellopontine angle tumors. Scandinavian Audiology, 12, 35–41.

Coats, A. C. (1981). The summating potential and Meniere's disease. Archives of Otolaryngology, 104, 199–208.

Coats, A. C. (1986). Electrocochleography: Recording techniques and clinical applications. Seminars in Hearing, 29, 247–266.

Coats, A. C., & Dickey, J. R. (1970). Non-surgical recording of human auditory nerve action potentials and cochlear microphonics. Annals of Otology, Rhinology and Laryngology, 29, 844–851.

Committee on Hearing and Equilibrium. (1995). Guidelines for the diagnosis and evaluation of therapy in Meniere's disease. American Academy of Otolaryngology—Head and Neck Surgery, 113, 181–185.

Cullen, J. K., Ellis, M. S., Berlin, C. I., & Lousteau, R. J. (1972). Human acoustic nerve action potential recordings from the tympanic membrane without anesthesia. Acta Otolaryngologica, 74, 15–22.

Dallos, P. (1973). The auditory periphery: Biophysics and physiology. New York: Academic Press.

Dallos, P. (1997, April). Outer hair cells: The inside story. Paper presented at the annual convention of the American Academy of Audiology.

Dallos, P., Schoeny, Z. G., & Cheatham, M. A. (1972). Cochlear summating potentials: Descriptive aspects. Acta Otolaryngologica, 301(Suppl.), 1–46.

Dauman, R., Aran, J. M., Sauvage, R. C., & Portmann, M. (1986). Clinical significance of the summating potential in Meniere's disease. American Journal of Otology, 9, 31–38.

Davis, H., Fernandez, C., & McAuliffe, D. R. (1950). The excitatory process in the cochlea. Proceedings of the National Academy of Sciences of the United States of America, 36, 580–587.

Deviah, A. K., Dawson, K. L., Ferraro, J. A., & Ator, G. (2003). Utility of area curve ratio: electrocochleography in early Meniere's disease. Archives of Otolaryngology Head and Neck Surgery, 129, 547–551.

Don, M., Kwang, B., & Tanaka, C. (2005). A diagnostic test for Meniere's disease and cochlear hydrops: Impaired high-pass noise masking of auditory brainstem responses. Otology and Neurotology, 26, 711–722.

Durrant, J. D. (1981). Auditory physiology and an auditory physiologist's view of tinnitus. Journal of Laryngology and Otology, 4(Suppl.), 21–28.

Durrant, J. D., & Dallos, P. (1972). Influence of direct current polarization of the cochlear partition on the summating potential. Journal of the Acoustical Society of America, 52, 542–552.

Durrant, J. D., & Ferraro, J. A. (1991). Analog model of human click-elicited SP and effects of high-pass filtering. Ear and Hearing, 12, 144–148.

Eggermont, J. J. (1976). Summating potentials in electrocochleography: Relation to hearing disorders. In R. J. Ruben, C. Elberling, & G. Salomon (Eds.), Electrocochleography (pp. 67–87). Baltimore, MD: University Park Press.

Evans, B., & Dallos, P. (1993). Stereocilia displacement induced somatic motility of cochlear outer hair cells. Proceedings of the National Academy of Sciences of the United States of America, 90, 8347–8351.

Ferraro, J. A. (1992). Electrocochleography: How, Part I. Audiology Today, 4, 26–28.

Ferraro, J. A. (1993). Electrocochleography: Clinical applications. Audiology Today, 5, 36–38.

Ferraro, J. A. (1997). Laboratory exercises in auditory evoked potentials. San Diego, CA: Singular Publishing Group.

Ferraro, J. A., Arenberg, I. K., & Hassanein, R. S. (1985). Electrocochleography and symptoms of inner ear dysfunction. Archives of Otolaryngologica, 111, 71–74.

Ferraro, J. A., Best, L. G., & Arenberg, I. K. (1983). The use of electrocochleography in the diagnosis, assessment and monitoring of endolymphatic hydrops. Otolaryngologic Clinics of North America, 16, 69–82.

Ferraro, J. A., Blackwell, W., Mediavilla, S. J., & Thedinger, B. (1994). Normal summating potential to tone bursts recorded from the tympanic membrane in humans. Journal of the American Academy of Audiology, 5, 17–23.

Ferraro, J. A., & Ferguson, R. (1989). Tympanic ECochG and conventional ABR: A combined approach for the identification of wave I and the I–V interwave interval. Ear and Hearing, 3, 161–166.

Ferraro, J. A., & Gaddam, A. (2004). ABR and CM recorded from the ear canal in newborns. Program of the 2004 International Conference on Newborn Hearing Screening Diagnosis and Intervention, 87 (A).

Ferraro, J. A., & Krishnan, G. (1997). Cochlear potentials in clinical audiology. Audiology and Neuro-otology, 2, 241–256.

Ferraro, J. A., & Ruth, R. A. (1994). Electrocochleography. In: J. Jacobson (Ed.), Auditory evoked potentials: Overview and basic principles (pp. 101–122). Boston: Allyn & Bacon.

Ferraro, J. A., Thedinger, B., Mediavilla, S. J., & Blackwell, W. (1994). Human summating potential to tone bursts: Observations on TM versus promontory recordings in the same patient. Journal of the American Academy of Audiology, 6, 217–224.

Ferraro, J. A., & Tibbils, R. (1997). SP/AP area ratio in the diagnosis of Meniere's disease. Abstracts of the Fifteenth Biennial Symposium of the International Evoked Response Audiometry Study Group, p. 13(A).

Fria, T. (1980). The auditory brainstem response: Background and clinical applications. Monographs of Contemporary Audiology, 2, 1–44.

Gerhardt, K. J., Melnick, W., & Ferraro, J. A. (1979). Reflex threshold shift in chinchillas following a prolonged exposure to noise. Journal of Speech and Hearing Research, 22, 63–72.

Gibson, W. P. R., & Arenberg, I. K. (1991). The scope of intraoperative electrocochleography. In I. K. Arenberg (Ed.), Proceedings of the Third International Symposium and Workshops on the Surgery of the Inner Ear (pp. 295–303). Amsterdam: Kugler Publications.

Gibson, W. P. R., Arenberg, I. K., & Best, L. G. (1988). Intraoperative electrocochleographic parameters following nondestructive inner ear surgery utilizing a valved shunt for hydrops and Meniere's disease. In J. G. Nadol (Ed.), Proceedings of the Second International Symposium on Meniere's Disease (pp. 170–171). Amsterdam: Kugler and Ghedini Publications.

Gibson, W. P. R., Moffat, D. A., & Ramsden, R. T. (1977). Clinical electrocochleography in the diagnosis and management of Meniere's disorder. Audiology, 16, 389–401.

Guinan, J., & Peake, W. (1967). Middle-ear characteristics of anesthetized cats. Journal of the Acoustical Society of America, 41, 1237–1261.

Hyde, M. L., & Blair, R. L. (1981). The auditory brainstem response in neuro-otology: Perspectives and problems. Journal of Otolaryngology, 10, 117–125.

Keith, R. W., Kereiakes, T. J., Willging, J. P., & Devine, J. (1992). Evaluation of cochlear function in a patient with "far-advanced" otosclerosis. American Journal of Otology, 13, 347–349.

Kiang, N. S. (1965). Discharge patterns of single nerve fibers in the cat's auditory nerve (Research Monograph 35). Cambridge, MA: MIT Press.

Kobayashi, H., Arenberg, I. K., Ferraro, J. A., & Van der Ark, G. (1993). Delayed endolymphatic hydrops following acoustic tumor removal with intraoperative and postoperative auditory brainstem response improvements. Acta Otolaryngologica, 504(Suppl.), 74–78.

Laureano, A. N., Murray, D., McGrady, M. D., & Campbell, K. C. M. (1995). Comparison of tympanic membrane-recorded electrocochleography and the auditory brainstem response in threshold determination. American Journal of Otology, 16, 209–215.

Levine, S. M., Margolis, R. H., Fournier, E. M., & Winzenburg, S. M. (1992). Tympanic electrocochleography for evaluation of endolymphatic hydrops. Laryngoscope, 102, 614–622.

Lilly, D. J., & Black, F. O. (1989). Electrocochleography in the diagnosis of Meniere's disease. In J. B. Nadol (Ed.), Meniere's disease (pp. 369–373). Berkeley, CA: Kugler & Ghedini.

Margolis, R. H., Rieks, D., Fournier, M., Levine, S. M. (1995). Tympanic electrocochleography for diagnosis of Meniere's disease. Archives of Otolaryngology—Head and Neck Surgery, 121, 44–55.

Mishler, E. T., Loosmore, J. L., Herzog, J. A., Smith, P. G., & Kletzker, G. K. (1994). The efficacy of electrocochleography in monitoring endolymphatic shunt procedures. Paper presented at the annual Meeting of the American Neuro-Otology Society.

Moller, A., & Janetta, P. (1983). Monitoring auditory functions during cranial nerve microvascular decompression operations by direct monitoring from the eighth nerve. Journal of Neurosurgery, 59, 493–499.

Morrison, A. W., Moffat, D. A., & O'Connor, A. F. (1980). Clinical usefulness of electrocochleography in Meniere's disease: An analysis of dehydrating agents. Otolaryngologic Clinics of North America, 11, 703–721.

Murphy, L. A., Ferraro, J. A., Chertoff, M., McCall, S., & Park, D. (1997, April). Issues in auditory evoked potentials. Paper presented at the annual meeting of the American Academy of Audiology, Ft. Lauderdale, FL.

Musiek, F. E., Borenstein, S. P., Hall, J. W. III, & Schwaber, M. K. (1994). Auditory brainstem response: Neurodiagnostic and intraoperative applications. In J. Katz (Ed.), Handbook of clinical audiology (4th ed., pp. 351–374). Baltimore, MD: Williams & Wilkins.

Orchik, J. G., Ge, X., & Shea, J. J. (1997). Action potential latency shift by rarefaction and condensation clicks in Meniere's disease. American Journal of Otology, 14, 290–294.

Perlman, M. B., & Case, T. J. (1941) Electrical phenomena of the cochlea in man. Archives of Otolaryngology, 34, 710–718.

Perlman, M. B., Kimura, R., & Fernandez, C. (1959). Experiments on temporary obstruction of the internal auditory artery. Laryngoscope, 69, 591–613.

Picton, T. W., Hillyard, S. H., Frauz, H. J., & Galambos, R. (1974). Human auditory evoked potentials. Electroencephalography and Clinical Neurophysiology, 36, 191–200.

Ruben, R., Sekula, J., & Bordely, J. E. (1960). Human cochlear responses to sound stimuli. Annals of Otorhinolaryngology, 69, 459–476.

Ruth, R. A., Lambert, P. R., & Ferraro, J. A. (1988). Electrocochleography: Methods and clinical applications. American Journal of Otology, 9, 1–11.

Schoonhoven, R., Fabius, M. A. W., & Grote, J. J. (1995). Input/output curves to tone bursts and clicks in extratympanic and transtympanic electrocochleography. Ear and Hearing, 16, 619–630.

Schwartz, D. M., & Berry, G. A. (1985). Normative aspects of the ABR. In J. T. Jacobson (Ed.), The auditory brainstem response (pp. 65–97). San Diego, CA: College Hill Press.

Sohmer, H., & Feinmesser, M. (1967). Cochlear action potentials recorded from the external canal in man. Annals of Otology, Rhinology and Otolaryngology, 76, 427–435.

Spoendlin, H. (1966). Organization of the cochlear receptor. Advances in Otorhinolaryngology, 13, 1–227.

Stapells, D., Picton, T. W., & Smith, A. D. (1982). Normal hearing thresholds for clicks. Journal of the Acoustical Society of America, 72, 74–79.

Starr, A., Sininger, Y., Nguyen, T., Michalewski, H. G., Oba, S., & Abdala, C. (2001). Cochlear receptor (microphonic and summating potentials, otoacoustic emissions) and auditory pathway (auditory brainstem potentials) activity in auditory. Ear and Hearing, 22, 91–99.

Stypulkowski, P. H., & Staller, S. J. (1987). Clinical evaluation of a new ECoG recording electrode. Ear and Hearing, 8, 304–310.

von Bekesy, G. (1950). DC potentials and energy balance of the cochlear partition. Journal of the Acoustical Society of America, 22, 576–582.

Wazen, J. J. (1994). Intraoperative monitoring of auditory function: Experimental observation, and new applications. Laryngoscope, 104, 446–455.

Yoshie, N., Ohashi, T., & Suzuki, T. (1967). Non-surgical recording of auditory nerve action potentials in man. Laryngoscope, 77, 76–85.

Chapter 20

The Auditory Brainstem Response

Sally A. Arnold

The auditory brainstem response (ABR) is one component of the auditory evoked potentials (AEPs), which also include electrocochleography, the auditory middle latency response, and the auditory late response. The term *auditory evoked potential* refers to electrical activity of the auditory system that occurs in response to an appropriate acoustic stimulus. One way to classify the AEPs is according to their time of occurrence (latency) following onset of the eliciting stimulus. The ABR is the group of potentials occurring within the first 10 msec following the stimulus. The ABR has also been called the brainstem evoked response (BSER), brainstem auditory evoked potential (BAEP), and brainstem auditory evoked response (BAER). Since its discovery over 35 years ago, the ABR has become a standard and valuable component of the audiologic test battery.

♦ General Description of the Auditory Brainstem Response

The Auditory Brainstem Response Waveform

The ABR consists of a series of seven positive-to-negative waves, occurring within ~10 msec following stimulus onset. Several systems of nomenclature have been devised for labeling the individual waveform peaks of the ABR, but the most popular convention in the United States is to label the positive peaks with Roman numerals: waves I to VII. Wave I occurs at ~1.5 to 2.0 msec following onset of the eliciting stimulus, depending on stimulus intensity, with the successive waves following at ~1 to 2 msec intervals. **Figure 20–1** shows the ABR waveform recorded from a normal subject, using a

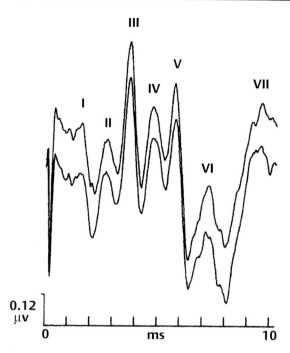

Figure 20–1 Two auditory brainstem response (ABR) waveforms, obtained from an adult subject using 80 dB nHL (normalized hearing level) clicks. The individual waves of the ABR are labeled with Roman numerals I to VII.

Information regarding the origin of individual wave components of the ABR has been provided by Moller and Jannetta (1985). In patients undergoing various neurosurgical procedures, the authors simultaneously measured electrical activity from exposed locations along the auditory brainstem pathway and the ABR recorded from the scalp in the standard manner. They were able to examine the temporal correspondence between the responses from these various intracranial sites and particular waves of the ABR. They concluded that both waves I and II arise from the auditory nerve—wave I from the distal portion and wave II from the proximal portion of the auditory nerve as it enters the brainstem. Wave III is generated mainly in the cochlear nucleus, and wave IV probably arises from the superior olivary complex. The sharp positive peak of wave V arises mainly from the lateral lemniscus; the following slow negative wave represents dendritic potentials in the inferior colliculus. Waves VI and VII appear to be generated in the inferior colliculus and perhaps the medial geniculate body.

Because it is overly simplistic to assume that each ABR component is derived from only a single structure, the above-mentioned sites should be viewed as primary, but not exclusive, generators. With the exception of waves I and II, which are derived solely from the auditory nerve, it is likely that activity from lower structures interacts with activity in higher structures to generate the successive ABR potentials.

high-intensity click stimulus (*click* is defined in a later section). Positive polarity is plotted in an upward direction. Two waveforms obtained under identical stimulus and recording conditions are shown. Note that the amplitudes of the peaks are extremely small (<1 μV). A desirable characteristic of the ABR is the high degree of repeatability between repetitions, as shown in this figure. The large negative deflection at the beginning of the waveform between 0 and 1 msec is stimulus artifact. This artifact can occur, particularly at high stimulus levels, because the earphones radiate electrical energy that may be picked up by the recording electrodes.

The full complement of seven waves shown in **Fig. 20–1** is not always present in the ABR waveform. A normal variant is for waves II, VI, and especially VII to be absent. Also, the morphology of waves IV and V varies considerably. These waves may occur separately as two distinct peaks (**Fig. 20–1**), they may be merged into a single peak, or they may occur together as the IV–V complex, in which one wave occurs in the form of a shoulder upon the other wave. Again, these variations in waveform morphology are considered normal.

Origins of the Auditory Brainstem Response

The ABR is generated by the auditory nerve and subsequent structures within the auditory brainstem pathways.

◆ Recording Techniques

Electrodes

The ABR is recorded from electrodes attached to various positions on the head. Typical electrodes are small metal cups or discs, coated with various materials such as silver, silver chloride, gold, tin, or platinum. Other electrode styles, such as self-adhesive disposables, ear clips, and ear canal electrodes, are also available. The electrodes are attached to insulated lead wires and connector pins that insert into electrode jacks.

The ABR is actually recorded by measuring the difference in electrical activity between two electrodes, a technique known as differential recording. One of the electrodes (the noninverting electrode) is usually placed on the vertex (on top of the head, at the center) or on the middle of the forehead just below the hairline. Another electrode (the inverting electrode) is usually placed on the earlobe or mastoid of the ipsilateral ear, that is, the ear receiving the stimulus. A third electrode, typically placed on the contralateral earlobe, contralateral mastoid, forehead, or nape of the neck, serves as the ground electrode.

Before attaching the electrodes, the skin must be thoroughly cleaned to remove excess oil, dead skin, and dirt to obtain a good contact between the skin and the electrode. Commercial cleansing preparations are available for this task. Next, the electrodes are filled with a conducting cream and taped into place. Once the electrodes have been applied, the adequacy of contact with the skin is assessed by measuring the electrical impedance between each electrode pair. For high-quality recordings, interelectrode impedances ≤ 6 kΩ are generally considered acceptable; impedances also should be fairly equal between electrode pairs. Low and balanced impedances will help reduce unwanted interference such as electrical noise and muscle artifact that can make waveform interpretation difficult.

Pearl

- If the impedance of one or more electrodes is discovered to be high, it can often be lowered by pressing on the electrode(s) for a few moments. If this is unsuccessful, the skin in the area of electrode placement may need to be rescrubbed to lower the impedance. This may be impractical in the case of an infant or young child who is already sleeping. Acceptable ABR recordings can often be obtained in these circumstances with much higher impedances, on the order of 10 to 12 kΩ, provided that the impedances are fairly balanced between electrode pairs and the recording environment is favorable.

Analysis Time Period

When recording the ABR, electrical activity from the electrodes is collected and analyzed over a certain time period, beginning at the onset of the stimulus and continuing long enough to encompass all of the response of interest. Although the entire ABR waveform occurs within the first 10 msec following stimulus onset for high-level clicks, the response will be considerably delayed at lower stimulus levels, for low-frequency stimuli, and when testing infants. To encompass the entire ABR under all of these various conditions, it is recommended to use a longer time window, of either 20 or 25 msec.

Processing of Electrical Activity

Electrical activity picked up by the recording electrodes within the specified time window must be processed through several stages to visualize the ABR waveform. This is because the ABR peaks are of extremely small voltage ($> 1 \mu V$) and are buried in a background of interference (termed *noise*), which includes ongoing electroencephalogram (EEG) activity, muscle potentials caused by movement or tension, and 60 Hz power-line radiation. The stages of processing include amplification, filtering, and signal averaging.

Amplification and Filtering

Because of small size of the ABR peaks, amplification is necessary to increase the magnitude of the electrical activity picked up by the electrodes. An amplifier gain of 10^5 is typically used.

The problem of interference obscuring the ABR can be diminished partially by filtering the electrical activity coming from the electrodes. Bandpass filters are used to accept energy only within the particular frequency band of interest and reject energy in other frequency ranges. For ABR recording, bandpass filter settings of 100 to 3000 Hz or 30 to 3000 Hz are commonly used. A filter setting of 30 to 3000 Hz is recommended to enhance the ABR when testing infants or when using low-frequency tone bursts or bone-conduction stimuli (see details below).

Filtering can only eliminate a portion of the interfering noise because of overlap between the frequency content of the ABR and the frequency of the interference. Therefore, another technique, called signal averaging, must be used to further reduce unwanted interference.

Signal Averaging

The ABR is very small, and even with filtering, it is buried in a background of noise. Signal averaging helps to reduce this noise so that the signal, in this case the ABR, can be detected. Signal averaging is possible because the ABR is time-locked to stimulus onset, whereas the noise interference occurs randomly. That is, the signal occurs at the same points in time following onset of the eliciting stimulus, but the noise has no regular pattern. In signal averaging, a large number of stimuli are presented, and the responses to each of the individual stimulus presentations (termed *sweeps*) are averaged together to obtain a final averaged waveform. By averaging, the random noise tends to cancel out, whereas the evoked potential is retained because it is basically the same in each sweep. The greater the number of stimulus presentations used, the greater the improvement in signal-to-noise ratio, and the more clearly the ABR can be visualized in the final averaged waveform. For ABR recording, between 1000 and 2000 sweeps are typically used. However, for efficient use of test time, averaging may be terminated before the specified number of sweeps is reached, as soon as a clear waveform is visualized in the averaged response. Conversely, a larger number of sweeps may be needed (e.g., 6000) near threshold where the amplitude of the response is small or when background noise is particularly high.

Even with signal averaging, the patient must be reclining or lying in a relaxed state without moving, or interference from muscle activity will make identification of the ABR difficult. For infants and young children, this generally requires that they be tested while asleep. A sedative such as chloral hydrate is often used to induce sleep.

◆ Stimulus Parameters

Stimulus Types

Clicks

The ABR is an onset response, meaning that it is generated by the onset of an auditory stimulus. The stimulus onset or rise time must be rapid to synchronize all the neurons contributing to the ABR. The ideal stimulus for eliciting the ABR is a click, which is a brief rectangular pulse of 50 to 200 μs duration, with an instantaneous onset. The rapid onset of the click provides good neural synchrony, thereby eliciting a clearly defined ABR.

Pitfall

There is a drawback to the use of click stimuli. Due to the reciprocal relationship between time and frequency of acoustic signals, a click is a broad-spectrum signal, containing energy across a wide range of frequencies. Because of this frequency spread, clicks cannot be used to assess sensitivity in specific frequency regions, but rather provide a gross estimate of hearing sensitivity.

Brief Tone Bursts

When assessing hearing sensitivity, it is desirable to take separate measurements within different frequency regions. To do this, one must use frequency-specific stimuli, or stimuli containing energy within a discrete band of frequencies. The pure-tone stimuli used for traditional audiometry, with long rise–fall times, are inappropriate for ABR because they are too slow to generate an onset response.

A stimulus used for ABR that represents a compromise between the desired frequency specificity and the required temporal brevity is the short duration tone burst (also termed *tone pip*). These stimuli are very brief tones with rise–fall times of only a few cycles and brief or no plateau duration. The so-called 2–1–2 tone burst is often used, which consists of 2 cycles of the tone in the rise–fall and 1 cycle in the plateau. The rise–fall time of the tone burst can be shaped with a nonlinear gating function such as a Blackman or cosine^2 window to reduce spectral splatter (i.e., sidebands of energy above and below the nominal frequency of the stimulus). Such tone burst stimuli are more confined in their frequency range than clicks, but they are considerably broader than the stimuli used for pure-tone audiometry.

Stimulus Polarity

Clicks

Most commercial evoked potential instruments allow a choice of rarefaction, condensation, or alternating rarefaction and condensation phase for the click onset. There is presently no consensus regarding which polarity is the best to use; however, most researchers recommend using either rarefaction or alternating phase. Rarefaction is the phase that stimulates the afferent dendrites of the auditory nerve and has been shown to produce shorter latencies and larger amplitudes of the major ABR waveform components in most individuals (Schwartz et al, 1990). Alternating phase is useful in reducing stimulus artifact, which may interfere with identification of wave I. The stimulus artifact follows the phase of the stimulus and therefore cancels out when opposite polarities are added together. Alternating phase, however, may degrade the clarity of the waveform, especially in the case of high-frequency hearing loss (Coats and Martin, 1977).

Tone Bursts

The difference between rarefaction and condensation phase is less important for tone bursts than clicks, because the stimulus rise time will include excursions of both polarities. Alternating phase can be used to cancel out the cochlear microphonic and stimulus artifact; however, for low-frequency tone bursts, alternating phase will broaden the ABR peaks and may degrade clarity of the waveform.

Stimulus Rate

During signal averaging, the stimulus must be presented at a specified rate, which must be slow enough to prevent the overlapping of responses that will occur if a new stimulus is presented before the response to the previous stimulus has been completed. For example, for a 10 msec time window, a rate of 100 per second would be the fastest rate possible. The choice of stimulus rate is a compromise between response clarity and test efficiency. A slower stimulus rate produces the most clearly defined waveform, but it increases the amount of time required to obtain a single average. A higher stimulus rate reduces test time, but it decreases the amplitude of the ABR, particularly the early components of the waveform. Stimulus rates of 17 to 20 per second are typically used clinically. Another clinical strategy is to use a slow rate (<20 per second) when clear definition of all waveform components is required, as for otoneurological assessment (see below), and to use a higher rate (e.g., 39 per second) when measuring wave V latency intensity functions (LIFs) for threshold estimation (see below), because wave V is most resistant to the effects of high stimulus rate.

Pearl

- An important factor to consider when choosing a stimulus rate is that the value should not be evenly divisible into 60, to avoid time-locking onto any 60 Hz electrical interference that may be present in the test environment. For maximum cancellation of 60 Hz artifact, an odd stimulus rate (e.g., 21.1 or 27.7 per second) is typically used.

Calibration of Stimulus Intensity

Unlike pure-tone audiometry, there are no standards for intensity calibration for the stimuli used in ABR measurement because of their short duration. A typical method of specifying intensity for both clicks and tone bursts is to find the average behavioral threshold for the stimulus in a group of normal adults. The average threshold is termed *0 dB normalized hearing level* (nHL). All intensities are then expressed in dB nHL relative to this previously determined zero point.

A physical measurement that is used to express intensity of clicks is the peak equivalent SPL (pe SPL). To measure this, the click is routed to an oscilloscope, and the peak amplitude or peak-to-peak amplitude is measured. Then, a sine wave is routed through the ABR earphone to the oscilloscope, and its amplitude is adjusted to equal that of the click. The SPL of the sine wave is measured with a sound level meter. The amplitude of the click can then be expressed as dB pe SPL re: frequency of the comparison sinusoid (Gorga et al, 1985). Generally, average behavioral threshold (0 dB nHL) will be ~30 dB pe SPL.

A sound level meter can be used to obtain a physical measurement of tone burst intensity by increasing the duration of the burst so that it is long relative to the response time of the meter. The intensity can then be measured and expressed in terms of dB SPL re: 20 μPa (Gorga, Abbas, and Worthington, 1985).

♦ Clinical Applications of the Auditory Brainstem Response

The ABR is used clinically both in the estimation of auditory sensitivity and in otoneurological assessment, that is, to detect lesions along the auditory nerve and brainstem pathways. It is by far the most widely used AEP in audiology. The popularity of the ABR stems from the fact that its characteristics are quite similar between people, making the response fairly easy to identify under most circumstances. It is also highly stable; that is, it is unaffected by subject state. Characteristics of the response do not vary between wakefulness and sleep and are not affected by most medications. This means that children may be tested reliably during natural or sedation-induced sleep.

Auditory Brainstem Response in Estimation of Auditory Sensitivity

ABR is an important tool for the evaluation of auditory sensitivity in those individuals who are not readily testable by conventional behavioral audiometric procedures. Such persons include infants, developmentally delayed children, multiply handicapped children and adults, autistic individuals, and persons suspected of pseudohypoacusis.

Click Stimuli

Historically, clicks were the first stimuli widely used clinically for threshold estimation, due to their ability to synchronize neurons, thus producing a clearly defined ABR waveform. The following discussion of ABR in estimation of auditory sensitivity will pertain to click stimuli. The use of frequency-specific stimuli will be described in a subsequent section.

In assessing hearing sensitivity, wave V of the ABR is used, because it is the most robust of the waves and the one best correlated with behavioral audiometric threshold. The full complement of ABR waves is seen only at intense click levels. As the level of the click decreases, most of the ABR

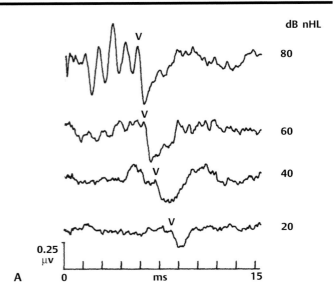

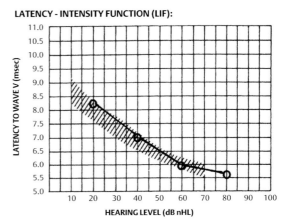

Figure 20–2 (A) Auditory brainstem response (ABR) intensity series, obtained from a normal adult subject, at click levels of 80 to 20 dB nHL (normalized hearing level). Wave V latency ranges from 5.64 msec at 80 dB to 8.28 msec at 20 dB nHL. **(B)** Wave V latency intensity function, plotted from the ABR intensity series.

waves disappear, except wave V, which generally can be elicited at intensity levels within 5 to 20 dB of behavioral threshold for the click. This can be seen in **Fig. 20–2A**, which shows a series of ABRs collected in a normal-hearing adult, at click levels from 80 to 20 dB nHL. Notice that as stimulus intensity decreases, the amplitude of wave V decreases, and its latency increases.

To estimate auditory sensitivity, ABR waveforms are obtained at a series of click levels, beginning at a moderate to high intensity (e.g., 60 dB nHL) and continuing down to lower levels until wave V is no longer seen. If there is no response at the starting level, then intensity must, of course, be increased. Wave V threshold is usually found to the nearest 5 or 10 dB. If wave V is present at 20 dB nHL, this is considered normal, and there is no need to test at lower levels. It is good clinical practice to obtain two waveforms at each stimulus level, especially near threshold, so that the repeatability of the waveform can be examined. This aids in determining whether or not wave V is present at a particular stimulus level.

Once the intensity series is obtained, the latency of wave V is measured at each stimulus level where present, and plotted on a graph known as a latency intensity function (LIF). **Figure 20–2B** shows the wave V LIF for the intensity series plotted at the top of the figure. The shaded area on the graph represents the adult normative wave V latency values (mean latency ± 2 standard deviations [SD]). The slope of the LIF, defined as latency change per dB, averages ~40 μs per decibel in normal subjects (Picton et al, 1981).

After the wave V intensity series is obtained, two factors are used in hearing estimation: wave V threshold and the LIF.

Wave V Threshold   The lowest click level at which wave V can be elicited provides information about the degree of hearing loss. It is well accepted that click threshold will be determined by auditory sensitivity within the mid- to high-frequency range, although there is some disagreement regarding the particular frequencies involved. Click threshold reportedly correlates best with hearing sensitivity between 2 and 4 kHz (Gorga, Worthington, et al, 1985; Picton et al, 1981) or between 1 and 4 kHz (Hyde, 1985; Jerger and Mauldin, 1978).

In normals and those with conductive hearing loss, click threshold will generally be ~10 to 20 dB higher than the best audiometric threshold within the mid- to high-frequency range. For cochlear losses, the difference between click threshold and audiometric thresholds is often reduced, and click threshold may be as close as 5 dB above best behavioral threshold. For convenience in the clinical setting, the behavioral threshold may be predicted to be a constant value (e.g., 10 dB) below click threshold. Due to individual variability, however, a constant correction factor will not be accurate in all cases.

The value of wave V threshold will range along a continuum, from ≤20 dB nHL (considered normal) to wave V absent at equipment limits. Because maximum output for clicks is limited to ~90 to 100 dB nHL (recall that 0 dB nHL =30 dB pe SPL), one will not always be able to differentiate between severe and profound losses.

Pitfall

- The absence of wave V to clicks does not imply the absence of hearing. Rather, it suggests a severe or profound degree of hearing loss within the mid- to high-frequency range. In one study (Rance et al, 1998), 25% of children with no click ABR at 100 dB nHL had useful residual hearing at all frequencies through 4 kHz.

Wave V Latency Intensity Function   The slope of the LIF for click stimuli and the position of the curve relative to normal provide some limited information concerning the type of hearing loss and the audiometric configuration. There are several characteristic LIF types that have come to be associated with certain audiometric patterns, as follows.

- *Conductive hearing loss*   In conductive hearing loss, the slope of the LIF typically is normal. However, the latency of wave V at each intensity will be prolonged, resulting in an LIF that runs parallel to the normal curve, but is shifted to the right. This occurs because conductive pathology primarily causes an attenuation of sound reaching the cochlea, thereby causing latency shifts as would be seen with lower stimulus intensities. **Figure 20–3** shows the audiogram and LIF for the right ear of a patient with a conductive hearing loss. The wave V threshold of 50 dB nHL is 10 dB above the best pure-tone threshold in the 1 to 4 kHz range (i.e., 40 dB at 2 kHz). At each stimulus level, wave V latency is quite prolonged, and the LIF parallels the normal curve.

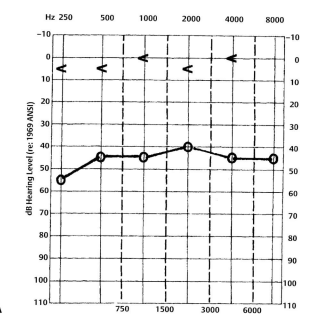

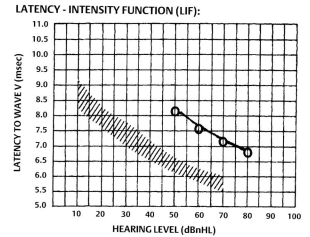

LATENCY - INTENSITY FUNCTION (LIF):

Figure 20–3 (A) Pure-tone audiogram and **(B)** wave V latency intensity function for a person with a right conductive hearing loss.

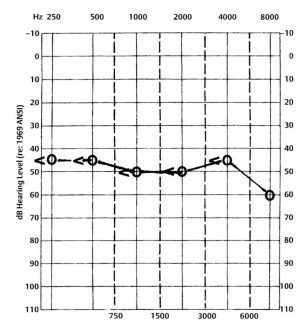

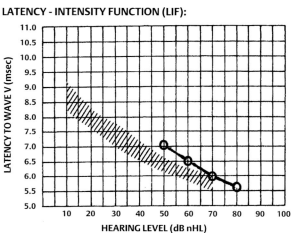

A

B

Figure 20–4 (A) Pure-tone audiogram and **(B)** wave V latency intensity function for a person with a right flat sensorineural hearing loss of cochlear origin.

♦ *Flat cochlear loss*   In cochlear losses having a flat audiometric configuration, wave V latencies may fall within the normal range for all intensities where present or may be slightly prolonged at levels near threshold. The prolongation will generally be less than seen for conductive losses. It should be noted, however, that there is no definitive value of latency shift that will consistently differentiate between cochlear and conductive losses. **Figure 20–4** shows the audiogram and corresponding LIF for a patient with a right flat cochlear loss. Here again, the wave V threshold is 50 dB nHL, which is 5 dB above the best threshold within the 1 to 4 kHz range (i.e., 45 dB at 4 kHz). Notice that the wave V latencies show less prolongation compared with the conductive loss in the previous example, resulting in an LIF that lies close to the normal curve.

♦ *Sloping high-frequency cochlear loss*   In sloping high-frequency cochlear hearing losses, the slope of the LIF is typically steeper than normal. A steep slope occurs when wave V latency is substantially prolonged at and near threshold but is normal or nearly normal at higher intensity levels. The steep slope is felt to be related to the configuration of the pure-tone audiogram (Gorga, Worthington, et al, 1985). That is, because wave V latency is determined in part by the region of the cochlea where the response is initiated, latency will be shorter when high-frequency fibers in the basal region are stimulated and longer when lower frequency fibers toward the apical region are stimulated. In sloping high-frequency losses, the basal portion of the cochlea contributes to the ABR only at high intensities, provided the stimulus exceeds the threshold for high-frequency fibers, whereas more apical regions contribute to the response for lower intensities. **Figure 20–5** shows an audiogram

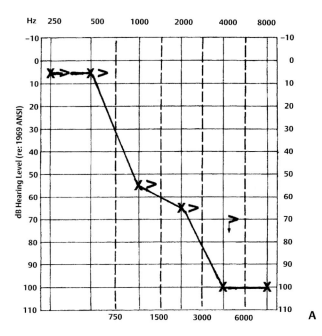

A

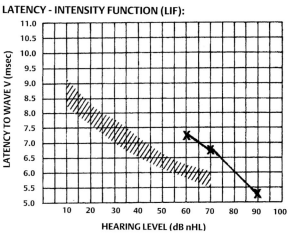

B

Figure 20–5 (A) Pure-tone audiogram and **(B)** wave V latency intensity function for a person with a left steeply sloping high-frequency sensorineural hearing loss of cochlear origin.

from the left ear of a patient with a sloping mid- to high-frequency sensorineural hearing loss, along with the wave V LIF for that ear. Note that wave V threshold is 60 dB nHL, which is 5 dB above the best threshold within the 1 to 4 kHz range (i.e., 55 dB at 1000 Hz). The slope of the LIF is steep compared with the normal curve.

In summary, ABR testing with click stimuli can predict auditory sensitivity within the 1 to 4 kHz range to within 5 to 20 dB. The wave V LIF can be somewhat helpful in ascertaining the type and configuration of the hearing loss. However, the reader should be cautioned that the relation between LIF and hearing loss is undoubtedly quite complex due to the myriad of possible audiometric contours. The LIF can only suggest audiometric patterns, which may not apply in individual cases.

A major limitation of click stimuli is that they are not frequency specific and therefore cannot provide information regarding the entire audiogram. Notice how, for the steeply sloping hearing loss shown in **Fig. 20–5**, the click threshold did not adequately describe the entire audiometric contour. Knowledge of the hearing loss configuration is important for hearing aid fitting and other (re)habilitation decisions. In addition, because click threshold gives an estimate of hearing within the mid- to high-frequency range, it is possible to have a normal ABR and still have significant hearing loss. Specifically, click ABR will not be sensitive to hearing loss below 1 kHz or above 4 kHz.

Pitfall

- A normal click ABR threshold does not necessarily imply normal hearing. Rather, it implies an area of normal sensitivity between 1 and 4 kHz. Many patterns of hearing loss (e.g., low-frequency rising, high-frequency notch, "island" of normal hearing) can yield normal click thresholds.

Frequency-Specific Stimuli

In attempting to approximate the behavioral pure-tone audiogram, it has become fairly common to include brief tone bursts as part of the test protocol. As previously stated, these stimuli have narrower frequency spectra than clicks, but are substantially broader than the pure-tone stimuli used for conventional audiometry, due to the brief rise–fall time. Brief tone bursts, especially with linear ramps, contain sidebands of energy at frequencies above and below the predominant energy peak. Because the sidebands are less intense than the peak of energy, the frequency spread is more of a problem at high levels of stimulation. With steeply sloping audiograms, this spread of stimulation may cause hearing loss in the frequency region under test to be underestimated, because neighboring frequency regions with better sensitivity will be stimulated, generating a response at a lower stimulus level. This frequency spread is more of a problem for low-frequency tone bursts than for mid- to high-frequency tone bursts.

Enhancement of Frequency Specificity The spectrum of brief tone bursts can be narrowed by shaping the rise–fall time with a nonlinear gating function. However, whether this actually enhances the frequency specificity of the ABR is questionable. For example, Purdy and Abbas (1989) showed no significant difference in ABR thresholds in hearing-impaired subjects for Blackman versus linear windows.

An alternative way to enhance frequency specificity of the ABR is to combine the tone bursts with notched noise masking presented to the same ear (Picton et al, 1981; Stapells et al, 1995). Notched noise is similar to wideband noise, containing energy across the frequency spectrum, except within a certain narrow range of frequencies (the notch). The frequency at which the notch occurs corresponds to the frequency of the tone burst being used. Thus, the sidebands of energy present in the tone burst are masked out, restricting the area of stimulation to the nominal frequency of the tone. This assures that the ABR is generated by neurons sensitive only to the test frequency. Notched noise-masking capability is presently available commercially from at least one manufacturer of ABR instrumentation (Intelligent Hearing Systems, Miami, FL).

Waveform Morphology The morphology of the ABR waveform elicited with high-frequency tone bursts is similar to that obtained using clicks. However, for tone burst frequencies of 1000 Hz and below, the early waveform components are not clearly seen, and wave V is broader than normal. This is related to the loss of neural synchrony in the apical, low-frequency region of the cochlea. A filter setting of 30 to 3000 Hz (rather than the typical 100–3000 Hz) is recommended when recording low-frequency ABRs to enhance wave V amplitude. The broad morphology and poor repeatability of the ABR to low-frequency stimuli can make wave V difficult to identify (Stapells et al, 1995), especially at low intensities, and considerable experience is necessary to accurately evaluate low-frequency ABR thresholds in the clinical setting. **Figure 20–6** shows examples of ABR waveforms obtained using 500, 1000, and 4000 Hz tone bursts from a normal adult subject. The location of wave V is labeled when present in a particular waveform. Note the broad morphology of wave V for the 500 and 1000 Hz stimuli.

Accuracy of Threshold Prediction The predictive accuracy of tone burst ABR has been studied extensively by Stapells and colleagues (Stapells et al, 1990, 1995) in populations of normal and hearing-impaired infants, children, and adults. They used tone bursts with linear rise–fall times, at frequencies between 500 and 4000 Hz, presented with notched noise to enhance frequency specificity. The authors found similar results for all age groups. About 98% of ABR thresholds were within 30 dB of pure-tone behavioral thresholds, 91 to 93% within 20 dB, and 66 to 69% within 10 dB. The average ABR threshold was ~10 dB higher for 500 Hz tone bursts than for higher frequencies.

Bone-Conduction Auditory Brainstem Response Testing

Several investigators have shown that it is feasible to do ABR testing with bone-conduction (B/C) stimulation, using both clicks (Cone-Wesson and Ramirez, 1997; Mauldin and Jerger, 1979; Yang et al, 1987) and tone bursts (Cone-Wesson and

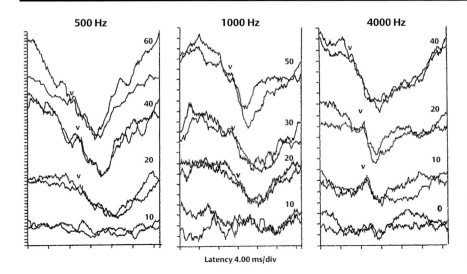

500 Hz   **1000 Hz**   **4000 Hz**

Latency 4.00 ms/div

Figure 20–6 Auditory brainstem response waveforms recorded from a normal adult with 500, 1000, and 4000 Hz Blackman-gated tone bursts. The number above each set of waveforms represents the intensity level in dB nHL (normalized hearing level).

Ramirez, 1997). As in pure-tone audiometry, B/C ABR testing is administered to estimate cochlear reserve in an attempt to define the type of hearing loss. It would typically be used when air-conduction (A/C) ABR thresholds are elevated and acoustic immittance results are abnormal or questionable. B/C ABR testing is particularly important for infants with ear canal atresia or other structural malformations of the external and/or middle ear when knowledge of cochlear status is crucial for planning habilitation.

Characteristics of the Auditory Brainstem Response to Bone-Conduction Stimulation   When B/C stimulation is used to elicit the ABR, wave V is the predominant component. The earlier waves, especially wave I, are often obscured by a large stimulus artifact. In adults, wave V latencies for B/C clicks are ~0.5 msec longer than latencies for A/C clicks at the same sensation level (Mauldin and Jerger, 1979), a difference that has been attributed to differences in the amplitude spectra of clicks for A/C and B/C (Mauldin and Jerger, 1979). In infants, in contrast, wave V latencies are shorter for B/C clicks than A/C clicks (Yang et al, 1987). Also, wave V thresholds for B/C are lower in infants than adults for both click and 500 Hz stimuli, with no difference seen for 4000 Hz stimuli (Cone-Wesson and Ramirez, 1997). Both the shorter latencies and lower thresholds for B/C in infants have been attributed to differences in skull characteristics between infants and adults (Yang et al, 1987) and to greater SPL values developed in the infant ear canal during B/C stimulation (Cone-Wesson and Ramirez, 1997).

Procedures for Recording the Auditory Brainstem Response with Bone-Conduction Stimulation   Details of recommended stimulus and recording parameters for B/C ABR testing have been reviewed by Cone-Wesson (1995). A basic description follows.

A vibrator placement on the temporal bone in the superoposterior auricular position (Yang et al, 1987) is recommended because it yields the lowest ABR threshold, particularly in infants. Yang and colleagues (1987) showed that wave V threshold was 30 to 40 dB higher in neonates using a forehead placement and 15 to 25 dB higher using an occipital bone placement, compared with a temporal bone placement. These differences were attributed to the fact that in infants, the skull sutures are not fused; therefore, the B/C stimulation is not efficiently conducted to the ear from the more remote locations. In adults, use of a forehead placement is not recommended because the behavioral threshold for B/C clicks in this location is ~10 dB higher than for a temporal bone placement, thereby reducing the maximum output available from the bone vibrator.

The vibrator may be held in place with the standard metal headband or a Velcro band placed around the head (Yang et al, 1987). It must be recognized, however, that securing the vibrator with a headband may be impractical in a sleeping infant. Use of a handheld vibrator is acceptable, provided that firm, consistent pressure is applied to the top of the vibrator with one finger only.

In recording B/C ABR, the inverting electrode should be placed at some distance from the oscillator to minimize stimulus artifact. Locations used include an inferior postauricular location, on the earlobe, in the ear canal, or low on the nape of the neck.

Both click and tone burst stimuli may be used for B/C ABR, as well as for A/C ABR. It is important to calibrate the B/C stimuli in terms of dB nHL. This is accomplished by finding the average behavioral threshold (0 dB nHL) for the B/C stimuli in a group of normal listeners, using the same oscillator placement as will be used for ABR testing. The 0 dB nHL value will be ~40 dB higher for B/C than A/C. This correction factor must then be applied to the intensity levels specified on the ABR instrumentation.

Analysis of test results involves comparing the wave V threshold for A/C and B/C stimuli to estimate the amount of air–bone gap. As for pure-tone audiometry, it is important to use masking in the contralateral ear when indicated.

Problems with Bone-Conduction Auditory Brainstem Response Testing   There are several problems related to B/C ABR testing that should be noted. At the higher stimulus levels, stimulus artifact from the oscillator can interfere with visualization of the ABR response, especially for tone burst stimuli. Stimulus artifact can be minimized by placing the oscillator high on the temporal bone and by using an earlobe, ear canal, or nape of neck location for the inverting electrode. The use of alternating phase stimuli will also minimize stimulus artifact, although this may substantially broaden the ABR response, especially for low-frequency tone bursts.

Another problem is that the maximum output of the BC vibrator is only ~45 to 55 dB nHL. This limits the ability to distinguish between mixed and sensorineural losses when A/C thresholds are elevated beyond the moderate loss range.

Suggested Diagnostic Protocol for Hearing Estimation

The diagnostic protocol should ideally combine ABR, otoacoustic emissions (OAE), and acoustic immittance measures (using a high-frequency probe tone for infants under 4 months of age) to maximize the information obtained regarding auditory status. For the ABR testing, first measure the click threshold and LIF in both ears. The click data provide a gross estimate of hearing sensitivity in the mid- to high-frequency range, as well as some insight into the type and configuration of hearing loss. In addition, analysis of the waveform at high click levels can be used to assess the integrity of the auditory brainstem (see section Otoneurological Assessment below). If click threshold and LIF are normal, and OAE are normal across the frequency range, then significant hearing loss can be ruled out in most cases. If click threshold and/or latencies are abnormal, or if OAE are abnormal, then frequency-specific ABR should be administered. A minimum of a low-frequency (e.g., 500 Hz) and a high-frequency (2000 or 4000 Hz) tone burst is needed to approximate the audiometric shape, which is essential prior to hearing aid fitting. If acoustic immittance results suggest evidence of middle ear abnormality, then B/C ABR should be administered (for at least one or two stimuli) to estimate the air–bone gap.

The duration of an ABR test session for infants and young children is limited by the amount of time they will remain sleeping. Because this time is unpredictable and may be quite short, the clinician must collect data in an efficient, judicious manner. Threshold search can be streamlined by beginning at a moderately high stimulus level (e.g., 60–70 dB nHL) and using bracketing to find wave V threshold in as few steps as possible. With experience, the clinician can learn to select test levels wisely, based on the appearance of the response at the current intensity level, to zero in on threshold in as few steps as possible. For example, a normal click LIF can be discerned using only 60 and 20 dB nHL test levels. Also, time may be saved by stopping the averaging if a response clearly emerges before the specified total number of sweeps is reached. The use of an automatic response detection procedure such as Fsp (described in the next section) can also save test time. If the child awakens before testing can be completed, a second diagnostic session should be scheduled as soon as possible.

Objective Auditory Brainstem Response Using the Fsp Procedure

When estimating hearing sensitivity using ABR threshold, one must determine the lowest stimulus level at which a response is present. This involves evaluating each waveform collected and deciding whether the ABR is present in the averaged waveform, or whether the average contains only noise. This judgment can be difficult at levels near threshold or when there is substantial noise in the average, especially for novice clinicians. Several statistical algorithms have been developed over the years to objectively analyze waveforms for response presence, thereby eliminating observer subjectivity. One such technique that is currently available commercially is the Fsp procedure, developed by Elberling and Don (1984).

In this procedure, the presence of the response is determined by comparing the overall amplitude of the averaged waveform to the background noise in the waveform. Overall amplitude is quantified by computing the variance across all points in the average, and background noise is quantified by computing the variance of a single point in the waveform over several sweeps. The two quantities are then compared in the form of a ratio to obtain the Fsp value. (F refers to the F ratio distribution, upon which the procedure is based; *sp* refers to "single point"). If the Fsp value exceeds a certain predetermined criterion, a response is judged to be present in the waveform.

An advantage of using the Fsp detection algorithm, in addition to eliminating observer subjectivity, is that it saves valuable test time because only one waveform needs to be collected at each stimulus level. Also, because Fsp is computed online during data collection, averaging can be stopped when the criterion value is reached, potentially saving additional test time.

Automated Auditory Brainstem Response Screening

In recent years, automated ABR instruments have been developed for screening newborns in a hospital setting. The need for such instrumentation arose because traditional ABR testing proved to be too expensive and time-consuming for mass screening of large numbers of infants.

ABR screeners use a single, low-level click stimulus (e.g., 35 dB nHL) to elicit the ABR. A computerized detection algorithm is employed to decide whether or not a response is present by comparing incoming data to a template of a normal waveform stored in memory. The result of this comparison yields a decision of either "pass" or "refer," depending on whether or not a response is detected. It is important to remember that, because a single click level is used, one cannot determine the degree of any existing hearing loss; rather, the test merely indicates which babies are in need of follow-up.

Because very little technical expertise is required to operate an ABR screener, testing can be accomplished by nonprofessionals such as technicians. This substantially reduces personnel costs for universal hearing screening programs.

Limitations of the Auditory Brainstem Response for Hearing Estimation

Although the ABR has proven to be a valuable clinical tool for auditory assessment, it does have limitations that must be kept in mind. First, because the ABR is generated subcortically, it does not truly measure "hearing." Rather, it assesses the integrity of the peripheral auditory system and auditory brainstem pathways, before sound is received by the cortex. Consequently, the ABR will not be sensitive to lesions above the midbrain level, which, if extensive, can impair hearing sensitivity. For example, in central deafness, due in most cases to bilateral temporal lobe lesions, persons typically show a normal ABR despite a severe to profound pure-tone hearing loss (Musiek et al, 2004). Though central deafness is relatively rare, clinicians need to be aware that the potential exists in certain pathological conditions for ABR to seriously underestimate the degree of hearing loss.

Additionally, ABR may overestimate the degree of pure-tone loss. In the recently recognized disorder termed *auditory neuropathy* (see, e.g., Berlin et al, 1998; Starr et al, 1996), the ABR waveform is absent or severely distorted and does not correspond to the behavioral pure-tone audiogram, which often shows only a mild or moderate degree of hearing loss. Speech recognition is typically poorer than would be expected based on the audiogram. Patients show normal outer hair cell function as evidenced by the presence of OAE and/or the cochlear microphonic. Auditory neuropathy is thought to be caused by a dysfunction of either auditory nerve fibers, inner hair cells, or the synapse between the two, which disrupts the neural synchrony necessary for ABR generation.

These cases highlight the importance of adhering to the cross-check principle by using a test battery diagnostic approach, including ABR, OAE, acoustic immittance, and behavioral audiologic testing when feasible, especially for individuals for whom amplification is contemplated.

Auditory Brainstem Response in Otoneurological Assessment

The ABR is useful not only in estimating auditory sensitivity but also in detecting retrocochlear lesions, that is, abnormalities along the auditory pathway beyond the cochlea, including the auditory nerve and various structures of the auditory brainstem.

Common examples of retrocochlear lesions are tumors of various types that may occur on the auditory nerve or within the auditory brainstem. Tumors originating outside the auditory brainstem can also affect the ABR if they grow large enough to exert pressure on the auditory brainstem pathways. Another type of retrocochlear lesion is demyelinating disease, most notably multiple sclerosis. The ABR has also proven useful in the detection of vascular lesions of the brainstem, including hemorrhage from a ruptured blood vessel or interruption of blood flow due to occlusion of a blood vessel.

In otoneurological applications, the ABR is useful in assessing the status of the auditory nerve and brainstem pathways because damage to these areas can alter the ABR in

characteristic ways. The location of the lesion will affect the ear in which ABR abnormalities are manifested. In general, a lesion of the auditory nerve will affect the ABR generated by stimulation of the ear ipsilateral to the lesion. In cases of large auditory nerve tumors located at the cerebellopontine angle, contralateral effects may also be seen due to compression of the brainstem. Lesions of the brainstem may cause ipsilateral, contralateral, or bilateral abnormalities of the ABR.

Pitfall

- It is not possible to diagnose the type of pathology causing the ABR abnormality (e.g., tumor vs vascular lesion). Abnormal findings merely indicate the possibility of a retrocochlear lesion, not the type of lesion.

In using ABR to assess the integrity of the central auditory pathways, click stimuli are generally used because they elicit the clearest waveform. Because information regarding auditory sensitivity is not of primary interest here, it is not necessary to find wave V threshold. Rather, the ABR is elicited at a fairly intense stimulus level, typically between 60 and 90 dB nHL, and various parameters of the ABR waveform are examined. Because peripheral hearing loss can confound the interpretation of many of the ABR parameters used in otoneurological assessment, the pure-tone audiogram should be obtained, when possible, before ABR testing for this purpose. Knowledge of the audiogram is also helpful in selecting the appropriate stimulus level. If hearing is normal, click levels of 60 to 70 dB nHL are typically used. If substantial high-frequency hearing loss exists, higher click levels may be needed to obtain useful data. If the ABR waveform is absent even at high click levels because of severe to profound peripheral hearing loss, then obviously the ABR cannot be used to detect retrocochlear pathology. The ABR parameters used in otoneurological assessment are described in the following sections.

Interpeak Latencies

The wave I–V interpeak latency (IPL) is the difference between the latency of wave I and the latency of wave V in a given waveform (**Fig. 20–7**). This IPL is often termed *central conduction time* or *brainstem transmission time*. Because Wave I is generated by the auditory nerve at the periphery of the auditory system, and wave V is presumably generated by lateral lemniscus fibers as they enter the inferior colliculus, the difference in latency between these waves is the time required for neural impulses to be conducted through the auditory brainstem. The normal wave I–V IPL is ~4.0 msec (Stockard et al, 1980). Retrocochlear lesions (e.g., a tumor causing pressure on the auditory nerve or brainstem) may slow neural conduction velocity and therefore increase the time between the ABR peaks. The IPL is usually considered abnormal if it is greater than 2.0 or 2.5 SDs above the mean.

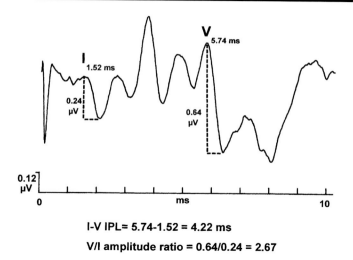

I-V IPL= 5.74-1.52 = 4.22 ms

V/I amplitude ratio = 0.64/0.24 = 2.67

Figure 20–7 Auditory brainstem response waveform from a normal adult, obtained with 80 dB nHL (normalized hearing level) clicks, showing calculation of the wave I–V interpeak latency and the wave V/I amplitude ratio. The absolute latencies and amplitudes of waves I and V are labeled on the waveform; the calculation of interpeak latency and amplitude ratio is shown below the tracings. IPL, interpeak latency.

Figure 20–8 (bottom) shows the ABR obtained from a patient with a surgically confirmed acoustic neuroma, compared with the ABR from a normal ear (top). Note that the wave V peak is prolonged in the tumor ear, thereby increasing the wave I–V IPL.

A further refinement of the IPL measure is to obtain the wave I–III and wave III–V IPLs as well. These measures are made in an attempt to more precisely pinpoint the location of the abnormality within the auditory pathway (Stockard et al, 1980).

In addition to comparing the IPLs to normative data, the IPLs may also be compared between ears in a given patient

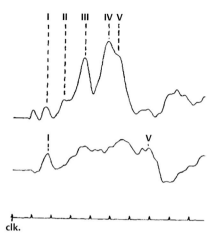

Figure 20–8 Auditory brainstem response (ABR) recorded from a patient with an acoustic neuroma (bottom) compared with the ABR from a normal ear (top). (From American Speech-Language-Hearing Association. (1987). The short latency auditory evoked potentials. Rockville Pike, MD: Author, with permission.)

for greater sensitivity. With retrocochlear pathology, the IPL may remain within normal limits, but may be longer in the affected ear compared with the other side.

Special Consideration

- It is important for the clinician to note that the wave I–V IPL can be influenced by the audiometric configuration. Specifically, high-frequency hearing loss of cochlear origin may prolong wave I more than wave V, resulting in a shortening of the wave I–V IPL (Coats and Martin, 1977). Thus, high-frequency cochlear loss can counteract the lengthening effect of retrocochlear pathology upon the wave I–V IPL, resulting in a false-negative outcome.

Absolute Latency of Wave V

Measurement of interpeak latencies depends on obtaining wave I, which usually appears in the ABR waveform only at moderate to high stimulus intensity levels. With significant hearing loss, it may not be possible to elicit wave I at the maximum stimulus level available, making calculation of the wave I–V IPL impossible. However, because a prolongation of the wave I–V IPL will also result in a prolongation of the wave V latency itself, some have used the wave V absolute latency in evaluating patients for retrocochlear lesions (Coats and Martin, 1977). A problem with using absolute latency is that hearing loss, both conductive and high-frequency sensorineural of cochlear origin, can cause some delay in the click-evoked wave V latency. Because many patients seen for otoneurological assessment will have concomitant hearing loss, this causes problems of interpretation and raises the possibility of excessive false-positive results. For this reason, the absolute latency of wave V is not typically used for otoneurological diagnosis.

Interaural Wave V Latency Difference

The interaural wave V latency difference is the difference in wave V latency, obtained at the same stimulus level, between the two ears. This measure is useful when inability to elicit wave I makes measurement of IPLs impossible. In normal-hearing individuals without neurological disease, the interaural wave V latency difference is typically 0 msec (± 0.2 msec). A latency difference greater than 0.2 to 0.4 msec between ears is generally considered abnormal (Bauch et al, 1996; Selters and Brackmann, 1977). As with the wave V absolute latency measure, there is a problem with false-positive results when using the interaural latency comparison if hearing loss is present. If a unilateral or asymmetrical hearing loss involving the high frequencies exists, wave V latency may be significantly prolonged in one ear simply because of the hearing loss, not because of retrocochlear pathology. Various correction factors have been proposed to compensate for the effects of hearing loss (Hyde, 1985; Selters and Brackmann, 1977), but none has gained universal acceptance. Another problem occurs when a retrocochlear lesion results in a bilateral prolongation of wave V. In this case, there may be no difference in wave V latency between ears, and the retrocochlear pathology will be missed.

Wave V/I Amplitude Ratio

Measures of absolute amplitude of the ABR waves have not proven to be useful clinically because amplitude is highly variable both within and between subjects and varies considerably with levels of physiological noise, electrode impedance, and electrode location. However, a relative amplitude measure, the wave V/I amplitude ratio, has proven to be useful in assessing brainstem integrity (Musiek et al, 1984; Stockard et al, 1977). To obtain this measure, the peak-to-peak amplitudes of waves I and V are measured (from the maximum positive peak to the following negative trough) and compared in the form of a ratio, as demonstrated in **Fig. 20–7**. In normal adults, wave V is larger than wave I, resulting in an amplitude ratio of > 1.0. Retrocochlear pathology may cause a decrease in wave V amplitude, resulting in a ratio of < 1.0.

Figure 20–9 shows the ABR obtained from the left and right ears of a patient with multiple sclerosis. Notice that, for right ear stimulation, wave V amplitude is less than wave I amplitude, resulting in an abnormal V/I amplitude ratio of < 1.0. The amplitude ratio for left ear stimulation is normal (> 1.0).

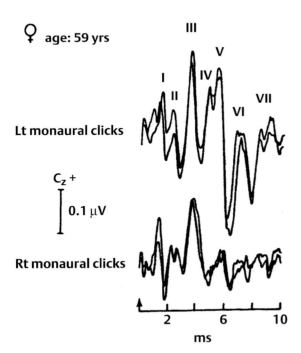

Figure 20–9 Auditory brainstem responses obtained from a 59-year-old patient with multiple sclerosis for left (top) and right (bottom) ear stimulation. Stimuli were 60 dB nHL (normalized hearing level) clicks. It can easily be seen that the wave V/I amplitude ratio is abnormally small for right ear stimulation. The latency of wave V is also slightly prolonged in the right ear relative to the left ear. (From Stockard, J. J., Stockard, J. E., & Sharbrough, F. W. (1977). Detection and localization of occult lesions with brainstem auditory responses. Mayo Clinic Proceedings, 52, 761–769, with permission.)

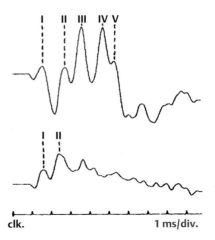

Figure 20–10 Auditory brainstem response (ABR) obtained from a patient with a meningioma in the cerebellopontine angle (bottom waveform) compared with a normal ABR (top). (From American Speech-Language-Hearing Association. (1987). The short latency auditory evoked potentials. Rockville Pike, MD: Author, with permission.)

Absent Waveform Components

Retrocochlear pathology may be severe enough to disrupt the generation of components of the ABR entirely, resulting in absent waves. The presence of a lesion at a given location can eliminate waves generated at the lesion site and rostral to the lesion. For example, with a tumor of the auditory nerve, wave I may be present because it is generated peripherally to the site of the tumor, while all the remaining waves may be absent. It is important to note that the absence of wave VI or VII is not diagnostically significant, because the presence of these waves is highly variable, even in normals. An example of missing ABR waves in a patient with a meningioma in the cerebellopontine angle is shown in **Fig. 20–10** (bottom). The ABR from a normal ear is shown in **Fig. 20–10** (top) for comparison. Note that only waves I and II are clearly present in the tumor ear.

Stacked Auditory Brainstem Response

A procedure called the stacked ABR has recently been developed by Don and colleagues (Don and Kwong, 2002) for detection of small tumors of the eighth cranial nerve (CN VIII). As noted by Don and Kwong (2002), standard ABR measures based on latency are quite sensitive to large CN VIII tumors, but they are less sensitive to tumors smaller than 1.0 cm. They speculate that this is because the latency of the standard ABR is dependent upon high-frequency auditory nerve fibers, whereas some tumors may affect only low- or midfrequency fibers in the early stages. The stacked ABR measures neural activity from all frequency regions of the cochlea, and thus has been shown to be more sensitive than traditional ABR methodology to tumors less than 1.0 cm (Don et al, 2005). A brief description of the stacked ABR procedure follows. The reader is referred to Don and Kwong (2002) for a more detailed explanation.

The ABR is obtained using click stimulation, first without masking, and then in the presence of high-pass noise masking at progressively lower cut-off frequency (8, 4, 2, 1, and 0.5 kHz).

In this manner, increasingly lower frequency regions of the cochlea are masked in each successive run. Next, the 8 kHz high-pass masked response is subtracted from the unmasked response to obtain the derived-band response from the area of the cochlea above 8 kHz. Similarly, the response masked with 4 kHz high-pass noise is subtracted from the 8 kHz masked response to obtain the derived-band ABR between 4 and 8 kHz. This procedure is continued for all of the masked responses, resulting in five derived-band ABRs spanning the length of the cochlea, each band approximately one octave wide. The latency of wave V will be progressively longer for each successive derived-band ABR, due in part to the traveling wave delay along the basilar membrane. Finally, the stacked ABR is constructed by time shifting all the derived-band waveforms so that their wave V latencies align temporally and summing the bands. The amplitude of wave V of the stacked ABR is then compared with normative data. A tumor is suspected if the amplitude is smaller than normal, based on an established criterion.

One limitation of this procedure is that cochlear loss can reduce the stacked ABR amplitude, resulting in a false-positive outcome (Don and Kwong, 2002). An automated version of the stacked ABR procedure is currently available from one evoked potential equipment manufacturer (Bio-logic Systems Corp., Mundelein, IL).

♦ Factors Affecting the Auditory Brainstem Response

The ABR is not affected by changes in the mental state of the subject, such as level of arousal or degree of attention paid to the eliciting stimulus. There is also no difference between waking and sleeping states, or with stages of sleep. For clinical use, the stability of the ABR across changes in mental state is an important advantage of the ABR over the later components of the auditory evoked potentials. There are, however, several subject factors that do influence characteristics of the ABR, including age, gender, pharmacological agents, and body temperature.

Age

Neonates and Young Children

The age of the patient must be considered in interpreting ABR results. ABR waveform morphology, peak latencies and peak amplitudes of neonates and young children differ from those of adults.

The ABR waveform in neonates consists primarily of three component peaks, corresponding to waves I, III, and V of the adult ABR (Jacobson et al, 1982; Salamy et al, 1975). During the first 18 months of life, the other component peaks of the ABR emerge, until the waveform assumes an adult morphology. The change in ABR waveform between newborn and adults is shown in **Fig. 20–11.**

Wave I amplitude in newborns is larger than in adults (Salamy et al, 1975), possibly because the recording electrode is closer to the cochlea due to the smaller head size of infants. On the other hand, wave V amplitude is smaller in

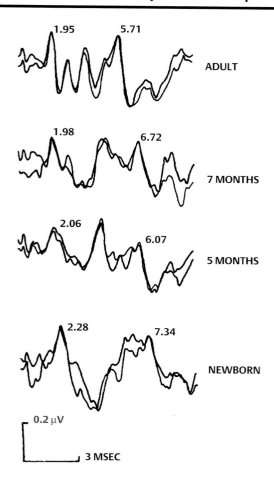

Figure 20–11 Auditory brainstem response (ABR) waveforms showing maturation of the response from newborn to adult. In each example, the latencies of waves I and V are indicated. Over time, the progressive emergence of waveform components, decrease in latencies, and change in amplitude ratio can be observed. (From Jacobson, J. T., & Hall, J. W. III. (1994). Newborn and infant auditory brainstem response applications. In J. T. Jacobson (Ed.), Principles and applications in auditory evoked potentials (pp. 313–344). Boston: Allyn & Bacon, with permission.)

infants than in adults. Therefore, the wave V/I amplitude ratio will be reduced for infants, often having a value less than 1.0 (Jacobson et al, 1982).

The latencies of the ABR waveform components are longer in neonates compared with adults and decrease progressively throughout the neonatal period due to maturation of the cochlea and brainstem. Wave I matures most rapidly, assuming an adult latency value by about 2 to 3 months of age (Jacobson et al, 1982; Salamy et al, 1982). Various reports show wave V assuming an adult value either by 12 to 18 months (Hecox and Galambos, 1974), by slightly over 2 years (Gorga et al, 1989), or as late as 2.5 years of age (Salamy et al, 1975). This differential maturation of waves I and V means that the wave I–V IPL progressively shortens as the infant grows. The wave I–V IPL decreases from ~5.0 msec at term to the adult value of ~4.0 msec by 12 to 18 months of age (Salamy et al, 1982). The time course of wave III maturation follows that of wave V.

The infant ABR is more vulnerable to the effects of increasing stimulus repetition rate. Consequently, slower rates of stimulus presentation may need to be used to maximize waveform clarity.

When testing infants from birth to ~18 to 24 months of age, it is important to use normative data appropriate for age, rather than adult values (see section Establishing Clinical Norms).

In premature infants, the ABR can be recorded as early as 27 to 30 weeks gestational age (Starr et al, 1977), although only at high stimulus intensity levels. As might be expected due to immaturity of the auditory system, latencies of waves I and V and the I–V IPL are prolonged in full-term infants, and decrease rapidly week by week until they reach full-term neonatal values at ~39 to 40 weeks of gestation (Starr et al, 1977). When testing premature infants, compensation must be made for the prematurity. The normative data used must be appropriate for conceptual age, which is the gestational age at birth plus the postnatal age. If premature infants are to be tested before they reach a conceptual age of 38 to 40 weeks (equivalent to full term), then norms must be established for various ages within the preterm period.

Older Adults

Some investigators have reported that ABR latencies increase with advanced age (e.g., Jerger and Hall, 1980). However, others have not found this effect of aging (e.g., Bauch et al, 1996).

> **Controversial Point**
>
> - The issue of whether it is necessary to establish separate normative data for older adults remains unresolved at this time.

Gender

A gender difference in ABR latencies and amplitude is well documented (Jerger and Hall, 1980; Stockard et al, 1979). Beginning at adolescence, females have slightly shorter wave III and V latencies than males. This difference is greatest for wave V, resulting in a wave I–V IPL ~0.1 to 0.2 msec shorter in females (Stockard et al, 1979). Females also show larger amplitudes for the later waves than males.

> **Controversial Point**
>
> - Some investigators (e.g., Don and Kwong, 2002) recommend establishing separate normative data for male and female adults to compensate for the gender difference. Others disagree (e.g., Bauch et al, 1996), feeling that any differences are not clinically significant.

Pharmacological Agents

Most sedatives, general anesthetics (with the exception of enflurane and isoflurane), and neuromuscular blocking agents have no effect on the ABR. This means that patients may be validly tested under sedation or anesthesia, a factor that makes the ABR particularly suited for clinical use.

Some drugs that have been shown to increase IPLs of the ABR are phenytoin, an anticonvulsant, and lidocaine, a local anesthetic that is used to treat cardiac arrhythmias. Alcohol intoxication has also been noted to increase IPLs, but some of this effect may be related to a concomitant decrease in body temperature (see next section).

Body Temperature

A decrease in body temperature below normal causes an increase in ABR IPLs (Stockard et al, 1980). This effect is thought to be due to slowed neural conduction velocity and synaptic transmission speed in hypothermia (Picton et al, 1981). Because low birth weight infants and comatose patients are prone to hypothermia, temperature should be measured prior to an ABR evaluation in these patients. One investigator (Hall, 1992) has published correction factors for the I–V IPL to compensate for the effects of hypothermia.

◆ Establishing Clinical Norms

When using ABR for threshold estimation and/or otoneurological assessment, it is vital to have appropriate normative values against which to compare patient data. Many of the ABR indices used clinically are dependent upon a host of stimulus and recording parameters, such as stimulus transducer type, stimulus intensity, stimulus polarity, stimulus presentation rate, tone burst frequency, tone burst rise–fall time, response filter settings, and electrode locations. Therefore, it is important to use norms that were obtained under conditions that are identical to the clinical protocol in use.

Because many ABR characteristics also vary with age, normative values must be established for all populations to be evaluated. When gathering norms, subjects are grouped by age intervals, which should be smallest where the expected rate of change in ABR parameters is largest. For example, if infants and young children are to be tested, an age grouping might be as follows: birth to 6 weeks, 7 weeks to 3 months, 4 to 6 months, 7 to 9 months, 10 to 12 months, and so on. If premature infants are to be tested before term, smaller age intervals should be used, for example, 31 to 32 weeks, 33 to 34 weeks, 35 to 36 weeks, 37 to 38 weeks, and so on, due to very rapid maturation during this period. If separate norms are to be established for older adults, the age groupings can be larger (e.g., 10-year intervals), beginning at about age 60, because the rate of change in the ABR is much slower. In addition to age-related norms, separate norms are sometimes established for male and female adults, due to gender differences in the ABR.

Normative values should be established for the following ABR parameters: absolute latencies (waves I, III, and V), interpeak latencies (I–V, I–III, and III–V), V/I amplitude ratio, wave V LIF for clicks, wave V threshold for B/C stimuli, and wave V threshold for tone burst stimuli.

The process of establishing normative data involves recording the ABR data of interest in a number of normal subjects, grouped within the preestablished age and gender categories.

For each group, the mean and SD of each ABR parameter are computed. The criterion for normality is typically considered to be within 2.0 or 2.5 SDs from the mean. The number of subjects required per group is not universally agreed upon. Many clinicians arbitrarily use 10 subjects per group, although there is no statistical basis for this practice. A better method has been described by Sklare (1987) for latency data, in which subjects are added to each group until the standard error of measurement for each ABR latency parameter is less than the time resolution of the response waveform. Using this approach, the number of subjects required per group will depend upon the variability in the data.

Gathering normative data can be a lengthy process. As an alternative, many sets of published norms are available (Cox, 1985; Gorga et al, 1987, 1989). One must be cautious, however, before using norms established at another facility. Clinicians need to be certain that stimulus and recording parameters for the published database, as well as characteristics of the normative population, are equivalent to their

particular clinical situation. If not, serious errors in interpretation of ABR data may arise.

♦ Summary

Auditory brainstem response testing is an important clinical tool for estimating hearing sensitivity and assessing the integrity of the auditory nerve and auditory brainstem pathways. This chapter has provided an overview of the ABR, including normative aspects of the waveform, recording procedures, clinical protocols, and interpretation. Numerous factors affecting the ABR, including stimulus and recording parameters, and pathologic and nonpathologic subject characteristics, have been described. It is important for the audiologist to be aware of these factors for accurate interpretation of ABR data in the clinical setting.

References

American Speech-Language-Hearing Association. (1987). The short latency auditory evoked potentials. Rockville Pike, MD: Author.

Bauch, C. D., Olsen, W. O., & Pool, A. F. (1996). ABR indices: Sensitivity, specificity, and tumor size. American Journal of Audiology, 5, 97–104.

Berlin, C. I., Bordelon, J., St. John, P., Wilensky, D., Hurley, A., Kluka, E., Hood, L. J. (1998). Reversing click polarity may uncover auditory neuropathy in infants. Ear and Hearing, 19(1), 37–47.

Coats, A. C., & Martin, J. L. (1977). Human auditory nerve action potentials and brain stem evoked responses Effects of audiogram shape and lesion location. Archives of Otolaryngology, 103, 605–622.

Cone-Wesson, B. (1995). Bone-conduction ABR tests. American Journal of Audiology, 4(3), 14–19.

Cone-Wesson, B., & Ramirez, G. M. (1997). Hearing sensitivity in newborns estimated from ABRs to bone-conducted sounds. Journal of the American Academy of Audiology, 8(5), 299–307.

Cox, L. C. (1985). Infant assessment: Developmental and age-related considerations. In J. T. Jacobson (Ed.), The auditory brainstem response (pp. 297–316). San Diego, CA: College Hill Press.

Don, M., & Kwong, B. (2002). Auditory brainstem response: Differential diagnosis. In J. Katz (Ed.), Handbook of clinical audiology (5th ed., pp. 274–297). Philadelphia: Lippincott Williams & Wilkins.

Don, M., Kwong, B., Tanaka, C., Brackmann, D., & Nelson, R. (2005). The stacked ABR: A sensitive and specific screening tool for detecting small acoustic tumors. Audiology and Neurotology, 10(5), 274–290.

Elberling, C., & Don, M. (1984). Quality estimation of averaged auditory brainstem responses. Scandinavian Audiology, 13, 187–197.

Gorga, M. P., Abbas, P. J., & Worthington, D. W. (1985). Stimulus calibration in ABR measurements. In J. T. Jacobson (Ed.), The auditory brainstem response (pp. 49–62). San Diego, CA: College-Hill Press.

Gorga, M. P., Kaminski, K. A., Beauchaine, W., Jesteadt, W., & Neely, S. T. (1989). Auditory brainstem responses from children three months to three years of age: Normal patterns of response. Journal of Speech and Hearing Research, 32, 281–288.

Gorga, M. P., Reiland, J. K., Beauchaine, K. A., Worthington, D. W., & Jesteadt, W. (1987). Auditory brainstem responses from graduates of an intensive care nursery: Normal patterns of response. Journal of Speech and Hearing Research, 30, 311–318.

Gorga, M. P., Worthington, D. W., Reiland, J. K., Beauchaine, K. A., & Goldgar, D. E. (1985). Some comparisons between auditory brain stem response thresholds, latencies and the pure-tone audiogram. Ear and Hearing, 6(2), 105–112.

Hall, J. W. III. (1992). Handbook of auditory evoked responses. Boston: Allyn & Bacon.

Hecox, K., & Galambos, R. (1974). Brain stem auditory evoked responses in human infants and adults. Archives of Otolaryngology, 99, 30–33.

Hyde, M. L. (1985). The effect of cochlear lesions on the ABR. In J. T. Jacobson (Ed.), The auditory brainstem response (pp. 133–146). San Diego, CA: College-Hill Press.

Jacobson, J. T., & Hall, J. W. III. (1994). Newborn and infant auditory brainstem response applications. In J. T. Jacobson (Ed.), Principles and applications in auditory evoked potentials (pp. 313–344). Boston: Allyn & Bacon.

Jacobson, J. T., Morehouse, C. R., & Johnson. J. (1982). Strategies for infant auditory brainstem response assessment. Ear and Hearing, 3, 263–270.

Jerger, J., & Hall, J. W. III. (1980). Effects of age and sex on auditory brainstem response (ABR). Archives of Otolaryngology, 106, 387–391.

Jerger, J., & Mauldin, L. (1978). Prediction of sensorineural hearing level from the brain stem evoked response. Archives of Otolaryngology, 104, 456–461.

Mauldin, L., & Jerger, J. (1979). Auditory brain stem evoked responses to bone-conducted signals. Archives of Otolaryngology, 105, 656–661.

Moller, A. R., & Jannetta, P. J. (1985). Neural generators of the auditory brainstem response. In J. T. Jacobson (Ed.), The auditory brainstem response (pp. 13–31). San Diego, CA: College-Hill Press.

Musiek, F. E., Charette, L., Morse, D., & Baran, J. A. (2004). Central deafness associated with a midbrain lesion. Journal of the American Academy of Audiology, 15, 133–151.

Musiek, F. E., Kibbe, K., Rackliffe, L., & Weider, D. J. (1984). The auditory brain stem response I–V amplitude ratio in normal, cochlear, and retrocochlear ears. Ear and Hearing, 5, 52–55.

Picton, T. W., Stapells, D. R., & Campbell, K. B. (1981). Auditory evoked potentials from the human cochlea and brainstem. Journal of Otolaryngology, 10(Suppl. 9), 1–41.

Purdy, S., & Abbas, P. J. (1989). Auditory brainstem response audiometry using linearly and Blackman-gated tonebursts. ASHA, 31, 115–116.

Rance, G., Dowell, R. C., Rickards, F. W., Beer, D. E., & Clark, G. M. (1998). Steady-state evoked potential and behavioral hearing thresholds in a group of children with absent click-evoked auditory brain stem responses. Ear and Hearing, 19(1), 48–61.

Salamy, A., McKean, C. M., & Buda, F. B. (1975). Maturational changes in auditory transmission as reflected in human brain stem potentials. Brain Research, 96, 361–366.

Salamy, A., Mendelson, T., & Tooley, W. H. (1982). Developmental profiles for the brainstem auditory evoked potential. Early Human Development, 6, 331–339.

Schwartz, D. M., Morris, M. D., Spydell, J. D., Brink, C. T., Grim, M. A., & Schwartz, J. A. (1990). Influence of click polarity on the auditory brainstem response (BAER) revisited. Electroencephalography and Clinical Neurophysiology, 77, 445–457.

Selters, W. A., & Brackmann, D. E. (1977). Acoustic tumor detection with brain stem electric response audiometry. Archives of Otolaryngology, 103, 181–187.

Sklare, D. A. (1987). Auditory brain stem response laboratory norms: When is the data base sufficient? Ear and Hearing, 8, 56–57.

Stapells, D. R., Gravel, J. S., & Martin, B. A. (1995). Thresholds for auditory brain stem responses to tones in notched noise from infants and young children with normal hearing or sensorineural hearing loss. Ear and Hearing, 16(4), 361–371.

Stapells, D. R., Picton, T. W., Durieux-Smith, A., Edwards, C. G., & Moran, L. M. (1990). Thresholds for short-latency auditory-evoked potentials to tones in notched noise in normal-hearing and hearing-impaired subjects. Audiology, 29, 262–274.

Starr, A., Amlie, R., Martin, W. H., & Sanders, S. (1977). Development of auditory function in newborn infants revealed by auditory brainstem potential. Pediatrics, 60, 831–839.

Starr, A., Picton, T. W., Sininger, Y., Hood, L. J., & Berlin, C. I. (1996). Auditory neuropathy. Brain, 119, 741–753.

Stockard, J. E., Stockard, J. J., Westmoreland, B. F., & Corfits, J. L. (1979). Brainstem auditory-evoked responses: Normal variation as a function of stimulus and subject characteristics. Archives of Neurology, 36(13), 823–831.

Stockard, J. J., Stockard, J. E., & Sharbrough, F. W. (1977). Detection and localization of occult lesions with brainstem auditory responses. Mayo Cinic Proceedings, 52, 761–769.

Stockard, J. J., Stockard, J. E., & Sharbrough, F. W. (1980). Brainstem auditory evoked potentials in neurology: Methodology, interpretation, clinical application. In M. J. Aminoff (Ed.), Electrodiagnosis in clinical neurology (pp. 370–413). New York: Churchill Livingstone.

Yang, E. Y., Rupert, A. L., & Moushegian, G. (1987). A developmental study of bone conduction auditory brain stem response in infants. Ear and Hearing, 8, 244–251.

Chapter 21

Middle and Long Latency Auditory Evoked Potentials

David L. McPherson, Bopanna B. Ballachanda, and Wafaa Kaf

The development of auditory evoked potentials (AEPs) closely follows advances in electronic technology. The earliest recording of a human AEP was accomplished by Vladimirovich Pravdich-Neminsky, a Russian scientist, in 1913 (Brazier, 1984). These recordings consisted of dim tracings on a cathode tube oscilloscope. Later, a camera would be used to take photographs of the cathode tube, and the waveforms that are "overlaid" would become dark because of the repetitive exposure of the cathode tube tracings on the film. The storage oscilloscope (i.e., the ability of an oscilloscope to "store" a recording without overwriting the previous tracing) coupled with a camera permitted an easier, more reliable means of reading the evoked potential recording.

During this same time, the recording oscilloscope, or what is more commonly called the strip-chart recorder, replaced the use of photographic film. However, it was the advent of the computer that brought AEPs out of the research laboratory and into the clinic. Allsion Laboratories was a pioneer in this area and manufactured the first commercial, clinical, evoked potential unit. Unfortunately, it was very expensive and short-lived. Interestingly, the early clinical use of AEPs faded because its use in establishing auditory thresholds was controversial and poorly defined. The discovery of auditory brainstem responses (ABRs) by Don Jewett in 1971 (Jewett and Williston, 1971) rekindled interest in the use of AEPs for estimating hearing sensitivity. The purpose of this chapter is to present material on the clinical use of middle and long latency AEPs.

♦ Recording Auditory Evoked Potentials

Some conventions used in this chapter need to be clarified. For example, the designation of polarity (positivity/negativity) may appear as positive up, negative down or negative up, positive down. These differences have a long history. In this chapter, the more conventional designation of positive up, negative down is used. However, in reading the literature, it is always important to refer to the figure designators and confirm the polarity of the waveforms.

Ferraro et al (1996) proposed a standard for presenting and specifying parameters in AEP testing and reporting. The tables in this chapter conform to those recommendations. Throughout this chapter, the designation dB nHL (normalized hearing level) is used as a reference to average behavioral threshold in normal subjects according to stimulus specifications.

Fig. 21–1 illustrates an overview of the morphological features of the AEPs discussed in this chapter. These were recorded from normal young adults (18–26 years old) without respect to gender. **Table 21–1** gives an overview of the description of the middle (MLAEPs) and long latency auditory evoked potentials (LLAEPs) discussed in this chapter. The reader is encouraged to use this chapter as a basis for further study and exploration into AEPs.

Electrodes

Electrodes consist of a metal alloy, the most common being tin, gold, silver, and silver-silver chloride (Ag-AgCl). For recording of responses whose frequencies are greater than ~100 Hz, the metal alloy is not particularly significant, especially for the ABR. Tin electrodes are frequently used in the clinical recording of the ABR unless extended recording times, beyond ~1 hour, are used. In such cases, both silver and gold electrodes have been found to be more stable. Low-frequency recordings, less than ~50 Hz, require stability as to changes in the surface potential between the electrode and the scalp. Gold electrodes tend to hold a potential and become polarized. Ag-AgCl electrodes are more stable, thus allowing long-term recordings of direct current (DC) potentials.

Because infection is always a possibility when abrading the skin as needed for electrode preparation, it is strongly recommended that disposable electrodes be used. In addition, skin preparation and electrode application should be performed with examining gloves.

It is common practice to use the linked earlobe, or linked mastoid, as a reference electrode site when recording many of the LLAEPs. This is particularly true for the P300 event-related potential (ERP). However, all electrode sites across the scalp are active. Therefore, one can expect electrical interactions of neural sites to bias the recordings obtained from other electrodes. This poses a particular problem in recordings, whereby the precise nature of the response across the scalp is desired, or in single-channel recordings, where hemispheric specificity is of interest.

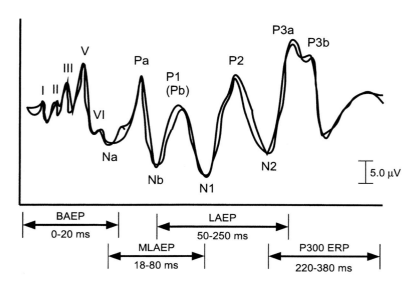

Figure 21–1 General morphological features of the auditory evoked potential (AEP) and the event-related potential (ERP). The auditory brainstem response (ABR) occurs between 0 and 20 msec post-stimulus; the middle latency auditory evoked potential (MLAEP), between 18 and 80 msec post-stimulus; the long latency auditory evoked potential (LAEP), between 50 and 250 msec post-stimulus; and the auditory ERP, between 220 and 380 msec post-stimulus. BAEP, brainstem auditory evoked response.

Table 21–1 Description of the Middle and Long Latency Auditory Evoked Potentials

Component	Classification	Latency (msec)	Amplitude (μV)	Response Features
Na	MLAEP exogenous	18–25	5–7	May be present even when the Pa is absent
Pa	MLAEP exogenous	24–36	8–12	
Nb	MLAEP exogenous	34–47	8–12	Not always fully developed until 8–10 years of age
Pb	MLAEP exogenous	55–80	5–7	Sensitive to changes in stimulus parameters (i.e., frequency, intensity, "on" and "off" effects); amplitude changes with sleep state
ASSR	Exogenous	9–38*	0.3–1.8*	This is a "frequency following" type of response using a combination of both AM and FM
P50 gating response	MLAEP exogenous/ gating response	40–70	3–8 (S1) 0–6 (S2)	S2 amplitude is 60% or less of the S1 amplitude in normal individuals; absent in ADHD and schizophrenia
P1	LLAEP† exogenous	55–80	5–7	Sensitive to changes in stimulus parameters (i.e., frequency, intensity, "on" and "off" effects); amplitude changes with sleep state
N1	LLAEP exogenous	80–150	5–10	Sensitive to changes in the acoustic features of the stimulus (i.e., spectrum); amplitude changes with sleep state and attention
P2	LAEP exogenous	145–180	3–6	Sensitive to changes in the acoustic features of the stimulus (i.e., spectrum); amplitude changes with sleep state and attention
N2	LLAEP endogenous	180–250	3–6	Sensitive to change in the acoustic features of the stimulus; amplitude significantly affected by attention as well as sleep state
MMN	Exogenous	200–300	30–50	Not affected by attention; subject sleep state will vary in both amplitude and latency
P300, P300a, P300b	Endogenous cognitive	220–380	12	P300a is related to stimulus novelty; P300b is related to task response; the amplitude is affected by attention as well as sleep state
N400	Endogenous linguistic	390–510	−10	Sensitive to linguistic content; amplitude changes with low versus high predictability sentences

* Designated as an MLAEP when labeled Pb. If labeled P1, then it is associated with the LLAEP.

† Designated as an LLAEP when labeled P1. If labeled Pb, then it is associated with the MLAEP.

Note: Amplitude and latency values vary with carrier frequency and type of modulation. For a detailed discussion, see Rodriquez et al (1986).

ADHD, attention deficit/hyperactivity disorder; AM, amplitude modulation; ASSR, auditory steady-state response; FM, frequency modulation; LLAEP, long latency auditory evoked potential; MLAEP, middle latency auditory evoked potential; MMN, mismatch negativity.

Pitfall

- Mixing electrode types will create unwanted electrical potentials and cause amplifier drift.

Electrode Montage

In referring to electrode montages, the 10 to 20 international system will be used (Jasper, 1958). The exception to this is when referring to mastoid placement of an electrode. Mastoid electrode placement will be abbreviated as M1 (left mastoid) and M2 (right mastoid). Also, Mi and Mc are used to designate ipsilateral mastoid (signal and electrode placement on the same side) and contralateral mastoid (electrode placement on the mastoid opposite the signal). Unless specifically stated as an exception, earlobe placement of an electrode (A1, A2) and mastoid placement of an electrode (M1, M2) are used interchangeably. However, the nonstandard use of a frontal electrode placement for the noninverting electrode instead of the vertex (Cz) electrode for ABRs, MLAEPs, and LLAEPs is not acceptable. This common, but technically incorrect, practice is discouraged.

All electrode sites across the scalp should be considered neural active sites. Wolpaw and Wood (1982) have clearly shown that the nasion, ear, and mastoid, as well as other cephalic locations, are in the auditory evoked field potential. Referential locations on or below the inferior neck provide the best and most accurate reference location. One of the most common locations is C7, located at the nape of the neck (McPherson and Starr, 1993).

Amplifiers

Considerable confusion exists over the use of amplifier and channel designations in evoked potentials. Much of the confusion is created by equipment manufacturers. The terms *noninverting* and *inverting* should be used in describing the amplifier inputs, and this convention has been used throughout this chapter. In general, the following are equated: (1) noninverting, positive, 1, active; and (2) inverting, negative, 2, reference. It is beyond the scope of this chapter to engage in a discussion of the technicalities of these terms. For a good discussion, readers are referred to Hall (1992) and McPherson (1996).

Many books and reference materials give gain specifications for the various AEPs. These are starting points. What is important is not so much the actual gain as a strong enough signal that meets the input requirements to the signal averager. It is also important to have a signal that does not overdrive the artifact reject. The best method to determine proper gain is to make an initial adjustment, and then, while viewing the raw unaveraged signal on the monitor, adjust the gain so that muscle movement will cause a reject. When the patient is quiet, the ongoing tracing will be relatively stable. Generally, a good starting for all AEPs is a gain setting somewhere between 10,000 and 20,000 times. Some manufacturers specify gain in terms of voltage per division. If a visual (i.e., screen) adjustment of gain is completed, it is a matter of adjusting the artifact to about three-quarters total screen excursion. Specifics need to be addressed based on the particular manufacturer.

Pearl

- Having the patient gently clench the teeth or lightly close the eyes is a good way to check the artifact reject setting.

Monitoring Eye Movement Artifact

Eye movement is a major known contaminant in the recording of AEPs, especially for low-frequency activity that is occurring beyond ~50 msec. This problem has two basic considerations. First, the amplitude and latency are such that not only may they obscure the desired response, but they may actually be mistaken for the response (Barrett, 1993; McPherson, 1996). Second, the eye blink is an easily conditioned response and may become synchronized with the auditory stimuli at a latency of ~250 msec.

An oblique electrode placement (**Fig. 21–2**) will permit the monitoring of both eye movement (i.e., electro-oculography) and eye blinks. The preferred situation is to activate the artifact rejection when the eye moves or blinks. An alternate procedure is to affix the electrode superior and lateral to the orbit of one eye and reference it to the contralateral mastoid (or earlobe). The bandpass of the amplifier should be approximately 0.1 to 30 Hz.

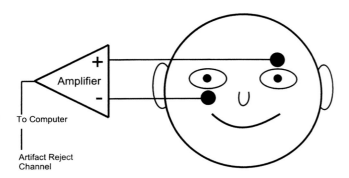

Figure 21–2 Placement of eye monitoring electrodes for eye muscle artifact. One electrode is placed above the orbit, and the second is placed below the orbit of the opposite eye. This permits both eye blinks and eye movement to be monitored and rejected from the recordings.

Postauricular Muscle Reflex

The postauricular muscle (PAM) is innervated by the posterior auricular branch of the facial nerve (seventh cranial nerve [CN VII]). The PAM contracts in response to moderately loud sounds and may become a conditioned reflex. Because of its timing (~18–30 msec), it may contaminate the MLAEP and be mistaken for a neural response within the MLAEP. The main feature in recognizing the PAM is that it is a very large negative response whose amplitude is not within the range of a known MLAEP. The PAM may easily be avoided by routinely using earlobe electrodes (A1, A2) instead of mastoid electrodes (M1, M2). If mastoid electrodes are used, placing the electrode on the head of the bony prominence will significantly reduce the probability of the PAM being recorded.

Repetition Rate and Interstimulus Interval

In most instances, the repetition rate (number of presentations per second) is the reciprocal of the interstimulus interval (ISI); the time between each individual stimulus presentation. However, in some instances, this is not the case, especially in paradigms that use paired or multiple stimuli. The ISI must be long enough to capture the entire desired response before the occurrence of the next trial.

Prestimulus Recording

We strongly recommend that all recordings include a prestimulus sample. That is, a sample that is ~10% of the sample window is obtained before the presentation of the acoustic event. This provides a better estimate of the baseline of the response and some indication of the noise present in the recording.

Pearl

- A good way to obtain an estimate of the noise level is to make a set of replicated averages with the stimulus off.

Subject State

The subject should be placed in a comfortable position with the neck at rest such that the muscles of the face and neck are in a relaxed position. The room should be sound isolated with no visual or other sensory distractions. A low light level is best. The person being tested should be instructed to be alert but not active. These instructions should be given for any of the recordings discussed in this chapter.

Controversial Point

- Although increasing the high-pass filter is frequently used in averaging techniques, this practice leads to distortion of the acquired waveform.

Attention

The effects of attention vary across components. In cochlear recordings and the ABR, it is not a significant factor. In the MLAEP, there is some indication that active attention may enhance the later components (Pb), but only to a very small degree. However, in the LLAEP and in auditory ERPs, the effect becomes significant, especially for responses occurring beyond ~150 msec.

Attention includes selective attention, whereby attention is maintained through an active discrimination task (i.e., same-difference task); active attention, whereby the observer is asked to respond to the stimuli (i.e., button push); passive attention, whereby the individual being tested is to be in an awake alert state but not necessarily attending to the stimuli; and an ignore condition, whereby the individual is being distracted from the stimuli. The effect of these various states of attention on the component varies with the component being measured.

Special Consideration

- In the original article on auditory neuropathy (Starr et al, 1991), it was noted that conditions exist whereby time-locked AEPs may be absent, such as in the ABR, as seen in auditory neuropathy, and cognitive AEPs may be present. This poses an interesting perspective on the interpretation of AEPs. It would appear that if the ABR is absent, one must ascertain whether the individual being tested fits this profile. Specifically, an auditory neuropathy is suspected when a percept of the auditory stimulus is present, but the ABR is absent despite the presence of the cochlear microphonic and otoacoustic emissions (OAE). If such is the case, then this significantly changes the interpretation of the AEPs. For example, if one is looking at a particular component of the MLAEP or LLAEP, and the components are absent or significantly abnormal, it becomes necessary to examine earlier components, especially wave I of the ABR. We strongly recommend the practice of preceding any AEP evaluation with both acoustic immittance measures, including tympanometry, and measures of OAE.

The use of the ABR for hearing screening and threshold estimation has been well established for almost 2 decades. It is primarily predicated on the observation that as intensity increases or decreases, latency demonstrates an inverse relationship. Wave V of the ABR is primarily used in this technique because it is very robust, stable, and repeatable (McPherson and Starr, 1993). Historically, the LLAEPs have not been used for hearing threshold assessment because latencies of these components generally do not show the same trend nor have they been considered as robust as the ABR (McPherson, 1996). Over the early years of developing the ABR as a measure of hearing amplitude, measures have been criticized as being unstable, especially across individuals. However, today these issues have changed, primarily because of changes in technology and a

better understanding of factors affecting these measures. It has clearly been established that the amplitude of the predominant AEP components are stable within the individual and that the changes seen in the amplitude with stimulus changes are consistent across individuals, although the absolute amplitude values across individuals may vary somewhat (McPherson, 1996).

Controversial Point

- The LLAEP is occasionally used to estimate hearing thresholds; however, because it has relatively high susceptibility to attention, the population it would be most helpful with is difficult to control for attention.

Although the amount of enhancement varies with each component, in general, it is important to realize that the greater a target signal is attended, the more robust the component is, with large effects of attention seen for the P300 and later responses (i.e., P300a, P300b, N400).

Calibration and Normal Values

Issues of stimulus calibration and specification are significant when recording and reporting AEPs, especially those discussed in this chapter. Significant differences exist between specifying a stimulus in dB HL (hearing level), dB nHL, dB SPL (sound pressure level), dB pe SPL (peak equivalent sound pressure level), and dB SL (sensation level). In some instances, the components will be more sensitive to threshold levels and SLs than to the actual SPLs. The reader is referred to Hall (1992), McPherson (1996), and Gorga and Neely (1994) for a more complete discussion on calibrating AEPs.

Peak latencies are fairly stable and robust in the major components of AEPs. Consequently, latency values may generally be used across studies and laboratories. This is not necessarily true for amplitude values. Electrode placement, filter settings, biological noise, stimulus specification, and subject state affect amplitude to a much greater extent than these factors affect latency. Although it is possible to use amplitude values from other studies and laboratories, it is absolutely necessary to maintain the exact stimulus and recording parameters as those that were used to obtain the normative data (**Table 21–2**). Even minor changes can affect the waveform. One of the greatest violations that occur in AEPs, and especially those using ABR, is adjusting filter settings and other parameters to obtain "better" waveforms. Indeed, such poor and naive techniques not only result in abuses of the procedure but also give the tester a false sense of obtaining reliable and meaningful test results. Unless one fully understands the consequences of changing a particular parameter, exact protocols should be followed. Clinicians should avoid using the phrase "In my clinical experience. . . ." This lead-in is commonly used as an excuse for the lack of rigor and understanding as related to established and proven procedures. The best procedure is to develop one's own normative data on the basis of the protocols chosen and keep within those protocols. Additionally, it is helpful to adopt published

Table 21-2   Summary of Auditory Evoked Potential Recording Parameters

Component	Montage[*],[†]	Time base (msec)	No. Averages	Filter	Stimuli (Type)	Level	Rate	ISI
MLAEP	Cz–Ai	80–100	500–1000	3–1500 Hz	Brief tones	75–80 dB nHL	5–11/s	90–200 msec (adult), 300–500 msec (young children)
ASSR	Cz–C7 or nape of neck	15–20	48–50	10–300 Hz	MM tones	10–120 dB HL	40–80 Hz	None (continuous tones)
P50	Cz–C7 or Ai	80	250–500	1–3000 Hz	Brief tone	70–75 dB nHL for both pairs	(see ISI)	S1-S2 interval, 500 ms S2-S1 interval, 10 s
LLAEP	Cz–Ai	300	200–250	1–300 Hz	Tone burst	75–80 dB HL	0.9–2.9/s	300 ms – 1.1 s
MMN	Fpz, F4, Fz, F3, C4, Cz, C3, Oz to tip of nose or C7	400	50–100	0.1–100.0 Hz	Oddball paradigm	75–80 dB HL	1/s	1000 ms
P300	Cz'–C7	500	200–250	0.05–50.0 Hz	Oddball paradigm	75–80 dB HL	0.9/s or less	1.1 s or longer
N400	Cz–C7	100 (pre) 750 (post)	100	0.05–50.0 Hz	Speech	75–80 dB HL	(see ISI)	1-2 s from end of sentence

[*] Montages are noted with the noninverting electrode stated first and the inverting electrode stated last (i.e., Cz–Mi, or Fpz, Cz–C7).

[†] A (earlobe) and M (mastoid) electrode designations are used interchangeably.

Ai, mastoid; ASSR, auditory steady-state response; Cz, vertex; Fpz, prefrontal area; Fz, frontal area; HL, hearing level; ISI, interstimulus interval; LLAEP, late latency auditory evoked potential; MLAEP, middle latency auditory evoked potential, MM, combination of both amplitude and frequency modulation; MMN, mismatch negativity; nHL, normal hearing level; Oz, occipital area.

data while maintaining the identical techniques that were used to collect the normative information.

Special Consideration

• At times, changes to protocol are necessary. Some information, after all, is better than nothing. As long as you know the factors induced in the changes to the protocol and clearly state the limitations on the report, such modifications are justifiable.

◆ Middle Latency Auditory Evoked Potentials

The MLAEPs consist of a biphasic waveform (**Fig. 21–3**), with a negative wave occurring at ~20 msec (Na), a positive wave occurring at ~30 msec (Pa), a second negative wave occurring at ~40 msec (Nb), and a second positive wave occurring at ~50 msec (Pb). The Pb component of the MLAEP is often identified as the P1 component of the LLAEP. However, because of the exogenous nature of the Pb, we prefer to classify it as an MLAEP. Further categorization of these components is seen because the Na–Pa wave has been identified as abnormal in temporal lobe lesions of the auditory system, and Pb has been reported as abnormal in schizophrenia, autism, stuttering, and attention deficit/hyperactivity disorder (ADHD). Buchwald and others have stated

that the Pb component of the MLAEP is related to activity of the reticular activating system and is responsible for the modulation of sensory stimuli (Buchwald et al, 1981; Erwin et al, 1991; Freedman et al, 1987; Hillyard and Kutas, 1983).

The MLAEPs represent primarily exogenous responses (i.e., those responses primarily generated by the physical characteristics of the stimulus) of the auditory system. The study of the generators of the MLAEP have given strong

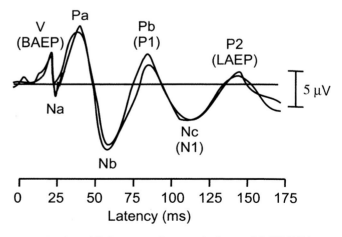

Figure 21–3 Middle latency auditory evoked potentials (MLAEPs) to a 2000 Hz pip presented at 70 dB nHL (normal hearing level). The components Pb and Nc are often considered part of the LAEPs. Wave V of the auditory brainstem response (ABR) and the P2 component of the late latency auditory evoked potential (LLAEP) are also shown to illustrate the distribution of the MLAEP. BAEP, brainstem auditory evoked potential.

support for thalamocortical projections to primary and secondary auditory cortices (Kraus, McGee, and Stein, 1994; McPherson and Starr, 1993; Parving et al, 1980; Di and Barth, 1992; Wolpaw and Wood, 1982; Wood and Wolpaw, 1982). However, clear evidence also exists that overlapping sources are present (Kraus, McGee, and Stein, 1994; McPherson and Davies, 1995; Wood and Wolpaw, 1982). Kraus and McGee (1995) suggest that the MLAEP pathways are sensory specific to the auditory stimulus, demonstrating a high degree of frequency specificity and temporal sequencing. Early portions of the MLAEP pathway are from the ventral portion of the medial geniculate with radiations into the primary auditory cortex. The MLAEP as recorded over the vertex is a mixture of both primary and secondary afferents, with the secondary afferents showing some state dependency, especially for sleep (Kraus and McGee, 1995).

Studies on the development of the middle latency response have yielded a variety of results and recommendations. The most important recommendation is that made by Kraus and McGee (1996), showing that to obtain reliable recordings of the middle latency response in infants, it is necessary to control and maintain subject sleep state. Specifically, these authors recommend that a constant state of light sleep or wakefulness be maintained throughout the testing. It is likewise necessary that this same state be maintained across subjects to develop and compare an individual recording to a set of age-matched norms.

Kraus and McGee (1996) have suggested that the middle latency response has a long developmental time course that is complete just after the first 10 years of life. The developmental aspects of the middle latency response appear to be related not only to amplitude and latency but also to the stability of the response and the effects of subject state. They attribute these factors to multiple generators of the MLAEP that may have different developmental sequences. Developmental studies by McPherson et al (1989) and Buchwald (1990b) have also shown that changes in morphology occur during development and that responses up to the Pb are usually present in the normal newborn period. The Na response is seen fairly consistently after the age of 8.

Pearl

- Light periodic fanning of a sleeping infant is enough to help keep the infant in a relatively stable and moderate state of sleep.

Filter settings are critical in the MLAEP, and incorrect filtering may provide false information, especially when using the MLAEP for maturation studies. Scherg (1982) observed waveform distortion in infants when filtering was narrowed, thus creating "phantom" peaks within the middle latency segment. Tucker and Ruth (1996) have shown that latency decreases and amplitude increases for the Pa component from birth (i.e., 24 hours postpartum) to adulthood. Most researchers agree that the MLAEP reaches adult values in the early teens.

Technical Specifications

The MLAEP is obtained with an 80 to 100 msec window. Between 500 and 1000 averages should be sufficient to collect replicable waveforms. A high-pass filter between 3 and 10 Hz and a low-pass filter between 1500 and 2000 Hz may be used (author preference is a bandpass of 3 to 1500 Hz). A presentation rate of ~5 per second will generally give good Na–Pa responses in adults; however, if the Na–Pa is not present or if young children or infants are being tested, it may be necessary to decrease the rate to 2 to 3 per second (**Table 21–3**). Unlike the Pa component that is present and is part of the primary auditory pathway, the later response, Pb, is part of the nonspecific auditory pathway and reticular activating system; thus, its presence and variation may depend on subject state.

Table 21–3 Middle Latency Auditory Evoked Potential Recording Parameters

Electrodes

Type	Ag-AgCl, silver, gold
Montage	Single channel
	Cz (noninverting)
	Ai (inverting)
	Fpz (ground)
	Multichannel (see text)
	Cz, T3, and T4 (noninverting)
	C7–noncephalic (inverting)
	Fpz (ground)

Recording Parameters

Channels	One channel is standard
	Two or more channels for hemispheric specificity
Time base	80–100 msec, with a 10 msec preanalysis
No. of averages	500–1000
Filter (bandpass)	3–1500 Hz
Artifact rejection	Three quarters maximum sampling amplitude

Stimuli

Type	100 msec acoustic clicks may be used but are not preferred
	Brief tone with a 2–1–2 cycle
	Blackman 5-cycle brief tone
Transducer	Tubal insert phones
	Calibrated earphones (e.g., TDH-39)
	Sound field speakers
Polarity*	Rarefaction
Level	75–80 dB nHL for a robust response showing all of the subcomponents
	Brief tones may be used to estimate hearing sensitivity, and the actual level would vary
Rate	Up to 11 per second, but lower rates are preferable (5 per second)
	In young children, rates as low as 2 to 3 per second yield best results
ISI	90–200 msec, with the longer ISI preferred
	300–500 msec in young children

* In children, it is sometimes necessary to reverse the polarity for better morphology.

ISI, interstimulus interval; nHL, normal hearing level.

Electrodes

The electrode type (i.e., Ag-AgCl, silver, or gold) is not critical, although tin is not recommended. The MLAEP does not require long time constants to record the response. Single-channel recordings are most common in the MLAEP. The MLAEP is maximally recorded over the vertex at Cz and referenced to the ipsilateral earlobe or mastoid. However, this gives a single vertex response (Cz) and does not provide information about interhemispheric responses. A more useful technique is to use three channels with electrodes located at Cz, T3, and T4 (noninverting), with a noncephalic electrode located at C7 or linked mastoids (A1 and A2). A ground, in either situation, is located at Fpz (prefrontal area). Similar montages have been consistently reported in the literature for use in measures of the middle latency auditory pathway function (Krause, McGee, and Stein, 1994; Kraus et al, 1982; McPherson and Starr, 1993).

Although the MLAEP does not have problems with eye movement contamination, it may become contaminated with activity of the PAM. This is no trivial matter and was the cause of extreme controversy in the early stages of evoked potential use. Contamination from the PAM may easily be reduced or resolved by using earlobe electrodes instead of mastoid electrodes (**Fig. 21–4**).

Recording Parameters

A 10 msec preanalysis baseline is obtained with an 80 msec post-stimulus recording. The signal is bandpass filtered between 3 and 1500 Hz, and 500 averages are obtained for each condition. An artifact reject is set to 75% maximum sampling amplitude to exclude the PAM reflex.

Stimuli

Oates and Stapells (1997a,b) demonstrated that the Na–Pa response of the MLAEPs, when using a derived band center frequency technique, showed good frequency specificity to brief tones. This would suggest that frequency specificity may be obtained in the MLAEP using brief tones with a linear 2–1–2 cycle window tone pip or a Blackman 5-cycle window tone pip. Both result in excellent frequency specificity for the MLAEPs.

Nelson et al (1997) showed that the variability of the Pb component of the MLAEP was reduced by using low-frequency (500 Hz) stimulation with a duration not less than ~60 msec and a repetition rate of 1.1 per second. The response was recorded optimally at Fz (frontal; inverting electrode) when a noncephalic reference (noninverting electrode) was used. They also reported that Pb had a larger amplitude and longer latency in children than adults. It should be realized, however, that a Cz placement is more common than Fz.

A rise–fall time of at least 2 msec is recommended to reduce spectral splatter and appears to maximize frequency specificity. Rise–fall times > 4 msec appear to significantly reduce the amplitude of the Na–Pa response. That is, the amplitude of the Na–Pa response increases for rise–fall

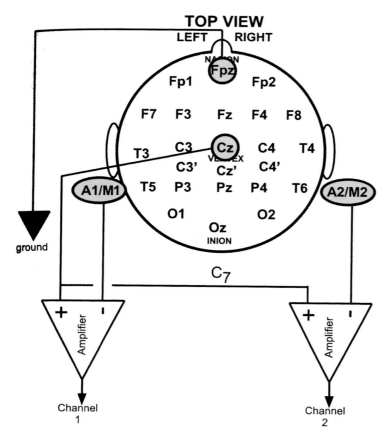

Figure 21–4 Electrode montage for the middle latency auditory evoked potential (Cz–A1 and Cz–A2).

times up to ~2 msec, asymptotes, and then shows a reduction in amplitude for rise–fall times > 2 msec. A rise–fall time of 4 cycles and a plateau time of 2 cycles is believed to be a good compromise in estimating an MLAEP threshold (Xu et al, 1997).

The stimulus may be presented in the sound field, through earphones, or through tubal insert phones. As previously noted, the intensity, except for threshold estimation, is usually at a moderately comfortable level (75–80 dB nHL). In adults, a rate of 5 per second gives the best results, but in young children and infants, a slower rate, between 2 to 3 per second, is necessary for reliable recordings.

Hearing threshold may be estimated by completing an intensity series beginning at 80 dB nHL and decreasing in either 10 or 15 dB steps. Threshold is estimated as the lowest level in which the Na–Pa response may be identified and is repeatable. Threshold estimation is completed by evaluating the changes in amplitude with intensity. Little or no latency change occurs with changes in the intensity of the acoustic stimulus.

The use of the MLAEP as a means of threshold estimation is extremely limited because of the necessity of controlling for sleep state, muscle contamination, and suppression of the MLAEP with sleep-enhancing drugs (i.e., chloral hydrate, barbiturates). The advantage, however, has been in the ability to obtain frequency-specific information, especially for the low frequencies where the use of click stimuli to obtain the ABR results in primarily mid- to high-frequency recordings. On the other hand, use of frequency-specific ABR techniques has greatly overcome this limitation in ABR (Oates and Stapells, 1997a,b).

Subject State and Variables

Kraus and McGee (1996) have shown that the MLAEP may be recorded in infants as long as the sleep state is controlled. These authors showed that the MLAEP is most consistent in the awake, stage 1, and rapid eye movement (REM) sleep conditions but extremely variable in stage 4 sleep. That is, changes occur in the morphology and detectability of the MLAEP as a function of sleep state. Consequently, it is necessary that a laboratory or clinic, when making these measurements in infants and very young children, be consistent in subject state. This necessitates the development of normative measures, group measures (e.g., age related), and repeated measures to be obtained in the same sleep state. It may be necessary to develop several sets of normative tables.

Litscher (1995) has shown that the amplitude of the Na–Pa component of the MLAEP decreases as body temperature decreases (similar to the amplitude and latency changes seen in the ABR). The author also demonstrated that increases in latencies and decreases in amplitudes of the MLAEP occurred during sedation of comatose patients. Although body temperature does not need to be monitored routinely, certain situations exist where this must be taken into account, such as coma or intraoperative monitoring of the MLAEP.

The MLAEP is suppressed with the patient under general anesthesia with the use of halothane, enflurane, isoflurane,

and desflurane (Schwender et al, 1996). The amount of suppression is dose-dependent and hence makes an excellent means of monitoring the depth of the anesthesia. Studies that have compared the electroencephalograph and the MLAEP during anesthesia have reported that the MLAEP is more sensitive to changes in the level of anesthesia (Plourde et al, 1997; Tatsumi et al, 1995).

Clinical Applications

Cottrell and Gans (1995) have reported significant differences in infants and children with multiple handicaps. Although no specific discriminant analysis or categorical profile was identified, the authors characterized the responses from these individuals as being "depressed" with substantial waveform variability.

Arehole et al (1995) recorded the MLAEP over the vertex and referenced the recordings to both the contralateral and ipsilateral mastoids in an attempt to obtain some hemispheric information on the MLAEP in a group of children classified as learning disabled. These authors reported abnormal recordings that varied with recording condition. The deviation from normal was varied, and no consistent trend was identified other than the MLAEP was abnormal, mostly for latency. Such inconsistencies are not surprising when one considers the observation that AEPs are not disorder-specific but appear to represent function.

Dietrich et al (1995) completed a study on 10 male stutterers and found that the latency of the Pb component of the MLAEP was significantly shorter than the age- and gender-matched controls, suggesting that some subcortical functional differences may be present in individuals who stutter.

The Pa component of the MLAEP has been used successfully in the establishment of threshold information and audiogram reconstruction. Although clicks have been used by some to obtain threshold estimates in the absence of ABRs (Kraus and McGee, 1990), tone pips provide a means to better assess the frequency response of the ear (Oates and Stapells, 1997a,b).

Controversial Point

- The use of clicks to obtain an MLAEP is widespread, especially among users of lower-end equipment. This practice results in poorer and more variable waveforms than the use of tone pips. Consequently, errors in diagnosis increase.

For example, the top panel of **Fig. 21–5** shows the morphological changes in the Pa–Nb waves for three frequencies as intensity is decreased. In the left panel, responses are seen at the lowest test level, 15 dB nHL. In the right panel, Pa–Nb is present at 15 dB nHL for the 500 Hz tone, 25 dB nHL for the 1000 Hz tone, and 45 dB nHL for the 4000 Hz tone. These have then been plotted as an amplitude-intensity function in the center panel. The bottom panel shows both the pure-tone audiogram and the evoked visual potential (EVP) thresholds plotted on a more traditional-looking

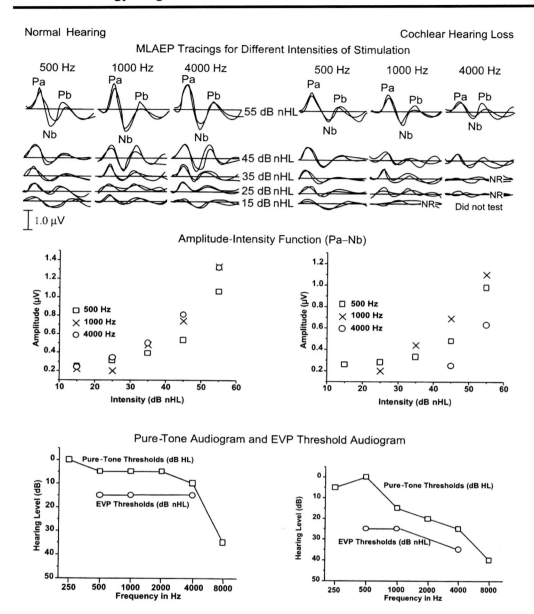

Normal Hearing   Cochlear Hearing Loss

Figure 21–5 Middle latency auditory evoked potentials (MLAEPs) in a normal ear (left side of figure) and in a cochlear hearing loss (right side of figure) for 500, 1000, and 4000 Hz tone pips. The top panel shows the averaged tracings for the Pa, Nb, and Pb components. The middle panel shows the amplitude-latency plots of the Pa–Nb components. The bottom panel shows both the pure-tone threshold audiogram and the reconstructed audiogram using the information obtained from the MLAEP. EVP, evoked visual potential; HL, hearing level; nHL, normal hearing level.

audiogram (remember that a difference in calibration does exist). The EVP thresholds overestimate the audiometric threshold by ~10 dB. Although this may seem excessive at first, it is better than no information and provides some frequency specificity. In using this information clinically, one takes into account the "average" difference.

Others have reported either absent or "abnormal" MLAEPs in (central) auditory processing disorders (C)APDs. These include Fifer and Sierra-Irizarry (1988), Özdamar and Kraus (1983), McPherson and Davies (1995), and Kraus and McGee (1996).

♦ P50 Gating Response

Two of the greatest challenges in audiology are the assessment of auditory thresholds in individuals in whom behavioral audiometric testing is either unreliable or not possible, and when the auditory disorder is not one of sensitivity but related to the processing of auditory information by the central nervous system (CNS). Sensory gating, which occurs in the MLAEP at ~50 msec after stimulus, has been found to be related to central auditory disorders, especially auditory attention.

Sensory gating in the auditory system is represented by a diminished response for repeated stimulation and appears to be necessary for targeted attention (Waldo et al, 1992). Auditory sensory gating uses a paired stimuli paradigm whereby two identical signals are separated by a short ISI (e.g., 500 msec), and the presentation of the pair has a much longer ISI (e.g., 10 seconds). The two stimuli presentations in the pair are averaged separately, and in the normal individual, the amplitude of the second paired stimulus will have a smaller amplitude, usually by ~40% (Nagamoto et al, 1989; Waldo et al, 1992).

The latency of the P50 auditory gating response occurs between 40 and 70 msec, suggesting a time window consistent with thalamic activity. Erwin et al (1991), in a study using a population of schizophrenic patients, stated that a sensory gating deficit is suggestive of subcortical dysfunction in the thalamus. However, Nagamoto et al (1989) believed that because gating depends on the interval between the paired stimuli and because responses in schizophrenic patients varied, multiple mechanisms were involved in sensory gating with various CNS pathways contributing to neuronal inhibition. Other areas, such as the temporal cortex and hippocampus, have been proposed, but the thalamic origin appears most likely at this time.

Technical Specifications

Electrodes

Because a relatively long time constant is used in the recording of the P50, it is recommended that Ag-AgCl electrodes be used. Other metals used in making electrodes tend to cause a shift in the DC potential gradient, thus giving rise to possible contamination from low-frequency artifact. A single-channel Cz–C7 (preferred) or Cz–Mi (mastoid) configuration is sufficient to record this response. A ground electrode may be placed at Fpz. In addition, eye movement must be monitored because the P50 response is in the general latency region of eye blinks that may become time locked to an acoustic event (**Fig. 21–6**). The signal is bandpassed between 1 and 3000 Hz (3 dB down, 12 dB/octave).

Pearl

- If excessive eye movement occurs, the use of cotton balls taped gently to the closed eyelid will provide enough light pressure to suppress involuntary eye movement.

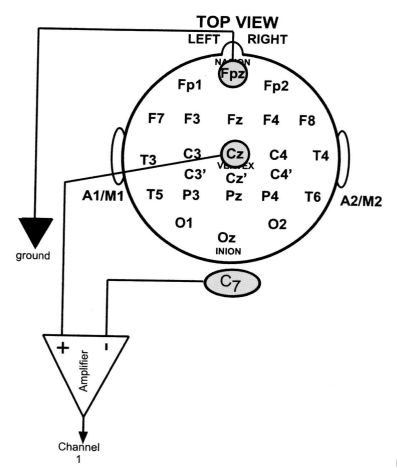

Figure 21–6 Electrode montage for the P50 (Cz–C7).

Recording Parameters

Although a single channel is used to record the P50 gating response to a paired stimuli paradigm, each stimulus (S1 and S2) must be averaged in separate buffers. Most commercial equipment allows for a P300 paradigm. The P50 protocol may be established by setting the P300 paradigm to identical stimuli, probability at 50%, nonrandom sequence, S1–S2 interval at 500 msec, and the ISI, or repeat cycle interval, at 10 seconds. This will permit the recording of the P50 on commercial equipment.

Each stimulus response, S1 and S2, is collected using an 80 msec sample window with a 10 msec preanalysis baseline. The signal is bandpassed between 1 and 3000 Hz, and an artifact reject is set on the eye blink channel.

Stimuli

Matched pairs of tone pips (i.e., S1 and S2) with a 2-cycle rise time, 1-cycle plateau time, and 2-cycle decay time (i.e., 2–1–2 cycle) are commonly used for these recordings (**Table 21–4**). Both S1 and S2 must be identical in frequency, intensity, temporal characteristics, and mode of presentation. That is, nothing can be different or novel between S1 and S2. Tubal insert phones or calibrated earphones, either a monaural or binaural (the latter being the most common), may be used. The stimulus should be presented at a moderate intensity, 70 to 75 dB nHL. A 500 msec ISI exists between S1 and S2 and a 10 second interval between the pairs. The 10 second interval is needed for the CNS to "forget" about the stimulus, whereas the shorter interval between S1 and S2 does not give the nervous system enough time to consider S2 a novel stimulus.

Pitfall

- Differences between S1 and S2 produce a mismatch negativity (MMN) and will be evaluated by the nervous system as two different stimuli, thus suppressing the gating response.

Subject State and Variables

No thorough or consistent studies have been done showing the effect of subject state on the response. However, active attention to the paired stimuli produces more consistent responses but does not account for the amount or frequency of suppression. Because this is a middle latency response, it must be assumed that, to a large extent, subject state considerations are similar for both types of responses.

Some aging effects appear on sensory gating. Freedman et al (1987) reported that in subjects younger than 18, the gating effect was more varied and perhaps absent before adolescence.

Other factors, such as attention (Jerger et al, 1992) and mood (Waldo and Freedman, 1986), do not affect sensory gating; however, anxiety, anger-hostility, and extreme tension tend to suppress the gating response.

Clinical Applications

It has been reported that, in normal subjects, the P50 amplitude of the second paired stimulus (S2) is ~5% of the P50 amplitude for the first paired stimulus (S1). The P50 may be completely absent in ~40 to 50% of those with normal auditory gating.

In our laboratory, for a vertex electrode recording, the upper limit for normal for the S2/S1 ratio is 0.68. For example, Boutros et al (1991) reported that the P50 to S2 will be completely absent (i.e., S2/S1 ratio of 0) in ~40% of the normal population. This is in contrast to schizophrenic patients, who will exhibit poorer suppression ratios of 95% or greater (Nagamoto et al, 1989), resulting in little or no suppression (**Fig. 21–7**). Similar findings are seen in adolescent males with ADHD.

Some have suggested that abnormal gating responses may be a genetic marker in schizophrenia. Siegel et al (1984) reported that ~50% of first-degree relatives of

Table 21–4   P50 Recording Parameters

Electrodes

Type	Ag-AgCl
Montage	Single channel
	Cz (noninverting)
	A11–A2, linked mastoid electrodes (inverting)
	FpZ (ground)
	Multichannel
	Cz (noninverting)
	C7–noncephalic (inverting
	Fpz (ground)
Eye movement (see text)	
Superior orbit of one eye to the inferior orbit of the opposite eye (polarity not specified)	

Recording Parameters

Channels	One channel is standard
	S1 and S2 must be averaged with equal trials, but separately
	Most equipment allows this by using a P300 paradigm with a probability of 50%
Time base	80 msec, with a 10 msec preanalysis
No. of averages	250–500
Filter (bandpass)	1–3000 Hz
Artifact rejection	Three quarters maximum sampling amplitude

Stimuli

Type	Brief tone with a 2–1–2 cycle
	Blackman 5-cycle brief tone
	Both S1 and S2 are matched identically
Transducer	Tubal insert phones
	Calibrated earphones (e.g., TDH-39)
Polarity*	Rarefaction
Level	70–75 dB nHL for both pairs
	Brief tones may be used to estimate hearing sensitivity, and the actual level would vary
Rate	See ISI for details
ISI	S1–S2 interval, 500 msec
	S2–S1 interval, 10 seconds

* In children, it is sometimes necessary to reverse the polarity for better morphology.

ISI, interstimulus interval; nHL, normal hearing.

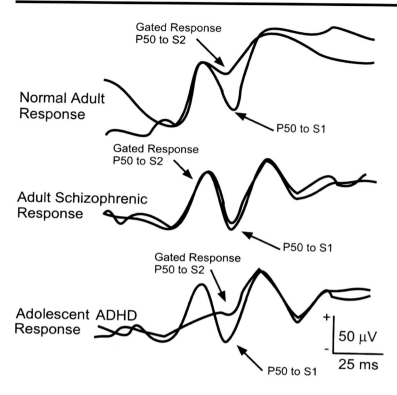

Figure 21–7 The P50 auditory gating response in a normal young adult male, a young adult female with schizophrenia, and a teenage male with attention deficit/hyperactivity disorder (ADHD). Notice on the top tracing that the S2 response is gated (i.e., a small amplitude negative wave) compared with the S1 response. Also, as noted in the bottom tracing, only partial gating has occurred to S2, illustrating the phenomenon that the amount of gating varies.

schizophrenic patients showed abnormalities in the gating response.

In addition to schizophrenia, the gating response has been found to change in manic depressive persons. Baker et al (1990) found that as depression increased, the ratio of the P50 auditory response increased (i.e., the amplitude of the P50 to S2 became larger). This type of graded response has not been observed in schizophrenic patients.

Special Consideration

- A neuropsychiatric history should be obtained before using this procedure.

◆ Long Latency Auditory Evoked Potentials

The LLAEPs traditionally have four components (**Fig. 21–8**): P1, occurring between 55 and 80 msec; N1, occurring between 90 and 110 msec; P2, occurring between 145 and 180 msec; and N2, occurring between 180 and 250 msec (McPherson, 1996). In some instances, the P1 of the LLAEP is also considered to be the Pb in the MLAEP.

The P1 response is primarily an exogenous potential (i.e., a response related strongly to stimulus parameters) occurring at ~60 msec. It is thought to represent late thalamic projections into the early auditory cortex and is part of the specific sensory system (Velasco et al, 1989). The P1 differs greatly from the N1, P2, and N2 components of the LLAEP

and consequently is considered, in general, to be part of the MLAEP. The N1 is also an exogenous potential, occurring at ~100 msec, and is associated with activity of the nonspecific multisensory system within the contralateral supratemporal auditory cortex (Knight et al, 1988). The P2 occurs at ~160 msec and is another exogenous potential of the nonspecific multisensory system demonstrating activity in the lateral-frontal supratemporal auditory cortex (Scherg et al, 1989). The N2 is the first of the endogenous potentials, occurring at ~200 msec. The N2 is part of the nonspecific multisensory system in the supratemporal auditory cortex (Velasco et al, 1989). The term *endogenous* refers to an ERP that is produced by the listener's internal processing of the stimulus. The N2 is highly related to attention, as is the entire N1–P2–N2 response, being related to the acoustic features of audition.

Technical Specifications

Electrodes

The LLAEP is maximal when recorded over the vertex at Cz. The typical recording is from Cz (noninverting electrode) to C7 (preferred) or the ipsilateral earlobe or mastoid (Ai) (inverting electrode). Hemispheric asymmetry measures may be obtained by using two channels, Cz–Ai and Cz–Ac (contralateral earlobe) (**Fig. 21–9**). Because the LLAEP may become contaminated with eye movement, as previously mentioned, it is necessary that eye movement be monitored by placing electrodes lateral to the orbit of one eye and superior to the orbit of the opposite eye. This will permit the simultaneous monitoring of vertical and horizontal eye movement and eye blinks.

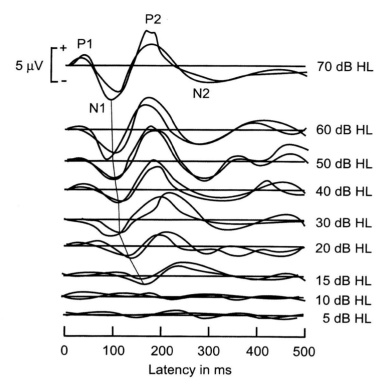

Figure 21–8 The long latency auditory evoked potential to different intensities. Notice that the latency of the response shows little variation at high to moderate levels, then quickly increases near threshold. In contrast, the amplitude shows a graded response with intensity.

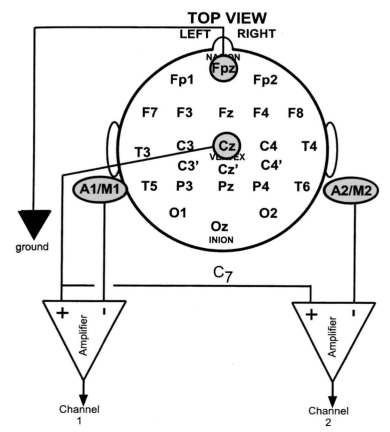

Figure 21–9 Electrode montage for the long latency auditory evoked potential (Cz–A1 and Cz–A2).

Recording Parameters

The most common type of recording is completed using a single channel. However, more useful information is obtained by the use of two or more channels. The recording should include a 50 msec preanalysis sample followed by a 300 msec post-stimulus sample (**Table 21–5**). A series of 200 to 250 artifact-free samples is obtained for each average, with a bandpass filter of 1 to 300 Hz.

Stimuli

The LLAEP, unlike the ABR, is not dependent on synchronous activity of the auditory nerve and brainstem. Consequently, more complex stimuli may be used in eliciting the LLAEP. The LLAEP is best recorded using tone bursts, speech, or speechlike stimuli. The response of the LLAEP is primarily to the acoustic features of audition, especially to the transition features. The most common, albeit the most simplistic, is a tone burst consisting of a rise–fall time between 5 and 10 msec and a plateau time between 25 and 50 msec. Speech material needs to have a total duration not greater than ~50 to 60 msec or minimally less than the first component of interest. Longer stimulus times will result in the recording of a sustained potential that may include stimulus artifact. For tonal stimulation, a rarefaction tone burst should be used, and in cases of poor morphological features, such as often seen in very young children, the polarity should be reversed between trials. The stimuli are presented at a rate between 0.9 and 2.9 per second, with the faster rates showing a reduction in the N1 amplitude.

Subject State and Variables

Both attention and subject state affect the LLAEPs. Attention appears to have its greatest effect on the N2 response, although the effects of subject and attention are similar. The amplitude of the N2 decreases when attention wanes. Subjects should be awake and attentive but not necessarily active in the task itself. Drugs that produce a central suppression of brain activity, such as barbiturates, will significantly influence and usually diminish the LLAEP.

Table 21–5   Long Latency Auditory Evoked Potential Recording Parameters

Electrodes

Type	Ag-AgC
Montage	Single channel
	Cz (noninverting)
	Ai (inverting)
	Fpz (ground).
	Multichannel (see text)
	Cz (noninverting)
	A1 (inverting)
	A2 (inverting)
	Fpz (ground)
Eye movement (see text)	
Superior orbit of one eye to the inferior orbit of the opposite eye (polarity not specified)	

Recording Parameters

Channels	One channel is standard
	Two or more channels for hemispheric specificity
Time base	300 msec, with a 50 msec preanalysis
No. of averages	200–250
Filter (bandpass)	1–300 Hz
Artifact rejection	Three quarters maximum sampling amplitude

Stimuli

Type	Tone bursts with a 5–10 msec rise–fall time and a 25–50 msec plateau time
	Brief duration speech material (i.e., CVC) may be used
Transducer	Tubal insert phones
	Calibrated earphones (e.g., TDH-39)
	Sound field speakers
Polarity*	Rarefaction
Level	75–80 dB nHL for a robust response showing all of the subcomponents
	Tone bursts may be used to estimate hearing sensitivity, and the actual level would vary
Rate	0.9–2.9 per second (we prefer the lower rate of about 0.9–1.3 per second)
ISI	300 msec–1.1 seconds, with the longer ISI preferred

* In children, it is sometimes necessary to reverse the polarity for better morphology.

CVC, consonant-vowel-consonant; ISI, interstimulus interval; nHL, normal hearing level.

Pearl

- A simple motivational technique for young children is to periodically award the child with tokens that may be exchanged for various rewards, such as toys, depending on the number of tokens accumulated throughout the test session.

Clinical Applications

The P1 is also discussed under the MLAEP Pb component because many of its characteristics are more representative of responses in that time domain. However, it is frequently designated as P1 in the clinical literature. Except for the P1, the LLAEP is usually seen as two distinct components: (1) the N1–P2 component, and (2) the P2–N2 or N2 component. We would like to suggest, however, that our preference for measurement is from baseline to the particular peak of the component (i.e., baseline–N1, baseline–P2). Because this is not a common convention in the clinical literature in the field of communicative disorders, we have chosen to use the more common method of amplitude measurement (i.e., peak-to-peak). The difficulty with peak-to-peak measures of the LLAEP components is that the amplitudes of the positive and negative peaks are not symmetrical, and each individual peak (i.e., positive peak, negative peak) varies. **Fig. 21–10** shows the N1–P2–N2 complex of the LLAEPs. Measurements include the N1–P2 peak-to-peak amplitude (10.7 mV), the P2 peak amplitude (7.2 mV), and the N1 peak amplitude (3.5 mV). As noted, the peaks are not symmetrical, with the positive

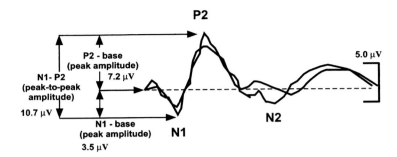

Figure 21–10 Long latency auditory evoked potential showing the measurement of the N1 peak amplitude, the P2 peak amplitude, and the N1–P2 peak-to-peak amplitude. Note the asymmetry in the amplitudes between the peak amplitudes of the N1 and P2.

peak having a greater amplitude. Because the generators and the stimulus response patterns are different between the individual peaks, using peak-to-peak measurements would reduce the value of the measurement.

Controversial Point

- In measuring the amplitude of a waveform, many studies may use a peak-to-peak measurement; however, it has been argued that the positive and negative peak may not necessarily represent the same set of generators and consequently behave differently. Therefore, a peak-to-baseline measurement may not only provide a more accurate measure but also be more sensitive to pathological changes.

P1 Component

The P1 has been shown to be useful in evaluating the development of the central auditory system and may be elicited in children with cochlear implants. Specifically, the P1 latency decreases as age increases, thus acting as an indicator of central auditory maturation (McPherson, 1996; Sharma et al, 2002).

One of the more interesting studies is that of Eggermont et al (1997) who used the P1 latency to study maturation of the auditory system in children with cochlear implants. These authors observed a graded maturation of the auditory system, as measured by changes in P1 with age. The normal-hearing group demonstrated a mature P1 by about age 15 years, whereas the children with cochlear implants showed a P1 delay in maturation about equal to the duration of the deafness. In earlier reports (Ponton, Don, Eggermont, Waring, Kwong, and Masuda, 1996; Ponton, Don, Eggermont, Waring, and Masuda, 1996), they were able to demonstrate that the regression line for development, as measured by P1, was interrupted in the deaf children but began after implant and eventually reached maturation, depending on the age at which the child received the cochlear implant. Similarly, Sharma and colleagues (Sharma, Dorman, and Kral, 2005; Sharma, Martin, et al, 2005) have demonstrated that there is a sensitivity period for central auditory development in young children, with children implanted

younger that ~3.5 years of age showing a strong development of the P1 waveform; those implanted later, after ~7 years of age, showed poorly developed P1 waveform morphology. There is good evidence to suggest that the P1 may be a "biological marker" of central auditory development and plasticity.

N1–P2 (N1) Component

Both the latency and amplitude of the N1–P2 response should be obtained. If one is interested in hemispheric asymmetries, the dominance (i.e., handedness) of the subject should be noted because ~27% of left-handed individuals will demonstrate a right hemisphere dominance (Knecht et al, 2000).

Because the latency of the N1–P2 is relatively stable within a variety of stimulus or pathological conditions, this measure may provide mean latencies within age groups. In children older than 5 and adults, we would expect to see this response out to ~195 msec. This would provide the following possibilities for the interpretation of latency: (1) normal (within age group), (2) maturational delay (below age group but older than 5), (3) prolonged latency (i.e., abnormal), and (4) absent.

Amplitude, unlike latency, varies considerably with both stimulus and pathological condition. Amplitude may also be expected to vary within the effect of age (i.e., increase with age to some extent). Stimulus intensity changes are also reflected in amplitude changes. As with the ABR, as the intensity of the stimulus decreases, the amplitude of the N1–P2 complex also decreases. However, latency remains stable except at and less than ~20 dB SL. Also, as the intensity becomes within ~10 to 15 dB of threshold, the P2 is no longer seen, and the N1 becomes the lowest observable response. This makes the N1–P2 a reasonable response for frequency-specific threshold information using an evoked potential paradigm. However, recording time becomes prolonged and, in individuals who are uncooperative, perhaps impossible due to movement artifact. Also, unlike the ABR, sedation cannot be used in recording the N1–P2 and may limit its use in obtaining frequency-specific threshold information in young children.

The N1–P2 reflects the acoustic characteristics of the acoustic stimulus. That is, it reflects changes in timing, the sequence of the event, and other physical dimensions, such as frequency and intensity. As a result, acoustic clicks, such as those used in the ABR, are poor stimuli.

P2–N2 (N2) Component

Similar to the N1–P2 component, both the latency and amplitude should be obtained for this response, along with information about dominance (i.e., handedness). Unlike the N1–P2, which is primarily exogenous, the N2 shows a greater influence of endogenous factors on the response than does the earlier N1–P2 component. In addition, the P2 shows a developmental sequence (**Fig. 21–11**). The P2 peak becomes larger and sharper with maturation (McPherson, 1996).

Intensity changes have little effect on the N2 for either latency or amplitude. However, significant changes are seen in the amplitude of the N2 for attention. Although the subject does not need to be actively attending to the task itself, the subject does need to be awake and alert (i.e., not drowsy). Active attention will slightly enhance the response.

The N2 first appears at ~3 years of age, with a latency between 200 and 280 msec, and reaches adult values by ~12 years of age, with a range from 185 to 235 msec. Because the changes in latency are not particularly outstanding with age, it is probably not a good measure of sensory maturation, although certainly the absence of the response in individuals older than 5 must be considered abnormal, particularly in light of the presence of earlier LLAEP components.

Similar to the latency of the N2, the amplitude is relatively stable and does not particularly vary with stimulus parameters. However, significant effects of amplitude have been seen in individuals with attention disorders. Specifically, the amplitude of the N2 shows approximately a 50% reduction of the N1/N2 ratio in these individuals.

The N2 is best obtained using a discrimination task of the acoustic aspects of the auditory event or a task requiring semantic discrimination. Hence, it may be used to evaluate such functions.

These measures have been used to study auditory function in cochlear implant patients. For example, Jordan et al (1997) studied the N1 and P300 in a group of cochlear implant patients. Findings revealed a general shortening of the latency of the N100 in the implant patients that began to approximate normal-hearing subjects. A two-tone perceptual task was used (i.e., detection of a 400 Hz vs 1450 Hz tone). Scalp distribution across the skull was broader for the implant patients than for the normal-hearing subjects. In addition, Micco et al (1995) reported, in a group of cochlear implant patients, no significant differences in the latency of the N1 and P2 when using the phonemes /da/ and /di/ as stimuli.

◆ Mismatch Negativity

Mismatch negativity is a recent introduction to the family of LLAEPs (Näätänen et al, 1978). The MMN is elicited by a physically deviant stimulus in a sequence of homogeneous, "standard" stimuli. The term *mismatch negativity* refers to the CNS's ability to compare a deviant stimulus to a previous standard set stored in short-term memory. It is assumed that MMN reflects an automatic mismatch process between the sensory inflow created by the deviant stimuli and the memory trace of the standard stimuli. These responses are automatic, not confounded by attention and cognitive factors, and can be observed even when the subject is not involved in the auditory task, such as while reading or performing visual discrimination. A typical response recorded from one subject is shown in **Fig. 21–12**. Responses to the deviant stimuli, that is, the infrequent and physically different stimuli, and for the sequence of the homogeneous standard stimuli are illustrated. The bottom trace labeled as MMN is derived by subtracting the responses to standard stimuli from that to the deviant

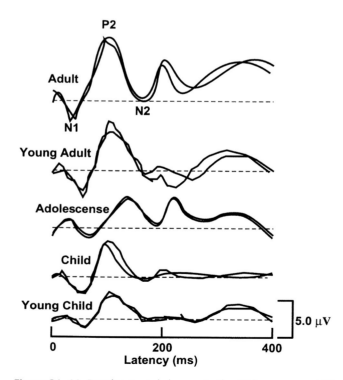

Figure 21–11 Developmental changes in the P2 from young child (~3 years old) to adult (~42 years old).

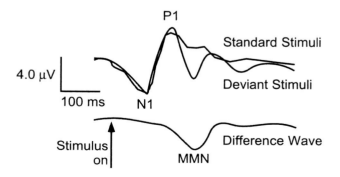

Figure 21–12 The mismatch negativity (MMN) to the phonemes /ba/ (standard stimulus) and /da/ (deviant stimulus). The bottom tracing shows the MMN as a difference wave; however, the MMN is clearly seen when the two waveforms (standard and deviant) are overlaid, as seen in the top tracing.

stimuli. The derived waveform (MMN) shows a clear negative deflection beginning at the N1 wave latency (~100 msec) and peaking later between 200 and 300 msec.

Amplitude and latency of the MMN are the most commonly measured parameters. Amplitude typically is measured between the positive peak and the following negative trough. The latency is measured from the time of stimulus onset to the initial peak of MMN waveform. In addition to these two measures, several researchers have used other analysis techniques to reflect other changes in the waveform. Most common is multiplying the peak amplitude of the MMN with its duration (Groenen et al, 1996). It is believed that this is a better indicator of the total amount of processing occurring in the MMN.

Studies investigating the scalp distribution of the MMN (Giard et al, 1990; Scherg et al, 1989), magnetic encephalography studies (Alho, 1995; Alho et al, 1994; Hari et al, 1984; Näätänen, 1992), intracranial studies in humans and animals (Csepe et al, 1987; Javitt et al, 1992; Kraus, McGee, Sharma, et al, 1992), and studies involving brain lesions in humans (Woods et al, 1993) have been used to identify the neural structures responsible for the generation of MMN. These studies indicate that the underlying neural structures contributing to the generation of the MMN are believed to lie in the auditory cortex. However, the exact location of MMN appears to change, depending on what aspect of the stimulus condition is varied (i.e., frequency, duration, intensity) and the complexity of the sounds (i.e., speech vs nonspeech sounds). In addition to the auditory cortex, strong indications show that frontal cortex activity contributes to the MMN, most probably related to automatic switching of attention from the standard signal to deviant stimuli. Animal studies suggest MMN subcomponents may be generated in the thalamus and hippocampus.

Technical Specifications

Electrodes

The most common electrode montage, recording parameters, and stimuli for MMN acquisition are listed in **Table 21–6**. Disk electrodes are used for MMN recordings, and Ag-AgCl electrodes are preferred to tin or gold-coated electrodes. No set montages, but good recordings, can be obtained by electrodes placed over the vertex (Cz), frontal area (Fz), parietal area (Pz), and, in some situations, over the occipital (Oz) and prefrontal (Fpz) areas. A single-channel recording may be obtaining by using an Fz electrode placement (**Fig. 21–13**). Electrodes placed at A1 or A2 produce a polarity reversal (Sandridge and Boothroyd, 1996), indicating variations in current density caused by dipole orientation. Electrode placements on the vertex and frontal cortex provide the best recording sites. The best recording site for the noninverting electrode is the tip of the nose. However, C7 as a noncephalic site is acceptable. The ground electrode can be placed on the forehead.

Recording Parameters

The number of electrodes can vary from three to seven, with three electrode recordings providing adequate

Table 21–6   Mismatch Negativity Recording Parameters

Electrodes	
Type	Ag-AgCl
Montage	Fpz, F4, Fz, F3, C4, C3, Oz (inverting)
	A1, A2, or tip of nose (noninverting)

Recording Parameters	
Channels	3–7
Time base	400 msec
No. of averages	50–100
Filter (bandpass)	0.1–100.0 Hz
	Artifact rejection

Stimuli	
Type	Oddball paradigm
Transducer	Tubal insert phones
	Calibrated earphones
Polarity	Not applicable
Level	75–80 dB HL
Rate	1 per second
ISI	1000 msec

HL, hearing level; ISI, interstimulus interval.

information. In addition to the scalp electrodes, two electro-oculogram electrodes should be used for monitoring eye movements. The time base of the recording window is usually set from 0 to 400 msec. A prestimulus baseline is recorded. Maturational studies require a wider recording window (**Table 21–6**).

Given that the MMN is part of the late evoked potentials, the amplitude values are considerably high. As a result, the number of averages can be as low as 50 or as high as 100. In addition, because the MMN contains very low frequency signals, the filters should be set between 0.1 and 100.0 Hz.

Stimuli

The stimulus condition applied to the recording of the MMN is a typical oddball paradigm using a probability for the deviant, or oddball, stimulus between .15 and .20 and the standard stimulus having a probability of .80 to .85. For example, given a deviant stimulus probability of .20, the standard stimulus probability would be .80. The MMN has been elicited by changes in stimulus parameters such as frequency (Sams et al, 1985), duration (Kaukoranta et al, 1989), intensity (Näätänen et al, 1987), and location (Paavilainen et al, 1989; Schroger, 1996). For example, the shorter the ISI, the larger the MMN amplitude (Näätänen, 1992). However, the MMN appears to be a suprathreshold phenomenon, and to elicit a robust MMN, stimuli must be presented at suprathreshold levels.

In addition to the tonal signals and their elementary variations, speech sounds have served to evaluate the discrimination abilities between categorical boundaries (Kraus et al, 1992, 1995), although they do not recognize categorical boundaries per se and have been used in newborns to determine simple discrimination abilities (Cheour-Luhtanen et al, 1995).

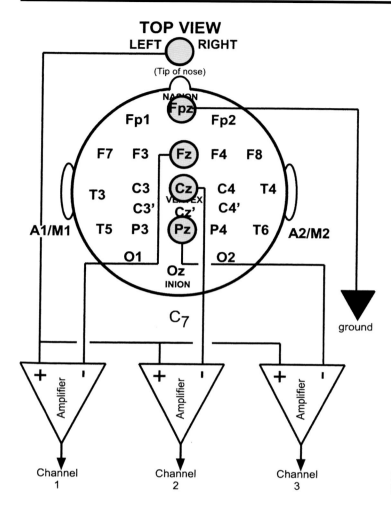

Figure 21–13 Electrode montage for the mismatch negativity (Fz, Cz, Pz–tip of nose).

Subject State and Variables

Unlike the late endogenous potentials, the MMN is not as affected by subject state, especially attention. Variations occur in individual MMN amplitudes and latencies across and within subjects. However, the amplitude variations seem to be greater than latency changes. Therefore, latency rather than amplitude appears to be a better indicator of the MMN response. The MMN amplitude and latency change with sleep level. When subjects are drowsy, amplitude and latency increase. For deep sleep, amplitude decreases, and the latency increases. Consequently, it is important for the subject to maintain alertness during the testing. Studies have also shown a positive relationship between MMN and drugs, with changes in waveforms noted with drugs, such as barbiturates, that have a general activating or deactivating effect on the CNS (Näätänen, 1992).

Clinical Applications

The MMN shows promise as a clinical tool in evaluating feature-specific testing of auditory functions in various hearing disorders. It can also be used to measure auditory analysis,

storing, and discrimination abilities. The advantages of the MMN are that it does not depend on attention and that it is a good technique to evaluate preattentive auditory discrimination processes and sensory memory.

Most of the clinical application is in the area of perceptual or processing abilities related to the psychophysical features of sound perception. The MMN has been used to examine the central auditory processing accuracy in patients with cochlear implants compared with normal-hearing subjects (Kraus et al, 1993a; Ponton and Don, 1995). In both of these studies, MMN findings suggest that the MMN can be used as an evaluation tool during rehabilitation.

Kraus and colleagues (Kraus et al, 1992; Kraus, McGee, Carrell, Sharma, Micco, and Nicol, 1993; Kraus, McGee, Carrell, Sharma, and Nicol, 1995), using a passive oddball paradigm and speech stimuli to obtain the MMN, were able to demonstrate that the MMN to speech stimuli provided a stable and reliable measure in school-age children and adults. They suggested that the MMN is a good tool for the study of central auditory function. In a subsequent study (Kraus, McGee, Litman, et al, 1994), the researchers reported on an adult with severely abnormal ABR in the presence of normal hearing. The MLAEPs, N1, P2, and

P300, were normal. However, the MMN was normal for speech stimuli in which the individual had relatively good speech perception but poorly defined when there was decreased speech perception. The case study points out the usefulness of the MMN and other AEPs in understanding auditory processing deficits. Other uses for the MMN have been in the study of voice onset time and central auditory plasticity (Tremblay et al, 1997), categorization of speech sounds (Sharma et al, 1993), and evaluation of speech in cochlear implant users (Kraus, Micco, et al, 1993). The latter study showed, using /da/ and /ta/ as paired stimuli, that the cochlear implant users were processing the speech stimuli the same as the normal-hearing individuals in the study. That is, essentially no difference was present in the MMN. The authors concluded that the MMN has potential as being an objective measure of cochlear implant function. Some controversy exists over its clinical adaptability because it is a derived waveform and not always easily identifiable.

The N1, P2, N2, P3, and MMN have been used to study auditory processing in individuals with cochlear implants. Kileny et al (1997) used intensity contrasts (1500 Hz for 75 vs 90 dB SPL), tonal contrasts (80 dB SPL for 1500 Hz vs 3000 Hz), and speech contrasts consisting of the words *heed* versus *who'd* in children with cochlear implants. Likewise, the MMN may provide an objective measure of speech perception in patients with cochlear implants. For example, both Ponton and Don (1995) and Groenen et al (1996) have shown that the MMN is a reliable tool for studying pitch and duration and that differences are seen in length of use of implant and implant effectiveness.

The MMN has also been shown to be useful in evaluating patients who are comatose, the aging population, those with Alzheimer's disease/dementia, those with Parkinson's disease, and in patients with CNS processing problems (for a review, see Csepe and Molnar, 1997).

◆ P300 Cognitive Auditory Evoked Potential

The P300 is a cognitive auditory ERP. It occurs in internal higher level brain processing associated with stimulus recognition and novelty. The P300 is classified as an endogenous auditory ERP and is non–sensory specific (i.e., it occurs with both unimodality and multimodality sensory stimulation). It occurs between ~220 and 380 msec. In some instances, it will be a bimodal peak with a P300a and P300b component (**Fig. 21–14**). The P300 is used in the study of memory disorder, information processing, and decision making.

The P300 has its maximum amplitude over the centroparietal areas at the midline. The generation sites of the P300 are complex, having multiple overlapping sites that appear to be simultaneously activated, especially in the frontal and temporal cortex. Activity is also seen in the temporoparietal association cortex. Other areas have included the primary auditory cortex and the multisensory association cortex (Buchwald, 1990a,b).

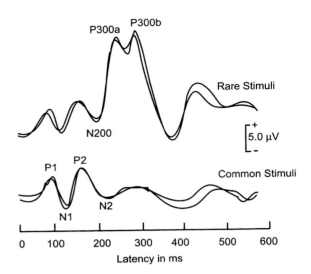

Figure 21–14 The P300 event-related auditory potential in response to the phoneme /ba/ (rare or oddball stimulus) and /da/ (common or frequent stimulus). The rare stimulus was presented with a probability of .20, and presentation of the stimulus did not occur in two consecutive trials.

Technical Specifications

Electrodes

The P300 may be recorded from an electrode placed between Cz and Pz, often referred to as Cz′, for the noninverting electrode, and C7 for the inverting electrode (**Fig. 21–15**). The ground may be placed at Fpz. A slightly normal variation appears in the maximum amplitude of the P300 from individual to individual between Cz and Pz. It is highly recommended that a three-channel system be used and that all three noninverting electrode positions be used (i.e., Fz, Cz, and Pz).

Eye movement can produce an artifact in the recording of the P300. The latency of this artifact is about the same as the P300. Therefore, protocol dictates that eye movement be monitored and that any such activity cause the sample to be discarded.

Recording Parameters

Although frequently used, single-channel recordings of the P300 are not recommended. This is primarily because of the normal variation of the response characteristics of the P300 along the midline. In the normal individual, the maximum may occur from Cz to Pz. The targets (rare stimuli) are averaged separately from the nontarget (standard or common stimuli) (see **Table 21–7** on p. 464).

A 500 to 800 msec epoch is recorded with a filter bandpass between 0.05 and 50.0 Hz. Two hundred artifact-free samples are collected consisting of 160 common samples and 40 rare samples. The amplitude of the P300 is enhanced by requiring the subject to actively attend to the rare stimulus. The two most common activities are to either have the subject count the rare stimuli or to push a button each time the rare stimulus occurs. **Fig. 21–14** is an example of a P300 recording.

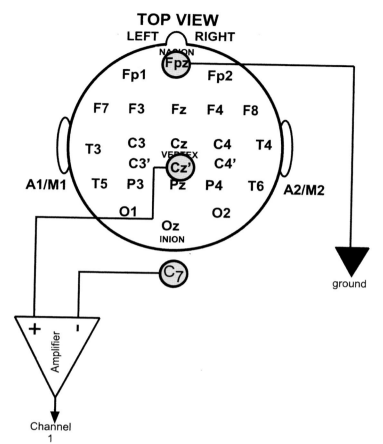

Figure 21–15 Electrode montage for the mismatch negativity (Cz–C7).

Special Consideration

- During active tasks, such as a button press, a premovement or premotor response may occur. This is called the Bereitschafts, or "readiness," potential. This is a slow negative potential that occurs up to 1 second before the onset of movement. In addition, two other potentials have been shown to occur just before motor movement. The characteristics of these potentials are such that they may both contaminate ERPs or be mistaken for an auditory neural response. The effect of these potentials becomes greater in conditioned response paradigms or where the subject has developed a sense of predictability in responding. Consequently, the more random and lower the probability of the oddball stimulus, the less these influences are observed in the recordings (a .20 probability of occurrence is optimum).

Stimuli

Tone bursts are the most common stimuli, having a rise–fall time of 10 msec and a plateau of 25 to 50 msec. Because stimulus novelty is paramount in obtaining a P300 response, two distinct tones should be used as the stimuli. This is referred to as an oddball paradigm, whereby one tone is the standard, common, or frequent, and the second tone is the deviant, oddball, or rare. Research has shown that the rare tone should randomly occur with a probability

not greater than .20 and should not occur twice in succession (McPherson, 1996). The response is not particularly affected by intensity, but differences in intensities between the two stimuli will affect the P300 response. Again, it is important to remember that it is the occurrence and recognition of stimulus differences that are the basis of the P300. An intensity level of 70 to 75 dB HL is sufficient to evoke a robust response.

Subject State and Variables

The significance, or task relevancy, is a key feature in the elicitation of the P300. Likewise, the occurrence of the rare, or target, stimulus must be uncertain. The more uncertainty or surprise (Donchin, 1981), the larger the amplitude of the P300. The P300 may be bimodal, having both an "a" and "b" component, depending on the particular paradigm being used. The "a" peak is present regardless of subject participation, whereas the "b" peak occurs when the subject is actively involved in the detection of the target stimuli, such as stimuli counting or button pushing (Michalewski et al, 1986). The amplitude of the P300 is primarily determined by two properties of the acoustic stimulus: the probability of occurrence and the meaning (i.e., perceived meaning) of the acoustic stimulus. Both of these factors need to be viewed relative to the subject's response (i.e., subjective probability and subjective meaning). It is the subjectiveness of these factors that makes the P300 so interesting and clinically useful.

Table 21–7   P300 Recording Parameters

Electrodes

Type	Ag-AgCl, gold (not preferred)
Montage	Single channel (not preferred)
	Cz' (noninverting)
	C7 (inverting)
	Fpz (ground)
	Multichannel (see text)
	Fz (noninverting)
	Cz (noninverting)
	Pz (noninverting)
	C7 (inverting)
	Fpz (ground)
Eye movement (see text)	
Superior orbit of one eye to the inferior orbit of the opposite eye (polarity not specified)	

Recording Parameters

Channels	One channel (not recommended)
	Three channels for best localization of the response
	The target, or oddball (rare), stimuli are averaged in one buffer, and the common or frequent stimuli are averaged in a second buffer
Time base	500 msec, with a 100 msec preanalysis
No. of averages	200–250
Filter (bandpass)	0.05–50.0 Hz
Artifact rejection	Three quarters maximum sampling amplitude

Stimuli

Type	Tone bursts with 10 msec rise/fall time and a 25–50 msec plateau time
	Brief duration speech material (i.e., CVC) may be used
	The target, or oddball (rare) stimuli, should occur not more than 20% of the time, randomly presented, and not occurring in succession
Transducer	Tubal insert phones
	Calibrated earphones (e.g., TDH-39)
	Sound field speakers
Polarity	Not specified
Level	75–80 dB nHL for a robust response showing all of the subcomponents
Rate	0.9 per second or less, depending on the stimulus length
ISI	1.1 seconds or longer, depending on the stimulus length

CVC, consonant-vowel-consonant; ISI, interstimulus interval; nHL, normal hearing level.

Picton and Hillyard (1974) have shown that the scalp distribution of the P300 shifts from a more frontal distribution to a more parietal distribution across the scalp as the task changes from active to passive participation. Consequently, a shift in the generators of the P300 is correlated with a shift in attention.

Special Consideration

- The use of tonal stimuli in a P300 paradigm is a simplistic type of task and is not as sensitive as using other stimuli, such as phonemes, that require more complex processing.

Clinical Applications

The clinical application of auditory P300 testing must begin with the fact that the P300 is task-relevant. Because of this, the P300 may be considered an index of stimulus processing and has great potential for studying higher level processing skills (McPherson, 1996).

In using an auditory continuous task paradigm, Salamat and McPherson (1999) found that the amplitude of the P300 in both a normal and adult ADHD population decreased as ISI decreased. However, the decrement of the P300 amplitude was greater in the ADHD adult population, suggesting that although the cognitive processes that are available in a normal population are present in an ADHD population, the degree of availability or quality of processes relevant to cognition is affected in the ADHD population. The use of P300 in trying to identify patients having ADHD versus ADHD-like behavior is useful in planning intervention schemes, especially because auditory attention disorders are generally present in ADHD populations, and treatment of auditory disorders with and without ADHD would vary. The latency of the P300 is more variable and longer in school-age children with confirmed ADHD than in age-matched, normal children when task difficulty was held constant and equal for both groups. P300 abnormalities in ADHD reflect processing as opposed to discrimination differences.

Kileny (1991) reported on the use of the P300 in the assessment of cochlear implant users as a means of determining cognition and discrimination. Likewise, others have shown its use in auditory discrimination tasks, including intensity (Hillyard et al, 1971), frequency, and duration (Polich, 1989b; Polich et al, 1985). In general, changes in frequency, intensity, and duration may be seen in changes in P300 latency. Frequency also affects amplitude of the P300.

Hurley and Musiek (1997) studied the effectiveness of central auditory processing tests in the identification of cerebral lesions in adults 22 to 73 years old. The P300 was recorded using an oddball paradigm, with a 1000 Hz tone as the frequent stimulus and a 2000 Hz tone as the oddball stimulus. The P300, using this paradigm, had a hit rate of ~59%. The researchers also reported a 98% probability of a patient not having a central auditory nervous system disorder when the P300 was normal.

The auditory P300 has been used to study auditory deprivation. Hutchinson and McGill (1997) looked at 17 children with profound bilateral deafness between the ages of 9 and 18 years who had been fitted with monaural hearing aids. An oddball paradigm using tonal stimulation revealed asymmetry in P300 results between ears and between an age-matched group of children with normal hearing. Although the purpose of the study was to show the importance of binaural amplification, the study illustrates the use of the P300 in the assessment of auditory function.

The use of P300 recordings in patients with cochlear implants has shown changes in the P300 consistent with behavioral performance in an oddball task. That is, patients who could behaviorally identify the oddball presentation showed a clear P300. In a few patients with cochlear implants who could behaviorally perform the oddball task, the P300 was absent (Jordan et al, 1997).

Micco et al (1995), using an oddball paradigm to synthesized phonemes of /da/ and /di/, reported that in the patients with cochlear implants, essentially no differences were seen in the P300 between the implant users and normal-hearing individuals. It was concluded that the P300 possibly may be a useful tool in evaluating cognitive function in cochlear implant users.

The P300 has been of greatest use in the study and diagnosis of dementia and Alzheimer's disease. The latency of the P300 is significantly increased for adjusted age level in dementia and shows both a decrease in amplitude and an increase in latency of the P300 in Alzheimer's disease. These differences, along with other clinical signs, help to distinguish Alzheimer's disease from dementia and other neuropsychiatric diseases, such as Korsakoff's psychosis (Barrett, 1993; Michalewski et al, 1986; Polich 1989a; St. Clair et al, 1988).

The amplitude and latency of the P300 are abnormal in several types of neuropsychiatric and behavioral disorders. The P300 has been found to demonstrate reduced amplitudes in autism and schizophrenia. An increase in the latency of the P300a and P300b, along with a decrease in the amplitude of the P300b, has been observed in ADHD. A decreased amplitude and increased latency of the P300 have been reported in children with (C)APDs (Allred et al, 1994; Goodin, 1990; Jirsa, 1992; Kraiuhin et al, 1990; Martineau et al, 1984, 1989; McPherson and Davies, 1995; Muir et al, 1988; Polich, 1989a; Polich et al, 1990; Satterfield et al, 1990; St. Clair et al, 1988).

◆ N400 Semantic Evoked Potential

Auditory evoked potentials occurring between 300 and 500 msec after stimulus onset are sensitive to lexical aspects of speech (Kutas and Hillyard, 1980). The N400 is an ERP that may be elicited after a semantically incorrect sentence, specifically one in which the ending is unexpected (**Fig. 21–16**). For example, the sentence "The dog bit the cat" has high contextual constraints, and the ending has a high probability of occurrence. This would be contrasted by the sentence "The dog bit the moon," whose ending would have a low probability of occurrence. The latter sentence would produce an N400. Terminal

words in spoken sentences with varying degrees of contextual constraint and probability will produce different amplitudes in the N400. Ending words with a high degree of expectation produce a low-amplitude N400, whereas ending words with a low degree of expectation produce a high-amplitude N400 (Connolly et al, 1990).

The latency of the N400 shifts with the complexity of the task (Connolly et al, 1992), whereas the amplitude of the N400 shifts inversely with the expectancy of the terminal word (Kutas and Hillyard, 1984). As can be understood from this brief discussion, the occurrence of an N400 requires a high level of linguistic processing, thus providing a mechanism of assessing brain processing of language.

The N400 demonstrates a centroparietal distribution in scalp topography (Connolly et al, 1990; Kutas and Hillyard, 1980, 1982). Similar to the P300, undoubtedly multiple, simultaneous overlapping generators exist.

Pitfall

- Lambda waves occur over the occipital region of the scalp in normal waking individuals have an amplitude between 20 and 50 mV and a frequency of ~8 to 12 Hz. Lambda is bilateral synchronous activity, lasting for ~200 to 300 msec, with a periodicity between 200 to 500 msec (Perez-Borja et al, 1962). Billings (1989) has shown that lambda waves may be time locked to both random and evoked saccadic eye movement and do not consistently appear in all recordings (Chatrian, 1976).

- Lambda waves cannot be elicited in darkness but may occur in darkness to eye blinks or eye movement (Niedermeyer, 1987). They have been reported during eye opening even in dimly lit situations and in the absence of eye movement.

- Lambda activity occurs in ~82% of children between 3 and 12 years of age, 72% of young adults between 18 and 30, and 36% of adults between 31 and 50 (Chatrian, 1976; Shih and Thompson, 1998).

- To prevent contamination from lambda activity, the ISI should be set to a time period that has a slight variation or to an odd-numbered value.

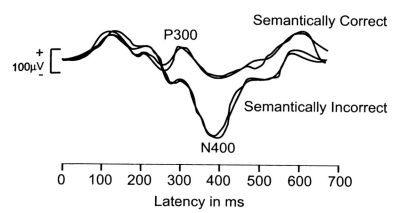

Figure 21–16 The N400 event-related potential to a semantically correct sentence ("The dog chewed the bone") and to a semantically incorrect sentence ("The dog chewed the green"). The N400 appears to the semantically incorrect sentence.

Technical Specifications

Electrodes are placed at Cz (noninverting) and referenced to C7 (**Fig. 21–17**). The signal is bandpass filtered between DC and 300 Hz. A 750 msec post-stimulus sample is acquired. Eye movement must be monitored.

Because the response diminishes rather quickly as a result of semantic adaptation, a total of 100 samples is obtained by collecting 50 trials of high-constraint, high-predictable sentences and 50 trials of low-constraint, low-predictable sentences (**Table 21–8**). The sentence presentations should be pseudorandomized. The sentences are presented at a comfortable level, ~70 dB HL in the binaural condition. A 1500 msec ISI is used. The subjects are merely instructed to listen carefully to the sentences. A good source for sentences is the SPIN test (Bilger et al, 1984). A subset of the sentences that have been found appropriate for first graders and above is as follows.

High-contextual constraint, high-predictability sentences:

1. The dog chewed on a bone.

2. Football is a dangerous sport.

3. A bicycle has two wheels.

Low-contextual constraint, low-predictability sentences:

1. Betty knew about the nap.

2. Jane has a problem with the coin.

3. They knew about the fur.

Subject State and Variables

The subjects must be awake and alert. They should be instructed to listen carefully to the sentences. Because eye movements may contaminate the results, they must be monitored. Because of the necessity of using a relatively small number of averages, eye movement artifact must be reduced and not just rejected by the averaging process.

Pearl

- Two basic mechanisms have varying degrees of success. The first is to have the individual focus on an object that is in the center of a relaxed visual field (but not fixate). The second is to have the individual gently close his or her eyes, place a cotton ball over the closed eyelid, and gently tape the cotton in place. Again, the problem of lambda wave contamination is of concern.

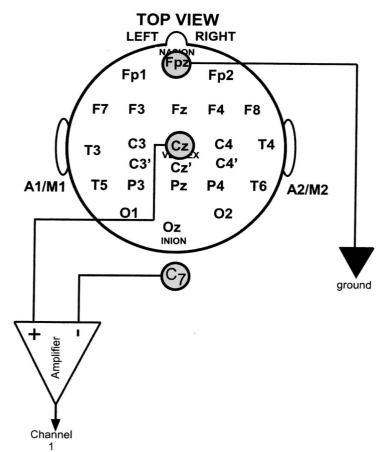

Figure 21–17 Electrode montage for the N400 (Cz–C7).

Table 21–8   N400 Recording Parameters

Electrodes

Type	Ag-AgCl
Montage	Single channel
	Cz (noninverting)
	C7 (inverting)
	Fpz (ground)
Eye movement (see text)	
Superior orbit of one eye to the inferior orbit of the opposite eye (polarity not specified)	

Recording Parameters

Channels	Single-channel response
	Each of the two stimuli, highly predictable and less predictable, are averaged in separate buffers
Time base	100 msec prestimulus
	750 msec post-stimulus
No. of averages	200 (100 for each stimulus)
	Presentations greater than 100/stimulus set will cause a diminished N400 (similar to habituation)
Filter (bandpass)	0.05–50.0 Hz
Artifact rejection	Three quarters maximum sampling amplitude

Stimuli

Type	Speech stimuli where S1 is a highly constrained and predictable sentence and S2 is a less constrained and less predictable sentence
	The sentences are pseudorandomized
Transducer	Tubal insert phones
	Calibrated earphones (e.g., TDH-39)
	Sound field speakers
Polarity	Not specified
Level	75–80 dB nHL for a robust response showing all of the subcomponents
Rate	See ISI
ISI	1–2 seconds from end of sentence

ISI, interstimulus interval; nHL, normal hearing level.

Clinical Applications

Kutas and Hillyard (1984) have shown that semantic "unexpectancy" results in the N400 and not a semantic "unrelatedness." Likewise, grammatical incongruities do not produce an N400; consequently, grammatical and semantic incongruities are not produced in the same manner.

The N400 does not appear to be part of the stimulus discrimination process associated with the N2. For example, in a phonological masking paradigm, Connolly et al (1992) showed the N400 latency increased for a phonologically correct masker. No changes were noted in the N2. The researchers concluded that their findings support a cognitive, semantic processing of the sentence.

The presence of an N400 depends on the complexity of the processing task, which shifts the latency of the N400, and the degree of expectancy of the terminal word, which is inversely related to the amplitude of the N400. In other words, amplitude shifts give information as to the ability to predict word usage from contextual cues, and latency shifts indicate the ability to process complex linguistic information.

Kutas and Hillyard (1983) reported on a series of school-age children that the N400 was present to semantic processing but was not present in sentences containing grammatical errors, thus concluding that grammatical errors are processed in a different manner than semantic incongruities.

Phonologically correct masking (i.e., 12 talker babble) was studied by Connolly et al (1992) using both the N200 and N400 ERPs. The N400 was affected by the presence of the phonological correct masking, whereas the N200 showed no effects, suggesting that the N400 responds to linguistic processing, and the N200 responds to the acoustic processing of the sentence. Because both potentials may be observed in the same recording, it is apparent that the N200 and N400 represent two distinct ERPs.

Other levels of language activity have also been studied. For example, syntactic anomalies, such as subcategorization, agreement violations, and tense violations, have been found to elicit a negative wave occurring between 300 and 500 msec, similar to the N400 but with a maximal amplitude over the frontal region of the scalp, as opposed to centroparietal distribution of the N400 (Connolly et al, 1990; Friederici et al, 1993; Kutas and Hillyard, 1980, 1982, 1983).

◆ Auditory Steady-State Response

The ASSR is an auditory evoked potential that uses continuous tonal auditory stimulation. It is considered an MLAEP and commonly termed the "40 Hz response" (Galambos et al, 1981). Early investigations of 40 Hz responses have shown that they are not reliable in infants because they are affected by sleep (Klein, 1983; Linden et al, 1985) and immaturity within the auditory system (Stapells et al, 1988). Currently, these limitations are somewhat overcome by recording the ASSR using higher modulation frequencies (80–110 Hz). Although these rapid rate responses are smaller in amplitude than the 40 Hz response, they are less affected by sleep and may be more reliably recorded in infants and sleeping children (Aoyagi et al, 1993; Cohen et al, 1991).

The ASSR reflects an ongoing response to continuous overlapping stimuli. This differs from the ABR, which uses a transient auditory stimulus, such as a click or tone burst/pip, which reflects immediate, transient response to a single stimulus. The ASSR may be elicited by amplitude modulation (AM), frequency modulation (FM), a combination of both AM and FM (MM), exponential amplitude modulation (AM^2), or independent amplitude and frequency modulation (IAFM). Mixed modulation stimuli are most commonly used and preferred because they produce the largest amplitude responses (Cohen et al, 1991; John et al, 2001; Petitot et al, 2005). **Fig. 21–18** illustrates both the time and frequency domain of an MM stimulus.

ASSR, when using a high modulation frequency, is capable of evaluating hearing sensitivity in individuals where reliable behavioral thresholds are not possible. Unlike the click ABR, which is unable to evaluate the low and midfrequencies for hearing, ASSR is capable of evaluating the four primary

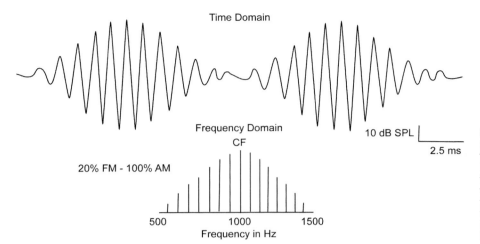

Figure 21–18 The top figure shows an amplitude modulation (AM) (100% modulation)/frequency modulation (FM) (20% modulation) tone with a 10 msec duration. The test frequency is 1000 Hz, with FM occurring between 800 and 1200 Hz. The AM occurs from full amplitude to zero amplitude. The bottom figure is a spectrum (fast Fourier transform [FFT]) of the stimulus shown in the top figure. SPL, sound pressure level.

audiologic frequencies—500, 1000, 2000, and 4000 Hz (Dimitrijevic et al, 2002; Herdman and Stapells, 2001, 2003; Kaf et al, 2006; Lins et al, 1995). The advantage of recording ASSR to multiple stimuli is an estimated 50% decrease in test time (John et al, 2002). In addition, the ASSR can assess thresholds up to the limits of most audiometers (~110 dB HL). This becomes important in the assessment of amplification, including cochlear implants (Rance and Rickards, 2002). Some reports, however, have shown conflicting responses when utilizing high stimulus levels and in cases with mixed hearing loss (Gorga et al, 2004; Jeng et al, 2004; Small and Stapells, 2004).

The click ABR provides a robust response, although it is not a frequency-specific response. Although there are techniques in ABR that permit a more frequency-specific recording, these are much more time consuming than utilizing ASSR and have a limited intensity range of ~90 dB nHL. Also, an important aspect of the ASSR is that the analysis is determined by well-founded analytical techniques (Aoyagi et al, 1993; Dobie and Wilson, 1996; Stapells et al, 1987; Valdes et al, 1997).

Pearl

- ASSR is valuable in assessing hearing thresholds and provides frequency-specific information in the speech frequency range.

Neural Generators

The ASSR is a neural response generated by repetition of the early and middle auditory evoked potentials elicited by a stimulus train, thus producing overlapping responses. The resulting ASSR is a neural response that is phase-locked to the modulation envelope of the acoustic stimuli.

There are conflicting opinions regarding the generator sites of the ASSR. Candidates include the cochlear nuclei, brainstem neural tracts, inferior colliculus, thalamocortical radiations, and auditory cortex (Pethe et al, 2001). The neural generators arise from multiple overlaying sources (Kiren et al, 1994; Tsuzuku, 1993) and differ at different modulation frequencies. According to Kuwada et al (1986), low modulation frequency

responses are generated by neuronal sources with long activation delays, and high modulation frequency responses are generated by neuronal sources with short activation delays. Kuwada et al (2002) have suggested that these sources may be in the midbrain or pons and the superior olivary complex or cochlear nucleus, depending on the modulated frequency. For low modulation frequencies, below 40 Hz, the cortex is involved in the generation of the ASSR, and for modulation frequencies ~40 to 60 Hz, the ASSR generators are believed to be subcortical, similar to those of MLAEPs. The ASSR with modulation above ~70 Hz has similar generators to those of the ABR (Herdman et al, 2002). Furthermore, ASSRs to high modulation frequencies have a shorter latency (7–9 msec) compared with ASSRs to low modulation frequencies (30 msec). This suggests that signals with low modulation frequencies travel farther and originate in the central auditory pathway, whereas higher modulation frequencies arise in the lower part of the central auditory pathway (Herdman et al, 2002; Kuwada et al, 1986). Because responses to higher modulation frequencies are subcortical, subject state is of less concern than with the MLAEP or LLAEP. Consequently, the ASSR is seen as peak responses situated around the rate of stimulation and its adjacent harmonics (**Fig. 21–19**).

Special Consideration

- The ASSR response to high-frequency modulation has essentially the same generators as the ABR, and hence subject state is of less concern than with low-frequency modulation.

Technical Specifications

Electrodes

Electrode locations are recommended based on the information about the best generator site(s). For example, Johnson et al (1988) recorded 40 Hz ASSR using a 21-channel topographic mapping. They found that front-central regions and the posterior neck elicit the largest 40 Hz ASSR. Thus, a

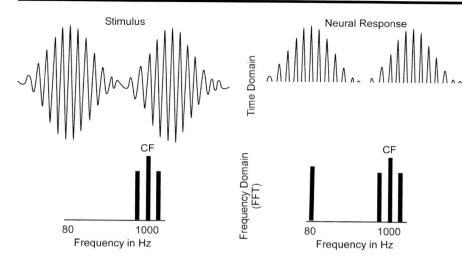

Figure 21–19 The top left figure shows the stimulus with a center frequency of 1000 Hz and a modulation rate of 80 Hz in the time domain, with the fast Fourier transform (FFT) of the stimulus seen in the bottom left. The neural response is represented in the top right (time domain) and the FFT of the neural response in the bottom right. Note that the top right represents the rectified response of the cochlear output. CF, carrier frequency. (Adapted from Luts, H. (2005). Diagnosis of hearing loss in newborns: Clinical application of auditory steady-state responses. Unpublished doctoral dissertation. Available at https://repository.libis.kuleuven.ac.be/dspace/bitstream/1979/75/2/ PhD+Heleen+Luts+2005.pdf, with permission.)

one-channel electrode montage would be between these two areas: midfrontal or vertex and the posterior neck. Although this montage provides a large response, it may be distorted by the myogenic noise from the posterior neck site. Van der Reijden et al (2001) suggested that the inion (Oz), rather than posterior neck, could be a better site to improve signal-to-noise ratio (SNR). Electrode position could be placed on the high forehead (Fz) and mastoid, with the low forehead (Fpz) as a common electrode site.

Similar to interference from the PAM frequently seen in ABR recordings of short latency, the 40 Hz response is prone to such influences for a mastoid-vertex electrode montage but not as prominent for the Cz and inion montage (**Fig. 21–20**; Picton et al, 2003).

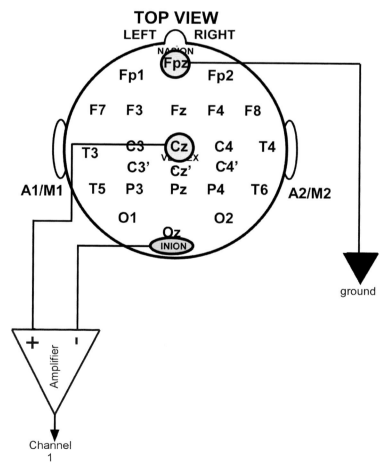

Figure 21–20 Recording montage for the auditory steady-state response (ASSR). This montage minimizes the influence of the postauricular muscle on the ASSR.

Recording Parameters

Stimulus

Amplitude modulation is a process by which the amplitude of a carrier wave is varied over time. This may occur through the use of two signals: a carrier signal, such as a pure tone, and a modulated signal. The modulated signal is a DC signal whose amplitude is varied over time and used to modulate the amplitude of the carrier signal. Typically, ASSR recordings use modulation frequencies between ~40 and 100 Hz and a modulation depth of 100% (i.e., the amplitude is varied between 0 and 100% amplitude).

Frequency modulation is characterized by variations in the frequency of a carrier wave over time that represents changes in the cochlear stimulation site resulting from the FM. This occurs when the carrier frequency (CF) is varied in direct proportion to changes in the amplitude of a modulating signal. Typically, ASSR recordings will modulate the frequency of the carrier wave by ~20% (i.e., the carrier wave will vary ± 20% around the CF).

The stimulus used for ASSR recordings consists of continuous AM and FM tones. **Table 21–9** shows the test parameters used for two commercial units: the MASTER, manufactured by Bio-logic Systems Corp. (Mundelein, IL), and the AUDERA, manufactured by VIASYS Healthcare (Warwick, UK). The approaches the two systems take are different, although they yield very similar results. The MASTER simultaneously presents the stimulus to both ears, whereas the AUDERA uses a monaural presentation. Although the degree of AM (100%) and FM (20%) are the same for the two instruments, the modulation frequencies vary. Luts and Wouters (2005) have reported that the MASTER requires a somewhat shorter test time; however, the ASSR thresholds are comparable and are within 5 to 15 dB (±7–12 dB SL) of the behavioral thresholds.

An AM tone will have its major energy at the CF, with side bands above and below the modulation frequency (MF), and the spectrum of the AM tone does not contain energy at the MF. For example, given a CF of 2000 Hz and an MF at 100 Hz, the peak energy will be at the CF of 2000 Hz, and the side bands at 1900 Hz (CF − MF) and 2100 Hz (CF + MF). Physiologically, the AM tone stimulates a specific area on the basilar membrane, resulting in depolarization and hyperpolarization of the hair cells. However, only depolarization stimulates the auditory nerve to fire and transmit action potentials. The electroencephalography (EEG) follows and synchronizes with the stimulus MF, rather than the CF. The resulting response is a quasi-sinusoidal response, consisting of a single peak in the spectrum at the MF.

Multiple AM stimuli presented simultaneously can be independently assessed if each stimulus is modulated at a different rate. Furthermore, the responses are detected at the MFs, not the CFs. These stimuli can be delivered effectively not only through earphones, including insert phones, but also in the sound field and through a bone-conduction vibrator. Picton et al (1998) reported that there are no significant differences between thresholds obtained using earphones versus sound field using multiple stimuli. The importance of this is the ability to use ASSR in children with hearing aids. This is possible because the periodicity of the

ASSR is not greatly affected by mild to moderate distortion that may be found in the sound field (Picton et al, 1998).

Subject State and Variables

Auditory evoked potentials that are generated at higher central auditory pathways are more affected by attention and sleep than those generated lower in the CNS. Consequently, sleep and attention have major impact on the ASSR amplitude to low MF and a lesser effect on ASSR amplitudes to high MF (Cohen et al, 1991; Levi et al, 1993; Lins and Picton, 1995; Picton, John, Purcell, and Plourde, 2003).

Several studies have shown that the response amplitudes to low MFs are significantly reduced during sleep compared with wakefulness (Cohen et al, 1991; Dobie and Wilson,

Table 21–9   Auditory Steady-State Response Recording Parameters

Electrodes

Type	Ag-AgCl
Montage	Monaural presentation
	Nasion (inverting)
	A1 (noninverting)
	A2 (noninverting
	Fpz (ground)
	Binaural presentation
	Cz (inverting)
	Nape of neck
	Cz (noninverting)
	Pz (noninverting)
	Fpz (ground)

Recording Parameters

Channels	2
Time base	15–20 seconds
No. of averages	48–50 sweeps
Filter (bandpass)	10–300 Hz
Artifact rejection	Three quarters maximum sampling amplitude

Stimuli*

Type	Modulated tones			
		AUDERA	MASTER	
	AM	100%	100%	
	FM	20%	20%	
	Presentation	Monaural	Binaural	
	CF (Hz)	MF (Hz)	MF (Hz)	
		Awake	Asleep	Right Ear	Left Ear
	500	46	74	86	82
	1000	46	81	94	90
	2000	46	88	102	98
	4000	46	95	110	106
Polarity	Not applicable			
Level	0−~110 dB HL (0−~100 dB SPL)			
Rate	See above MFs			
ISI	None (continuous tones)			
Transducer	Tubal insert phones			
	Calibrated earphones			
Response	F-test ($p < .05$) (MASTER) and phase coherence ($p < .01$) detection (AUDERA)			

* The following serve as examples of what is available on commercial units.

AM, amplitude modulation; AUDERA, VIASYS Healthcare (Warwick, UK); CF, carrier frequency; FM, frequency modulation; HL, hearing level; ISI, interstimulus interval; MASTER, Bio-logic Systems Corp., Mundelein, IL; MF, modulation frequency; SPL, sound pressure level.

1998). The degree of amplitude reduction during sleep differs among studies (Galambos et al, 1981; Shallop and Osterhammel, 1983); however, this is most likely due to variations and control of sleep stages and cycles. Nevertheless, the ASSR may be reliably recorded during sleep.

The effect of drug-induced sleep, diazepam, on ASSR amplitudes to low and high modulation rates was investigated by Pethe et al (2001). They found a decrease in the amplitude of the 40 Hz response of the ASSR, whereas the amplitude of the 80 Hz response showed no significant effect from sleep. However, this point is somewhat controversial. Earlier studies have suggested that sleep improves ASSR thresholds to low MFs. Linden et al (1985) reported that, in adults, the estimated hearing thresholds using 40 Hz ASSR were lower during stage 4 sleep (REM) than during more awake stages. It has been suggested that the improvement seen during sleep may be attributed to reduced background noise during sleep, resulting in a better SNR, thus improving detection thresholds by ~10 dB (Picton et al, 1987). High MF ASSRs, though, appear not to be affected by sleep or attention in the same manner it has on low MF ASSRs. Lins and Picton (1995) reported that wakefulness or sleep has little effect on the 80 Hz response amplitude in comparison to the 40 Hz response amplitude of the ASSR.

In the awake state, the 40 Hz ASSR latency is longer (34 msec) than during sleep (27 msec) (Lins and Picton, 1995; Stapells et al, 1984). The shorter latency during sleep provides support for a cortical origin of the 40 Hz ASSR. Because sleep has an inhibitory effect on the cortex, as opposed to the brainstem, the cortical component of the response decreases, thus resulting in a reduction in the latency of ASSR. When a higher modulation rate (e.g., 80 Hz) is used, the latency of the ASSR appears to be stable in both the awake and sleep conditions.

Controversial Point

- There is no definitive conclusion on the effects of either drug-induced sleep or natural sleep on the ASSR. Studies vary somewhat in their findings, and their conclusions are somewhat hypothetical based on the difference in origins of the 40 versus 80 Hz ASSR.

Selective attention has been investigated using the 40 Hz ASSR. In general, the response amplitudes are larger during active attention, with greater responses seen over the left hemisphere, as well as over the left frontal and central areas (Ross et al, 2004; Tiitinen et al, 1993).

Clinical Applications

The most significant application of ASSR is its use in objective audiometry for estimating audiometric threshold when reliable behavioral thresholds cannot be obtained (Aoyagi et al, 1994; Cone-Wesson, Dowell, et al, 2002; Cone-Wesson, Parker, et al, 2002a; Lins et al, 1996; Perez-Abalo et al, 2001; Picton et al, 1998; Rance et al, 1995). Several studies have shown the accuracy of 80 Hz ASSR thresholds in estimating the behavioral hearing thresholds on normal-hearing

adults. The findings were consistent and showed that ASSR thresholds gave an accurate and valid estimation of behavioral thresholds. However, given that the 40 Hz ASSR is large when subjects are awake and alert, it is suggested that 40 Hz ASSR be used in adults when objective audiometry is needed and subject state is not a concern.

ASSR has been used in selecting candidates for cochlear implants and to measure performance in both hearing aid and cochlear implant users, especially in young children (Picton et al, 1998).

Because of the complex stimuli used in obtaining an ASSR and because of the relationship between this type of neural decoding and the type of neural decoding that occurs in speech within the auditory system, studies have investigated the relationship between the ASSR and word recognition scores (WRSs; Dimitrijevic et al, 2001, 2004). Results showed, for normal-hearing individuals, a correlation coefficient between .74 and .65. Dimitrijevic et al (2004) concluded that the number of responses is correlated with WRS. This finding could be used as an objective measurement to assess suprathreshold auditory processes, such as those necessary for speech perception and sound discrimination.

The 40 Hz ASSR is also considered a useful tool for monitoring level of anesthesia during surgery. Plourde and Boylan (1991) recorded the 40 Hz ASSR amplitude before induction of anesthesia, 5 to 10 minutes after induction, and when patients started to recover from anesthesia. They reported a gradual diminution of the 40 Hz amplitudes, with absence of the response when the patients lost consciousness. Five to 10 minutes following unconsciousness, the response amplitude reappeared and remained at a low level during the remainder of the surgical operation. The 40 Hz ASSR amplitude gradually increased postanesthesia until it reached its preanesthesia amplitude (Madler et al, 1991; Plourde and Picton, 1990; Schwender et al, 1994).

Adults

Various studies have shown the efficacy of the ASSR using modulation rates around 80 Hz as a relatively valid measure of auditory sensitivity (Dimitrijevic et al, 2002; Herdman and Stapells, 2001, 2003; Kaf et al, 2006).

Rance et al (1995) compared the ASSR hearing thresholds to 90 Hz MF between two hearing-impaired groups (35 adults and 25 children). They reported that the estimated thresholds were close to the behavioral thresholds with better prediction for higher frequencies and for profound hearing losses than for lower frequencies and moderate hearing losses. No statistically significant difference in the prediction of hearing thresholds was obtained between adults and children.

Lins et al (1996) investigated ASSR thresholds of 10 normal-hearing adults and 21 normal 1- to 10-month-old infants. ASSR thresholds in adults range from 29 to 39 dB HL, with a mean threshold of 12 dB above behavioral threshold. In infants, the ASSR thresholds were between 26 and 45 dB HL. The amplitudes of the adult responses were significantly larger than those of the infants. Herdman and Stapells (2001) examined 10 normal-hearing adults and reported that ASSR thresholds were within 5 to 15 dB of the behavioral thresholds. Similarly, Kaf et al (2006) found that ASSR thresholds were comparable with behavioral thresholds and N1–P2 thresholds when using normal-hearing individuals and simulating hearing loss. The researchers also reported that ASSR thresholds followed behavioral audiometric configurations, except for the mildest degree of simulated hearing loss.

Studies using bone-conduction vibrators have been neither reliable nor overly encouraging (Gorga et al, 2004; Jeng et al, 2004; Picton and John, 2004; Small and Stapells, 2004). This is mostly due to the nature of using transducers that radiate large amounts of magnetic artifact and have long-time constants.

Given that the 40 Hz auditory steady-state responses are large when individuals are awake and alert, it is suggested that the 40 Hz ASSR be used in adults.

Children

ASSRs in children have been found to overestimate behavioral thresholds between 6 to 15 dB for frequencies of 500, 1000, 2000, and 4000 Hz (Stueve and O'Rourke, 2003; Swanepoel et al, 2004;). The actual difference varies as a function of frequency, with 500 Hz having the greatest variability. The variability is somewhat reduced when hearing loss is present as opposed to normal hearing. For normal hearing, ASSR seems to show a variation between 5 and 15 dB above behavioral threshold (Perez-Abalo et al, 2001; Rance et al, 1998), which is quite similar to ABR estimates of thresholds. ASSR, however, is more frequency specific than ABR and, when using frequency-specific ABR techniques, has a shorter acquisition time.

Infants

One of the clinical utilities of AEPs, in general, is estimation of behavioral hearing thresholds in children and difficult-to-test subjects. ASSR is a technique that provides an objective measure for estimating hearing sensitivity in infants. To avoid the effect of sleep and sedation on the ASSR, high-frequency modulation should be used (70–100 Hz). ASSR threshold estimates in normal-hearing infants are poorer compared with those in normal-hearing adults (Cone-Wesson, Dowell, et al, 2002; Cone-Wesson et al, 2002a,b; Lins et al, 1996; Rance et al, 2005; Rickards et al, 1994). Lins et al (1996) showed that the ASSR amplitudes in normal-hearing infants are one third to one half smaller than the response amplitudes observed in normal-hearing adults. Rance and Rickards (2002) reported a 6 to 10 dB difference between ASSR thresholds and behavioral thresholds in infants with a moderate hearing loss. Infants with severe to profound hearing loss had about a 5 dB difference, with behavioral thresholds being reported as better than ASSR thresholds.

As noted in most studies of AEPs, OAE, and similar techniques, amplitude and threshold of the ASSR increase as a function of age (John et al, 2001). Several studies have shown that ASSR thresholds are lower at high frequencies (25–40 dB HL) compared with the low to midfrequencies (35–45 dB HL) (Cone-Wesson, Dowell, et al, 2002; Levi et al, 1995; Rance et al, 2005). Rance and Tomlin (2006) reported that the ASSR thresholds at 500 Hz were greater than those found for 4000 Hz for infants up to 6 weeks of age.

♦ Summary

The purpose of this chapter is to introduce practitioners to MLAEPs and LLAEPs. These potentials are not considered as mainstream electrophysiological tests in routine audiology practice. However, they promise to be a valuable tool in diagnosing various auditory processing problems. Therefore, the orientation of this chapter is toward clinical applications relevant to audiology practice. It is anticipated that future developments in auditory electrophysiology will prove the value of late auditory evoked responses in clinical applications.

Acknowledgments   Appreciation is expressed to Lisa Mullins, Department of Communication Disorders, Brigham Young University, for reviewing and helping with this chapter. Partial funding for this work was provided by a grant from the David O. McKay School of Education and the Office of Research and Creative Works, Brigham Young University.

References

Alho, K. (1995). Cerebral generators of mismatch negativity (MMN) and its magnetic counterpart (MMN) elicited by sound changes. Ear and Hearing, 16, 38–51.

Alho, K., Woods, D. L., Algazi, A., Knight, R. T., & Näätänen, R. (1994). Lesions of frontal cortex diminish the auditory mismatch negativity. Electroencephalography and Clinical Neurophysiology, 91, 353–362.

Allred, C., McPherson, D. L., & Bartholomew, K. (1994). Auditory training in a patient with severe dysfunction in auditory memory and figure ground. Paper presented at the annual meeting of the Academy of Rehabilitative Audiology. Salt Lake City, UT.

Aoyagi, M., Furuse, H., Yokota, M., Kiren, T., Suzuki, Y., & Koike, Y. (1994). Detectability of amplitude-modulation following response at different carrier frequencies. Acta Otolaryngologica Supplementum, 511, 23–27. (Stockholm)

Aoyagi, M., Fuse, T., Suzuki, Y., Yoshinori, K., & Koike, Y. (1993). An application of phase spectral analysis to amplitude-modulation following response. Acta Otolaryngologica Supplementum, 504, 82–88.

Arehole, S., Augustine, L. E., & Simhadri, R. (1995). Middle latency response in children with learning disabilities: Preliminary findings. Journal of Communication Disorders, 28, 21–38.

Baker, N. J., Staunton, M., Adler, L. E., et al. (1990). Sensory gating deficits in psychiatric inpatients: Relation to catecholamine metabolites in different diagnostic groups. Biological Psychiatry, 27, 519–528.

Barrett, G. (1993). Clinical applications of event-related potentials. In A. M. Halliday (Ed.), Evoked potentials in clinical testing (pp. 589–633). London: Churchill Livingstone.

Bilger, R. C., Nuetzel, J. M., Rabinowitz, W. M., & Rzeczkowski, C. (1984). Standardization of a test of speech perception in noise. Journal of Speech and Hearing Research, 27, 32–48.

Billings, R. J. (1989). The origin of the initial negative component of the averaged lambda potential recorded from midline electrodes. Electroencephalography and Clinical Neurophysiology, 72, 114–117.

Boutros, N. N., Zouridakis, G., & Overall, J. (1991). Replicating and extension of P50 findings in schizophrenia. Clinical Electroencephalography, 22(1), 40–45.

Brazier, M. A.B. (1984). Pioneers in the discovery of evoked potentials. Electroencephalography and Clinical Neurophysiology, 59, 2–8.

Buchwald, J. S. (1990a). Animal models of event-related potentials. In J. Rohrbaugh, R. Parasuraman, and R. Johnson (Eds.), Event-related potentials of the brain (pp. 57–75). New York: Oxford Press.

Buchwald, J. S. (1990b). Comparison of plasticity in sensory and cognitive processing systems. Clinical Perinatology, 17, 57–66.

Buchwald, J. S., Hinman, C., Norman, R., Huang, C., & Brown, K. (1981). Middle and long latency auditory evoked responses recorded from the vertex of normal and chronically lesioned cats. Brain Research, 205, 91–109.

Chatrian, C. E. (1976). The lambda waves. In A. Remond (Ed.), Handbook of electroencephalography and clinical neurophysiology (Vl. 6A, pp. 123–149). Amsterdam: Elsevier.

Cheour-Luhtanen, M., Alho, K., Kujala, T., et al. (1995). Mismatch negativity indicates vowel discrimination in newborns. Hearing Research, 82, 53–58.

Cohen, L. T., Rickards, F. W., & Clark, G. M. (1991). A comparison of steady-state evoked potentials to modulated tones in awake and sleeping humans. Journal of the Acoustical Society of America, 90, 2467–2479.

Cone-Wesson, B., Dowell, R. C., Tomlin, D., Rance, G., & Ming. W. J. (2002). The auditory steady-state response: 1. Comparisons with the auditory brainstem response. Journal of the American Academy of Audiology, 13, 173–187.

Cone-Wesson, B., Parker, J., Swiderski, N., & Rickards, F. (2002a). The auditory steady-state response: 2. Full-term and premature neonates. Journal of the American Academy of Audiology, 13, 260–269.

Cone-Wesson, B., Parker, J., Swiderski, N., & Rickards, F. (2002b). The auditory steady-state response: 3. Clinical observations and applications in infants and children. Journal of the American Academy of Audiology, 13, 270–282.

Connolly, J. F., Phillips, N. A., & Stewart, SH. (1990). The effects of processing requirements on neurophysiological responses to spoken sentences. Brain and Language, 39, 302–318.

Connolly, J. F., Phillips, N. A., Stewart, S. H., & Brake, W. G. (1992). Event-related potential sensitivity to acoustic and semantic properties of terminal words in sentences. Brain and Language, 43, 1–18.

Cottrell, G., & Gans, D. (1995). Auditory evoked response morphology in profoundly-involved multi-handicapped children: Comparisons with normal infants and children. Audiology, 34, 189–206.

Csepe, V., Karmos, G., & Molnar, M. (1987). Evoked potential correlates of stimulus deviance during wakefulness and sleep in the cat: Animal model of mismatched negativity. Electroencephalography and Clinical Neurophysiology, 66, 571–578.

Csepe, V., & Molnar, M. (1997). Towards the possible clinical application of the mismatch negativity component of event-related potentials. Audiology and Neurootology, 2, 354–369.

Di, S., & Barth, D. S. (1992). The functional anatomy of middle-latency auditory evoked potentials: Thalamocortical connections. Journal of Neurophysiology, 68, 425–431.

Dietrich, S., Barry, S., & Parker, D. (1995). Middle latency auditory responses in males who stutter. Journal of Speech and Hearing Research, 38, 5–17.

Dimitrijevic, A., John, M. S., van Roon, P., & Picton, T. W. (2001). Human auditory steady-state responses to tones independently modulated in both frequency and amplitude. Ear and Hearing, 22, 100–111.

Dimitrijevic, A., John, S., Van Roon, P., et al. (2002). Estimating the audiogram using multiple auditory steady-state responses. Journal of the American Academy of Audiology, 13, 205–224.

Dimitrijevic, A., John, S. J., & Picton, T. W. (2004). Auditory steady-state responses and word recognition scores in normal-hearing and hearing-impaired adults. Ear and Hearing, 25, 68–84.

Dobie, R. A., & Wilson, M. J. (1998). Low-level steady-state auditory evoked potentials: Effects of rate and sedation on detectability. Journal of the Acoustical Society of America, 104, 3482–3488.

Dobie, R. A., & Wilson, M. J. (1996). A comparison of t test, F test, and coherence methods of detecting steady-state auditory evoked potentials, distortion-product otoacoustic emissions, or other sinusoids. Journal of the Acoustical Society of America, 100, 2236–2246.

Donchin, E. (1981). Surprise! Surprise? Psychophysiology, 18, 493–513.

Eggermont, J. J., Ponton, C. W., Don, M., Waring, M. D., & Kwong, B. (1997). Maturational delays in cortical evoked potentials in cochlear implant users. Acta Otolaryngologica, 117, 161–163.

Erwin, R. J., Mawhinney-Hee, M., Gur, R. C., & Gur, R. E. (1991). Midlatency auditory evoked responses in schizophrenics. Biological Psychiatry, 30, 430–442.

Ferraro, J. A., Durrant, J. D., Siniger, Y. S., & Campbell, K. (1996). Recommended guidelines for reporting AEP specifications. American Journal of Audiology, 5, 35–37.

Fifer, R. C., & Sierra-Irizarry, B. (1988). Clinical applications of the auditory middle latency response. American Journal of Otology, 9, 47–56.

Freedman, R., Adler, L. E., & Waldo, M. (1987). Gating of the auditory evoked potential in children and adults. Psychophysiology, 24, 223–227.

Friederici, A. D., Pfeifer, E., & Hahne, A. (1993). Event-related brain potentials during natural speech processing: Effects of semantic, morphological and syntactic violations. Brain Research and Cognitive Brain Research, 1, 183–192.

Galambos, R., Makeig, S., & Talmachoff, P. J. (1981). A 40-Hz auditory potential recorded from the human scalp. Proceedings of the National Academy of Sciences of the United States of America, 78, 2643–2647.

Giard, M. H., Perrin, F., Pernier, J., & Bouchet, P. (1990). Brain generators implicated in processing of auditory stimulus deviance: A topographic event-related potential study. Psychophysiology, 27, 627–640.

Goodin, D. S. (1990). Clinical utility of long latency "cognitive" event-related potentials (P3): The pros. Electroencephalography and Clinical Neurophysiology, 76, 2–5.

Gorga, M., & Neely, S. T. (1994). Stimulus calibration in auditory evoked potential measurements. In J. T. Jacobson (Ed.), Principles and applications in auditory evoked potentials (pp. 85–98). New York: Allyn & Bacon.

Gorga, M. P., Neely, S. T., Hoover, B. M., Dierking, D. M., Beauchaine, K. L., & Manning, C. (2004). Determining the upper limits of stimulation for auditory steady-state response measurements. Ear and Hearing, 25, 302–307.

Groenen, P., Snik, A., & van den Broek, P. (1996). On the clinical relevance of mismatch negativity: Results from subjects with normal-hearing and cochlear implant users. Audiology and Neurootology, 1, 112–124.

Hall, J. W. (1992). Handbook of auditory evoked potentials. Boston: Allyn & Bacon.

Hari, R., Hamalainen, M., Ilmoniemi, R., et al. (1984). Responses of the primary auditory cortex to pitch changes in a sequence of tone pips: Neuromagnetic recordings in man. Neuroscience Letters, 50, 127–132.

Herdman, A. T., Lins, O., Van Roon, P., Stapells, D. R., Scherg, M., & Picton, T. W. (2002). Intracerebral sources of human auditory steady-state responses. Brain Topography, 15, 69–86.

Herdman, A. T., & Stapells, D. R. (2001). Thresholds determined using the monotic and dichotic multiple auditory steady-state response technique in normal hearing subjects. Scandinavian Audiology, 30, 41–49.

Herdman, A. T., & Stapells, D. R. (2003). Auditory steady-state response thresholds of adults with sensorineural hearing impairments. International Journal of Audiology, 42, 237–248.

Hillyard, S. A., & Kutas, M. (1983). Electrophysiology of cognitive processing. Annual Review of Psychology, 34, 33–61.

Hillyard, S. A., Squires, K. C., Bauer, J. W., & Lindsay, P. H. (1971). Evoked potential correlates of auditory signal detection. Science, 172, 1357–1360.

Hurley, R. M., & Musiek, F. E. (1997). Effectiveness of three central auditory processing (CAP) tests in identifying cerebral lesions. Journal of the American Academy of Audiology, 8, 257–262.

Hutchinson, K. M., & McGill, D. J. (1997). The efficacy of utilizing the P300 as a measure of auditory deprivation in monaurally aided profoundly hearing-impaired children. Scandinavian Audiology, 26, 177–185.

Jasper, H. H. (158). Report on Committee on Methods of Clinical Examination in Clinical Electroencephalography. Electroencephalography and Clinical Neurophysiology, 10, 370–375.

Javitt, D. C., Schroeder, C. E., Steinschneider, M., Arezzo, J. C., & Vaughan, H. G., Jr. (1992). Demonstration of mismatch negativity in the monkey. Electroencephalography and Clinical Neurophysiology, 83, 87–90.

Jeng, F. C., Brownt, C. J., Johnson, T. A., & Vander Werff, K. R. (2004). Estimating air–bone gaps using auditory steady-state responses. Journal of the American Academy of Audiology, 15, 67–68.

Jerger, K., Biggins, C., & Fein, G. (1992). P50 suppression is not affected by attentional manipulations. Biological Psychiatry, 31(4), 365–377.

Jewett, D. L., & Williston, J. S. (1971). Auditory evoked far fields recorded from scalp of humans. Brain, 94, 681–696.

Jirsa, R. E. (1992). The clinical utility of the P3 AERP in children with auditory processing disorders. Journal of Speech and Hearing Research, 35, 903–912.

John, M. S., Dimitrijevic, A., van Roon, P., & Picton, T. W. (2001). Multiple auditory steady-state responses to AM and FM stimuli. Audiology and Neurootology, 6, 12–27.

John, M. S., Purcell, D. W., Dimitrijevic, A., & Picton, T. W. (2002). Advantages and caveats when recording steady-state responses to multiple simultaneous stimuli. Journal of the American Academy of Audiology, 13, 246–259.

Johnson, B. W., Weinberg, H., Ribary, U., Cheyne, D. O., & Ancill, R. (1988). Topographic distribution of the 40 Hz auditory evoked-related potential in normal and aged subjects. Brain Topography, 1, 117–121.

Jordan, K., Schmidt, A., Plotz, K., von Specht, H., Begali, K., Roth, N., & Scheich, H. (1997). Auditory event-related potentials in post- and prelingually deaf cochlear implant recipients. American Journal of Otology, 18(6, Suppl.), 116–117.

Kaukoranta, E., Sams, M., Hari, R., Hamalainen, M. & Naatanen, R. (1989). Reactions of human auditory cortex to a change in tone duration. Hearing Research, 41(1), 15–21.

Kileny, P. R. (1991). Use of electrophysiologic measures in the management of children with cochlear implants: Brain stem, middle latency, and cognitive (P300) responses. American Journal of Otology, 12(Suppl.), 37–42.

Kileny, P. R., Boerst, A., & Zwolan, T. (1997). Cognitive evoked potentials to speech and tonal stimuli in children with implants. Otolaryngology—Head and Neck Surgery, 117(3, Pt. 1), 161–169.

Kiren, T., Aoyagi, M., Furuse, H., & Koike, Y. (1994). An experimental study on the generator of amplitude-modulation following response. Acta Otolaryngologica Supplementum, 511, 28–33.

Klein, A. J. (1983). Properties of the brain-stem response slow-wave component. Archives of Otolaryngology, 109, 6–12.

Knecht, S., Dräger, B., Deppe, M., et al. (2000). Handedness and hemispheric language dominance in healthy humans. Brain, 123, 2512–2518.

Knight, R. T., Scabini, D., Woods, D. L., & Clayworth, C. (1988). The effects of lesions of superior temporal gyrus and inferior parietal lobe on temporal and vertex components of the human AEP. Electroencephalography and Clinical Neurophysiology, 70, 499–509.

Kraiuhin, C., Gordon, E., Stanfield, P., Meares, R., & Howson, A. (1990). Normal latency of the P300 event-related potential in mild-to-moderate Alzheimer's disease and depression. Biological Psychiatry, 28, 372–386.

Kraus, N., & McGee, T. (1990). Clinical applications of the middle latency response. Journal of the American Academy of Audiology, 1, 130–133.

Kraus, N., & McGee, T. (1995). The middle latency response generating system. Electroencephalography and Clinical Neurophysiology Supplement, 44, 76–92.

Kraus, N., & McGee, T. (1996). Auditory development reflected by middle latency response. Ear and Hearing, 17, 419–429.

Kraus, N., McGee, T., Carrell, T., King, C., Littman, T., & Nicol, T. (1994). Discrimination of speech-like contrasts in the auditory thalamus and cortex. Journal of the Acoustical Society of America, 96(5, Pt. 1), 2758–2768.

Kraus, N., McGee, T., Carrell, T., Sharma, A., Micco, A., & Nicol, T. (1993). Speech evoked cortical potentials in children. Journal of the American Academy of Audiology, 4, 238–248.

Kraus, N., McGee, T., Carrell, T., Sharma, A., & Nicol, T. (1995). Mismatch negativity to speech stimuli in school-age children. Electroencephalography and Clinical Neurophysiology Supplement, 44, 211–217.

Kraus, N., McGee, T., Ferre, J., Hoeppner, J. A., Carrell, T., Sharma, A., & Nicol, T. (1993). Mismatch negativity in the neurophysiologic/behavioral evaluation of auditory processing deficits: A case study. Ear and Hearing, 14, 223–234.

Kraus, N., McGee, T., Litman, T., Nicol, T., & King, C. (1994). Non-primary auditory thalamic representation of acoustic change. Journal of Neurophysiology, 72, 1270–1277.

Kraus, N., McGee, T., Sharma, A., Carrell, T., & Nicol, T. (1992). Mismatch negativity event-related potential elicited by speech stimuli. Ear and Hearing, 13, 158–164.

Kraus, N., McGee, T., & Stein, L. (1994). The auditory middle latency response: Clinical uses, development, and generating system. In J. T. Jacobson (Ed.), Principles and applications in auditory evoked potentials (pp. 155–178). Needham Heights, MA: Simon & Schuster.

Kraus, N., Micco, A. G., Koch, D. B., et al. (1993). The mismatch negativity cortical evoked potential elicited by speech in cochlear-implant users. Hearing Research, 65, 118–124.

Kraus, N., Özdamar, Ö., Hier, D., & Stein, L. (1982). Auditory middle latency responses (MLRs) in patients with cortical lesions. Electroencephalography and Clinical Neurophysiology, 54, 275–287.

Kutas, M., & Hillyard, S. A. (1980). Reading senseless sentences: Brain potentials reflect semantic incongruity. Science, 207, 203–205.

Kutas, M., & Hillyard, S. A. (1982). The lateral distribution of event-related potentials during sentence processing. Neuropsychologia, 20, 579–590.

Kutas, M., & Hillyard, S. A. (1983). Event-related brain potentials to grammatical errors and semantic anomalies. Memory and Cognition, 11, 539–550.

Kutas, M., & Hillyard, S. A. (1984). Brain potentials during reading reflect word expectancy and semantic association. Nature, 307, 161–163.

Kuwada, S., Batra, R., & Maher, V. L. (1986). Scalp potentials of normal and hearing-impaired subjects in response to sinusoidally amplitude-modulated tones. Hearing Research, 21, 179–192.

Kuwada, S., Anderson, J. S., Batra, R., Fitzpatrick, D. C., Teissier, N., & D'Angelo, W. R. (2002). Sources of the scalp-recorded amplitude-modulation following response. Journal of the American Academy of Audiology, 13, 188–204.

Levi, E. C., Folsom, R. C., & Dobie, R. A. (1993). Amplitude-modulation following response (AMFR): Effects of modulation rate, carrier frequency, age and state. Hearing Research, 68, 42–52.

Levi, E. C., Folsom, R. C., & Dobie, R. A. (1995). Coherence analysis of envelop-following responses (EFRs) and frequency-following responses (FFRs) in infants and adults. Hearing Research, 89, 21–27.

Linden, R. D., Campbell, K. B., Hamel, G., & Picton, T. W. (1985). Human auditory steady state potentials during sleep. Ear and Hearing, 6, 167–174.

Lins, O. G., & Picton, T. W. (1995). Auditory steady-state responses to multiple simultaneous stimuli. Electroencephalography and Clinical Neurophysiology, 96, 420–432.

Lins, O. G., Picton, T. W., Boucher, B. L., et al. (1996). Frequency-specific audiometry using steady-state responses. Ear and Hearing, 17, 81–96.

Lins, O. G., Picton, P. E., Picton, T. W., Champagne, S. C., & Durieux-Smith, A. (1995). Auditory steady-state responses to tones amplitude-modulated at 80–110 Hz. Journal of the Acoustical Society of America, 97, 3051–3063.

Litcher, G. (1995). Middle latency auditory evoked potentials in intensive care patients and normal controls. International Journal of Neuroscience, 83, 253–267.

Luts, H. (2005). Diagnosis of hearing loss in newborns: Clinical application of auditory steady-state responses. Unpublished doctoral dissertation. Available at https://repository.libis.kuleuven.ac.be/dspace/bitstream/1979/75/2/PhD+Heleen+Luts+2005.pdf.

Luts, H., & Wouters, J. (2005). Comparison of MASTER and AUDERA for measurement of auditory steady-state responses. International Journal of Audiology, 44, 244–253.

Martineau, J., Barthelemy, C., Roux, S., Garreau, B., & Lelord, G. (1989). Electrophysiological effects of fenfluramine or combined vitamin B6 and magnesium on children with autistic behaviour. Developmental Medical Child Neurology, 31(6), 721–727.

Martineau, J., Garreau, B., Barthelemy, C., & Lelord, G. (1984). Evoked potentials and P300 during sensory conditioning in autistic children. Annals of New York Academy of Sciences. 425, 362–369.

McPherson, D. L. (1996). Late potentials of the auditory system. San Diego, CA: Singular Publishing Group.

McPherson, D. L., & Davies, K. (1995). Binaural interaction in school age children with attention deficit hyperactivity disorder. Journal of Human Physiology, 21(1), 47–53.

McPherson, D. L., & Starr, A. (1993). Auditory evoked potentials in the clinic. In A. M. Halliday (Ed.), Evoked potentials in clinical testing (pp. 359–381). New York: Churchill Livingstone.

McPherson, D. L., Tures, C., & Starr, A. (1989). Binaural interaction of the auditory brain stem potentials and middle latency auditory evoked potentials in infants and adults. Electroencephalography and Clinical Neurophysiology, 74, 124–130.

Madler, C., Keller, I., Schwender, D., & Poppel, E. (1991). Sensory information processing during general anaesthesia: effect of isoflurane on auditory evoked neuronal oscillations. British Journal of Anaesthesia, 66, 81–87.

Micco, A. G., Kraus, N., Koch, D. B., et al. (1995). Speech-evoked cognitive P300 potentials in cochlear implant recipients. American Journal of Otology, 16, 514–520.

Michalewski, H. J., Rosenberg, C., & Starr, A. (1986). Event-related potentials in dementia. In R. Q. Cracco & I. Bodis-Wollner (Eds.), Evoked potentials (pp. 521–528). New York: Alan R. Liss.

Muir, W. J., Squire, I., Blackwood, D. H., Speight, M. D., St Claire, D. M., Oliver, C., & Dickens, P. (1998). Auditory P300 response in the assessment of Alzheimer's disease in Down's syndrome: A 2-year follow-up study. Journal of Mental Deficiencies Research, 32, 455–463.

Näätänen, R. (1992). Attention and brain function. Hillsdale, NJ: Lawrence Erlbaum.

Näätänen, R., Gaillard, A. W. K., & Mantysalo, S. (1978). Early selective attention effect on evoked potential reinterpreted. Acta Psychologica (Amsterdam), 42, 313–329.

Näätänen, R., Paavilainen, P., Alho, K., Reinikainen, K., & Sams, M. (1987). The mismatch negativity to intensity changes in an auditory stimulus sequence. Electroencephalography and Clinical Neurophysiology Supplement, 40, 125–131.

Nagamoto, H. T., Adler, L. E., Waldo, M. C., & Freedman, R. (1989). Sensory gating in schizophrenics and normal controls: Effects of changing stimulation interval. Biological Psychiatry, 25, 549–561.

Nelson, M. D., Hall, J. W. III, & Jacobson, J. T. (1997). Factors affecting the recordability of auditory evoked response component Pb (P1). Journal of the American Academy of Audiology, 8, 89–99.

Niedermeyer, E. (1987). The normal EEG in the waking adult. In E. Niedermeyer & F. Lopes da Silva (Eds.), Electroencephalography (pp. 110–112). Munich: Urban & Schwarzenberg.

Oates, P., & Stapells, D. (1997a). Frequency specificity of the human auditory brain stem and middle latency responses to brief tones: 1. High-pass noise masking. Journal of the Acoustical Society of America, 102, 3597–3608.

Oates, P., & Stapells, D. (1997b). Frequency specificity of the human auditory brain stem and middle latency responses to brief tones: 2. Derived responses. Journal of the Acoustical Society of America, 102, 3609–3619.

Özdamar, Ö., & Kraus, N. (1983). Auditory middle latency responses in humans. Audiology, 22, 34–49.

Paavilainen, P., Karlsson, M. L., Reinikainen, K., & Näätänen, R. (1989). Mismatch negativity to change in spatial location of an auditory stimulus. Electroencephalography and Clinical Neurophysiology, 73, 129–141.

Parving, A., Salomon, G., Elberling, C., Larsen, B., & Lassan, N. A. (1980). Middle components of the auditory evoked response in bilateral temporal lobe lesions. Scandinavian Audiology, 9, 161–167.

Perez-Abalo, M. C., Savio, G., Torres, A., Martin, V., Rodriguez, E., & Galán, L. (2001). Steady state response to multiple amplitude-modulated tones: An optimized method to test frequency-specific thresholds in hearing-impaired children and normal-hearing subjects. Ear and Hearing, 22, 200–210.

Perez-Borja, C., Chatrian, G. E., Tyce, F. A., & Rivers, M. H. (1962). Electrographic patterns of the occipital lobes in man: A topographic study based on use of implanted electrodes. Electroencephalography and Clinical Neurophysiology, 14, 171–182.

Pethe, J., Von Specht, H., Muhler, R., & Hocke, T. (2001). Amplitude modulation following responses in awake and sleeping humans—a comparison for 40 Hz and 80 Hz modulation frequency. Scandinavian Audiology Supplementum, 52, 152–155.

Petitot, C., Collett, L., & Durrant, J. D. (2005). Auditory steady-state responses (ASSR): Effects of modulation and carrier frequencies. International Journal of Audiology, 44, 567–573.

Picton, T. W., Durieux-Smith, A., Champagne, C., Whittingham, J., Moran, L. M., Giguere, C., & Beauregard, Y. (1998). Objective evaluation of aided thresholds using auditory steady-state responses. Journal of the American Academy of Audiology, 9, 315–331.

Picton, T. W., & Hillyard, S. A. (1974). Human auditory evoked potentials: 2. Effects of attention. Electroencephalography and Clinical Neurophysiology, 36, 191–199.

Picton, T. W., & John, M. S. (2004). Avoiding electromagnetic artifacts when recording auditory steady-state responses. Journal of the American Academy of Audiology, 15, 541–554.

Picton, T. W., John, M. S., Dimitrijevic, A., & Purcell, D. (2003). Human auditory steady-state responses. International Journal of Audiology, 42, 177–219.

Picton, T. W., John, M. S., Purcell, D. W., & Plourde, G. (2003). Human auditory steady-state responses: The effects of recording technique and state of arousal. Anesthésie et Analgésie, 97, 1396–1402.

Picton, T. W., Skinner, C. R., Champagne, S. C., Kellett, A. J. C., & Maiste, A. C. (1987). Potentials evoked by the sinusoidal modulation of the amplitude or frequency of a tone. Journal of the Acoustical Society of America, 82, 165–178.

Plourde, G., Baribeau, J., & Bonhomme, V. (1997). Ketamine increases the amplitude of the 40-Hz auditory steady-state response in humans. British Journal of Anaesthesia, 78, 524–529.

Plourde, G., & Boylan, J. F. (1991). The auditory steady state response during sufentanil anaesthesia. British Journal of Anaesthesia, 66, 683–691.

Plourde, G., & Picton, T. W. (1990). Human auditory steady state responses during general anesthesia [in French]. Anesthésie et Analgésie, 71, 460–468.

Polich, J. (1989a). P300 and Alzheimer's disease. Biomedicine and Pharmacotherapy, 43, 493–499.

Polich, J. (1989b). Frequency, intensity, and duration as determinants of P300 from auditory stimuli. Journal of Clinical Neurophysiology, 6(3), 277–286.

Polich, J., Howard, L., & Starr, A. (1985). Stimulus frequency and masking as determinants of P300 latency in event-related potentials from auditory stimuli. Biological Psychology, 21, 309–318.

Polich, J., Ladish, C., & Bloom, F. E. (1990). P300 assessment of early Alzheimer's disease. Electroencephalography and Clinical Neurophysiology, 77, 179–189.

Ponton, C. W., & Don, M. (1995). The mismatch negativity in cochlear implant users. Ear and Hearing, 16, 131–146.

Ponton, C. W., Don, M., Eggermont, J. J., Waring, M. D., Kwong, B., & Masuda, A. (1996). Auditory system plasticity in children after long periods of complete deafness. Neuroreport, 8(1), 61–65.

Ponton, C. W., Don, M., Eggermont, J. J., Waring, M. D., & Masuda, A. (1996). Maturation of human cortical auditory function: Differences between normal-hearing children and children with cochlear implants. Ear and Hearing, 17, 430–437.

Rance, G., Dowell, R. C., Rickards, F. W., Beer, D. E., & Clark, G. M. (1998). Steady-state evoked potential and behavioral hearing thresholds in a group of children with absent click-evoked auditory brain stem response. Ear and Hearing, 19, 48–61.

Rance, G., & Rickards, F. (2002). Prediction of hearing threshold in infants using auditory steady-state evoked potentials. Journal of the American Academy of Audiology, 13, 236–245.

Rance, G., Rickards, F. W., Cohen, L. T., De Vidi, S., & Clark, G. M. (1995). The automated prediction of hearing thresholds in sleeping subjects using auditory steady-state evoked potentials. Ear and Hearing, 16, 499–507.

Rance, G., Roper, R., Symons, L., et al. (2005). Hearing threshold estimation in infants using auditory steady-state responses. Journal of the American Academy of Audiology, 16(5), 293–302.

Rance, G., & Tomlin, D. (2006). Maturation of auditory steady-state responses in normal babies. Ear and Hearing, 27, 20–29.

Rickards, F. W., Tan, L. E., Cohen, L. T., Wilson, O. J., Drew, J. H., & Clark, M. (1994). Auditory steady-state evoked potentials in newborns. British Journal of Audiology, 28, 327–337.

Rodriguez, R., Picton, J., Linden, D., Hamel, G., & Laframboise, G. (1986). Human auditory steady state responses: Effects of intensity and frequency. Ear and Hearing, 7(5), 300–313.

Ross, B., Picton, T. W., Herdman, A. T., & Pantev, C. (2004). The effect of attention on the auditory steady-state response. Neurology and Clinical Neurophysiology, November 30, 22.

Salamat, M. T., & McPherson, D. L. (1999). Interactions among variables in the P300 response to a continuous performance task. Journal of the American Academy of Audiology, 10, 379–387.

Sams, M., Paavilainen, P., Alho, K., & Naatanen, R. (1985). Auditory frequency discrimination and event-related potentials. Electroencephalography Clinical Neurophysioly, 62(6), 437–448.

Sandridge, S. A., & Boothroyd, A. (1996). Using naturally produced speech to elicit the mismatch negativity. Journal of the American Academy of Audiology, 7, 105–112.

Satterfield, J. H., Schell, A. M., Nicholas, T. W., Satterfield, B. T., & Freese, T. E. (1990). Ontogeny of selective attention effects on event-related potentials in attention-deficit hyperactivity disorder and normal boys. Biological Psychiatry, 28, 879–903.

Scherg, M. (1982). Distortion of middle latency auditory response produced by analog filtering. Scandinavian Audiology, 11, 57–60.

Scherg, M., Vajsar, J., & Picton, T. (1989). A source analysis of the late human auditory evoked potentials. Journal of Cognitive Neuroscience, 1, 3336–3355.

Schroger, E. & Wolff, C. (1996). Mismatch response of the human brain to changes in sound location. Neuroreport, 7(18), 3005–3008.

Schwender, D., Madler, C., Klasing, S., Peter, K., & Poppel, E. (1994). Anesthetic control of 40 Hz brain activity and implicit memory. Consciousness and Cognition, 3, 129–147.

Schwender, D., Klasing, S., Conzen, P., Finsterer, U., Poppel, E., & Peter, K. (1996). Midlatency auditory evoked potentials during anesthesia with increasing end expiratory concentrations of desflurane. Acta Anaesthesiologica Scandinavica, 40, 171–176.

Shallop, J. K., & Osterhammel, P. A. (1983). A comparative study of measurements of SN 10 and the 40/sec middle latency response in newborns. Scandinavian Audiology, 12, 91–95.

Sharma, A., Dorman, M. F., & Spahr, A. J. (2002). A sensitive period for the development of the central auditory system in children with cochlear implants: Implications for age of implantation. Ear and Hearing, 23, 532–539.

Sharma, A., Dorman, M. F., & Kral, A. (2005). The influence of a sensitive period on central auditory development in children with unilateral and bilateral cochlear implants. Hearing Research, 203, 134–143.

Sharma, A., Kraus, N., McGee, T., Carrell, T., & Nicol, T. (1993). Acoustic versus phonetic representation of speech as reflected by the mismatch negativity event-related potential. Electroencephalography and Clinical Neurophysiology, 88, 64–71.

Shih, J. J., & Thompson, S. W. (1998). Lambda waves: Incidence and relationship to photic driving. Brain Topography, 10, 265–272.

Siegel, C., Waldo, M., Mizner, G., Adler, L. E., & Freedman, R. (1984). Deficits in sensory gating in schizophrenic patients and their relatives: Evidence obtained with auditory evoked responses. Archives of General Psychiatry, 41, 607–612.

Small, S. A., & Stapells, D. R. (2004). Artifactual responses when recording auditory steady-state responses. Ear and Hearing, 25, 611–623.

St. Clair, D., Blackburn, I., Blackwood, D., & Tyrer, G. (1988). Measuring the course of Alzheimer's disease. A longitudinal study of neuropsychological function and changes in P3 event-related potential. British Journal of Psychiatry, 152, 48–54.

Stapells, D. R., Galambos, R., Costello, J. A., & Makeig, S. (1988). Inconsistency of auditory middle latency and steady-state responses in infants. Electroencephalography and Clinical Neurophysiology, 71, 289–295.

Stapells, D. R., Linden, D., Suffield, J. B., Hamel, G., & Picton, T. W. (1984). Human auditory steady state potentials. Ear and Hearing, 5, 105–113.

Stapells, D. R., Makeig, S., & Galambos, R. (1987). Auditory steady-state responses: Threshold prediction using phase coherence. Electroencephalography and Clinical Neurophysiology, 67, 260–270.

Starr, A., McPherson, D., Patterson, J., et al. (1991). Absence of both auditory evoked potentials and auditory percepts dependent on timing cues. Brain, 114, 1157–1180.

Stueve, M. P., & O'Rourke, C. A. (2003). Estimation of hearing loss in children: Comparison of auditory steady-state response, auditory brainstem response, and behavioral test methods. American Journal of Audiology, 12, 125–136.

Swanepoel, D., Hugo, R., & Roode, R. (2004). Auditory steady-state responses for children with severe to profound hearing loss. Archives of Otolaryngology—Head and Neck Surgery, 130, 531–535.

Tatsumi, K., Hirai, K., Furuya, H., & Okuda, T. (1995). Effects of sevoflurane on the middle latency auditory evoked response and the electroencephalographic power spectrum. Anesthésie et Analgésie, 80, 940–943.

Tiitinen, H., Sinkkonen, J., Reinikainen, K., Alho, K., Lavikainen, J., & Näätänen, R. (1993). Selective attention enhances the auditory 40-Hz transient response in humans. Nature, 364(6432), 59–60.

Tremblay, K., Kraus, N., Carrell, T., & McGee, T. (1997). Central auditory system plasticity: Generalization to novel stimuli following listening training. Journal of the Acoustical Society of America, 102, 3762–3773.

Tsuzuku, T. (1993). 40-Hz steady state response in awake cats after bilateral chronic lesions in auditory cortices or inferior colliculi. Auris, Nasus, Larynx, 20, 263–274.

Tucker, D. A., & Ruth, R. A. (1996). Effects of age, signal level, and signal rate on the auditory middle latency response. Journal of the American Academy of Audiology, 7, 83–91.

Valdes, J. L., Perez-Abalo, M. C., Martin, V., Savio, G., Sierra, C., Rodriguez, E., & Lins, O. (1997). Comparison of statistical indicators for the automatic detection of 80 Hz auditory steady state responses. Ear and Hearing, 18, 420–429.

Van der Reijden, C. S., Mens, L. H. M., & Snik, A. F. M. (2001). Comparing signal-to-noise ratios of amplitude modulation following responses from four EEG derivations in awake normally hearing adults. Audiology, 40, 202–207.

Velasco, M., Velasco, F., & Velasco, A. L. (1989). Intracranial studies on potential generators of some vertex auditory evoked potentials in man. Stereotactic and Functional Neurosurgery, 53, 49–73.

Waldo, M. C., & Freedman, R. (1986). Gating of auditory evoked responses in normal college students. Psychiatry Research, 19, 233–239.

Waldo, M., Gerhardt, G., Baker, N., Drebing, C., Adler, L., & Freedman, R. (1992). Auditory sensory gating and catecholamine metabolism in schizophrenic and normal subjects. Psychiatry Research, 44, 21–32.

Wolpaw, J. R., & Wood, C. C. (1982). Scalp distribution of human auditory evoked potentials: 1. Evaluation of reference electrode sites. Electroencephalography and Clinical Neurophysiology, 54, 15–24.

Wood, C. C., & Wolpaw, J. R. (1982). Scalp distribution of human auditory evoked potentials: 2. Evidence for overlapping sources and involvement of auditory cortex. Electroencephalography and Clinical Neurophysiology, 54, 25–38,

Woods, D. L., Knight, R.T., & Scabini, D. (1993). Anatomical substrates of auditory selective attention: Behavioral and electrophysiological effects of posterior association cortex lesions. Brain Research and Cognitive Brain Research, 1, 227–240.

Xu, Z. M., Cawenberge, K., Vinck, D., & De Vel, E. (1997). Choice of a tone-pip envelope for frequency-specific threshold evaluations by means of the middle-latency response: Normally hearing subjects and slope of sensorineural hearing loss. Auris, Nasus, Larynx, 24, 333–340.

Chapter 22

Otoacoustic Emissions

Theodore J. Glattke and Martin S. Robinette

The discovery of otoacoustic emissions (OAE) by David Kemp in 1977 created the basis for changes in our understanding of how the auditory system is able to respond to the minute energy levels that are required to reach the threshold of perception of humans. The report by Kemp (1978) on stimulated or evoked otoacoustic emissions (EOAE) and his later description of spontaneous otoacoustic emissions (SOAE) (Kemp, 1979) provided important evidence that fueled the development of modern auditory theory and offered important clues regarding the future applications of OAE measurement in clinical situations. Contemporary theory is an amalgamation of elements proposed by von Helmholtz (1863) more than 100 years ago, Békésy (1928) nearly 80 years ago, and Gold (1948) nearly 60 years ago. Von Helmholtz's theory called for the existence of precise resonators that are tuned to individual frequencies. The resonators were thought to respond to the motion of the basilar membrane and to vibrate in and of themselves. Von Helmholtz's resonance theory of hearing was the first modern explanation to predict that tonotopic organization of the cochlea would be arranged with representation of high-frequency stimuli at the base and low-frequency stimuli at the apex of the cochlea. Békésy's report of a traveling wave disturbance that progressed along the cochlea's basilar membrane from base to apex had a

profound effect on auditory theory. Békésy (1928) was critical of von Helmholtz's theory because he believed that the resonators that were proposed by von Helmholtz could not be tuned with sufficient precision to explain precipitous high-frequency hearing loss that had been reported clinically. It is ironic that the lack of precision in the traveling wave formed the basis for later criticisms of Békésy's theory of cochlear analysis.

Gold (1948) examined the theories of von Helmholtz and Békésy and the data on auditory perception that had accumulated and concluded that the sharply tuned resonators proposed by von Helmholtz and the mechanical activity recorded by Békésy were both important components of the response of the inner ear to sound. In addition, he argued that some form of positive feedback, or amplification, must be in place to allow humans to respond to low energy levels and do so with great sensitivity to small changes in stimulus frequency. Gold recognized that the positive feedback mechanism might reveal itself through episodes of oscillation like the audible tonal feedback associated with hearing aids and public address systems. He also considered that it should be possible to detect the presence of the amplifier mechanism through detection of the oscillation. Today, we routinely record SOAE that were predicted by Gold.

The mechanism of emission production is not known. However, the discovery of outer hair cell motility (Brownell, 1983), coupled with recordings of enhanced basilar membrane vibration in response to low-intensity stimulation (Johnstone et al, 1986; Ruggero and Rich, 1991), has led to a consensus that the outer hair cells (OHCs) supply the driving force for the emissions and the "cochlear amplifier" described by Davis (1983). The discovery of the protein dubbed *prestin* that contributes to the motility of the hair cells has increased our understanding of phenomena that were not conceived by the mainstream researchers through much of the 20th century (Dallos and Fakler, 2002).

Pearl

- *Prestin,* the name given to the protein that enables the hair cells to change dimension quickly, is after the Italian word *presto,* meaning "fast." *Presto* is a term familiar to musicians: it indicates a speedy execution.

Today, the Békésy traveling wave is thought to be the basis for the spatial representation and temporal dispersion of the inner ear's response to sound, and micromechanical activity originating in the OHCs is thought to provide the threshold sensitivity and tuning that characterize normal hearing (Dallos, 1992). Hearing loss of cochlear origin in the mild to moderate range now is thought to be due to the loss of the biomechanical amplifier system rather than the reduction in sensitivity of sensory cells. Because OAE are intimately related to the operation of the OHCs and because those cells are critical components in the normal cochlear response to sound, it follows that OAE properties are sensitive to the presence of hearing loss caused by hair cell abnormalities.

◆ Detection and Measurement of Otoacoustic Emissions

The emissions are low-intensity sounds that may be detected in the external ear canal by a microphone. They offer a glimpse of the motion that originates within the cochlea. Force created in the cochlea arrives at the stapes footplate and is changed to acoustic energy because the middle ear apparatus functions like a loudspeaker diaphragm system. If the middle ear system is compromised, it is likely that the acoustic energy detected in the ear canal will also be compromised. In addition, the action of the middle ear muscles can be expected to influence the characteristics of OAE (e.g., Margolis and Trine, 1997). Outer hair cells receive a rich efferent innervation from the central nervous system (CNS; see, e.g., Warr, 1992), and the interaction of OAE with external stimulation reflects the influence of the CNS on the operation of the cochlear biomechanical system.

As Probst (1990) stated, any sound that is produced by the cochlea and detected in the ear canal is an otoacoustic emission. The various types of OAE share several common features:

1. They are low-intensity sounds, ranging from the noise floor of the instrumentation (approximately –20 dB sound pressure level [SPL]) to a maximum between 20 and 30 dB SPL. The amplitude of an EOAE is related to the stimulus amplitude in a complex manner. Early investigations (e.g., Wilson, 1980) demonstrated that EOAE obtained in response to near-threshold click stimuli contained more energy than was present in the stimulus. EOAE reach saturation for stimuli in the middle-intensity range. A click stimulus at peak amplitude of 80 dB SPL will produce an emission with amplitude that is ~50 to 70 dB below the stimulus amplitude. Similar results occur for continuous tonal stimuli presented at moderate intensities. For example, the distortion product signal created using routine forms of primary tone stimulation is expected to be found at an SPL that is ~55 dB below the primary tone levels.

2. The temporal and spectral characteristics of the emission will reflect the region of the cochlea that produces it. In a healthy ear, EOAE will mirror the stimulus: click stimuli will produce emissions with complex waveforms and spectra that extend over a broad frequency range, tone bursts elicit brief tonal emissions, and continuous tones produce continuous emissions at frequencies predicted by the frequency of the tonal stimuli.

3. Emissions can be suppressed or reduced in amplitude by presentation of ipsilateral or contralateral stimuli.

4. Emission properties are altered in the presence of slight hearing loss (Harris and Probst, 1991), and the probability of detecting an emission in the frequency region where hearing loss exceeds 30 dB HL varies inversely with the amount of hearing loss (Harris and Probst, 1997).

5. Emissions are extracted from the background noise in the external ear canal by sampling the sound in the ear canal to develop an average time waveform, or a spectral analysis, or a combination of temporal and spectral averaging techniques.

Otoacoustic emissions typically are classified after Probst (1990) according to the stimuli used to produce them (**Table 22–1**).

Spontaneous Otoacoustic Emissions

As the name implies, SOAE occur without intentional stimulation of the ear. When detected in the absence of any external stimulus, they are registered through the use of spectral analysis of the sound in the external ear canal. **Fig. 22–1** provides an illustration of the typical representation of an SOAE.

There is no intentional auditory stimulation, but, of course, the ambient noise in the external ear canal can be substantial. A spectral analysis of the signal detected in the ear canal

Table 22–1 Types of Otoacoustic Emissions

Type of Emission	Stimulus	Recording/Analysis
Spontaneous (SOAE)	None	Narrowband signal detected by high-resolution spectral averaging
Synchronized spontaneous (SSOAE)	Click	Time-locked averaging over a window of (SSOAE) ~80 msec after the stimulus. A spectral analysis conducted on the 60-80 msec window reveals the emission(s) as line(s) in the spectrum.
Transient evoked (TEOAE)	Click or brief tone burst	Time-locked averaging over a window of 12.5 to 20.0 msec (depending on software). Response waveforms stored in two memory locations (A and B) for correlation analysis. See text for explanation.
Stimulus frequency (SFOAE)	Sinusoid	SPL in ear canal is monitored as stimulus (SFOAE) is swept through frequency region of interest at fixed SPL. Fluctuations in SPL are combinations of incident and emission energy.
Distortion product (DPOAE)	Paired sinusoids at F1 and F2	Signal from microphone is submitted to time averaging followed by spectral analysis. Energy at 2F1-F2 is considered to be the emission.

SPL, sound pressure level.

reveals the presence of one or more narrowband signals emerging above the noise floor in any given frequency region. Measures of SOAE include (1) peak frequency; (2) sound pressure level (SPL); and (3) signal-to-noise ratio (SNR), where the noise is estimated at a frequency region adjacent to the SOAE. This form of emission was anticipated by Gold's (1948) prediction that the ear must incorporate an active feedback system. The active feedback of the type Gold predicted can produce oscillations at discrete frequencies (in essence, spontaneous emissions).

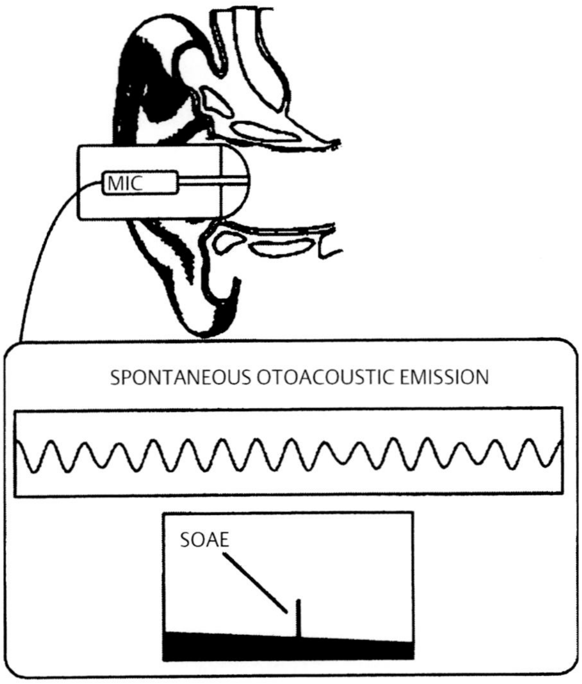

Synchronized Spontaneous Otoacoustic Emissions

SOAE can be synchronized with an external stimulus, and, when recorded this way, they are designated as synchronized spontaneous otoacoustic emissions (SSOAE) (Prieve and Falter, 1995). As illustrated in **Fig. 22–2**, the synchronous behavior of the emission allows the SSOAE to be captured using time-averaged sampling to improve the SNR of the recording. In the usual SSOAE recording, a low-intensity transient signal

Figure 22–1 Representation of a spontaneous otoacoustic emission (SOAE). The signal in the ear canal is detected by a miniature microphone and submitted to spectral analysis. The SOAE is evident as a narrowband, tonelike signal that emerges from the background noise.

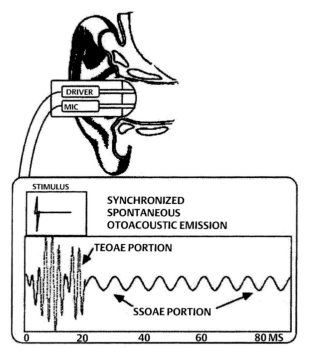

Figure 22–2 Representation of a synchronized spontaneous otoacoustic emission (SSOAE). The SSOAE is captured by repeated sampling of sound in the ear canal after presentation of a low-intensity transient stimulus. The transient evoked otoacoustic emission (TEOAE) persists for ~20 msec, but the SSOAE continues, time-locked to the stimulus. A spectral analysis of the 60 to 80 msec portion of the response waveform reveals the frequencies present in the SSOAE.

is used to elicit a transient evoked otoacoustic emission (TEOAE), but the recording time window is increased to 80 msec post-stimulus onset. The synchronized (time-locked) SSOAE emerges from the recording after the more robust TEOAE decays. A spectral analysis of the waveform captured in the 60 to 80 msec time window confirms the presence of the synchronized emission. Pacheco (1997) replicated earlier findings of Wable and Collete (1994) by analyzing more than 200 SOAE and SSOAE records obtained in a large population of listeners with normal OAE responses. She determined that the two recording techniques identify the same emissions and that the SSOAE method represents the emission and noise floor more favorably because of the time-averaging process. As is the case with SOAE, fundamental measures of SSOAE include frequency, amplitude, and SNR.

As reviewed by Bright (1997), SOAE occur more frequently in women than in men and more often in the right ear than in the left. SOAE range from the noise floor of the recording system to ~20 to 30 dB SPL. Although it occurs only rarely, it is possible for a person presenting with a spontaneous emission to actually hear the emission signal (Fritsch et al, 2001; Oostenbrink and Verhaagen-Warnaar, 2004). Early speculation that routine recordings of emissions could offer evidence of the presence of tinnitus has not been supported by investigations that reveal the loss of emissions with the onset of tinnitus because of aspirin ingestion (Penner and Coles, 1992). Virtually all published investigations suggest that SOAE obtained from the right ear are larger than those obtained from the left and that those obtained from women are larger than those obtained from men (Bright, 1997). SOAE are stable over long periods of time, but they are not used in clinical screening programs because they may be absent in nearly 50% of ears with normal pure-tone thresholds.

Transient Evoked Otoacoustic Emissions

Evoked otoacoustic emissions occur either during long-term stimulation or after a brief stimulus. Responses to brief stimuli are known as transient evoked otoacoustic emmisions (TEOAE). An example of a typical TEOAE recording is illustrated in **Fig. 22–3**.

The probe apparatus includes a miniature loudspeaker and microphone. The signal in the ear canal is sampled for ~20 msec after the stimulus is presented to the ear. Although important exceptions exist (Gorga et al, 1993; Prieve et al, 1993), most of the published data regarding TEOAE have been obtained through the use of hardware and software supplied by Otodynamics Ltd. (Hatfield, Hertfordshire, UK) and known as ILO-88. The typical TEOAE stimulus is a brief, broad-spectrum click, but tone bursts also may be used to elicit the response (Xu et al, 1994). The response follows the stimulus with a latency that is determined by cochlear traveling wave dynamics. As illustrated in **Fig. 22–3**, high-frequency components appear with a shorter latency than lower frequency components. This time delay reflects cochlear dynamics and anatomy: the traveling wave response is much more rapid for high-frequency stimulus components than for low-frequency components.

The TEOAE response is recorded through the use of techniques that are identical to those used to record the short latency auditory evoked potentials, or auditory brainstem response (ABR). Approximately 1000 stimuli are presented to improve the SNR of the response in each of two (A and B) average waveforms. As is the case for electrophysiological recordings, the repeated sampling reduces the random variance in the signal by an amount predicted by the square root of the sample size. The effect of this is to reduce the noise by ~30 dB, allowing an emission to be extracted from the ambient noise in the ear canal. The typical clinical recording involves stimulation at a level of 80 dB peak equivalent SPL (pe SPL), or ~40 dB spectrum level (see, e.g., Glattke, 1983), and response amplitudes are typically at levels ~60 to 70 dB below the level of the stimulus.

Stimulus Frequency Otoacoustic Emissions

Stimulus frequency otoacoustic emissions (SFOAE) occur during stimulation of the ear with tonal stimuli. As illustrated in **Fig. 22–4**, they appear at the frequency of the external stimulus; consequently, it is difficult to separate the response and the stimulus (Kemp and Chum, 1980). SFOAE result from energy leaking back into the ear canal from the cochlear amplifier. When recorded simultaneously with the arriving stimulus, the stimulus frequency emission may interact with the incident energy in a complex way, resulting in fluctuations in the SPL recorded in the external ear canal. Because SFOAE are intimately related to the function of the

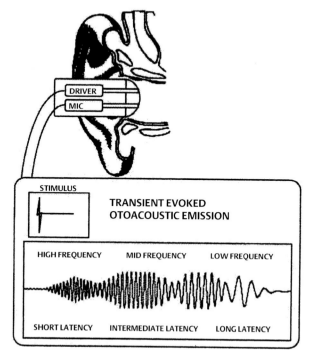

Figure 22–3 Representation of a transient evoked otoacoustic emission (TEOAE). The acoustic signal in the external ear canal is sampled for ~20 msec for 2000 replications of an abrupt stimulus. The stimulus artifact is eliminated from the first 2 to 3 msec of the recording, and the remaining complex waveform mirrors the mechanical response of the outer hair cells of the cochlea.

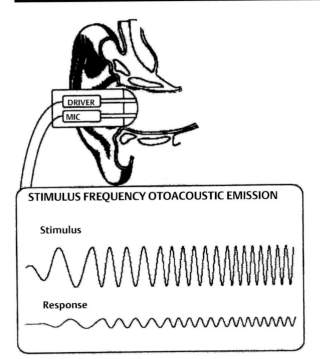

Figure 22–4 Example of a stimulus frequency otoacoustic emission (SFOAE). The SFOAE is recorded using a continuous tone. When swept across frequencies, the cochlear response includes a tone that is delayed in time due to cochlear mechanical events. The addition of the emission and the incident tone is recorded as fluctuations of sound pressure level in the external ear canal.

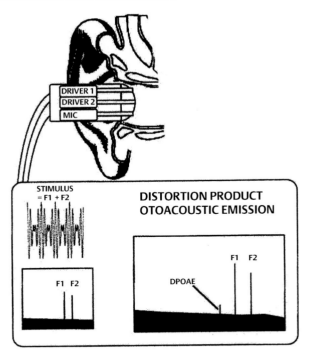

Figure 22–5 Representation of a distortion product otoacoustic emission (DPOAE). The acoustic probe system must include two independent loudspeakers so that any distortions that occur are produced in the ear, not in the signal generation equipment. The primary tones are set at two known frequencies (F1 and F2), and the DPOAE of interest occurs at a frequency of 2F1–F2.

cochlear amplifier, their relative contribution to the SPL in the ear canal increases as the external or incident stimulus energy is attenuated. Hence, wide fluctuations are recorded for incident stimuli near the threshold of hearing. Because of the difficulty associated with recording and interpreting SFOAE, they have not been used in clinical investigations.

Pearl

- If you want to hear distortion product otoacoustic emissions, listen to a good-quality recording of Giuseppe Tartini's *Il trillo del Diavolo*. He discovered the acoustic phenomenon of resultant tones, which he dubbed terzo *suono* ("third sound"). For even more fun, travel to Pirano, Istria, and check out his statue near the edge of the Adriatic.

Distortion Product Otoacoustic Emissions

Distortion product otoacoustic emissions (DPOAE) also occur simultaneously with a stimulus. Examples of the stimulus response waveform and response spectra associated with DPOAE are illustrated in **Fig. 22–5**. DPOAE are relatively easy to detect because they occur at frequencies that are different than the stimulus frequencies. They represent distortions of the stimulus, hence their name. DPOAE are recorded clinically in response to the presentation of a pair of primary

tones, called F1 and F2. Distortion products appear at several frequencies when the two primary tones are applied to the ear. The most robust is located at a frequency equal to 2F1–F2. In a practical situation, the DPOAE frequency is found to be as far below F1 as F2 is above F1. The DPOAE response appears at a level that is ~50 to 60 dB below the level of the primary stimulus, and it occurs only when the primary stimuli are located in a region of the cochlea that responds normally. For example, a DPOAE produced by primary tones at 4000 (F1) and 4800 Hz (F2) will be detected only if the region of the cochlea responding to F1 and F2 is functioning normally. The actual distortion product will be at 3200 Hz in this instance, but its presence does not reflect the function of the portion of the cochlea that normally responds to 3200 Hz. If the distortion product at 3200 Hz were absent for the primary stimuli at 4000 and 5000 Hz, one would expect cochlear dysfunction at the sites where F1 and F2 interact. This precise location remains to be determined but is in the region of the F2 "place" in the cochlea.

Special Consideration

- Increasing evidence supports the concept that DPOAE and TEOAE may be produced by different cochlear mechanisms. Complete agreement between TEOAE and DPOAE results should not be expected under all circumstances.

Recent work of several investigators (Shera, 2004; Shera and Guinan, 2003; Siegel et al, 2005) suggest that OAE may arise from two different mechanisms within the cochlea. SOAE and TEOAE appear to be highly dependent upon reflections from discontinuities along the length of the organ of Corti. DPOAE are more intimately related to nonlinear processes inherent in the biological amplifier system. The taxonomy provided by Shera and others helps to explain the discrepancies that have been reported regarding the vulnerability of various types of OAE to the compromise of the auditory system and, indirectly, to the differences in prevalence and characteristics of OAE in various species.

In summary, OAE are small signals that depend on the integrity of the entire auditory periphery, including the external and middle ear apparatus, as well as the cochlea and its interactions with the CNS. No responsible author has suggested that OAE can be used to estimate the amount of hearing loss with great precision, but it is clear that clinical recordings of OAE are important elements in the audiologist's toolbox.

♦ Interpretation of Transient Evoked Otoacoustic Emissions

Fig. 22–6 is a printout of a TEOAE recording obtained using Otodynamics ILO-92 software. The components of the display and many of the algorithms employed by the ILO software have been incorporated into more recent software releases by other manufacturers.

The discussion that follows reviews the information contained in the display seen in **Fig. 22–6**.

1. *Stimulus* The panel labeled *Stimulus* includes an illustration of the stimulus waveform that was sampled before the onset of data collection. The display spans a total time period of 5 msec. The amplitude scale is indicated in pascals (Pa). A value of 0.3 Pa is equivalent to 83.5 dB SPL. In this instance, the peak SPL was detected at 80.4 dB SPL.

2. *Patient/software* The center panels identify the version of the software used to display the data and information about the patient, ear tested, and stimulus mode. The designation MX NONLIN CLIKN indicates that the ILO default nonlinear stimulus mode was used to obtain the data. Responses are gathered for sets of four stimuli. Three are presented in one phase at the indicated amplitude and the fourth is presented in the opposite phase at a level that is 3 times greater than each of the three previous stimuli (i.e., it is 10 dB greater). The sum of the response to the four stimuli consists of waveforms that follow the stimulus precisely (linear components) and components that do not change in a simple fashion with stimulus intensity or phase (nonlinear components). Kemp et al (1986) estimated that the linear stimulus artifacts and response components could be reduced by 40 dB, whereas the desired nonlinear portion of the emission would be reduced by only 6 dB with this stimulus method. In the default setting, the ILO-88 software stores the average response to one half of the stimuli in a memory buffer identified as "A." The response for other stimuli is stored in a buffer, "B." The sampling process continues until responses from 260 sets of stimuli have been stored in each of the two memory areas. Therefore, the A and B waveforms each represent the mean of responses to 260 × 4 transients, or 1040 stimuli, and the total number of stimuli used in the default condition is 2080.

3. *Response waveform* The display illustrates the time-averaged waveforms sampled for a 20.48 msec period after the onset of the transient stimulus. Tracings are plotted for the "A" and "B" memory locations, and each tracing consists of 512 data points. Each data point corresponds to a time period of 40 μs. The first 2.5 msec, or 63 data points, have been eliminated to reduce the contribution of a stimulus artifact to the average response waveform. The sensitivity of the vertical scale in the response waveform panel is 60 dB greater than the scale used to represent the click stimulus in the upper left-hand panel. Put another way, the stimulus waveform in the upper left panel is actually ~1000 times the peak pressure level of the response (stimulus = ~80 dB pe SPL, response = ~20 dB SPL).

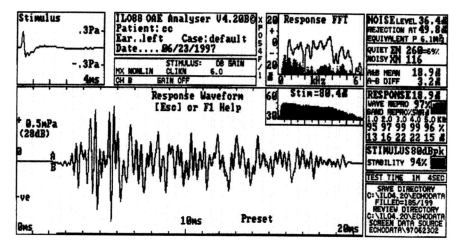

Figure 22–6 Transient evoked otoacoustic emission response obtained from a young adult with normal hearing thresholds.

4. *Response FFT*   This display provides illustrations of the fast Fourier transforms (FFTs) that are based on the A and B waveforms. The resolution of the FFT analysis is ~49 Hz per line. The open histogram reflects the spectrum of the response that is common to the A and B tracings. The cross-hatched display represents the spectrum of the difference between the A and B waveforms or the noise that remains in the average waveform. The horizontal scale extends from 0 to 6000 Hz. The vertical scale extends from less than −20 dB SPL to approximately +20 dB SPL.

5. *Stim*   This display provides a tabular representation of the pe SPL of the stimulus at the onset of the sampling. The spectrum of the stimulus is illustrated by the solid histogram. The horizontal scale of the stimulus spectrum is identical to the horizontal scale for the response FFT. The vertical scale extends from 30 dB SPL to > 60 dB SPL. For a typical transient stimulus with a peak level of 80 dB SPL, the spectrum level (or level per cycle) will be 40 to 45 dB SPL. As may be determined, the energy is spread across the spectrum, with a gradual loss in the high-frequency region.

6. *Noise*   The tabular value of the noise is the average SPL detected by the microphone during the samples that were not rejected by the software. The noise level in this instance was ~36 dB. The signal averaging process allows the emission, with overall level of ~18 dB, to be extracted from the background noise.

7. *Rejection at ___ dB*   The software permits the examiner to select a rejection threshold to reduce unwanted noise. The default rejection threshold is 47 dB SPL, and the range available to the examiner extends from 24 to 55 dB SPL. The rejection level can be adjusted continuously throughout the sampling period, and the tabular value is the threshold selected by the examiner at the end of the sampling. The rejection threshold value also is shown in millipascals.

8. *Quiet ΣN*   This entry is the number of responses accepted for the A and B waveforms. The percentage of all samples ultimately selected for the average waveform also is listed in tabular form.

9. *Noisy XN*   This entry is a tally of the number of response sets that were rejected during the sampling procedure. Approximately 30% of the samples were rejected due to noise.

10. *A&B Mean*   This is the sound pressure level of the average of the A and B waveforms. In this instance, the value is 18.9 dB.

11. *A–B Diff*   This is the average difference between the A and B waveforms and is the level of energy represented by the cross-hatched area of the Response FFT window. It is computed by taking the differences between the A and B waveforms on a point-by-point basis, less 3 dB. In this case, the A–B value of 3.2 dB is 15.7 dB less than the average power of the A and B waveforms. The A–B Diff value is the residual "noise" in the Responses FFT window.

12. *Response*   This value is the overall level of the correlated portions of the A and B response waveforms and is obtained from the FFT displayed in the Response FFT window. The large difference between the A&B Mean (18.9 dB) result and the A–B Diff (3.2 dB) windows means that there was little effect of the residual noise (difference between A and B) on the final response. The 15.9 dB difference between the A&B Mean and the A–B Diff windows corresponds to a power ratio of ~40:1. Said another way, the energy in the residual noise is only ~2.25% of the average response waveform, and when subtracted from the average response, the 2.25% amounts to less than 1 dB. Hence, there is no difference between the A&B Mean and the Response values.

13. *Wave Repro*   This is known as "whole-wave reproducibility." The entry is actually the value of the cross-correlation between the A and B waveforms expressed as a percentage. The correlation is recomputed after every 20 stimulus sets, and the value of the correlation is represented in the small histogram to the right of the percent value. The result in this case is 97%, reflecting a near-perfect correlation, which is compatible with the small A–B Diff value.

14. *Band Repro % SNR dB*   The reproducibility and signal-to-noise ratio values are listed below column headings of 1 through 5 kHz. To obtain these results, the A and B waveforms are filtered into bandwidths of ~1000 Hz centered at the indicated frequencies. The correlations are recomputed, and the difference between the powers computed for the FFTs represented by the open and cross-hatched histograms in the Response FFT window are represented as the SNR at each frequency.

15. *Stimulus ___ dB pk*   The stimulus intensity is measured after every 16 stimulus sets. The tabular value listed at this location is the result of the final computation. The final result may be different than the value obtained at the outset of the sampling procedure. The initial value is tabulated in the portion of the display containing the stimulus spectrum (see no. 5).

16. *Stability ___ %*   This entry and the accompanying histogram reflect changes that occur in the stimulus intensity. The single entry expresses the greatest difference throughout the sampling period as a percentile rather than dB value (1 dB is ~10%). In this case, the stability, at 94%, means that the maximum fluctuation was less than 1 dB throughout the sampling procedure. The small histogram to the right of the entry chronicles the history of the stimulus intensity measurements.

17. *Test time*   This entry records the duration of the test, in this instance, 64 seconds.

Figs. 22–7 through **22–9** are included to help the reader understand the computations involved in determination of the TEOAE response characteristics.

The reader will find that the tabular data in **Fig. 22–7** are identical to those in **Fig. 22–6**. The waveform illustrated in

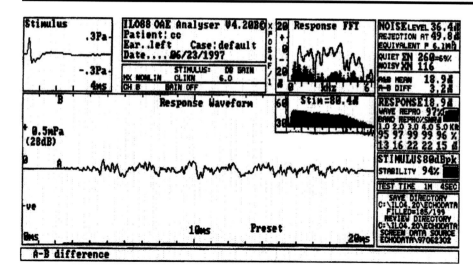

Figure 22–7 The A–B difference tracing based on the data illustrated in **Fig. 22–6.**

the Response window of **Fig. 22–7** is the point-by-point difference between the A and B memory waveforms illustrated in the previous figure. In this instance, the total power is 3.2 dB SPL (see A–B Diff tabular amount). The spectrum of this difference waveform is illustrated as the solid histogram in the Response FFT window. Most of the energy is in the low-frequency region, below 2000 Hz. Occasional peaks occur at 3500 and 4500 Hz.

The data in **Fig. 22–8** are the same as those in **Fig. 22–6,** but the response waveforms were intentionally shifted in the computer memory so that there is little overlap between the A and B memories. As the reader can determine, the A&B Mean window indicates a drop to 13.8 dB, the A–B Diff window shows a dramatic rise to 20.4 dB, and the Response FFT window now suggests that the bulk of the data contained in the Response Waveform window is "noise." A few, slow changes in the waveform are misinterpreted as reliable response components, a phenomenon

that Harris and Probst (1991) identified many years ago. In general, the reproducibility scores have fallen to 0, and the SNR data reflect the fact that the waveforms now are interpreted as noise.

Fig. 22–9 provides the basis for the new interpretation of the data that were shifted in time.

In this final figure, the "difference tracing" appears as if it is a strong TEOAE response. It was computed on the basis of the time-shifted waveforms reviewed in **Fig. 22–8** and represents the moment-to-moment difference in the amplitude of the response waveforms, or the noise in the FFT response spectrum. Note that the difference tracing appears as if it were a normal TEOAE response. The waveform represents a very slight shift in the A and B memories, but the original data are precisely the same as those in **Fig. 22–6.** Thus, we have made "noise" out of what had been a nearly perfect replication of the response in the A and B memories.

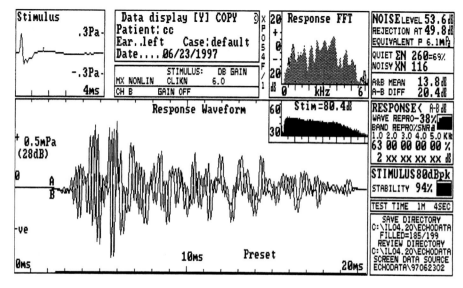

Figure 22–8 Previous transient evoked otoacoustic emission data with artificial shift in memory locations. Note that there is little overlap between the A and B memories.

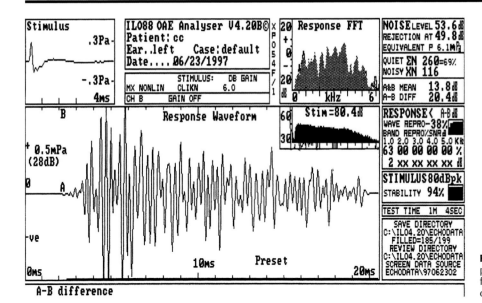

Figure 22–9 The "difference" data from the previous screen **(Fig. 22–8).** Note that the difference appears to be a strong transient evoked otoacoustic emission response.

♦ Transient Evoked Otoacoustic Emissions in Practice

Clinical evaluation of electrophysiological responses, such as the ABR or electrocochleographic (ECoG) recordings obtained from the eighth cranial nerve (CN VIII), rely on estimates of response threshold, latency, and amplitude, to estimate the integrity of the auditory system. More recently, studies of the auditory steady-state response (ASSR) have relied on spectral and phase measurements to help identify the presence of responses and track them to threshold levels. Measures of OAE include all of the observations made of electrophysiological responses. At the outset of studies of emissions, Kemp (1978) observed the highly nonlinear nature of the response, and he and his coworkers reported that the minimum intensity at which a TEOAE can be detected rarely corresponds with perceptual threshold (e.g., Kemp et al, 1990). Kemp warned that the apparent "threshold" of the response is critically dependent on the noise in the recording situation and the status of the ear under test. For example, although a newborn may have robust emissions, physiological noise produced by the neonate may preclude detection of the emissions at levels corresponding to the infant's auditory threshold. An ear with strong emission responses may reveal little attenuation of the response with significant reductions of the stimulus intensity, as little as 0.1 dB per 1 dB change (Kemp et al, 1990). Thus, it is impossible to estimate the threshold of hearing from the apparent threshold of the emission response or extrapolate from detected responses to presumed threshold on the basis of amplitude measurements. Kemp (1978), Prieve et al (1993, 1997), Grandori and Ravazzani (1993), Stover and Norton (1993), and Prieve and Falter (1995) are among the investigators who have examined the complex interaction between click stimulus intensity and response characteristics, including threshold. In the most general terms, it is impossible to estimate audiometric threshold from any characteristic of the TEOAE. As

Robinette (2003) has reviewed, the probability that a TEOAE will be present in any given frequency region is related to the audiometric threshold in the frequency region of interest, but threshold cannot be predicted with precision. As Kemp et al (1990) suggested, we are far from having a standard against which response threshold, latency, and growth characteristics can be evaluated in a clinical setting. In this sense, interpretation of OAE shares difficulties encountered in the interpretation of cochlear microphonic (CM) potentials, which, like the emissions, are intimately related to the status of the hair cells in the cochlea (e.g., Glattke, 1983).

The most common clinical application of TEOAE involves click stimuli presented at moderate intensities, 80 dB peak equivalent SPL or ~45 dB greater than perceptual threshold. The default stimulus used by the ILO-88 equipment was selected to screen for hearing loss: if no response can be obtained, then it is possible that a hearing loss is present. In the most general sense, the spectrum of a TEOAE elicited from a healthy ear reflects the spectrum of the stimulus. TEOAE obtained in response to click stimuli are expected to have broad response spectra. The amplitudes of TEOAE vary directly with the amplitudes of the stimuli, but the relationships between stimulus and response are complicated by the fact that TEOAE result from highly nonlinear phenomena. From the outset, reports of properties of TEOAE elicited from normal ears have emphasized the idiosyncratic nature of the responses. Unfortunately, few studies have provided tabular summaries of the data provided by the ILO-88 software or grouped data in terms of subject characteristics such as age, gender, and right/left differences. The data that are summarized in the sections that follow were obtained using ILO-88 default stimulus conditions: (1) 80 μs transients, (2) nominal stimulus level of 80 to 83 dB pe SPL, and (3) nonlinear mode, unless stated otherwise.

Although several studies have described the properties of OAE in healthy infants and children, there are few large-scale studies of emission characteristics in children whose audiometric status has been documented by behavioral tests (e.g., Glattke et al, 1995). One report of the results of a newborn screening program, in which control for sensitivity and specificity of the screening procedure was evaluated, has appeared in the literature (Lutman et al, 1997). The salient property of TEOAE obtained from healthy newborns is a robust response amplitude. Kok et al (1993) reported that the median response amplitude for infants is ~20 dB SPL, and the response reproducibility is directly related to response amplitude. As Prieve et al (1997) found, the largest changes in TEOAE amplitude appear to occur between birth and 4 years of age. The average amplitude of the response to default stimuli (80 dB) declines from 20 to ~15 dB for preschool children and to 10 dB for adults.

Glattke and Robinette (1997) and Prieve and Falter (1995) have reported that TEOAE amplitude does not decrease with age when the responses obtained from older adults are compared with those obtained from young adults, so long as adequate control is provided for normal-hearing thresholds. Glattke and Robinette (1997) and Robinette (2003) observed a continuing attenuation of response with age when "normal" thresholds were defined as 25 dB HL or better. If the "normal" criterion was adjusted to 15 dB HL or better, then no age correction was needed. Prieve and Falter (1995) noted that the presence of SOAE was associated with a robust TEOAE, regardless of age of the subject.

Other measures of TEOAE proposed for clinical measurements include response reproducibility and SNR as a function of frequency. A reproducibility score of 50% or greater signals the presence of an emission in the frequency region of interest (Kemp et al, 1990). The signal-to-noise computed by the ILO software is based on a comparison of the power of the reproducible portion of the A and B response waveforms, with the power in a waveform that is computed as the difference between the A and B memories. A reproducibility score of 50% or greater usually is associated with an SNR of 3 dB or more, but the relationship between the reproducibility and signal-to-noise measures is complex.

◆ Distortion Product Otoacoustic Emissions in Practice

DPOAE are attractive as clinical tools because the frequency at which the response occurs is predicted exactly by the frequencies of the primary tones. The relationship among the primary stimuli and the frequency at which the distortion product is located helps to reduce the ambiguity in determining whether or not a response is present. A typical DPOAE display (DP-gram) is illustrated in **Fig. 22–10**. Primary tone frequency is plotted on the horizontal axis. Put another way, the abscissa is a representation of the region of the cochlea stimulated by the primary tones. The display may be arranged in terms of value of F2 and F1, or some intermediate frequency. The ordinate of the illustrations depicts SPL.

The manufacturers of DPOAE systems use several algorithms to create stimuli and sample the sound present in the ear canal during stimulation. In general terms, DPOAE data are obtained by presenting the primary tones through

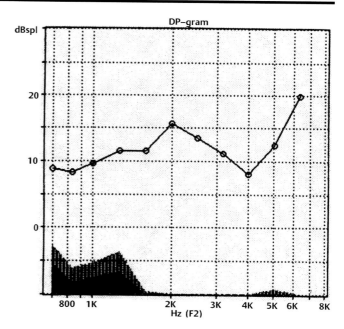

Figure 22–10 Example of DP-gram. The horizontal axis represents the frequency of the stimulus signal, usually F2 (the higher of two primary tones). The vertical axis corresponds to sound pressure level (SPL). In this instance, the graph reveals the SPL of the distortion product created with F2 at the indicated frequency. The solid and striated portions of the figure indicate the average value of the noise floor plus 1 standard deviation (solid) and 2 standard deviations (striated).

independent transducers to reduce the possibility of distortion caused by the instrumentation. The waveform of the sound in the ear canal is submitted to time-averaging procedures that are synchronized to the stimuli. This has the effect of reducing background noise. The averaged waveform is submitted to a spectral analysis to determine the SPL at the DPOAE frequency and the background noise at frequencies near the DPOAE. The resolution (bin width) of the spectral analysis is an important factor in determining the precision and SNR associated with DPOAE measurements.

Regardless of the sampling and analysis methods, the display typically represents the magnitude of the DPOAE and the noise present in the ear canal in the frequency region of the DPOAE. Responses that are obtained from ears with normal audiometric thresholds are influenced by (1) stimulus amplitude (designated as L, for level), (2) relative amplitude of F1 (L1) and F2 (L2), and (3) ratio of F2 and F1 frequencies.

The optimal intensities for stimuli to elicit DPOAE from ears with normal audiometric thresholds are between 50 and 70 dB SPL, with L2 ~10 or 15 dB below L1 (Prieve et al, 1997). The optimal ratio of F2/F1 is ~1.2:1, which places the DPOAE at a point that is one-half octave below F2 (Lonsbury-Martin et al, 1997). Under stimulus conditions such as these, the DPOAE response amplitude is ~10 dB SPL in children and adults (Pafitis et al, 1994) and at ~15 dB SPL in infants (Prieve et al, 1997). As illustrated in the example in **Fig. 22–10**, the typical response pattern reveals a slight reduction in DPOAE amplitude when the primary tones are in the midfrequency (2–5 kHz) region. This finding has been replicated in virtually all studies that have presented group data from ears with normal audiometric thresholds (Lonsbury-Martin et al, 1997). As is the case with TEOAE, an individual's DPOAE response is idiosyncratic; consequently, clinical measurements have no universally accepted norms. For example, some protocols require that the response be at least 10 dB above the noise floor to be considered valid. Others require a response-to-noise ratio of 3 or 1 dB. In the example illustrated in **Fig. 21–10**, the DPOAE amplitude is more than 10 dB above the noise floor for every data point.

Gorga et al (1993) and Prieve et al (1997) have provided data that are important to the development of response norms. The relationship between the stimulus and response amplitudes may signal the presence of cochlear abnormalities (e.g., Harris and Probst, 1997). DPOAE response latency measures may provide important information about the status of the ear (Lonsbury-Martin et al, 1997), but no large-scale studies of response latency properties in normal and disordered populations have been completed to date.

Attempts to predict pure-tone thresholds from DPOAE thresholds, input/output functions, SNR, or other measures have enjoyed some success in large population studies when the high-frequency region was examined, but estimating audiometric thresholds with precision remains elusive (Boege and Janssen, 2002; Janssen et al, 2005).

♦ Clinical Examples

TEOAE and DPOAE responses are indices of a cochlear phenomenon, the electromotile activity of outer hair cells in response to acoustic stimuli. Although recent experimental evidence suggests that the two types of emissions may result from different specific mechanisms, the correlation of TEOAE and DPOAE measures is generally robust (Balatsouras et al, 2006). The choice between TEOAE and DPOAE instrumentation may be influenced by the frequency range of interest. In terms of separating patients with normal-hearing sensitivity (20 dB or better) from those with mild or greater hearing loss, TEOAE are more sensitive at 1000 Hz, TEOAE and DPOAE are essentially equivalent for 2000 and 3000 Hz, and DPOAE are more sensitive from 4000 through 6000 Hz (Gorga et al, 1993, 1997; Prieve et al, 1993).

The preferred EOAE stimulus levels that optimize the separation between patients with normal versus impaired cochlear function are 80 to 82 dB pe SPL for click stimuli used for TEOAE measures and pure-tone stimulus levels of L1 and L2 at 65 and 55 dB SPL, respectively, for DPOAE measures. Under these conditions, the tests are effective in separating patients with pure-tone hearing sensitivity of 20 to 25 dB HL or better from patients with hearing losses of 35 dB HL or poorer (Gaskill and Brown, 1990; Gorga et al, 1993, 1997; Prieve et al, 1993; Probst and Harris, 1993; Robinette, 1992; Stover et al, 1996).

The probability of obtaining EOAE as a function of hearing loss of cochlear origin has been estimated by Harris and Probst (1997), Robinette and Glattke (2000), and Robinette (2003). If a patient has hearing thresholds better than 25 dB HL, there is an excellent chance (99% or better) that he or she

will produce measurable TEOAE responses in the frequency region where hearing is normal. If a patient has a hearing loss greater than 40 dB HL, there is a very low probability of detecting a TEOAE response. The range of uncertainty for TEOAE stimuli is in the region of 20 to 40 dB HL. The region of uncertainty for DPOAE may range from 20 to 50 dB HL. The difference in outcomes for TEOAE and DPOAE may be explained in part by the relative amount of energy in the stimulus used to detect each type of response. In the case of TEOAE, the stimulus is a broadband click with peak intensity of ~80 dB SPL or a spectrum level (energy per cycle) of ~40 dB SPL. In the case of DPOAE, the primary stimuli are at 65 and 55 dB SPL, typically. The increase in energy at specific stimulus frequencies may make the DPOAE result less vulnerable to small changes in status of the outer hair cells. This uncertainty can make interpretation of DPOAE measures more difficult, especially as a screening test for the identification of hearing loss. It is suggested that initial DPOAE measures be completed with low-level stimulation. If DPOAE are absent for low-level stimulation but present for high-level stimulation, an interpretation of mild cochlear hearing loss is defensible.

As mentioned previously, it is not appropriate to estimate pure-tone hearing sensitivity (audiometric thresholds) from EOAE data. EOAE show evidence of normal to near-normal middle ear and cochlear function but do not reflect hearing thresholds. Although trends from group data suggest that EOAE amplitudes are inversely related to audiometric thresholds within the normal range (Gaskill and Brown, 1993; Gorga et al, 1993; LePage and Murray, 1993), the between-subject variability of EOAE amplitudes is substantial. As Lapsley-Miller et al (2004) have reported, it is premature to use TEOAE and DPOAE measures to replace hearing tests in hearing conservation programs.

Pearl

- The presence of EOAE tells the examiner that the middle ear is functioning well enough to transmit the stimulus to the inner ear, that sufficient energy is generated in the inner ear, and that the middle ear is functioning well enough to transmit the response back to the recording microphone.

Influence of the Middle Ear

As Margolis and Trine (1997) have reviewed, the influence of middle ear status on the EOAE is significant. Ambient middle ear pressure, middle ear effusion, and any other factor that can influence the loading of the tympanic membrane are likely to influence EAOE results. Glattke and colleagues (1995) reported that tympanometric configuration has a significant impact on OAE outcomes, independent of the amount of conductive hearing loss that might be present. The TEOAE and DPOAE data in **Fig. 22–11** provide examples of the potential impact of slight/mild conductive hearing loss. There is a 30 dB air–bone gap closing at 4000 Hz on the right, accompanied by a flat tympanogram, and a 15 dB air–bone gap closing at 1000 Hz on the left, accompanied by an asymmetric tympanogram

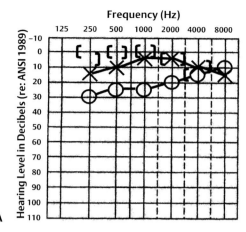

A

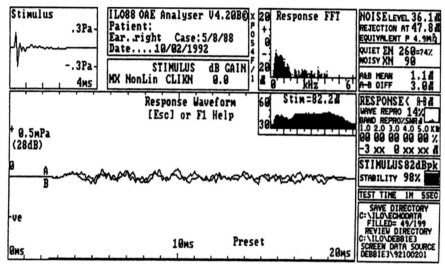

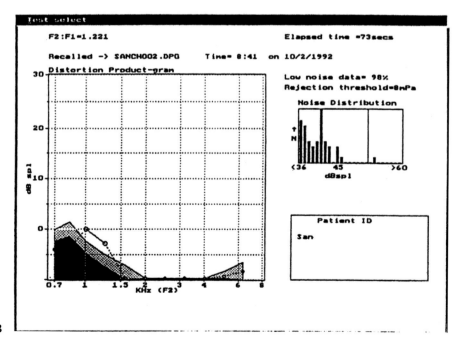

B

Figure 22–11 (A) Audiogram for patient with bilateral conductive hearing loss. **(B)** Transient evoked otoacoustic emission (TEOAE) and distortion product otoacoustic emission (DPOAE) results for the right ear with conductive hearing loss.

(continued)

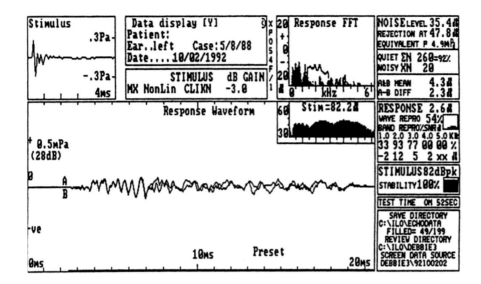

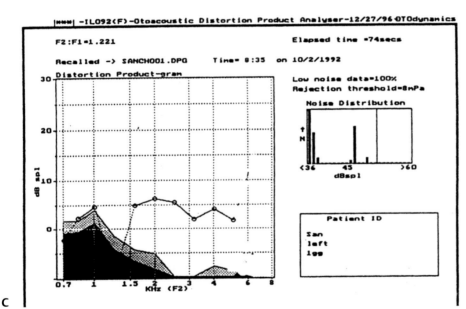

Figure 22-11 *(Continued)* **(C)** TEOAE and DPOAE results for the left ear with conductive hearing loss.

C

with peak pressure at –200 daPa. TEOAE and DPOAE energy emerges from background noise in the midfrequency region for the left ear, but there is no response apparent for the right ear, despite the fact that thresholds in the high-frequency region are essentially identical for the right and left ears.

Cochlear Hearing Loss

A high correlation has been observed between the frequencies of pure-tone hearing loss and frequency region of decreased or absent EOAE (Bonfils and Uziel, 1988; Harris, 1990; Harris and Probst, 1991; Johnsen et al, 1993; Kemp et al, 1986; Lind and Randa, 1989; Probst et al, 1987; Robinette, 1992). Studies of the relationship between DPOAE amplitude and temporary threshold shift (TTS) reveal that, for both animal and human models, the DPOAE amplitude decrease is frequency specific. The greatest reduction in amplitude occurred approximately half an octave above the frequency of the fatiguing stimuli (Engdahl and

Kemp, 1996; Martin et al, 1987). This reduction in response is similar to that demonstrated by psychoacoustic measurements in humans that also reveal the greatest TTS at one-half octave above the frequency of the fatiguing stimulus (David et al, 1950). Robinette (2003) has published composite audiograms obtained from more than 150 patients seen at the Mayo Clinic to illustrate the probability of the presence of TEOAE coincident with high-frequency hearing loss. As others, such as Harris and Probst (1991), had demonstrated, there is an excellent "fit" between the audiometric configuration on the one hand and the TEOAE (or DPOAE) configuration on the other. EOAE often tend to decrease about a half-octave below the frequency at which the hearing loss exceeds 30 dB HL (Avan et al, 1995; Harris, 1990; LePage and Murray, 1993; Reshef et al, 1993).

Fig. 22-12 provides an example of TEOAE and DPOAE frequency specificity for a reverse-slope hearing loss of cochlear origin. The results were obtained from a 13-year-old with bilateral low-frequency sensorineural hearing loss

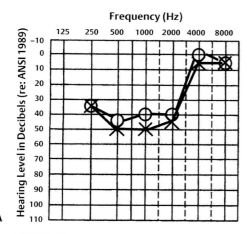

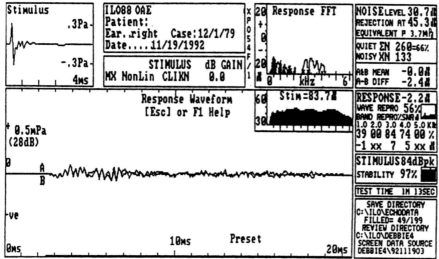

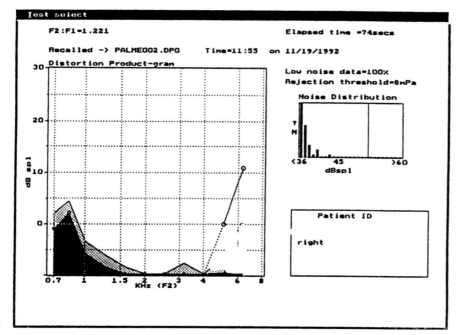

Figure 22–12 (A) Audiogram with sensorineural hearing loss and reverse-slope configuration. **(B)** Transient evoked otoacoustic emission (TEOAE) and distortion product otoacoustic emission (DPOAE) results for the right ear audiogram with reverse-slope configuration.

(continued)

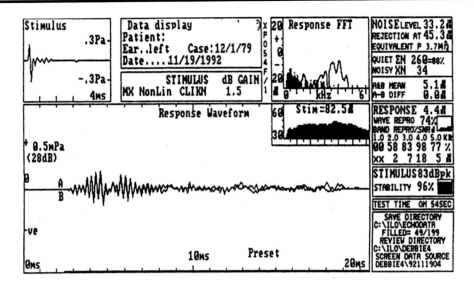

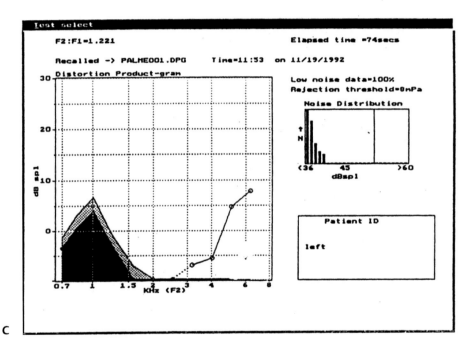

Figure 22–12 *(Continued)* **(C)** TEOAE and DPOAE results for the left ear audiogram with reverse-slope configuration.

C

averaging between 40 and 50 dB through 2000 Hz. The TEOAE and DPOAE results both mirror the audiometric configuration, although there is a partial dissociation between the magnitude of the OAE responses and the magnitude of hearing loss. Magnitude of noise levels, magnitude of response amplitudes, and magnitude of hearing loss were all slightly greater on the left than on the right.

Special Consideration

- Measures of OAE may provide information leading to a differential diagnosis that can identify disorders specific to outer hair cell function.

Differential Diagnosis

The diagnostic implications of OAE are of considerable interest. Classically, audiologic tests separate hearing loss into two categories: conductive and sensorineural. EOAE can provide an objective measure of preneural cochlear function and assist in the discrimination among pathological conditions that result in OHC dysfunction. For patients with moderate to profound hearing loss, the presence of EOAE supports the diagnosis of retrocochlear hearing loss. Reports in the literature generally are focused on four patient groups: those with acoustic neuromas (Bonfils and Uziel, 1988; Cane et al, 1994; Durrant et al, 1993; Prasher et al, 1995; Robinette et al, 1992; Robinette and Durrant, 1997; Telischi, Roth, et al, 1995), those with idiopathic sudden hearing loss (Cevette et al, 1995; Nakamura et al, 1997;

Robinette and Facer, 1991; Sakashita et al, 1991; Truy et al, 1993), those with auditory neuropathy (Hood et al, 1994; Starr et al, 1996; Stein et al, 1996), and those with pseudohypoacusis (Durrant et al, 1997; Kvaerner et al, 1996; Musiek et al, 1995). In addition, several case studies have been published to highlight the contribution of EOAE to the evaluation of retrocochlear hearing disorders (Cevette and Bielek, 1995; Doyle et al, 1996; Gravel and Stapells, 1993; Katona et al, 1993; Konradsson, 1996; Laccourreye et al, 1996; Lutman et al, 1989; Monroe et al, 1996; Robinette, 1992).

Acoustic Neuroma

For patients with acoustic neuromas, EOAE have been used as a diagnostic indicator for intraoperative monitoring and to provide preoperative and postoperative information on cochlear reserve. The diagnostic value of EOAE in identification of acoustic neuromas is limited. From a review of several reports, Robinette and Durrant (1997) found that only 20% of 316 patients with surgically confirmed CN VIII tumors had mild or greater hearing loss with EOAE present to support the diagnosis of retrocochlear hearing loss. This lack of diagnostic precision may be attributed to cochlear hearing losses that frequently accompany CN VIII tumors. The cochlear loss is thought to be due to the restriction of the blood supply to the cochlea related to tumor growth (Levine et al, 1984). Intraoperative monitoring of cochlear function by EOAE during acoustic tumor removal has been demonstrated and found to provide evidence of cochlear compromise before changes are detected in the ABR (Cane et al, 1992; Telischi, Widick, et al, 1995).

The measurement of EOAE preoperatively and postoperatively, in conjunction with other tests, is helping to define the site of surgical insult when hearing is decreased or not preserved (Robinette et al, 1992; Robinette and Durrant, 1997). From a group of 11 patients with hearing preservation after acoustic neuroma removal, about half of the patients had poorer hearing postoperatively. Neural function was improved postoperatively for most patients (as measured by ABR), whereas cochlear function was decreased for most patients postoperatively (as measured by EOAE; Robinette and Durrant, 1997). These data suggest that neural function is often improved when the auditory nerve is preserved with tumor pressure removed, but subsequent hearing loss may be related more to cochlear damage from vascular compromise during surgery. Therefore, even though EOAE may have a limited role in the diagnosis of acoustic neuromas, they do have promise as a measure of preoperative, perioperative, and postoperative cochlear function.

Sudden Hearing Loss

Some patients with sudden idiopathic hearing loss (ISHL) have EOAE despite significant hearing loss. Sakashita et al (1991) reported on two groups of patients with moderate to severe sensorineural hearing loss. About 50% of the group with ISHL had measurable EOAE, whereas none of the group with long-standing hearing loss had EOAE. They concluded that for many patients in the ISHL group, the inner ear injury was not to the OHCs but to other cochlear structures.

Of course, sudden hearing loss may also involve the CN VIII or central auditory tracts.

Auditory Neuropathy

As mentioned previously, OAE can be suppressed by ipsilateral or contralateral sound stimulation. Ipsilateral suppression studies have demonstrated the precision of tuning in the auditory periphery and probable contributions of the uncrossed olivocochlear efferent neural supply to the cochlea (e.g., Harris and Glattke, 1992). In addition, several investigations have demonstrated that contralateral stimuli of low or moderate intensity are effective in reducing the amplitude of OAE; although, the question of tuning of the contralateral effect remains controversial. The primary effect of contralateral stimulation with broadband noise is a slight reduction in the amplitude of the emission (Collet et al, 1990). *Auditory neuropathy* is a relatively new term used to categorize patients with a triad of symptoms: (1) mild to profound behavioral hearing loss on the basis of audiometric thresholds; (2) normal cochlear OHC function, as evidenced by the presence of EOAE or CMs; and (3) abnormal auditory pathway function, as shown by absent or abnormal auditory brainstem evoked potentials, elevated or absent acoustic reflex thresholds, and absent contralateral suppression of TEOAE (Sininger et al, 1995; Starr et al, 1996). Before the use of EOAE as an objective clinical measure of cochlear function leading to the identification of auditory neuropathy, patients with absent auditory evoked potentials and mild-to-moderate hearing loss were considered a curious paradox (Davis and Hirsh, 1979; Hildesheimer et al, 1985; Kraus et al, 1984; Lenhardt, 1981; Worthington and Peters, 1980). Cases of auditory neuropathy are relatively uncommon, but they highlight the value of EOAE in clinical assessment.

Pitfall

- The absence of OAE does not allow the clinician to conclude that a hearing loss is present. Additional information must be gathered to rule out contributions of the middle ear to the negative outcome. Similarly, the presence of OAE does not guarantee that auditory function is normal. It may be necessary to employ electrophysiological measures to rule out auditory neuropathy.

Pseudohypoacusis

The audiology literature is replete with descriptions of methods for identification of pseudohypoacusis. The Stenger test is the procedure of choice in detecting unilateral pseudohypoacusis (Robinette and Gaeth, 1972). Cases of bilateral pseudohypoacusis are more difficult to document by objective procedures, with auditory evoked potential testing being the most reliable (Sanders and Lazenby, 1983). However, even evoked potentials may be misleading under some conditions (Glattke, 1983). EOAE have been found to be a quick and reliable screening test of both unilateral and bilateral pseudohypoacusis (Durrant et al, 1997; Kvaerner et al, 1996; Musiek et al, 1995; Robinette, 1992).

◆ Summary

The discovery of OAE by David Kemp in 1978 has led to dramatic changes in our understanding of the physiology of auditory perception of exquisitely soft sounds by humans. In the clinical setting, the methods of assessing evoked emissions by both TEOAE and DPOAE provide the opportunity to assess sensory function and, specifically, to document normal to near-normal cochlear function. An additional value is that the clinical measurement is objective, efficient, and noninvasive, which is very appealing in screening the hearing of newborns and other populations unable to provide reliable behavioral responses. The disadvantage, however, is that the absence of EOAE does not reflect the actual magnitude of the hearing loss (i.e., mild, moderate, severe, or profound) or the site of the disorder leading to the loss. Even with this limitation, EOAE have great value as a part of the diagnostic test battery. Researchers and clinicians have much to learn about this new clinical tool as applications continue to open our professional eyes.

References

Avan, P., Bonfils, P., Loth, D., Elbez, M., & Erminy, M. (1995). Transient-evoked otoacoustic emissions and high-frequency acoustic trauma in the guinea pig. Journal of the Acoustical Society of America, 97, 3012–3020.

Balatsouras, D. G., Kaberos, A., Koustos, G., Economou, N. C., Sakellariadis, V., Fassolis, A., Korres, F. G. (2006). Correlation of transiently evoked to distortion-product otoacoustic emission measures in healthy children. International Journal of Pediatric Otorhinolaryngology, 70, 89–93.

Békésy, G. (1960). Vibratory pattern of the basilar membrane. In E. G. Wever (Trans.), Experiments in hearing (pp. 404–429). New York: McGraw-Hill. (Original work published 1928).

Boege, P., & Janssen, T. (2002). Pure tone threshold estimation from extrapolated distortion product otoacoustic emission I/O functions in normal and cochlear hearing loss ears. Journal of the Acoustical Society of America, 111, 1810–1818.

Bonfils, P., & Uziel, A. (1988). Evoked otoacoustic emissions in patients with acoustic neuromas. American Journal of Otology, 9, 412–417.

Bright, K. (1997). Spontaneous otoacoustic emissions. In M. S. Robinette & T. J. Glattke (Eds.), Otoacoustic emissions: Clinical applications (pp. 46–62). New York: Thieme Medical Publishers.

Brownell, W. E. (1983). Observations on a motile response in isolated outer hair cells. In R. W. Webster & L. E. Aitken (Eds.), Mechanisms of hearing (pp. 5–10). Clayton, Australia: Monash University Press.

Cane, M. A., Lutman, M. E., & O'Donoghue, G. M. (1994). Transiently evoked otoacoustic emissions in patients with cerebellopontine angle tumors. American Journal of Otology, 15, 207–216.

Cane, M. A., O'Donoghue, G. M., & Lutman, M. E. (1992). The feasibility of using evoked otoacoustic emissions to monitor cochlear function during acoustic neuroma surgery. Scandinavian Audiology, 21, 173–176.

Cevette, M. J., & Bielek, D. (1995). Transient evoked and distortion product otoacoustic emissions in traumatic brain injury. Journal of the American Academy of Audiology, 6, 225–229.

Cevette, M. J., Robinette, M. S., Carter, J., & Knops, J. L. (1995). Otoacoustic emissions in sudden unilateral hearing loss associated with multiple sclerosis. Journal of the American Academy of Audiology, 6, 197–202.

Collet, L., Kemp, D. T., Veuillet, E., Duclaux, R., Moulin, A., & Morgon, A. (1990). Effect of contralateral auditory stimuli on active cochlear micromechanical properties in human subjects. Hearing Research, 43, 251–262.

Dallos, P. (1992). The active cochlea. Journal of Neuroscience, 12, 4575–4585.

Dallos, P., & Fakler, B. (2002). Prestin, a new type of motor protein. Nature Reviews: Molecular Cell Biology, 3, 104–111.

David, H., Morgan, C. T., Hawkins, J. E., Galambos, R., & Smith, F. K. (1950). Temporary deafness following exposure to loud tones and noise. Acta Otolaryngologica, 88(Suppl.), 1–57.

Davis, H. (1983). An active process in cochlear mechanics. Hearing Research, 9, 79–90.

Davis, H., & Hirsh, S. K. (1979). A slow brain stem response for low-frequency audiometry. Audiology, 18, 445–461.

Doyle, K. J., Fowler, C., & Starr, A. (1996). Audiologic findings in unilateral deafness resulting from contralateral pontine infarct. Otolaryngology—Head and Neck Surgery, 114, 482–486.

Durrant, J. D., Kamerer, D. B., & Chin, D. (1993). Combined OAE and ABR studies in acoustic tumor patients. In D. Hochmann (Ed.), EcoG, OAE and intraoperative monitoring (pp. 231–239). Amsterdam: Kugler.

Durrant, J. D., Kesterson, R. K., & Kamerer, D. B. (1997). Evaluation of the nonorganic hearing loss suspect. American Journal of Otology, 18, 361–367.

Engdahl, B., & Kemp, D. T. (1996). The effect of noise exposure on the details of distortion product otoacoustic emissions in humans. Journal of the Acoustical Society of America, 99, 1573–1587.

Fritsch, M. H., Wynne, M. K., Matt, B. H., Smith, W. L., & Smith, C. M. (2001). Objective tinnitus in children. Otology and Neurotology, 22, 644–649.

Gaskill, S. A., & Brown, A. M. (1990). The behavior of the acoustic distortion product, 2f1-f2, from the human ear and its relation to auditory sensitivity. Journal of the Acoustical Society of America, 88, 821–839.

Gaskill, S. A., & Brown, A. M. (1993). Comparing the level of the acoustic distortion product, 2f1-f2, with behavioral threshold audiograms from normal-hearing and hearing-impaired ears. British Journal of Audiology, 27, 397–407.

Glattke, T. J. (1983). Short latency auditory evoked potentials. Baltimore, MD: University Park Press.

Glattke, T. J., Pafitis, I., Cummiskey, C., & Herer, G. (1995). Identification of hearing loss in children and young adults using measures of transient otoacoustic emission reproducibility. American Journal of Audiology, 4, 71–86.

Glattke, T. J., & Robinette, M. S. (1997). Transient evoked otoacoustic emissions. In M. S. Robinette & T. J. Glattke (Eds.), Otoacoustic emissions: Clinical applications (pp. 63–82). New York: Thieme Medical Publishers.

Gold, T. (1948). Hearing: 2. The physical basis of the action of the cochlea. Proceedings of the Royal Society of London, Series B, 135, 492–498.

Gorga, M. A., Neely, S. T., Bergman, B. M. Beauchaine, K. L., Kaminski, J. R., Peters, J., Schultes, L., & Jesteadt, W. (1993). A comparison of transient evoked and distortion product otoacoustic emissions in normal-hearing and hearing-impaired subjects. Journal of the Acoustical Society of America, 94, 2639–2648.

Gorga, M. P., Neely, S. T., Dorn, P. A., & Hoover, B. M. (2003). Further efforts to predict pure tone thresholds from distortion product otoacoustic emission input/output functions. Journal of the Acoustical Society of America, 113, 3275–3284.

Gorga, M. P., Neely, S. T., Ohlrich, B., Hoover, B., Redner, J., & Peters, J. (1997). From laboratory to clinic: A large scale study of distortion product otoacoustic emissions in ears with normal hearing and ears with hearing loss. Ear and Hearing, 18, 440–455.

Grandori, F., & Ravazzani, P. (1993). Non-linearities of click-evoked otoacoustic emissions and the derived non-linear response. British Journal of Audiology, 27, 97–102.

Gravel, J. S., & Stapells, D. R. (1993). Behavioral, electrophysiologic, and otoacoustic measures from a child with auditory processing dysfunction: Case report. Journal of the American Academy of Audiology, 4, 412–419.

Harris, F. P. (1990). Distortion-product otoacoustic emissions in humans with high-frequency sensorineural hearing loss. Journal of Speech and Hearing Research, 33, 594–600.

Harris, F. P., & Glattke, T. J. (1992). The use of suppression to determine the characteristics of otoacoustic emissions. Seminars in Hearing, 13, 67–80.

Harris, F. P., & Probst, R. (1991). Reporting click-evoked and distortion-product otoacoustic emission results with respect to the pure tone audiogram. Ear and Hearing, 12, 399–405.

Harris, F., & Probst, R. (1997). Otoacoustic emissions and audiometric outcomes. In M. S. Robinette & T. J. Glattke (Eds.), Otoacoustic emissions: Clinical applications (pp. 151–180). New York: Thieme Medical Publishers.

Hildesheimer, M., Muchnik, C., & Rubinstein. M. (1985). Problems in interpretation of brain stem-evoked response audiometry results. Audiology, 24, 374–379,

Hood, L. J., Berlin, C. I., & Allen, P. (1994). Cortical deafness: A longitudinal study. Journal of the American Academy of Audiology, 5, 330–342.

Janssen, T., Gehr, D. D., Klein, A., & Muller, J. (2005). Distortion product otoacoustic emissions for hearing threshold estimation and differentiation between middle ear and cochlear disorders in neonates. Journal of the Acoustical Society of America, 117, 2969–2979.

Johnsen, N. J., Parbo, J., & Elberling, C. (1993). Evoked acoustic emissions from the human ear: 6. Findings in cochlear hearing impairment. Scandinavian Audiology, 22, 87–95.

Johnstone, B. M., Patuzzi, R., & Yates, G. K. (1986). Basilar membrane measurements and the traveling wave. Hearing Research, 22, 147–153.

Katona, G., Buki, B., Farkas, Z., Pytel, J., Simon-Nagy, E., & Hirschberg, J. (1993). Transitory evoked otoacoustic emission (TEOAE) in a child with profound hearing loss. International Journal of Pediatric Otorhinolaryngology, 26, 263–267.

Kemp, D. T. (1978). Stimulated acoustic emissions from within the human auditory system. Journal of the Acoustical Society of America, 64, 1386–1391.

Kemp, D. T. (1979). Evidence of mechanical nonlinearity and frequency selective wave amplification in the cochlea. Archives of Otorhinolaryngology, 224, 37–46.

Kemp, D. T., Bray, P., Alexander, L., & Brown, A. M. (1986). Acoustic emission cochleography: Practical aspects. Scandinavian Audiology Supplementum, 25, 71–95.

Kemp, D. T., & Chum, R. (1980). Properties of the generator of stimulated acoustic emissions. Hearing Research, 2(3–4), 212–232.

Kemp, D. T., Ryan, S., & Bray, P. (1990). A guide to the effective use of otoacoustic emissions. Ear and Hearing, 11, 93–105.

Kok, M. R., Van Zanten, G. A., Brocaar, M. P., & Wallenburg, H. C. S. (1993). Click-evoked otoacoustic emissions in 1036 ears of healthy newborns. Audiology, 32, 213–223.

Konradsson, K. S. (1996). Bilaterally preserved otoacoustic emissions in four children with profound idiopathic unilateral sensorineural hearing loss. Audiology, 35, 217–227.

Kraus, N., Ozdamar, V., Stein, L., & Reed, N. (1984). Absent auditory brain stem response: Peripheral hearing loss or brain stem dysfunction? Laryngoscope, 94, 400–406.

Kvaerner, K. J., Engdahl, B., Aursnes, J., Arnesen, A. R., & Mair, I. W. S. (1996). Transient evoked otoacoustic emissions: Helpful tool in the detection of pseudohypoacusis. Scandinavian Audiology, 25, 173–177.

Laccourreye, L., Francois, M., Huy, E. T. B., & Narcy, P. (1996). Bilateral evoked otoacoustic emissions in a child with bilateral profound hearing loss. Annals of Otology, Rhinology and Laryngology, 105, 286–288.

Lapsley-Miller, J. A., Marshall, L., & Heller, L. M. (2004). A longitudinal study of changes in evoked otoacoustic emissions and pure tone thresholds as measured in a hearing conservation program. International Journal of Audiology, 43, 307–322.

Lenhardt, M. L. (1981). Childhood central auditory processing disorder with brain stem evoked response verification. Archives of Otolaryngology, 107, 623–625.

LePage, E. L., & Murray, N. M. (1993). Click-evoked otoacoustic emissions: Comparing emission strengths with pure tone audiometric thresholds. Australian Journal of Audiology, 15, 9–22.

Levine, R. A., Ojemann, R. G., Montgomery, W. W., & McGaffigan, P. M. (1984). Monitoring auditory evoked potentials during acoustic neuroma surgery: Insights into the mechanism of the hearing loss. Annals of Otology, Rhinology and Laryngology, 93, 116–123.

Lind, O., & Randa, J. (1989). Evoked acoustic emissions in high-frequency vs. low/medium-frequency hearing loss. Scandinavian Audiology, 18, 21–25.

Lonsbury-Martin, B. L., Martin, G. K., & Whitehead, M. L. (1997). Distortion product otoacoustic emissions. In M. S. Robinette & T. J. Glattke (Eds.), Otoacoustic emissions: Clinical applications (pp. 83–109). New York: Thieme Medical Publishers.

Lutman, M. E., David, A. C., Fortnum, H. M., & Wood, S. (1997). Field sensitivity of targeted neonatal hearing screening by transient evoked otoacoustic emissions. Ear and Hearing, 18, 265–276.

Lutman, M. E., Mason, S. M., Sheppard, S., & Gibbin, K. P. (1989). Differential diagnostic potential of otoacoustic emissions: A case study. Audiology, 28, 205–210.

Margolis, R. H., & Trine, M. B. (1997). Influence of middle-ear disease on otoacoustic emissions. In M. S. Robinette & T. J. Glattke (Eds.), Otoacoustic emissions: Clinical applications (pp. 130–150). New York: Thieme Medical Publishers.

Martin, G. K., Lonsbury-Martin, B. L., Probst, R., Scheinin, S. A., & Coates, A. C. (1987). Acoustic distortion products in rabbit ear canal: 2. Sites or origin revealed by suppression contours and pure tone exposures. Hearing Research, 28, 191–208.

Monroe, J. A. B., Krauth, L., Arenberg, I. K., Prenger, E., & Philpot, P. (1996). Normal evoked otoacoustic emissions with a profound hearing loss due to a juvenile pilocytic astrocytoma. American Journal of Otology, 17, 639–642.

Musiek, F. E., Bornstein, S. P., & Rintelmann, W. F. (1995). Transient evoked otoacoustic emissions and pseudohypoacusis. Journal of the American Academy of Audiology, 6, 293–301.

Nakamura, M., Yamasoba, T., & Kaga, K. (1997). Changes in otoacoustic emissions in patients with idiopathic sudden deafness. Audiology, 36, 121–135.

Oostenbrink, P., & Verhaagen-Warnaar, N. (2004). Otoacoustic emissions. American Journal of Electroneurodiagnostic Technology, 44, 189–198.

Pacheco, M. (1997). A comparison of SOAEs and SSOAEs. Unpublished senior honor's thesis, University of Arizona.

Pafitis, I., Cummiskey, C., Herer, G., & Glattke, T. J. (1994). Detection of hearing loss using otoacoustic emissions. Proceedings of Internoise, 94, 763–768.

Penner, M. J., & Coles, R. R. (1992). Indications for aspirin as a palliative for tinnitus caused by SOAEs: A case study. British Journal of Audiology, 26, 91–96.

Prasher, D. K., Tun, T., Brooks, G. B., & Luxon, L. M. (1995). Mechanisms of hearing loss in acoustic neuroma: An otoacoustic emission study. Acta Otolaryngologica, 115, 375–381.

Prieve, B. A., & Falter, S. R. (1995). COAEs and SSOAEs in adults with increased age. Ear and Hearing, 16, 521–528.

Prieve, B. A., Fitzgerald, T. S., & Schulte, L. E. (1997). Basic characteristics of click-evoked otoacoustic emissions in infants and children. Journal of the Acoustical Society of America, 102, 2860–2870.

Prieve, B. A., Gorga, M. P., Schmidt, A., Neely, S., Peters, I., Schultes, L., & Jesteadt, W. (1993). Analysis of transient-evoked otoacoustic emissions in normal-hearing and hearing-impaired ears. Journal of the Acoustical Society of America, 93, 3308–3319.

Probst, R. (1990). Otoacoustic emissions: An overview. Advances in Otorhinolaryngology, 44, 1–91.

Probst, R., & Harris, F. P. (1993). Transiently evoked and distortion-product otoacoustic emissions: Comparison of results from normally hearing and hearing-impaired human ears. Archives of Otolaryngology—Head and Neck Surgery, 119, 858–860.

Probst, R., Lonsbury-Martin, B. L., & Coats, A. (1987). Otoacoustic emissions in ears with hearing loss. American Journal of Otolaryngology, 8, 73–81.

Reshef, I., Attias, J., & Furst, M. (1993). Characteristics of click-evoked otoacoustic emissions in ears with normal-hearing and with noise-induced hearing loss. British Journal of Audiology, 27, 387–395.

Robinette, M. S. (1992). Clinical observations with transient evoked otoacoustic emissions with adults. Seminars in Hearing, 13, 23–36.

Robinette, M. S. (2003). Clinical observations with evoked otoacoustic emissions at Mayo Clinic. Journal of the American Academy of Audiology, 14, 213–224.

Robinette, M. S., Bauch, C. B., Olsen, W. O., Harner, S. G., & Beatty, C. W. (1992). Use of TEOAE, ABR, and acoustic reflex measures to assess auditory function in patients with acoustic neuroma. American Journal of Audiology, 1, 66–72.

Robinette, M. S., & Durrant, J. D. (1997). Contributions of evoked otoacoustic emissions in differential diagnosis of retrocochlear disorders. In M. S. Robinette & T. J. Glattke (Eds.), Otoacoustic emissions: Clinical applications (pp. 205–232). New York: Thieme Medical Publishers.

Robinette, M. S., & Facer, G. W. (1991). Evoked otoacoustic emissions in differential diagnosis: A case report. Otolaryngology–Head and Neck Surgery, 105, 120–123.

Robinette, M. S., & Gaeth, J. H. (1972). Diplacusis and the Stenger test. Journal of Audiology Research, 12, 91–100.

Robinette, M. S., & Glattke, T. J. (2000). Otoacoustic emissions. In R. J. Roeser, M. Valente, & H. Hosford-Dunn (Eds.), Audiology: Diagnosis (pp. 503–526). New York: Thieme Medical Publishers.

Ruggero, M. A., & Rich, N. C. (1991). Application of a commercially manufactured Doppler shift laser velocimeter to the measurement of basilar membrane vibration. Hearing Research, 51, 215–230.

Sakashita, T., Minowa, W., Hachikawa, K., Kubo, T., & Nakai, Y. (1991). Evoked otoacoustic emissions from ears with idiopathic sudden deafness. Acta Otolaryngologica Supplementum, 486, 66–72.

Sanders, J. W., & Lazenby, P. B. (1983). Auditory brain stem response measurement in the assessment of pseudohypoacusis. American Journal of Otology, 4, 292–299.

Shera, C. A. (2004). Mechanisms of mammalian otoacoustic emission and their implications for the clinical utility of otoacoustic emissions. Ear and Hearing, 25(2), 86–97.

Shera, C. A., & Guinan, J. J. (2003). Stimulus-frequency-emission group delay: A test of coherent reflection filtering and a window on cochlear tuning. Journal of the Acoustical Society of America, 113, 2762–2772.

Siegel, J. H., Cerka, A. J., Recio-Spinoso, A., Temchin, A. N., van Dijk, P., & Ruggero, M A. (2005). Delays of stimulus-frequency otoacoustic emissions and cochlear vibrations contradict the theory of coherent reflection filtering. Journal of the Acoustical Society of America, 118, 2434–2443.

Sininger, Y. S., Hood, L. J., Starr, A., Berlin, C. I., & Picton, T W. (1995). Hearing loss due to auditory neuropathy. Audiology Today, 7, 10–13.

Starr, A., Picton, T. W., Sininger, Y., Hood, L. J., & Berlin, C. I. (1996). Auditory neuropathy. Brain, 119, 741–753.

Stein, L., Tremblay, K., Pasternak, J., Banerjee, S., Lindemann, K., & Kraus, N. (1996). Brain stem abnormalities in neonates with normal otoacoustic emissions. Seminars in Hearing, 17, 197–213.

Stover, L., Gorga, M. P., Neely, S. T., & Montoya, D. (1996). Towards optimizing the clinical utility of distortion product otoacoustic emission measurements. Journal of the Acoustical Society of America, 100, 956–967.

Stover, L., & Norton, S. J. (1993). The effects of aging on otoacoustic emissions. Journal of the Acoustical Society of America, 94, 2670–2681.

Telischi, F. F., Roth, J., Lonsbury-Martin, B. L., & Balkany, T. J. (1995). Patterns of evoked otoacoustic emissions associated with acoustic neuroma. Laryngoscope, 105, 675–682.

Truy, E., Veuillet, E., Collete, L., & Morgon, A. (1993). Characteristics of transient otoacoustic emissions in patients with sudden idiopathic hearing loss. British Journal of Audiology, 27(6), 379–385.

von Helmholtz, H. L. F. (1863). On the sensations of tone as a physiological basis for the theory of music. Translated by A. J. Ellis, (1885). London: Longman.

Wable, J., & Collete, L. (1994). Can synchronized otoacoustic emissions really be attributed to SOAEs? Hearing Research, 80, 141–145.

Warr, W. B. (1992). Organization of olivocochlear efferent systems in mammals. In D. B. Webster, A. N. Popper, & R. R. Fay (Eds). The mammalian auditory pathway: Neuroanatomy (Vol. 1., pp. 410–488). New York: Springer-Verlag.

Wilson, J. P. (1980). Evidence for a cochlear origin for acoustic re-emissions, threshold fine structure and tonal tinnitus. Hearing Research, 2, 233–252.

Worthington, D. W., & Peters, J. F. (1980). Quantifiable hearing and no ABR: Paradox or error? Ear and Hearing, 1, 281–285.

Xu, L., Probst, R., Harris, F. P., & Roede, J. (1994). Peripheral analysis of frequency in human ears revealed by tone burst evoked otoacoustic emissions. Hearing Research, 74, 173–180.

Chapter 23

Neonatal Hearing Screening, Follow-up, and Diagnosis

Lynn G. Spivak

Hearing loss in newborns is the most common birth defect detectable in the neonatal period (Centers for Disease Control and Prevention, 2003). Recognition of the developmental consequences of undetected, congenital hearing loss and technological advances that have made mass screening for hearing loss feasible and cost effective have provided the impetus for the development of efforts to screen all newborns for hearing loss. In 1993, when the U.S. National Institutes of Health (NIH) Consensus Conference on Early Identification of Hearing Impairment in Infants and Young Children issued its position statement, there were no mandated universal hearing screening programs in the United States. By 2004, however, 38 states had passed legislation mandating newborn hearing screening, and an additional 4 states were operating voluntary programs. This chapter will trace the development of newborn hearing screening, explain the rationale for screening all newborns for hearing impairment, and describe methods and protocols for screening, follow-up, and diagnosis that will lead to early detection and intervention of hearing loss in infants.

◆ Background

The 1993 NIH Consensus Conference on Early Identification of Hearing Impairment in Infants and Young Children was the catalyst that drove the adoption and eventual proliferation of universal newborn hearing screening programs in the United States. An interdisciplinary group of researchers consisting of representatives from the professions of audiology, speech-language pathology, otology, pediatrics, child development, and epidemiology addressed the specific issues of the conference that included the advantages of early identification of hearing loss, the appropriate target population for screening, and an appropriate screening model. Among the landmark decisions of the NIH panel was the much discussed and debated recommendation that all newborns, regardless of the presence of risk factors, be screened for hearing loss within the first 3 months of life. This recommendation was a significant departure from the more common practice at the time of screening only those babies who were considered to be at risk for hearing loss.

Risk-Based versus Universal Screening

Rationale for risk-based hearing screening is based on the higher yield and greater cost effectiveness of this approach as compared with universal screening. In 1970, the interdisciplinary group known as the Joint Committee on Infant Hearing (JCIH) issued its first position paper recognizing the need for early identification of hearing loss but concluded that mass screening of newborns was not justified (JCIH, 1976). Instead, the JCIH recommended screening those infants who presented with one or more risk factors, which were published in a supplement (**Table 23–1**). These

Table 23–1   Risk Factors for Hearing Loss in Newborns

- History of hereditary childhood hearing impairment
- Rubella or other nonbacterial intrauterine fetal infection (i.e., cytomegalovirus and herpes)
- Defects of the ear, nose, or throat; malformed, low-set, or absent pinnae; cleft lip or palate (including submucous cleft); and residual abnormality of the otorhinolaryngeal system
- Birth weight less than 1500 g
- Bilirubin level greater than 20 mg/100 mL serum

Source: Joint Committee on Infant Hearing. (1974). Supplementary statement of the Joint Committee on Infant Hearing Screening. ASHA, 16, 160.

risk factors became known as the High Risk Register (JCIH, 1974).

The most compelling reason for limiting screening to infants at risk for hearing loss is the low prevalence of significant hearing loss among infants who are not at risk. Although reports vary, it has been estimated that the prevalence of congenital, sensorineural hearing loss is between 1 and 3 per 1000 in the general population. Estimates of hearing loss among high-risk infants, however, range from 2 to 4 per 100, or approximately 10 times greater than the general population (Mehl and Thomson, 2002; Prieve and Stevens, 2000). It was argued that, by focusing screening efforts on high-risk infants, the positive predictive value and the cost effectiveness of screening would be significantly increased. It was also believed that the majority of infants with congenital hearing loss would be identified.

The inadequacy of a risk-based approach to newborn hearing screening became apparent with increasing evidence from numerous researchers that this approach misses ~50% of congenitally hearing-impaired infants (Mehl and Thomson, 2002). In other words, half of all hearing-impaired infants demonstrate no risk factors for hearing loss and, therefore, would not be identified by the screening program. It is clear from these data that, to achieve the goal of 100% detection of hearing loss in the neonatal period, it is necessary to screen all newborns for hearing loss.

In the past, the high cost associated with available methods for newborn screening was a major obstacle for implementing mass screening of newborns. Technological advances including the development of automated test equipment, however, significantly reduced the cost of screening and weakened this argument.

In 1994, a year after the NIH consensus statement, the JCIH endorsed universal detection of hearing loss within the first 3 months after birth but stopped short of recommending direct screening of every newborn. The recommendation for universal newborn hearing screening was not to come until 2000, when the JCIH published a new set of guidelines for early hearing detection and intervention. The recommendation was based on emerging clinical evidence that (1) early identification of hearing loss and intervention leads to better speech and language outcomes and (2) ~50% of congenitally hearing-impaired infants have no risk factors for hearing loss. The 2000 JCIH guidelines included a modified list of risk indicators for neonates from birth to 28 days that was intended for use where universal newborn hearing screening was not available. A second list of 10 risk

Table 23–2   Risk Indicators for Hearing Loss in Infants

Birth through 28 Days

1. Illness or condition requiring admission of 48 hours or more to the NICU
2. Stigmata or other findings associated with hearing loss
3. Family history of permanent childhood hearing loss
4. Craniofacial anomalies, including those affecting the pinna and ear canal
5. In utero infection, such as cytomegalovirus, herpes, toxoplasmosis, or rubella

29 Days through 2 Years

1. Parental or caregiver concern regarding hearing, speech, language, and/or developmental delay
2. Family history of permanent childhood hearing loss
3. Stigmata or other findings associated with hearing loss
4. Postnatal infections associated with sensorineural hearing loss
5. In utero infection
6. Neonatal indicators: hyperbilirubinemia requiring exchange transfusion, persistent pulmonary hypertension associated with mechanical ventilation, and conditions requiring extracorporeal membrane oxygenation
7. Syndromes associated with progressive hearing loss
8. Neurodegenerative or sensory motor neuropathies
9. Head trauma
10. Recurrent or persistent otitis media with effusion for 3 months or more

NICU, neonatal intensive care unit.

Source: Joint Committee on Infant Hearing. (2000). Year 2000 position statement: Principles and guidelines for early hearing detection and intervention programs. Pediatrics, 106, 798–817.

indicators for infants from 29 days through 2 years of age was included to guide ongoing surveillance of infants who may be at risk for late onset or progressive hearing loss that is not detected in the neonatal period. The 2000 JCIH risk indicators are listed in **Table 23–2**.

Justification for Newborn Hearing Screening

To determine if any screening program is justified, it is necessary that certain criteria be met (Northern and Downs, 1991):

1. There is high prevalence or serious consequences of not detecting the disease.

2. There must be an available screening test.

2. There must be availability of follow-up and effective treatment.

4. Cost of the screening must be reasonably commensurate with benefits to the individual.

The rationale for newborn hearing screening can be evaluated with regards to these principles.

Prevalence and Consequences of Undetected Hearing Loss

In addition to being the most prevalent disorder in newborns, it is widely recognized that undetected hearing loss has profound implications for development of speech and language in infants and young children. Because audition is the primary channel for speech and language learning, normal development will not occur in the presence of hearing loss. It has been shown that even mild and moderate hearing loss, although not completely depriving the infant of sound, will have a negative impact on speech and language development (Bess et al, 1998).

Availability of a Screening Test

The introduction of automated hearing screening instruments in the 1980s heralded the age of efficient, cost-effective implementation of newborn hearing screening on a large scale in hospital nurseries. Automated auditory brainstem response (A-ABR) equipment can be reliably operated by nonprofessional personnel, making the gold standard physiologic test for infant hearing available for mass screening (Jacobson et al, 1990). Ten years after the development of the A-ABR, the otoacoustic emission test (OAE) was introduced as a new tool for the assessment of hearing and was quickly adopted for newborn hearing screening (White et al, 1993). Automation of the OAE test further increased its efficiency and popularity as a tool for newborn screening.

Availability of Follow-up and Treatment

Standardized and accepted methods and protocols for diagnosis of congenital hearing loss in early infancy are available (American Speech-Language-Hearing Association [ASHA], 2004). Successful treatment of congenital hearing loss includes early fitting with hearing aids and early speech and language therapy. Recent evidence suggests that early detection and intervention for hearing loss, preferably before an infant's 6 month birthday, are effective in preventing delays commonly seen in congenitally hearing-impaired children (Moeller, 2000; Yoshinaga-Itano et al, 1998). Furthermore, it has been demonstrated that universal newborn hearing screening is successful in decreasing the age of diagnosis and intervention for infants with congenital hearing loss and is, therefore, instrumental in improving outcomes (Harrison et al, 2003; Mehl and Thomson, 2002).

Controversial Point

- Research evidence in favor of universal newborn hearing screening is accumulating; however, there still remain significant gaps in the scientific literature that reports the benefits of newborn screening. Although studies clearly indicate that newborn screening leads to a decrease in the average age of identification and intervention, there is insufficient research evidence to definitively support significant improvement in speech and language outcomes at age 3, due to limitations in the research design of existing studies. This issue will be resolved only with well-controlled, longitudinal studies of speech and language development in early identified hearing-impaired infants.

Costs

Costs of screening programs have been analyzed by individual hospital programs as well as by statewide programs (Grosse, 1997; Lemons et al, 2002). For example, the first statewide universal hearing screening program in the United States, the Rhode Island Hearing Assessment Project (RIHAP), reported a cost of $25 per infant screened (White et al, 1993). Other reports of birth admission screening costs ranged from under $10.00 to $33.30 per infant, depending on the technology used and the type of personnel performing the screen. Overall cost for identification of infants with congenital hearing loss has been reported to be comparable with costs for identifying other routinely screened congenital disorders (Mehl and Thomson, 2002). When compared with the costs to the individual and society associated with late detection of hearing loss (e.g., delayed language development, need for special education, reduced earning potential), the cost of newborn hearing screening can be easily justified (Johnson, Mauk, et al, 1993).

♦ Early Hearing Detection and Intervention

Goals

Early hearing detection and intervention (EHDI) programs promote screening of all infants and timely provision of intervention to avoid the developmental sequelae associated with late-diagnosed hearing loss. The U.S. Center for Disease Control and Prevention cites seven national goals for EHDI programs throughout the country (National Center on Birth Defects and Developmental Disabilities, 2005). These goals are listed in **Table 23–3**. The first three goals have come to be known as the "1-3-6 plan":

1. *All newborns will be screened before the age of 1 month.* This includes the birth admission screen and outpatient rescreen of all infants who failed or missed the birth admission screen.

2. *All infants who fail the screen will have a diagnostic audiologic evaluation by 3 months of age.* The diagnostic evaluation consists of physiologic tests and should be

Table 23–3 National Early Hearing Detection and Intervention Goals

1. All newborns will be screened by 1 month of age.
2. All infants with a positive screen will have a diagnostic audiologic evaluation by 3 months of age.
3. All infants with hearing loss will receive appropriate early intervention services by 6 months of age.
4. All infants and children with late-onset, progressive, or acquired hearing loss will be identified at the earliest possible time.
5. All infants with hearing loss will have a Medical Home.
6. Every state will have a complete early hearing detection and intervention (EHDI) tracking and surveillance system to minimize loss to follow-up.
7. Every state will have a comprehensive system that monitors and evaluates progress toward the EDHI goals and objectives.

performed by an audiologist who is experienced in infant assessment.

3. *All infants with a hearing loss will receive appropriate early intervention services by 6 months of age.* Part C of the Individuals with Disabilities Act (IDEA) provides funding for statewide early intervention programs to make services available for infants from birth to 3 years of age at no cost to the families. Federal regulations require that a child who is either experiencing a developmental delay or has a diagnosed condition with a high probability of resulting in a developmental delay be eligible to receive services under the state's early intervention program. Hearing loss identified in infancy is considered by early intervention programs in most states to constitute automatic eligibility for Part C services (White et al, 2005). This facilitates early access to a timely and comprehensive multidisciplinary evaluation and implementation of an individual family service plan (IFSP) that details all the needed services for effective habilitation of infants with hearing loss.

Pearl

• *Healthy People 2010* (U.S. Department of Health and Human Services, Office of Disease Prevention and Health Promotion, n.d.) describes the national health objectives designed to identify and reduce preventable threats to health. The goals of objective 28–11 of *Healthy People 2010* are to increase the proportion of newborns that are screened for hearing loss by the age of 1 month, that receive audiologic evaluation by the age of 3 months, and that are enrolled in appropriate intervention by the age of 6 months.

The EHDI goals are actively promoted by the American Academy of Pediatrics (AAP). In 2001, the AAP implemented a program to increase involvement of the primary care physician in early detection and intervention of hearing loss. This program, called Improving the Effectiveness of Newborn Hearing, Diagnosis and Intervention through the Medical Home, is overseen by an AAP-appointed task force. A key component of the program is the concept of the Medical Home, in which every child has a primary health care provider who serves as the coordinator for all medical services required by the child. According to the AAP, all children should have a Medical Home in which care is "accessible, family centered, continuous, comprehensive, compassionate and culturally competent" (American Academy of Pediatrics, 2002). The involvement of the pediatrician in the process of identification and diagnosis, as well as intervention in, congenital hearing loss is the key to achieving the goals set forth by the EHDI program.

Implementation of the Early Hearing Detection and Intervention Plan

Program Goals and Quality Assurance

A successful newborn screening program will have clearly defined goals and a process in place to monitor attainment of the goals. Therefore, before implementation, the specific performance standards that the program is expected to meet, as well as a method to measure program performance, must be known. The quality of a screening program can be assessed by comparing performance to standards, or benchmarks. The benchmarks define the minimum performance levels for each goal of the EHDI program:

• Screen all newborns.

• Identify all newborns with hearing loss.

• Minimize false-positive rates.

• Confirm hearing loss by 3 months of age.

• Initiate intervention by 6 months of age.

Benchmarks are established by regulatory agencies and/or professional organizations. Recommended benchmarks based on published data from large screening programs have been established for both the screening and follow-up phases of EHDI programs (American Academy of Pediatrics, 1999; JCIH, 2000). These benchmarks call for a screening rate of 95% or more of newborns, with a referral rate for audiologic and medical evaluation of no more than 4%. The benchmark for a successful rescreen phase of the program is the return of at least 70% of the infants who were referred for follow-up services.

JCIH (2000) proposed benchmarks for the confirmation of hearing loss and recommended, in the absence of published guidelines, that the goal be to provide services to 100% of the infants who require them. The benchmarks for this phase of the program include coordination of services through the infant's Medical Home, provision of audiologic and medical evaluation by 3 months of age or 3 months after discharge, referral of infants with confirmed hearing loss for otologic evaluation, and enrollment in the state's early intervention program.

Measurement of program performance and attainment of the benchmarks is accomplished with quality indicators that focus on key processes that are relevant to the patient, staff, and program budget (Moore, 1998). Quality indicators are an objective way to evaluate care and achieve the following:

• Standardization and uniformity of care

• Quantification of care that can be tracked and trended

• Definition of problems for performance improvement and measurement of improvement

• Increased accountability of the caregiver and improvement of clinical practice (Dlugacz et al, 2004).

Quality indicators for newborn hearing screening programs are listed in **Table 23–4**.

Quality management ensures the effectiveness of the screening program and protects its credibility. An ongoing quality monitoring system provides continuous feedback that will quickly identify weak points in the program and allow for timely intervention to resolve system breakdowns (Moore, 1998).

Table 23–4 Quality Indicators for Newborn Hearing Screening Programs

Screening Phase

1. Percentage of infants screened during the birth admission
2. Percentage of infants screened before 1 month of age
3. Percentage of infants who do not pass the birth admission screen
4. Percentage of infants who do not pass the birth admission screen and return for follow-up
5. Percentage of infants who do not pass the birth admission or outpatient screens who are referred for audiologic and medical evaluation
6. Percentage of families who refuse hearing screening on birth admission

Confirmation of Hearing Loss Phase

1. Percentage of infants and families whose care is coordinated between the Medical Home and related professionals
2. Percentage of infants whose audiologic and medical evaluations are obtained before 3 months of age
3. Percentage of infants with confirmed hearing loss referred for otologic evaluation
4. Percentage of families who accept audiologic and evaluation services
5. Percentage of families of infants with confirmed hearing loss that have a signed IFSP by the time the infant reaches 6 months of age

IFSP, individual family service plan.

Source: Joint Committee on Infant Hearing. (2000). Year 2000 position statement: Principles and guidelines for early hearing detection and intervention programs. Pediatrics, 106, 798–817.

Newborn Hearing Screening Tests

The purpose of a screening test is to separate a population into two groups: those who are normal and those who are affected by the targeted disorder. How well a hearing test achieves this purpose will be influenced by the performance characteristics of the test chosen, the pass/fail criterion, and the targeted hearing loss.

Performance Characteristics: Sensitivity and Specificity A perfect screening test would pass all individuals who are normal (i.e., 100% specificity) and fail all individuals who have the targeted disorder (i.e., 100% sensitivity). No screening test is perfect, however, and we must accept a compromise between sensitivity and specificity. The performance characteristics of a screening test can be demonstrated by constructing a 2 × 2 matrix and charting the outcomes of the test (**Table 23–5**). The accuracy of a screening test is measured by the proportion of outcomes that fall into the upper left and lower right boxes of the

matrix. The number of individuals who fail the screen and are positive for the disorder (upper left box) are true-positives; the number of individuals who pass the screen and are normal (lower right box) are true-negatives. Incorrect and missed identifications of the disorder are represented in the remaining two boxes. Individuals who are normal but fail the screen (upper right box) are false-positives, and those who have the disorder but pass the screen (lower left box) are false-negatives.

Assignment of screening results into the appropriate category (i.e., true-positive, false-negative, etc.) assumes that the actual condition of each individual undergoing the screen is known. In the case of infant hearing loss, this knowledge is obtained from the outcomes of follow-up evaluations designed to determine the infant's true hearing status. The specificity of a screening protocol can be readily determined because infants who fail the screen are likely to be retested in the follow-up phase of the program. Therefore, the number of normal infants who failed the screen (false-positives) is known. Sensitivity, in contrast, is more difficult to assess. Infants who pass the screening test usually do not return for follow-up; therefore, it is not known how many infants in the "pass" group may actually be hearing impaired. The RIHAP study, for example, calculated sensitivity and specificity data by assuming that all babies who passed the screen had normal hearing (White et al, 1993). Sensitivity of the screen was 100% by default. The literature now contains reports of screening programs that followed infants who passed as well as those who failed the newborn screen. When screening outcomes of all infants were compared with the gold standard behavioral hearing test (visual response audiometry) at 6 to 12 months of age, it was found that a small percentage of hearing-impaired infants who initially passed the birth admission hearing screen had permanent hearing loss (Johnson et al, 2005; Norton et al, 2000b). Thus, although the false-negative rate is low, no screening test currently in use will detect 100% of hearing-impaired newborns.

Pearl

- According to Johnson et al (2005; p. 671), "It is critically important to continue to emphasize to families and physicians that passing a hospital-based hearing screening test does not eliminate the need to monitor language development and consistently conduct additional hearing screening. Parents are the front-line defense and at every opportunity should be provided with understandable information regarding language milestones and anticipatory guidance."

Table 23–5 Matrix Analysis of Screening Test Performance*

	Hearing Impaired	Normal
Fail	True-positive	False-positive
Pass	False-negative	True-negative
Total	Total hearing Impaired	Total normal

* Sensitivity = true-positives/total hearing impaired; specificity = true-negatives/total normal hearing.

An efficient screening program requires that false-negative and false-positive results be kept to a minimum. A false-negative result is particularly problematic because a hearing-impaired newborn will be missed by the program, and intervention will be delayed. Although the consequences of a false-positive are not as serious, incorrectly identifying a normal-hearing infant as potentially hearing impaired impacts screening costs by increasing the number of infants who must be tracked and retested in the follow-up phase of the program. False-positives also cause unnecessary anxiety for new parents and reduce confidence in the program.

Controversial Point

- Opponents of universal newborn hearing loss have cited parental anxiety as a potential adverse effect of a false-positive result. Although surveys have found that the majority of parents are supportive of newborn hearing screening and understand the benefits of early identification of hearing loss, a small percentage of parents have reported ongoing anxiety and a change in the parent–infant relationship as a result of learning that their infant did not pass the screen.

Pass/fail criteria. Performance characteristics, or the balance between sensitivity and specificity, will be influenced by the pass/fail criteria of the test being used. On the one hand, a lax pass criterion, set inappropriately high (e.g., 50 dB for a pure-tone screen), would pass all babies with normal hearing, but would also pass some babies with hearing loss (low sensitivity). This test would result in missing hearing-impaired infants and not achieving the goals of the EHDI program. A strict pass criterion set inappropriately low (e.g., 0 dB for a pure-tone screen), on the other hand, would fail all infants with hearing loss, but would also fail some babies with normal hearing (low specificity). The consequences of such a screening test would be a large number of false-positives that would lower the efficiency and increase the cost of the program. For a comprehensive analysis of pass/fail criteria for screening technology currently in use, the reader is referred to a series of articles on the results of a multicenter study of newborn hearing screening (Gorga et al, 2000; Norton et al, 2000a; Sininger et al, 2000).

Targeted Hearing Loss   Recognizing the limitations of screening technology and the need to minimize false-positive results, the JCIH (2000) recommended that screening programs target permanent bilateral or unilateral hearing loss of 30 to 40 dB or greater in the audiometric frequencies important for speech recognition (500–4000 Hz). Results of large, multicenter studies by Norton et al (2000b) and Johnson et al (2005) that examined the effectiveness of various screening modalities and protocols to identify hearing loss in newborns indicated that identification of mild hearing loss is not consistently attainable. Norton et al (2000b) found that the three screening technologies used in their study—ABR, transient evoked otoacoustic emissions (TEOAE), and distortion product otoacoustic emissions (DPOAE)— were equally effective in identifying moderate or greater hearing loss but could not reliably differentiate between normal hearing and mild hearing loss. Similarly, Johnson et al (2005) found that a small percentage of infants with mild hearing loss were missed by the multistage screening protocol (otoacoustic emissions [OAE]

followed by A-ABR) examined in their study. Therefore, although mild hearing loss in newborns is known to have potentially negative developmental consequences, detection of mild hearing loss may not be practical or cost effective given the current state of the art.

Birth Admission Screen

The first goal of the EHDI program is to screen all newborns for hearing impairment within the first month of life. Establishing the screening program in the hospital nursery and performing the screen prior to discharge will best accomplish this goal. This strategy ensures access to all infants born in the hospital and avoids the need for time-consuming, expensive, and often unsuccessful tracking of large numbers of infants after they leave the hospital. There are a variety of options available for implementation of a successful in-hospital screening program. The following discussion will explore those options and consider the pros and cons of each, as well as the factors that come into play that will determine which choices are most appropriate.

Well Baby Nursery versus Neonatal Intensive Care Unit

By definition, universal newborn hearing screening requires administration of the screen in the well baby nursery (WBN) as well as the neonatal intensive care unit (NICU). Each nursery presents its own set of challenges for administration of a newborn hearing screening program.

Well Baby Nursery   The WBN is characterized by relatively large volume and short length of stay, typically 48 hours or less in which to accomplish the screen. Further compressing the time frame for screening is the recommendation that screening be delayed until newborns are 24 hours old, when they are more likely to pass the screen (Vohr, 1998). Because infants can be discharged from the WBN at any hour and any day of the week, screening in the WBN will need to be a 7 day a week operation to ensure that no newborn is missed by the program. A positive aspect of the WBN is that mothers, who are generally discharged at the same time as their newborns, are available on the postpartum unit, facilitating communication of screen results and scheduling of follow-up appointments, if necessary. Additionally, the prevalence of hearing loss in the WBN population is low, and healthy newborns are likely to pass the screen on the first attempt (Spivak and Sokol, 2004).

Neonatal Intensive Care Unit   Whenever possible, NICU infants should be screened close to discharge when they are medically stable and no longer require monitoring equipment, ventilators, oxygen, or other means of life support. Close coordination with the primary neonatal nurse for each infant is essential in this regard because he or she is in the best position to know the infant's schedule and can determine the best time to perform the screen. Although infants in the NICU have longer lengths of stay, as can be seen in **Fig. 23–1**, the miss rate can be higher than in the WBN primarily because the discharge date is unpredictable

Fail & Miss Rates WBN vs. NICU

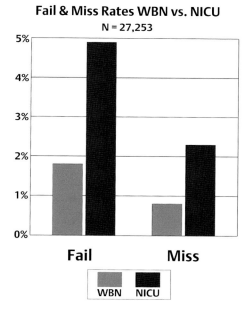

Figure 23–1 Comparison of fail and miss rates in the well baby nursery (WBN) and the neonatal intensive care unit (NICU).

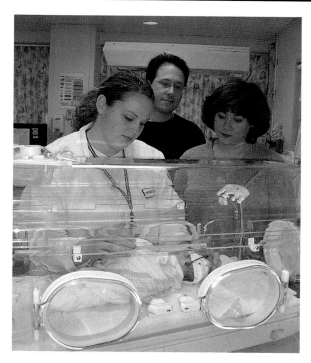

Figure 23–2 A premature infant is screened in the neonatal intensive care unit (NICU) with parents looking on. The NICU environment is not ideal for hearing screening. Screeners must contend with high noise levels, electrical artifact from electronic equipment, and fragile infants.

(Spivak et al., 2000). In some cases, critically ill infants are transferred to other facilities for surgery or treatment before they are stable enough to be screened. Good documentation and a means for tracking are essential to ensure that these infants are eventually screened before they are discharged to home (Vohr, 1998).

Fail rates are higher in the NICU than in the WBN for several reasons (**Fig. 23–1**). First of all, prevalence of hearing loss in the NICU is approximately 10 times higher than in the WBN. Second, high levels of ambient, electrical, and physiologic noise that are routinely encountered in the NICU also contribute to the higher fail rate in NICU screening programs (**Fig. 23–2**). Third, higher incidence of middle ear effusion has been reported in NICU infants, which could contribute to the higher fail rate within this population (Balkany et al, 1978). Unlike in the WBN, parents of NICU infants are not always present when the screen is performed. Therefore, a reliable method of communicating with parents regarding test results and need for follow-up must be established.

Personnel

Personnel required for newborn hearing screening include professional, technical, and support staff to carry out the various components of the program. These components include management and supervision, provision of the in-hospital screening test, data management and record keeping, infant tracking, and case management. The size of the screening program will determine the type and number of personnel involved. In large programs, there may be staff dedicated solely to the screening program, whereas in smaller programs, screening duties will constitute only a portion of the job description.

Audiologists The audiologist has an essential role in newborn hearing screening that is recognized and endorsed by the JCIH (2000). In most hospital programs, it is not cost effective for the audiologist to directly screen newborns. With the advent of automated newborn hearing screening instruments, the skills of the audiologist are not required to perform the screen and are better used in management and supervision of the program (Johnson, Maxon, et al, 1993; Orlando and Sokol, 1998). The audiologist is the most appropriate professional to provide supervision and training to technical staff, oversee data management and documentation, and manage quality assurance. As professionals who are expert in the diagnosis and management of childhood hearing loss, audiologists are needed to conduct the follow-up evaluation and plan the habilitation of infants referred from the birth admission screen. The audiologist also serves as service coordinator for families of infants requiring follow-up and provides the link between the hospital program and provision of diagnostic and habilitative services. In this role, audiologists serve as a liaison between the screening program and the community and can provide the necessary education and outreach to facilitate effective follow-up (Finitzo et al, 1998; Orlando and Sokol, 1998).

Nurses Nurses are experts in infant care and handling, and are present in the nursery 24 hours a day. They are, therefore, by virtue of training and logistics, an excellent choice of personnel to perform the newborn hearing screening test. An additional advantage of using nurses as hearing screeners is that this task becomes part of the job responsibilities of an existing employee and avoids the need to hire additional staff.

Nurses have performed well as hearing screeners in many programs; however, there are issues and potential conflicts that may arise that need to be recognized and managed to assist nurses in their role as hearing screeners. Very often, nurses will view newborn hearing screening as just another duty added to their already overly busy schedule. It is essential, therefore, that nurses support the goals of the program and understand its importance to their patients. This can be accomplished through in-service education prior to the program's initiation. Furthermore, the tendency for screening duties to be shared by many nurses among several shifts can result in newborns being missed. Another issue that arises in large programs where many nurses share the job of screening, as well as in small programs with low birth census, is that an individual nurse infrequently performs the screen. Thus, nursing staffs do not have the opportunity to practice and maintain a high level of competence in screening newborns. Under these circumstances, the rate of referral to the follow-up phase of the program will be high and ultimately result in an increase in the cost of the program (Finitzo et al, 1998; Johnson, Maxon, et al, 1993; Spivak et al, 2000). This problem can be avoided by appropriate program design that will be discussed later in this chapter.

Technicians   Universal newborn hearing screening in large birthing hospitals will require dedicated screening technicians to handle the volume of babies born. The use of technicians is made possible by automated screening technology that does not require clinical decision making on the part of the tester. Use of technicians instead of professional personnel reduces the cost of the program. It is very important, however, that technicians be trained and supervised and that their performance be monitored by audiologists to guarantee quality (Johnson, Maxon, et al, 1993; Orlando and Sokol, 1998). Dedicated screeners who screen large numbers of newborns on a consistent basis develop excellent skills that help to keep fail rates at a minimum.

Support Staff   Clerical staff is required for a variety of support functions, including maintaining records, tracking infants, scheduling follow-up appointments, and sending out reminder notices. In large screening programs, it is usually the job of a secretary to input screening and follow-up results into a database. Use of a computerized database is essential to facilitate infant tracking and compliance with the follow-up program, as well as enable the development of state- and nationwide data tracking systems (Finitzo et al, 1998; JCIH, 2000; Moore, 1998). The clerical worker who has responsibility for continually updating the database is in the best position to monitor compliance with follow-up and focus efforts on families who are resistant to returning for follow-up.

Screening Technology

The essential requirements for screening equipment are accuracy, ease of use, and speed. Because most newborn

hearing screenings will be performed by nonaudiologists (i.e., nurses, technicians, or other personnel), it is necessary that the equipment be automated and self-scoring, thereby not requiring any clinical decision making on the part of the tester. Results of the screening test should be a clear "pass" or "refer." Keeping in mind that the screen is not a diagnostic test, "pass" is interpreted as meaning that no further follow-up is indicated, and "refer" indicates the need for additional testing to determine hearing status. Establishing threshold or site of lesion is beyond the scope of a screening test.

Early attempts to use behavioral techniques to screen the hearing of infants proved to be ineffective and inaccurate. Physiologic tests of hearing are the only acceptable methods for newborn screening today (ASHA, 2004). Both ABR and OAE have been demonstrated to be effective and efficient techniques for screening the hearing of newborns. Moreover, manufacturers have incorporated both ABR and OAE tests into compact, automated units that are designed for fast and efficient crib-side testing in newborn nurseries.

Auditory Brainstem Response   The ABR has been the gold standard physiologic test of infant hearing since its introduction in the early 1970s. Studies have demonstrated that the sensitivity, specificity, and reliability of the ABR test in newborn screening are high; thus, refer rates will be low, and missing a true hearing loss will be rare (Jacobson et al, 1990). Conventional ABR, however, was found to be impractical for screening in the nursery because of the complexity of test administration, the need for professional interpretation of test results, and the time required to perform the test. Automation of ABR solved many of these problems and made it practical for use in the newborn nursery (**Fig. 23–3**). Test administration was simplified, interpretation of results was automated, and test time was shortened. Automated screening equipment uses a statistical model to determine the presence or absence of a response. Most A-ABR screening units deliver a 35 dB nHL (normalized hearing level) click and are capable of detecting moderate hearing loss (Johnson

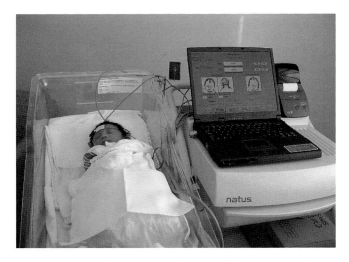

Figure 23–3 A newborn is screened in the well baby nursery using automated auditory brainstem response equipment.

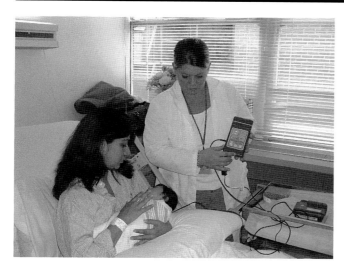

Figure 23–4 A technician uses a handheld transient evoked otoacoustic emissions hearing screener to test a newborn as she sleeps in her mother's arms.

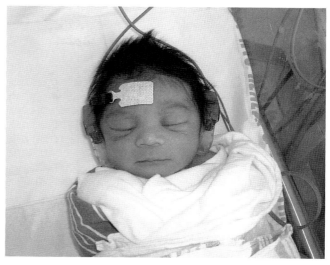

Figure 23–5 The picture shows a newborn prepared for automated auditory brainstem response testing. Preparation involves cleaning the electrode sites, attaching disposable electrodes (forehead, nape of neck, and shoulder), and placing disposable ear couplers over the newborn's ears.

et al, 2005; Norton et al, 2000b). Results of A-ABR have been shown to compare well with results of conventional ABR (Jacobson et al, 1990).

Otoacoustic Emissions   When OAE became available for clinical use in the early 1990s, the application of this new technology for newborn screening quickly became apparent. Efficacy of TEOAE for screening newborns was first demonstrated by the RIHAP study (Johnson, Maxon, et al, 1993). The OAE response is large and robust and easily detectable in the normal-hearing infant. OAE responses are present in neonates when hearing levels are ~30 dB HL (hearing level) or better and absent when hearing levels exceed mild hearing loss levels (Bergman et al, 1995). Results of the OAE test naturally fall into one of two categories, present or absent, generating the dichotomous outcome that is desirable in a screening test. Both TEOAE and DPOAE have been used successfully for newborn screening with comparable results (Norton et al, 2000b). The OAE test is relatively easy to administer and, in the hands of a well-trained tester, can be performed quickly and efficiently (**Fig. 23–4**).

Otoacoustic Emissions versus Auditory Brainstem Response

Each technology has its advantages as well as its limitations. Managers who are charged with choosing a screening tool must weigh the benefits and the liabilities of each technology and match the tool to the particular nursery environment and the goals of the program. The following discussion will focus on factors that should be considered in the decision-making process.

Test time. Although automation of the ABR significantly reduced the time it takes to perform a click ABR screen, the average A-ABR screen takes longer to administer than an OAE screen. Unlike the OAE test, A-ABR requires preparation of the infant, including cleansing of electrode sites, attaching electrodes, and positioning earphones, all of which will

add to the time involved in performing the test (**Fig. 23–5**). Norton et al (2000b) reported that preparation of the infant added an average of 6 minutes to the A-ABR test time. There is also the risk that the greater amount of infant handling required in A-ABR test preparation may wake a lightly sleeping infant and further delay the test. Although test time will vary depending on the state of the infant, hearing status, and ambient noise, the average test time for A-ABR has been reported to be ~12 minutes (Gabbard et al, 1999). Time required to position the probe and perform an OAE screen, in contrast, has been reported to be ~2 minutes per infant for TEOAE screens and, depending on the pass criteria chosen, ~5 minutes per infant for DPOAE screens (Gorga et al, 2000; Norton et al, 2000a; see **Fig. 23–6**). It should be kept in mind that a restless newborn or noisy environment will increase the test time for any screening method.

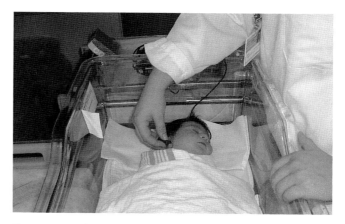

Figure 23–6 The otoacoustic emissions (OAE) probe is placed carefully in the newborn's ear canal to create an airtight seal. Good probe placement is the key to successful OAE screening.

False-Positive Rate   It is known that refer rates can differ markedly depending on the technology used. Although sensitivity of OAE testing has been found to be high, programs using this technology tend to have a greater number of false-positive results as compared with programs using A-ABR. A report of the outcomes of screening programs in Colorado, for example, showed that the average refer rate for hospitals using OAE was 11%, whereas the average refer rate for hospitals using A-ABR was 1.2% (Mehl and Thomson, 2002). Similar differences between A-ABR and OAE refer rates have been reported by other investigators (Finitzo et al, 1998; Grosse, 1997; Lemons et al, 2002; Spivak et al, 2000).

The primary reason for the higher number of false-positives from OAE screens is the presence of transient conditions such as vernix blocking the ear canal and middle ear fluid that can reduce the amplitude of the OAE and preclude obtaining a pass result (Chang et al, 1993). Another significant source of over-referral from OAE screening is poor technique on the part of the tester. Obtaining a pass result on a normal-hearing infant requires selection of the proper-size probe tip and correct positioning of the probe with an airtight seal between the probe and ear canal wall.

Pitfall

- Poor test technique is the Achilles' heel of many OAE screening programs. Unfortunately, the simplicity of OAE testing has been overstated by manufacturers as well as by some professionals, without enough emphasis on the need for proper staff training, skill development, and practice.

A third factor affecting successful recording of OAE is ambient noise levels. The presence of background room noise can increase both the duration of the OAE screen and the number of fails (Headley et al, 2000). This is especially problematic for implementation of OAE screening in the NICU, where noise levels are typically high.

Detection of Auditory Neuropathy/Dys-synchrony   Although the exact prevalence of auditory neuropathy/dys-synchrony is unknown, it has been estimated that neuropathy affects up to 10% of the deaf population (Berlin et al, 2003). Because the site of lesion of auditory neuropathy is the auditory nerve and not cochlear outer hair cells, newborns with neuropathy will pass an OAE screen, but they will fail an A-ABR screen. If a goal of the screening program is to detect auditory neuropathy, A-ABR must be incorporated into the protocol. JCIH (2000) recognizes the need for surveillance of infants for signs of auditory neuropathy and suggests that future screening programs may need to adjust their protocols to detect neuropathy in the neonatal period. Factors frequently associated with auditory neuropathy such as hyperbilirubinemia and prematurity increase the risk of finding neuropathy among newborns treated in the NICU (Madden et al, 2002). Therefore, some hospitals prefer to use A-ABR in addition to or as an alternative to OAE in the NICU screening program.

Inpatient Cost   The inpatient cost per infant will be dictated by the cost of the equipment, supplies, and personnel used to perform the screen. The advent of automated screening equipment allowed for rapid testing by nonprofessional staff that reduced the cost of screening and made it feasible for mass screening programs. There are, nonetheless, significant differences in the cost of each screening method for the inpatient phase of a program. Initial capital expense for A-ABR screening equipment is roughly 4 times higher than for OAE screening equipment. Additionally, cost of disposable supplies for A-ABR can be as much as $10.00 per infant compared with disposable ear tips for the OAE test that cost approximately $1.00 per infant. A comparative cost analysis performed by the Centers for Disease Control and Prevention (CDC) showed that the average cost to perform TEOAE screening was $17.96 per infant, and the average cost to perform A-ABR was $26.03 (Grosse, 1997). However, the higher cost of the A-ABR screening may be offset in the follow-up phase.

Follow-up Cost   In determining true costs of a screening program, the cost of the follow-up as well as the inpatient portion of the program must be considered. The number of infants referred from the birth admission screen will drive follow-up costs. The accuracy and efficiency of the in-hospital screening procedure, then, are critical to determining the cost of the follow-up program. As discussed earlier, OAE fail rates tend to be higher than A-ABR fail rates. It follows, then, that the number of infants that will need follow-up services will be larger in programs using OAE technology than in programs using A-ABR. A study by Lemons et al (2002) compared the refer rates and program costs of two similar-size screening programs, one using TEOAE and the other using A-ABR as the screening tool. The TEOAE program referred 240 infants (16%), and the A-ABR program referred 92 infants (7%). Because of the larger number of babies who required outpatient rescreening in the TEOAE program, total cost to perform the outpatient rescreen was higher for the TEOAE program ($35,590) than for the A-ABR program ($13,643). With ~10% of all rescreened babies in each program requiring further diagnostic testing, the total postdischarge cost for the TEOAE programs was $39,527, as compared with $17,186 for the A-ABR programs. The conclusion that can be drawn from this study is that, when the cost of the follow-up phase of the program is considered, an OAE screening program will cost more than an A-ABR program because of the larger number of infants that will be referred from an OAE program and require follow-up. Thus, savings realized on the inpatient side will ultimately be offset by higher costs on the outpatient side.

Efficiency   Based on the results of the multicenter study conducted by Norton and colleagues (2000b), it can be concluded that currently available screening tools—TEOAE, DPOAE, and A-ABR—are equally good at differentiating normal from moderately hearing-impaired newborns. The selection of a screening tool, then, depends on its efficiency within the context of the specific screening environment in which it will be used. It has been demonstrated, for example, that OAE fail rates meeting or exceeding the accepted benchmark are attainable in large screening programs in which screening staff are well trained and have sufficient opportunity to practice and maintain their skills (Spivak and Sokol, 2004). As mentioned earlier, in small programs, programs with high turnover of personnel, or programs in which many individuals share the responsibility for screening, good OAE testing skills are not likely to be acquired, leading to excessively high refer rates. Administration of A-ABR does not require the probe placement skill that is so critical in obtaining a valid OAE measurement. Therefore, when screening personnel test infrequently or test small numbers of newborns, better results are obtained with A-ABR. **Fig. 23–7** shows outcomes from two small community hospitals in which nurses performed the birth admission screen. Hospital 1, with 555 births per year, used an automated transient OAE screener for 2 years and had an average fail rate of 9%. When the hospital switched to A-ABR, the fail rate dropped to 1%, significantly exceeding the benchmark. Hospital 2, with an annual birth rate of 379 newborns, used A-ABR exclusively in its screening program and maintained an excellent fail rate of less than 1%.

Auditory Steady-State Response

A test modality that is gaining acceptance in infant auditory assessment is the auditory steady-state response (ASSR). Although not currently in use in newborn hearing screening programs, it is included here because the technique has potential for use in screening programs in the future. The ASSR is a scalp recorded auditory evoked potential that is phase locked to a frequency and/or amplitude modulated pure-tone stimulus. High rates of stimulation (70–100 Hz) used in ASSR evoke responses from generators within the brainstem. Good correlation between ASSR thresholds and behavioral thresh-

olds in infants has been demonstrated (Rance et al, 2005). ASSR technology has several characteristics that make its potential application to newborn hearing screening promising: the test is relatively fast; commercially available equipment incorporates automated response detection; and results are frequency specific, a feature that current screening modalities lack. Evidence to date, however, demonstrates that ASSR does not perform as well as either A-ABR or OAE in the screening situation, indicating that more research and test development will be needed before ASSR can be adopted as a viable newborn hearing screening tool (Cone-Wesson et al, 2002).

Screening Protocols

An effective strategy to reduce refer rates from a newborn hearing screening program is to rescreen all infants who fail the screen before discharge. The rationale for rescreening is that the transient conditions that may have caused an initial screen failure (middle ear fluid, vernix blocking the ear canal, infant irritability, and high ambient noise) may resolve before discharge, at which point the newborn will pass the screen. A multistage program can be developed using a single technology, in which the same test is repeated, or may combine OAE and ABR in a two-technology screening protocol.

Multistage/Single-Technology Protocol   Either A-ABR or OAE may be chosen for a multistage/single-technology protocol. Repeating the A-ABR screen on newborns who fail the initial screen at a later time before discharge from the nursery has been shown to further improve refer rates from A-ABR screening programs (Connolly et al, 2005). OAE screening performance can also be significantly improved by incorporating OAE into a multistage protocol. **Fig. 23–8** illustrates the improvement in fail rate when a second OAE

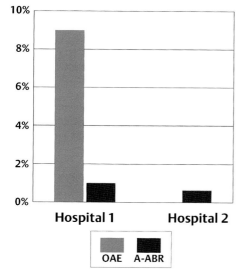

Fail Rates From 2 Small Screening Programs

Figure 23–7 Screen fail rates from two small community hospitals in which nurses perform the screen. Hospital 1 experienced high fail rates using otoacoustic emissions (OAE). Fail rates were significantly reduced after switching to automated auditory brainstem response (A-ABR). Low fail rates were also achieved by Hospital 2 using A-ABR as their screening method.

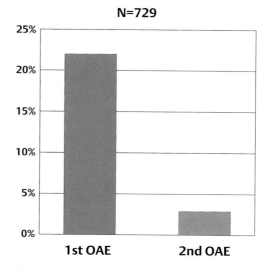

One vs. Two Stage OAE Protocol

N=729

Figure 23–8 Fail rate resulting from the administration of one otoacoustic emissions (OAE) screen was 22%. Infants who failed the initial OAE screen received a second OAE screen prior to discharge, resulting in a decrease in the fail rate to 2.9%.

NIH Recommended
2 Stage Screening Protocol

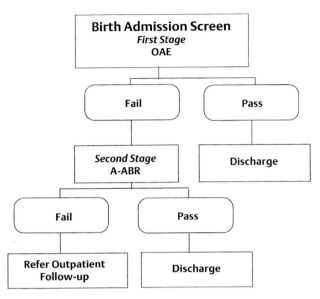

Figure 23–9 Flow chart illustrating the two-stage screening protocol (otoacoustic emissions [OAE] followed by auditory brainstem response [ABR]) endorsed by the National Institutes of Health at the 1993 consensus meeting.

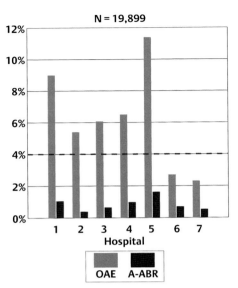

Figure 23–10 Screen outcomes from seven hospitals (Northshore-Long Island Jewish Health System) using a two-stage, two-technology protocol. Fail rates for the first-stage otoacoustic emissions (OAE) screen is represented by the light bars; fail rates for the second-stage automated auditory brainstem response (A-ABR) screen is represented by the dark bars. Hospitals are ranked according to size, ranging from 555 births per year (hospital 1) to 6117 births per year (hospital 7). Nurses perform the screen in the smaller hospitals (1–5) and achieve the benchmark of 4% (indicated by the broken line) after the second-stage A-ABR screen. Dedicated screening technicians in hospitals 6 and 7 achieve the benchmark with the first-stage OAE screen and reduce the fail rate even further with the second-stage A-ABR.

screen is performed on newborns who failed their initial OAE screen. In a group of 726 newborns from the WBN, repeating the OAE test prior to discharge reduced the initial fail rate of 22% to an acceptable 2.9% (Spivak and Sokol, 2004).

Multistage/Two-Technology Protocol   A strategy that takes advantage of the low cost and speed of the OAE screen, as well as the lower refer rate of the A-ABR screen, is to rescreen infants who fail the OAE screen with A-ABR. This is the protocol that was recommended by the NIH consensus meeting in 1993 and has been adopted by many hospital screening programs (**Fig. 23–9**). The improvement in fail rate using OAE followed by A-ABR compared with using OAE alone is demonstrated in the data collected over a 1 year period from seven hospitals that use the multistage/two-technology protocol. **Fig. 23–10** shows the fail rates for the OAE screen compared with the fail rates when newborns who failed the OAE screen were rescreened using A-ABR.

There are drawbacks to the two-technology protocol, however. First, this protocol obviously requires the purchase and maintenance of two pieces of equipment and their associated disposable supplies, which increases the costs of the in-hospital phase of the program. Second, screening personnel must attain and maintain competence in each technology. Third, the test time for infants requiring the second-stage screen is necessarily increased. Nevertheless, the overall benefit in reducing the number of infants referred from the program usually outweighs the disadvantages.

◆ Follow-up

Newborn hearing screening is only the first step toward providing early intervention. Identification of hearing impairment at birth serves no purpose and will not benefit an infant unless a well thought out and effective follow-up program is in place. Planning for follow-up must coincide with planning for the inpatient program to ensure seamless transition of infants from screening to diagnosis. An effective follow-up program allows for early confirmation of hearing loss and timely initiation of intervention.

Obstacles to Effective Follow-up

Those involved with newborn hearing screening can attest to the fact that follow-up is the most difficult part of an EHDI program. It is, therefore, very important that obstacles to follow-up be identified and ways to eliminate barriers be found. By far, the greatest obstacle to compliance with follow-up is tracking infants once they leave the hospital. Therefore, the best technique for improving follow-up efficiency is to reduce the number of infants who require follow-up by improving the efficiency of the birth admission screening program.

Metropolitan areas with large transient populations pose a particular problem for follow-up efforts. Results of the New York State demonstration project revealed significantly lower compliance with follow-up from urban hospitals as compared with suburban hospitals (Prieve et al, 2000); Folsom et al, (2000) found that low socioeconomic status and social risk factors were the most common causes of noncompliance with follow-up in their study. Other factors, including accessibility of follow-up facilities; financial burdens imposed by travel, babysitters, or time off from work; busy family schedules; and a lack of appreciation of the importance of the follow-up evaluation, can also lead to noncompliance with the follow-up program.

Pitfall

- In an effort to allay parental alarm about a newborn's failed screen, screening personnel must be careful not to underemphasize the significance of the test result and the need for prompt follow-up testing.

The most effective tool for improving compliance with follow-up is good communication with parents so that they understand the importance of the follow-up visit. Audiologists are typically not present when screening is performed in the nursery and, therefore, must rely on others to communicate information to parents about seeking follow-up services. Nurses, screening technicians, and pediatricians who understand the consequences of undetected hearing loss are in an excellent position to emphasize this point prior to the infant's discharge. In this context, the Medical Home becomes a valuable resource that can facilitate delivery of follow-up care to infants at risk for hearing loss.

An effective strategy that is implemented in some hospitals is to make the appointment for the follow-up audiologic evaluation prior to discharge, either immediately after the screening is completed or as part of the discharge planning conference. This practice avoids problems associated with contacting families after discharge (wrong or changed phone numbers and addresses, unanswered messages, language barriers, etc.) and guarantees that the infant will be scheduled in a timely fashion. Close communication between the nursery and the hospital department or outside facility that provides the follow-up services is crucial to make sure that appointments are kept and missed appointments are rescheduled.

Postdischarge Evaluation

The postdischarge, follow-up evaluation should include all infants who are identified by the birth admission screen as well as those infants who were discharged before hearing screening could be performed. The goals of the EHDI program require that the diagnostic evaluation occur by 3 months of age.

Pearl

- An advantage to performing the diagnostic evaluation by 3 months of age is that infants in this age group can usually be tested in natural sleep. Older infants may require sedation to complete physiologic tests.

Ideally, the follow-up evaluation of infants who are at risk for hearing loss will take place in the Audiology Home, that is, a facility that is designed to meet all the service needs of hearing-impaired infants and their families (Jerger et al, 2001). Staffed by professionals with expertise in childhood hearing loss, the Audiology Home offers the full spectrum of family-oriented services, including audiologic assessment, intervention, and management, as well as counseling, community outreach, and education. Services offered in the Audiology Home provide the continuity of care that facilitates timely diagnosis of hearing loss and maximizes the outcomes of intervention.

Follow-up Models

There are two schools of thought concerning the best approach to the initial follow-up visit to accomplish the goals of the EHDI program. In model 1, a repeat screening test is administered within 1 month of discharge at the first outpatient visit. Infants who pass the rescreen are discharged from the program; infants who fail the outpatient rescreen are referred for complete audiologic evaluation within the 3 month time frame. The rationale for readministering the screening test is based on the fact that a majority of infants who do not pass the birth admission screen will pass a repeat screen at 1 month of age. Results of the Newborn Hearing Screening Demonstration Project in New York State, for example, showed that 79% of infants who returned for their follow-up visit passed the outpatient rescreen and did not require a diagnostic evaluation (Prieve et al, 2000). This follow-up model is a cost- and time-efficient way to eliminate infants from the follow-up program who may have failed the inpatient screen because of transient conditions that resolve shortly after discharge. Thus, many false-positive referrals will be eliminated from the diagnostic phase of the EHDI program. This is an effective model for larger screening programs that could become overburdened with a large number of expensive and time-consuming diagnostic evaluations.

Model 2 calls for full diagnostic evaluation at the initial outpatient visit. This model requires that infants who do not pass the birth admission screen be referred immediately to an audiologist in the hospital or community for follow-up evaluation. Proponents of this approach argue that it increases compliance with follow-up, streamlines the process by eliminating a step in the follow-up procedure, and takes full advantage of the opportunity to obtain a maximum amount of information about the infant's hearing status in one visit (Kileny and Lesperance, 2001). This model may be favored by hospitals in remote areas where patients need to travel long distances to obtain services. It is also a useful model for hospitals with a preponderance of patients who are difficult to track or resistant to compliance with the hospital's follow-up efforts.

Diagnostic Evaluation

As stated above, depending on the model adopted by the screening program, the diagnostic evaluation may be

Table 23–6   Objectives of Audiologic Assessment

Audiologic assessment for children from birth to 5 years of age is designed to serve the following purposes:

- to determine the status of the auditory mechanism
- to identify the type, degree, and configuration of hearing loss for each ear
- to characterize associated disability and potentially handicapping conditions
- to access the ability to use auditory information in a meaningful way
- to identify individual risk factors and the need for surveillance of late-onset or progressive hearing loss
- to access candidacy for sensory devices
- to refer for additional evaluation and intervention services when indicated
- to provide culturally and linguistically sensitive counseling for families/caregivers
- to communicate findings and recommendations, with parental consent, to other professionals
- to consider the need for additional assessments and/or screenings (i.e., speech-language, cognitive, behavioral)

Source: American Speech-Language-Hearing Association. (2004). Guidelines for the audiologic assessment of children from birth to 5 years of age. Available at http://www.asha.org/NR/rdonlyres/0BB7C840-27D2-4DC6-861B-1709ADD78BAF/0/v2GLAudAssessChild.pdf.

administered at the first outpatient visit or after failure of an outpatient rescreen. Either way, in keeping with the EHDI goals, infants will be scheduled for the diagnostic evaluation by 3 months of age. ASHA (2004) published updated guidelines detailing the appropriate protocol for the evaluation of infants in this age group. The guidelines were based on research evidence and clinical experience and were intended to serve as a "bridge" between newborn screening and early intervention (**Table 23–6**).

Behavioral measures of hearing, such as visual response audiometry, have been shown to be unreliable in infants < 5 months of age and are not recommended for the assessment of hearing in this age group (ASHA, 2004). The diagnostic evaluation of infants referred at the recommended age from the screening program, therefore, consists of a battery of physiologic measures. The components of the physiologic test battery evaluation are ABR, OAE, and immittance measurements.

Auditory Brainstem Response

The twofold purpose of the ABR test is to provide information about the neural integrity of the infant's auditory system and an objective measurement of hearing sensitivity. To accomplish this purpose, the ABR is obtained using both click and tonal stimuli.

Click-Evoked Auditory Brainstem Response   There are two advantages to obtaining the ABR latency-intensity series in response to click stimuli. First, moderate intensity clicks (60–70 dB nHL) produce an organized, easily visualized

waveform, allowing for identification of peaks I, III, and V. Thus, results of the click ABR are useful for assessing neural conduction through the brainstem auditory pathway. Second, a click ABR threshold can be quickly obtained and provides a ballpark estimate of overall response thresholds. This will help to guide subsequent tonal ABR testing in which waveforms are typically less clear and robust than click-evoked waveforms.

Tone Burst–Evoked Auditory Brainstem Response   Evaluation with tonal stimuli is necessary to provide frequency-specific assessment of hearing. It is well known that, because of the wide spectrum of the click stimulus, click ABR can underestimate thresholds in certain frequency regions where hearing loss exists (Oates and Stapells, 1998). In contrast, it has been established that tonal ABR thresholds correlate well with behavioral thresholds in infants and, therefore, can be used reliably for assessing hearing levels and predicting the audiogram (Stapells and Oates, 1997). The frequency-specific threshold information obtained from tone burst ABR will be required for hearing aid fitting.

Because tone burst ABR waveforms are smaller in amplitude and less distinct than responses to click stimuli, it is often necessary to replicate responses to tonal stimuli more than once. Tone burst ABR testing, therefore, is usually more time consuming than the click latency intensity function.

Bone-Conduction Auditory Brainstem Response   Bone-conduction ABR is useful to determine cochlear reserve and to help differentiate between sensorineural and conductive hearing loss in infants who have elevated air-conduction thresholds. Both click and tonal stimuli have been used for bone-conduction ABR (Foxe and Stapells, 1993; Yang et al, 1993). Differences between bone-conduction responses obtained from infants and adults, due to differences in skull transmission, have been documented and must be accounted for in bone-conduction ABR measurements in infants (Stuart et al, 1993). Several test protocols for obtaining bone-conduction ABR thresholds in infants have been proposed. These include comparison of air- and bone-conduction ABR latencies and thresholds, bone-conduction recordings in the presence of masking noise (sensorineural acuity level [SAL] technique), and interear differences in bone-conduction latencies to determine the ear with the better cochlear reserve (see Cone-Wesson, 1995, for a review of bone-conduction techniques).

Although ABR is considered to be the gold standard of threshold assessment for young infants, there are a variety of factors that may compromise the information obtained from the ABR and influence its interpretation. These factors may be technological in nature, such as the presence of electrical or myogenic artifact, or pathological in nature, such as the presence of middle ear effusion, a blocked ear canal, or auditory neuropathy/dys-synchrony.

Otoacoustic Emissions   The presence of OAE is indicative of intact cochlear outer hair cell function and is consistent with hearing thresholds of 30 dB HL or better. OAE do not provide a means of threshold prediction but are useful in the diagnostic evaluation as a cross-check on results obtained from the ABR test.

Pearl

- The cross-check principle is well known in pediatric audiology and states that diagnosis should be based on a pattern of diagnostic data that emerge from the results of a battery of tests, not on one test alone (Jerger and Hayes, 1976).

Agreement between ABR and OAE results increases the level of confidence in the diagnosis. Disagreement between results of ABR and OAE, in contrast, indicates the need for further evaluation to uncover the cause. For example, normal ABR results with absent OAE may indicate the presence of a small conductive component. It may also signal a technical error such as poor probe placement that prevented recording the OAE. It is also possible that ABR results were misinterpreted (e.g., artifact in a noisy waveform identified as a response). At the very least, a second look at test results and perhaps repeat testing are indicated when such discrepancies exist.

Special Consideration

- Auditory neuropathy/dys-synchrony is an example of a pathology that requires the results of both ABR and OAE for accurate diagnosis. Normal OAE in the presence of abnormal ABR results is the hallmark of auditory neuropathy. Thus, when auditory neuropathy is present, results of ABR alone might be incorrectly interpreted as evidence of severe to profound sensorineural hearing loss. The differentiation of auditory neuropathy from sensorineural hearing loss is critical to ensure the initiation of an appropriate plan of habilitation that would be markedly different for each pathology.

Acoustic Immittance   When elevated ABR thresholds are obtained, tympanometry can be a valuable tool in the test battery to assess middle ear status and to help determine the type of hearing loss. However, poor validity of tympanometry using low-frequency probe tones (226 Hz) in infants has been documented (Holte et al, 1991). Therefore, it is recommended that tympanometry be performed using high-frequency probe tones such as 660 or 1000 Hz in infants younger than 5 months (ASHA, 2004).

Obstacles to Intervention

Timely evaluation and diagnosis do not necessarily guarantee that intervention will follow the recommended time course. There are still potential obstacles that can delay the initiation of intervention services that must be negotiated following diagnosis. In a survey conducted by Harrison et al (2003), it was found that ~50% of respondents reported encountering a time lag of 1 month or more between diagnosis and fitting of hearing aids. There were four primary reasons cited for the delay in obtaining early intervention:

- Scheduling problems
- Need for repeat testing
- Suspicion of auditory neuropathy
- Financial issues

Interestingly, the barriers to timely initiation of early intervention services that were identified by Harrison et al in 2003 were similar to those reported by the first two authors some 6 years earlier (Harrison and Roush, 1996). It can be concluded, then, that in spite of technological advances and an increasingly friendly environment for the growth of newborn hearing screening programs, the socioeconomic issues as well as technical problems associated with obtaining a reliable diagnosis in young infants continue to be significant impediments to early intervention. It is clear that future efforts need to focus on improving follow-up effectiveness and timely access to services so that all infants will enjoy the benefits of early detection and intervention of hearing loss.

◆ Summary

The evolution of technology that can reliably and inexpensively detect hearing loss in newborns and the accumulating research evidence demonstrating the benefits of early detection and intervention have combined to create an environment in which newborn screening has become the standard of care in most hospital nurseries. The potential benefits of early detection can only be realized if there is an effective follow-up program in place that makes certain that all infants who are referred from the newborn hearing screening program are retested and that those who are found to be hearing impaired are enrolled in a program of habilitation. The success of EHDI programs is responsible for the growing number of hearing-impaired children who are enrolled in mainstream classrooms, achieving speech, language, and academic performance comparable to their hearing peers.

References

American Academy of Pediatrics Task Force on Newborn and Infant Hearing. (1999). Newborn and infant hearing loss: Detection and intervention. Pediatrics, 103, 527–530.

American Academy of Pediatrics. (2002). Policy statement: The medical home. Pediatrics, 110, 184–186.

American Speech-Language Hearing Association. (2004). Guidelines for the audiologic assessment of children from birth to 5 years of age. Available at http://www.asha.org/NR/rdonlyres/0BB7C840-27D2-4DC6-861B-1709ADD78BAF/0/v2GLAudAssessChild.pdf.

Balkany, T. J., Berman, S. A., Simmons, M. A., & Jafek, B. W. (1978). Middle ear effusions in neonates. Laryngoscope, 88(3), 398–405.

Bergman, B. M., Gorga, M. P., Neely, S. T., Kaminski, J. R., Beauchaine, K. L., & Peters, J. (1995). Preliminary descriptions of transient-evoked and distortion-product otoacoustic emissions from graduates of an intensive care nursery. Journal of the American Academy of Audiology, 6, 150–162.

Berlin, C. I., Hood, L., Morlet, T., Rose, K., & Brashears, S. (2003). Auditory neuropathy/dys-synchrony: Diagnosis and management. Mental Retardation and Developmental Disabilities Research Reviews, 9(4), 225–231.

Bess, F. H., Dodd-Murphy, J., & Parker, R. A. (1998). Children with minimal sensorineural hearing loss: Prevalence, educational performance, and functional status. Ear and Hearing, 19, 339–354.

Centers for Disease Control and Prevention. (2003). Infants tested for hearing loss: United States, 1999–2001. MMWR Morbidity and Mortality Weekly Report, 52(41), 981–984.

Chang, K. W., Vohr, B. R., Norton, S. J., & Lekas, M. D. (1993). External and middle ear status related to evoked otoacoustic emission in neonates. Archives of Otolaryngology—Head and Neck Surgery, 119, 276–282.

Cone-Wesson, B. (1995). Bone-conduction ABR tests. American Journal of Audiology, 4, 14–18.

Cone-Wesson, B., Parker, J., Swiderski, N., & Rickards, F. (2002). The auditory steady- state response: Full-term and premature neonates. Journal of the American Academy of Audiology, 13(5), 260–269.

Connelly, J. L., Carron, j. D, & Roark, S. D., (2005). Universal newborn hearing screening: Are we achieving the Joint Committee on Infant Hearing (JCIH) objectives? Laryngoscope, 11, 232–236.

Dlugacz, Y. D., Restifo, A., & Greenwood, A. (2004). The quality handbook for health care organizations. San Francisco: Josey-Bass.

Finitzo, T., Albright, K., & O'Neal, J. (1998). The newborn with hearing loss: Detection in the nursery. Pediatrics, 102, 1452–1460.

Folsom, R. C., Widen, J. E., Vohr, B. R., Cone-Wesson, B., Gorga, M. P., Sininger, Y. S., & Norton, S. J. (2000). Identification of neonatal hearing impairment recruitment and follow-up. Ear and Hearing, 21, 462–470.

Foxe, J. J., & Stapells, D. R. (1993). Normal infant and adult auditory brainstem responses to bone-conducted tones. Audiology, 32, 95–109.

Gabbard, S. A., Northern, J., & Yoshinaga-Itano, C. (1999). Hearing screening in newborns under 24 hours of age. Seminars in Hearing, 20, 291–304.

Gorga, M. P., Norton, S. J., Siniger, Y. S., et al. (2000). Identification of neonatal hearing impairment: Distortion product otoacoustic emissions during the perinatal period. Ear and Hearing, 21, 400–424.

Grosse, S. (1997). The costs and benefits of universal newborn hearing screening. Paper presented at the Joint Committee for Infant Hearing, Alexandria, VA.

Harrison, M., & Roush, J. (1996). Age for suspicion, identification, and intervention for infants and young children with hearing loss: A national study. Ear and Hearing, 17, 55–62.

Harrison, M., Roush, J., & Wallace, J. (2003). Trends in age of identification and intervention in infants with hearing loss. Ear and Hearing, 24, 89–95.

Headley, G. M., Campbell, D. E., & Gravel, J. S. (2000). Effect of neonatal test environment on recording transient-evoked otoacoustic emissions. Pediatrics, 105(6), 1279–1285.

Holte, L., Margolis, R. H., & Cavanaugh, R. M. (1991). Developmental changes in multifrequency tympanograms. Audiology, 30(1), 198–210.

Jacobson, J. T., Jacobson, C. A., & Spahr, R. C. (1990). Automated and conventional ABR screening techniques in high-risk infants. Journal of the American Academy of Audiology, 1, 187–195.

Jerger, J. F., & Hayes, D. (1976). The cross-check principal in pediatric audiometry. Archives of Otolaryngology, 102, 614–620.

Jerger, S., Roeser, R. J., & Tobey, E. A. (2001). Management of hearing loss in infants: The UTD/Callier Center position statement. Journal of the American Academy of Audiology, 12, 329–336.

Johnson, J. L., Mauk, G. W., Takekawa, K. M., Simon, P. R., Sia, C. C. J., & Blackwell, P. M. (1993). Implementing a statewide system of services for infants and toddlers with hearing disabilities. Seminars in Hearing, 14, 105–118.

Johnson, M. J., Maxon, A. B., White, K. R., & Vohr, B. R. (1993). Operating a hospital-based universal newborn hearing screening program using transient evoked otoacoustic emissions. Seminars in Hearing, 14, 46–55.

Johnson, J. L., White, K. R., Widen, J. E., et al. (2005). A multicenter evaluation of how many infants with permanent hearing loss pass a two-stage otoacoustic emissions/automated auditory brainstem response newborn hearing screening protocol. Pediatrics, 116(3), 663–672.

Joint Committee on Infant Hearing. (1976). 1970 Statement on Neonatal Screening for Hearing Impairment. Available at: www.jcih.org/JCIH1971.pdf

Joint Committee on Infant Hearing. (1974). Supplementary statement of the Joint Committee on Infant Hearing Screening. ASHA, 16, 160.

Joint Committee on Infant Hearing. (2000). Year 2000 position statement: Principles and guidelines for early hearing detection and intervention programs. Pediatrics, 106, 798–817.

Kileny, P. R., & Lesperance, M. M. (2001). Evidence in support of a different model of universal newborn hearing loss identification. American Journal of Audiology, 10(2), 65–67.

Lemons, J., Fanaroff, A., Stewart, E. J., Bentkover, J. D., Murray, G., & Diefendorf, A. (2002). Newborn hearing screening: Costs of establishing a program. Journal of Perinatology, 22, 120–124.

Madden, C., Rutter, M., Hilbert, L., Greinwald, J. H., Jr., & Choo, D. I. (2002). Clinical and audiological features in auditory neuropathy. Archives of Otolaryngology—Head and Neck Surgery, 128(9), 1026–1030.

Mehl, A. L., & Thomson, V. (2002). The Colorado newborn hearing screening project, 1992–1999: On the threshold of effective population-based universal newborn hearing screening. Pediatrics, 109(1), E7.

Moeller, M. P. (2000). Early intervention and language development in children who are deaf and hard of hearing. Pediatrics, 106(3), 43.

Moore, P. E. (1998). Data and quality management. In L. G. Spivak (Ed.), Universal newborn hearing screening (pp. 167–186). New York: Thieme Medical Publishers.

National Center on Birth Defects and Developmental Disabilities. (2005). Early hearing detection and intervention program. Available at http://www.cdc.gov/ncbddd/ehdi/ehdi.htm.

National Institutes of Health. (1993). Early Identification of Hearing Impairment in Infants and Young Children. NIH Consensus Statement, 11, 1–24.

Northern, J., & Downs, M. (1991). Hearing in children (pp. 232–233). Baltimore, MD: Williams & Wilkins.

Norton, S. J., Gorga, M. P., Widen, J. E., et al. (2000a). Transient evoked otoacoustic emissions during the perinatal period. Ear and Hearing, 21, 425–442.

Norton, S. J., Gorga, M. P., Widen, J. E., et al. (2000b). Identification of neonatal hearing impairment: Evaluation of transient evoked otoacoustic emission, distortion product otoacoustic emission and auditory brain stem response test performance. Ear and Hearing, 21, 508–528.

Oates, P., & Stapells, D. R. (1998). Auditory brain stem response estimates of the pure tone audiogram: Current status. Seminars in Hearing, 10, 61–85.

Orlando, M. S., & Sokol, H. (1998). Personnel and supervisory options for universal newborn hearing screening. In L. G. Spivak (Ed.), Universal newborn hearing screening (pp. 67–86). New York: Thieme Medical Publishers.

Prieve, B., Dalzell, L., Berg, A., et al. (2000). The New York State universal newborn hearing screening demonstration project: Outpatient outcome measures. Ear and Hearing, 21(2), 104–117.

Prieve, B. A., & Stevens, F. (2000). The New York State universal newborn hearing screening demonstration project: Introduction and overview. Ear and Hearing, 21, 85–91.

Rance, G., Roper, R., Symons, L., Moody, L. J., Povlis, C., Dourlay, M., & Kelly, T. (2005). Hearing threshold estimation in infants using auditory steady-state responses. Journal of the American Academy of Audiology, 16(5), 291–300.

Sininger, Y. S., Cone-Wesson, B., Folsom, R. C., et al. (2000). Identification of neonatal hearing impairment: Auditory brain stem responses in the perinatal period. Ear and Hearing, 21(5), 383–399.

Spivak, L., Prieve, B., Dalzell, L., et al. (2000). The New York State universal newborn hearing screening demonstration project: Inpatient outcome measures. Ear and Hearing, 21(2), 92–103.

Spivak, L. G., & Sokol, H. (May 2004). Factors affecting effectiveness of newborn hearing screening protocols. Paper presented at NHS 2004 International Conference on Newborn Hearing Screening, Diagnosis and Intervention, Milan, Italy.

Stapells, D. R., & Oates, P. (1997). Estimation of pure-tone audiogram by the auditory brainstem response: A review. Audiology and Neurootology, 2(5), 257–280.

Stuart, A., Yang, E. Y., Stenstrom, R., & Reindorp, A. G. (1993). Auditory brainstem response thresholds to air and bone conducted clicks in neonates and adults. American Journal of Otology, 14(2), 176–182.

U.S. Department of Health and Human Services, Office of Disease Prevention and Health Promotion. (n.d.). Healthy people 2010. Available at http://www.healthypeople.gov/document/html/objectives/28-11.htm.

Vohr, B. R. (1998). Practical medical issues when screening infants. In L. G. Spivak (Ed.), Universal newborn hearing screening (pp. 145–166). New York: Thieme Medical Publishers.

White, K. R., Vohr, B. R., & Behrens, T. R. (1993). Universal newborn hearing screening using transient otoacoustic emissions: Results of the Rhode Island Hearing Assessment Project. Seminars in Hearing, 14, 18–29.

White, K. R., Shisler, L., & Watts, K. (2005, February). The status of EHDI programs in the United States. Paper presented at the 2005 National Early Hearing Detection and Intervention Conference, Atlanta.

Yang, E. Y., Stuart, A., Mencher, G. T., Mencher, L. S., & Vincer, M. J. (1993). Auditory brainstem responses to air and bone-conducted clicks in the audiological assessment of at-risk infants. Ear and Hearing, 14, 175–182.

Yoshinaga-Itano, C., Sedey, A. L., Coulter, D. K., & Mehl, A. L. (1998). Language of early and later identified children with hearing loss. Pediatrics, 102(5), 1161–1171.

Chapter 24

Intraoperative Neurophysiologic Monitoring

Aage R. Møller

Operations that involve the nervous system always involve risks of death and neurologic deficits. Such risks can never be eliminated because not all factors that are involved can be controlled, and the possibility always exists that mistakes may be made or that unforeseen circumstances can cause injuries or death. If it is physically possible to make a mistake, it will be made eventually, but the likelihood that a mistake occurs can be reduced. It is the goal of procedures in the operating room to make the likelihood of mistakes as small as possible. Intraoperative neurophysiologic monitoring is one of many means that can reduce the likelihood of mistakes that

can lead to injury and permanent postoperative neurologic deficits, but it cannot eliminate surgically induced deficits.

Intraoperative (neurophysiologic) monitoring (IOM) is based on the assumption that recordable neuroelectric potentials change because of an injury to the nervous system and that the injury can be reversed before the severity of the injury has reached the level where permanent deficits result. Besides reducing the risk of permanent deficits, IOM may give the surgeon an increased feeling of security and can often help the surgeon in identifying neural structures that are not directly visible. In some operations, these electrophysiologic methods can help the surgeon achieve the therapeutic goal of an operation.

This type of monitoring uses recordings of neuroelectric potentials, such as sensory evoked potentials and electromyographic (EMG) potentials, to detect changes in the function of specific systems. Far-field sensory evoked potentials and near-field potentials recorded directly from nerves, nuclei, and muscles are now commonly monitored in the operating room. Electrical stimulation of neural structures in the operative field is used for identifying specific nerves. EMG activity elicited by surgical manipulations of motor nerves is used as an indicator of activation of motor nerves and to detect injuries to them. Electrophysiologic recordings from deep brain structures are used to guide placement of lesions and for implantation of electrodes for deep brain stimulation (DBS).

IOM is now recognized as a medical subspecialty, and it has its own society, the American Society of Neurophysiological Monitoring (ASNM), and an organization, the American Board of Neurophysiologic Monitoring (ABNM), that provides board certification of candidates. The exam has two parts, written and oral. After passing the written exam, which has 250 questions, candidates are eligible for the oral exam; after passing that, they become diplomats of ABNM.

◆ History

It was not until the early 1970s that IOM came into general use, first for monitoring the integrity of the spinal cord in operations for scoliosis (Brown and Nash, 1979) and later for monitoring of the auditory nerve (Grundy, 1983) and cranial motor nerves (Møller, 1987). But it was perhaps preservation of the facial nerve in operations for vestibular schwannomas that first demonstrated the benefits from the use of electrophysiologic methods in the operating room. Such methods made it possible to assist in finding the facial nerve to remove vestibular schwannomas and test its function. Being able to find the facial nerve, naturally, is a prerequisite for being able to preserve its function. Krauze (1912) is reported to have used electrical stimulation of the facial nerve in the operative field during removal of vestibular schwannomas. Only a few reports on the use of facial nerve monitoring appeared in the 1960s (Hilger, 1964; Jako, 1965), and monitoring of facial function in operations for vestibular schwannoma did not gain common use in such operations until the late 1970s (Delgado et al, 1979; Harner et al, 1988; Kartush and Bouchard, 1992; Lanser et al, 1992; Møller and Jannetta, 1984; Prass and Lueders, 1986; Sugita and Kobayashi, 1982; Yingling and Gardi, 1992). (For details, see Møller, 2006b.)

Monitoring the function of the auditory nerve in microvascular decompression operations for hemifacial spasm and for face pain was described in the 1980s (Fischer, 1989; Friedman et al, 1985; Grundy, 1983; Linden et al, 1988; Møller et al, 1983; Radtke et al, 1989; Raudzens, 1982) and

gained general use during the following decade. During that period, the use of electrophysiologic methods for preserving neural function increased rapidly.

Besides the facial nerve and the auditory-vestibular nerve, which are at risk in operations in the cerebellopontine angle (CPA), several cranial nerves are at risk of being injured in operations to remove large tumors of the brain that are located near the base of the skull (skull base tumors). When operations were developed to treat skull base tumors other than vestibular schwannomas (Sekhar and Møller, 1986; Sekhar and Schramm, 1987), IOM helped to reduce the risks of neurologic deficits (Møller, 1987; Yingling, 1994; Yingling and Ashram, 2005). These major neurosurgical operations involve a high risk of permanent neurologic deficit from surgical injuries to many different kinds of neural tissue. The development of the surgical technique used in these operations also benefited from the use of the electrophysiologic methods intraoperatively because such techniques can identify specific neural structures. That was important because the normal anatomy was often distorted by such tumors (for details about monitoring in skull base operations, see Møller, 2006b).

◆ Principles of Intraoperative Monitoring

The use of intraoperative monitoring as a means to decrease the risk of postoperative neurologic deficits is based on the assumption that surgical manipulations cause measurable changes in conduction in nerves and fiber tracts before permanent injuries to the nerve fibers occur. In a similar way, it is assumed that synaptic transmission becomes impaired and may even cease to occur before permanent injury to the nerve cells in question occurs. To reduce the risk of permanent injury, changes in neural function are detected as soon as possible after the injury has occurred and before they reach a level where the injury leads to permanent neurologic deficits.

Conduction in nerves and fiber tracts in the brain and synaptic transmission in nuclei can be monitored intraoperatively by recording sensory evoked potentials or by recording evoked responses directly from exposed neural tissue. Nerve conduction in peripheral nerves can be monitored by electrically stimulating a nerve and recording compound action potentials (CAPs) from the nerve. The function of motor nerves can be monitored by recording EMG potentials from the muscles they innervate.

The person who performs the monitoring must inform the surgeon when a change in function has occurred, and that person must describe which neural structures are affected and what surgical manipulations caused the injury to occur. That emphasizes the importance of informing the surgeon as soon as possible after a change in function has occurred. The recording techniques used in the operating room must be chosen with this in mind. It is important that the recorded neuroelectric potentials reflect the function of the structures that are at risk.

◆ Monitoring Sensory Systems

The auditory nerve is at risk in many neurosurgical operations that involve the CPA. Microvascular decompression (MVD) operations for hemifacial spasm and trigeminal neuralgia involve a risk of injuring the intracranial portions of the auditory (and vestibular) nerves. More common are operations for vestibular schwannomas (earlier known as acoustic tumors or vestibular neurinomas) where the auditory nerve is at risk because it is directly involved in the tumor. Many patients with vestibular schwannomas already have hearing loss. Preservation of hearing is feasible in operations for small vestibular schwannomas if the patient has good hearing before the operation. However, many of the reports on statistics of preserving hearing in small vestibular neurinomas only concern the pure-tone thresholds, and many of these patients have poor speech discrimination and often worse tinnitus following surgery. Monitoring of auditory evoked potentials is also used in operations where the brainstem is being manipulated.

The somatosensory system is monitored in connection with operations on peripheral nerves and on the central nervous system (CNS), such as for aneurysms. Monitoring of the visual system is rarely done, but it has some value in operations for pituitary tumors. Monitoring of the somatosensory and visual systems will not be further discussed in this chapter, and interested readers are referred to Møller (2006b).

Most of the electrophysiologic methods used in IOM are similar to those used for diagnostic purposes. However, the fact that the records obtained in the operating room must be interpreted as soon as they are available requires that the person who performs the IOM be capable of interpreting the recordings that are obtained. It is also important that the surgeon can identify which step in the operation caused the change in function.

Recording Sensory Evoked Potentials in the Operating Room

Sensory evoked potentials such as the auditory brainstem response (ABR) and somatosensory evoked potentials (SSEPs) are far-field potentials that are recorded from electrodes placed on the scalp. The amplitude of such potentials is small, and much smaller than the ongoing electroencephalographic (EEG) activity that is also picked up by the recording electrodes. To make far-field sensory evoked potentials interpretable, the responses to many stimuli must be added (signal averaging). That takes time and thus means a delay in interpretation. Such delay may not be of any great importance when evoked potentials are used in the clinic, but it is a serious obstacle to their use in the operating room for monitoring. A long delay between an injury and its detection may cause the injury to become permanent before it can be reversed. It is difficult to identify which surgical manipulation caused the injury when the time between the occurrence of an injury and its detection is long.

The following list summarizes the factors that are important for obtaining a clean interpretable record in as short a time as possible:

1. Decrease the electrical interference that reaches the recording electrodes.
2. Use an optimal stimulus repetition rate.
3. Use optimal stimulus strength.
4. Use optimal filtering of the recorded potentials.
5. Use optimal placement of recording electrodes.
6. Use quality control that does not require replicating records.

◆ Monitoring Auditory Brainstem Responses

Under the best circumstances, it takes at least 20 seconds to obtain an interpretable ABR record in an individual with normal hearing if the electrical interference is reduced to negligible values and optimal stimulus parameters are used together with aggressive (digital) filtering of the recorded responses. In patients with hearing loss, the time it takes to obtain an interpretable record becomes longer than it is in patients with normal hearing. Electrical interference can make it necessary to average many more responses, which can further increase the time it takes to obtain an interpretable record.

Thus, optimizing stimulation to increase the amplitude of the potentials, selection of optimal recording parameters, and reduction of electrical interference are all factors that can shorten the time it takes to obtain an interpretable record.

Electrical and Magnetic Interference

Electrical interference in the operating room is often large because of all the electronic equipment used, but interference from biological potentials (such as ongoing brain activity, EEG potentials, and electromyographic potentials generated by muscles) may also be noticeable. Alternating magnetic fields such as those produced by power transformers can induce electrical current in electrode leads and thereby appear as electrical interference. Methods for reducing the electrical interference from other equipment are described in detail elsewhere (Møller, 2006b) and will not be repeated here. The interference from muscles is not a problem when the patient is paralyzed, but muscle relaxants cannot be used in operations where EMG potentials are recorded, such as in monitoring the facial nerve.

Filtering

Optimal filtering of the recorded evoked potentials can shorten the time it takes to obtain an interpretable result because it reduces the number of responses that must be collected to obtain an interpretable record (Møller, 2006b).

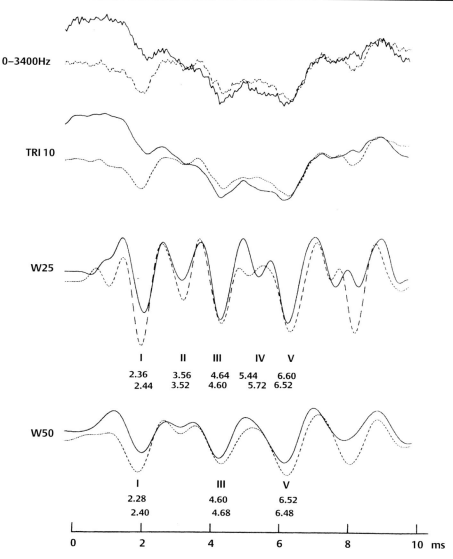

0–3400Hz

TRI 10

W25

I	II	III	IV	V
2.36	3.56	4.64	5.44	6.60
2.44	3.52	4.60	5.72	6.52

W50

I	III	V
2.28	4.60	6.52
2.40	4.68	6.48

0   2   4   6   8   10 ms

Figure 24–1 Effects on the waveform of the auditory brainstem response (ABR) of different types of digital filters. The upper tracing was filtered with electronic filters only; the second tracing from the top (TRI10) shows the same recordings after low-pass filtering with a digital filter that had a triangular weighing function with a base length of 0.4 msec. The two lower tracings show the effects of filtering the same record with two different digital bandpass filters (W25 and W50) that had W-shaped weighing functions (similar to a truncated sin(x)/x function), with the base length being 1 and 2 msec, respectively. The numbers on the two bottom curves are the latency values obtained using computer programs that automatically identified peaks of the ABR and printed their latencies. The two tracings (solid and dashed) show replications. (From Møller, A. R. (1988). Evoked potentials in intraoperative monitoring. Baltimore, MD: Williams & Wilkins, with permission.)

Interpretation of evoked potentials does not require that all the information contained in evoked potentials be preserved. Filtering can eliminate unnecessary parts of the recorded potentials, and that can reduce the number of responses that need to be collected because more noise is eliminated. Modern digital filters, such as zero-phase finite impulse response filters, offer much more flexibility than electronic filters, and it is possible to enhance certain portions of a record that are important for interpretation (Møller, 2006b). **Fig. 24–1** illustrates what can be accomplished by optimal filtering. A clean record allows computer programs to identify the peaks and automatically print out their latencies in ABRs. This can be done without operator intervention, such as using a cursor to identify the peaks and valleys.

Quality Control

Replication of records is the common method for quality control of evoked potentials in the clinic. However, if that method is used in the operating room, it will increase the time it takes to detect changes in function because two interpretable records must be obtained. Better ways of quality control that do not require replication of records have been devised (Hoke et al, 1984; Schimmel, 1967), and such methods are suitable for use in the operating room.

These matters are discussed in detail elsewhere (Møller, 2006b).

Stimulation

The optimal stimuli for recording of the ABR in the operating room are clicks presented at a rate of 30 to 40 per second at an intensity of 100 to 105 dB peak equivalent sound pressure level (pe SPL), corresponding to 65 to 70 dB hearing level (HL) when presented at a rate of 20 clicks per second. The most suitable earphones are the insert type (e.g., the tubephone) or the miniature stereo earphones used in connection with portable tape players (Møller, 2006b). Either rarefaction or condensation clicks should be used. It is not a good idea to use clicks with alternating polarity because the response to condensation and rarefaction clicks is different, particularly in individuals with hearing loss.

Pitfall

- Using clicks with alternating polarity may result in adding responses that may have different waveforms, which decreases the amplitude of the response and can make individual peaks become broader than the peaks elicited by either rarefaction or condensation clicks.

Recording Electrodes

Needle electrodes are more suitable for ABR recordings in the operating room than the conventional surface electrodes, such as gold cup electrodes. It is common to use subdermal platinum needle electrodes such as the Grass Instrument Co. type E2 (Gross Technologies, AST-MED, West Warwick, RI). These are equipped with a lead to connect to the electrode box of the amplifier. The electrodes should be inserted after the patient is anesthetized, and they should be secured by adhesive tape of good quality.

All modern recording amplifiers record the difference between the potentials that are applied to their two inputs. The usual way to record ABRs in the clinic uses an electrode montage, with one electrode placed at the vertex and the other at the ipsilateral earlobe. It is advantageous to use two channels of recordings. The electrodes of one channel should be connected to electrodes placed on the earlobes, and the other channel should record from the vertex and upper neck.

Amplifiers and Filters

Recording electrodes are connected to the main amplifiers through an electrode box. Some modern recording equipment has a preamplifier located in the electrode box. Some types have an analog-to-digital converter located in the electrode box that is connected to the main amplifier via a fiberoptic cable, which is insensitive to electrical or magnetic interference.

The amplification should be set at 50,000×. Use of higher amplification may prolong stimulus artifacts and other interference signals because of overloading. If only electronic filters are used, a setting of 150 to 1500 Hz is suitable. If digital filters are used, the electronic filters in the amplifiers should be set at 10 to 3000 Hz, and the digital filters should be set to enhance the peaks of the ABR (Møller, 2006b).

Interpretation of the Auditory Brainstem Response

The ABR is characterized by a series of peaks and valleys. Interpretation of abnormalities in the ABR has mainly concerned the vertex positive peaks that are traditionally labeled using Roman numerals. The two earliest peaks (I and II) are generated by the distal and the proximal portion of the auditory nerve, respectively. The auditory nerve is ~2.5 cm long (Lang, 1985), and the conduction velocity of the auditory nerve is ~20 m per second (Møller, Colletti, and Fiorino, 1994). This explains the interval of 1.0 to 1.2 msec between peaks I and II. In operations involving the CPA, peak I is not likely to change, but peak II and all following peaks will be affected. Because the changes in the latency of earlier peaks are imposed on later peaks, it is most convenient to use the latency of peak V or III as an indicator of changes in the conduction time in the auditory nerve. The large amplitudes of peaks III and V make them easy to identify, and their latencies can be accurately determined. The amplitude of these peaks is also affected by injuries to the auditory nerve, but the large variability of their amplitudes has detracted from using changes in amplitude as an indicator of trauma. Although it is mainly the latencies of the peaks that have been used as indicators of injuries, studies have shown that the change in amplitude may be a valuable indicator of changes in neural conduction of the auditory nerve (Hatayama and Møller, 1988).

◆ Monitoring Brainstem Structures by Recording the Auditory Brainstem Response

Surgical manipulations of the brainstem may occur in operations of larger tumors of the CPA, such as large vestibular schwannomas. Such manipulations have traditionally been detected by observing changes in cardiovascular parameters, such as heart rate and blood pressure. However, the systems that control the heart are under the influence of feedback systems that tend to keep conditions stable. Therefore, blood pressure and heart rate may not change noticeably until rather large surgical manipulations have been made. Monitoring of the ABR elicited by stimulation of the ear contralateral to the operated side can give earlier warnings about manipulations of the brainstem than observations of cardiac parameters (Angelo and Møller, 1996; Kalmanchey et al, 1986).

When ABR is used to monitor neural conduction in the auditory nerve in the CPA, all peaks except peak I are expected to change when the neural conduction in the auditory nerve is affected and is at risk of being surgically injured. The question is more complex when recording of ABR is used to monitor specific structures of the brainstem. For that use, it is important to know which anatomical structures generate the different components of the ABR.

Neural Generators of the Auditory Brainstem Response

As mentioned above, the earliest two vertex positive peaks of the ABR (peaks I and II) are generated by the auditory nerve. These are the only components of the ABR that have single generators. The subsequent peaks have contributions from more than one structure. Peak III and the following trough (negative peak) are generated mostly by the cochlear nucleus. Less is known about the generators of peak IV, but evidence has been presented that they are located close to the midline (Møller, 2006a), probably the superior olivary complex. The sharp tip of peak V is generated mainly by the lateral lemniscus, probably where it terminates in the inferior colliculus. The slow negative wave that follows peak V (Davis et al, 1979) is probably generated by dendrites in the inferior colliculus. The subsequent peaks of the ABR (VI and VII) may be generated by cells in the inferior colliculus and the brachium of the inferior colliculus, and perhaps by neurons in the medial geniculate body (MGB).

Pearl

- The fact that peaks I and II are generated by the auditory nerve shows that a nerve in the auditory system can generate stationary peaks in recordings made at a long distance from the auditory nerve (far field). It may also be assumed that fiber tracts of the ascending auditory pathway can generate stationary peaks in the ABR. It is less certain, however, that cells in nuclei can generate noticeable far-field potentials, but it has been convincingly demonstrated that the inferior colliculus can generate slow far-field potentials (i.e., a broad peak in the ABR). This component is known as the SN_{10}, for slow negative at 10 msec. (For further details about the neural generators of the ABR, see Møller, 2006a.)

Directly Recording from the Auditory Nervous System

To provide the surgeon with timely information about injuries to the auditory nerve, it is important to obtain an interpretable record in as short a time as possible. Even when all efforts are made to optimize recordings of ABR and under the best circumstances, it takes at least 20 seconds to obtain an interpretable ABR record in an individual with normal hearing. In patients with hearing loss, it may take several times longer. The problems in obtaining an interpretable record in a short time can be overcome by recording evoked potentials directly from exposed portions of the nervous system, because the amplitude of such near-field evoked potentials is much larger than that of the ABR. In fact, the amplitude of the evoked potentials recorded directly from the auditory nerve and the cochlear nucleus are large enough to be interpreted directly, or after only a few responses have been added together (Møller, 2006b). Changes can therefore be detected almost immediately when they occur, which makes it possible to provide the surgeon with nearly instantaneous information

about the function of the auditory nerve. Recordings of the CAPs from the intracranial portion of the auditory nerve is now in routine use (Colletti et al, 1994; Linden et al, 1988; Silverstein et al, 1984) in operations for vestibular schwannomas and in other operations in the CPA (Møller, 2006b). Evoked potentials recorded from the cochlear nucleus (Møller and Jannetta, 1983a; Møller, Jannetta, and Jho, 1994) are also used in other operations where the auditory nerve is at risk of being injured, such as MVD of cranial nerves.

Recording Electrodes

Recordings of evoked potentials from the intracranial portion of the exposed eighth cranial nerve (CN VIII) for monitoring purposes employ a monopolar recording electrode (Møller, 2006b; Møller and Jannetta, 1981, 1983b) that is placed directly on the exposed nerve. The recording electrode should be placed as close to the brainstem as possible because it must be located proximally to the parts of the auditory nerve that are at risk of being injured. The electrode wire should be tucked under the sutures that hold the dura open (**Fig. 24–2**) to minimize the risk that surgical manipulations dislocate the recording electrode.

A suitable monopolar recording electrode can be made from a multistrand Teflon-insulated silver wire with a small cotton wick sutured to its uninsulated tip, which is bent over, using a 5–0 silk suture (**Fig. 24–2**). The purpose of the cotton wick is to reduce the risk of injury to the auditory nerve and to obtain more stable recordings than can be obtained by using a metal electrode in direct contact with the auditory nerve. It is imperative that the cotton be sutured well to the wire so that it is not lost inside the brain. If that is a concern, cotton can be replaced by shredded Teflon felt, which does not cause inflammatory reactions if accidentally left in the brain. It is important that the wire be flexible so that it does not injure the nerve on which it is placed, yet stiff enough that it will remain in position.

Pearl

- When recording from neural tissue for research purposes, bipolar recording electrodes are often used because such electrodes are more spatially selective (i.e., record from more specific neural structures). Bipolar recording electrodes have been used in recordings from the auditory nerve for research purposes and for finding the cleavage plane between the vestibular and auditory nerves (Møller et al, 1994b; Rosenberg et al, 1993). However, there is little reason to use bipolar electrodes for monitoring neural conduction in the auditory nerve because other neural structures that might contribute to the response are located anatomically far from the auditory nerve, and their contributions to the recordings from the auditory nerve using a monopolar electrode are small. It is more difficult to place a bipolar recording electrode on the exposed CN VIII.

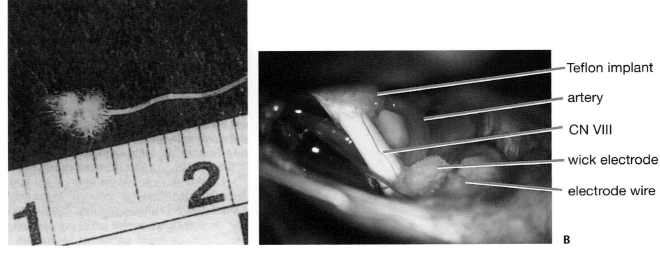

Figure 24–2 (A) Wick electrode used for intracranial recordings. The small divisions on the scale are millimeters. (From Møller, A. R. (1988). Evoked potentials in intraoperative monitoring. Baltimore, MD: Williams & Wilkins, with permission) **(B)** Placement of a wick recording electrode on the eighth cranial nerve (CN VIII) for an operation to relieve hemifacial spasm. (From Møller, A. R. (2006). Intraoperative neurophysiologic monitoring (2nd ed.). Totowa, NJ: Humana Press, with permission.) **(See Color Plate 24–2B.)**

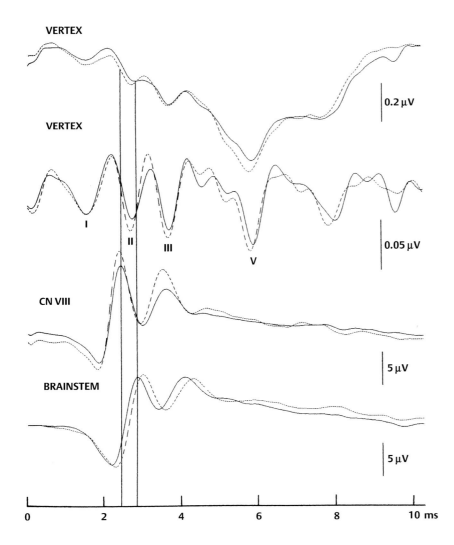

Figure 24–3 Comparison of the auditory brainstem responses recorded from electrodes placed on the vertex without digital filtering (upper tracings) and with digital filtering (second tracings). Vertex positivity is a downward deflection. Compound action potentials are recorded from the exposed eighth cranial nerve (CN VIII) at two different locations, near the porus acusticus and near the brainstem. Solid lines indicate the responses to rarefaction clicks; dashed lines, the responses to condensation clicks (105 dB peak equivalent sound pressure level [pe SPL]). The results were obtained in a patient with normal hearing undergoing a microvascular decompression operation.

Amplifiers

The recording electrode should be connected to the inverting input so that a negative potential results in an upward deflection. The other input to the amplifier should be connected to a needle electrode (reference electrode) placed in the wound. The shielded cable should be anchored at the drape with a towel clip so that accidental pulling of that cable will not dislocate the electrode. The filters should be set at 30 to 3000 Hz, and no digital filtering is required.

Stimuli

The same stimuli as used for recording ABR are suitable for eliciting direct-recorded evoked potentials from the auditory nerve.

Responses

A CAP recorded from the exposed auditory nerve in response to click stimulation is shown in **Fig. 24–3**, together with the simultaneously recorded ABR. The CAP has a triphasic waveform, typical for the response recorded with a monopolar electrode from a long nerve, in which a brief depolarization travels past the recording electrode. The initial positive deflection is generated when the region of depolarization approaches the recording electrode, and the main negative peak occurs when the depolarization passes under the recording electrode. The positive deflection that follows is generated when the depolarization moves away from the location of the recording electrode (Lorente de No, 1947[l]; Møller, 2006b). The latency of the large negative peak of the CAP is approximately the same as peak II of the ABR (**Fig. 24–3**). The latency of the CAP increases with decreasing stimulus intensity, and the amplitude decreases (**Fig. 24–4**).

Interpreting Potentials Recorded from the Auditory Nerve

The waveform of the CAP is closely related to the discharge pattern of auditory nerve fibers (Goldstein, 1960) and thus provides more direct information about abnormalities in the discharge pattern than the ABR.

When a monopolar recording electrode is placed on CN VIII close to the brainstem, passively conducted potentials from the cochlear nucleus may contribute to the recorded potentials, but these potentials will have longer latencies than those caused by propagated neural activity in the auditory nerve. Comparison between bipolar and monopolar recordings from the exposed CN VIII have confirmed that the CAP recorded by a monopolar electrode for the most part reflects propagated neural activity in the auditory nerve (Møller, 2006b; Møller et al, 1994b). The slow deflection seen to occur at latencies longer than that of the initial triphasic waveform probably has noticeable contributions from the cochlear nucleus. These components are more prominent in the responses to low-intensity clicks, and they are probably generated by dendrites of cochlear nucleus cells and conducted passively to the recording site on CN VIII from the cochlear nucleus (**Fig. 24–4**). Many

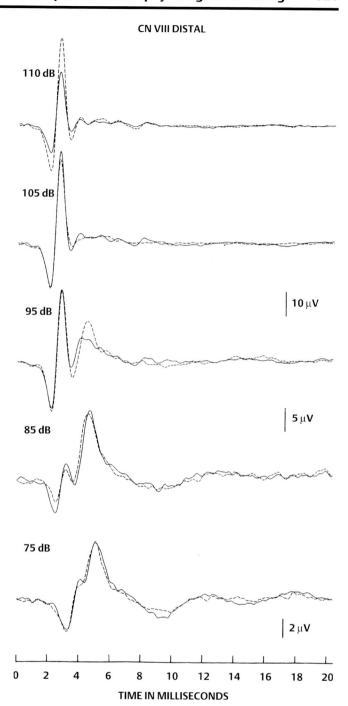

CN VIII DISTAL

Figure 24–4 Compound action potentials recorded from the intracranial portion of the eighth cranial nerve (CN VIII) in a patient with normal hearing undergoing a microvascular decompression operation for trigeminal neuralgia. The stimuli were rarefaction clicks (solid lines) and condensation clicks (dashed lines). The stimulus intensity is given by legend numbers, in dB pe SPL (peak equivalent sound pressure level). (From Møller, A. R. (1993). Direct eighth nerve compound action potential measurements during cerebellopontine angle surgery. In D. Hoehmann (Ed.), Proceedings of the First International Conference on EcoG, OAE, and Intraoperative Monitoring (pp. 275–280). Amsterdam: Kugler, with permission.)

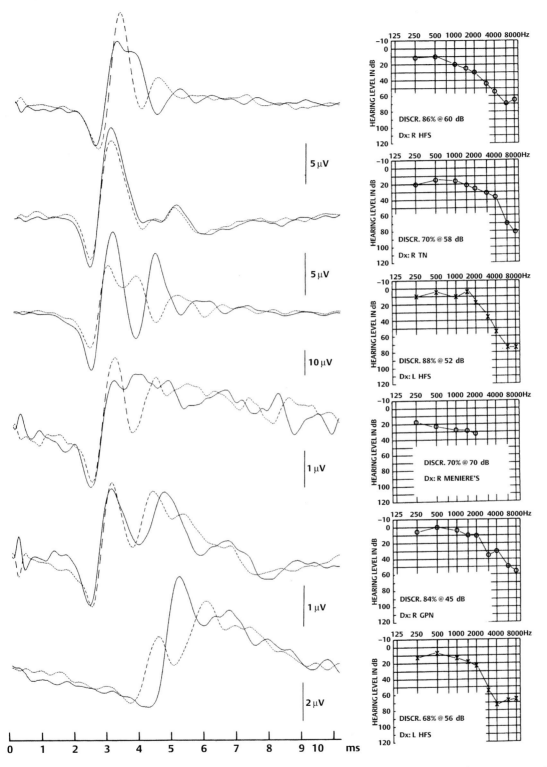

Figure 24–5 Examples of recordings from the exposed intracranial portion of the eighth cranial nerve (CN VIII) in patients with different degrees of hearing loss. The recordings were obtained during microvascular decompression operations before CN VIII was manipulated. The diagnosis is given below the pure-tone audiograms. (From Møller, A. R., & Jho, H. D. (1991). Effect of high frequency hearing loss on compound action potentials recorded from the intracranial portion of the human eighth nerve. Hearing Research, 55, 9–23, with permission.)

patients who are operated upon have hearing loss before the operation, and that can affect the waveform of the CAP, which depends on the degree of hearing loss (**Fig. 24–5**) and the nature of the pathology that causes the hearing loss. Additionally, the waveform of the CAP in response to condensation and rarefaction clicks is similar in patients with normal hearing, but it is often very different in patients with hearing loss. The amplitude and the waveform of the responses to clicks of opposite polarity may differ considerably in patients with hearing loss, and in some individuals, the CAP in response to clicks exhibits several waves (damped oscillations) that may last more than 10 msec (**Fig. 24–5;** see Møller and Jho, 1991b). The waveform of such prolonged oscillations reverses with reversing click polarity, suggesting that these waves are the result of abnormal motion of the basilar membrane and not a sign of abnormal neural conduction in the auditory nerve.

Pearl

- Action potentials of auditory nerve fibers are initiated mainly when the basilar membrane is deflected in one direction. Therefore, potentials that are related to the discharges in the auditory nerve, such as the CAP recorded from the intracranial portion, will also be related to the deflection of the basilar membrane. The CAP is the sum of the neural activity in many nerve fibers, and CAPs with large amplitudes are associated with simultaneous discharges in many nerve fibers. The normal traveling wave motion of the basilar membrane does not generate such synchronous activity, only the initial deflection of the basilar membrane. That is the reason the normal CAP is a single peak (N1). Only when large parts of the basilar membrane vibrate in phase can prolonged oscillations occur. A standing wave motion, caused by reflections from a certain point on the basilar membrane, is a plausible explanation for these prolonged oscillations.

Changes in the Compound Action Potentials from Injury to the Auditory Nerve

Injury from surgical manipulations of CN VIII that cause changes in neural conduction result in different kinds of changes in the CAP when recorded from a point that is central to the location of the injury. Such an injury may occur from a slight stretching of the auditory nerve, causing a slowing of neural conduction (decrease in conduction velocity) and an increase in the latency of the CAP (**Fig. 24–6**). The auditory nerve is particularly sensitive to injury from stretching at the point at which it passes through the area called the cribrosa. Even slight stretching may cause small bleedings in the nerve in that region (Sekiya and Møller, 1987). More severe stretching also causes broadening of the negative peak of the CAP and decreased amplitude, because the increase in conduction time is different for different nerve fibers. More severe injuries may cause some nerve fibers to cease conducting nerve impulses, which results in an increase in the amplitude of the initial positive deflection and a decrease in the

amplitude of the negative peak (**Fig. 24–6**). (Notice the difference in the response to condensation and rarefaction clicks that is typical in patients with hearing loss.) If all fibers cease to conduct nerve impulses at a location that is distal to the recording electrode, the CAP will become reduced to a single positive deflection (**Fig. 24–7**). This is what is known as a "cut end" potential, which can be recorded from a nerve that has been cut or crushed (Lorente de No, 1947; Møller, 2006b).

Severe injury to the auditory nerve that causes arrest of neural propagation (**Fig. 24–7**) can be caused by heat transferred from electrocoagulation of a vein close to the auditory nerve. Bipolar radiofrequency coagulation that is now the standard form of electrocoagulation used in the brain leaks only a very small amount of radiofrequency current, compared with monopolar electrocoagulation, which was previously used. However, bipolar electrocoagulation does use heat to coagulate tissue, which may be transferred to neural tissue and cause irreversible damage. The transfer of heat can be reduced by placing heat-insulating material between the nerve and the site of coagulation or by using the coagulator at the lowest possible setting. Coagulating in several short spurts instead of one long burn is also effective in reducing the injury to nervous tissue.

Directly Recording Potentials from the Cochlear Nucleus

When recording directly from the auditory nerve during operations for vestibular schwannomas, it may be difficult to keep the recording electrode in its correct position because of its proximity to the tumor. A better solution to direct recording is to place the recording electrode on (or close to) the surface of the cochlear nucleus (Kuroki and Møller, 1995; Møller and Jannetta, 1983a; Møller, Jannetta, and Jho, 1994). The surface of the cochlear nucleus is the floor of the lateral recess of the fourth ventricle, and a recording electrode placed here will record evoked potentials from the cochlear nucleus (Møller and Jannetta, 1983a). The electrode can be placed so that it will not be dislocated by surgical manipulations in removing a tumor from CN VIII. This is the main advantage of recording from the cochlear nucleus over recording from the exposed auditory nerve.

Recording Electrodes

The same wick electrode as described above for recording from the exposed auditory nerve is also suitable for recordings from the cochlear nucleus. The lateral recess can be reached through the foramen of Luschka, which is located dorsal to the entrance of CN IX and X (Kuroki and Møller, 1995; Møller, Jannetta, and Jho, 1994). Often, a small tuft of choroid plexus can be seen protruding from that opening, but it may be shrunk by electrocoagulation to make room for the recording electrode. In fact, suitable recordings can be obtained by placing the recording electrode on the brainstem, dorsal to the entrance of CN IX and X.

BEFORE MANIPULATION

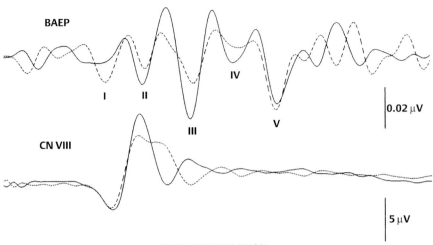

BAEP

I   II   IV   V

III

0.02 μV

CN VIII

5 μV

AFTER MANIPULATION

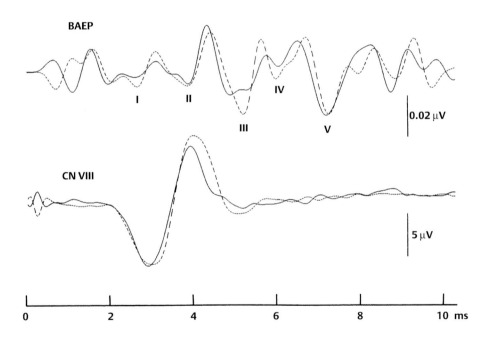

BAEP

I   II   IV   V

III

0.02 μV

CN VIII

5 μV

0   2   4   6   8   10 ms

Figure 24–6 Comparison of the auditory brainstem response (ABR) and the compound action potential recorded from the exposed eighth cranial nerve (CN VIII) before (top tracing) and after (bottom tracing) the eighth nerve was stretched to show the effect of slight injury to the auditory nerve and to the ABR. Top recordings were obtained in the beginning of the operation, and the bottom recordings were obtained after surgical manipulations of the eighth nerve. BAEP, brainstem auditory evoked potential. (From Møller, A. R., & Jannetta, P. J. (1983). Monitoring auditory functions during cranial nerve microvascular decompression operations by direct recording from the eighth nerve. Journal of Neurosurgery, 59, 493–499, with permission.)

When the electrode wire is placed along the caudal wall of the wound and tucked under the dura sutures, it is far away from the area of operation and is not at risk of being dislocated or caught by the drill used on the wall of the porus acusticus (see **Fig. 24–8**, p. 526).

Responses

The recorded potentials from the cochlear nucleus have nearly the same amplitude as those recorded from the exposed auditory nerve (see **Fig. 24–9**, p. 526). The response to transient sounds consists of an initial positive-negative deflection that signals the arrival of a volley of nerve impulses from the auditory nerve, followed by a slow nega-

tive deflection that represents electrical activity from cells in the cochlear nucleus. Recordings from the cochlear nucleus reflect injuries to the auditory nerve in a similar way as those recorded from the proximal portion of the auditory nerve. The initial positive-negative deflection is probably a better indicator of injury to the auditory nerve than the slow potential that follows.

Use of Electrocochleography to Monitor Auditory Function

As a means of obtaining auditory evoked potentials of larger amplitude than the ABR, some investigators have used recordings of electrocochleography (ECoG) potentials for monitoring purposes (Levine et al, 1984; Sabin et al,

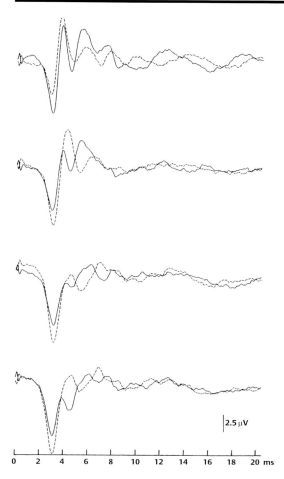

Figure 24–7 The effect of heating from electrocoagulation on the compound action potential recorded from the exposed intracranial portion of the eighth cranial nerve (CN VIII) in an individual with preoperative hearing loss. The top recording was obtained before coagulation, and the recordings below that were obtained with short time intervals during electrocoagulation of a vein close to CN VIII. The solid line indicates responses to rarefaction clicks; dashed lines indicate responses to condensation clicks. (From Møller, A R. (1988). Evoked potentials in intraoperative monitoring. Baltimore, MD: Williams & Wilkins, with permission.)

1987) However, ECoG potentials only reflect the neural activity in the most distal portion of the auditory nerve. The intracranial portion of the auditory nerve can therefore be injured without any noticeable change in the ECoG.

Pitfall

- The intracranial portion of the auditory nerve can be injured and even severed without any detectable change occurring in the electrocochleogram (ECoGm). Only if the blood supply to the cochlea is compromised will the ECoG potentials change noticeably. That means recording of ECoG potentials is not suitable for monitoring neural conduction in the auditory nerve in operations where the intracranial portion of the auditory nerve is at risk.

◆ Monitoring the Vestibular Nerve

The vestibular nerve cannot be monitored as readily as the auditory nerve, but protecting the auditory nerve from injury can also help to protect the vestibular nerve from injuries because these two nerves are close to each other. Manipulations that affect the auditory nerve will most likely also affect neural conduction in the vestibular nerve. The postoperative consequences of injuries to the vestibular nerve are not as obvious as those that follow from injuries to the auditory nerve, but many people with surgically induced hearing loss also experience vestibular symptoms, indicating that the vestibular nerve has been injured in addition to the injury of the auditory nerve (Sekiya et al, 1991).

◆ Monitoring Cranial Motor Nerves

Cranial motor nerves are at risk in surgical operations to remove tumors located at the base of the skull (there are 12 cranial nerves—some are sensory nerves, some are motor nerves, and some are part of the autonomic nervous system; see **Table 24–1**). The most common skull base tumor is the vestibular schwannoma, and operations to remove vestibular schwannomas place the auditory and facial nerves at risk. The facial nerve runs close to the auditory-vestibular nerve, and it is at eminent risk of being injured during removal of vestibular schwannoma. In addition to protecting the auditory nerve, it is always important to reduce the risks of injuries to the facial nerve that may result in facial weakness, synkinesis, or facial palsy. Impairment or loss of facial function has severe consequences and affects the entire life of a person.

Monitoring the Facial Nerve in Operations to Remove Vestibular Schwannomas

Intraoperative monitoring of the facial nerve has been the model for monitoring other cranial motor nerves. The methods used for stimulation have been little changed, but the methods for detecting when the facial muscles contract have been different. Earlier, the patient's face was observed by the surgeon or by an assistant. This was replaced by the use of electronic sensors introduced by Sugita and Kobayashi (1982) and further developed by other investigators (Silverstein et al, 1984). Later, the use of recordings of EMG potentials became the method of choice for detecting contraction of facial muscles (Møller, 2006b; Møller and Jannetta, 1984; Prass and Lueders, 1986; Yingling and Gardi, 1992).

Special Consideration

- Efforts have been made to develop methods for monitoring neural conduction in the facial nerve using other techniques than recordings of muscle contractions, but so far none of these methods have reached a level of development that make any of them a practical alternative.

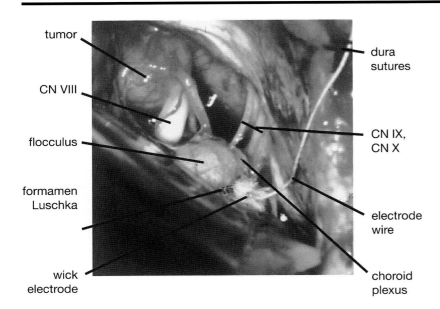

tumor

CN VIII

flocculus

formamen
Luschka

wick
electrode

dura
sutures

CN IX,
CN X

electrode
wire

choroid
plexus

Figure 24–8 Placement of the recording electrode in the lateral recess of the fourth ventricle. (From Møller, A. R., Jho, H. D., & Jannetta, P. J. (1994). Preservation of hearing in operations on acoustic tumors: An alternative to recording BAEP. Neurosurgery, 34, 688–693, with permission.) *(See Color Plate 24-8.)*

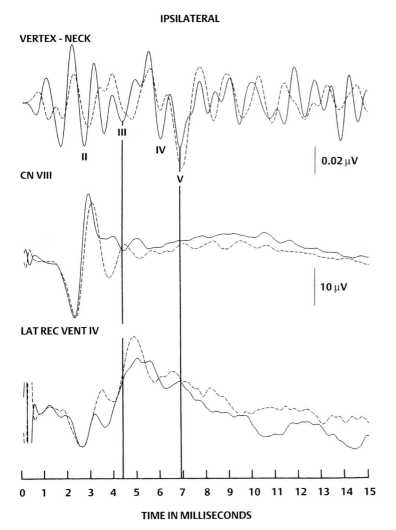

IPSILATERAL

VERTEX - NECK

III

II   IV

V

0.02 µV

CN VIII

10 µV

LAT REC VENT IV

0 1 2 3 4 5 6 7 8 9 10 11 12 13 14 15

TIME IN MILLISECONDS

Figure 24–9 Comparison of the auditory brainstem response (upper tracings: digitally filtered as in **Fig. 24–6**), together with the responses recorded from the exposed eighth cranial nerve (CN VIII; middle tracings) and the responses recorded from an electrode placed in the lateral recess of the fourth ventricle (lower tracings), as shown in **Fig. 24–8.** Solid line indicates responses to rarefaction clicks; dashed line indicates responses to condensation clicks. All recordings were obtained at about the same time during an operation to relieve hemifacial spasm. (From Møller, A. R., Jho, H. D., & Jannetta, P. J. (1994). Preservation of hearing in operations on acoustic tumors: An alternative to recording BAEP. Neurosurgery, 34, 688–693, with permission.)

Table 24–1   The Main Functions of Cranial Nerves

Nerve	Type	Function	Description
I	Olfactory	Sensory	Smell
II	Optic	Sensory	Vision
III	Oculomotor	Motor	Eye movements: innervates all extraocular muscles, except the superior oblique and lateral rectus muscles; innervates the striated muscle of the eyelid
		Autonomic	Mediates pupillary constriction and accommodation for near vision
IV	Trochlearis	Motor	Eye movements: innervates the superior oblique muscle
V	Trigeminal	Sensory	Mediates cutaneous and proprioceptive sensations from skin, muscles, and joints in the face and mouth, including the teeth, and from the anterior two thirds of the tongue
		Motor	Innervates muscles of mastication
VI	Abducens	Motor	Eye movements: innervates the lateral rectus muscle
VII	Facial	Motor	Innervates muscles of facial expression
		Autonomic	Lacrimal and salivary glands
		Sensory	Mediates taste and possibly sensation from part of the face (behind the ear)
	Nervous intermedius		Pain around the ear; possibly taste
VIII	Vestibulocochlear	Sensory	Hearing
			Equilibrium, postural reflexes, orientation of the head in space
IX	Glossopharyngeal	Sensory	Taste
		Sensory	Swallowing: mediates Innervates taste buds in the posterior third of the tongue visceral sensation from palate and posterior third of the tongue; innervates the carotid body
		Motor	Muscles in posterior throat (stylopharyngeal muscle)
		Autonomic	Parotid gland
X	Vagus	Sensory	Mediates visceral sensation from the pharynx, larynx, thorax, and abdomen
			Innervates the skin in the ear canal and taste buds in the epiglottis
		Autonomic	Contains autonomic fibers that innervate smooth muscle in heart, blood vessels, trachea, bronchi, esophagus, stomach, and intestine
		Motor	Innervates striated muscles in the soft palate, pharynx, and larynx
XI	Spinal accessory	Motor	Innervates the trapezius and sternocleidomastoid muscles
XII	Hypoglossal	Motor	Innervates intrinsic muscles of the tongue

From Møller, A. R. (1995). Intraoperative neurophysiologic monitoring. Luxembourg: Harwood Academic Publishers.

Stimuli

A handheld stimulating electrode is used to probe the operative field. A return electrode is placed in the wound. Electrical stimulation of a nerve can use constant current, constant voltage, or a mixture of these two (Møller, 2006b; Møller and Jannetta, 1984; Yingling, 1994; Yingling and Gardi, 1992). Constant current means that the stimulator delivers electrical current that is independent of the resistance of the tissue that is being stimulated. An electrode connected to a constant voltage stimulator applies a constant voltage to the tissue with which the stimulating electrode is in contact. This means that the current that flows through the tissue that is being stimulated depends on the electrical resistance of the tissue. For stimulating the facial nerve in the operative field during removal of vestibular schwannomas, it is preferable to use constant (or semiconstant) voltage rather than constant current

because constant voltage stimulation will deliver a stimulus to the facial nerve that is less dependent on how wet the operative field is. The current delivered to a nerve using constant current stimulation will vary with the electrical conductivity of the surrounding media (Møller, 2006b; Møller and Jannetta, 1984; Yingling, 1994; Yingling and Gardi, 1992).

Recording EMG Potentials

As for recording the ABR, needle electrodes are preferred to surface electrodes for recording of EMG potentials because they provide a stable recording condition over a longer period (Møller, 2006b; Møller and Jannetta, 1984). Some investigators have advocated recording from muscles of the upper and lower face separately by using two amplifiers. One is connected to electrodes placed in the forehead and the orbicularis oculi (the muscle around the eye); the other is connected to electrodes placed in the orbicularis oris (the muscle around the mouth) and in the nasal fold. Because the objective is not to differentiate between contractions of muscles of the upper and lower face, some experts recommend recording EMG potentials in only one channel with electrodes placed in the upper and lower face (Møller, 2006b; see **Fig. 24–10**). Such recordings will reveal contractions of most muscles of the face, including the masseter and temporalis muscles. The motor portion of the trigeminal nerve innervates these muscles; thus, stimulation of the trigeminal nerve will result in EMG activity that might be misinterpreted as arising from stimulation of the facial nerve. However, the EMG response from the facial nerve can easily be distinguished from that of the trigeminal nerve because of the much longer latency of the response from facial muscles compared with those innervated by the trigeminal nerve (6.5–8.0 msec vs 1.5–2.0 msec; **Fig. 24–11**). A second amplifier may become more useful when connected to electrodes placed in the masseter muscle (**Fig. 24–10**) to record from muscles innervated by the (motor) trigeminal nerve. This makes it easier to differentiate between the responses from muscles innervated by the facial and the trigeminal nerves, including activity elicited by mechanical stimulation of the respective nerves, as well as activity caused by injuries to these nerves.

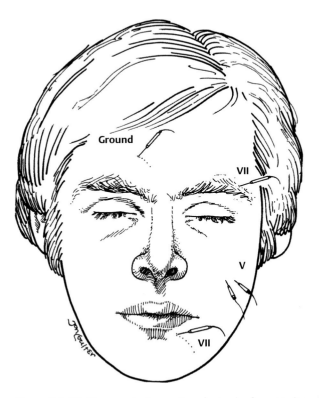

Figure 24–10 Placement of recording electrodes for recording electromyographic potentials from face muscles. Also shown is how recording can be done from the masseter muscle. V, fifth cranial nerve; VII, seventh cranial nerve. (From Møller, A. R. (1995). Intraoperative neurophysiologic monitoring. Luxembourg: Harwood Academic Publishers, with permission.)

Pearl

- It is now common to make the EMG potentials audible through a loudspeaker (Møller and Jannetta, 1984; Prass and Lueders, 1986) so that the surgeon can hear when electrical stimulations cause a contraction of facial muscles. Some commercial equipment uses the recorded EMG potentials to trigger a tone to signal that muscle contractions have occurred. However, the EMG signal contains valuable information that is lost if it is used to trigger a tone. When the recorded EMG potentials are made audible, the stimulus artifacts will be disturbing and could mask the sound of the EMG potentials. The stimulus artifact can, however, be easily prevented from reaching the audio amplifier by a suitable gating circuit (Møller and Jannetta, 1984).

Practical Aspects of Monitoring the Facial Nerve in Operations to Remove Vestibular Schwannomas

Monitoring of the facial nerve in operations for vestibular schwannomas has three purposes: finding areas of the tumor where there is no part of the facial nerve present, identifying the anatomical location of the facial nerve, and detecting when the facial nerve has been injured.

Finding Areas of a Tumor Where There Is No Part of the Facial Nerve Present   When operating on a large vestibular schwannoma, the first use of facial nerve monitoring is to identify regions of the tumor where there are no parts of the facial nerve present. This is done by probing the regions of the tumor with the handheld stimulating electrode. It should be done immediately after the tumor has been exposed and before any part of the tumor is being removed, while observing facial muscle contractions. When the parts of the tumor where there is no response have been identified, indicating that there is no part of facial nerve in the tumor mass that is probed, they can be removed safely. This form of monitoring allows the surgeon to remove large volumes of the tumor without risk of injuring the facial nerve, shortening the operation. It also gives the surgeon an increased feeling of security, in addition to decreasing the risk of permanent postoperative impairment of facial function.

At this point in a surgical procedure, preservation of the facial nerve depends on the absence of a response. Unfortunately, the absence of a response can also be caused by malfunction of equipment, including recording and stimulating electrodes, and by using too low a stimulus intensity. Therefore, this form of electrical stimulation places a greater demand on the settings of the stimulus intensity and on the reliability of electrodes and electronic equipment. The stimulus strength must be sufficient to activate the facial nerve at a small distance, but the stimulus strengths should not be so strong that it activates the facial nerve at too large a distance, because that would result in a response from large parts of the tumor where there is no nerve present. The greatest risk is to have too low a stimulus strength, because that might

STIM
CN VII

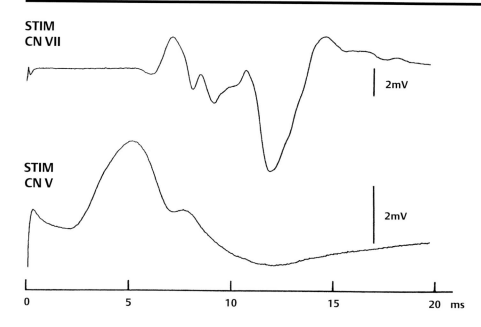

2mV

STIM
CN V

2mV

Figure 24–11 Electromyographic potentials recorded from electrodes placed on the face, as shown in **Fig. 24–10**, when the intracranial portion of the facial nerve (seventh cranial nerve, CN VII) was stimulated electrically (upper tracing) and when the portio minor of the fifth cranial nerve (CN V) was stimulated (lower tracing). (From Møller A. R. (1995). Intraoperative neurophysiologic monitoring. Luxembourg: Harwood Academic Publishers, with permission.)

0   5   10   15   20   ms

lead to the conclusion that a certain amount of tumor tissue could be safely removed, when in fact it might contain parts of the facial nerve that then would be destroyed.

Equipment failure or misplacement of recording electrodes that prevent recording of facial muscle contractions would give the surgeon the impression that no facial nerve was present in the tumor volume probed, when in actuality the nerve was present. Extracting a portion of the tumor that contains parts of the facial nerve would cause severe injury to the facial nerve. To reduce that risk, the recording and stimulation system must be tested meticulously before its use. The best way of testing the facial nerve monitoring equipment is to stimulate the facial nerve before tumor removal begins. This can be done in operations for tumors that do not reach the brainstem and where the facial nerve can be observed before it enters the tumor. It is usually not possible in operations for large tumors, so other methods must be used. Observation of the stimulus artifact in the EMG recording displayed on a computer screen is a useful indicator that the stimulator is delivering a current and that the EMG amplifier is working, but it does not guarantee that the stimulation is sufficient to elicit a facial muscle contraction or that the amplifiers of the EMG potentials work correctly. One common cause of failure is when the return electrode for the stimulator, usually a needle placed in the wound, becomes dislocated. That would eliminate any stimulus current to be delivered by the handheld probe, but it may not necessarily abolish the stimulus artifact.

Another serious risk of failure to elicit a muscle contraction is that the patient has inadvertently been paralyzed, a situation that would not be revealed by observing the stimulus artifact. This risk is reduced when the team that is performing the intraoperative monitoring keeps in close contact with the anesthesia team, allowing the monitoring team to know if changes were made in administering anesthesia, such as adding neuromuscular blocking agents.

Identifying the Anatomical Location of the Facial Nerve
When the bulk of a large tumor has been removed, the task

of facial nerve monitoring is to help find the facial nerve so that the surgeon knows at all times where it is located. Probing the surgical field with the handheld electrical stimulator can help identify the anatomical location of the facial nerve. If moving the stimulating electrode results in an increase in the amplitude of the recorded EMG response, then the facial nerve is located in the direction the electrode was moved. If moving the electrode results in a smaller response, the electrode was moved away from the nerve. The use of this method requires frequent adjustments of the stimulus strength to keep the response below its maximal amplitude, and it requires a close collaboration between the person who does the monitoring and the surgeon.

The facial nerve is often divided in several parts, and it should therefore not be assumed that the entire facial nerve has been found when a response to electrical stimulation has been obtained. The entire operative field must be explored with the facial nerve stimulator so that all parts of the facial nerve can be found.

Pitfall

- Probing the surgical field with a surgical instrument to find the location of the facial nerve should never be used as a substitute for probing the surgical field with a handheld electrical stimulation electrode. The reason that surgical manipulations of the facial nerve often elicit facial muscle activity is most likely that the nerve is injured. A normal nerve has a low degree of sensitivity to mechanical manipulations.

Testing the Integrity of the Facial Nerve   Testing the integrity of the facial nerve can be done by stimulating the facial nerve with the handheld probe and examining the EMG response. It is a sign of deteriorating function when the amplitude of the EMG response decreases and its latency increases. The threshold of the facial nerve for electrical stimulation may increase when the nerve is injured, but it may also decrease, which means that threshold is not a valuable measure of the integrity of the nerve. When the facial nerve's integrity is tested, it must be stimulated at its most proximal location close to the brainstem.

Continuous Monitoring of Facial Muscle Activity   Methods for continuous monitoring of the integrity of the facial nerve, such as is done for the auditory nerve, have not been described. Monitoring of the activity-evoked facial nerve can be a great help in reducing the risk of injury to the facial nerve. Continuous monitoring of EMG activity without electrical stimulation of the facial nerve is valuable for identifying manipulations that may cause injuries to the facial nerve. Removing parts of a tumor that adhere to the facial nerve is a challenge because it can cause injury to the nerve. Safe removal of such tumor tissue is facilitated by listening to the EMG activity that is elicited by the surgical manipulations of the facial nerve or activity elicited by injury to the facial nerve. Such activity may have several different forms, and the nature of the sound generated by the EMG activity provides information about the risks of postoperative impairments of facial function. The activity that causes the least concern is the EMG activity that is a direct response to touching the nerve with a surgical instrument and that stops immediately when the manipulation stops. The activity that continues after the manipulation is stopped may suggest a greater risk of permanent impairment of facial function. The risk of permanent impairment increases with the length of time that such activity lasts and by the number of times during the operation that surgical manipulations of the facial nerve have caused such activity. Surgically induced muscle activity should therefore be reduced as much as possible. That can best be achieved by making the EMG activity audible so that the surgeon can hear the activity and moderate the surgical manipulations accordingly (Møller, 2006b; Møller and Jannetta, 1984; Prass and Lueders, 1986). It is also important that the EMG activity of all facial muscles is represented in the audible EMG so that manipulations of all parts of the facial nerve are covered.

Pearl

- The most critical part of operations to remove large vestibular schwannomas regarding preservation of the facial nerve occurs when tumor tissue is removed from near the facial nerve where it emerges from the internal auditory meatus and turns downwards. That part of the facial nerve is often severely injured by the tumor, and it is often spread out to form a thin sheath of nerve tissue that has the consistency of wet tissue paper. It is therefore extremely fragile, and even the slightest manipulation can destroy the nerve. Continuous monitoring of facial muscle EMG through a loudspeaker can facilitate safe removal of tumor tissue from such an injured facial nerve without causing further injury to the nerve.

Another critical part of operations for vestibular schwannomas occurs when a tumor is to be removed from the facial nerve or the vicinity along its course inside the internal auditory meatus (IAC). Drilling of the bone of the IAC generates heat than can injure the facial nerve. Monitoring of EMG activity from facial muscles can detect such injuries, and the surgeon should be encouraged to make pauses in manipulations or drilling that elicit such activity. Use of irrigation to cool the bone may help reduce the risk from drilling.

IOM of the facial nerve is now in common use in operations for vestibular schwannomas, and its use has been supported by an official statement by the National Institutes of Health (NIH, 1991):

> There is a consensus that intraoperative real-time monitoring improves the surgical management of vestibular schwannoma, including the preservation of facial nerve function, and possibly improves hearing preservation by use of intraoperative auditory brainstem response monitoring. New approaches to monitoring auditory nerve function may provide more rapid feedback to the surgeon, thus enhancing their usefulness. Intraoperative monitoring of cranial nerves V, VI, IX, X, and XI also has been described, but the full benefits of this monitoring remains to be determined.

Less than 20 years ago, facial nerve function was rarely preserved in operations for vestibular schwannomas. Now, facial function can be preserved most times. Several factors, in addition to the introduction of IOM, have contributed to the improvement in preservation of the facial nerve. Many tumors that are surgically removed are smaller now than they were some years ago because they are often detected earlier as a result of better diagnostic methods. The introduction of better operating equipment and the refinement of surgical technique have also contributed to a higher success rate in preserving function of these two nerves.

Other Cranial Nerves May Be Involved in Vestibular Schwannomas   Large vestibular schwannomas may extend to the location of CN V. Electrically stimulating CN V elicits contractions of the temporalis and the masseter muscles because they are innervated by the motor portions of the trigeminal nerve. EMG electrodes placed on the face for recording EMG potentials from facial muscles will also pick up activity from the masseter and temporalis muscles. The latency of the EMG potentials recorded from these two muscles in response to stimulation of the motor portion of the trigeminal nerve is much shorter than that of the facial muscles in response to stimulation of the facial nerve intracranially. This means that the nerve that is stimulated can be distinguished on the basis of the latency of the EMG responses (**Fig. 24–11**). Determining the latency of the EMG responses from these muscles requires that the responses be displayed on a computer screen. If two recording channels for EMG potentials are available, one channel may be used to record EMG potentials from the masseter muscles (**Fig. 24–10**), which makes it possible to easily distinguish between the EMG activity elicited by electrical as well as mechanical stimulation of the facial and trigeminal nerves.

Large vestibular schwannomas that extend caudally may involve the glossopharyngeal and vagus nerves and sometimes even the spinal accessory nerve (CN IX, X, and XI). Monitoring of these nerves can be done using similar methods as for monitoring the facial and trigeminal nerves.

Monitoring Other Cranial Motor Nerves in Operations to Remove Skull Base Tumors

Although vestibular schwannomas are the most common neoplasm in the CPA, a variety of tumors may occur near the base of the skull. These tumors are often benign, and they may grow to large sizes before they give noticeable symptoms. At that stage, such tumors may affect several cranial nerves, and they may extend inside the cavernous sinus. Surgical removal of such tumors can place several cranial nerves at risk of being injured or destroyed. The nerves of the extraocular muscles are often displaced, and it may be difficult to find these nerves by visual inspection of the surgical field. Tumors (chordomas) found adjacent to the base of the skull (clivus) may involve lower cranial nerves, such as the hypoglossal (CN XII), the loss of which may have severe and even life-threatening consequences. Loss of CN V results in numbness in the face and degeneration of mastication muscles.

Removal of other skull base tumors, such as those invading the cavernous sinus, may place several cranial nerves in jeopardy, particularly those that innervate the extraocular muscles (CN III, IV, and VI). Loss of function of CN III makes the eye essentially useless because that nerve, in addition to controlling three of the five extraocular muscles, controls accommodation and the size of the pupil. Impairment of the function of the other two nerves, CN IV (trochlearis) and VI (abducens), causes noticeable disturbances. Loss of function of the lateral rectus muscle, innervated by CN VI, makes it impossible to move the eye laterally from the midline. Loss of function of CN IV, which innervates the superior oblique muscle, has the least severe consequences but makes it difficult to look down (see **Table 24–1**).

Loss of function of CN V (trigeminal) causes loss of sensation in the face (the sensory portion of the nerve) and loss of function of mastication (the motor portion of the nerve). Skull base tumors that extend caudally on the clivus (the downward sloping surface of the base of the skull to the foramen magnum) may be close to the lower cranial nerves, which may become at risk of being injured during removal of such tumors. Although loss of function of CN IX on one side will affect swallowing, loss of that nerve bilaterally is life threatening because of its role in controlling blood pressure. The most noticeable deficits from loss of function of CN X (vagus) on one side is probably disturbance of closure of the vocal cords and consequently impairment of speech. Bilateral loss of function of the vagus nerve is life threatening. Loss of function of CN XII on one side paralyzes one side of the tongue and affects swallowing, and bilateral loss of function of CN IX, X, or XII may be life threatening.

As for monitoring the facial nerve, it is important to be able to find the anatomical location of these motor nerves. That can be done by using a handheld stimulating probe while observing the EMG potentials that are recorded from the muscles that are innervated by these nerves. Intraoperative monitoring using a handheld stimulating electrode in connection with recording of EMG potentials from the muscles they innervate is often the only way to find these nerves. The principles of monitoring these cranial motor nerves intraoperatively are similar to that of monitoring the facial nerve, as described earlier in this chapter.

Examination of the pattern of the spontaneous activity of the muscles that a motor nerve innervates provides important information about the degree of injury to the nerve. Injured nerves are more likely to respond to mechanical stimulation than uninjured nerves, and the sensitivity to mechanical stimulation can therefore provide information about the extent to which a nerve is injured. A motor nerve may have been injured before the operation started as a result of a tumor or other disease process, and it may be useful to have preoperative tests of the function of the motor nerves that can be monitored during an operation.

Pitfall

- A prerequisite of using these methods to monitor and find motor nerves is that the patient is not paralyzed. Because muscle-relaxing agents are common components of modern anesthesia techniques, the anesthesia often has to be modified to accommodate intraoperative monitoring of muscle contractions using EMG potentials or any other means of detecting contractions of muscles.

◆ Monitoring the Nerves of the Extraocular Muscles

The principles of monitoring these cranial motor nerves intraoperatively are similar to those for monitoring the facial nerve as described above.

Recording Electrodes

EMG potentials from the extraocular muscles can be recorded by placing needle electrodes through the skin (percutaneously) into these muscles or their close vicinity (**Fig. 24–12**; Møller, 1987, 2006b; Sekhar and Møller, 1986; Yingling and Ashram, 2005). Only one electrode is placed in each muscle, and the reference electrodes for all the recording electrodes should be placed on the forehead on the opposite side to avoid the interference from facial muscle contractions on the operated side. This technique has a low risk, provided that it is done by a person who is trained in the procedure and well acquainted with the anatomy. It should only be done after the patient is anesthetized, and the electrodes should be carefully removed before the patient wakes up. Such recordings yield EMG potentials of sufficient amplitude to make them visible and

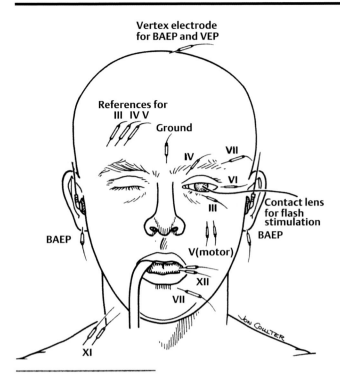

Figure 24–12 Electrode placements for recording electromyographic potentials from the extraocular muscles (III, IV, VI), the masseter muscle (V motor), the facial muscles (VII), the shoulder muscles (XI), and the tongue (XII). Electrode placement for recording auditory brainstem response and a contact lens for delivering visual stimuli for recording visual evoked potentials are also shown. BAEP, brainstem auditory evoked potential; VEP, visual evoked potential. (From Møller, A. R. (1990). Intraoperative monitoring of evoked potentials: An update. In R. H. Wilkins & S. S. Rengachary (Eds.), Neurosurgery update: Diagnosis, operative technique, and neuro-oncology (Vol. 1, pp. 169–176). New York: McGraw-Hill, with permission.)

interpretable without averaging (**Fig. 24–13**). EMG potentials can also be recorded from the extraocular muscles using noninvasive recording electrodes in the form of small wire rings placed under the eyelids (Sekiya et al, 1993).

♦ Monitoring the Sensory Portion of the Trigeminal Nerve

Monitoring of the sensory portion of the trigeminal nerve can be done by recording evoked potentials from electrodes placed on the scalp. However, these potentials are affected by common anesthetics, which, together with uncertainties regarding the neural generators of these potentials, have prevented the general use of trigeminal evoked potentials in intraoperative monitoring.

Recordings from the three branches of the trigeminal nerve while the intracranial portion is being stimulated electrically are used for identifying the three branches of the trigeminal nerve root (Stechison et al, 1996). Such recordings are used in operations for sectioning of specific parts of the nerve.

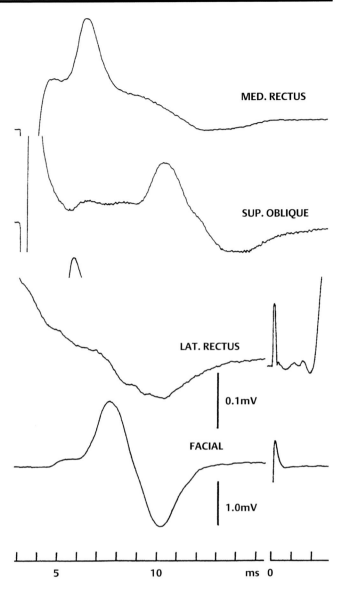

Figure 24–13 Recordings from the extraocular muscles and from facial muscles with electrodes placed as shown in **Fig. 24–12**. The muscles contractions were elicited by electrical stimulation of the respective motor nerves intracranially. Electrode placement for recording the auditory brainstem response is also shown. (From Møller, A. R. (1987). Electrophysiological monitoring of cranial nerves in operations in the skull base. In L. N. Sekhar & V. L. Schramm, Jr. (Eds.), Tumors of the cranial base: Diagnosis and treatment (pp. 123–132). Mt. Kisco, NY: Futura Publishing, with permission.)

♦ Monitoring the Optic Nerve

Intraoperative monitoring of the optic nerve has gained some usage. Visual evoked potentials recorded from electrodes placed on the scalp have been the most common method for such monitoring, but evoked potentials have also been recorded directly from the exposed optic nerve and optic tract (Møller, 1987). However, several technical factors have made it difficult to use visual evoked potentials in intraoperative monitoring. Clinical studies have shown that the optimal stimulus for eliciting visual evoked potentials to detect pathologies of the optic nerve is a reversing pattern of a checkerboard. Because the use of such stimulation requires that a pattern can be focused on the retina, it cannot be used in an anesthetized patient; the only stimuli that can be used in anesthetized individuals are light flashes. It has been shown that changes in the visual evoked potentials elicited by light flashes are not generally good indicators of intraoperative injuries to the optic nerve and optic tract (Cedzich et al, 1988), in agreement with clinical experience. More recently, it has been indicated that visual evoked potentials elicited by high-intensity light flashes are better indicators of pathology than potentials evoked by flashes from light-emitting diodes (Pratt et al, 1994). Therefore, it may be recommended that monitoring of the optic nerve be performed using high-intensity light flashes.

◆ Monitoring the Lower Cranial Motor Nerves

Several of the lower cranial nerves (CN IX, X, XI, and XII; **Table 24–1**) are mixed nerves, and it is the motor portion that is monitored. It is easier to monitor the motor portions of these nerves than the sensory parts, and it is assumed that preserving the motor portions also indicates preservation of the sensory portions. In general, the same principles can be used for preserving these nerves as described for preservation of the function of the facial nerve. Thus, the motor portion of the glossopharyngeal (CN IX) can be monitored by recording EMG potentials from muscles in the posterior palate (Lanser et al, 1992; Møller, 2006b; Yingling, 1994). This nerve should be stimulated cautiously because of its possible effect on circulation (blood pressure) and the heart. When stimulating that nerve, the anesthesia team should be informed and encouraged to watch the patient's blood pressure and heart rate.

The motor portion of the vagal nerve (CN X) can be monitored by recording EMG potentials from larynx muscles (Lanser et al, 1992; Møller, 2006b; Stechison, 1995; Yingling, 1994). The recording electrodes may be inserted in the vocal folds under laryngoscopic guidance, percutaneously, or by using a tracheal tube with conductive rings that act as recording electrodes. The spinal accessory nerve (CN XI) can be monitored by placing EMG recording electrodes in muscles innervated by that nerve, such as the shoulder muscles (**Fig. 24–12**).

The hypoglossal nerve (CN XII) is very small and difficult to find by visual observation, but it is easily located by probing the surgical field with a handheld electrical stimulating electrode. Its motor portion can be monitored by placing EMG recording electrodes in the lateral side of the tongue (Lanser et al, 1992; Møller, 2006b; Sekhar and Møller, 1986; Yingling, 1994; **Fig. 24–12**).

Amplifiers

One amplifier and display are required for each muscle from which EMG recordings are to be made. In most skull base operations, it is also justified to record from muscles innervated by four to eight motor nerves, a technique that may require many recording channels with simultaneously displayed outputs. The option to mix all channels for making the EMG potentials audible or to listen to a selected channel should be available. Filter settings should be 30 to 3000 Hz.

Stimuli

As described for monitoring of the facial nerve, a handheld electrical stimulating electrode can be used for finding areas of a tumor where none of these other nerves are present. Identification of the location of motor nerves and monitoring of the neural conduction in individual nerves can be done by using the same methods as described earlier for the facial nerve. The vagus nerve should be stimulated with caution, and it is particularly important that a high rate of stimulation be avoided. Use of stimulus rates of 5 pulses per second (pps) or lower seems safe, but the anesthesia team must be informed when electrical stimulation is to be done. Caution should be exercised when stimulating CN XI because it innervates large muscles, which may be injured if all motor nerve fibers are activated at the same time and at a high rate.

The EMG activity elicited by mechanical stimulation of these motor nerves or elicited by injury to the nerve can be monitored in the same way as described above for the facial nerve.

◆ Monitoring the Peripheral Portion of the Facial Nerve

Monitoring of the peripheral portion of the facial nerve can be done using similar methods as described for monitoring of the intracranial portion of the facial nerve in operations of the skull base. Such monitoring is of value in several kinds of operations of the face, such as operations on the parotid gland and in reconstructive and cosmetic operations of the face. Usually only one branch of the facial nerve is affected, and EMG potentials should be recorded from muscles innervated by that branch. The wound can be probed by an electrical stimulating electrode in the same way as described for removal of vestibular schwannomas. The latencies of the responses are shorter than those of the responses elicited by stimulation of the intracranial portion of the facial nerve, which must be taken into account when setting the duration of the suppression of the stimulus artifact.

◆ Doing Interoperative Monitoring

Intraoperative monitoring should not be regarded as a method for providing warnings of imminent disasters, but as a source of information that can help the surgeon carry out the operation in the safest way possible, reducing the likelihood of emergency situations. To fulfill that goal, it is important that the individuals who are responsible for the monitoring be knowledgeable about the physiology of the systems that are monitored and understand what signs indicate a change in neural function. The person who conducts the monitoring must also have good knowledge about the operation and be present in the operating room at all times when there is risk of injury to neural tissue. It is also essential that frequent contact with the surgeon and the anesthesia team be maintained. The latter is especially important in monitoring of motor nerves. It is not only surgical manipulations that can cause change in the potentials that are monitored, and the person who is responsible for monitoring must be able to discriminate significant from insignificant changes.

The success of intraoperative monitoring depends on several practical matters. It is important that monitoring be well planned so that the individuals responsible for monitoring know which organ systems are to be monitored and how to do that (placement of electrodes, stimulus and recoding parameters, etc.). It is also essential that all necessary equipment be available immediately whenever it is needed and that contingency plans be in place for covering equipment failure, including having spare electrodes available.

Clinical use of electrophysiologic tests, such as evoked potentials, customarily involves comparison of the obtained results with a standard that is the average of results obtained in many individuals without known pathologies. Intraoperative recordings instead compare the obtained responses with the patient's own preoperative test results. That provides a higher sensitivity, which means that smaller changes in the recorded potentials can be used as signs of injuries than what would be the case if the results were compared with a laboratory standard. The baseline recording of evoked potentials, such as the ABR, is preferably obtained after the patient is anesthetized but before the operation is started.

Although recordings of sensory evoked and EMG potentials done in the clinic and the operating room are similar in many ways, they are also different. One important difference is that the recordings in the operating room must be interpreted immediately. Another difference is that it is the deviation from an individual patient's own recordings that is important in the operating room and not deviations from a standard. These matters must be taken into account when planning and performing intraoperative monitoring. Yet another difference involves the fact that recordings in unconscious individuals are naturally different from clinical tests of awake patients.

It has often been claimed that the large amount of electrical equipment in the operating room produces so much electrical interference that it is difficult (or even impossible) to record small electrical potentials such as the ABR. However, it is possible to reduce the effect of such interference to a degree that makes it possible to obtain high-quality evoked potentials, even when the amplitude is small, as with the ABR. It is important that the techniques for reducing the electrical interference in the operating room are in place and that the people who do monitoring

have the skills to search for the sources of electrical interference and can take appropriate action. It is also important that the individuals who perform intraoperative monitoring can obtain recordings of good quality and know how to solve problems regarding electrical and other kinds of interference that may occur at any time during an operation.

The techniques for reducing interference to obtain optimal recording conditions are described in detail elsewhere (see, e.g., Møller, 2006b).

Electrodes placed on the head are usually out of reach after the patient has been draped. Therefore, it is important that recording electrodes be secured so that they will not come off during the operation. Having extra electrodes placed can be valuable in ensuring that monitoring does not need to be aborted because an electrode fails. Needle electrodes usually provide a stable recording condition over many hours, whereas surface electrodes may be dislocated or change their recording conditions over time. Needle electrodes, however, involve a small risk of causing burns when electrocautery is used. It is mainly older electrocautery equipment that poses such a risk. Burns may also occur if the return electrode of the electrocautery is faulty. Such unfortunate events are extremely rare when modern equipment is used (see Møller, 2006b).

The Effect of Anesthesia

Anesthesia does not affect auditory evoked potentials (ABR or CAP recorded from the auditory nerve or the cochlear nucleus), but a common component of anesthesia, namely, the muscle relaxant, makes it impossible to record EMG potentials from muscles. That means that the anesthesia regimen must often be altered when recordings are to be made from muscles. When monitoring depends on recording of muscle contractions using EMG or other methods, arrangements must be made with the anesthesiologist before the operation, preferably the preceding day, to ensure that the patient will not be paralyzed.

When Preoperative and Postoperative Tests Are Important

Patients who are to be monitored in an operation should have preoperative tests of the systems that are to be monitored. If it is not possible to obtain a response before the operation, it is unlikely that it will be possible in the operating room, and it would be wasted effort to try. Failure to obtain a response in the operating room in patients who had satisfactory sensory evoked potentials before the operation could be a result of equipment failure, and that should be remedied. For similar reasons, it is important to test motor systems that are to be monitored preoperatively.

The preoperative evoked potential recordings may be used as baseline for the intraoperative recordings, but it is better to obtain a baseline recording after the patient is anesthetized but before the operation begins.

Which Changes Should Be Reported to the Surgeon?

It has been suggested that the surgeon should only be informed when changes in the recorded potentials indicate that there would be a high likelihood that the patient would suffer permanent neurologic deficits if the manipulation that caused the changes was not reversed. Other investigators have found evidence that it is preferable to inform the surgeon immediately when a change has occurred that was larger than the normal small variations (Møller, 2006b; Møller and Møller, 1989). Early information about changes in recorded potentials makes it easy for the surgeon to identify the cause, and it gives him or her several options. One is to do nothing and wait to see if the changes increase. If the surgeon knows what caused the change, the manipulation may be reversed at any time. Another (and better) option is to immediately reverse the manipulation, which means that the surgeon does not need to be concerned about the problem in the future. If the surgeon is not informed until the change has reached a dangerous level, his or her options become limited. It may not be known what has caused the change because of the time that has elapsed between the occurrence of the change in function and the time the surgeon was informed. If attempts to reverse the injury are unsuccessful, the patient may have permanent postoperative neurologic deficit. Experience has shown that surgeons who choose to reverse an injury immediately after it has been discovered have far fewer incidents of permanent neurologic deficits than those who choose the "wait and see" option (Møller, 2006b). In a consecutive series of 350 microvascular decompressions of CN V, VII, and VIII, a surgeon who used these criteria had no incidence of postoperative hearing loss, defined as 20 dB or more at two frequencies (Møller, 2006b).

Which Operations Should Be Monitored?

Use of intraoperative neurophysiologic monitoring that is aimed at reducing the risk of surgically induced injuries to neural tissue should be considered in all operations where neural tissue is to be surgically manipulated. Because risk involved in different operations varies, and because the reduction of the risks of postoperative permanent deficits that can be achieved by IOM varies between different kinds of operations, it has been thought to be unnecessary to monitor some operations. The risks and benefits of IOM also vary between surgeons with different degrees of training and experience. The selection of operations for monitoring must depend on the risk without monitoring and the reduction in risks that can be achieved with monitoring. Most risk calculations, however, show that IOM is economically sound because of large costs involved in caring for people with neurologic deficits (Møller, 2006b). From a human perspective, the advantages of IOM are even greater and may serve as an example of a situation where suffering can be reduced by a small economic sacrifice. IOM can also act as a teaching aid because electrophysiologic recordings can point to which surgical manipulations cause injuries and therefore which manipulations should be avoided.

Which Surgeons May Benefit from Monitoring?

Intraoperative neurophysiologic monitoring is likely to benefit surgeons in different ways, depending on their level of experience. Also, surgeons may benefit from different aspects of intraoperative monitoring. Monitoring of the facial nerve in operations for vestibular schwannomas serves as an example. An extremely experienced surgeon may feel more comfortable by having IOM available to help confirm the anatomy, even if it provides only a modest reduction of facial nerve injuries. The slightly less experienced surgeon may have a greater reduction in facial nerve injuries because of the use of IOM and will be able to complete the operation in a considerably shorter time. The moderately experienced surgeon will always benefit from confirmation of the anatomical location of the facial nerve and will benefit from knowing when surgical manipulations cause injuries.

Pearl

- Many highly experienced surgeons refuse to operate without the aid of intraoperative monitoring because they believe that IOM reduces the risks of complications and gives them a feeling of security..

Determining the Benefits of Intraoperative Monitoring

For several reasons, it has been difficult to do controlled studies of the benefits of IOM. Ethical reasons and the surgeons' reluctance to deprive their patients of the benefit of IOM have made it difficult to do studies using randomly selected patients for monitoring. Studies based on comparisons between the rate of complications before and after the introduction of monitoring have been published (Møller and Møller, 1989; Radtke et al, 1989), but they have been criticized because it has been claimed that other improvements in surgery could have accounted for the lower rate of complications. The fact that different surgeons achieve different degrees of reduction of complications, depending on their experience, also adds to the difficulty in determining what operations would benefit from IOM. This is one reason why IOM has been officially regarded as beneficial in relatively few operations, but as indispensable by most individual surgeons who perform the operations. IOM for preservation of facial function during operations for vestibular schwannomas is an exception because it has received official recommendation (National Institutes of Health, 1991).

The economic aspects of the use of intraoperative monitoring has been analyzed only in connection with a few types of operations. One example is placement of pedicle screws in operations on the spine (Toleikis, 2002). In these studies, it was convincingly shown that the inclusion of IOM was economically beneficial in that it reduces the risks of intraoperative injuries that could cause lengthy suffering and neurologic deficits (Møller, 2006b).

◆ Intraoperative Monitoring as an Aid to the Surgeon in Carrying Out Operations

In a few operations, intraoperative neurophysiologic recordings can help the surgeon carry out the operation so that the therapeutic goal is achieved. One example of that is recordings of the abnormal muscle response in operations for hemifacial spasm using the MVD technique (Haines and Torres, 1991; Møller and Jannetta, 1987). Another example is from operations where the vestibular nerve is to be cut to treat disorders caused by hyperactivity of the vestibular organ. Recordings from CN VIII can help find the cleavage plane between the auditory and vestibular nerves in operations where the vestibular nerve is to be sectioned (Rosenberg et al, 1993). Operations aimed at specific neural tissue that may not be identified visually in the surgical field may benefit from electrophysiologic recordings. Considerable individual variations in anatomy are easily overlooked and may lead to mistakes. The risk of errors may be reduced by using electrophysiologic methods as an aid in finding the anatomical location of specific neural tissue.

Vestibular Nerve Section

Vestibular nerve section is an example of an operation in which electrophysiologic identification may help to perform a selective section of the vestibular nerve without injuring the auditory nerve (Rosenberg et al, 1993). The superior vestibular and auditory nerves have a slight difference in grayness, but it may be difficult to distinguish between these two parts of CN VIII from visual inspection. Recording of auditory evoked potentials using a bipolar recording electrode can help in identifying the demarcation line between these two nerves (Møller et al, 1994b; Rosenberg et al, 1993; **Fig. 24–14**). The evoked potentials change as the recording electrode is moved around the circumference of the intracranial portion of CN VIII, and the best separation between recordings from these two nerves is achieved when a low stimulus sound intensity is used (Rosenberg et al, 1993).

Hemifacial Spasm

Hemifacial spasm is characterized by involuntary contractions of muscles in one side of the face. Moving a blood vessel off the intracranial portion of the facial nerve root (MVD operation) can cure the spasm. The operation has a success rate of ~85% (Barker et al, 1995, 1996). The reason for failure is almost always the inability to identify the blood vessel that is the cause of the spasm. Monitoring the abnormal muscle response can help identify the vessel that causes the disorder. It can ensure that the therapeutic goal of the operation has been reached before the operation is ended. The abnormal muscle response is believed to be specific for patients with hemifacial spasm and can be demonstrated by electrically stimulating one branch of the face while recording the EMG response from a muscle innervated by another

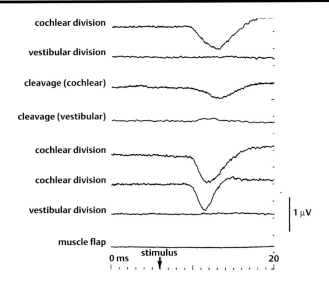

Figure 24–14 Bipolar recordings of auditory evoked potentials from the intracranial portion of the eighth cranial nerve. The stimuli were clicks at 25 dB above threshold for the auditory brainstem response. (From Rosenberg, S. I., Martin, W. H., Pratt, H., Schwegler, J. W., & Silverstein, H. (1993). Bipolar cochlear nerve recording technique: A preliminary report. American Journal of Otology, 14, 362–368, with permission.)

branch (Møller and Jannetta, 1987; **Fig. 24–15**). It can be recorded during surgical anesthesia, provided that muscle relaxants are not used. This response disappears totally when the blood vessel that is related to the spasm is moved off the facial nerve. The success rate increased considerably after the recording method was introduced as part of routine monitoring during MVD operations for hemifacial spasm (Haines and Torres, 1991; Møller and Jannetta, 1987). Introduction of these electrophysiologic techniques has nearly eliminated the need for reoperations. In addition to increasing the success rate, such monitoring gives the surgeon an increased feeling of security. It has shortened the operating time because it makes it unnecessary to look for other vessels once the one that caused this abnormal muscle response has been found.

Implantations of Electrodes for Deep Brain Stimulation

The advent of techniques that require either small lesions to be made in specific structures in the CNS or placement of stimulating electrodes has created the need for recording from electrodes that are placed deep in the brain. These techniques are used in the treatment of movement disorders, such as Parkinson's disease, and chronic pain. The lesions or the stimulating electrodes are placed in structures of the basal ganglia or the thalamus. Stereotactic techniques, based on magnetic resonance imaging, are used to insert the electrodes, but their precision is insufficient. The fine placement of the lesions or the implanted electrodes is done on the basis of the results of recordings from the inserted electrodes. These techniques are described in detail in other books (see, e.g., Møller, 2006b) and will not be discussed further here.

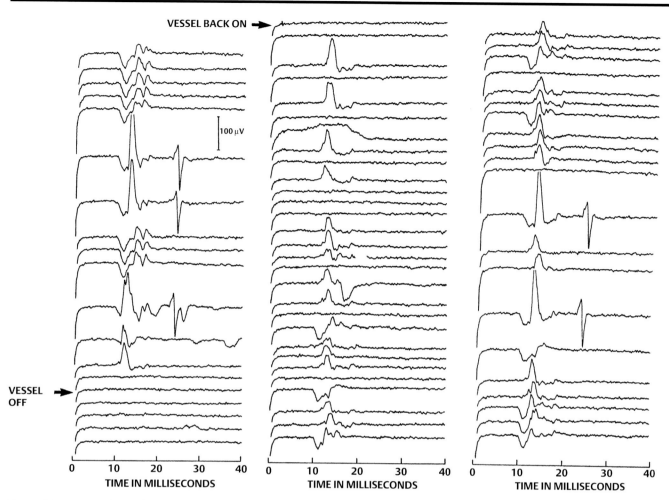

VESSEL BACK ON ➡

100 μV

VESSEL
OFF ➡

0   10   20   30   40
TIME IN MILLISECONDS

0   10   20   30   40
TIME IN MILLISECONDS

0   10   20   30   40
TIME IN MILLISECONDS

Figure 24–15 Recordings of the abnormal muscle response from the mentalis muscle in response to electrical stimulation of the peripheral portion of the zygomatic branch of the facial nerve presented at a rate of 10 pps, obtained in a patient undergoing a microvascular decompression operation for hemifacial spasm. The top part of the left column shows consecutive EMG recordings before the offending blood vessel was lifted off the facial nerve. At the arrow, the vessel was lifted off the nerve and it fell back on the nerve as marked at the top of the middle column. (From Møller, A. R., & Jannetta, P. J. (1985). Microvascular decompression in hemifacial spasm: Intraoperative electrophysiological observations. Neurosurgery, 16, 612–618, with permission.)

◆ Risks Involved in Intraoperative Monitoring

Intraoperative monitoring that is intended to reduce risk can itself be a risk, much like medication may have side effects that can cause pathologies. In general, mistakes may not necessarily be avoidable, but the probability of their occurrence can be decreased. Inadvertently stimulating nervous tissue with too high an electrical current, for example, can only be avoided if the stimulating equipment is not able to deliver currents that pose risks, but adequate training of the people who operate the equipment can reduce the likelihood of the occurrence. Another risk is to monitor the wrong system, which could cause changes from surgical manipulations to appear unnoticed. An example of that is placing the EMG recording electrodes on the wrong side of the face in an operation for a vestibular schwannoma. The use of checklists can help to reduce the occurrence of mistakes.

◆ Summary

Intraoperative neurophysiologic monitoring can help to reduce the risk of permanent neurologic injuries in surgical procedures that affect the nervous system. It is a unique addition to the operating room because its main purpose is to reduce the risk of iatrogenic injuries, thus reducing the risk of harm in surgical treatment. This means that IOM reduces the incidences of suffering to patients. Intraoperative electrophysiologic recordings can help the surgeon to carry out an operation with greater ease, and they can reduce operating time. IOM is useful in developing better operating techniques and in teaching surgical residents. In some operations, electrophysiological methods can help surgeons identify specific structures and achieve therapeutical goals. IOM is essential in identifying the correct placement of lesions in specific structures in the brain. Implantations of electrodes for stimulation of specific structures of the basal ganglia and the thalamus for treating movement disorders and pain also benefit from electrophysiologic recordings. These benefits are difficult to evaluate quantitatively, but they should not be ignored when the value of IOM is assessed.

References

Angelo, R., & Møller, A. R. (1996). Contralateral evoked brainstem auditory potentials as an indicator of intraoperative brainstem manipulation in cerebellopontine angle tumors. Neurological Research, 18, 528–540.

Barker, F. G., Jannetta, P. J., Bissonette, D. J., Larkins, M. V., & Jho, H. D. (1996). The long-term outcome of microvascular decompression for trigeminal neuralgia. New England Journal of Medicine, 334, 1077–1083.

Barker, F. G., Jannetta, P. J., Bissonette, D. J., Shields, P. T., & Larkins, M. V. (1995). Microvascular decompression for hemifacial spasm. Journal of Neurosurgery, 82, 201–210.

Brown, R. H., & Nash, C. L. (1979). Current status of spinal cord monitoring. Spine, 4, 466–478.

Cedzich, C., Schramm, J., Mengedoht, C. F., & Fahlbusch, R. (1988). Factors that limit the use of flash visual evoked potentials for surgical monitoring. Electroencephalography and Clinical Neurophysiology, 71, 142–145.

Colletti, V., Bricolo, A., Fiorino, F. G., & Bruni, L. (1994). Changes in directly recorded cochlear nerve compound action potentials during acoustic tumor surgery. Skull Base Surgery, 4, 1–9.

Davis, H., & Hirsh, S. K. (1979). A slow brain stem response for low-frequency audiometry. Audiology, 18, 441–465.

Delgado, T. E., Bucheit, W. A., Rosenholtz, H. R., & Chrissian, S. (1979). Intraoperative monitoring of facial muscle evoked responses obtained by intracranial stimulation of the facial nerve: A more accurate technique for facial nerve dissection. Neurosurgery, 4, 418–421.

Fischer, C. (1989). Brainstem auditory evoked potential (BAEP) monitoring in posterior fossa surgery. J. Desmedt (Ed.), Neuromonitoring in surgery (pp. 191–218). Amsterdam: Elsevier Science Publishers.

Friedman, W. A., Kaplan, B. J., Gravenstein, D., & Rhoton, A. L. (1985). Intraoperative brain-stem auditory evoked potentials during posterior fossa microvascular decompression. Journal of Neurosurgery 62, 552–557.

Goldstein, M. H., Jr. (1960). A statistical model for interpreting neuroelectric responses. Information and Control, 3, 1–17.

Grundy, B. L. (1983). Intraoperative monitoring of sensory evoked potentials. Anesthesiology, 58(1), 72–87.

Haines, S. J., & Torres, F. (1991). Intraoperative monitoring of the facial nerve during decompressive surgery for hemifacial spasm. Journal of Neurosurgery, 74(2), 254–257.

Harner, S. G., Daube, J. R., Beatty, C. W., & Ebersold, M. J. (1988). Intraoperative monitoring of the facial nerve. Laryngoscope, 98(2), 209–212.

Hatayama, T., & Møller, A. R. (1988). Correlation between latency and amplitude of peak V in brainstem auditory evoked potentials: Intraoperative recordings in microvascular decompression operations. Acta Neurochirurgica, 140, 681–687.

Hilger, J. (1964). Facial nerve stimulator. Transactions—American Academy of Ophthalmology and Otolaryngology, 68, 74–76.

Hoke, M., Ross, B., Wickesberg, R., & Luetkenhoener, B. (1984). Weighted averaging—Theory and application to electrical response audiometry. Electroencephalography and Clinical Neurophysiology, 57, 484–489.

Jako, G. (1965). Facial nerve monitor. Transactions—American Academy of Ophthalmology and Otolaryngology, 69, 340–342.

Kalmanchey, R., Avila, A., & Symon, L. (1986). The use of brainstem auditory evoked potentials during posterior fossa surgery as a monitor of brainstem function. Acta Neurochirurgica, 82, 128–136.

Kartush, J., & Bouchard, K. (1992). Intraoperative facial monitoring: Otology, neurotology, and skull base surgery. In J. Kartush, & K. Bouchard (Eds.), Neuromonitoring in otology and head and neck surgery (pp. 99–120). New York: Raven Press.

Krauze, F. (1912). Surgery of the brain and spinal cord (1st English ed.). New York: Rebman Company.

Kuroki, A., & Møller, A. R. (1995). Microsurgical anatomy around the foramen of Luschka with reference to intraoperative recording of auditory evoked potentials from the cochlear nuclei. Journal of Neurosurgery, 82(6), 933–939.

Lang, J. (November 1985). Anatomy of the brain stem and the lower cranial nerves, vessels, and surrounding structures. American Journal of Otology, Supplement, 1–19.

Lanser, M., Jackler, R., & Yingling, C. (1992). Regional monitoring of the lower (ninth through twelfth) cranial nerves. In J. Kartush & K. Bouchard (Eds.), Intraoperative monitoring in otology and head and neck surgery (pp. 131–150). New York: Raven Press.

Levine, R. A., Ojemann, R. G. Montgomery, W. W., & McGaffigan, P. M. (1984). Monitoring auditory evoked potentials during acoustic neuroma surgery: Insights into the mechanism of the hearing loss. Annals of Otology, Rhinology, and Laryngology, 116–123.

Linden, R., Tator, C., Benedict, C., Mraz, C., & Bell, I. (1988). Electro-physiological monitoring during acoustic neuroma and other posterior fossa surgery. Journal des Sciences Neurologiques, 15, 73–81.

Lorente de No, R. (1947). Analysis of the distribution of action currents of nerve in volume conductors. Studies of the Rockefeller Institute for Medical Research, 132, 384–482.

Møller, A. R. (1987). Electrophysiological monitoring of cranial nerves in operations in the skull base. In L. N. Sekhar & V. L. Schramm, Jr. (Eds.), Tumors of the cranial base: Diagnosis and treatment (pp. 123–132). Mt. Kisco, NY: Futura Publishing.

Møller, A. R. (1988). Evoked potentials in intraoperative monitoring. Baltimore, MD: Williams & Wilkins.

Møller, A. R. (1990). Intraoperative monitoring of evoked potentials: An update. In R. H. Wilkins & S. S. Rengachary (Eds.), Neurosurgery update: Diagnosis, Operative Technique, and Neuro-oncology (Vol. 1, pp. 169–176). New York: McGraw-Hill.

Møller, A. R. (1995). Intraoperative neurophysiological monitoring. Luxembourg: Harwood Academic Publishers.

Møller, A. R. (2006a). Hearing: Anatomy, physiology and disorders of the auditory system (2nd ed.). Amsterdam: Academic Press.

Møller, A. R. (2006b). Intraoperative neurophysiological monitoring (2nd ed.). Totowa, NJ: Humana Press.

Møller, A. R., Colletti, V., & Fiorino, F. (1994). Click evoked responses from the exposed intracranial portion of the eighth nerve during vestibular nerve section: Bipolar and monopolar recordings. Electroencephalography and Clinical Neurophysiology, 92, 17–29.

Møller, A. R., Colletti, V., & Fiorino, F. G. (1994). Neural conduction velocity of the human auditory nerve: Bipolar recordings from the exposed intracranial portion of the eighth nerve during vestibular nerve section. Electroencephalography and Clinical Neurophysiology, 92, 316–320.

Møller, A. R., & Jannetta, P. J. (1981). Compound action potentials recorded intracranially from the auditory nerve in man. Experimental Neurology, 74, 862–874.

Møller, A. R., & Jannetta, P. J. (1983a). Auditory evoked potentials recorded from the cochlear nucleus and its vicinity in man. Journal of Neurosurgery, 59, 1013–1018.

Møller, A. R., & Jannetta, P. J. (1983b). Monitoring auditory functions during cranial nerve microvascular decompression operations by direct recording from the eighth nerve. Journal of Neurosurgery, 59, 493–499.

Møller, A. R., & Jannetta, P. J. (1984). Preservation of facial function during removal of acoustic neuromas: Use of monopolar constant voltage stimulation and EMG. Journal of Neurosurgery, 61, 757–760.

Møller, A. R., & Jannetta, P. J. (1985). Microvascular decompression in hemifacial spasm: Intraoperative electrophysiological observations. Neurosurgery, 16, 612–618.

Møller, A. R., & Jannetta, P. J. (1987). Monitoring facial EMG during microvascular decompression operations for hemifacial spasm. Journal of Neurosurgery, 66, 681–685.

Møller, A. R., Jannetta, P. J., & Jho, H. D. (1994). Click-evoked responses from the cochlear nucleus: A study in human. Electroencephalography and Clinical Neurophysiology, 92, 215–224.

Møller, A. R., & Jho, H. D. (1991). Effect of high frequency hearing loss on compound action potentials recorded from the intracranial portion of the human eighth nerve. Hearing Research, 55, 9–23.

Møller, A. R., & Møller, M. B. (1989). Does intraoperative monitoring of auditory evoked potentials reduce incidence of hearing loss as a complication of microvascular decompression of cranial nerves? Neurosurgery, 24, 257–263.

National Institutes of Health. (December 1991). Consensus statement. Consensus Development Conference. Washington, DC: Author.

Prass, R. L., & Lueders, H. (1986). Acoustic (loudspeaker) facial electromyographic monitoring (Part 1). Neurosurgery, 392–400.

Radtke, R. A., Erwin, W., & Wilkins, R. H. (1989). Intraoperative brainstem auditory evoked potentials: Significant decrease in post-operative morbidity. Neurology, 39, 187–191.

Raudzens, R. A. (1982). Intraoperative monitoring of evoked potentials. Annals of the New York Academy of Sciences, 388, 308–326.

Rosenberg, S. I., Martin, W. H., Pratt, H., Schwegler, J. W., & Silverstein, H. (1993). Bipolar cochlear nerve recording technique: A preliminary report. American Journal of Otology, 14, 362–368.

Sabin, H. I., Bentivoglio, P., Symon, L., Cheesman, A. D., Prasher, D., & Momma, F. (1987). Intraoperative electrocochleography to monitor cochlear potentials during acoustic neuroma excision. Acta Neurochirurgica, 85, 110–116.

Schimmel, H. (1967). The (+/−) reference: Accuracy of estimated mean components in average response studies. Science, 157, 92–94.

Sekhar, L. N., & Møller, A. R. (1986). Operative management of tumors involving the cavernous sinus. Journal of Neurosurgery, 64(6), 879–889.

Sekhar, L. N., & Schramm, V. L., Jr. (1987). Tumors of the cranial base: Diagnosis and treatment. Mt. Kisco, NY: Futura Publishing.

Sekiya, T., Hatayama, T., Iwabushi, T., & Maeda, S. (1993). Intraoperative recordings of evoked extraocular muscle activities to monitor ocular motor function. Neurosurgery, 32, 227–235.

Sekiya, T., Iwabuchi, T., Hatayama, T., & Shinozaki, N. (1991). Vestibular nerve injury as a complication of microvascular decompression. Neurosurgery, 29(5), 773–775.

Sekiya, T., & Møller, A. R. (1987). Avulsion rupture of the internal auditory artery during operations in the cerebellopontine angle: A study in monkeys. Neurosurgery, 21, 631–637.

Silverstein, H., Norrell, H., & Hyman, S. (1984). Simultaneous use of CO2 laser with continuous monitoring of eight cranial nerve action potential during acoustic neuroma surgery. Otolaryngology and Head and Neck Surgery, 92, 80–84.

Stechison, M. T. (1995). Vagus nerve monitoring: A comparison of percutaneous versus vocal fold electrode recording. American Journal of Otology, 16(5), 703–706.

Stechison, M. T., Møller, A. R., & Lovely, T. J. (1996). Intraoperative mapping of the trigeminal nerve root: Technique and application in the surgical management of facial pain. Neurosurgery, 38, 76–82.

Sugita, K., & Kobayashi, S. (1982). Technical and instrumental improvements in the surgical treatment of acoustic neurinomas. Journal of Neurosurgery, 57(6), 747–752.

Toleikis, J. R. (2002). Neurophysiological monitoring during pedicle screw placement. In V. Deletis & J. L. Shils (Eds.), Neurophysiology in neurosurgery (pp. 231–264). Amsterdam: Elsevier.

Yingling, C. (1994). Intraoperative monitoring in skull base surgery. In R. K. Jackler & D. E. Brackmann (Eds.), Neurotology (pp. 967–1002). St. Louis, MO: Mosby.

Yingling, C. D., & Ashram, Y. A. (2005). Intraoperative monitoring of cranial nerves in skull base surgery. In R. K. Jackler & D. E. Brackmann (Eds.), Neurotology (2nd ed., pp. 958–993). Philadelphia: Elsevier-Mosby.

Yingling, C., & Gardi, J. (1992). Intraoperative monitoring of facial and cochlear nerves during acoustic neuroma surgery. Otolaryngology Clinics of North America, 25 (2), 413–448.

Chapter 25

Assessment of Vestibular Function

Richard E. Gans and M. Wende Yellin

According to the National Institutes of Health (NIH), 90 million Americans will experience dizziness, vertigo, or imbalance sometime in their lives. Equilibrium disturbance in the form of dizziness, vertigo, or poor balance affects people of all ages and walks of life. The onset of symptoms may be sudden or gradual, and the symptoms may range from mild, lasting only seconds, to severe, lasting hours to days and resulting in total incapacity. In addition to dizziness, individuals may experience visual disturbances; headaches and muscle aches; motion sickness, nausea, and vomiting; and fatigue and loss of stamina (Goebel, 2001). Equilibrium disturbance is the third most common complaint reported by patients of all ages to physicians, preceded only by headache and lower back pain, and for individuals over 70 years of age, dizziness is the leading medical complaint.

For older individuals, balance problems pose a serious health risk both in morbidity and mortality because falls can lead to serious injuries, such as fractures of the femur and hip, as well as traumatic brain injury (TBI). Falls are the leading cause of accidental injury death in persons over age 65 years. In 2000 alone, falls in the elderly accounted for 1.6 million emergency room visits and over 10,000 deaths. It is predicted that as the population of the United States ages, the number of individuals seeking medical attention for dizziness will dramatically increase, escalating costs to Medicare and Medicaid programs and society as a whole (Gans, 1999; NIH, 1993). Direct costs alone are anticipated to exceed $32 billion by 2020, leading the NIH to identify dizziness and balance disorders as a national health care crisis (Keeping Seniors Safe from Falls Act, 109th Congress, 2005).

Normal equilibrium is dependent on accurate information from the visual, somatosensory, and vestibular systems being correctly processed and integrated by the central nervous system (CNS). A disorder in any one peripheral system or in the central nervous pathways may induce dizziness, vertigo, or disequilibrium. However, compensatory contributions from the unaffected systems may obscure the true site of lesion. Evaluation of patients reporting vertigo, dizziness, imbalance, or a history of falls, therefore, is complicated and complex. The challenge faced in evaluating vestibular function lies in differentiating the integrity of the input received from each system and determining the area of dysfunction.

Audiologists play a major role in evaluating equilibrium disorders because conditions causing vertigo and balance dysfunction often also cause auditory symptoms. A thorough evaluation of the dizzy patient, therefore, should include assessment of the complete audiovestibular system to provide a comprehensive analysis of the patient's condition (Gans, 1999; Goebel, 2001). This responsibility often lies with the audiologist because of the anatomical and physiological relationship between the auditory and vestibular systems and the audiologist's expertise in these areas. The American Academy of Audiology (AAA) and American Speech-Language-Hearing Association (ASHA) have recognized vestibular assessment as being as within the audiologist's scope of practice (AAA, 2004; ASHA, 2004).

This chapter will provide a comprehensive overview of procedures involved in the clinical assessment of vestibular function. The purpose is to familiarize audiologists with tests available to assess the balance system and to describe practical aspects of integrating these tests into the clinical workup of the patient with dizziness.

◆ Patient History

The causes of dizziness, vertigo, and balance disorder are numerous and considerable, so assessment of the vestibular system should begin with a complete medical history to explore the presence of precipitating disorders or illnesses

(Furman and Cass, 2003; Hester and Silverstein, 2002). The most common pathological conditions associated with equilibrium disturbance are categorized in **Table 25–1**.

Pearl

- A thorough patient history and interview will provide invaluable information regarding the nature of the patient's problem and exacerbating conditions. Understanding the specific situations and conditions that cause the symptoms will provide guidance in test selection and patient triage.

After obtaining the medical history, it is important for the patient to define and explain the symptoms comprehensively. Areas explored should include onset of symptoms, characteristics of symptoms at onset, the progression of symptoms over time, current symptoms, the nature and duration of typical spells, and past or current medications and treatment strategies (Baloh and Honrubia, 2001). Patients with vestibular disorders have a deficit in their spatial orientation mechanism, which often makes it difficult for them to describe exactly what they are feeling, especially as it relates to direction of motion. Although dizziness generally refers to one's perception of the body in space, and vertigo refers to the sensation or hallucination of movement, the patient should be encouraged to provide a more precise description using his or her own terms. The patient may report experiencing giddiness, wooziness, faintness, or light-headedness, feeling a spinning sensation (subjective vertigo), or feeling that the environment is spinning (objective vertigo). The patient may describe symptoms of clumsiness, swaying, instability, stumbling, or falling. It is important to include the history of falls in the description, because falls occurring within the home suggest a more severe problem. Defining the patient's symptoms in a variety of ways, therefore, provides a better understanding of the total disability.

Table 25–1 Causes of Equilibrium Disturbances

Otologic Conditions	Neurologic Conditions	Trauma	Other
Benign paroxysmal positional vertigo	Migraine	Head or cervicospinal injury	Tumors; cerebellopontine angle, and posterior fossa cysts
Vestibular neuronitis	Stroke	Labyrinthine concussion	Chiari malformations type I and II
Labyrinthitis	Seizure disorders	Barotrauma	Aging; sensory loss, cerebral hypoxia, and deconditioning
Meniere's disease	Multiple sclerosis		Medication: prescription, over-the-counter, supplements, and polypharmacy
Superior canal dehiscence	Spinocerebellar degeneration		Ocular disorders; glaucoma, refractive errors, and low vision
Perilymph fistula			Metabolic disorders; diabetes, hypoglycemia, and thyroid disease
Vestibular schwannoma			Cardiovascular; aortic stenosis, low cardiac output, peripheral arterial disease, and postural hypotension
Acoustic neuroma			Musculoskeletal and orthopedic problems; anxiety and psychiatric disorders

The impact of the symptoms on the patient's daily activities is another area to be discussed. Transitory symptoms may be a mere annoyance to one person but debilitating to another. To evaluate the functional, physical, and emotional effects of balance disturbance on the patient, the Dizziness Handicap Inventory (DHI) was developed (Jacobson and Newman, 1990; Jacobson et al, 1991). The DHI consists of 25 items requiring a "yes," "no," or "sometimes" response (see the appendix). Responses provide insight into the patient's perception of the balance disturbance and its effect on the quality of his or her life.

Once the patient's symptoms have been clarified and their impact determined, a patient profile develops, and differential diagnosis begins (Baloh and Honrubia, 2001; Goebel, 2001). In general, dizziness accompanied by light-headedness or floating indicates a nonvestibular balance disorder. These symptoms tend to be continuous and constant, can be precipitated by stress, and exacerbate in specific situations. Episodic vertigo or spinning is usually consistent with a vestibular site of the disorder. Accompanying the vertigo are sensations of drunkenness or motion sickness and feelings of falling to one side or tilting. Severe vertigo associated with hearing loss, tinnitus, nausea, and vomiting is usually of peripheral origin, whereas vertigo with neurologic symptoms of diplopia, dysarthria, numbness, or weakness is of central origin. Once symptoms are categorized, formal assessment begins.

♦ Pretest Preparation

For convenience to the patient and consistency of results, all balance function tests should be scheduled during a single block of time. The length of the complete evaluation will depend on whether the patient has previously undergone audiological testing, including electrophysiological assessment, and radiographic studies. In general, patients undergoing the complete battery should be prepared for 2 to 3 hours of testing.

To ease anxiety, the patient should receive information about the tests ordered prior to the appointment. This information should include the name and purpose of the test, a brief description of test procedures, and expectations of the patient. The description and explanations should be in consumer-friendly, simple-to-understand language. When the patient understands the nature of the tests and the procedures that are included, anxiety can be reduced.

Instructions should include information regarding test day protocol. The patient should be told to wear loose, comfortable clothing; women should wear slacks instead of dresses or skirts. Women also should not wear makeup, and both men and women should not apply oil to their skin the day of the test. The patient should not consume any caffeinated drinks, such as coffee and cola beverages, or use tobacco the day of the test. Because some of the tests may cause dizziness and/or nausea, the patient should have little or nothing to eat for 4 hours prior to testing. If a morning appointment is scheduled, and some nourishment is neces-

sary, only toast and juice should be allowed. If an afternoon appointment is scheduled, the patient should eat breakfast early in the morning and skip lunch. However, the individual health needs of the patient must always be considered, and fasting may be medically contraindicated for some patients, including those with diabetes and hypoglycemia. These patients should be asked to refrain from eating a greasy or dairy-rich meal and encouraged to eat a light meal, such as clear broth or a dry sandwich.

Instructions must be provided to the patient concerning the use of medications and alcohol before testing because the presence of medications or alcohol in the patient's system may affect test results and inaccurately indicate brainstem-cerebellar, CNS, or vestibular system dysfunction. In general, medications taken for heart problems, high blood pressure, diabetes, or other medical conditions should not be interrupted. Tranquilizers, sedatives, and vestibular suppressants should be stopped 48 hours prior to testing. Although medications for seizure or anxiety disorders should not be taken prior to testing, the patient's physician should be consulted before discontinuing these medications. Alcohol should be discontinued for at least 48 hours before testing (Cass and Furman, 1993; Goebel, 2001). Oftentimes, use of medications cannot be abruptly halted. If discontinuing any medication is medically contraindicated or impractical, the patient should be allowed to take the medication, but its use should be included in the report; results should be cautiously reviewed and interpreted, indicating the possible influence of the medications on all findings.

♦ Eye Movement and Vestibular Evaluation

Recording eye movement provides valuable information when evaluating the vestibular system because many eye movement abnormalities are specific to certain pathophysiological or pharmacological influences. Eye movement is easy to record, quantify, and interpret because it is limited to movement in the horizontal, vertical, and rotational planes, and the movement itself either shifts vision during head movement or stabilizes vision. The vestibular system stabilizes vision with head movement. The mechanoreceptors of the labyrinth sense the direction and speed of head acceleration and move the eyes accordingly. When disease affects a particular semicircular canal within the labyrinth, nystagmus may occur in the plane of the involved canal. It is this anatomical and physiological relationship of the vestibulo-ocular reflex (VOR) that makes its assessment so important.

Special Consideration

- If a patient is blind in one eye or has an ocular prosthesis, or if the clinician notes disconjugate eye movements, this should be carefully noted, as test procedures may need to be modified. Such factors will affect the interpretation of all eye movement tests.

Electronystagmography and Videonystagmography

One of the oldest tests developed to evaluate vestibular function is electronystagmography (ENG), which is based on electro-oculography, a technique that objectively records eye movements by measuring the corneoretinal potential. ENG can provide important information often missed in more recently developed imaging and electrophysiological procedures. It continues to be an essential part of the diagnostic battery of inner ear function. Because of the complex organization of the vestibulo-ocular system, innervation of the semicircular canal receptors influences eye motion on the horizontal plane. When the head is rotated, movement of the endolymph causes the normal individual to produce compensatory eye movements away from the fluid motion. The eyes will move slowly until they reach maximum deviation, then return quickly back into position because of CNS correction before repeating the compensatory motion. This activity generated by the VOR is identified as nystagmus.

Recordings of nystagmus have a sawtooth appearance. The slow phase represents eye motion induced by inner ear fluid movement; the fast phase reflects CNS correction. Nystagmus is identified by the direction of the fast phase of the eye movement, being left or right beating on the horizontal plane and up or down beating on the vertical plane (**Fig. 25–1**). The intensity of nystagmus is determined by measuring the slow phase angle of nystagmus, known as the slow phase velocity (SPV), and reporting the SPV in degrees of rotation per second.

Recently, videonystagmography (VNG) has emerged as a more popular and diagnostically efficient recording method. VNG is a highly effective and noninvasive method of recording linear and torsional eye movement (Vitte and Semont, 1995). Before this procedure was available, torsional eye movements could only be detected with research sclera coils, or 3 dB HL (hearing level) analysis, and these procedures were not available at most facilities. By using infrared video cameras, both linear and torsional eye movements can be visualized and recorded. However, it should be noted that the recording capability of most clinical systems is still limited to the linear aspect of eye movement.

VNG is significantly different from traditional ENG, which measures the corneoretinal potential or the eye's batterylike effect. With ENG, the eyes' side-to-side and up-and-down movements stimulate the corneoretinal potential; the positive and negative discharge of this potential is recorded by electrodes placed around the eyes (**Fig. 25–2**). With VNG technology, infrared cameras mounted in goggles track eye location and movement using the center of the pupil as a guide. There are two types of VNG equipment. In the first type, the camera is mounted directly in front of one eye, and the patient uses the other eye to follow targets. This monocular approach is not ideal because it does not allow for binocular tracking and limits the recording to only one eye. If the patient has a unilateral neuro-ophthalmic track involvement and recordings are made of the uninvolved eye, the abnormality can be missed. The other type, which is preferable, uses dichotic filters inside the goggles. These goggles act like two-way mirrors that reflect the infrared light and allow the patient

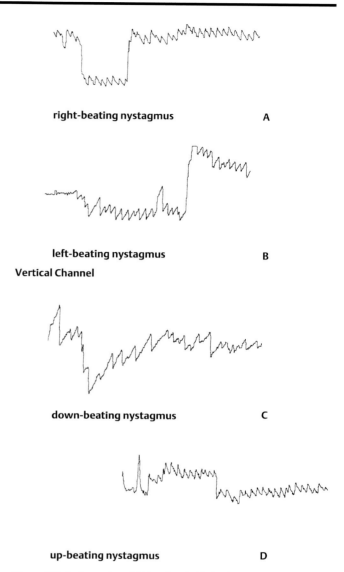

right-beating nystagmus   A

left-beating nystagmus   B

Vertical Channel

down-beating nystagmus   C

up-beating nystagmus   D

Figure 25–1 Examples of **(A)** right-, **(B)** left-, **(C)** up-, and **(D)** down-beating nystagmus.

to see normally (**Fig. 25–3**). Computer algorithms then analyze the position of the eyes.

The most advantageous and efficient video-oculographic system uses two cameras to record and analyze movement for each eye, a protocol that cannot be adapted to single camera VNG or ENG. This type of analysis is of particular importance in the oculomotor test subsets, which include saccadic, pendular, and optokinetic pursuit tasks. Identification of abnormalities in precision (gain or accuracy), latency, or peak velocity can provide the clinician and referring physicians with important differential diagnostic information regarding neural ophthalmic tract involvement. For peripheral vestibular lesions, which produce positional or positioning nystagmus in nonstabilized, noncompensated unilateral vestibular dysfunction, or benign paroxysmal positional vertigo (BPPV), differences in the strength and nature of nystagmus of the undermost versus uppermost ear

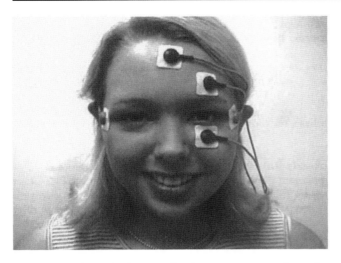

Figure 25–2 Electrode placement for electronystagmography testing.

during positional and positioning tasks can be observed and recorded. With BPPV of the posterior canal (BPPV-PC), the eye of the undermost (involved) ear will show a stronger rotatory-torsional component, whereas the eye of the contralateral (noninvolved) ear will have a more linear-vertical component. It should be remembered, however, that although these systems can record the rotatory-torsional nystagmus, the ability to quantitatively analyze is not available in most commercial systems. The advantages and disadvantages of VNG testing are listed in **Table 25–2.**

VNG and ENG evaluation protocols are essentially the same. Prior to initiating any tests, the equipment must be calibrated so the computerized system can set the requite gain of the eye movement. Depending on the equipment

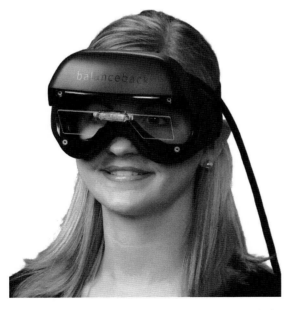

Figure 25–3 Video goggles with binocular infrared light for videonystagmography testing.

Table 25–2 Advantages and Disadvantages of Videonystagmography Testing

Advantages

1. Allows visual observation and videorecording of actual eye movement; advantageous for differential diagnosis of BPPV variants and visualization of rotatory-torsional nystagmus
2. Two-camera VNG systems provide evaluation of the ocular motility of each eye independently.
3. Does not require patient preparation and electrode placement
4. Does not require calibrations, as are necessary with traditional ENG corneoretinal-based technology
5. Patient is not required to close eyes, eliminating Bell's phenomenon and need for tasking.
6. No need to maintain darkened test room environment
7. Preferable for pediatric testing
8. Allows correlation between actual eye movement and graphic algorithm analysis
9. Provides increased educational/clinical understanding of the neurophysiologic and neuromuscular basis of eye movement

Disadvantages

1. Video goggles can be weighty or slightly uncomfortable for some patients.
2. Positioning of patient may require adjustment of camera angle(s).
3. Patients with dark eyelashes and blepharochalasis (drooped eyelids) may require their eyes to be taped open.
4. Ophthalmic hemorrhages may pose difficulty for the camera's tracking of the pupil.

BPPV, benign paroxysmal positional vertigo; VNG, videonystagmography.

manufacturer, calibration may be in the form of a shortened saccadic or smooth pursuit task. Once calibration has been successfully completed, the actual testing process may begin. In general, the battery of subtests consists of measurements of spontaneous nystagmus, the saccade test, smooth pursuit test, optokinetic test, gaze test, headshake test, modified Dix-Hallpike positioning tests, positional nystagmus tests, bithermal caloric tests, and assessment of the ability to suppress caloric-induced nystagmus by fixation (American Academy of Neurology, 1996; Brookler, 1991; Gans and Roberts, 2006; Resnick and Brewer, 1983). The VNG test battery and an overview explanation of VNG results are given later in this chapter and listed in **Table 25–3**.

Spontaneous Nystagmus

Spontaneous nystagmus is involuntary, unprovoked, repetitive eye movement that can appear in any direction or be rotary. It is present in all head positions when the eyes are closed or opened. Spontaneous nystagmus must be measured early in the VNG evaluation because its presence can influence the interpretation of all subsequent test results.

Pearl

- Eye blinks may appear as right- or left-beating nystagmus in the horizontal channel. If horizontal nystagmus is observed, check the vertical channel response for the presence of sharp, eye-blink movements.

Table 25–3 Videonystagmography Test Battery and Description of Findings

Test	Abnormality	Interpretation
Spontaneous nystagmus test	Involuntary, unprovoked nystagmus that can appear in any direction	Indicates the presence of pathological condition within the peripheral or central vestibular system
Saccade test	Ocular dysmetria, characterized by overshoot, undershoot, glissades, pulsions occurring over 50% of the time in the recording	CNS pathological condition, involving the cerebral cortex, brainstem, or cerebellum
Smooth pursuit test	Breakup of smooth pursuit	Cerebellar dysfunction, eye, and neurological disorder, as well as systemic conditions affecting the CNS
Optokinetic test	Asymmetry in amplitude of response	CNS pathological condition or uncompensated vestibular
Gaze test	Persistent nystagmus recorded for ocular displacements of 20 degrees or less	Peripheral or CNS pathological condition, indicating brainstem or cerebellar disturbance
Headshake test	Provocable nystagmus following 20 seconds of head shaking	Peripheral lesions tend to produce a fast phase away from involved ear; CNS lesions may cause nystagmus toward or away from the lesion
Modified Dix-Hallpike positioning test	Onset of rotary nystagmus ~10 seconds after positioning, then diminishes	Peripheral site of disorder consistent with posterior canal benign paroxysmal positional vertigo
Positional nystagmus test	Nystagmus provoked by static position; may be in any direction	Consistent with lesions in the peripheral or central vestibular pathway, or both
Bithermal caloric tests	UW: SPV differs by 20–30% or more between ears DP: Nystagmus in one direction is more intense than responses in the other direction; if no UW, a difference of 20% or more between right- and left-beating nystagmus is significant; if UW is present, a difference of 30% or more right- and left-beating nystagmus is significant BW: SPV on each side is less than ~12 degrees per second	UW: Peripheral (nerve and/or end-organ) vestibular site of lesion DP: Finding suggesting either a peripheral or central vestibular abnormality BW: Either CNS disorder or peripheral vestibular abnormality
Fixation suppression	Inability of CNS to attenuate caloric nystagmus with vision enabled	Brainstem and/or cerebellar disease

BW, bilateral weakness; CNS, central nervous system; DP, directional preponderance; SPV, slow phase velocity; UW, unilateral weakness.

To evaluate for spontaneous nystagmus, the patient is seated upright with the back supported. Ocular movements are recorded continuously for ~20 seconds with vision denied by closing the cover on the VNG goggles. If a spontaneous nystagmus is detected with vision denied, recordings are made for an additional 20 seconds with vision enabled (cover removed) to determine if the nystagmus is suppressed with vision. The presence of spontaneous nystagmus is consistent with pathology within the peripheral or central vestibular system (Brandt, 1993). In acute stages of peripheral vestibular disease, spontaneous horizontal nystagmus appears toward the unaffected ear; in later stages, the nystagmus may reverse itself or diminish. If spontaneous nystagmus is maintained when the eyes are open, or if direction-changing spontaneous nystagmus is observed, it is indicative of a CNS disorder.

Controversial Point

- Modern theory of vestibular test interpretation acknowledges that the presence of nystagmus of any degree is not normal and requires further evaluation. Historically, prior to the advent of magnetic resonance imaging, it was believed that low-intensity nystagmus was normal in the general population.

Saccade Test

The saccade test is one of three ocular motor pursuit function tests. For pursuit function tests, a visual stimulus/target, which is controlled by the computer program, is projected on a wall by a liquid crystal display (LCD) or is on a light bar. Light bar testing is limited to horizontal and vertical eye movements; the bar must be manually rotated to move from horizontal to vertical testing. A projected or full-screen stimulus, therefore, is preferred.

The saccade is the most rapid movement the oculomotor system is capable of performing. The saccade test evaluates the eyes' ability to shift the point of visual fixation (Evans and Melancon, 1989). To perform the test, the patient is seated upright facing the stimulus with the back supported. The patient is asked to follow and fixate on a single target that randomly moves horizontally, vertically, and/or diagonally, for distances ranging from 5 to 20 degrees. The patient must fixate for several seconds on a point, rapidly switch to a new point when the stimulus moves, then fixate for several seconds at the new point without any head movement.

Eye motion is evaluated for latency, velocity, and accuracy of the response (Honrubia, 1995). Normal tracings are rectangular in shape and occur within a specified latency. An example of saccade test results are shown in **Fig. 25–4**. In pathological cases, the patient is unable to follow the target accurately. The four most common patterns of saccadic inaccuracy are undershoot dysmetria, overshoot

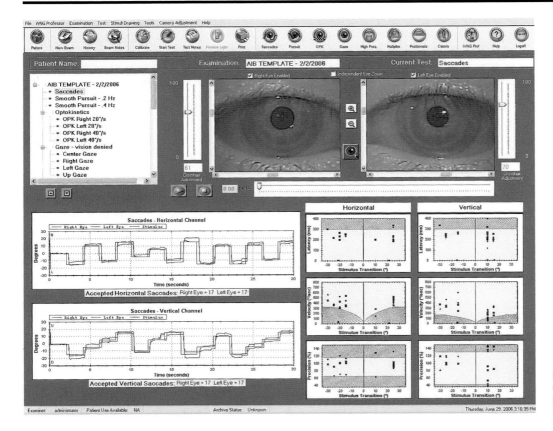

Figure 25–4 Results from saccade test showing normal accuracy, latency, and peak velocity. *(See Color Plate 25–4.)*

dysmetria, glissades, and pulsions (Hain, 1993). Although these patterns are sometimes observed transiently in normal patients, they are considered abnormal if they occur more than 50% of the time in the recording. The presence of ocular dysmetria indicates a CNS pathological condition involving the cerebral cortex, brainstem, or cerebellum (Konrad, 1991; Sataloff and Hughes, 1988).

Smooth Pursuit Test

The smooth pursuit test examines the ocular smooth pursuit system. To perform the test, the patient is seated upright facing the stimulus with the back supported. The patient is instructed to fixate on a target moving in a sinusoidal pattern that extends 20 degrees to the right and left from center without moving the head. The target movement progresses from low frequency (slow moving) to high frequency (fast moving).

Normal sinusoidal tracking responses are characterized by smooth, sinusoidal movements whose amplitudes correspond to the motion of the target (**Fig. 25–5**). The most common abnormality observed is breakup of smooth pursuit, which suggests cerebellar dysfunction. Abnormal patterns have also been associated with eye disease, neurological disorders, and systemic conditions affecting the CNS (Evans and Melancon, 1989; Hain, 1993). Results from this test, however, must be interpreted with caution because performance is strongly affected by attention and does degenerate as a function of age.

Optokinetic Test

The optokinetic test measures nystagmus elicited by watching repetitive stimulus movement across the visual field. The test has been compared with watching cars on a moving train because the stimuli used for testing are constantly moving checkerboards or stripes. To truly test the optokinetic pursuit system, the visual field must be at least 80% filled, which cannot be accomplished using a light bar (Baloh and Honrubia, 2001). Therefore, optokinetic testing can only be accomplished using a stimulus projected on a large screen or presented within an enclosure.

To perform the test, the patient is seated upright facing the stimulus with the back supported. Stimuli are presented horizontally, moving from right to left for ~20 seconds, then left to right for 20 seconds. The stimuli are presented in each direction at a slow speed (20 degrees per second) and at a fast speed (40 degrees per second). Stimuli may be presented vertically, moving from bottom to top for ~20 seconds, then top to bottom for ~20 seconds, but because abundant research does not indicate significant pathological findings, vertical optokinetic testing is often omitted.

Results of the optokinetic test are analyzed for symmetry in each direction of pursuit (**Fig. 25–6**). If asymmetry is observed, responses are considered abnormal and indicative of either a CNS pathological condition or a peripheral lesion when the stimulus moves in the direction of an

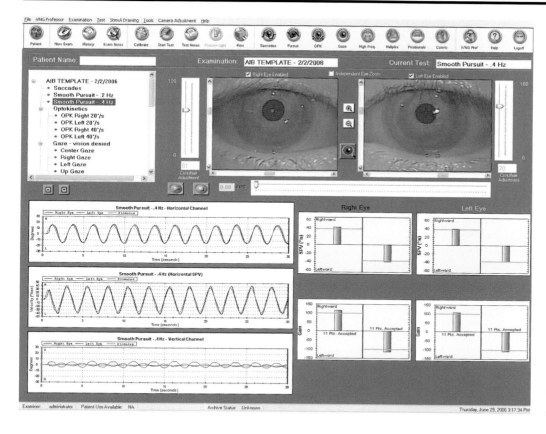

Figure 25–5 Results from smooth pursuit test showing normal gain and peak velocity. *(See Color Plate 25–5.)*

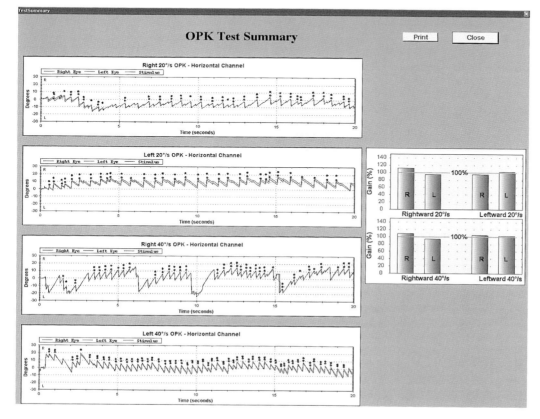

Figure 25–6 Results from bidirectional, slow- and fast-speed optokinetic (OPK) test showing normal gain. *(See Color Plate 25–6.)*

uncompensated or active unilateral vestibular weakness (Leigh and Zee, 1999). The asymmetry observed is due to the integration of both vestibular and visual stimuli within the vestibular nucleus, a primary locus of central compensation (Honrubia, 2002).

Gaze Test

The gaze test records any nystagmus that is present when the head is stable and upright and the eyes are in a fixed position. To perform the test, the patient is seated upright with the back supported and with vision denied (goggles cover on). Five separate, 20 second recordings are made as the patient fixates at a target placed at 0 degree azimuth, displaced 20 degrees to the right of center, 20 degrees to the left of center, 20 degrees above center, and 20 degrees below center. Any persistent nystagmus recorded for ocular displacements of 20 degrees or less is considered abnormal. In those conditions where nystagmus is recorded, the test is repeated with vision enabled (cover off) to see if vision will suppress the nystagmus.

The presence of gaze nystagmus is consistent with acute or recent peripheral lesions, congenital nystagmus, or CNS pathological conditions, indicating brainstem or cerebellar disturbance (Baloh and Honrubia, 2001; Sataloff and Hughes, 1988). The direction of the nystagmus and nature of the gaze evoked pattern will help differentiate the origin of the lesion. For example, vertical nystagmus is typically associated only with CNS lesions, whereas horizontal nystagmus may indicate either peripheral or CNS lesions. Suppression of horizontal nystagmus with vision usually suggests a peripheral origin.

Headshake Test

The headshake test records nystagmus that is elicited after the patient performs 20 seconds of head shaking. To perform the test, the patient is seated upright with the back supported and without vision (cover on) to minimize visual suppression. The required side-to-side head movement at a frequency of ~2 Hz per second is demonstrated, and the patient performs the test within a comfortable cervicospinal range of motion (ROM); frequency of head movement is important, not ROM. The patient should be cued by an automated stimulus tone or by instruction throughout the 20 second time to ensure active head movement at the proper speed.

The appearance of post-headshake nystagmus has been attributed to both peripheral and CNS origins (Palla et al, 2005; Stockwell and Bojrab, 1993). The provocation of nystagmus post-headshake is attributed to an asymmetrical status within the velocity storage mechanism located in the brainstem. In active or uncompensated peripheral lesions, the nystagmus will tend to follow Ewald's law and beat away from the lesion. In some cases of recovering vestibular function, the nystagmus will first beat away from the lesion, then reverse and beat toward it. This is referred to as a recovery nystagmus. In CNS lesions, the direction of the nystagmus may be less predictable. Although the presence of postheadshake nystagmus is abnormal, it cannot absolutely

differentiate the nature of the lesion and must be used in conjunction with other test findings (Palla et al, 2005; Perez et al, 2004).

Modified Dix-Hallpike Positioning Tests

The Dix-Hallpike positioning tests are designed to elicit nystagmus and subjective vertigo that are caused by BPPV. BPPV is the result of dislodged otoconia settling in the posterior semicircular canal, generating a gravity-dependent cupula deflection. Symptoms of BPPV-PC include brief and transient onset of nystagmus and vertigo that are precipitated by positioning of the patient's head so the undermost ear, specifically the posterior semicircular canal, is gravity dependent. It is important to remember that the Dix-Hallpike maneuver evaluates only BPPV-PC, which is the most prevalent (90–95%) type of BPPV due to the location of the posterior canal just inferior to the utricle. Possible migration of otoconial debris into the horizontal semicircular canal (BPPV-HC) is evaluated during the positional testing, and will be discussed later in this chapter.

Testing for BPPV should always be performed with the patient's eyes open to allow for direct observation. Unlike other forms of peripherally generated nystagmus, nystagmus induced by BPPV will not be suppressed by vision. The traditional Dix-Hallpike maneuver was performed with the examiner standing to the side of the patient throughout the test (Dix and Hallpike, 1952). This position was cumbersome to both the patient and the examiner when performing the maneuver and observing the patient. For greater ease, the modified Dix-Hallpike has been described and recommended (Gans and Harrington-Gans, 2002). In this procedure, the examiner stands behind the patient. The patient turns the head slightly toward the test ear, and the examiner supports the patient's neck and back while the patient is lowered into the provoking supine position with the neck slightly hyperextended and off the examination table (**Fig. 25–7A–C**). Because the provocation of symptoms is gravity based and due to changing positions of the involved posterior canal, rapid positioning is not required. Once in the supine position, the examiner has a clear view of the patient's eyes.

Although the modified Dix-Hallpike maneuver is appropriate for the general population, another modification has been described that is more appropriate for the older population. BPPV is common in patients over 50 years of age, but it is even more prevalent in the older population (Korres et al, 2002). The older population may have comorbid factors that must be considered, including vertebrobasilar insufficiency, cervical spondylosis, and limited ROM. The Dix-Hallpike maneuver is contraindicated in these patients because it results in hyperextension of the neck. Humphriss et al (2003) described a modification of Dix-Hallpike that uses a side-lying maneuver. In this modification, the head and neck of the patient are fully supported on the examining table (see **Fig. 25–8A,B**, p. 550). Humphriss et al (2003) reported positive results when using this positioning procedure, which was also supported by Cohen (2004) as an appropriate alternative for patients with these comorbid conditions.

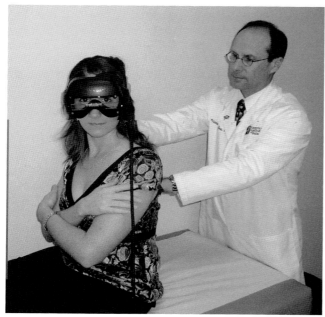

A

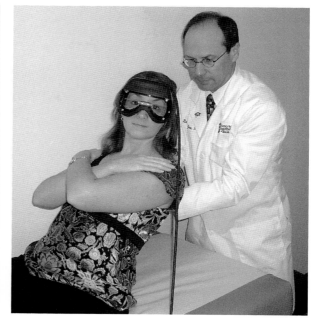

B

C

Figure 25–7 (A–C) Modified supported Dix-Hallpike maneuver.

Pitfall

- The patient must be screened for a history of neck or back injury or impairment before performing the modified Dix-Hallpike maneuver and positional tests. If the patient reports any such problems, select the modified procedure that is most biomechanically safe and comfortable for the patient.

Positional Nystagmus Tests

Positional testing is performed to determine if nystagmus can be elicited or if previously elicited nystagmus can be changed when the head and body are placed in static positions. Positional testing is performed following the modified Dix-Hallpike maneuver so BPPV does not contaminate the positional tests as positions are changed and to prevent a reduced BPPV response from occurring due to displacement of the otoconia prior to performing the modified Dix-Hallpike.

To perform the positional tests, the patient is placed in the following positions: supine, head/body right, and head/body left. When placed in the head/body left and right positions, the head must be rotated 90 degrees so the ear is perpendicular with the ground. If the patient is unable to assume this position, a body lateral position rather than a head turning position should be performed. Recordings

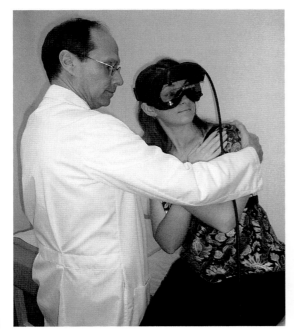
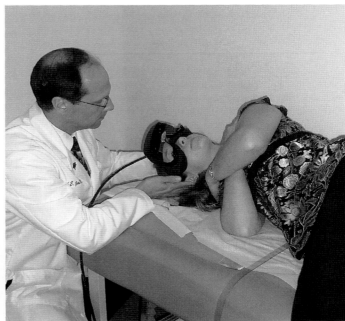

A   B

Figure 25–8 **(A,B)** Modified side-lying Dix-Hallpike maneuver.

should be obtained for 20 seconds in each position with vision denied (cover on). If nystagmus is detected in any position, recording should be performed again with vision enabled (cover off) to evaluate for suppression of nystagmus with vision.

Nystagmus in positional tests is described by the direction of its fast phase, being either toward the ground (geotropic) or away from the ground (ageotropic). Geotropic nystagmus is most often attributed to peripheral lesions, whereas ageotropic is most often correlated with CNS, pharmacological, or alcohol influences. Geotropic nystagmus, which suppresses with vision, is most likely related to a peripheral origin, with the exception of BPPV-HC, which, like BPPV-PC, does not suppress with vision (Roberts et al, 2006). The presence of up- or down-beating vertical positional nystagmus is usually indicative of brainstem, midbrain, or cerebellar lesions (Kanaya et al, 1994; Parker, 1993).

The duration of the nystagmus and whether it is persistent or transient provide additional diagnostic information. Persistent nystagmus suggests CNS pathology; transient nystagmus suggests a peripheral site of disorder. The presence of nystagmus in positional tests should always be correlated with any other report of symptoms by the patient, such as vertigo or nausea. It is also important to note any subjective vertigo or nausea described by the patient in the absence of nystagmus.

Bithermal Caloric Tests

Bithermal caloric testing is often considered the most important part of the VNG battery because it specifically isolates and evaluates the ability of each horizontal semicircular canal to respond to a stimulus. Irrigating the external

auditory canal (EAC) warms or cools the skin of the EAC and tympanic membrane, transmitting a temperature change to the endolymph in the horizontal semicircular canal (Jacobson and Newman, 1993). This temperature change causes induction currents in the horizontal semicircular canals, simulating endolymphatic fluid movements like those that occur during head rotation. Warm stimulation causes ampullopetal (toward the ampulla) movement of the horizontal canal cupula, and cool stimulation causes ampullofugal (away from the ampulla) movement of the cupula. In response to this movement, hair cell activity in the crista increases and generates nystagmus. The expected physiological responses to thermal stimulation are left-beating nystagmus to right cool stimulation, right-beating nystagmus to left cool stimulation, left-beating nystagmus to left warm stimulation, and right-beating nystagmus to right warm stimulation. By stimulating each external auditory canal with a warm stimulus and a cool stimulus, the physiological integrity of the left and right horizontal semicircular canals can be evaluated separately and compared.

> **Pearl**
>
> • To help remember the expected direction of nystagmus induced by caloric stimulation, the acronym COWS is used: cold (stimulation) = opposite (direction nystagmus); warm (stimulation) = same (direction nystagmus).

Before testing begins, instructions should be given to prepare the patient for the test. Begin by explaining that this part of the VNG isolates the contributions of each inner ear system to balance function. Each system will be presented a cool stimulus followed by a warm stimulus to change the temperature of the inner ear fluids, and responses will be measured and compared to determine whether each system is responding and whether the contribution from each system is "equal." It is helpful to show the patient the irrigator that will be used to induce the temperature changes. Continue by more specifically explaining that each system will be measured separately, starting with a cool stimulus to the right ear, then to the left ear, followed by a warm stimulus to the left ear and finally to the right ear. Five to 10 minute breaks will be taken between each stimulation to allow the inner ear fluids to return to their normal temperature. The patient is to stay relaxed throughout testing with eyes open inside the goggles with the cover on. A light will appear at some time following the conclusion of the irrigation, and the patient is to fixate on the light. The patient should be told that caloric stimulation may induce the sensation of turning or floating, so the patient will not be alarmed if symptoms occur. This sensation diminishes as the inner ear fluids return to their normal temperature.

Two types of irrigators are currently available for caloric stimulation. A third type, called the closed-loop system, is no longer commercially available. The water irrigator consists of two baths containing warm or cool water, temperature-sensing devices, thermostats to heat the water, a switch that gates water flow controlled by an activator switch that controls the volume of water flow, and a delivery system that presents the water in the EAC. The main disadvantages of water irrigation include the inconvenience of purging the system before each caloric stimulation to ensure correct water temperature, the need to recover water flowing out of the EAC, the possibility of water contamination, and the potential for electrical shock. The second type of irrigation system, which is becoming increasingly popular, is the air caloric irrigator. The air irrigator consists of an air flow regulator, a heater, a thermostat, and a hose or speculum through which air is delivered to the EAC. The advantages of air stimulation are the ability to visualize the tympanic membrane during stimulation, convenience, lack of hygiene issues, and a more comfortable patient experience. If using air stimuli, the air can be blown on the patient's hand prior to testing to reduce any apprehension. Temperature of the irrigations will differ based on the stimuli. Water irrigations are performed at 30 and 44°C and air irrigations at 24 and 50°C, respectively.

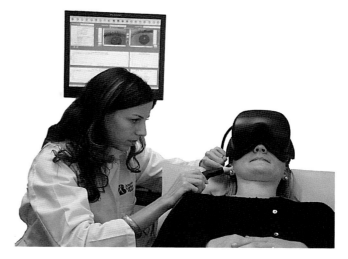

Figure 25–9 Photograph of caloric testing with the patient's head elevated 30 degrees with vision denied. (Courtesy of Balanceback, Boca Raton, FL.)

(**Fig. 25–9**). Recordings should begin prior to the irrigation to record any spontaneous nystagmus. The irrigation is initiated, and the stimulus is presented to the ear. Stimulation will continue for 30 seconds when using water and 60 seconds when using air calorics. Once stimulation ends, the patient maintains his or her position with the eyes opened to ensure the infrared cameras are recording eye movements. A fixation light inside the goggle will typically be set to turn on at ~40 seconds after the conclusion of the irrigation, which should be at the time of maximum amplitude of the nystagmus. Once fixation is obtained, testing is completed, recording stops, and the patient may relax until the next stimulation.

The SPV of the induced nystagmus is the most useful variable for quantifying the caloric response. For each caloric stimulation, the SPV is quantified by averaging 10 consecutive beats of nystagmus at the peak of the caloric response. Right ear responses are compared with left ear responses to determine unilateral weakness (UW) or canal paresis, and right-beating nystagmus is compared with left-beating nystagmus to determine directional preponderance (DP; Gans and Roberts, 2006).

Results from the caloric test can identify several abnormalities (Evans and Melancon, 1989; Jacobson et al, 1993). A UW is present when the SPV differs by 20 to 30% or more between ears and suggests a peripheral (nerve and/or end-organ) vestibular site of the lesion. A BW is demonstrated when the SPV induced from caloric irrigations on each side is less than ~12 degrees per second. BW can be caused by both CNS disorders and peripheral vestibular abnormalities. The presence of a BW, therefore, must be interpreted with information from other diagnostic procedures. A DP is identified when responses in one direction of nystagmus are more intense than responses in the other direction. If no UW is present, a difference of 20% or more between right- and left-beating nystagmus is considered significant; if a UW is present, a difference of 30% or more between

---

Pitfall

- The EAC and tympanic membrane must be examined for abnormalities before caloric stimulation. If the patient has a perforation of the tympanic membrane, air calorics must be used to prevent water from entering the middle ear space. Warm air irrigation of a moist EAC or middle ear mucosa has an evaporative or cooling effect, which may result in a reversal of the anticipated nystagmus direction.

To perform the test, the patient is placed in a supine position with the head elevated and resting at a 30 degree angle. The eyes are open within the covered goggles

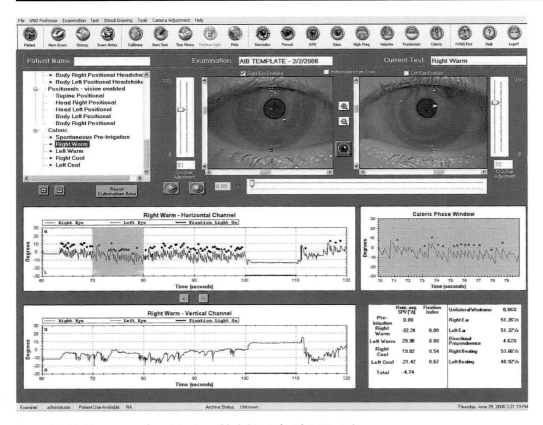

Figure 25–10 Nystagmus when vision is enabled. *(See Color Plate 25–10.)*

right- and left-beating nystagmus is considered significant. The presence of a DP suggests either a peripheral or central vestibular abnormality. The most common cause of a DP is a preexisting or spontaneous nystagmus that occurs prior to irrigation. Fixation suppression evaluates the ability of the CNS to control vestibular nuclei and attenuate caloric nystagmus when the eyes are opened (**Fig. 25–10**). Failure of fixation suppression suggests brainstem and/or cerebellar disease. **Fig. 25–11** shows the nystagmus from each irrigation, the culmination period, SPVs, calculations for UW and DP, and graphic representations of the data.

Advantages and Disadvantages of Videonystagmography

VNG offers several advantages over other measures of balance function. First, because nystagmus is the only physical sign uniquely linked to the vestibular system, VNG is a crucial tool in evaluating the vestibular system. Second, VNG recordings can be made with and without vision, which becomes critical when it is realized that pathologically significant nystagmus is completely suppressed by visual fixation. Third, VNG is capable of detecting subtle abnormalities of both volitional and reflex eye movement controlled at the brainstem and higher levels that cannot be detected by any other techniques. Thus, VNG may provide the only substantial and documentable evidence of brainstem dysfunction. Fourth, VNG is the only clinical test that can unequivocally

isolate one labyrinth from its contralateral partner. Finally, VNG provides a permanent, objective video and graphic recording that can be reviewed after it was made and compared with new tracings to establish a serial record of the evolution of dysfunction or to document improvement.

Despite these advantages, the test has some limitations. The caloric part of VNG testing is not a true physiological stimulus because caloric irrigation is not a natural occurrence as is head movement. The caloric stimulus is also subject to a variety of variables that are not under the examiner's control. Such variables include the shape and size of the individual patient's EAC, the thickness and position of the tympanic membrane, the size of the tympanic cavity, and the thickness of bone and pneumatization of the patient's middle ear and mastoid. Most importantly, the test evaluates only the horizontal semicircular canals and at an ultra low frequency of 0.003 Hz (Jacobson et al, 1993), which is well below the frequency of everyday active head movement.

Pitfall

- Although VNG testing is the cardinal test of peripheral vestibular function, its sensitivity and specificity are significantly improved when findings are correlated with patient history and symptoms and other available vestibular function tests.

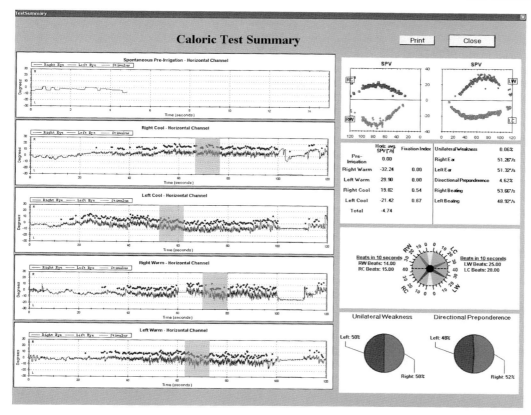

Figure 25–11 Caloric test summary page showing nystagmus from each irrigation, the culmination period, slow phase velocity (SPV), calculations for unilateral weakness (UW) and directional preponderance (DP), and graphic representations of the data. *(See Color Plate 25–11.)*

◆ Vestibular Evoked Myogenic Potentials

Vestibular evoked myogenic potential (VEMP) testing is based on the vestibulocollic reflex (VCR), which occurs between the saccule otolith organ and the sternocleidomastoid (SCM) muscle. Specifically, the response pathway is from the saccule to the lateral vestibular nucleus via the inferior vestibular portion of the eighth cranial nerve (CN VIII). The pathway then extends to the lateral vestibulospinal tract. The reflex arc is completed with the innervations of the SCM by CN XI, the accessory nerve (Colebatch and Halmagyi, 1992). The benefit of measuring VEMPs is an ability to identify lesions of the saccule, inferior vestibular nerve, and descending vestibulospinal pathways, including the lower brainstem.

Because the VEMP is actually a myogenic recording from the large SCM muscle, as shown in **Fig. 25–12**, it is easy to produce a response with clear P13 and N23 components. When compared with other evoked potentials, such as the auditory brainstem response (ABR), whose amplitude is < 1 μV, the VEMP is robust, with an amplitude of ~200 μV. The test is most commonly performed with a click or tone burst stimulus but has also been observed using a nonacoustic tapping technique.

Based on a unique ability to assess the VCR pathway, the recording of VEMPs has provided useful diagnostic information on both otologic and neurologic conditions. VEMP findings have been reported in a variety of pathologies, ranging from otologic disorders such as Meniere's disease, superior canal dehiscence syndrome (SCDS), and vestibular neuritis, to neurologic disorders such as multiple sclerosis, spinocerebellar degeneration, and migraine (Colebatch and Halmagyi, 1992; Liao and Young, 2004; Zapala and Brey, 2004). This sound-evoked potential is an especially useful clinical tool because it appears robust even when there is significant sensorineural hearing loss; however, the patient must have a normally functioning middle ear system to elicit this response.

Interpretation of VEMPs may be based on latency or amplitude. As waveform labeling suggests, typical P13 absolute latency is 13 msec, whereas N23 absolute latency is 23 msec. Many laboratories advocate use of an asymmetry ratio calculated as

$$100(Amplitude_{Left} - Amplitude_{Right})/(Amplitude_{Left} + Amplitude_{Right})$$

An amplitude asymmetry > 30 to 47% is considered clinically significant.

Depending on the disorder, P13–N23 responses may be absent, delayed in latency, reduced in amplitude, or elevated in amplitude. Liao and Young (2004) described results from VEMP studies in patients with migraine. They found

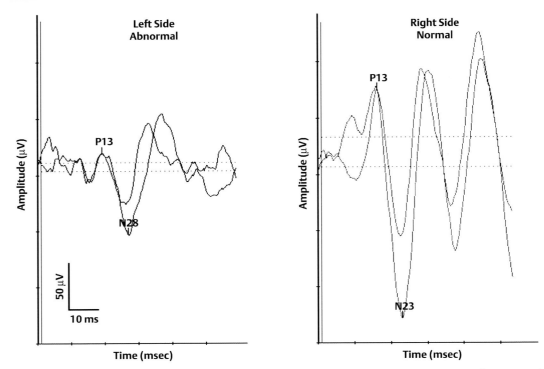

Figure 25–12 Vestibular evoked myogenic potential responses obtained from a patient diagnosed with Meniere's disease. Results with stimulation to the left ear (involved ear) were reduced in amplitude relative to responses obtained with stimulation to the right ear.

absent or delayed responses for many of the patients. Following 3 months of medical intervention, normal VEMPs were obtained in 90% of the migraine patients.

Intense stimulus levels of 95 to 100 dB nHL (normalized hearing level) are typically needed to record VEMPs in the normal population, but for certain disorders, reliable responses have been recorded at much lower levels. Brantberg et al (1999) reported replicable VEMPs in patients with SCDS for stimulus levels as low as 70 to 75 dB nHL.

Young et al (2002) reported that augmented VEMPs could be obtained in patients with Meniere's disease as the fluid-distended saccule is in closer proximity to the stapes footplate. This is thought to increase the effective stimulus level reaching the saccule.

Patient Preparation

Before testing can begin, the patient's skin needs to be prepared, and electrodes must be placed. The patient's skin should be cleansed with alcohol, with no abrading necessary, followed by placement of electrodes. Large pregelled electrodes, which are used for cardiac and myogenic recordings, are recommended. It is easier to prepare the patient and place electrodes bilaterally, even when using a one-channel system (rather than cleaning, prepping, and running the right ear, then the left). Electrode placement may be as follows: ground–low forehead; active (noninverting)–point of SCM attachment at the collarbone and sternum or high forehead; and reference (inverting)–on the belly of the SCM muscle. There is some variance among laboratories in terms of placement for the active (noninverting)

and reference (inverting) electrodes, and although the positive and negative peaks and troughs will invert, latency remains unaffected.

To identify the SCM muscle and allow appropriate electrode placement, the patient should lie in the supine position. The patient's head should be elevated several inches, then rotated to the right, causing a clearly visible contraction of the SCM muscle (**Fig. 25–13**). Once the electrodes have been placed on the right SCM, the procedure can be

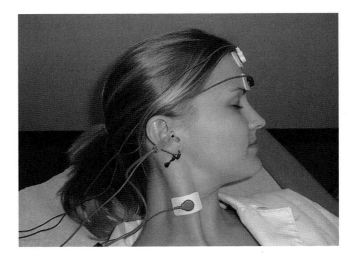

Figure 25–13 Photograph of vestibular evoked myogenic potential (VEMP) electrode montage and contraction of the right sternocleidomastoid muscle.

repeated with contraction of the left SCM for appropriate electrode placement on the left SCM.

Recordings can be made using either a one- or two-channel ABR system. When using a one-channel system, test one side, then change the electrodes in the preamplifier box to the other set of electrodes to test the other side. When using a two-channel system, record/test the ipsilateral side using channel 1, and monitor the contralateral SCM muscle activity on channel 2. Because there is no sound presented to the contralateral side, a VEMP should not be observed.

Protocols

Most auditory evoked potential systems should be able to perform this test. The system will present the stimuli and record the SCM muscle response. Either insert or traditional headphones may be used. No masking is necessary in the nontest (contralateral) ear. As with most electrophysiologic recordings, fluorescent lights should be off, and the patient should close his or her eyes during data collection. Background or ambient noise is less of an issue with this large amplitude response when compared with ABR testing.

The test is conducted ipsilaterally. When recording the contraction of the right SCM muscle, the acoustic stimulus is delivered to the right ear, and the patient must turn his or her head to the left to cause the proper right SCM contraction. When recording the contraction of the left SCM muscle, the acoustic stimulus is delivered to the left ear, and the patient must turn his or her head to the right to cause the proper left SCM contraction. The patient must maintain an appropriate level of SCM muscle contraction ipsilateral to the stimulus during the data collection period. Some authors advocate monitoring of SCM activation during recording to maintain a target level of ~50 μV, but this monitoring may not be feasible in all laboratories. We have successfully recorded reliable VEMPs with the patient lifting and rotating the head away from the test ear while lying in a supine position. If the patient becomes fatigued, gentle cuing is usually sufficient to maintain the muscle contraction.

Pearl

- VEMP testing may be used with neonates and infants who have been identified as hearing impaired as a screening test of vestibular function. It is reported that 30 to 40% of children with sensorineural hearing loss also have a vestibular deficit (Kelsch et al, 2006; Sheykholesami et al, 2005).

◆ Dynamic Visual Acuity Tests

Patients with vestibular dysfunction who are uncompensated following an acute vestibular event commonly report unstable gaze during active head movement (Bhansali et al, 1993; Longridge and Mallinson, 1987). This symptom was termed *oscillopsia* by Brickner (1936). Patients with bilateral or unilateral vestibular impairment may demonstrate a functional VOR deficit on tests measuring dynamic visual acuity (Roberts et al, 2006; Schubert et al, 2002). For these patients, simple tasks such as reading signs while walking or driving may be difficult.

Numerous tests of dynamic visual acuity (DVA) have been reported in the literature as a means of assessing the impact of impaired VOR function (Roberts et al, 2006; Schubert et al, 2002). Several of the tests are commercially available for clinical use. These tests are generally scored by comparing a baseline visual acuity score obtained with no head movement to a DVA score with head movement in the vertical and/or horizontal planes. Patients with normal VOR function exhibit little degradation in visual acuity for these conditions. Patients with uncompensated VOR dysfunction, however, exhibit degradation in visual acuity with head movement compared with the baseline score.

Although scoring is similar among tests, there is some variability in the tests themselves. For example, patients may be asked to read the letters on a Snellen eye chart (Bhansali et al, 1993) or to read computer-presented number stimuli on a computer screen (Hillman et al, 1999; Roberts et al, 2006) or even to read the optotype *E* (Herdman et al, 1998; Schubert et al, 2002). Some investigators have used a treadmill to provide a natural head movement for the dynamic condition (Hillman et al, 1999), whereas others have simply used volitional head movement with or without an auditory cuing tone (Bhansali et al, 1993; Herdman et al, 1998; Hillman et al, 1999; Roberts et al, 2006; Schubert et al, 2002). Herdman et al (1998) and Schubert et al (2002) used a rate sensor to monitor head movement and restrict testing to movements within the VOR range.

Advantages and Disadvantages of Dynamic Visual Acuity Tests

The use of DVA testing helps identify whether a VOR deficit exists and provides additional insight into which direction of head movement is most problematic. The results may be correlated with the patient's reported symptoms and provide a functional measurement to identify patients who would benefit from vestibular rehabilitation therapy (VRT). Pre- and post-VRT testing will demonstrate treatment efficacy and VOR recovery. The primary disadvantages of DVA testing are it requires the patient's volitional head movement to be maintained at a consistent speed; some patients are somewhat rhythmically challenged and have difficulty with the necessary coordinated movement; and patients with bi- or trifocal refractive lenses must keep the visual target inside the appropriate visual field during testing.

◆ Vestibular Autorotation Test

The vestibular autorotation test (VAT) was developed in 1986 (Fineberg et al, 1987) to test VOR function encountered during normal active movements at frequencies of 2 to 6 Hz. Although VNG and ENG test VOR function, testing is limited because only horizontal canal function is assessed at the ultra-low-frequency sensitivity of 0.003 Hz. Likewise, sinusoidal harmonic acceleration (SHA) testing is limited to the horizontal plane, and its upper limit frequency is 0.64 Hz, well below that of most normal everyday head movement. Because natural active head movement occurs in the range of 2 to 6 Hz, it is possible for a high-frequency vestibular lesion to go undetected if testing the full range of VOR sensitivity is not performed; thus the development of VAT.

Patient Preparation and Test Protocol

The patient is seated with the back supported facing a 1 cm diameter target placed on a wall ~60 inches from his or her position. Five electro-oculographic (EOG) electrodes are placed at the outer canthi of each eye, on the forehead, and above and below one eye. This montage is exactly the same as that for the montage used in ENG testing. The electrodes are connected to the preamplifier on a headband worn by the patient. All electrodes and leads are secured with tape to prevent movement artifact during head shaking. The headband is adjusted for a tight but comfortable fit.

Two instructions are given to the patient: stare at the target spot on the wall, and move your head in time to the computer-generated auditory cue. Each test lasts 18 seconds. A computer-generated auditory cue paces head movements at ~0.5 Hz during the first 6 seconds, then sweeps progressively faster over a range from 1 to 6 Hz during the remaining 12 seconds. Horizontal (side-to-side) head testing is done first, followed by vertical (nose up–nose down)

testing. It is helpful to demonstrate the test for the patient and to let him or her practice prior to recording. It is important that the patient move only his or her head within a comfortable cervicospinal ROM. The frequency of head movement is critical, not the patient's ROM.

Test results are analyzed and displayed on the monitor for previewing and later plotted on a printer for clinical documentation. The multiple tests from each patient are combined statistically as means and standard deviations, and compared with data from 100 normal subjects, as shown in **Fig. 25–14**. The five graphs used for reporting are horizontal VOR gain, phase, and asymmetry, and vertical VOR gain and phase. Gains and phases are plotted versus frequency from 2 to 6 Hz. Asymmetry is computed and plotted from frequency harmonics from 2 to 10 Hz.

Advantages and Disadvantages of Vestibular Autorotation Testing

VAT testing allows for evaluation of VOR function in both the horizontal and vertical planes of head movement at frequencies encountered in everyday life. It also provides objective physiological data that may be correlated with the patient's subjective report of symptoms. This information can be used diagnostically and as a pretherapy baseline and post–vestibular rehabilitation therapy (VRT) guide to demonstrate successful treatment outcomes. Recovery of VOR function is seen as gain, phase, symmetry return within normal parameters. The disadvantage of VAT testing is similar to that of DVA testing. It is a volitional test that requires the patient to move his or her head cooperatively at the appropriate

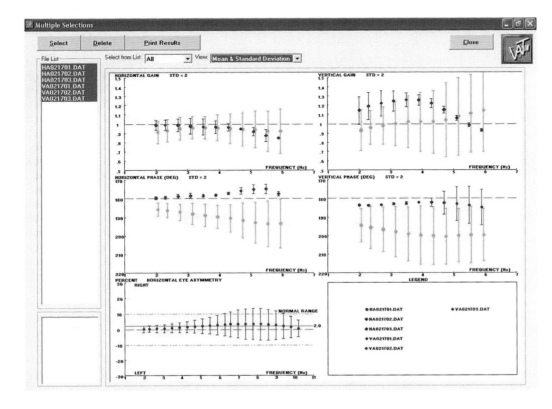

Figure 25–14 Vestibular autorotation test (VAT) summary page showing normal horizontal and vertical gain, phase, and symmetry. **(See Color Plate 25–14.)**

frequencies. If the patient is unable to do so, because he or she is not sufficiently coordinated or motivated, the results will not be reliable.

◆ Sinusoidal Harmonic Acceleration Test

Sinusoidal harmonic acceleration (SHA) testing assesses balance function by measuring eye movements (nystagmus) induced in response to back-and-forth sinusoidal movement of a motorized chair. Barany (1907) first demonstrated the presence of nystagmus after rapidly turning a patient from side to side, but research was limited because of difficulties controlling chair acceleration and deceleration and the inability to measure eye movements effectively.

The development of torque-driven motors to control chair rotation and computer software to record nystagmus led to renewed interest in rotational testing. Because SHA testing simulates natural environmental motion to evaluate vestibular function, it has become an integral part of the standard balance function protocol.

When the head is rotated on the vertical axis, the horizontal semicircular canals on each side of the head are simultaneously stimulated (Jacobson and Newman, 1991). This activity is complementary but proportional. Head movements to the right increase neural discharge from the right labyrinth and decrease neural discharge from the left labyrinth, whereas head movement to the left increases left labyrinth neural activity and decreases right labyrinth neural activity. These changes in discharge rate induce nystagmus. By measuring the VOR response, information can be obtained concerning the activity and interactions of the right and left vestibular systems.

The SHA test may be performed using VNG infrared goggles, which eliminates the need for a darkened test chamber. If an ENG recording technique is used, the chair must be located in a darkened concentric booth to prevent visual input. A seatbelt is worn for safety. With the aid of a sculpted cushion and head band, the patient's head is fixed and tilted at a 30 degree angle to provide maximum stimulation of the horizontal semicircular canals.

Instructions to the patient should include the following: the SHA test is an attempt to simulate everyday head motion in a controlled manner. The chair will be rotated at several different speeds, with short rest periods between each rotational speed. The first rotation will be very slow, turning the chair 360 degrees in both directions. The speed of rotation will be progressively faster until the final rotation, which results in a back-and-forth, sinusoidal motion. The patient should be told to relax in the chair and keep his or her eyes open while the test is being performed and to participate in concentration tasks. It is essential that the clinician watch the patient through the infrared monitor and be diligent performing the alerting tasks to ensure that the nystagmoid response is not suppressed. The clinician should also tell the patient when rotation has stopped because there may be a lag between cessation of movement and perception of cessation of movement by the patient.

A minimum of five test frequencies is incorporated into SHA testing to evaluate vestibular output over a wide operating range. Testing at only one frequency would be equated to performing a hearing test at only one frequency to assess hearing sensitivity. Frequencies commonly used are 0.01, 0.02, 0.04, 0.08, 0.16, 0.32, and 0.64 Hz (Hamid et al, 1986; Hirsch, 1986; Jacobson and Newman, 1991). At 0.01 Hz, 0.01 cycle is completed in 1 second, taking 100 seconds to complete 1 cycle; at 0.16 Hz, 0.16 cycle is completed in 1 second, taking 6.25 seconds to complete 1 sinusoidal cycle. For each frequency, the chair reaches a maximum velocity of 50 degrees per second, whereas the rate of acceleration depends on the frequency of rotation (Wolfe et al, 1978).

After stimulation at the five frequencies indicated, fixation support to rotational testing is evaluated. The chair is again rotated at the two highest frequencies of rotation, first at 0.32 Hz, then at 0.64 Hz, and the patient is instructed to fixate on a light located at eye level directly in the forward visual field. During this part of the testing, no alerting tasks are performed so the patient can concentrate on suppressing the nystagmoid response.

Rotation on a vertical axis generates compensatory eye movements in the direction opposite rotation; saccadic eye movement brings the eyes back into the central position. These nystagmoid movements are recorded, then analyzed using fast Fourier transform (FFT) to remove the fast phase component of the movement. The SPV of the eyes can then be compared with the velocity of the head movement controlled by the rotating chair. The parameters used to analyze the nystagmoid movements are phase, gain, and symmetry (**Fig. 25–15**; Hamid et al, 1986; Hirsch, 1986; Li et al, 1991). In general, low-frequency rotations reveal abnormal phase and gain responses, whereas high-frequency rotations demonstrate asymmetries (Stockwell and Bojrab, 1993).

Phase analysis measures the temporal relationship between the initiation of changes in head (chair) movement velocity and changes in eye movement velocity. As chair movement is initiated, eye movement is elicited after a known latency that depends on the frequency of the rotation. Although the induced eye movement is opposite in direction to the movement of the head (chair), responses are inverted so that latencies can be compared.

Phase abnormalities represent differences in how long after the start of the stimulus (change in head movement) the compensatory eye movement occurs. When eye movement velocity occurs later in time with respect to head (chair) movement, phase lag occurs. When eye movement occurs earlier in time to head (chair) movement, phase lead occurs. Most peripheral vestibular disorders have been associated with phase abnormalities, characterized by pronounced phase differences at low frequencies that improve to near normal phase values at high frequencies (Hamid et al, 1986; Hirsch, 1986; Li et al, 1991). The phase pattern often remains abnormal for years despite successful physiological adaptation and compensation, making phase evaluation beneficial when assessing chronic vestibular disorder (Jacobson and Newman, 1991; Parker, 1993). When phase abnormality is the same over all measured frequencies or shows increased abnormality as rotation frequency increases, CNS dysfunction should be suspected (Gresty et al, 1977).

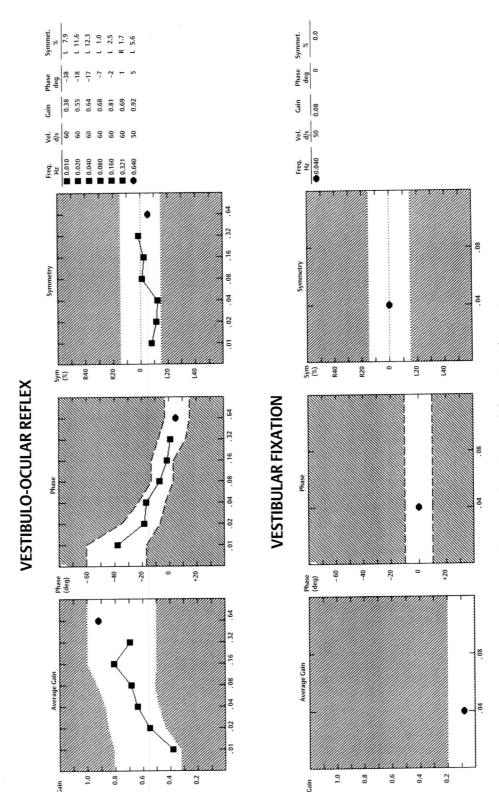

Figure 25–15 Results from sinusoidal harmonic acceleration test illustrating normal phase, gain, and symmetry.

Symmetry evaluates and compares clockwise and counterclockwise eye displacements or nystagmus. When the head (chair) is rotated in the clockwise direction, counterclockwise eye movements are induced, whereas head (chair) rotation in the counterclockwise direction induces clockwise eye movements. Symmetry is determined by comparing the peak SPV generated by right movement to the peak SPV generated by left movement and calculating the percentage difference or DP (Hirsch, 1986).

Before interpreting symmetry, the influence of underlying spontaneous nystagmus must be examined. If a patient has a 10 degree right-beating spontaneous nystagmus, responses to left rotations, which elicit right-beating nystagmus, will be enhanced 10 degrees per second, whereas responses to right rotations, which elicit left-beating nystagmus, will be reduced 10 degrees per second. It will appear to the clinician that the individual's eyes "prefer" to beat to the right, and a right DP is present. However, this bias is not due to rotational stimulation. The clinician must calculate the influence of spontaneous nystagmus on the response; once the influence of spontaneous nystagmus has been ruled out or clarified, symmetry results can be interpreted.

In the early stages of acute, peripheral lesions, significant asymmetry will be observed but will not necessarily indicate the side of disorder because both systems are stimulated simultaneously. Studies have shown that active Meniere's disease may cause increased response toward the diseased ear, whereas responses after labyrinthectomy or removal of acoustic neuroma will show increased responses toward the normal ear (Hirsch, 1986; Parker, 1993). Therefore, early on, only if phase lag is observed in conjunction with an asymmetry can the side of vestibular loss be deduced (Hamid, 1991). In later stages of peripheral vestibular disorder, asymmetry disappears as compensation takes place, whereas phase lag remains, limiting the usefulness of symmetry results when evaluating patients with chronic vestibular dysfunction. However, patients with central lesions demonstrate persistent low-level asymmetry that is associated with minimal changes in symptoms (Hamid et al, 1986).

Gain measures the amplitude of eye movements induced in response to head movement and depends on the velocity of rotation (Hirsch, 1986). When head (chair) velocity is low, compensatory eye movements are small because the stimulus is not strong enough to elicit a strong eye response. As head (chair) velocity increases, eye velocity increases, and at high velocities, eye movement velocity approaches chair velocity. For example, if the amount of eye movement induced by a given degree of rotation (in degrees per second) were exactly the same as the magnitude of the chair rotation (also in degrees per second), the gain would be 1.0; if the induced eye movements were half as large, the gain would be 0.5; and if the induced eye movement were twice as large, the gain would be 2.0. It is not surprising that the amplitude of gain depends on the velocity of rotation. Very slow rotational movements induce relatively small eye movements, with a typical gain of 0.5 for 0.01 Hz stimuli. As rotation speed increases, eye movement similarly increases but at a faster rate, so that at a rotational speed of 0.16 Hz, normal gains are in the 0.7 range.

Gain results must be considered before interpreting any SHA results. When gain is low, the vestibular system has not been stimulated sufficiently to provide meaningful data. Therefore, phase and symmetry calculations cannot be interpreted. Low gains are usually a consequence of bilateral chronic vestibular weakness. In fact, patients with bilateral vestibular paresis who demonstrate no measurable response to bithermal caloric stimulation may actually respond to higher frequency rotations, providing evidence of remaining vestibular function (Furman and Kamerer, 1989; Parker, 1993). However, low gains occasionally occur in response to acute unilateral labyrinthine lesions when the cerebellum deliberately suppresses output from all vestibular nuclei to minimize symptoms of rotation, nausea, and vomiting (Hirsch, 1986; Jacobson and Newman, 1991). In such cases, obvious signs of acute vestibular pathological conditions will generally be present, especially spontaneous nystagmus. Individuals with CNS injury occasionally show increased gain because of the absence of descending inhibition (Baloh et al, 1981). Such increased gain is similar to other varieties of "release" pathological neurological symptoms. However, it is essential to interpret gain with caution because it is highly variable and is significantly influenced by the alertness of the patient (Möller et al, 1990).

Fixation suppression must be considered separately from all other SHA results. In normal individuals, staring at a fixed point during rotation results in suppression of the nystagmoid response. Gain scores will be low or at least 50% less than the gain observed at the corresponding rotational frequency speed. Inability to suppress nystagmus while fixating during rotational testing is consistent with CNS pathological conditions (Baloh and Furman, 1989).

Advantages and Disadvantages of Sinusoidal Harmonic Acceleration Testing

SHA testing has several advantages over the more traditional tests of vestibular function, such as VNG (Hirsch, 1986; Parker, 1993). First, because the stimulus that initiates the VOR is mechanically generated by the chair in which the patient sits, the stimulus can be precisely and accurately controlled and modified. The clinician does not need to be concerned about adequate transfer of thermal energy through skin tissue and bone, as in bithermal calorics, to adequately stimulate each inner ear system. Second, the stimulus used in SHA is physiological, simulating the sort of rotational movement one might encounter in everyday life. The semicircular canals are therefore stimulated in a more natural way. Third, compensation and adaptation (or its lack) can be confirmed by monitoring changes in symmetry. Fourth, SHA testing may be performed immediately after ear surgery because direct stimulation of the ear canal is not necessary. Fifth, SHA testing can be performed when the patient is taking vestibular suppressant drugs because the VOR is not affected by such medications, and phase relationships will not be altered. Finally, SHA testing is more comfortable and acceptable to the patient because it does not induce the nausea and vertigo of caloric stimulation.

SHA testing, though, has two distinct disadvantages. First, both labyrinths are tested simultaneously during sinusoidal testing, preventing ear-specific information and making it more difficult to obtain unequivocal side-of-lesion data. Second, the test requires the installation of expensive, fixed equipment, resulting in limited clinical application.

Pearl

- SHA testing is highly advantageous when testing infants, young children, and adults who may not be able to tolerate the caloric portion of the VNG test. Patients who have had unpleasant experiences with prior caloric testing usually are quite comfortable with SHA testing. It is also a useful objective test for patients who are involved in litigation and may be uncooperative in more behaviorally based assessment procedures.

◆ Computerized Dynamic Platform Posturography

Computerized dynamic platform posturography (CDP) is a systematic test of balance function that assesses the patient's ability to use sensory input to coordinate the motor responses necessary to maintain balance (Nashner and Peters, 1990). Although other tests of balance function concentrate on evaluating the integrity of the vestibular system by assessing peripheral and central components of the vestibulo-ocular system, CDP assesses the individual's ability to use information from the vestibular, somatosensory, and visuosensory systems, both singly and together, to coordinate motor responses to maintain center of gravity (COG) and balance (Nashner, 1971; Nashner et al, 1982).

To understand CDP, the contributions of each sensory system to balance function must be understood (Nashner and McCollum, 1985; Nashner et al, 1982). Visual input orients the eyes and head and is derived from sway-dependent motions of the head relative to the visual surround. Somatosensory input orients body parts and is derived from the forces and motions exerted by the feet on the support surface. Vestibular input measures gravitational, linear, and angular accelerations of the head in relation to inertial space and is derived from head motions related to active or passive body sway in reference to gravity. When the visual field is stable and the support surface is fixed, vision and somatosensation dominate balance control because they are sensitive to subtle changes in body position. Specifically, the somatosensory system is sensitive to rapid changes, whereas the visual system is sensitive to slower changes in body orientation.

Inaccurate sensory information provides conflicting input to the brain that must be compensated for. Sensory breakdown can occur when objects in the visual field are moving, when the eyes are closed and visual information is absent, or when the support surface is compliant or moving. When

visual and somatosensory information is conflicting or insufficient, the vestibular system resolves the situation and sends accurate information to the brain (Black and Nashner, 1984). If an abnormality or lesion occurs in any of the sensory systems, this coordination of compensating activity will be affected, resulting in disequilibrium and balance disorders.

To perform CDP, as shown in **Fig. 25–16**, the patient must be able to stand erect and unassisted with eyes open for periods of at least 1 minute. During testing, the clinician should watch for signs of fatigue and give breaks if necessary. Shoes must be removed, although socks or stockings may be worn. The patient should be told that balance will be assessed while standing on a movement-sensitive platform. At times, the platform and visual surround will move in response to patient movements, whereas at other times, platform movement will cause the patient to move. The battery of tests begins with easy tasks that become progressively more difficult. A description of each subtest and instructions to the patient will be provided before each trial.

For safety, the patient wears a parachute-type harness connected to an overhead bar. The harness should be adjusted so that the patient's weight is transferred through the patient's lower trunk rather than the upper trunk and shoulders. The straps connecting the harness to the overhead bar must allow for complete freedom of motion within the limits of normal stability. If the overhead straps are too tight, they may hold the patient up when extreme sway or even a fall would have occurred. They may also interfere with the patient's movement strategy.

Once instructions have been given and the harness has been adjusted, the patient's feet must be positioned on the

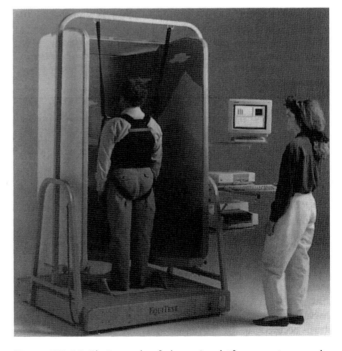

Figure 25–16 Photograph of dynamic platform posturography. (Courtesy of NeuroCom International, Inc., Clackamas, OR.)

force plate. To ensure proper alignment, the medial malleolus of the ankle joint (the bone protruding from the ankle on the inside of the foot) should be centered directly over a marking stripe that transects the two footplates. To ensure this alignment, the clinician's hand may be vertically positioned from the bone to the stripe. Once the patient is in place, testing begins.

The CDP test battery is divided into two parts (Hunter and Balzer, 1991; Nashner, 1993). The sensory organization test (SOT) assesses the patient's ability to integrate correct sensory information while ignoring inaccurate sensory cues. These findings isolate the site of breakdown and contribute to overall diagnosis of the disorder. The motor control test (MCT) measures the patient's ability to adapt to increasing anterior and posterior rocking and body sway.

Pitfall

• Patients who have biomechanical, orthopedic, or neuromuscular involvements will pose a greater challenge during CDP or Clinical Test of Sensory Integration of Balance (CTSIB) testing. Profiles should be cautiously interpreted for patients with these comorbidities.

Sensory Organization Test

The SOT assesses the patient's stability under six conditions of increasing difficulty (**Fig. 25–17**). Conditions 1 and 2 are essentially Romberg tests. In condition 1, the patient stands on the force plate with eyes open, whereas in condition 2, the eyes are closed, preventing the reception of visual input. In condition 3, the eyes are open, and the force plate is stable, but the visual surround moves, providing inaccurate visual input. In condition 4, the eyes are open, and the visual surround is stationary, but the support surface moves, providing inaccurate proprioceptive input. In condition 5, the eyes are closed while the force plate moves. The patient is deprived of visual information, and somatosensory input is inaccurate, so the patient is completely dependent on vestibular information. In condition 6, the eyes are open, but both the visual surround and the force plate move, providing inaccurate visual and somatosensory information and forcing the patient to, again, rely on vestibular information to maintain balance. The patient is assessed in each condition with three separate 20 second trials.

Motor Control Test

The MCT assesses the patient's responses to perturbations of the force plate. Two types of perturbations are used. In the first part of the test, random small, medium, and large forward-and-backward translations in the horizontal direction are presented. The size of the translation is based on the patient's height. The patient's ability to adapt to these sudden, quick movements is measured. In the second part of the test, the patient's ability to adapt when the support

surface is disrupted at an angle, forcing the toes up or down, is measured. Each translation stimulus consists of three presentations, and results are averaged to characterize the response.

Abnormalities in MCT results can be due to a variety of problems and can contribute to the diagnosis of balance dysfunction (Hunter and Balzer, 1991; Nashner and Peters, 1990). Before analyzing results for evidence of automatic postural response abnormalities, the influence of orthopedic and/or musculoskeletal problems such as peripheral muscle atrophy and unilateral hip disease must be ruled out because these disorders produce abnormal response patterns. In general, prolonged latencies for either leg to forward or backward translations is indicative of a pathological condition within the long-loop automatic response pathways and demonstrate extravestibular CNS lesions (Nashner et al, 1983; Voorhees, 1989). Abnormally large strength differences between the two legs indicate long-loop automatic response abnormality (Nashner et al, 1983). Patients with CNS abnormalities caused by multiple sclerosis or spinocerebellar degeneration exhibit characteristic MCT abnormality patterns (Williams et al, 1997).

Responses from the MCT also describe the patient's ability to perform and adapt in a complex environment and provide insight into a patient's ability to perform daily balance tasks (Horak et al, 1988). Amplitude scaling scores indicate whether the patient's responses to external perturbations are too strong or too weak. Overreactions are characterized by extreme sway to maintain balance, whereas underreactions disrupt the patient's ability to return to a balanced position. Adaptation indicates a patient's ability to adjust to uneven or compliant walking surfaces. Low scores suggest that the patient is unable to suppress the influence of disruptive stimuli to maintain balance. This information can be used in the development of rehabilitation programs and to monitor progress during rehabilitation efforts.

Interpretation of Computerized Dynamic Platform Posturography

Interpretation of CDP results is based on response patterns of the SOT and MCT. Decreased performance on conditions 5 and 6, condition 5 only, and condition 6 only of the SOT suggests peripheral vestibular deficits, because visual and somatosensory input is inaccurate, and the patient is depending on correct vestibular information to maintain balance (Dickins et al, 1992; Keim et al, 1990). Decreased performance on several conditions simultaneously indicates multisensory abnormalities and can be interpreted in several ways (Nashner and Peters, 1990). If scores in conditions 4, 5, and 6 are abnormal, the patient is dependent on somatosensory information; if scores in conditions 2, 3, 5, and 6 are abnormal, the patient is dependent on visual information. The inability to effectively use two of the three available senses to maintain balance is indicative of vestibular and extravestibular central disorders (Keim et al, 1990). If scores in conditions 2, 3, 4, 5, and 6 are abnormal, the patient is dependent on a combination of visual and somatosensory inputs, another

SENSORY ORGANIZATION TEST

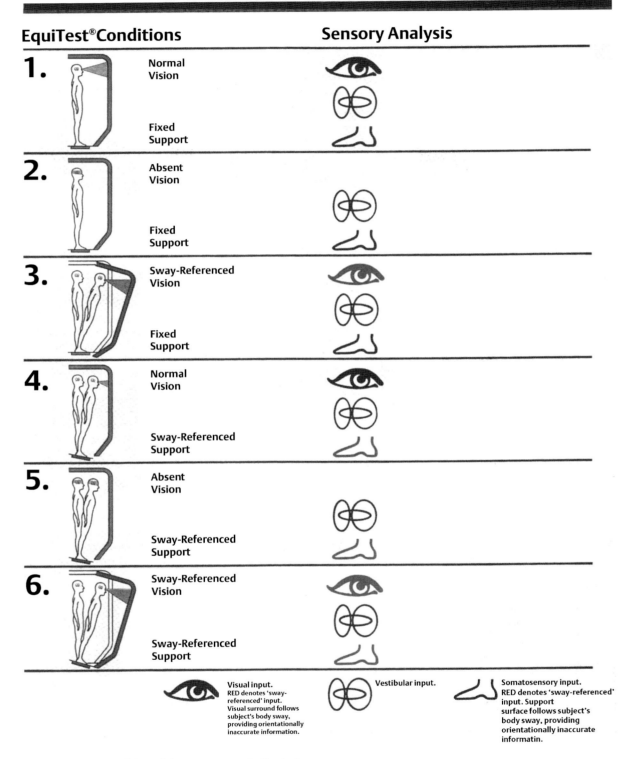

Figure 25–17 Six conditions of the sensory organization test.

indication of vestibular and extravestibular central pathological conditions (Nashner and Peters, 1990). When scores on conditions 4, 5, and 6 are equal to or better than scores on conditions 1, 2, and 3, results are physiologically inconsistent and suggest either patient anxiety or exaggeration of disability (Nashner and Peters, 1990). Prolonged latencies and/or strength asymmetries for either leg in either direction of the MCT indicate a pathological condition within the long-loop automatic response pathways and suggest extravestibular CNS lesions (Nashner et al, 1983; Voorhees, 1989).

Advantages and Disadvantages of Computerized Dynamic Platform Posturography

Results from CDP provide unique information that can be reviewed with other tests of balance function to qualitatively determine the nature of a balance disorder (DiFabio, 1995; Nashner and Peters, 1990). In general, if vestibular function tests indicate normal peripheral input and CDP indicates balance abnormality, a central pathological condition localized to central vestibular and/or extravestibular pathways and to the long-loop motor pathways of the brainstem, spinal cord, and peripheral nerves is suspected. When tests of vestibular function are abnormal, indicating peripheral vestibular disorder, and CDP is normal, it is assumed that the patient has adapted to and compensated for the peripheral lesion. Abnormal vestibular function tests and abnormal CDP are indicative of a central and/or peripheral pathological condition.

The primary disadvantages of CDP are the size and cost of the equipment. For facilities that do not have access to a CDP system, an alternative SOT evaluation procedure has been suggested (Shumway-Cook and Horak, 1986). The CTSIB uses six sensory conditions. These are two Romberg conditions on a static surface, eyes open and closed; two dynamic conditions (patient standing on foam) eyes open, then closed; and a sway-referenced condition with eyes open on static and dynamic surfaces while wearing a visual surround. Most clinicians have limited the procedure to the first four conditions. Similar to the CDP, with the CTSIB, patients with vestibular loss or dysfunction demonstrate an inability to maintain postural stability on dynamic surface conditions without vision (condition 4 of the CTSIB).

◆ Summary

Balance is an extremely complex process that involves reception of input from the vestibular, somatosensory, and visual systems, processing and integration of this sensory input, and coordination of motoric responses to maintain balance. No single procedure can identify the site of the lesion and assess the impact of balance disturbance on a patient's quality of life. Therefore, the development of clinical pathways utilizing patient history, symptoms, and evidence-based test procedures that provide a comprehensive evaluation of peripheral, central vestibular, and equilibrium function is critical. The diagnostic tests described in this chapter evaluate components involved in vestibular and balance function separately and together to determine where in the system dysfunction or loss occurs. Once the evaluation and tests are completed, a patient profile begins to emerge. The profile can be used to confirm diagnosis, recommend further assessment with imaging techniques, or help determine whether medical or surgical intervention is necessary. Perhaps the most valuable aspect of the evaluative-diagnostic process is the identification and triage of patients with vestibular and balance disorders who would benefit from treatment for BPPV, uncompensated symptomatic vestibular dysfunction, or increased risk of falls through canalith repositioning, vestibular rehabilitation, or balance retraining (Gans, 2002).

Audiologists' critical role in performing electrophysiological studies of the audiovestibular system and considerable expanding knowledge and expertise in vestibular and balance testing will continue to be in the forefront of this increasingly important clinical science.

Pearl

- Explanation and interpretation of test results should be provided to both referring physicians and patients in a clear and concise manner. Recommendations for treatment of BPPV and uncompensated vestibular deficits with VRT or balance retraining should be thoroughly explained as well as providing patients with realistic expectations of outcomes.

Appendix

The Dizziness Handicap Inventory

(Reprinted with permission)

Instructions: The purpose of this scale is to identify difficulties that you may be experiencing because of your dizziness or unsteadiness. Please answer "yes," "no," or "sometimes" to each question. Answer each question as it pertains to your dizziness or unsteadiness problem only.

P1.   Does looking up increase your problem?

E2.   Because of your problem do you feel frustrated?

F3.   Because of your problem do you restrict your travel for business or recreation?

P4.   Does walking down the aisle of a supermarket increase your problem?

F5.   Because of your problem do you have difficulty getting into or out of bed?

F6.   Does your problem significantly restrict your participation in social activities such as going out to dinner, movies, dancing, or parties?

F7.   Because of your problem do you have difficulty reading?

P8.   Does performing more ambitious activities like sports, dancing, and household chores such as sweeping or putting dishes away increase your problem?

E9.   Because of your problem are you afraid to leave your home without having someone accompany you?

E10. Because of your problem have you been embarrassed in front of others?

P11. Do quick movements of your head increase your problem?

F12. Because of your problem do you avoid heights?

P13. Does turning over in bed increase your problem?

F14. Because of your problem is it difficult for you to do strenuous housework or yardwork?

E15. Because of your problem are you afraid people may think you are intoxicated?

F16. Because of your problem is it difficult for you to go for a walk by yourself?

P17. Does walking down a sidewalk increase your problem?

E18. Because of your problem is it difficult for you to concentrate?

F19. Because of your problem is it difficult for you to walk around your house in the dark?

E20. Because of your problem are you afraid to stay home alone?

E21. Because of your problem do you feel handicapped?

E22. Has your problem placed stress on your relationships with members of your family or friends?

E23. Because of your problem are you depressed?

F24. Does your problem interfere with your job or household responsibilities?

P25. Does bending over increase your problem?

A "yes" response is scored 4 points. A "sometimes" response is scored 2 points. A "no" response is scored 0 point.
F represents an item contained on the functional subscale, *E* represents an item contained on the emotional subscale, and *P* represents an item contained on the physical subscale.

References

American Academy of Audiology. (2004). Audiology: Scope of practice. Available at www.audiology.org.

American Academy of Neurology, Therapeutics and Technology Subcommittee. (1996). Assessment: Electronystagmography. Neurology, 46, 1763–1766.

American Speech-Language-Hearing Association. (2004). Scope of practice in audiology. ASHA 24(Suppl.).

Baloh, R. W., & Furman, J. M. R. (1989). Modern vestibular function testing. Western Journal of Medicine, 150, 59–67.

Baloh, R. W., & Honrubia, V. (2001). Clinical neurophysiology of the vestibular system (3rd ed.). New York: Oxford University Press.

Baloh, R. W., Yee, R. E., Kimm, J., & Honrubia, V. (1981). The vestibulo-ocular reflex in patients with lesions of the vestibulocerebellum. Experimental Neurology, 72(1), 141–152.

Barany, R. (1907). Physiologie und Pathologie des Bogengangapparates biem Menschen. Vienna: Franz Deuticke.

Bhansali, S. A., Stockwell, C. W., & Bojarb, D. I. (1993). Oscillopsia in patients with loss of vestibular function. Otolaryngology—Head and Neck Surgery, 109, 120–125.

Brickner, R. (1936). Oscillopsia: A new symptom commonly occurring in multiple sclerosis. Archives of Neurology and Psychiatry, 36, 586–589.

Black, F. O., & Nashner, L. M. (1984). Postural disturbance in patients with benign paroxysmal positional nystagmus. Annals of Otology, Rhinology and Laryngology, 93, 595–599.

Brandt, T. (1993). Background, technique, interpretation, and usefulness of positional and positioning testing. In G. P. Jacobson, C. P. Newman, & J. M. Kartush (Eds.), Handbook of balance function testing (pp. 123–155). St. Louis, MO: Mosby–Year Book.

Brantberg, K., Bergenius, J., & Tribukait, A. (1999). Vestibular-evoked myogenic potentials in patients with dehiscence of the superior semicircular canal. Acta Otolaryngologica, 119, 633–640.

Brookler, K. H. (1991). Standardization of electronystagmography. American Journal of Otology, 12, 480–483.

Cass, S. P., & Furman, J. M. R. (1993). Medications and their effects on vestibular function testing (ENG report). Chicago: ICS Medical Corp.

Cohen, H. S. (2004). Side-lying as an alternative to the Dix-Hallpike test of the posterior canal. Otology and Neurotology, 25, 130–134.

Colebatch, J. G., & Halmagyi, G. M. (1992). Vestibular evoked potentials in human neck muscles before and after unilateral vestibular deafferentation. Neurology, 42, 1635–1636.

Dickins, J. R. E., Cyr, D. G., Graham, S. S., Winston, M. E., & Sanford, M. (1992). Clinical significance of type 5 patterns in platform posturography. Otolaryngology—Head and Neck Surgery, 107, 1–6.

Di Fabio, R. P. (1995). Sensitivity and specificity of platform posturography for identifying patients with vestibular dysfunction. Physical Therapy, 75, 290–305.

Dix, M. R., & Hallpike, C. S. (1952). The pathology, symptomatology and diagnosis of certain common disorders of the vestibular system. Annals of Otology, Rhinology and Laryngology, 61, 987–1016.

Evans, K. M., & Melancon, B. B. (1989). Back to basics: A discussion of technique and equipment. Seminars in Hearing, 10, 123–140.

Fineberg, R., O'Leary, D. P., & Davis, L. L. (1987). Use of active head movements for computerized vestibular testing. Archives of Otolaryngology—Head and Neck Surgery, 113, 1063–1065.

Furman, J. M., & Cass, S. P. (2003). Vestibular disorders: A case study approach (2nd ed.). New York: Oxford University Press.

Furman, J. M., & Kamerer, D. B. (1989). Rotational responses in patients with bilateral caloric reduction. Acta Otolaryngologica, 108, 355–361.

Gans, R. E. (1999, June). Evaluating the dizzy patient: Establishing clinical pathways. Hearing Review, 45–47.

Gans, R. (2002). Vestibular rehabilitation: Critical decision analysis. Seminars in Hearing, 23, 149–159.

Gans, R., & Harrington-Gans, P. (2002). Treatment efficacy of benign paroxysmal positional vertigo (BPPV) with canalith repositioning maneuver and Semont liberatory maneuver in 376 patients. Seminars in Hearing, 23, 129–142.

Gans, R., & Roberts, R. A. (2006). VNG handbook: A clinical guide. Seminole, FL: AIB Education Press.

Goebel, J. A. (2001). Practical management of the dizzy patient. Philadelphia: Lippincott Williams & Wilkins.

Gresty, M. A., Hess, K., & Leech, J. (1977). Disorders of the vestibulo-ocular reflex producing oscillopsia and mechanisms of compensating for loss of labyrinthine function. Brain, 100, 693–716.

Hain, T. C. (1993). Interpretation and usefulness of ocular motility testing. In G. P. Jacobson, C. P. Newman, & J. M. Kartush (Eds.), Handbook of balance function testing (pp. 101–122). St. Louis, MO: Mosby–Year Book.

Hamid, M. A. (1991). Determining side of vestibular dysfunction with rotatory chair testing. Otolaryngology—Head and Neck Surgery, 105, 40–43.

Hamid, M. A., Hughes, G. B., Kinney, S. E., & Hanson, M. R. (1986). Results of sinusoidal harmonic acceleration test in one thousand patients: Preliminary report. Otolaryngology—Head and Neck Surgery, 94, 1–5.

Herdman, S. J., Tusa, R. J., Blatt, P., Suzuki, A., Venuto, P., & Roberts, D. (1998). Computerized dynamic visual acuity test in assessment of vestibular deficits. American Journal of Otology, 19, 790–796.

Hester, T. O., & Silverstein, H. (2002). Patient interview: History of symptoms and definitions of common vestibular disorders. Seminars in Hearing, 23, 107–111.

Hillman, E. J., Bloomberg, J. J., McDonald, P. V., & Cohen, H. S. (1999). Dynamic visual acuity while walking in normals and labyrinthine-deficient patients. Journal of Vestibular Research, 9(1), 49–57.

Hirsch, B. E. (1986). Computed sinusoidal harmonic acceleration. Ear and Hearing, 7, 198–203.

Honrubia, V. (2002). Quantitative vestibular function tests and the clinical examination. In: S. Herdman (Ed.), Vestibular rehabilitation (2nd ed., pp. 105–171). Philadelphia: F. A. Davis.

Honrubia, V. (1995). Contemporary vestibular function testing: Accomplishments and future perspectives. Otolaryngology—Head and Neck Surgery, 112, 64–77.

Horak, F. B., Shumway-Cook, A., Crowe, T. K., & Black, F. O. (1988). Vestibular function and motor proficiency of children with impaired hearing, or with learning disability and motor impairments. Developmental Medicine and Child Neurology, 30, 64–79.

Humphriss, R. L., Baguley, D. M., Sparkes, V., Peerman, S. E., & Moffat, D. A. (2003). Contraindications to the Dix-Hallpike maneuver: A multidisciplinary review. International Journal of Audiology, 42, 166–173.

Hunter, L. L., & Balzer, G. K. (1991). Overview and introduction to dynamic platform posturography. Seminars in Hearing, 12, 226–247.

Jacobson, G. P., & Newman, C. W. (1990). The development of the dizziness handicap inventory. Archives of Otolaryngology—Head and Neck Surgery, 116, 424–427.

Jacobson, G. P., & Newman, C. W. (1991). Rotational testing. Seminars in Hearing, 12, 199–225.

Jacobson, G. P., & Newman, C. W. (1993). Background and technique of caloric testing. In G. P. Jacobson, C. P. Newman, & J. M. Kartush (Eds.), Handbook of balance function testing (pp. 156–192). St. Louis, MO: Mosby–Year Book.

Jacobson, G. P., Newman, C. W., Hunter, L., & Balzer, G. K. (1991). Balance function test correlates of the dizziness handicap inventory. Journal of the American Academy of Audiology, 2, 253–260.

Jacobson, G. P., Newman, C. W., & Peterson, E. L. (1993). Interpretation and usefulness of caloric testing. In G. P. Jacobson, C. W. Newman, & J. M.

Kartush (Eds.), Handbook of balance function testing (pp. 193–233). St. Louis, MO: Mosby–Year Book.

Kanaya, T., Nonaka, S., Kamito, M., Unno, T., Sako, K., & Takei, H. (1994). Primary position upbeat nystagmus localizing value. ORL Journal for Oto-rhino-laryngology and Its Related Specialties, 56, 236–238.

Keim, R. J., Dickins, J. R.E., & Nashner, L. M. (1990). Computerized dynamic posturography: Fundamentals and clinical applications. Instructional course presented at the Annual Convention of the American Academy of Otolaryngology–Head and Neck Surgery, San Diego, CA.

Kelsch, T. A., Schaefer, L. A., & Esquivel, C. R. (2006). Vestibular evoked myogenic potentials in young children: Test parameters and normative data. Laryngoscope, 116, 895–900.

Konrad, H. R. (1991). Clinical application of saccade-reflex testing in man. Laryngoscope, 101, 1293–1302.

Korres, S., Balatsouras, D., Kaberos, A., Economou, C., Kandiloros, D., & Ferekidis, E. (2002). Occurrence of semicircular canal involvement in benign paroxysmal positional vertigo. Otology and Neurotology, 23, 926–932.

Leigh, J. R., & Zee, D. S. (1999). The neurology of eye movements (3rd ed.). New York: Oxford University Press.

Li, C. W., Hooper, R. E., & Cousins, V. C. (1991). Sinusoidal harmonic acceleration testing in normal humans. Laryngoscope, 101, 192–196.

Liao, L. J., & Young, Y. H. (2004). Vestibular evoked myogenic potentials in basilar artery migraine. Laryngoscope, 114, 1305–1309.

Longridge, N. S., & Mallinson, A. I. (1987). The dynamic illegible E (DIE) test: A simple technique for assessing the ability of the vestibulo-ocular reflex to overcome vestibular pathology. Journal of Otolaryngology, 16, 97–103.

Möller, C., Ödkvist, L., White, V., & Cyr, D. (1990). The plasticity of compensatory eye movements in rotary tests. Acta Otolaryngologica, 109, 15–24.

Nashner, L. M. (1971). A model describing vestibular detection of body sway motion. Acta Otolaryngologica, 72, 429–436.

Nashner, L. M. (1993). Computerized dynamic posturography. In G. P. Jacobson, C. P. Newman, & J. M. Kartush (Eds.), Handbook of balance function testing (pp. 280–307). St. Louis, MO: Mosby–Year Book.

Nashner, L. M., Black, F. O., & Wall, C. III. (1982). Adaptation to altered support and visual conditions during stance: Patients with vestibular deficits. Journal of Neuroscience, 2, 536–544.

Nashner, L. M., & McCollum, G. (1985). The organization of human postural movements: A formal basis and experimental synthesis. Behavioral and Brain Sciences, 8, 135–172.

Nashner, L. M., & Peters, J. F. (1990). Dynamic posturography in the diagnosis and management of dizziness and balance disorders. Neurologic Clinics, 8, 331–350.

Nashner, L. M., Shumway-Cook, A., & Marin, O. (1983). Stance posture control in selected groups of children with cerebral palsy: Deficits in sensory organization and muscular coordination. Experimental Brain Research, 49(3), 393–409.

National Institute on Deafness and Other Communication Disorders, U.S. Department of Health and Human Services, National Institutes of Health. (1995). The national strategic research plan (Rep. 97–3217, pp. 77–110). Washington, DC: Authors.

Palla, A., Marti, S., & Straumann, D. (2005). Head-shaking nystagmus depends on gravity. Journal of the Association for Research in Otolaryngology, 6, 1–8.

Parker, S. W. (1993). Vestibular evaluation—electronystagmography, rotational testing, and posturography. Clinical Electroencephalography, 24, 151–158.

Perez, P., Lorente, J. L., Gomez, J. R., del Campo, A., Lopez, A., & Suarez, C. (2004). Functional significance of peripheral head shaking nystagmus. Laryngoscope, 114, 1078–1084.

Resnick, D. M., & Brewer, C. C. (1983). The electronystagmography test battery: Hit or myth? Seminars in Hearing, 4, 23–32.

Roberts, R. A., Gans, R. E., Johnson, E. L., & Chisolm, T. H. (2006). Computerized dynamic visual acuity with volitional head movements in patients with vestibular dysfunction. Annals of Otology, Rhinology and Laryngology, 115(9), 658–666.

Roberts, R. A., Gans, R. E., & Kastner, A. H. (2006). Differentiation of migrainous positional vertigo (MPV) from horizontal canal benign paroxysmal positional vertigo (HC-BPPV). International Journal of Audiology, 45, 224–226.

Sataloff, R. T., & Hughes, M. E. (1988). How I do it: An easy guide to electronystagmography interpretations. American Journal of Otology, 9(2), 144–151.

Schubert, M. C., Herdman, S. J., & Tusa, R. J. (2002). Vertical dynamic visual acuity in normal subjects and patients with vestibular hypofunction. Otology and Neurotology, 23(3), 372–377.

Sheykholesami, K., Kaga, K., Megerian, C. A., & Arnold, J. E. (2005). Vestibular-evoked myogenic potentials in infancy and early childhood. Laryngoscope, 115, 1440–1444.

Shumway-Cook, A., & Horak, F. B. (1986). Assessing the influence of sensory interaction on balance: Suggestions from the field. Physical Therapy, 66, 1548–1550.

Stockwell, C. W., & Bojrab, D. I. (1993). Background and technique of rotational testing. In G. P. Jacobson, C. P. Newman, & J. M. Kartush (Eds.). Handbook of balance function testing (pp. 237–258). St. Louis, MO: Mosby–Year Book.

Vitte, E., & Semont, A. (1995). Assessment of vestibular function by videonystagmoscopy. Journal of Vestibular Research, 5(5), 1–7.

Voorhees, R. L. (1989). The role of dynamic posturography as a screening test in neurotologic diagnosis. Laryngoscope, 99, 995–1001.

Williams, N. P., Roland, P. S., & Yellin, W. (1997). Vestibular evaluation in patients with early multiple sclerosis. American Journal of Otology, 18, 93–100.

Wolfe, J. W., Engelken, E. J., Olson, J. E., & Kos, C. M. (1978). Vestibular responses to bithermal caloric and harmonic acceleration. Annals of Otology, Rhinology and Laryngology, 87, 861–867.

Young, Y. H., Wu, C. C., & Wu, C H. (2002). Augmentation of vestibular evoked myogenic potentials: An indication for distended saccular hydrops. Laryngoscope, 112(3), 509–512.

Zapala, D. A., & Brey, R. H. (2004). Clinical experience with the vestibular evoked myogenic potential. Journal of the American Academy of Audiology, 15, 198–215.

Index

Page numbers followed by *f* or *t* indicate entries in figures or tables, respectively.

Amplitude modulated signals
 auditory cortex sensitivity to, 56
 in auditory steady-state response, 467, 468f, 470
Ampulla of semicircular duct, 67, 68f, 70, 71
Anesthesia
 auditory steady-state response monitoring of, 471
 effects on intraoperative monitoring, 534
Angular gyrus, 48f, 49
 vascular anatomy of, 56
Animal models, genetic, 108–110
Anomic aphasia, 328t
Anotia, 84–85
ANSI/ISO Hearing Level, 202
ANSI S3.1-1999 standard, 223–224, 223t
ANSI S3.6-1996 standard, 196
ANSI S3.6-2004 standard, 196, 197–199
ANSI S3.39-1987 standard, 196, 220
Antagonist, 160
Anterior commissure, 51f
Anterior ventral cochlear nucleus (AVCN), 39, 40f
Anteroinferior cerebellar artery, 45, 45f
 compression by, 98–99
Anticancer drugs, ototoxicity of, 36, 93–94, 163–164
Antidepressants, for tinnitus, 78
Antihistamines, blood–brain barrier and, 158
Antihypertensive drugs, and vertigo, 80
Antimalarial drugs, ototoxicity of, 93–94, 165–166
Antiphasic condition, 351
AOM. *See* Acute otitis media
APD. *See* Auditory processing disorder
Aperiodic signals, 172–173
 Fourier integral of, 173–174
Aphasia syndromes, 327–328, 328t
AP-N$_1$ latency difference, in electrocochleography, 414–415, 415f
Arborization, 59
Arcuate fasciculus, 50
Articulation index (AI), 290, 299–301, 301f
Artifacts, in immittance testing, 223
Artificial ear (NBS 9-A coupler), 202
Artificial headbone, 204
Ascending reticular activating system (ARAS), 44–45
Ascending threshold technique, 247–248
ASHA. *See* American Speech–Language–Hearing Association
Aspartate, in auditory neurotransmission, 57–58
Aspergillosis, 84
Aspirin
 ototoxicity of, 93–94, 162, 165
 pharmacodynamics of, 161
 and tinnitus, 78, 93–94, 165
Association areas of auditory cortex, 47
Association studies, 111–112
ASSR. *See* Auditory steady-state response
Atmospheric pressure, and immittance instruments, 220
Atoh1 gene, 119
Atropine, and hearing in noise, 57
Attention, 189–190
 and auditory evoked potentials, 447
 and auditory steady-state response, 470–471
 and sensory gating, 452–453, 455
Attention deficit/hyperactivity disorder (ADHD), 336
 audiological evaluation in, 326
 versus auditory processing disorder, 336, 337t, 343, 349
 checklist for, 343
 DSM-IV-TR criteria for, 326, 336, 336t
 P50 gating response in, 454

P300 cognitive auditory evoked potential in, 464–465
 symptoms of, 326, 326t
Attenuation, interaural, 264–266
Attenuator, of audiometers, 242t, 243, 243t
Attenuator linearity, of audiometers, 210, 218, 230
Attic cholesteatoma, 131
AUDERA, 470
Audibility of speech, 292, 292f
Audiogram, 252, 253f
 Count-the-Dot, 299–301, 301f, 302f
 descriptions of, 257–258, 257t, 258t
Audiological diagnosis, *versus* medical diagnosis, 14–15
Audiologists
 diagnosis of hearing loss by, 14
 neonatal screening by, 503
Audiology. *See also specific entries*
 definition of, 1
 patients *versus* clients in, 15
 scope of practice, 1–2, 2t, 14–15, 541
Audiology Home, 315–316
Audiometers, 197–202, 240–245. *See also specific types*
 amplifier of, 242t, 243
 attenuator linearity of, 210, 218, 230
 attenuator of, 242t, 243, 243t
 battery-powered, 202
 bone-conduction oscillators of, 199, 201, 201f, 241t, 245, 251–252
 calibration of, 202–206, 228–233, 245
 components of, 241f, 242–245, 242t
 correction card for, 207–208, 207f, 215
 diagnostic, 241
 earphones for, 199, 200–201, 241t, 244–247, 244f
 ear selection for, 247
 electrical safety of, 202
 frequency of, 210–211, 215–216, 218, 230, 233
 frequency selector dial of, 242t, 243
 general requirements for, 201–202
 harmonic distortion in, 211–212, 216, 231
 humidity output of, 201–202
 infection control with, 249
 inspection checks of, 216–218, 217f
 instruction manual for, 202
 listening checks of, 216, 217f, 218–219
 loudspeakers of, 199, 201, 241t, 245
 marking or labels of, 202
 masking level controller of, 241f, 242t, 243–244
 maximum hearing levels of, 197, 199t
 minimum required features of, 197, 198t, 199t
 noise of, 218
 output levels of, 206–210, 206t, 214–215
 performance characteristics of, 206–216
 power (on/off) switch of, 242, 242t
 reference signals for, 198t, 213
 screening, 258–259, 259t
 signal route switch of, 242t, 243
 signal selection switch of, 241t, 245
 signal switching in, 198t, 212–213
 speech, 6–8
 standards for, 196, 197, 226–227
 temperature output of, 201–202
 tone interrupter (tone reverse) switch of, 242t, 243
 transducers for, 199–201
 types of, 197–199, 241–242
Audiometric symbols, 252, 253f
Audiometric test rooms, 223–225
Audiometry. *See also specific tests*
 Békésy (self-recording), 4–5